Neonatal
and Pediatric
Respiratory Care

Neonatal and Pediatric Respiratory Care

FOURTH EDITION

Brian K. Walsh, BS, MBA, RRT-NPS, RPFT, ACCS, FAARC
Clinical Research Coordinator
Boston Children's Hospital
Department of Anesthesia
Division of Critical Care

Research Associate in Anaesthesia
Harvard Medical School

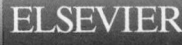

ELSEVIER
SAUNDERS

3251 Riverport Lane
St. Louis, Missouri 63043

Content Manager: Billi Sharp
Senior Content Development Specialist: Charlene Ketchum
Publishing Services Manager: Catherine Jackson
Project Manager: Sara Alsup
Design Direction: Teresa McBryan, Jessica Williams

Printed in Canada

Last digit is the print number: 9 8 7 6 5 4 3 2

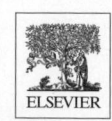 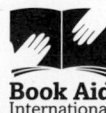

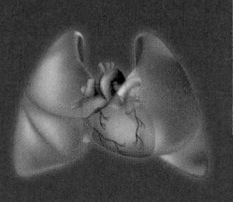

To all the students and pediatric respiratory care providers, may this book add knowledge to your wisdom. To the contributors and reviewers that have made this book what it is today, I could not have done it without you. Finally, to my parents, Kenneth and Brenda Walsh, who pushed me to believe that I can do anything if I am willing to work hard and never give up.
BKW

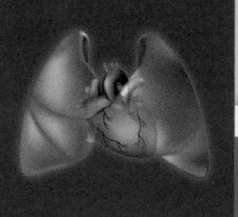

Arzu Ari, PhD, RRT, PT, CPFT, FAARC
Associate Professor
Department of Respiratory Therapy
Georgia State University
Atlanta, Georgia

Peter Betit, RRT-NPS, FAARC
Director Respiratory Care and ECMO Program
Boston Children's Hospital
Boston, Massachusetts

Amy C. Brenski, MD
Assistant Professor
University of Texas Southwestern Medical School
Children's Medical Center
Dallas, Texas

Ira M. Cheifetz, MD, FCCM, FAARC
Professor of Pediatrics
Interim Chair, Department of Pediatrics
Interim Chief Medical Officer, Children's Services
Chief, Pediatric Critical Care Medicine
Director, Pediatric Critical Care Services
Duke Children's Hospital
Durham, North Carolina

Nana E. Coleman, MD, EdM
Assistant Professor of Pediatrics
Division of Pediatric Critical Care Medicine
Weill Cornell Medical College
New York, New York

Adriann Combs, RN
Regional Perinatal Center Coordinator
Stonybrook University Hospital
Stonybrook, New York

Danielle Corrigan, MD
Division of Pediatric Pulmonology
University of Texas Southwestern
Dallas, Texas

Kevin L. Crezeé, BS, RRT-NPS
Respiratory NICU Coordinator
Respiratory Care, Primary Children's Medical Center
Salt Lake City, Utah

Michael D. Davis, RRT, BS
Project Director—Exhaled Breath Research
Adult Health and Nursing, Virginia Commonwealth
  University
Richmond, Virginia

Ashok Deorari, MD, FAMS
Professor
Department of Pediatrics, Division of Neonatology
Coordinator, WHO-CC for Training and Research in
  Newborn Care
All India Institute of Medical Sciences
Ansari Nagar, New Delhi, India

Rania A. El-Farrash, MD
Assistant Professor of Pediatrics
Children's Hospital—Neonatology Division
Ain Shams University
Cairo, Egypt

James B. Fink, PhD, RRT-NPS, FAARC
Adjunct Professor
Georgia State University
Atlanta, Georgia

Alessandra C. Gasior, DO
Pediatric Surgery Critical Care Fellow
Children's Mercy Hospital
Kansas City, Missouri

Michael L. Green, MD
Assistant Professor, Department of Pediatrics
Division of Critical Care Medicine
University of Texas Southwestern Medical Center
Dallas, Texas

Ann-Janette Griffin, RRT
Clinical Director
Home Ventilator Program Manager
Cherub Medical Supply
Merriam, Kansas

Kristen Hood, RRT-NPS
Clinical Educator
Children's Medical Center Dallas
Dallas, Texas

Katrina M. Hynes, RRT, CPFT
Assistant Supervisor
Pulmonary Function Laboratory
Mayo Clinic
Rochester, Minnesota

Kensho Iwanaga,MD, MS
Health Sciences Assistant Clinical Professor
Division of Pediatric Pulmonology
Department of Pediatrics
University of California, San Francisco School of
    Medicine
San Francisco, CA

Patrice Johnson, MBA, RRT-NPS
Director, Respiratory Care Services
Children's Mercy Hospitals & Clinics
Kansas City, Missouri

Robert L. Joyner, Jr., PhD, RRT, FAARC
Associate Dean Richard A. Henson School of Science
    and Technology
Director, Respiratory Therapy Program
Salisbury University
Salisbury, Maryland

David Alan Kaufman, MD
Professor
Department of Pediatrics, Division of Neonatology
University of Virginia School of Medicine
Charlottesville, Virginia

Nina Kowalczyk, PhD, RT(R)(CT)(QM), FASRT
Assistant Professor
School of Health and Rehabilitation Sciences, College
    of Medicine
The Ohio State University
Columbus, Ohio

Jan Hau Lee, MBBS, MRCPCH
Associate Consultant
Children's Intensive Care Unit, KK Women's and
    Children's Hospital
Singapore
Duke-NUS Graduate School of Medicine
Singapore

Peter M. Luckett, MD, FCCP
Professor of Pediatrics
University of Texas Southwestern Medical Center
Medical Director, Respiratory Care Department
Children's Medical Center Dallas
Dallas, Texas

George B. Mallory, Jr., MD
Medical Director, Lung Transplant Program
Texas Children's Hospital
Professor of Pediatrics
Baylor College of Medicine
Houston, Texas

Carl D. Mottram, BA, RRT, RPFT, FAARC
Technical Director, Mayo Clinic Pulmonary Function
    Laboratories and Pulmonary Rehabilitation
Associate Professor of Medicine
Mayo Clinic College of Medicine
Rochester, Minnesota

Linda Allen Napoli, MBA, RRT-NPS, RPFT
Director, Respiratory Care, Neurodiagnostics, Pulmonary
    Function and Sleep Labs, Neurodiagnostics,
    ECMO, Transport Team and Apnea Monitoring
The Children's Hospital of Philadelphia
Philadelphia, Pennsylvania

Syed Kamal Naqvi, MD
Medical Director, Sleep Disorders Center
Children's Medical Center Dallas
Assistant Professor of Pediatrics
University of Texas Southwestern Medical Center
Dallas, Texas

Sean T. Nguyen, PharmD, BCPS
Senior Clinical Pharmacist
Pediatric Infectious Diseases
Children's Medical Center Dallas
Dallas, Texas

J. Gerald Quirk, MD, PhD
Professor of Obstetrics, Gynecology & Reproductive
    Medicine
Stony Brook Medicine
Stony Brook, New York

Marc G. Schecter, MD
Medical Director, Pediatric Lung Transplant Program
Cincinnati Children's Hospital Medical Center
Cincinnati, Ohio

Kurt P. Schropp, MD, FACS
Associate Professor of Surgery and Pediatrics
Kansas University Medical Center
Kansas City, Kansas

Paul W. Sheeran, MD
Attending Anesthesiologist, Attending Pediatric Intensivist
University of Texas Southwestern Medical Center
Dallas, Texas

Steven E. Sittig, RRT-NPS, C-NPT, FAARC
Neonata/Pediatric Transport Clinical Specialist
Assistant Professor of Anesthesia—Mayo Clinic College
    of Medicine
Mayo Clinic
Rochester, Minnesota

Anthony D. Slonim, MD, DrPH
Executive Vice President/Chief Medical Officer
Barnabas Health
West Orange, New Jersey

Craig D. Smallwood, BS, RRT
Coordinator of Respiratory Research
Respiratory Care Department
Boston Children's Hospital
Boston, Massachusetts

Paul C. Stillwell MD
Senior Instructor, Department of Pediatrics
University of Colorado School of Medicine, Anschutz
    Medical Campus
Pediatric Pulmonologist
Children's Hospital Colorado
Aurora, Colorado

W. Gerald Teague, MD
Professor of Pediatrics
Director, Division of Respiratory Medicine, Allergy, and
    Immunology
Department of Pediatrics
University of Virginia School of Medicine
Charlottesville, Virginia

Denise Thompson-Batt, RRT
Clinical Research Coordinator
Division of Respiratory Medicine, Allergy, and
    Immunology
Department of Pediatrics
University of Virginia School of Medicine
Charlottesville, Virginia

Anu Thukral, DM, MNAMS
Senior Research Associate
Department of Pediatrics, Division of Neonatology
All India Institute of Medical Sciences
Ansari Nagar, New Delhi, India

Lisa M. Tyler, MS, RRT-NPS, CPFT
Manager
Respiratory Care Department, the Children's Hospital
    of Philadelphia
Philadelphia, Pennsylvania

Jennifer Watts, MD, MPH
Pediatric Emergency Medicine
Assistant Professor of Pediatrics
Children's Mercy Hospital and Clinics
Kansas City, Missouri

Santina A. Zanelli, MD
Assistant Professor of Pediatrics
University of Virginia Medical School
Charlottesville, Virginia

EVOLVE CONTRIBUTOR

Ruben D. Restrepo, MD, RRT, FAARC
Professor of Respiratory Care
Director, Bachelor's Completion Program
The University of Texas Health Science Center at
    San Antonio
San Antonio, Texas

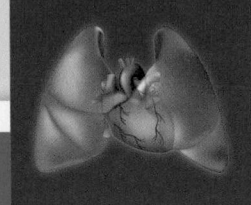

Reviewers

Shelley P. Ahrens, CNP, CNS
Pediatric Nurse Practitioner
Mayo Clinic
Rochester, Minnesota

Michelle Barker, BA, RRT-NPS
Assistant Professor, Respiratory Care Program
Tarrant County College
Hurst, Texas

Margaret-Ann Carno, PhD, MBA, RN, CPNP, D, ABSM, FNAP, FAAN
Associate Professor of Clinical Nursing and Pediatrics
University of Rochester, School of Nursing
Rochester, New York

Shauna L. Cilberg, MEd, RRT-NPS
Respiratory Care Instructor
Francis Tuttle Technology Center
Oklahoma City Community College
Oklahoma City, Oklahoma

Patricia Conlon, MS, RN, CNS, CNP
Pediatric Clinical Nurse Specialist
Mayo Clinic Children's Center
Rochester, Minnesota

Dana Evans, MHA, RRT-NPS
Respiratory Care Manager
Mercy Children's Hospital—St. Louis
Mercy Hospital—St. Louis
St. Louis, Missouri

Karen Goeke, RN, MS, CCNS
Neonatal Clinical Nurse Specialist
Mayo Clinic
Rochester, Minnesota

Robert L. Joyner, Jr., PhD, RRT, FAARC
Associate Dean Richard A. Henson School of Science and Technology
Director, Respiratory Therapy Program
Salisbury University
Salisbury, Maryland

Norma L. Lahart-Cloyd, BS, RRT-NPS
Respiratory Care Instructor
Alvin Community College
Alvin, Texas

Bernard Lee, PharmD, BCPS
Clinical Manager, Pediatrics
Department of Pharmacy
UNC Hospitals—Children's Hospital of North Carolina
Chapel Hill, North Carolina

Ruben D. Restrepo, MD, RRT, FAARC
Professor of Respiratory Care
Director, Bachelor's Completion Program
The University of Texas Health Science Center at San Antonio
San Antonio, Texas

Narciso E. Rodriquez, BS, RRT-NPS, RPFT, AE-C
Assistant Professor and Program Director
Respiratory Care Program
UMDNJ School of Health Related Professions
Newark, New Jersey

Jerelyn M. Sehl, M.S., R.N.
Perinatal Clinical Nurse Specialist
Department of Nursing
Instructor in Nursing
Mayo Clinic College of Medicine
Rochester, Minnesota

Robert A. Sinkin, MD, MPH, FAAP, FATS
Charles Fuller Professor of Neonatology
Department of Pediatrics
University of Virginia Children's Hospital
Division Head, Neonatology
Medical Director for Newborn Services
Charlottesville, Virginia

Margaret Waters, MAT, RRT
Respiratory Care Instructor
Respiratory Care Program
Henry Ford Community College
Dearborn, Michigan

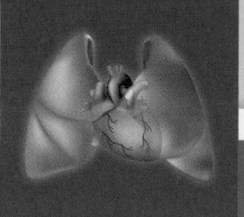

Since the first edition was published in 1995, *Perinatal and Pediatric Respiratory Care* has been a foundational neonatal and pediatric respiratory care textbook. We are proud to continue that tradition with the fourth edition. For this edition, we have changed the title to *Neonatal and Pediatric Respiratory Care* to better reflect the title of the national Neonatal/Pediatric Specialty (NPS) credentialing exam, which has become a requirement in many children's hospitals.

The fundamental role of the pediatric respiratory therapist (RT) continues to be redefined on a daily basis. Dr. Dean Hess, editor-in-chief of the journal *Respiratory Care,* has described today's respiratory therapist as "a technologist, a clinician, and a physiologist." RTs specializing in the care of children are an integral part of an autonomous health care team. As our health care system changes, these individuals will need to be highly professional, have critical thinking skills, and be more involved in critical roles as experts in critical and acute care, extracorporeal membrane oxygenation (ECMO), air and ground transport, discharge coordination, home care, education, health care quality, and research. All roles that encompass the respiratory care of children require an individual who remains current with the changing face of this profession. The proliferation of new surgical interventions, discoveries in applied translational and clinical research, devices and mechanical ventilator technologies, and strategies that are currently being implemented into practice require dynamic, self-driven clinicians, and lifelong learners who are dedicated to providing the highest quality care possible. Increases in premature and multiple births, as well as paradigm shifts in strategies focused at reducing hospital costs and health care spending, have led to the growth and development of many neonatal special care or intensive care units across the nation. RTs working outside of free-standing children's and university hospitals, many of whom have typically cared for adults, are now often called to support newborns at high-risk deliveries or to manage pediatric patients in respiratory distress. With advance practice roles becoming the norm, practitioners are faced with more challenging decisions that require collaboration, teamwork, and sharp critical thinking skills. These attributes, coupled with a better understanding of evidence-based practice and technologically advanced equipment, will positively affect patient outcomes and raise future ethical debates.

We believe that *Neonatal and Pediatric Respiratory Care,* fourth edition, will provide you with the tools and knowledge to improve the respiratory care of neonates, infants, and children regardless of your education, experience, or the environment in which you work.

AUDIENCE

Although principally designed as a textbook for the respiratory care student and practitioners new to the field, this book is also intended to be detailed enough to serve as a current desktop reference for the experienced practitioner engaged in mastering the practice of respiratory care in infants and children, regardless of professional discipline. This textbook may also serve as a study guide for the National Board for Respiratory Care's (NBRC) specialty examination concerning the respiratory care of neonatal and pediatric patients. For convenience, the Evolve Resources for this edition include a correlation guide for the NBRC's Neonatal/Pediatric Respiratory Care Specialty Examination.

New to this Edition

The publisher and editors of this textbook have taken a more focused approach to satisfying some of the essential features that are needed to help guide educators and students at the collegiate level. This fourth edition introduces the following:

- The text is now presented in full color with major updates to the art program.
- The combination of several chapters create a compressive look at several diseases or themes.
- Revisions to all the chapters reflect the latest updates in scientific literature.
- A new chapter titled "Quality and Safety" has improved the well-rounded character of the book.
- Measurable learning objectives, key terms, and key points have been added to each chapter. The objectives are designed to succinctly guide the student to key areas of importance and mastery of chapter content.
- Each chapter concludes with a series of multiple-choice assessment questions. Answers can be found on the Evolve website at http://evolve.elsevier.com/Walsh/neonatal.

LEARNING AIDS

Evolve Resources—http://evolve.elsevier.com/Walsh/neonatal

Evolve is an interactive learning environment designed to work in conjunction with this text. Instructors may use Evolve to provide an Internet-based course component that reinforces and expands the concepts presented in class. Evolve may be used to publish the class syllabus, outlines, and lecture notes; set up "virtual office hours" and e-mail communication; share important dates and information through the online class calendar; and encourage student participation through chat rooms and discussion boards. Evolve allows instructors to post exams and manage their grade books online.

For the Instructor

For the instructor, Evolve offers valuable resources to help them prepare their courses, including the following:
- PowerPoint lecture for each chapter
- A test bank of approximately 800 questions in ExamView
- An image collection of the figures from the book available in PowerPoint presentations for each chapter
- National Board for Respiratory Care (NBRC) Neonatal/Pediatric Respiratory Care Specialty (NPS) examination correlation guide

For Students

For students, Evolve offers valuable resources to help them succeed in their courses, including the following:
- Answers to Assessment Questions and Case Studies
- NBRC Neonatal/Pediatric Respiratory Care Specialty (NPS) examination correlation guide

  For more information, visit http://evolve.elsevier.com/Walsh/neonatal or contact an Elsevier sales representative.

ACKNOWLEDGMENTS

I thank all the contributors to this edition of *Neonatal and Pediatric Respiratory Care*. It is their work that yet again laid the foundation for this edition. I thank them for their patience and the professional quality of each chapter's content. I also thank Dr. Ruben Restrepo for his work writing the test bank and PowerPoint presentations for the accompanying Evolve instructor resources.

I also must include a special and warm appreciation for Sherry L. Barnhart, Michael Czervinske, and Robert DiBlasi as previous editors of this book who could no longer participate as editors. They have my gratitude for making this book what it is today. None of this would have been possible without their knowledge, dedication, and drive.

Additionally I thank the developmental publishing staff, especially Senior Content Development Specialist Charlene Ketchum, who tirelessly attempted to keep the contributors and me in line and on target for publication. I continue to be awed by your wonderful attitude and never-ending supply of positive instruction, in spite of many delays and changes along this journey. I also thank Billie Sharp, Content Manager, for her calm patience and attention to detail.

Last, but by no means least, I especially thank my wife, Stephanie, for her endless love, patience, support, and encouragement to persevere through this project. I am blessed beyond words.

Brian K. Walsh

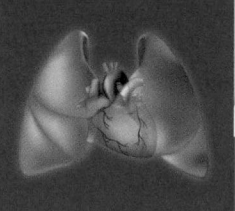

Contents

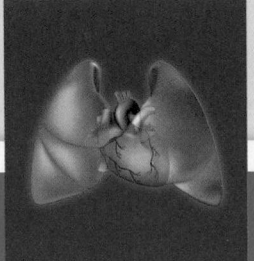

Chapter 1

Fetal Lung Development

ROBERT L. JOYNER, JR.

LEARNING OBJECTIVES

After reading this chapter the reader will be able to:

1. List the five stages of fetal lung development and the gestational age at which they occur
2. Explain the key steps of each stage of fetal development
3. Identify the gestational age during which extrauterine viability occurs, and explain why it cannot occur earlier
4. Identify several conditions that lead to abnormal lung development and injury
5. Discuss the role of the type II pneumocyte in surfactant production
6. Discuss the various physiological functions of surfactant
7. Explain how fetal lung liquid differs from amniotic fluid and describe how it is cleared during and after labor

KEY TERMS

Fetal lung fluid
Lamellar bodies
Oligohydramnios
Primary germ layers

Pseudoglandular
Pulmonary acinar units
Pulmonary hypoplasia
Saccules

Secondary crests
Surfactant

At birth, the lungs become the source for gas exchange between the external environment and the blood. External respiration through the lungs becomes essential to the survival of the newborn. Fetal lung development is progressive, and at birth the lungs have reached only that degree of morphological, physiological, and biochemical maturity required for basic functioning to support extrauterine life. In other words, lung development is not complete at birth: The newborn lung continues to undergo differentiation and growth well beyond birth.[1,2] Fetal lung development is not considered complete until the alveoli possess an adequate surface area for gas exchange. The pulmonary vascular system must also have sufficient capacity to transport an adequate amount of blood through the lungs for carbon dioxide and oxygen exchange. The alveoli need to be structurally and functionally stable and sufficiently elastic and resilient to endure the cyclical stretching associated with tidal breathing and crying.

What is known about the normal development of the human lung originates from Reid's anatomical description of the developing human lung. From this description the following can be ascertained:

The bronchial tree develops by week 16 of intrauterine life.

After birth the alveoli develop in increasing numbers until the age of 8 years and increase in size until growth of the chest wall is finished.

Preacinar arteries and veins develop after the airway has been established; intra-acinar vessels develop after the alveoli are generated.[3]

Although the criteria listed here are generally agreed on, research interest in the mechanics of fetal lung development continues to be kindled by the desire to prevent acute and chronic lung injury in premature infants. This interest is currently centered on the biochemical and genetic mechanisms of cellular repair in the immature lung that permit recovery of injured lungs in premature infants. Another topic of focus concerns the complex process of geometric growth and alveolar development.[4-6]

As stated earlier, birth does not signal the end of lung development. A remarkably complex process of growth occurs after birth, accommodating differing proportions of airway size, alveolar size, and surface area. The full-term infant, with an estimated 50 million alveoli, has the potential to add another 250 million alveoli and increase its total alveolar surface area from approximately 3 to 70 m^2 at maturity. More than 40 different cell types, with many different functions, are found in the lung. Adding to this complexity are growth factors, which are responsible for normal cell and structural development and affect various aspects of prenatal and postnatal lung function, growth, and structure.

PHASES OF LUNG DEVELOPMENT

In humans there are five well-recognized phases of lung development: embryonal, pseudoglandular, canalicular, saccular, and alveolar (Table 1-1).[7-9] Next you will find a description and important milestones of progression for each phase.

TABLE 1-1

Classification of Phases of Human Intrauterine Lung Growth

Stage	Time of Occurrence	Significance
Embryonal	Day 26 to day 52	Development of trachea and major bronchi
Pseudoglandular	Day 52 to week 16	Development of remaining conducting airways
Canalicular	Week 17 to week 26	Development of vascular bed and framework of respiratory acini
Saccular	Week 26 to week 36	Increased complexity of saccules
Alveolar	Week 36 to term	Development of alveoli

Embryonal Phase

The embryonal phase includes primitive lung development and is generally regarded to encompass the first 2 months of gestation. The lung begins to emerge as a bud from the pharynx 26 days after conception (Figure 1-1). This lung bud elongates and forms two bronchial buds and the trachea, which then separate from the esophagus through the development of the tracheoesophageal septum. Further subdivisions occur in an irregular, dichotomous way until the end of the embryonal stage. By this time, the major airways have developed. Various growth factors and fibroblasts mediate morphogenesis of the tubular epithelium, which results in airway branching: 10 on the right and 9 on the left.[1] The left and right pulmonary arteries form plexuses even before the heart descends into the thorax. Left and right pulmonary veins start to develop at about week 5 as a single evagination in the sinoatrial portion of the heart.

Within the embryonal phase, the respiratory epithelium develops from an area of the endoderm referred to as the foregut bud. The endoderm is the innermost layer of the three **primary germ layers** (i.e., endoderm, mesoderm, and ectoderm). The foregut bud interacts with the bronchial mesoderm (the middle primary germ layer) and through a number of complex embryonic development processes, this interaction eventually gives rise to the pulmonary interstitium, smooth muscle, blood vessels, and cartilage.[10] The mesenchyme, a network of undifferentiated embryonic connective tissue cells, determines the nature of airway branching by a complex interaction of epithelial cells with the bronchial mesoderm.[11] The mesenchyme and epithelium are separated from each other by a basal lamina containing type I collagen at the sites of airway branching.

The diaphragm also develops during the embryonal stage of lung development. Complete development of the diaphragm occurs by approximately week 7 of gestation.

Pseudoglandular Phase

The pseudoglandular phase, named after the distinct glandular appearance of the developing lung, extends to week 16 of gestation, during which time the conducting airways continue to develop. In this phase there is extensive subdivision of the conducting airway system. The branching pattern that occurs in both lungs determines the pattern in the adult lung.[12] The subsequent growth of these airways is in size only. The most distal structures are the terminal bronchioles, which likely differentiate into the respiratory bronchioles and alveolar ducts.[13] Once the pattern is laid, the subsequent growth of these airways is in size only. The gas-exchanging part of the lung, consisting of the pulmonary acini, or terminal respiratory units, may also be laid down completely during the pseudoglandular phase. Various growth factors and chemical mediators also begin to transdifferentiate the primordial tracheal epithelium into respiratory type II epithelial cells required for alveolar development.[1]

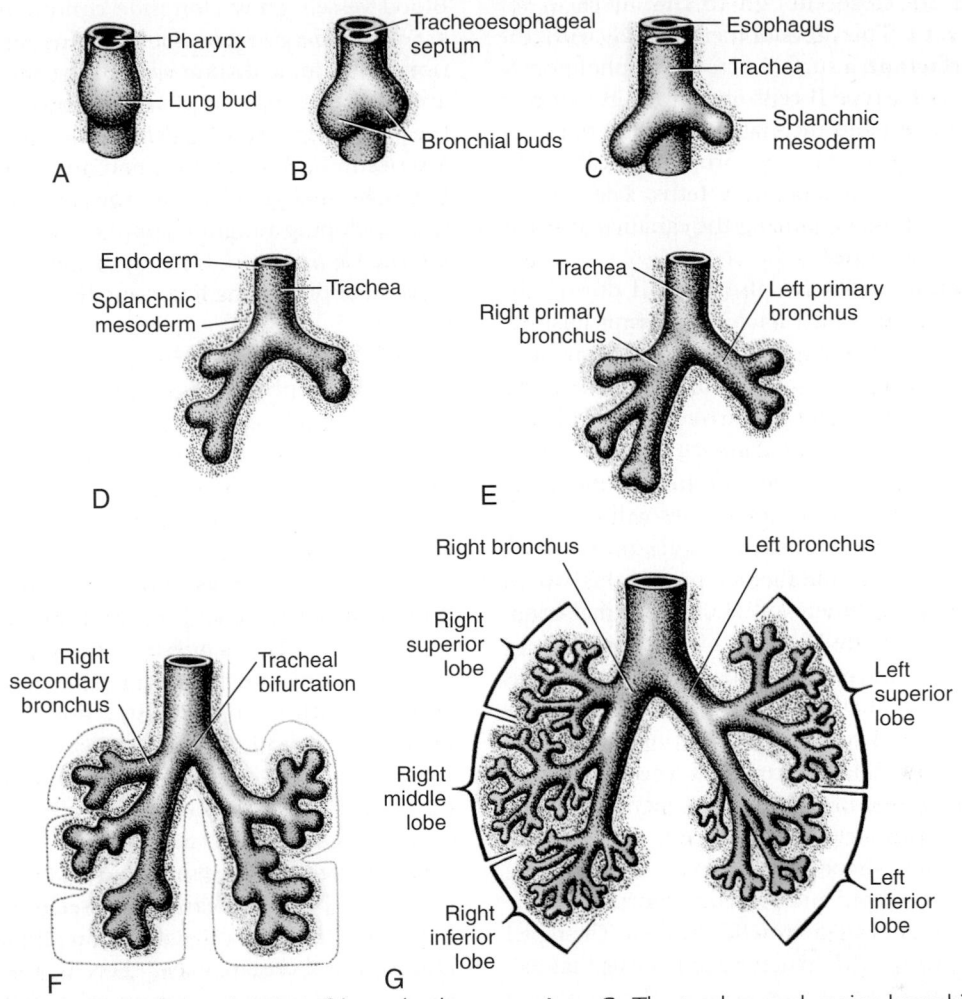

FIGURE 1-1 Embryonal stage of lung development. **A** to **C,** The trachea and major bronchi at 4 weeks; **D** and **E,** 5 weeks; **F,** 6 weeks; **G,** 8 weeks.

During the pseudoglandular phase, cilia appear on the surface of the epithelium of the trachea and the mainstem bronchi at 10 weeks of gestation and are present on the epithelial cells of the peripheral airways by 13 weeks of gestation. Goblet cells appear in the bronchial epithelium at 13 to 14 weeks of gestation, and submucosal glands arise as solid buds from basal layers of the surface epithelium at 15 to 16 weeks of gestation. Smooth muscle cells derived from the primitive mesenchyme surrounding the airways can be seen at the end of week 7 of gestation and by week 12 form the posterior wall of the large bronchi. The development of cartilage has been documented at 24 weeks of gestation and may be present earlier. Cartilage may be present in about 10 to 14 airway generations at 24 weeks of gestation. The cartilage is immature at this stage. Lymphatics appear first in the hilar region of the lung during week 8 of gestation and in the lung itself by week 10. This phase has been termed **pseudoglandular** because random histologic sections show the appearance of multiple round structures resembling glands. They are separated from each other by mesenchyme and its derivatives. The cells lining the spaces are columnar and contain glycogen. By the end of this stage, airways, arteries, and veins have developed in the pattern corresponding to that found in the adult.

Maturation of the immune system begins before birth. By 14 weeks' gestation, T lymphocytes can be found in the respiratory system. Fetal immune responses to allergens develop early and can be detected in cord blood. The potential routes of exposure are via the placenta (transplacental) or the fetal gut (by the swallowing of amniotic fluid). However, the relative importance of the two is not fully understood.[3]

Canalicular Phase

The canalicular phase follows the pseudoglandular phase and lasts from approximately 17 weeks to about 26 weeks of gestation. This phase is so named because of the appearance of vascular channels, or capillaries, which begin to grow by forming a capillary network around the air passages.[14] Some of the capillaries extend into the epithelium. The capillaries develop at 20 weeks of gestation and by 22 weeks have increased in number. Satisfactory gas exchange cannot occur until the capillaries have sufficient surface area and are close enough to the airspaces for efficient gas transfer. This development, along with the appearance of **surfactant,** a surface-active phospholipoprotein formed by alveolar type II cells important in reducing alveolar surface tension and ultimately reducing the work required for breathing in the newborn, is critical to the extrauterine survival of the immature fetus. The survival of the fetus becomes possible during the canalicular stage, at 22 to 24 weeks of gestation.

Pulmonary acinar units are also formed during the canalicular period (Figure 1-2). Each acinar unit (also referred to as an acinus) consists of a respiratory bronchiole (which contains no cartilage in its wall), alveolar ducts, and alveolar sacs. It follows that primitive lobules will have formed by the beginning of the canalicular phase. Each lobule will contain three to five terminal bronchioles; approximately 25,000 terminal bronchioles will be found in the adult lung. If the primitive acinar units are all formed by the end of the canalicular phase, this would imply that the full complement of 25,000 terminal bronchioles should be present by 28 weeks of gestation.

Thinning of the extracellular matrix, or mesenchyme, continues through the canalicular phase. By 20 to 22 weeks of gestation, two types of cells can be identified within the developing human lung. These distinct cell types are referred to as type I pneumocyte and type II pneumocyte epithelial cells. Within the canalicular phase the type II pneumocytes retain their cytoplasmic shape of their precursors and contain concentric layers of lipid and protein important for the production of surfactant called **lamellar bodies.** The type I pneumocytes will provide the structural apparatus that will become the alveoli and begin this process by flattening and elongating during this phase of development. The conducting airways have now developed smooth muscle.

By the end of the canalicular phase, the developing air–blood barrier is thin enough to support gas exchange.

Blood vessels grow alongside conducting airways, which are also undergoing muscularization, to a peripheral position that is more distant than in the adult.[15] The bronchial artery system may be as critical for lung development as the pulmonary arteries, although the role of the bronchial arteries in lung differentiation and growth is not clear.[16] It has been suggested that the most peripheral parts of the developing lung are supplied only by the pulmonary arterial vasculature.[15] The epithelial cells at this point are capable of producing fetal lung liquid.

Saccular Phase

The saccular phase was formerly thought to be the last stage of lung development before birth. However, because alveoli are now known to form before birth, the termination of the saccular period is arbitrarily set at 35 to 36 weeks of gestation. At the beginning of this phase, about 26 weeks of gestation, the terminal structures are referred to as **saccules** and are relatively smooth-walled, cylindrical structures. They then become subdivided by ridges known as **secondary crests** (Figure 1-3). As the crests protrude into the saccules, part of the capillary net is drawn in with them, forming a double capillary layer.[17,18] Further septation between the crests results in smaller spaces, which have been termed subsaccules. Exactly when these subsaccular structures become alveoli is a matter of debate (Figure 1-4). Some have advocated that any structure bordered on three sides should be termed an alveolus. Alveoli can be seen as early as 32 weeks of gestation and are present at 36 weeks of gestation in all fetuses (Figure 1-5). During the saccular phase, there is a marked increase in the potential gas-exchanging surface area.

Alveolar Phase

Distinction between the saccular and alveolar phases is somewhat arbitrary. Hislop, Wigglesworth, and Desai[19]

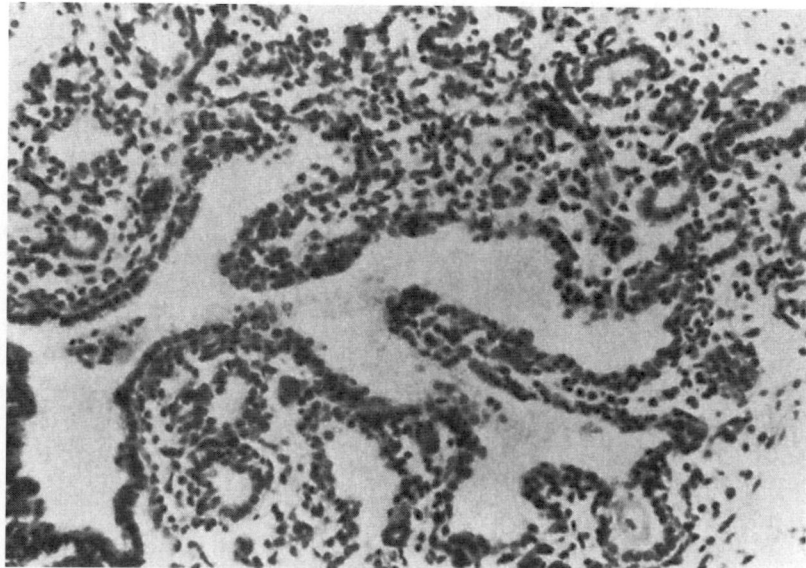

FIGURE 1-2   Canalicular stage of lung development at 22 weeks of gestation. A terminal bronchiole *(bottom left)* leads into a prospective acinus. Note that branches are sparse.

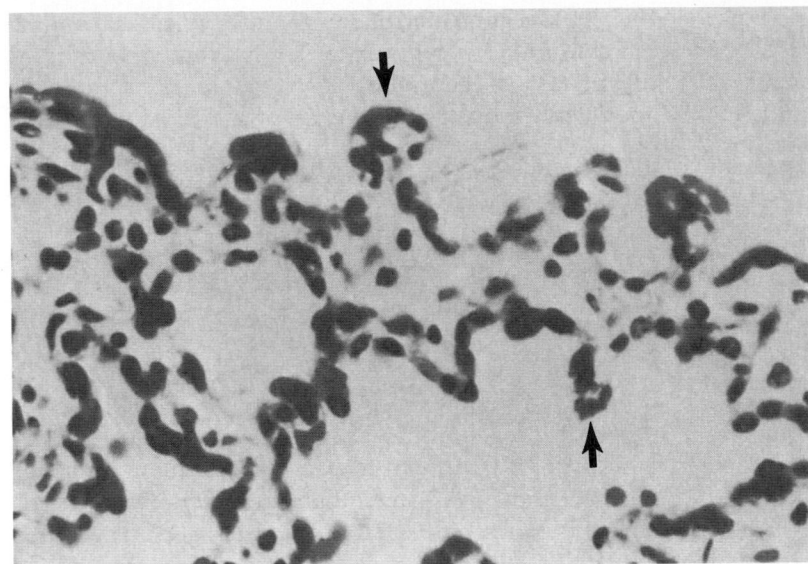

FIGURE 1-3 Saccular stage of lung development at 29 weeks of gestation. Secondary crests *(arrows)* begin to divide saccules into smaller compartments.

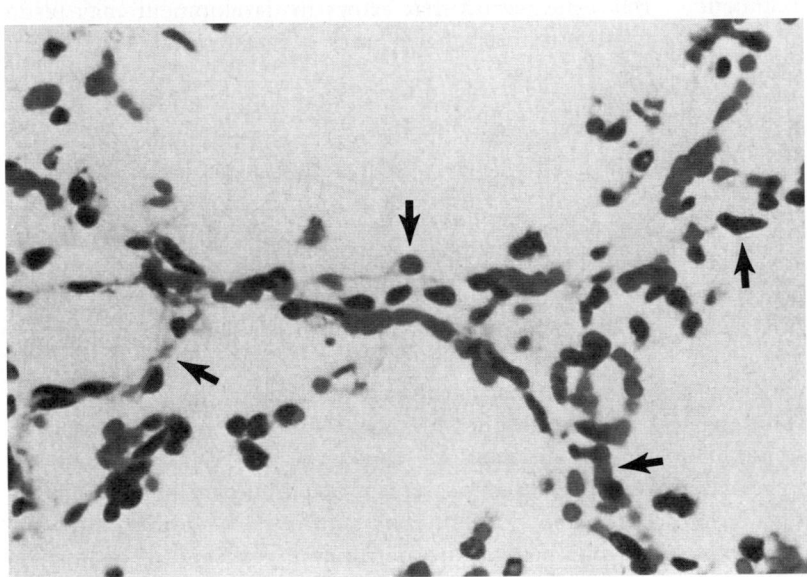

FIGURE 1-4 Alveolar stage of lung development at 36 weeks of gestation. Note the double capillary network *(solid arrows, center and right)* and the single capillary layer *(arrow at left)*.

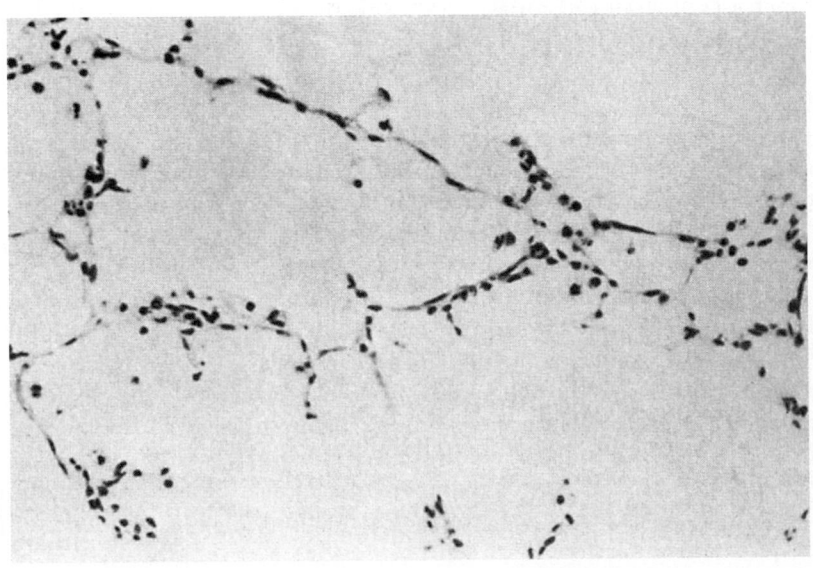

FIGURE 1-5 Alveolar stage of lung development at 36 weeks of gestation: Thin-walled alveoli are present.

claim that alveoli are present at 29 weeks of gestation; Langston and coworkers[7] believe that 36 weeks of gestation is the earliest point at which subsaccules and alveoli can be distinguished. Alveolar maturation and proliferation are primarily a postnatal event, extending beyond birth with rapid growth up to 18 months postgestation.[1] Alveologenesis is characterized by a complex interaction of epithelial, fibroblast, and vascular growth factors with extracellular matrix components.

At birth, the number of alveoli is highly variable, ranging from 20 to 150 million. The accepted mean number of alveoli, as described in the literature, is also variable, given as 50 million by Langston and colleagues[7] and 150 million by Hislop, Wigglesworth, and Desai.[19] It has been estimated that only 15% to 20% of the adult number of alveoli are present at birth, and thus alveologenesis is largely a postnatal event. Hislop, Wigglesworth, and Desai[19] believe that almost half the total number of alveoli are present at birth. The important point is that alveolarization is rapidly progressing during the period of development from late fetal to early neonatal life and may be complete by a year or so after birth.

POSTNATAL LUNG GROWTH

Normal lung growth is a continuous process that begins early in gestation and extends through infancy and childhood. Major structural development occurs in late gestation and continues over the first few years of postnatal life.[20,21] As stated earlier, estimates of alveolar number at birth vary widely, and the average of 50 million is generally accepted. These alveoli provide a total gas-exchanging surface of approximately 3 to 4 m^2. More than 80% of the eventual total number of alveoli—about 300 million—will form after birth. Lung volume will increase 23-fold, alveolar number will increase 6-fold, alveolar surface area will increase 21-fold, and lung weight will increase 20-fold. Lung volume increases disproportionally to alveolar number.

As the human infant doubles in body weight by 6 months and triples by 1 year, oxygen uptake increases proportionally; this is achieved by an increase in alveolar growth. The area of the air–tissue interface increases in a linear relationship to body surface area.[22] Alveolar volume and alveolar surface area increase in proportion to each other. However, alveolar number and alveolar diameter do not change proportionally. Most of the postnatal formation of alveoli in the infant occurs over the first 1.5 years of life.[23,24] Thereafter, the lung continues to grow in proportion to body growth.

Boyden and Tompsett[25] have described a mechanism of alveolar formation that includes extension of the gas-exchange region by transformation of the respiratory bronchioles into alveolar ducts and terminal bronchioles into respiratory bronchioles. Lateral pouches from these transformed respiratory bronchioles formed new alveoli. It has been proposed that new alveolar formation occurs in

this manner into later childhood and that this is the likely mechanism for new alveolar formation throughout life. At 2 years of age, the number of alveoli varies substantially among individuals. After 2 years of age, males have more alveoli than do females. After the end of alveolar multiplication, the alveoli continue to increase in size until thoracic growth is completed.[21]

FACTORS AFFECTING PRENATAL AND POSTNATAL LUNG GROWTH

Success of each phase of lung development, as previously defined, requires the precise interaction of numerous complex physiological mechanisms to result in the production of a flawless maturing lung at birth. It is understandable that occasionally there are problems that arise in the developmental process of the fetal lung that can affect prenatal lung growth. Development of the initial structures of the pulmonary tree occurs in the embryonal stage. It is during this time period that errors in development may result in laryngeal, tracheal, or esophageal atresia or stenosis may develop.[26] **Pulmonary hypoplasia,** an incomplete development of the lungs characterized by an abnormally low number and/or size of bronchopulmonary segments and/or alveoli, can develop during the pseudoglandular phase.[27] If the fetus is born during the cannicular phase (i.e., prematurely), severe respiratory distress can be expected as the inadequately developed airways and insufficient and immature surfactant production by alveolar type II cells lead to the constellation of problems know as infant respiratory distress syndrome.[28]

Developmental abnormalities of other organ systems can also affect lung development in the fetus. For example, abnormalities of the chest wall and renal hypoplasia can result in varying severities of pulmonary hypoplasia, the latter known as Potter's syndrome.[29,30] Additionally, some complex genetic disorders may also affect lung growth.[31]

Other clinical factors have been cited as causing diminished lung growth. These conditions can be divided into four categories:

· Chest wall compression as occurs in diaphragmatic hernia—that is, an abnormal opening in the prenatal diaphragm that allows some of the abdominal organs to move into the chest and exert pressure on the developing lungs; chest wall abnormalities; and probably hydrops fetalis—that is, abnormal fluid accumulation in the fetus, often resulting in hydrothorax and ascites—have all been implicated in diminished lung growth.[32]

· **Oligohydramnios,** a reduced quantity of amniotic fluid present for an extended period, with or without renal anomalies, is associated with lung hypoplasia.[33-35] The mechanisms by which amniotic fluid volume influences lung growth remain unclear. Possible explanations include mechanical restriction of the chest wall, interference with fetal breathing, and/or failure to produce fetal lung liquid. These clinical and experimental observations possibly point to a common denominator, lung stretch, as being a major growth stimulant.

· Diminished respiration has been shown to have a severe effect on lung growth. This effect could be mediated through a lack of stretch of the developing lung parenchyma.[36]

· A variety of hormonal or metabolic abnormalities may alter lung growth and structure. Leprechaunism, associated with abnormal carbohydrate metabolism, results in dysmorphic lungs with a decreased number of terminal bronchioles, dilated alveolar ducts and saccules, and enlarged airspaces.[37] Experimental diabetes produced by streptozotocin administration to 3-week-old rats resulted in diminished airspace size, increased alveolar number, and a marked effect on pulmonary connective tissue metabolism.[38,39]

An example of altered lung development is seen in children with Down syndrome. Although fetal lung growth is normal, postnatal lung growth is characterized by larger and fewer alveoli than normal.[40]

ABNORMAL LUNG DEVELOPMENT

Structural development of the lung may be altered by a number of conditions affecting the lungs in utero or by postnatal events.[41,42] Complex relationships exist among humoral, hormonal, and physical forces acting on the developing lung, altering its growth in ways that are poorly understood. Growth retardation of the fetal lung may affect size and weight but not maturation of airways and alveoli, whereas malnutrition may slow functional rather than structural maturation.[41]

Timing or dating of adverse events influencing fetal lung development is important in considering the approach to treatment and prognosis. Abnormalities occurring in the embryonic period are often associated with renal agenesis or dysplastic kidneys; branching of the lungs may also be affected. Abnormalities occurring later in development, such as diaphragmatic hernia, may affect the lungs during the pseudoglandular period, or before 16 weeks of gestation, and thereby decrease airway branching. If abnormalities occur during the second trimester of pregnancy, completion of pulmonary vascularization and acinar development may not proceed and hypoplasia in the gas-exchanging area may result. Problems occurring in the perinatal period, such as premature birth and bronchopulmonary dysplasia, may alter subsequent alveolar growth and differentiation, ultimately leading to a decrease in alveolar number.

PULMONARY HYPOPLASIA

Pulmonary hypoplasia, or failure of the lungs to develop in utero, is a relatively common abnormality of lung development, with a number of clinical associations and anatomical correlates. Hypoplasia may be considered to be present when there are too few cells, too few alveoli, or too few airways. The incidence of pulmonary hypoplasia diagnosed at autopsy is between 10% and 25% of all cases.[42-45]

The best-studied condition associated with hypoplasia is diaphragmatic hernia. The incidence of diaphragmatic hernia is about 1 in 4000 births. The range of abnormalities reported is wide and is probably related to variations in the severity and timing of the onset of lung compression.[46] Compression of the lung before 16 weeks of gestation causes incomplete branching of the conducting airways, terminal airways, or both. Early and severe compression results in severe hypoplasia can reduce the weight of the affected lung to less than half that of the contralateral lung. The affected lung demonstrates fewer, smaller alveoli, a decreased surface area for gas-exchange, and a proportional decrease in pulmonary vasculature.

Other forms of lung compression may result in hypoplasia. Causes include osteogenesis imperfecta, hypophosphatasia,[47] and thoracic dystrophies. In addition to chest wall anomalies, pleural effusion, ascites, intrathoracic tumors, and extralobar sequestration may cause lung compression.

Pulmonary hypoplasia occurs in oligohydramnios as a result of leakage of amniotic fluid. It was first described by Potter in association with renal agenesis.[33] Experimental evidence supports the conclusion that the amount of lung liquid present in the fetus is a major determinant of lung growth, because chronic tracheal drainage produces pulmonary hypoplasia and tracheal ligation produces lungs with increased tissue mass.[48] It has been shown that experimental oligohydramnios causes pulmonary hypoplasia, which can be more or less severe depending on its timing.[43,49]

Several experimental studies suggest that lung growth alteration may be caused by various hormonal imbalances.[50-54] Changes caused by endocrine effects may cause lung compression or diminished lung liquid and respiration. Glucocorticoid administration has been shown to accelerate lung maturation but may also affect lung growth. Type II epithelial cell maturation is induced both functionally and anatomically by this drug. Depending on the dose, glucocorticoids may reduce the rate of DNA synthesis and thus produce hypoplasia. Thyroidectomy in fetal sheep produces pulmonary hypoplasia and diminished type II cell differentiation. Maternal growth hormone apparently plays little role in fetal growth, but the effect of maternal administration of growth hormone on fetal lung growth has not been studied. Maternal experimental diabetes results in diminished tissue maturity in the fetus.[55]

ALVEOLAR CELL DEVELOPMENT AND SURFACTANT PRODUCTION

As the primordial epithelium evolves, the epithelial lining undergoes cellular division and differentiation into the highly specialized type I and type II pneumocytes. Type I pneumocytes are flat (squamous) cells serving as a thin, gas-permeable membrane for the diffusion of gases and as a barrier against water and solute leakage.[56] They account for more than 97% of the alveolar surface area, primarily as a result of their size, shape, and large cellular surface.[57]

Despite its smaller surface area, the cuboidal-appearing type II pneumocyte is the principal cell involved in surfactant production, storage, secretion, and reuse. Surfactant storage occurs in the lamellar bodies inside type II pneumocytes. An additional function of the type II pneumocyte is its ability to differentiate into type I pneumocytes.[58]

Type II pneumocytes contain the precursors required for surfactant synthesis and osmiophilic lamellar bodies that function as the storage apparatus for the synthesized surfactant.[9,57] Through a continuous process of exocytosis, the lamellar bodies release their contents of tubular myelin into the alveolar hypophase (the thin liquid lining of the internal surface of the alveoli). The liberated tubular myelin unravels and disperses to form a monolayer at the air–liquid interface.[58]

The primary role of mammalian surfactant is to lower the surface tension within the alveolus, specifically at the air–liquid interface. This allows the delicate structure of the alveolus to expand when filled with air. Without surfactant, the alveolus remains collapsed because of the high surface tension of the moist alveolar surface. Surfactant is composed predominantly of an intricate blend of phospholipids, neutral lipids, and proteins. See Chapter 14 (Surfactant Replacement) for more information about surfactant composition.

Of clinical relevance during late gestation, analysis of amniotic fluid for the concentration of phosphatidylglycerol and phosphatidylcholine has been shown to be a sensitive indicator of the state of fetal lung maturity.[59] In addition, various chemical and mechanical stimulatory mechanisms leading to increased surfactant precursor (and presumably mature surfactant) production have been identified and include, but are not limited to, β-adrenergic agonists, prostaglandins, epidermal growth factor, and mechanical ventilation.

FETAL LUNG LIQUID

Fetal lungs are secretory organs that make breathing-like movements but serve no respiratory function before birth. They secrete about 250 to 300 ml of liquid per day. Thus the fetal airways are not collapsed but filled with fluid from the canalicular phase until delivery and the initiation of ventilation. This liquid flows from the terminal respiratory units through the conducting airways and into the oropharynx, where it is either swallowed or expelled into the amniotic sac. The presence of **fetal lung fluid** is essential for normal lung development. This luminal fluid is high in chloride and low in bicarbonate, with a negligible concentration of protein.[60,61] Active transport of chloride

ions across the fetal pulmonary epithelium generates an electric potential difference and causes liquid to flow from the lung microcirculation through the interstitium and into the airspaces.[62] The pulmonary circulation, rather than the bronchial circulation, is the major source of this liquid. The balance between production and drainage of this liquid has an important effect on lung development. During fetal breathing, there is a small but steady movement of fluid outward from the trachea. The net movement of fluid away from the lungs has been measured at about 15 ml/hr and was about five times higher during periods of fetal breathing than during apnea.[63] Prolonged outflow obstruction expands the lungs and leads to a decrease in type II cells.[64] In contrast, unimpeded removal of lung liquid decreases lung size, increases apparent tissue density, and stimulates proliferation of type II cells.[48]

The clearance of fetal lung fluid is essential for normal neonatal respiratory adaptation. However, several studies have shown that both the rate of liquid formation and the volume within the lumen of the fetal lung normally decrease before birth.[65-67] It is unknown what causes the reduction in fetal lung secretions before birth. Hormonal changes, which occur in the fetus just before and during labor, may have an important role in triggering this process. The influence of catecholamines on fetal lung liquid volume has been investigated. It has been shown that injecting β-adrenergic agonists into pregnant rabbits reduces the amount of water in the lungs of their pups.[68] Epinephrine has been shown to inhibit secretion of fetal lung liquid.[69] Other hormones, such as arginine vasopressin and prostaglandin E_2, which are secreted around the time of birth, may reduce production of lung luminal liquid.[70,71]

Removal of lung liquid continues after birth. When breathing begins, air inflation shifts residual liquid from the lumen into distensible perivascular spaces around large pulmonary blood vessels and bronchi. Accumulation of liquid in these connective tissue spaces, which are distant from the sites of respiratory gas exchange, allows time for small blood vessels and lymphatics to remove the displaced liquid with little or no impairment of neonatal lung function at this critical juncture.[72,73] The clearance of the fluid from the interstitial spaces occurs over many hours.

KEY POINTS

- Each developmental phase of the fetal lung is defined by its characteristic anatomical growth and maturation.
- A thorough understanding of each stage of fetal lung development is an important basis for identifying problems occurring during fetal lung development as well as helping to prepare for the delivery and care of the premature infant.
- Fetal survival outside the uterus becomes possible at approximately 24 weeks' gestation. Survival outside

the uterus before this is not possible because the pulmonary capillary system is not sufficient to support gas exchange.

- Abnormal lung development can occur at any point during gestation.
  - Early developmental problems can be associated with abnormalities of other organ systems (e.g., renal agenesis associated lung branching abnormalities).
  - Other developmental problems can occur as through the direct hindrance of proper gestational growth (e.g., congenital diaphragmatic hernia with direct compression to the developing lung inhibits normal growth.)
- By 22 weeks' gestation, the cytoplasm within the alveolar type II cells begins to contain lamellar bodies, which are important in the production of surfactant.
- Surfactant produced by alveolar type II cells is a phospholipoprotein important for reducing alveolar surface tension. This reduction in surface tension reduces the work of breathing in a spontaneously breathing newborn.
- Fetal lung fluid is secreted by cells of the fetal airways. This fluid flows from the distal terminal airways toward the pharynx and eventually is either swallowed or expelled as a constituent of the amniotic fluid.
- During the birthing process, production of fetal lung fluid is slowed, and after birth the fetal lung fluid is cleared by the lymphatic system of the lung.

ASSESSMENT QUESTIONS

See Evolve Resources for answers.

1. Which of the following are phases of human lung development?
   I. Embryonal
   II. Canalicular
   III. Blastocystic
   IV. Chorionic
   V. Saccular
      A. I, III, and III
      B. I, II, and V
      C. II and IV
      D. III and V
      E. I, IV, and V

2. The initial lung bud emerges from which of the following?
   A. Esophagus
   B. Trachea
   C. Umbilical cord
   D. Pharynx
   E. Mesoderm layer

3. The bronchial tree is formed at which gestational phase of lung development?
   A. Embryonal
   B. Canalicular
   C. Pseudoglandular
   D. Saccular
   E. Alveolar

4. The alveolar epithelial lining undergoes cell division into type I and type II pneumocytes. Which of the following correctly describe the pneumocytes?
   I. Type I pneumocytes account for more than 97% of the alveolar surface area.
   II. Type II pneumocytes form a gas-permeable membrane for diffusion of gases.
   III. Surfactant production occurs in the lamellar bodies of type II pneumocytes, which release surfactant by exocytosis.
   IV. Type I pneumocytes are responsible for surfactant production and storage.
   V. Type I pneumocytes are squamous shaped and optimized for gas exchange; type II pneumocytes are cube shaped and may differentiate into type I cells.
      A. I, II, IV, and V
      B. I, III, and V
      C. I, IV, and V
      D. II, IV, and V
      E. III and IV

5. What are the minimal developmental features required for an immature human fetus to survive outside the uterus?
   I. 32 weeks of gestation
   II. Sufficient alveolar and vascular surface area for gas exchange
   III. Sufficient endoplasmic reticulum production
   IV. 22 to 24 weeks of gestation
   V. Near completion of the canalicular stage of lung development
      A. I, II, III, and IV
      B. I and V
      C. II, III, and V
      D. II, IV, and V
      E. III, IV, and V

6. Which of the following best describe(s) fetal lung liquid?
   A. It lowers surface tension within the alveoli.
   B. It maintains the structure of the airway lumen and developing alveoli, preventing complete collapse.
   C. With fetal breathing movement it continuously flows out of the lungs and is swallowed or excreted into the amniotic fluid.
   D. A and B
   E. B and C

7. Estimates of the exact number of alveoli at birth vary widely, but investigators agree that
   A. The surface area of gas exchange increases inversely with age.
   B. Normal structural development is complete before the first breath.
   C. Normal lung growth is a continuous process that extends into adulthood.
   D. Gas exchange surface area grows proportionally with an increase in oxygen consumption and body surface area.
   E. Extension of gas exchange occurs with transformation of alveolar ducts and terminal bronchioles into respiratory bronchioles.

8. Which is the lung development stage formerly thought to be the last stage before birth, and characterized by relatively smooth-walled, cylindrical structures subdivided by ridges known as secondary crests?
   - A. Alveolar phase
   - B. Saccular phase
   - C. Terminal phase
   - D. Trophoblast phase
   - E. Canalicular phase

9. Pulmonary hypoplasia is a relatively common abnormality of lung development with a number of clinical associations, including which of the following?
   - A. Lung tissue compression
   - B. Oligohydramnios
   - C. Maternal diabetes
   - D. All of the above
   - E. A and C only

10. Which of the following statements represent Reid's laws of human lung development?
    - I. The bronchial tree develops by week 16 of intrauterine life.
    - II. Preacinar vasculature develops after the airway has been established, and intra-acinar vasculature develops after the alveoli are generated.
    - III. Alveolar development is complete when there is sufficient gas exchange surface area to support extrauterine life.
    - IV. The esophageal lung bud arises from the embryonic mesoderm to form the tracheal bronchial tree.
    - V. Alveoli increase in number until 8 years of age and grow in size until chest wall growth is complete.
      - A. I and IV
      - B. I, II, and V
      - C. I, III, IV, and V
      - D. II and III
      - E. II, III, and V

References

1. Burri P: Structural aspects of prenatal and post natal development and growth of the lung. In McDonald J, editor: *Lung growth and development*, New York, 1997, Marcel Dekker, pp 1–35.
2. Boyden E: Development and growth of the airways. In Hodson W, editor: *Development of the lung*, New York, 1977, Marcel Dekker, pp 3–35.
3. Reid L: The embryology of the lung. In DeReuck A, Porter R, editors: *Development of the lung*, Boston, 1967, Little Brown, pp 109–130.
4. Sheffield M, Mabry S, Thibeault DW, Truog WE: Pulmonary nitric oxide synthases and nitrotyrosine: findings during lung development and in chronic lung disease of prematurity, *Pediatrics* 118(3):1056, 2006.
5. Kreiger PA, Ruchelli ED, Mahboubi S, Hedrick H, Scott Adzick N, Russo PA: Fetal pulmonary malformations: defining histopathology, *Am J Surg Pathol* 30(5):643, 2006.
6. Bourbon J, Boucherat O, Chailley-Heu B, Delacourt C: Control mechanisms of lung alveolar development and their disorders in bronchopulmonary dysplasia, *Pediatr Res* 57(5 Pt 2):38R, 2005.
7. Langston C, Kida K, Reed M, Thurlbeck WM: Human lung growth in late gestation and in the neonate, *Am Rev Respir Dis* 129(4):607, 1984.
8. Liggins GC: Growth of the fetal lung, *J Dev Physiol* 6(3):237, 1984.
9. Xu J, Tian J, Grumelli SM, Haley KJ, Shapiro SD: Stage-specific effects of cAMP signaling during distal lung epithelial development, *J Biol Chem* 281(50):38894, 2006.
10. Loosli CG, Potter EL: Pre- and postnatal development of the respiratory portion of the human lung with special reference to the elastic fibers, *Am Rev Respir Dis* 80(1, Part 2):5, 1959.
11. Spooner BS, Wessells NK. Mammalian lung development: interactions in primordium formation and bronchial morphogenesis, *J Exp Zool* 175(4):445, 1970.
12. Hislop A, Reid L: Growth and development of the respiratory system: anatomical development. In Davies J, Dobbing J, editors: *Scientific foundation of paediatrics*, London, 1974, Medical Books, pp 214–254.
13. Itoh K, Itoh H: A study of cartilage development in pulmonary hypoplasia, *Pediatr Pathol* 8(1):65, 1988.
14. Thurlbeck WM: Prematurity and the developing lung, *Clin Perinatol* 19(3):497, 1992.
15. Hilslop A, Reid L: Formation of the pulmonary vasculature. In Hodson W, editor: *Development of the lung*, New York, 1979, Marcel Dekker, pp 37–86.
16. Boyden EA: The time lag in the development of bronchial arteries, *Anat Rec*, 166(4):611, 1970.
17. Cooney TP, Thurlbeck WM: The radial alveolar count method of Emery and Mithal: a reappraisal 2—intrauterine and early postnatal lung growth, *Thorax* 37(8):580, 1982.
18. Bruce MC, Honaker CE, Cross RJ: Lung fibroblasts undergo apoptosis following alveolarization, *Am J Respir Cell Mol Biol* 20(2):228, 1999.
19. Hislop AA, Wigglesworth JS, Desai R: Alveolar development in the human fetus and infant, *Early Hum Dev* 13(1):1, 1986.
20. Reid L: 1976 Edward B.D. Neuhauser lecture: the lung: growth and remodeling in health and disease, *AJR Am J Roentgenol* 129(5):777, 1977.
21. Thurlbeck WM: Postnatal growth and development of the lung, *Am Rev Respir Dis* 111(6):803, 1975.
22. Dunnill M: Postnatal growth of the lung, *Thorax* 17(4):329, 1962.
23. Zeltner TB, Burri PH: The postnatal development and growth of the human lung. II. Morphology, *Respir Physiol* 67(3):269, 1987.
24. Zeltner TB, Caduff JH, Gehr P, Pfenninger J, Burri PH: The postnatal development and growth of the human lung. I. Morphometry, *Respir Physiol* 67(3):247, 1987.
25. Boyden EA, Tompsett DH: The changing patterns in the developing lungs of infants, *Acta Anat (Basel)* 61(2):164, 1965.
26. Berrocal T, Madrid C, Novo S, Gutierrez J, Arjonilla A, Gomez-Leon N: Congenital anomalies of the tracheobronchial tree, lung, and mediastinum: embryology, radiology, and pathology, *Radiographics* 24(1):e17, 2004.
27. Kotecha S: Lung growth: implications for the newborn infant, *Arch Dis Child Fetal Neonatal Ed* 82(1):F69, 2000.
28. Wirbelauer J, Speer CP: The role of surfactant treatment in preterm infants and term newborns with acute respiratory distress syndrome, *J Perinatol* 29(Suppl 2):S18, 2009.
29. Fraga JR, Mirza AM, Reichelderfer TE: Association of pulmonary hypoplasia, renal anomalies, and Potter's facies, *Clin Pediatr (Phila)* 12(3):150, 1973.

30. Swischuk LE, Richardson CJ, Nichols MM, Ingman MJ: Bilateral pulmonary hypoplasia in the neonate, *AJR Am J Roentgenol* 133(6):1057, 1979.

31. Nogee LM, de Mello DE, Dehner LP, Colten HR: Brief report: deficiency of pulmonary surfactant protein B in congenital alveolar proteinosis, *N Engl J Med* 328(6):406, 1993.

32. Karamanoukian HL, O'Toole SJ, Holm BA, Glick PL: Making the most out of the least: new insights into congenital diaphragmatic hernia, *Thorax* 52(3):209, 1997.

33. Potter EL: Bilateral renal agenesis, *J Pediatr* 29:68, 1946.

34. King JC, Mitzner W, Butterfield AB, Queenan JT: Effect of induced oligohydramnios on fetal lung development, *Am J Obstet Gynecol* 154(4):823, 1986.

35. Perlman M, Williams J, Hirsch M: Neonatal pulmonary hypoplasia after prolonged leakage of amniotic fluid, *Arch Dis Child* 51(5):349, 1976.

36. Nagai A, Thurlbeck WM, Deboeck C, Ioffe S, Chernick V: The effect of maternal CO_2 breathing on lung development of fetuses in the rabbit. Morphologic and morphometric studies, *Am Rev Respir Dis* 135(1):130, 1987.

37. Thurlbeck WM, Cooney TP: Dysmorphic lungs in a case of leprechaunism: case report and review of literature, *Pediatr Pulmonol* 5(2):100, 1988.

38. Ofulue AF, Kida K, Thurlbeck WM: Experimental diabetes and the lung. I. Changes in growth, morphometry, and biochemistry, *Am Rev Respir Dis* 137(1):162, 1988.

39. Ofulue AF, Thurlbeck WM: Experimental diabetes and the lung. II. In vivo connective tissue metabolism, *Am Rev Respir Dis* 138(2):284, 1988.

40. Cooney TP, Wentworth PJ, Thurlbeck WM: Diminished radial count is found only postnatally in Down's syndrome, *Pediatr Pulmonol* 5(4):204, 1988.

41. Lipsett J, Tamblyn M, Madigan K, Roberts P, Cool JC, Runciman SI, et al: Restricted fetal growth and lung development: a morphometric analysis of pulmonary structure, *Pediatr Pulmonol* 41(12):1138, 2006.

42. Reale FR, Esterly JR: Pulmonary hypoplasia: a morphometric study of the lungs of infants with diaphragmatic hernia, anencephaly, and renal malformations, *Pediatrics* 51(1):91, 1973.

43. Moessinger AC, Abbey-Mensah M, Driscoll JM, Blanc WA: Pulmonary hypoplasia, a disorder on the rise? [abstract], *Pediatr Res* 17:327A, 1983.

44. Moessinger AC, Collins MH, Blanc WA, Rey HR, James LS: Oligohydramnios-induced lung hypoplasia: the influence of timing and duration in gestation, *Pediatr Res* 20(10):951, 1986.

45. Page DV, Stocker JT: Anomalies associated with pulmonary hypoplasia, *Am Rev Respir Dis* 125(2):216, 1982.

46. George DK, Cooney TP, Chiu BK, Thurlbeck WM: Hypoplasia and immaturity of the terminal lung unit (acinus) in congenital diaphragmatic hernia, *Am Rev Respir Dis* 136(4):947, 1987.

47. Silver MM, Vilos GA, Milne KJ: Pulmonary hypoplasia in neonatal hypophosphatasia, *Pediatr Pathol* 8(5):483, 1988.

48. Alcorn D, Adamson TM, Lambert TF, Maloney JE, Ritchie BC, Robinson PM: Morphological effects of chronic tracheal ligation and drainage in the fetal lamb lung, *J Anat* 123 (Pt 3):649, 1977.

49. Blachford KG, Thurlbeck WM: Lung growth and maturation in experimental oligohydramnios in the rat, *Pediatr Pulmonol* 3(5):328, 1987.

50. Crone RK, Davies P, Liggins GC, Reid L: The effects of hypophysectomy, thyroidectomy, and postoperative infusion of cortisol or adrenocorticotrophin on the structure of the ovine fetal lung, *J Dev Physiol* 5(5):281, 1983.

51. Erenberg A, Rhodes ML, Weinstein MM, Kennedy RL: The effect of fetal thyroidectomy on ovine fetal lung maturation, *Pediatr Res* 13(4 Pt 1):230, 1979.

52. Liggins GC, Kitterman JA, Campos GA, Clements JA, Forster CS, Lee CH, et al: Pulmonary maturation in the hypophysectomised ovine fetus. Differential responses to adrenocorticotrophin and cortisol, *J Dev Physiol* 3(1):1, 1981.

53. Morishige WK, Joun NS: Influence of glucocorticoids on postnatal lung development in the rat: possible modulation by thyroid hormone, *Endocrinology* 111(5):1587, 1982.

54. Pinkerton KE, Kendall JZ, Randall GC, Chechowitz MA, Hyde DM, Plopper CG: Hypophysectomy and porcine fetal lung development, *Am J Respir Cell Mol Biol* 1(4):319, 1989.

55. Sosenko IR, Frantz ID 3rd, Roberts RJ, Meyrick B: Morphologic disturbance of lung maturation in fetuses of alloxan diabetic rabbits, *Am Rev Respir Dis* 122(5):687, 1980.

56. Schneeberger EE: Alveolar type I cells. In Crystal RG, West JB, editors: *The lung: scientific foundations*, New York, 1991, Raven Press, pp 1677–1685.

57. Notter RH, Shapiro DL: Lung surfactants for replacement therapy: biochemical, biophysical, and clinical aspects, *Clin Perinatol* 14(3):433, 1987.

58. Adamson IY, Bowden DH: The type 2 cell as progenitor of alveolar epithelial regeneration. A cytodynamic study in mice after exposure to oxygen, *Lab Invest* 30(1):35, 1974.

59. Kresch MJ, Gross I: The biochemistry of fetal lung development, *Clin Perinatol* 14(3):481, 1987.

60. Mescher EJ, Platzker AC, Ballard PL, Kitterman JA, Clements JA, Tooley WH: Ontogeny of tracheal fluid, pulmonary surfactant, and plasma corticoids in the fetal lamb, *J Appl Physiol* 39(6):1017, 1975.

61. Adams FH, Fujiwara T, Rowshan G: The nature and origin of the fluid in the fetal lamb lung, *J Pediatr* 63:881, 1963.

62. Olver RE, Strang LB: Ion fluxes across the pulmonary epithelium and the secretion of lung liquid in the foetal lamb, *J Physiol* 241(2):327, 1974.

63. Harding R, Sigger JN, Wickham PJ, Bocking AD: The regulation of flow of pulmonary fluid in fetal sheep, *Respir Physiol* 57(1):47, 1984.

64. Carmel JA, Friedman F, Adams FH: Fetal tracheal ligation and lung development, *Am J Dis Child* 109:452, 1965.

65. Kitterman JA, Ballard PL, Clements JA, Mescher EJ, Tooley WH: Tracheal fluid in fetal lambs: spontaneous decrease prior to birth, *J Appl Physiol* 47(5):985, 1979.

66. Dickson KA, Maloney JE, Berger PJ: Decline in lung liquid volume before labor in fetal lambs, *J Appl Physiol* 61(6):2266, 1986.

67. Brown MJ, Olver RE, Ramsden CA, Strang LB, Walters DV: Effects of adrenaline and of spontaneous labour on the secretion and absorption of lung liquid in the fetal lamb, *J Physiol* 344:137, 1983.

68. Enhorning G, Chamberlain D, Contreras C, Burgoyne R, Robertson B: Isoxsuprine-induced release of pulmonary surfactant in the rabbit fetus, *Am J Obstet Gynecol* 129(2):197, 1977.

69. Lawson EE, Brown ER, Torday JS, Madansky DL, Taeusch HW Jr: The effect of epinephrine on tracheal fluid flow and surfactant efflux in fetal sheep, *Am Rev Respir Dis* 118(6):1023, 1978.

70. Bland RD, Fike CD, Teague WG, Braun D, Keil LC: Vasopressin decreases lung water in fetal lambs [abstract], *Pediatr Res* 19(4):399A, 1985.

71. Kitterman JA: Fetal lung development, *J Dev Physiol* 6(1):67, 1984.

72. Bland RD, Hansen TN, Haberkern CM, Bressack MA, Hazinski TA, Raj JU, et al: Lung fluid balance in lambs before and after birth, *J Appl Physiol* 53(4):992, 1982.

73. Bland RD, McMillan DD, Bressack MA, Dong L: Clearance of liquid from lungs of newborn rabbits, *J Appl Physiol* 49(2):171, 1980.

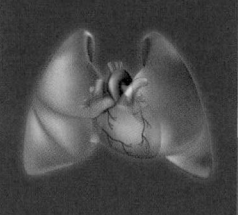

Chapter 2

Fetal Gas Exchange and Circulation

ROBERT L. JOYNER, JR.

OUTLINE

Embryological Overview
    Fertilization to Implantation
    Maternal Fetal Gas Exchange
Cardiovascular Development
    Early Development

    Chamber Development
    Maturation
Fetal Circulation and Fetal Shunts
Transition to Extrauterine Life

LEARNING OBJECTIVES

After reading this chapter the reader will be able to:

1. Discuss the identifiable stages of heart development and explain the development of the heart chambers
2. Name the three fetal shunts and discuss their role during fetal circulation
3. Explain the direction of blood flow and relative vascular pressures in the placenta, umbilical vein, three fetal shunts, right-side heart chambers, left-side heart chambers, pulmonary artery, lungs, aorta, and umbilical arteries
4. Describe the cardiac and pulmonary sequences of events that occur when transitioning from fetal to extrauterine life, including the changes in fetal shunts

KEY TERMS

Angiogenic clusters
Aorticopulmonary septum
Atrial bulge
Blastocyst
Bulboventricular loop
Bulbus cordis
Chorion
Chorionic membrane

Chorionic villi
Dextral looping
Ectoderm
Embryonic disk
Endocardial cushions
Endoderm
Foramen ovale
Intimal mounds

Mesoderm
Placenta
Septum primum
Septum secundum
Trophoblast
Ventricular bulge
Wharton's jelly
Zygote

What initially may seem like a remote concept for respiratory care practitioners—a basic understanding of embryology—is essential to understanding the care of the newborn. Whether care is being provided to a premature newborn with respiratory distress syndrome as a result of insufficient or poorly functioning surfactant or to a newborn afflicted with persistent pulmonary hypertension resulting from severe meconium staining, all respiratory care practitioners working with infants must have a breadth of knowledge of embryology and fetal development that provides them with an understanding of

normal development and what to expect when something goes awry.

EMBRYOLOGICAL OVERVIEW

The rapidly growing embryo and fetus must develop a vascular network to circulate nutrients and provide gas exchange. The fetus depends on the mother's circulation for nutrient and gas exchange; however, the maternal and fetal vascular networks are separate systems, and no blood is shared between the two. By day 22 of gestation the primitive fetal heart begins to beat, with myocardial pump function to support fetal circulation beginning on day 27 to day 29.[1]

Fertilization to Implantation

As the fertilized egg, or **zygote,** travels to the uterus, it undergoes numerous iterations of cell division but has no nutrient source, as in a bird egg. The ball of developing cells, at this point termed the **blastocyst,** must attach itself and implant in the uterine lining for nourishment. The outer surrounding layer of the blastocyst is the **trophoblast,** which combines with tissues from the endometrium to form the **chorionic membrane** around the blastocyst.[2] Inside the blastocyst, a group of cells arrange on one side in the shape of a figure eight. The central portion is the **embryonic disk,** which forms the three embryonic germ layers: the **ectoderm** and the **endoderm,** followed by the **mesoderm.**[3] Box 2-1 lists the tissue systems that arise from the three germ layers.

The outer or top loop of the figure eight envelops the embryonic structure and forms the amniotic sac, while the inner or bottom loop forms the yolk sac. The yolk sac soon degenerates and incorporates into the embryo, giving way for the amniotic sac to grow. Suspended in the cavity of the blastocyst, the amniotic sac then surrounds the entire embryo. The embryo attaches to the outer layer through the umbilical stalk, which later becomes the umbilical cord.

Maternal–Fetal Gas Exchange

As the umbilical cord matures, finger-like projections extend into the outer lining of the **chorion,** or **chorionic villi** (Figure 2-1). Within the chorionic villi a capillary network forms and connects to the umbilical stalk. The villi intertwine into the blood-filled lacunar cavities of the endometrium of the maternal uterus.[2] Oxygen, carbon dioxide, and nutrients diffuse through the vast capillary surface area of this indirect connection between mother and fetus. As fetal development continues, the region of this interface becomes limited to the discus-shaped **placenta,** because the amniotic sac completely fills the chorionic cavity. The umbilical cord connects the placenta to the fetus with one large vein and two smaller arteries. As the cord grows, the vessels tend to spiral.[4] **Wharton's jelly,** a gelatinous substance inside the umbilical cord, helps protect the vessels and may prevent the cord from kinking.

Box 2-1	Origin of the Various Tissue Systems from the Three Embryonic Germ Layers

ECTODERM
- Central nervous system: brain and spinal cord
- Peripheral nervous system: cranial nerves and spinal nerves
- Sensory epithelia of the eyes, inner ears, and nose
- Glandular tissues: posterior pituitary gland, adrenal medulla
- Skin: epidermal layer
- Specializations of the skin: sweat and sebaceous glands, hair follicles, nails, mammary glands
- Teeth: enamel

MESODERM
- Cardiovascular system: heart and blood vessels
- Lymphatic system vessels
- All connective tissue: general connective tissue, and cartilage, bone, bone marrow, and blood cells
- All muscle tissue: skeletal, cardiac, and smooth
- Skin: dermis and hypodermis
- Kidneys and ureters, spleen
- Reproductive tissues (not including the germ cells)
- The three major body cavities: pericardium, left and right pleura, and peritoneum
- Serous linings of organs within the body cavities
- Teeth: dentine, cementum, and pulp

ENDODERM
- Digestive system: stomach, small and large intestines, and epithelial lining of the entire digestive system except parts of the mouth and pharynx, and anus (which are supplied by the ectoderm)
- Respiratory system: pharynx, lungs, and epithelial lining of the trachea and lungs
- Urinary system: bladder, and lining of the urethra
- Liver and pancreas and epithelial lining of all glands that open into the digestive system
- Tonsils, thymus, thyroid, parathyroid
- Epithelial lining of auditory tube and tympanic cavity

Adapted from Moore KL, Persaud TVN, editors: *The developing human: clinically oriented embryology,* ed 6, Philadelphia: WB Saunders, 1998, pp 63-82.

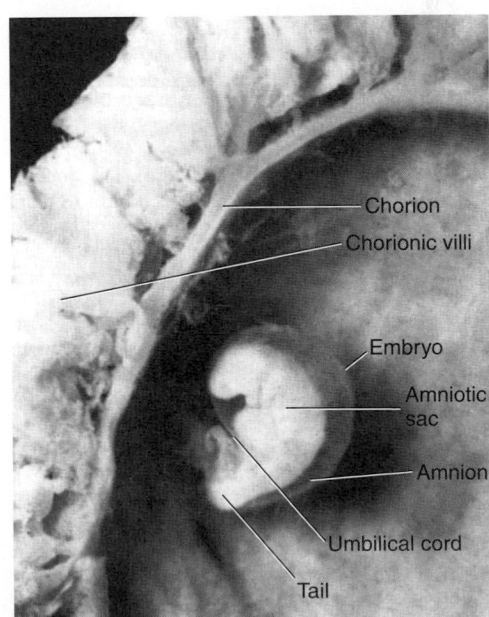

FIGURE 2-1 Implanted human embryo, approximately day 28, showing the relationship of the chorion, amnion, and chorionic villi. The umbilical cord and tail are difficult to differentiate in this view.

CARDIOVASCULAR DEVELOPMENT

During the third week of gestation, the heart is fully formed. The heart is considered to be the first complete organ formed. By 8 weeks of gestation, the fetal heart is fully functional, complete with all chambers, valves, and major vessels. In addition, the fetal heart must accommodate the circulatory configuration required to support a fetus that is residing, growing, and maturing enclosed within a fluid-filled environment. The anatomical solutions to circulate oxygenated blood cannot be the same in the placenta-respiring fetus as it is in the air-breathing newborn. As the embryonic heart changes are described, note which of them may result in the cardiac anomalies discussed in Chapter 24 (Congenital Cardiac Defects). Table 2-1 lists the timing of the key cardiac developments.

Early Development

During early embryonic development, small cellular pools, referred to as **angiogenic clusters** or blood islands, supply nutrition to the growing embryo. These clusters coalesce to form two heart tubes lined with specialized myocardial tissue.[5] On approximately day 18, the heart tubes fold into

TABLE 2-1

Timetable of Significant Events During Fetal Heart Development

Time of Gestation	Event
Early Development	
Week 3	
Day 16	Angiogenic clusters (blood islands) appear
Day 18	Heart tubes form
Day 21	Heart tubes fuse
Chamber Development	
Week 4	
Day 22	Fusion of heart tubes complete
	Heart begins to beat
	Bidirectional blood flow begins
Day 23	Folding, looping, ballooning begin
Day 25	Atrial septation begins with growth of septum primum
Day 28	Ventricular septation starts
	Endocardial cushions form
	Unidirectional blood flow begins
Week 5	
Day 32	Septum secundum starts
Week 6	
Day 37	Foramen ovale complete
Maturation	
Day 46	Ventricle formation complete
Day 49	Four chambers complete
	Valve formation matures
Week 8	
Day 52	Aorta/pulmonary artery complete separation
Day 56	Valve formation complete

what will become the thoracic cavity. At this point, they become close enough to fuse, and grow into a complete single-chamber tubular structure by day 21. The cardiovascular system forms primarily from the mesoderm layer, but myocardial tissue has a diverse origin related to the recruitment of myocytes from surrounding tissue types during embryogenesis.[6] By day 22 cardiac contractions are detectable and bidirectional tidal blood flow begins.[4]

Chamber Development

Dramatic changes begin to occur during the fourth week of gestation. The heart tubes continue to merge into three identifiable structures called the **bulbus cordis,** the **ventricular bulge,** and the **atrial bulge.** These structures empty into the sinus venosus, which also receives blood from three additional sources: the vitelline veins (arising from the yolk sac), the common cardinal veins (from the embryo), and the umbilical veins (from the primitive placenta) (Figure 2-2).[7] These structures continue to bend, fold, and dilate by incorporating components from surrounding tissue structures as the truncus arteriosus (which connects the heart to the future arterial system) becomes recognizable.[8] Note that initially the atrial bulge is inferior to the ventricular bulge. Between days 23 and 28 a process referred to as **dextral looping** occurs, whereby the ventricular bulge balloons into a C-shaped loop that pushes the atrial bulge in a superior direction (see Figure 2-2). Subsequently, the embryonic heart appears as a twisted S shape, and the ventricular structure merges with the bulbus cordis to form a one-ventricle structure known as the **bulboventricular loop,** which continues to dilate.[9]

Simultaneous with the external changes, the **septum primum** begins the separation of the primitive atrium, followed shortly by growth of the **endocardial cushions,** which will separate the atria from the ventricles. During this time, the left atrium incorporates the primordial pulmonary veins as four pulmonary veins empty into the primordial left atrium. The right horn of the sinus venosus grows in dominance and merges into the future right atrium from the inferior and superior vena cavae. By the end of the fourth week, the dilating ventricular spaces fold into each other and force the ventricular septal bud upward at the base of the bulboventricular loop (Figure 2-3).[4] By this time, blood flow matures into a unidirectional path as the myocardium continues to strengthen by recruiting myocytes from the surrounding mesenchymal tissue.[3, 6]

During weeks 5 and 6 the internal and external structures continue to mature rapidly. Between the atria, the **septum secundum** begins to appear. By week 6, the septum secundum and a flap from the septum primum form the **foramen ovale,** one of the fetal shunts discussed later in this chapter (Figures 2-4 and 2-5). The atrioventricular canal continues to mature, and the endocardial cushions separate the ventricular spaces from the atrium. The muscular portion of the ventricular septum continues to grow into the ventricular space as the two ventricles

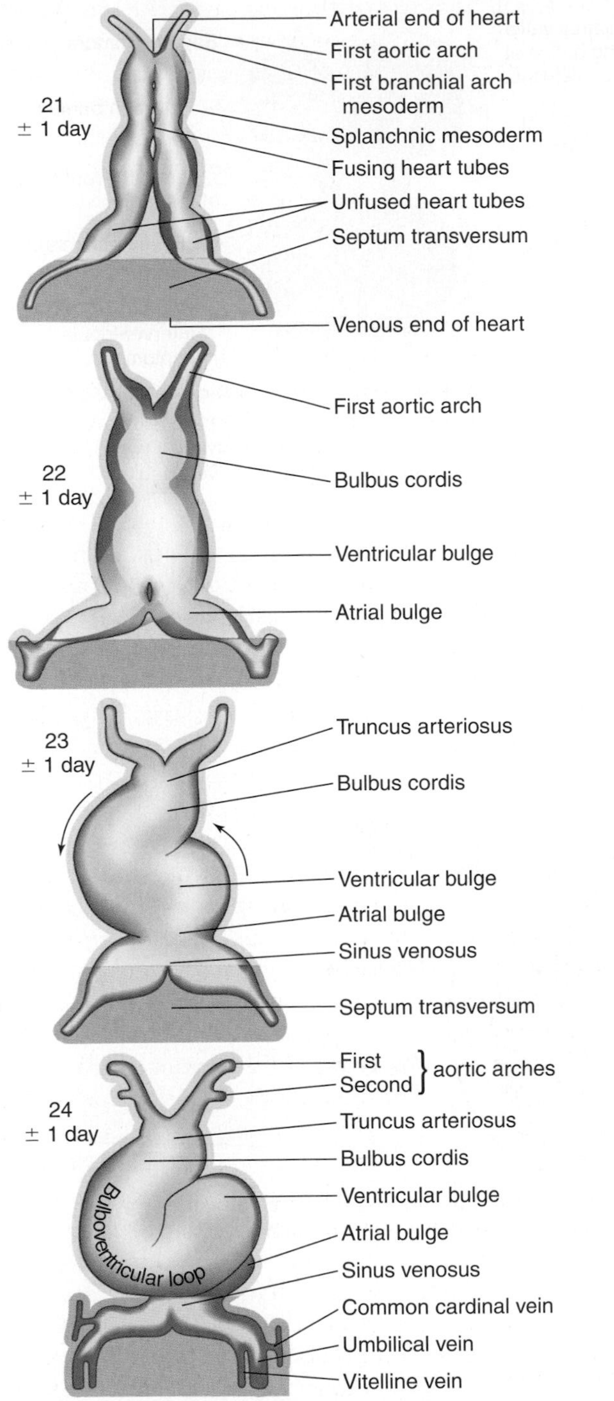
21
± 1 day
Arterial end of heart
First aortic arch
First branchial arch mesoderm
Splanchnic mesoderm
Fusing heart tubes
Unfused heart tubes
Septum transversum
Venous end of heart
22
± 1 day
First aortic arch
Bulbus cordis
Ventricular bulge
Atrial bulge
23
± 1 day
Truncus arteriosus
Bulbus cordis
Ventricular bulge
Atrial bulge
Sinus venosus
Septum transversum
24
± 1 day
First
Second
aortic arches
Truncus arteriosus
Bulbus cordis
Ventricular bulge
Atrial bulge
Sinus venosus
Common cardinal vein
Umbilical vein
Vitelline vein
Bulboventricular loop

FIGURE 2-2 Formation of the primordial heart chambers after fusion of the heart tubes at a gestational age of 3 weeks.

dilate. Ridges also appear opposite each other in the bulbus cordis and truncus. They grow toward each other and fuse into a spiraling **aorticopulmonary septum,** which ultimately separates into the aorta and pulmonary arteries.[3] A fetal heart rate of about 95 beats per minute becomes discernible during this period and increases by approximately 4 beats per day until heart development is complete.[10]

Maturation

Continuing maturation of the internal and external structures characterizes weeks 7 and 8. The ventricles finish forcing the ventricular septum up from its base. A small intraventricular foramen remains, and blood flows between the two ventricles until the endocardial cushions fuse with the ventricular septum (see Figure 2-4). At the end of the seventh week, tissue from remnants of the bulbus cordis and tissue from the endocardial cushions grow into the ventricular foramen, closing it as they merge with the muscular ventricular septum. The tricuspid and mitral valves form from specialized tissue surrounding the two atrioventricular openings. The aorticopulmonary septum divides the bulbus cordis and truncus into an aortic and pulmonary trunk. As these outflow tracts continue to mature, the semilunar valves form at the base of each structure.[8] Early in the eighth week the outflow tracts and valves are completely developed. At this stage, development of the cardiac structures is complete and blood flows through the fetal circulation pathway. The heart continues to develop, increasing proportionately more in length than width, paralleling embryonic growth.[11,12]

FETAL CIRCULATION AND FETAL SHUNTS

Fetal circulation necessarily differs from circulation after the infant is birthed because external respiration by the fetus does not occur within the lungs. Figure 2-6 illustrates fetal circulation and the three shunts present in the fetus that close soon after birth. The mother's lungs and liver perform most of the metabolic functions required by the same organs of the fetus. The fetal circulation pathway allows blood flow to be shunted around the fetal liver and lungs. Shunting most of the blood volume through the fetal heart, bypassing the lungs, facilitates pumping the required large quantities of fetal blood to the placenta, which is the gas, nutrient, and waste exchange interface between the maternal and fetal organ systems.[11]

Oxygenated blood travels from the placenta to the fetus through the umbilical vein. The *ductus venosus,* the first fetal shunt, appears continuous with the umbilical vein, shunting approximately 30% to 50% of the oxygen-rich blood directly to the inferior vena cava, effectively bypassing the fetal liver. The amount of shunting through the ductus venosus appears to decrease with gestational age.[13] The oxygen-rich blood within the umbilical vein empties into the inferior vena cava and mixes with oxygen-depleted systemic venous blood as it flows to the right atrium. Even though some admixture occurs, the blood entering the right atrium contains the highest oxygen saturations available to the fetus.

In the right atrium most of the blood flow from the inferior vena cava crosses through a hole within the atrial septum, called the foramen ovale, into the left

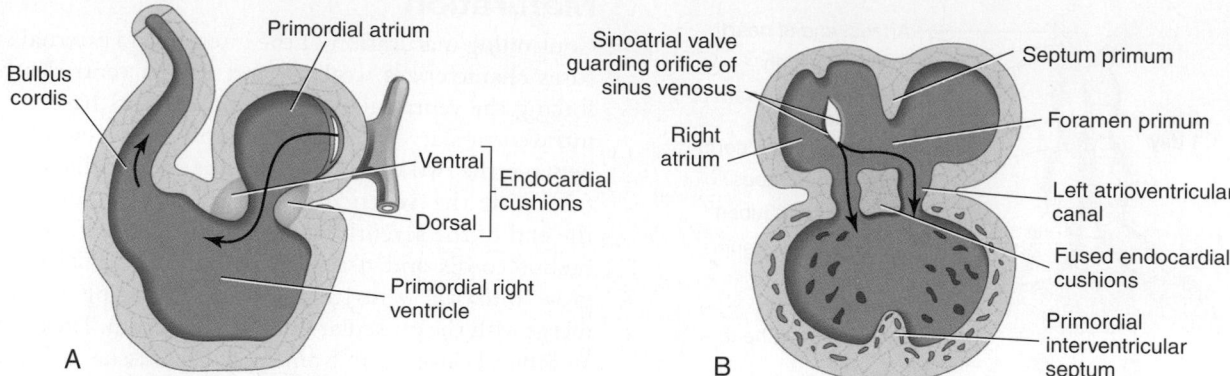

FIGURE 2-3 **A,** Sagittal view of the developing heart during week 4, showing the position of the atrium, bulbus cordis, ventricles, and endocardial cushions merging from the ventral and dorsal sides. **B,** Traditional view of the developing heart during weeks 4 to 5, showing budding interventricular septum, fused endocardial cushions, septum primum, and the left and right atria. The ventricular septum continues to fold and grow upward between the ventricles.

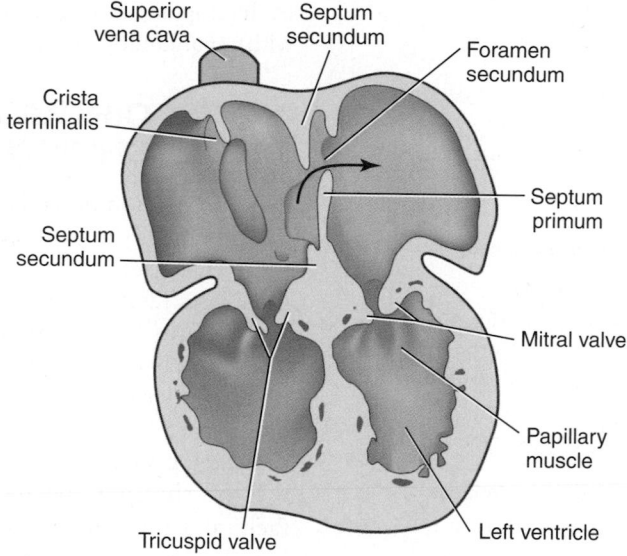

FIGURE 2-4 Frontal view of the fetal heart between weeks 5 and 6, showing the development of the four chambers nearing completion. The *arrow* shows the one-way path through the foramen ovale.

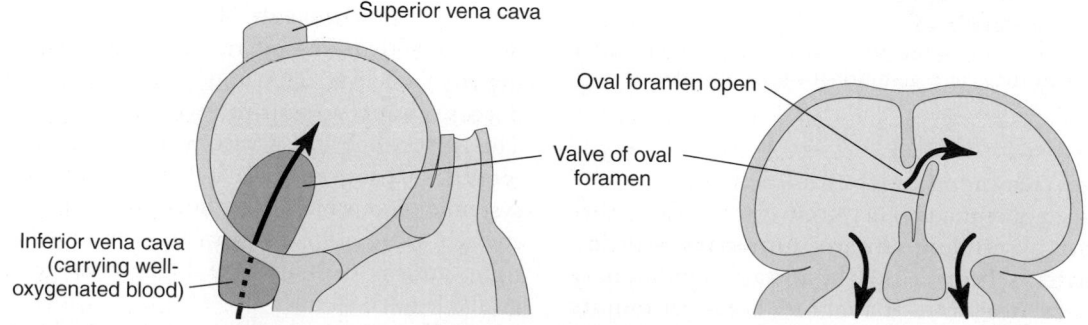

FIGURE 2-5 Frontal view *(right)* and side view *(left)* schematics of the foramen ovale. The septum primum forms the flap, and the septum secundum remains open to form the foramen ovale. The *arrows* show the one-way path through the foramen ovale.

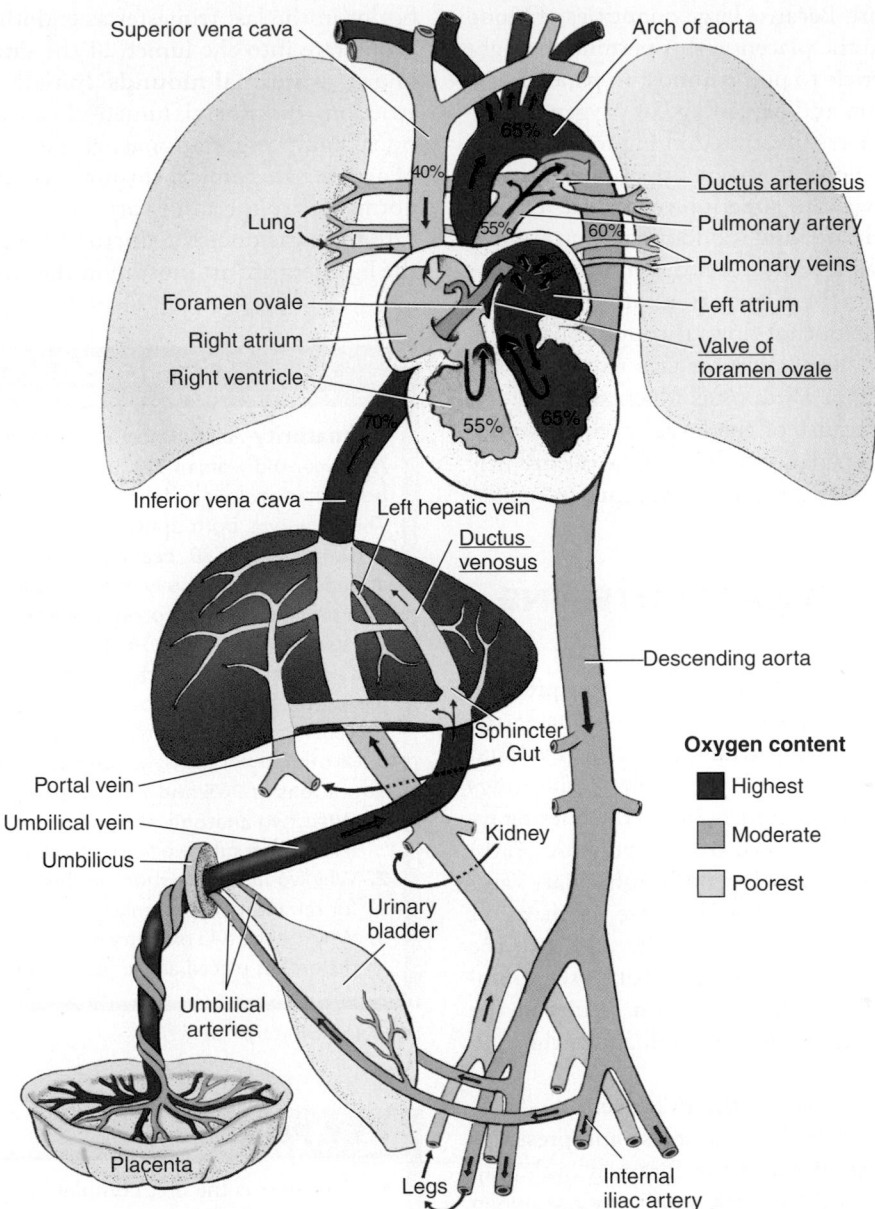

Superior vena cava

Arch of aorta

Lung

Ductus arteriosus

Pulmonary artery

Pulmonary veins

Foramen ovale

Left atrium

Right atrium

Right ventricle

Valve of foramen ovale

Inferior vena cava

Left hepatic vein

Ductus venosus

Descending aorta

Sphincter

Gut

Portal vein

Umbilical vein

Umbilicus

Kidney

Oxygen content

Highest

Moderate

Poorest

Urinary bladder

Umbilical arteries

Legs

Internal iliac artery

Placenta

FIGURE 2-6 A diagram of the fetal circulation showing blood containing oxygen and nourishment moving from the placenta to the fetal heart and through the three fetal shunts: the ductus venosus, the foramen ovale, and the ductus arteriosus.

atrium. The foramen ovale, the second fetal shunt, is formed during septation of the atria as described previously. The septum primum acts as a one-way valve over the ostium secundum (see Figure 2-5). The remainder of the blood in the right atrium mixes with desaturated blood from the superior vena cava and drains into the right ventricle. Blood in the right ventricle contains slightly higher oxygen content than blood from the superior vena cava and is pumped into the pulmonary artery to the developing lungs.

The pulmonary vascular resistance (PVR) in utero is high. Likely mechanisms include physical compression of the vessels resulting from relatively low lung volumes and hypoxic pulmonary vasoconstriction resulting from the low partial pressure of oxygen within the alveolus of the fetus. Both mechanisms help induce chemical mediators that maintain a high resistive tone in the pulmonary vascular bed.[14] Up to 13% to 25% of the fetal blood flow presented to the right atrium reaches the lungs.[11,15]

Blood from the pulmonary veins empties into the left atrium and then flows into the left ventricle, out the aortic valve, and into the ascending aorta, where it supplies blood with the highest oxygen content to the head, right arm, and coronary circulation. The high PVR causes most of the blood flowing through the pulmonary artery from the right ventricle to pass through the less resistant *ductus arteriosus,* the third fetal shunt, directly into the aorta. This allows blood within the pulmonary artery to bypass the lungs and left heart. Because large quantities of blood are required to flow to the placenta, this permits the right ventricle and left ventricle to pump almost in parallel. The path of fetal circulation and percentage of oxygen saturation in various locations is illustrated in Figure 2-6.[16]

The deoxygenated blood from the upper torso returns to the right atrium via the superior vena cava. Finally, blood in the descending and abdominal aorta flows through common iliac arteries to two umbilical arteries and back to the placenta for oxygenation.[17] Initially 17% to 20% of the fetal cardiac output flows through the umbilical arteries, but as the fetus matures this rises to 33%.[18] At any point, the placenta contains as much as half of the fetal blood volume. Because of the large vascular surface area of the placenta, impedance to blood flow is extremely low, allowing blood flow through the placenta to remain consistent and stable.[11]

TRANSITION TO EXTRAUTERINE LIFE

Clamping the umbilical vessels removes the low-pressure system of the placenta from fetal circulation. During the first breath, several factors drastically reduce the PVR and increase pulmonary blood flow.[19] Inflation of the lungs initiates gas exchange, which in turn dilates the pulmonary arterioles. Rising systemic arterial oxygen pressure (PaO_2) also stimulates the release of endogenous pulmonary vasodilating cytokines that act locally to increase the diameter of the pulmonary arterial vasculature.[20] Stretching of the pulmonary parenchyma also physically expands the vasculature. Besides vasodilation, lung inflation results in the inhibition of vasoconstricting agents produced by the lung to facilitate fetal circulation.[19]

Once the cord is clamped and the PVR decreases, pressures in the right side of the heart decrease and pressures in the left side increase. Because the foramen ovale flap allows blood to flow only from right to left, it closes when the pressures in the left atrium become greater than those in the right atrium. Closing the foramen ovale further facilitates the increase of blood flow to the lungs during the transitional period and is necessary to maintain normal extrauterine circulation.

Because the pressure in the aorta also increases and becomes greater than the pressure in the pulmonary artery, the amount of shunting through the ductus arteriosus decreases. The functional closure of the ductus arteriosus occurs as a result of being exposed to an increase in PaO_2, a decrease in PVR leading to the reduction in blood pressure within the ductal lumen, a decrease in the local production of prostaglandins, and a reduction in the number of prostaglandin receptors within the tissue of the ductus arteriosus.[21,22] Normally, constriction of the ductus arteriosus starts to occur at birth, and 20% of the ductus closes within 24 hours, with 80% closed in 48 hours and 100% by 96 hours after birth.[23] Anatomical closure of the ductus arteriosus

begins in the last trimester as endothelial tissue begins to proliferate into the lumen of the ductus, forming bulges known as **intimal mounds**. Initially assisted by vasoconstriction, the ductal lumen closes completely as gestational and postgestational age advances.[24] By 2 to 4 weeks of age, the anatomical closure is complete and blood flow normalizes to the adult pattern of circulation.[23] The structure that was once the ductus arteriosus is referred to as the ligamentum arteriosum in the adult.

CASE STUDY

Prematurity-Associated Respiratory Distress

A 32-year-old woman has just given birth to a 38-week newborn after prolonged labor as a result of shoulder dystocia. The baby was born apneic, with minimal muscle tone and a heart rate of 80 beats per minute. The newborn was attended to immediately by the neonatal resuscitation team, who provided positive pressure ventilation for approximately 30 seconds. The newborn began breathing spontaneously and was transferred to the intensive care nursery on supplemental oxygen. Three hours later, despite the supplemental oxygen the baby was still cyanotic. The physician ordered pulse oximetry of the right hand and left foot, which revealed saturations of 96% and 75%, respectively.

1. What two anatomical shunts normally present in the fetus can result in persistent cyanosis in the newborn?
2. Why would the newborn in this case example be at risk for refractory hypoxemia?
3. Why are the two oximetry readings necessary, and why are the probes placed at the sites specified by the physician?

See Evolve Resources for answers.

KEY POINTS

- The heart is the first complete organ formed. Identifying the stages of development of the heart is important in understanding congenital problems that can occur when development does not proceed as expected.
- The ductus venousus, foramen ovale, and ductus arteriosus are the anatomical shunts present in the fetus that allow fetal circulation. These shunts are essential to the proper nutrient and gas exchange in the fetus.
- The three anatomical shunts and the pressure gradients induced by the circulatory systems (e.g., placental, pulmonary, and systemic) are all necessary to ensure proper directional blood flow through the fetus. This provides for gas and nutrient exchange and appropriate distribution of blood through the fetus.
- Transition from fetal circulation to adult circulation during the birthing process is a complex event that seems to take place effortlessly in nearly every birth. Recognizing the signs and symptoms of inappropriate transition is important to ensure that the right care is quickly delivered.

ASSESSMENT QUESTIONS

Select the best answer. See Evolve Resources for answers.

1. Which of the following are true statements concerning the development of the circulatory system?
   I. Heart development is completed by about 32 weeks of gestation.
   II. Heart development, other than growth, is complete when valve formation is complete.
   III. Angiogenic clusters supply nutrition in the earliest stages of the growing embryo.
   IV. The right-side myocardial fibers begin contracting before the left side to provide blood flow to the lungs.
   V. At about 3 weeks, two heart tubes fuse into what will become the basic structure of the four-chamber heart.
   A. I, III, and V
   B. II and III
   C. II, III, and IV
   D. II, III, and V
   E. III and IV

2. Which of the following are recognizable structures during development of the heart after the heart tubes fuse?
   I. Sinus venosus
   II. Bulbus cordis
   III. Atrial bulge
   IV. Ventricular bulge
   V. Truncus arteriosus
   A. I and III
   B. I, II, IV, and V
   C. II, III, and IV
   D. II, III, IV, and V
   E. III, IV, and V

3. The oxygenated blood leaves the placenta and travels to the fetus through the _____.
   A. Aortic artery
   B. Umbilical vein
   C. Umbilical artery
   D. Spiral artery
   E. Ductus arteriosus

4. Most of the fetal blood entering the main pulmonary artery is shunted to the aorta through the _____?
   A. Foramen ovale
   B. Ductus venosus
   C. Ductus arteriosus
   D. Superior vena cava
   E. Iliac arteries

5. Most of the fetal blood entering via the umbilical vein is shunted to the inferior vena cava through the _____?
   A. Foramen ovale
   B. Ductus venosus
   C. Ductus arteriosus
   D. Superior vena cava
   E. Iliac arteries

6. Normal circulatory changes occurring within the transitional stage at birth include which of the following?
   I. A decrease in pulmonary vascular resistance
   II. A decrease in systemic vascular resistance
   III. A decrease in pulmonary artery pressure
   IV. An increase in left ventricular pressure
   V. An increase in pulmonary blood
   A. I and IV
   B. I, II, IV, and V
   C. I, III, IV, and V
   D. II, III, and V
   E. III, IV, and V

7. Most of the fetal blood entering via the right atrium is shunted to the left atrium through the _____?
   A. Foramen ovale
   B. Ductus venosus
   C. Ductus arteriosus
   D. Superior vena cava
   E. Aortoiliac shunt

8. When discussing fetal circulation, which of the following is true?
   A. Fetal shunts help to shunt the best oxygenated blood to the head.
   B. Pressure gradients related to blood flow are the opposite of those in an adult.
   C. Fetal shunts help to bypass the lungs.
   D. The placenta has low vascular resistance.
   E. All of the above

9. What *one* set of actions causes the systemic circulation to transition from a low-resistance system to a high-resistance system?
   A. Clamping the umbilical cord and creating a short period of hypoxia
   B. Getting a higher concentration of oxygen into the lungs with the first breath
   C. Clamping the umbilical cord, thus preventing blood flow to the placenta
   D. Pulmonary hypertension from a change in blood flow direction
   E. Expulsion of the placenta at birth

10. Anatomical narrowing of the ductus arteriosus begins in the last trimester by which process?
    A. The formation of bulges known as intimal mounds
    B. The release of tolazoline compounds
    C. Ductal termination
    D. The formation of the aortic valve
    E. Activating thrombokinins

References

1. Pensky B: *Review of medical embryology*, New York, 1982, McMillan, pp 291–335.
2. Kingdom JC, Kaufmann P: Oxygen and placental vascular development, *Adv Exp Med Biol* 474:259, 1999.
3. Moore KL, Persaud TVN, editors: *The developing human: clinical oriented embryology*, Philadelphia, 1998, WB Saunders, pp 63–82.
4. England MA, editor: *Color atlas of life before birth: normal fetal development*, Chicago, 1996, Year Book Medical, pp 102.

5. Gourdie RG, Kubalak S, Mikawa T: Conducting the embryonic heart: orchestrating development of specialized cardiac tissues, *Trends Cardiovasc Med* 9(1–2):18, 1999.

6. Eisenberg LM, Markwald RR: Cellular recruitment and the development of the myocardium, *Dev Biol* 274(2):225, 2004.

7. Abdulla R, Blew GA, Holterman MJ: Cardiovascular embryology, *Pediatr Cardiol* 25(3):191, 2004.

8. Moorman A, Webb S, Brown NA, Lamers W, Anderson RH: Development of the heart: (1) formation of the cardiac chambers and arterial trunks, *Heart* 89(7):806, 2003.

9. Bartman T, Hove J: Mechanics and function in heart morphogenesis, *Dev Dyn* 233(2):373, 2005.

10. Tezuka N, Sato S, Kanasugi H, Hiroi M: Embryonic heart rates: development in early first trimester and clinical evaluation, *Gynecol Obstet Invest* 32(4):210, 1991.

11. Kiserud T, Acharya G: The fetal circulation, *Prenat Diagn* 24(13):1049, 2004.

12. Marecki B: The formation of heart-proportion in fetal ontogenesis, *Z Morphol Anthropol* 79(2):197, 1992.

13. Kiserud T: Fetal venous circulation—an update on hemodynamics, *J Perinat Med* 28(2):90, 2000.

14. Heymann MA: Control of the pulmonary circulation in the fetus and during the transitional period to air breathing, *Eur J Obstet Gynecol Reprod Biol* 84(2):127, 1999.

15. Lakshminrusimha S, Steinhorn RH: Pulmonary vascular biology during neonatal transition, *Clin Perinatol* 26(3):601, 1999.

16. Rudolph AM: *Congenital diseases of the heart*, Chicago, 1974, Year Book Medical.

17. Sharma A, Ford S, Calvert J: Adaptation for life: a review of neonatal physiology, *Anaesth Intensive Care Med* 12(3): 85, 2011.

18. Goldkrand JW, Moore DH, Lentz SU, Clements SP, Turner AD, Bryant JL: Volumetric flow in the umbilical artery: normative data, *J Matern Fetal Med* 9(4):224, 2000.

19. Rudolph AM: The development of concepts of the otogeny of the pulmonary circulation. In Weir EK, Archer SL, Reeves JT, editors: *The fetal and neonatal pulmonary circulations*. Armonk, NY, 2000, Futura Publishing.

20. Hageman JR, Caplan MS: An introduction to the structure and function of inflammatory mediators for clinicians, *Clin Perinatol* 22(2):251, 1995.

21. Clyman RI: Mechanisms regulating the ductus arteriosus, *Biol Neonate* 89(4):330, 2006.

22. Hammerman C: Patent ductus arteriosus. Clinical relevance of prostaglandins and prostaglandin inhibitors in PDA pathophysiology and treatment, *Clin Perinatol* 22(2):457, 1995.

23. Lim MK, Hanretty K, Houston AB, Lilley S, Murtagh EP: Intermittent ductal patency in healthy newborn infants: demonstration by colour Doppler flow mapping, *Arch Dis Child* 67(10 Spec No):1217, 1992.

24. Mirro R, Gray P: Aortic and pulmonary blood velocities during the first 3 days of life, *Am J Perinatol* 3(4):333, 1986.

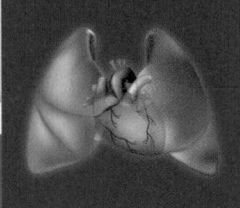

Chapter 3

Antenatal Assessment and High-Risk Delivery

ADRIANN COMBS, J. GERALD QUIRK

OUTLINE

Maternal and Perinatal Disorders
　Diabetes Mellitus
　Infectious Diseases
　Toxic Habits in Pregnancy
High-Risk Conditions
　Hypertension and Preeclampsia
　Fetal Membranes, Umbilical Cord, and Placenta
　Disorders of Amniotic Fluid Volume
　Preterm Birth
　Cervical Insufficiency
　Postterm Pregnancy

Antenatal Assessment
　Ultrasound
　Amniocentesis
　Nonstress Test and Contraction Stress Test
　Fetal Biophysical Profile
　Mode of Delivery
Intrapartum Monitoring
Fetal Transition to Extrauterine Life

LEARNING OBJECTIVES

After reading this chapter the reader will be able to:
1. Identify various high-risk conditions that may adversely affect pregnancy outcome
2. Describe current methods used for antenatal and intrapartum assessment of fetal well-being
3. Explain preterm labor and postterm pregnancy evaluation and management
4. Describe the current recommendations for assisting the newborn from intrauterine to extrauterine life

KEY TERMS

Anencephaly
Biophysical profile (BPP)
β-Mimetic drugs
Bronchopulmonary dysplasia (BPD)
Cervical cerclage
Cervical dilation
Cervical effacement
Cervical insufficiency
Contraction stress test (CST)
Doppler ultrasonography
Endomyometritis
Esophageal atresia
Fetal alcohol syndrome
Fetal fibronectin
Germinal matrix
Gestational diabetes mellitus
Group B *Streptococcus* (GBS)

Growth restriction
Hepatitis B virus (HBV)
Herpes simplex virus (HSV)
Human immunodeficiency virus (HIV)
Hydrops fetalis
Intrauterine growth restriction (IUGR)
Intraventricular hemorrhage (IVH)
Laminaria tent
Listeria monocytogenes
Macrosomia
Meconium aspiration
Necrotizing enterocolitis (NEC)
Nonstress test (NST)
Oligohydramnios
Oxytocin

Placenta previa
Placental abruption
Polyhydramnios
Potter's syndrome
Preeclampsia
Preterm delivery
Premature rupture of membranes (PROM)
Respiratory distress syndrome (RDS)
Retinopathy of prematurity (ROP)
Sudden infant death syndrome (SIDS)
Syphilis
Teratogen
Tocolytic
Velamentous cord insertion

The transition from intrauterine life to the outside world is a critical process that involves major physiological changes and may require medical attention for an optimal outcome. Cooperation and communication among all members of the health care team are essential to identify potential problems and to intervene in a timely manner. That team includes obstetricians, pediatricians, nurses skilled in obstetrics and neonatology, anesthesiologists, and respiratory therapists. Maternal history, antenatal assessment (as dictated by maternal–fetal risk factors), and intrapartum monitoring are all-important in identifying the fetus or newborn at risk of decompensation during the perinatal period. This chapter outlines the essentials of antenatal assessment and touches briefly on the management of some high-risk conditions: preterm delivery, post-term pregnancy, and extrauterine transition of the fetus. The following sections will also discuss some commonly encountered risk factors associated with pregnancy and delivery. Comorbidities of the mother and abnormalities of the pregnancy that contribute significantly to compromised fetal well-being and preterm delivery are described. The chapter concludes with a section on assisting the fetus to extrauterine life.

MATERNAL AND PERINATAL DISORDERS

At the initial prenatal visit, the obstetrical care provider obtains a comprehensive maternal history and performs a physical examination. Disorders that place a pregnancy at increased risk for adverse pregnancy outcome are identified and included in an initial problem list that serves as a quick summary for future reference. Subsequent periodic visits serve the purpose of identifying new obstetrical risks that may necessitate special interventions. The following sections discuss commonly encountered maternal–fetal risk factors and their impact on obstetrical care and perinatal outcome.

Diabetes Mellitus

Diabetes in pregnancy is classified broadly as pregestational or gestational.

Pregestational Diabetes Mellitus. Women whose diabetes was diagnosed before the onset of pregnancy (pregestational diabetes) are at significant risk for adverse maternal and fetal outcomes. Adverse maternal outcomes include increased risk of developing diabetic ketoacidosis, proliferative retinopathy, and preeclampsia/eclampsia. Close maternal metabolic surveillance focused on attaining normal blood glucose levels throughout pregnancy has significantly decreased the frequency of these outcomes.

Adverse fetal outcomes include unexplained fetal death in the third trimester of pregnancy and major fetal structural malformations. Close maternal metabolic surveillance coupled with close fetal biophysical evaluation has significantly decreased the risk of fetal death and the necessity of delivering a fetus prematurely because of abnormal test results. The rate of fetal structural malformations in infants born to pregestational diabetic women can be as high as 10% to 15%, compared with a rate of 1% to 2% for infants of otherwise healthy women. The most commonly encountered defects are malformations of the cardiovascular system, including both the heart and great vessels, and the central nervous system, including the brain and spinal cord. No amount of maternal metabolic surveillance or fetal biophysical assessment after the period of fetal organogenesis will decrease this risk. Therefore it is recommended strongly that women with diabetes mellitus receive counseling and treatment with the goal of achieving optimal glycemic control before they become pregnant.

Gestational Diabetes Mellitus. Gestational diabetes mellitus (GDM) is abnormal glucose tolerance of variable degree that occurs or is first recognized during pregnancy. The frequency of this disorder varies according to body mass index, maternal age, and the ethnic background of the woman and is said to complicate about 3% to 8% of pregnancies in the United States. Poor blood sugar control in these women is associated with an increased risk of **macrosomia** (birth weight greater than 4000 g), traumatic vaginal delivery, and preterm delivery and a small risk of fetal death in some women. After delivery, the infants are at increased risk for metabolic disturbances in the neonatal period; these include hypoglycemia, hypocalcemia, hyperkalemia, hyperbilirubinemia, and idiopathic respiratory distress syndrome. In the long term, women with GDM are at risk of developing type 2, or adult-onset, diabetes; nearly 50% will be diagnosed with type 2 diabetes within 10 years.

Among pregnant women, selective screening based on risk factors identifies only half. Thus, at the present time, it is recommended that all pregnant women be screened for gestational diabetes. Traditionally, patients have been screened with the 1-hour glucose challenge test administered between 24 and 28 weeks of gestation. For those with an abnormal screening result, the diagnosis of GDM is made when there are two abnormal values on a 3-hour, 100-g oral glucose tolerance test. The American Diabetes Association now recommends performing a 2-hour, 75-g oral glucose tolerance test between 24 and 28 weeks in all pregnant women not previously diagnosed with diabetes mellitus.[1]

Maternal glycemic control and fetal biophysical status are monitored in a manner similar to protocols for managing the pregnancy complicated by pregestational diabetes (see Table 3-1). With good maternal glycemic control, pregnancies complicated by GDM can proceed to full term with a normal delivery; cesarean delivery is reserved for traditional obstetrical indications. Insulin has traditionally been the drug of choice for achieving glycemic control in patients with gestational diabetes. More recently, glyburide, a sulfonylurea analog that

TABLE 3-1

Criteria for the Diagnosis of Diabetes Mellitus Using Oral Glucose Tolerance Testing

Glucose Load Time	100 g Glucose		75 g Glucose	
	SERUM GLUCOSE MG/DL	MMOL/L	SERUM GLUCOSE MG/DL	MMOL/L
Fasting	95	5.3	92	5.1
1 hour	180	10.0	180	10.0
2 hours	155	8.6	153	8.5
3 hours	140	7.8		

The diagnosis of diabetes during pregnancy is based on the serum glucose after ingestion of an oral glucose load. The diagnosis is made when two serum glucoses are elevated after ingestion of the 100-gram load or one elevated serum glucose after ingestion of the 75-gram load. American Diabetes Association. Postpartum statement: diagnosis and classification of diabetes mellitus, *Diabetes Care* 2011;34:s562.

stimulates the release of insulin from beta cells in the pancreas, has come into use in the treatment of gestational diabetes. It appears to be free of adverse perinatal effects and is as effective as insulin, especially is women whose fasting glucose is 110 mg/dl (5.5 mmol/L) or less.[2]

Infectious Diseases

A number of infectious agents can affect pregnancy outcome. Among the most important in the United States are **group B** Streptococcus **(GBS), herpes simplex virus (HSV), human immunodeficiency virus (HIV),** and **hepatitis B virus (HBV).**

Group B Streptococcus

As many as 10% to 40% of pregnant women are colonized with GBS. Their infants are at risk for death or severe morbidity if they are born prematurely or after prolonged rupture of the fetal membranes.

In the past, two approaches were adopted for the prevention of early-onset GBS disease: culture-based and risk-based approaches. More recently, and based on a large retrospective cohort study, the American College of Obstetricians and Gynecologists recommends the culture-based approach because of its superiority in prevention of GBS disease.[3]

Vaginal/rectal cultures are usually obtained at 35 to 37 weeks of gestation. Patients with positive cultures should be treated with antibiotics from the time of membrane rupture or from the onset of labor. Penicillin is the drug of choice, with ampicillin being a good alternative. In the case of allergy to penicillin, sensitivity studies for clindamycin and erythromycin should be performed. Vancomycin is indicated in the case of resistance to clindamycin and erythromycin or in case of absent sensitivity studies. Patients who present in labor or with rupture of membranes with unknown GBS status should be given antibiotic prophylaxis in case of intrapartum fever, prolonged membrane rupture (more than 18 hours), or

preterm **delivery** (less than 37 weeks of gestation). Note finally that antibiotic prophylaxis for GBS disease should be given to all patients with GBS bacteriuria during the current pregnancy or with a previous infant with invasive GBS disease.[3]

Herpes Simplex Virus

Genital HSV infection is perhaps the most common sexually transmitted disease. Women who have primary or recurrent HSV outbreaks during pregnancy risk infecting their baby if there is viral shedding as evidenced by herpetic lesions in the vagina or on the vulva at the time of membrane rupture or the onset of labor. In these circumstances, the virus can ascend to infect the fetus; therefore cesarean delivery is undertaken as soon as possible after membrane rupture or after the onset of labor. If clinical shedding occurs earlier in pregnancy, the woman can be treated according to Centers for Disease Control and Prevention (CDC) guidelines with acyclovir with no risk to the fetus.[4] It is now well established that, for women who experience frequent outbreaks of HSV shedding, continuous suppression with acyclovir beginning at 36 weeks of gestation results in fewer outbreaks at term and a decreased need for cesarean delivery.[5]

Human Immunodeficiency Virus and Hepatitis B Virus

At this time, all pregnant women enrolled in prenatal care are screened for HIV and HBV infection. Both viruses can cause disease in the fetus.

HIV. In the general obstetrical population in the United States, the frequency of HIV infection is about 1 per 1000. The prevalence is as high as 1% to 1.5% in inner-city populations.[6] Approximately 30% of the exposed fetuses will also acquire the infection.[7] Zidovudine (an antiretroviral drug) used during pregnancy, during labor, and as chemoprophylaxis for 6 weeks in exposed newborns is associated with a decrease in perinatal HIV transmission to 8.3%.[8] When care includes both zidovudine therapy and a scheduled cesarean delivery, the risk is approximately 2%.[9] Nursing should be discouraged in HIV-positive women because the virus is secreted in breast milk.

HBV. Around the world some 2 billion individuals have been infected with HBV and 350 million remain chronically infected. In the United States 0.5% of the population test positive for the hepatitis B surface antigen and are thus chronically infected.[10] Infants of women infected with HBV are at high risk of becoming infected at delivery. When these infants are treated with anti–hepatitis B immunoglobulin and are begin vaccination within the first 12 hours of life, 95% of neonatal infections are prevented. Cesarean delivery of these newborns provides no protection at delivery.[11]

Cytomegalovirus, rubella, *Toxoplasma gondii, Listeria monocytogenes,* mycobacterial species, and *Treponema pallidum* (**syphilis**) can all significantly affect the mother, fetus, and fetoplacental unit. Early diagnosis and treatment of the pregnancy complicated by infection with *Listeria, Toxoplasma,* or syphilis can result in normal pregnancy outcomes.

Toxic Habits in Pregnancy

Maternal habits should be assessed early in the course of gestation. Smoking, alcohol use, and illicit drug use in pregnancy can cause well-described adverse effects on the fetus. The American College of Obstetricians and Gynecologists (Washington, DC) estimates that the prevalence of substance abuse in pregnant women is about 10%.[12]

Alcohol

Alcohol is a potent **teratogen,** an agent or factor that causes malformation of the fetus. **Fetal alcohol syndrome,** first described in 1973 by Jones and colleagues[13] and associated with maternal use of alcohol during pregnancy, is characterized by mental retardation and prenatal and postnatal growth restriction, as well as by brain, cardiac, spinal, and craniofacial anomalies. It is usually seen among children of women who consume four to six drinks daily throughout pregnancy.[14] However, no safe range for drinking alcohol during pregnancy has been established.

Smoking

Smoking during pregnancy can cause several adverse effects. Carbon monoxide and nicotine, the main ingredients responsible, mediate their effects by decreasing the availability of oxygen to the fetus and placenta. A strong association occurs between cigarette smoking and lower birth weight.[15] The mean birth weight of infants of women who smoke during pregnancy is about 200 g less than that of infants of nonsmokers. Smoking is also associated with a higher incidence of preterm **premature rupture of membranes** (**PROM,** i.e., rupture of the membranes before the onset of labor before 37 weeks of gestation),[16] placental abruption (i.e., separation of the placenta before birth of the newborn), and placenta previa (i.e., when the placenta partially or completely covers the cervix),[17] and risk of infant death from **sudden infant death syndrome,** the unexplained death of an infant under 1 year of age.[18]

Cocaine

Cocaine has a potent sympathomimetic action and hence is a potent constrictor of blood vessels. It can cause numerous maternal medical complications that include myocardial infarction, stroke, seizures, bowel ischemia, and death. Cocaine is also associated with adverse pregnancy sequelae: placental abruption, preterm delivery, birth of an infant more than 20 weeks and less than 37 weeks of gestation, and **growth restriction** (estimated fetal weight less than the tenth percentile for gestational age).[19] It is also thought to cause congenital malformations of the limbs, heart, brain, and genitourinary tract.

Other Substances

Finally, infants born to women who abuse opiates or amphetamines during pregnancy tend to have significant withdrawal symptoms after birth and to be small for gestational age. The obstetrical care provider can have an impact on prevention of substance abuse in pregnancy by identifying patients at risk, educating patients about the effects of drugs, and referring patients already abusing drugs.

HIGH-RISK CONDITIONS

Hypertension and Preeclampsia

Hypertensive disease complicates 12% to 22% of pregnancies in the United States and is second only to pulmonary embolism as a cause of maternal mortality.[9,20] Perinatal morbidity and mortality are increased secondary to **intrauterine growth restriction (IUGR),** placental abruption, and preterm delivery. **Preeclampsia** is a pregnancy-specific multisystem disorder traditionally diagnosed as the onset or exacerbation of hypertension, proteinuria, and edema in the second half of pregnancy. It complicates approximately 5% to 8% of pregnancies. Predisposing factors for the development of preeclampsia are listed in Box 3-1.

Preeclampsia remains a poorly understood disease despite extensive research. Immunological mechanisms, genetic predisposition, dietary deficiencies, vasoactive substances, and endothelial dysfunction have all been implicated in the pathophysiology of preeclampsia.[21] The diagnosis of severe preeclampsia (Box 3-2) generally mandates immediate delivery whether or not the fetus is mature.

Definitive treatment of preeclampsia is by delivery of the fetus and placenta. Magnesium sulfate is used to prevent seizures, and antihypertensive agents such as hydralazine and labetalol are usually used to control severe hypertension. The recurrence rate of preeclampsia is about 25%.[22] Calcium, magnesium, and zinc supplementation and use of low-dose aspirin have been studied for prevention of pregnancy-induced hypertension, with conflicting results thus far.

Box 3-1	**Predisposing Factors for the Development of Preeclampsia**

- Nulliparity (never having given birth to a child)
- Advanced maternal age
- Chronic hypertension
- Chronic renal disease
- Diabetes mellitus
- Twin gestation
- Molar pregnancy (gestational trophoblastic disease)
- Hydrops fetalis (total body edema [anasarca] with pleural and pericardial effusion)

Box 3-2	Criteria for the Diagnosis of Severe Preeclampsia

Clinical criteria for the diagnosis of severe preeclampsia is diagnosed in the presence of the following:
- Systolic blood pressure higher than 160 mm Hg
- Diastolic blood pressure higher than 110 mm Hg
- Proteinuria: more than 5 g per 24-hour urine collection
- Pulmonary edema
- Intrauterine growth restriction
- Oliguria: urine output less than 500 ml in 24 hours
- Thrombocytopenia: platelet count less than 100,000/ml
- Headache
- Visual disturbances: scotomata, blindness
- Epigastric or right upper quadrant abdominal pain
- Hepatocellular dysfunction
- Grand mal seizure: definition of eclampsia

Fetal Membranes, Umbilical Cord, and Placenta

In utero the fetus is contained in the sterile, fluid-filled amniotic sac. If the membranes that compose the external lining of the amniotic sac rupture before term (before 37 weeks of gestation) or before the onset of normal labor at term, the fetal environment is no longer sterile, increasing the risk of fetal infection. At the same time, the volume of fluid in the sac decreases. This may cause compression of the umbilical cord, resulting in compromised blood flow between the placenta and fetus. The causes of premature rupture of the fetal membranes are generally not known but are responsible for 35% to 40% of preterm births in the United States. Preterm rupture of the fetal membranes can be seen as being responsible for all the problems faced by most prematurely born infants.

Abnormalities of the umbilical cord and placenta can have profound effects on fetal development and pregnancy outcome. The umbilical cord has a mean length of 55 cm and contains three vessels: two arteries and one vein. The two arteries arising from the end of the fetal aorta bring relatively deoxygenated blood from the fetus to the placenta, and the single umbilical vein returns oxygenated blood from the placenta to the fetus. In 3% of pregnancies, the umbilical cord contains a single umbilical artery. A single umbilical artery is associated with fetal structural and chromosomal anomalies as well as fetal growth restriction.[23]

The length of the umbilical cord has long been recognized to be of clinical significance. A short cord predisposes to placental abruption and uterine inversion. A long cord is associated with cord prolapse (delivery of the cord before the infant, with compromise of blood flow from compression), cord knots, and nuchal cords (cord wrapped around the infant's neck). Marginal cord insertion (on the edge of the placenta) is of little clinical importance. **Velamentous cord insertion** (in which the umbilical vessels cross the fetal membranes unsupported by placenta or cord structure) may be associated with risk of rupture of a fetal vessel at the time of rupture of membranes, resulting in fetal exsanguination.

Placental abruption is separation of the placenta from its implantation anytime before delivery of the fetus. Abruption complicates 1:180 deliveries. Partial or complete separation results in abrupt cessation of gas exchange between the mother and fetus with rapidly evolving fetal hypoxia, acidosis and fetal death. In addition, the mother can suffer life-threatening hemorrhage and coagulopathy.

It is usually associated with the following[24]:
- Hypertensive disease in pregnancy
- Advanced maternal age
- Multiparity
- Preterm premature rupture of membranes
- Trauma
- Cigarette smoking
- Cocaine abuse
- Uterine leiomyoma (benign tumor of the uterus) behind the placental implantation site

Placenta previa occurs when the placenta implants over or close to the internal cervical os. Placenta previa complicates nearly 1:300 deliveries. Cesarean delivery is usually required. Placenta previa is associated with the following:
- Advanced maternal age
- Multiparity
- Prior cesarean delivery
- Multiple gestation

Disorders of Amniotic Fluid Volume

Early in pregnancy, amniotic fluid is derived from the fetal periderm (the as yet noncornified fetal skin) and the fetal membranes that compose the amniotic sac. Later, the majority of amniotic fluid is the product of fetal urination, with little contribution from the now cornified fetal skin. Fetal swallowing is an important mechanism for absorption of amniotic fluid. The fetal lungs help circulate the amniotic fluid. The amniotic fluid index (AFI) is calculated by measuring the depth of the largest vertical pocket of fluid in each of the four equal uterine quadrants at the time of ultrasound examination. It is the most commonly used method for quantification of amniotic fluid volume.

Oligohydramnios, too little amniotic fluid or an AFI below 5 cm, is usually associated with congenital anomalies (especially renal agenesis or urinary tract obstruction), fetal growth restriction or demise, postterm pregnancy (pregnancy continuing beyond 42 weeks from the first day of the pregnant woman's last menstrual period [more than 294 days]), ruptured membranes, uteroplacental insufficiency, and use of prostaglandin synthase inhibitors. When oligohydramnios occurs early in gestation, it can cause lung hypoplasia and limb deformities. When renal agenesis occurs in association with oligohydramnios, it is called **Potter's syndrome** and is always fatal. Later in gestation, oligohydramnios is usually associated with adverse perinatal outcomes secondary to compression of the umbilical cord. In labor there is an increase in variable decelerations (as a result of cord compression) and an increase in cesarean delivery rates.[25]

Polyhydramnios, too much amniotic fluid or an amnAFI greater than 24 cm, is often associated with fetal malformations that might affect swallowing of amniotic fluid (e.g., **anencephaly;** congenital absence of the cranial vault; **esophageal atresia;** and tracheoesophageal fistula, connection between the trachea and esophagus). It is also associated with **hydrops fetalis,** effusions within the pericardial, pleural and peritoneal space of the fetus with fetal edema, twin gestation (with twin–twin transfusion syndrome), and maternal diabetes. Polyhydramnios overdistends the uterus and can lead to premature rupture of membranes, preterm labor, and cord prolapse.

Preterm Birth

Preterm birth is the greatest cause of infant mortality in the otherwise normal newborn. In the United States, 12% to 14% of neonates are born preterm and are at risk for significant morbidities, including **sepsis; respiratory distress syndrome (RDS); intraventricular hemorrhage (IVH);** bleeding into the ventricular system of the brain; **retinopathy of prematurity (ROP);** disorganized retinal vascular growth, which can lead to retina scarring and blindness; **bronchopulmonary dysplasia (BPD),** a chronic pulmonary disease associated with oxygen and positive pressure ventilation and **necrotizing enterocolitis (NEC),** a bacterial infection of the intestinal wall; visual and hearing problems; and cerebral palsy. The smaller the infant, the greater are the risks for mortality and morbidity[26] (Table 3-2).

Box 3-3 lists some specific medical risk factors for preterm labor and delivery. Preterm birth can also be seen as the consequence of four broad categories of events (Figure 3-1). The baseline risk that any pregnant woman will experience preterm labor leading to the delivery of a

Box 3-3	**Medical Risk Factors Associated with Preterm Labor and Delivery**

- Previous preterm delivery
- Premature rupture of membranes
- Genital infections: *Chlamydia trachomatis, Gardnerella vaginalis*
- Nongenital infections: pyelonephritis, pneumonia
- Chorioamnionitis: infection of fetal membranes and amniotic fluid
- Conditions that overdistend the uterus: multiple gestations, increased amount of amniotic fluid
- Bleeding in the first trimester of pregnancy
- Placental conditions: placental abruption or placenta previa
- Abnormalities of the uterine cavity: uterine septum or fibroids
- Fetal anomalies
- Cervical insufficiency
- Short interval between pregnancies
- Lifestyle factors:
  - Smoking
  - Illicit drug use
  - Inadequate weight gain
  - Obesity
  - Young or advanced maternal age
  - Poverty
  - Short stature
- Occupational factors:
  - Prolonged standing or walking
  - Strenuous work conditions
  - Long work hours

TABLE 3-2

Infant Mortality Rates in the United States, 2008

	Live Births No. (%)	Infant Death No. (%)	Infant Mortality Rate*
Total Infants	4,247,726 (2)	28,075	6.61
<32 weeks	84,230 (1.6)	14,778 (53)	175.45
32-33 weeks	66,648 (2)	1172 (4)	17.58
34-36 weeks	372,162 (9)	2753 (10)	7.40
37-41 weeks	3,478,057 (82)	8470 (30)	2.44
≥42 weeks	240,795 (6)	648 (2)	2.69
Unknown	5834 (0.1)	255 (1)	

*Deaths of children up to 1 year of age per 1000 live births.
From Mathew TJ, Mac Dorman MF. Infant mortality statistics from the 2008 period: linked birth/ infant death data set, *Natl Vital Stat Rep* 2012;60(5).

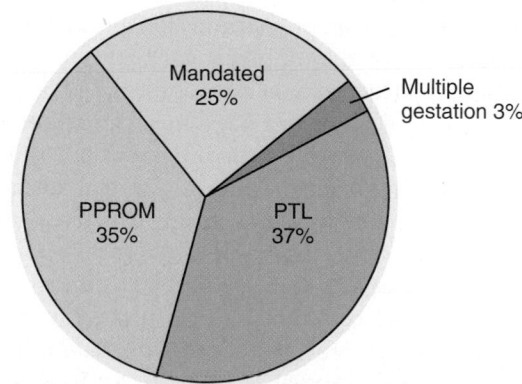

Reasons for preterm birth

FIGURE 3-1   A pie chart of the four most common reasons for preterm birth.

preterm infant is about 5.6%. A history of spontaneous preterm labor with delivery is one of the most important risk factors for subsequent preterm labor. With one prior preterm birth, a woman carries a 15% risk of subsequent preterm delivery; this risk increases to 32% with a history of two previous preterm births.[27]

Signs of preterm labor include back pain, menstrual-like pains, pelvic heaviness, vaginal discharge, and vaginal bleeding. Diagnosis of labor is based on having six contractions in a 1-hour period associated with cervical changes: **cervical dilation** (opening wider) and **cervical effacement** (thinning out). Several approaches to prevention of preterm labor have been studied. These include serial cervical examinations, home uterine activity monitoring, prophylactic use of oral **tocolytics** (an agent used to arrest uterine contractions), and bed rest. None has been shown to be clearly effective.

Fetal fibronectin (a glycoprotein produced in the chorion) is expressed in cervical and vaginal secretions in most cases of preterm labor. It has been studied as a marker of preterm labor in symptomatic patients. The absence of fetal fibronectin is a strong predictor that preterm delivery is unlikely to happen within 1 to 2 weeks, with a negative predictive value exceeding 95% in some studies.[28] Its use may be beneficial in providing reassurance to asymptomatic women who have high-risk factors for preterm delivery.[29]

Once preterm labor is diagnosed, prompt measures should be taken to try to stop labor and prevent an early delivery. Intravenous hydration is commonly the first approach used. It does not seem to be of clinical significance in a well-hydrated patient.[30] Excessive hydration should be avoided, because it can potentiate the risk of pulmonary edema that is usually associated with tocolytic use. Commonly used tocolytics:

· Magnesium sulfate
· β-Mimetic agents
· Indomethacin (a prostaglandin inhibitor)

Less commonly used tocolytics:

· Nifedipine (calcium channel blocker)
· Nitroglycerin (nitric oxide donor drug)
· Atosiban (oxytocin antagonist)
· Combination therapy

Magnesium sulfate is usually given as an initial intravenous bolus of 4 g to 6 g followed by intravenous infusion at 2 to 4 g/hr. Its main mechanism of action is decrease free intracellular calcium ion concentration, resulting in decreased electrical potential of the cell. Magnesium sulfate is contraindicated in patients with hypocalcemia, renal failure, and myasthenia gravis. Potential toxic effects include pulmonary edema, respiratory depression, cardiac arrest, muscular paralysis, and profound hypotension.[31] Loss of deep tendon reflexes usually precedes the previously mentioned complications. Deep tendon reflexes are frequently checked to monitor patients receiving therapy. Magnesium blood level can also be assessed. Toxic effects are rarely seen with levels less than 8 mg/dl or in patients with deep tendon reflexes.

β-Mimetic drugs (e.g., terbutaline and ritodrine), agents that mimic naturally occurring hormones that stimulate the β-adrenergic receptor, can also cause uterine relaxation. They decrease the electrical potential of the cell by increasing calcium binding to the intracellular sarcoplasmic reticulum, an effect mediated by cyclic adenosine monophosphate. They are contraindicated in patients with poorly controlled diabetes, thyrotoxicosis, and maternal cardiac disease. Potential side effects include hyperglycemia, hypokalemia, hypotension, pulmonary edema, arrhythmias, and myocardial ischemia. β-Mimetic drugs are administered intravenously. The rate of infusion is slowly titrated upward until a clinical response is obtained. Maternal pulse rate correlates with the blood concentration of the drug and is typically used to assess the adequacy of the dosage. A pulse rate higher than 120 beats per minute should be avoided. This class of tocolytic drugs is infrequently used because of the significant complications associated with their use.

Indomethacin (a prostaglandin inhibitor) reduces the synthesis of prostaglandins by inhibiting cyclooxygenase. It is contraindicated in patients with asthma, gastrointestinal bleeding, renal failure, coronary artery disease, and oligohydramnios. Its major potential complications include renal failure, gastrointestinal bleeding, and hepatitis (with chronic use). It can cause oligohydramnios and when used after 32 weeks of gestation it may induce closure of the ductus arteriosus in the fetus, leading to heart failure and hydrops. Indomethacin is used orally or via the rectal route. Ultrasound is used to periodically assess the amniotic fluid volume when indomethacin is used.

Tocolytics are widely used for the treatment of preterm labor. Studies have failed to show much success beyond delaying delivery for 48 hours.[32] Adjunctive therapy with corticosteroids for induction of fetal lung maturity is beneficial and justifies the use of tocolytics.

All women between 24 and 34 weeks of gestation with preterm labor and intact membranes are candidates for antenatal corticosteroid therapy.[33] Patients with preterm labor and ruptured membranes benefit from corticosteroid therapy between 24 and 32 weeks of gestation. Betamethasone and dexamethasone are most commonly used for antenatal corticosteroid therapy. Maximal benefit occurs 48 hours after initiation of therapy and lasts for 7 days. Corticosteroids reduce respiratory distress syndrome and neonatal morbidity by 50%.[34] This effect is due to induction of proteins that regulate the production of surfactant by type II cells in the fetal lungs. Corticosteroids also decrease the incidence of intracranial hemorrhage, probably by promoting maturation of the **germinal matrix,** a highly cellular and vascularized region of the brain that produces both neurons and glial cells that migrate to the cerebral cortex. Repeated corticosteroid courses should not be used routinely because of the possible risk of adverse neurodevelopmental outcome.[33]

Prevention of preterm delivery in patients with previous preterm deliveries is currently being studied. A study using weekly intramuscular injection of 17α-hydroxyprogesterone caproate showed promising results in decreasing the rate of recurrent preterm birth.[35] Other progesterone formulations and other routes of administration are being studied. Preliminary results are promising. Long-term safety studies are under way.

Cervical Insufficiency

Cervical insufficiency is defined as painless dilation of the uterine cervix in the second trimester of pregnancy. This may progress to prolapse of the fetal membranes through the cervix into the vagina with delivery of an immature newborn. There is no consensus at this time concerning the causes of cervical insufficiency. Some have implicated prior surgery of the cervix, such as cone biopsy, and trauma to the cervix from mechanical dilation or birth-associated lacerations. The patient with risk factors for cervical insufficiency is generally evaluated by transvaginal ultrasound examination of the cervix at intervals starting at 16 weeks of gestation to identify changes in cervical length and dilation (Figure 3-2). If cervical shortening or funneling of the cervix is diagnosed at any time into the late second trimester (22 to 24 weeks of gestation), a **cervical cerclage** is offered.[36] The most commonly performed cerclage is simply a purse-string suture placed as high as possible around the cervix. For women with a history of pregnancy loss caused by cervical insufficiency, elective cerclage is usually performed at 14 weeks of gestation after confirmation by ultrasound of the absence of gross congenital anomalies in the fetus.[37]

Postterm Pregnancy

Postterm pregnancy complications occur in 3% to 12% of pregnancies. The most common reason for a diagnosis of postdate gestation is inaccurate dating because of either irregular ovulation or inaccurate recall of last menstrual period. Inaccurate dating is often encountered in patients who become pregnant after discontinuation of birth control pills. These patients tend to experience a delay in ovulation of 2 or more weeks. Less common causes of

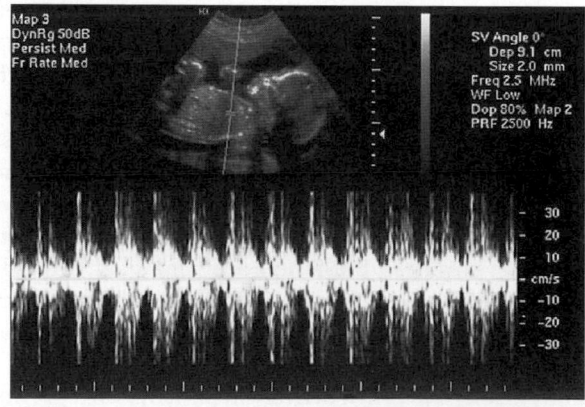

FIGURE 3-2   Ultrasound picture of a fetus at 23 weeks of gestation *(top)*, with a Doppler study of the fetal heart *(bottom)*. *Dop,* Doppler; *Fr,* frame; *Freq,* frequency; *PRF,* pulse-repetition frequency; *SV,* sample volume; *WF,* wall filter. (Courtesy Frank Fox, RDMS.)

posterm pregnancy are fetal anencephaly, placental sulfatase deficiency, and abdominal pregnancy. Most postterm pregnancies are of unknown cause; deficiency of prostaglandin production or refractoriness of the cervix to endogenous prostaglandins could be the cause.[38] An emerging modifiable risk factor associated with postterm pregnancy is obesity.[39]

Posterm pregnancy may be associated with maternal and neonatal problems. A woman may suffer from anxiety when she is past her due date and still undelivered. She is at higher risk of obstetrical trauma (e.g., vaginal and cervical laceration) from delivery of a large infant. Physically she is at increased risk of long-term sequelae such as incontinence and pelvic relaxation. The infant may suffer from oligohydramnios, macrosomia, **meconium aspiration** (inhalation of fetal fecal discharge into the fetal lungs), and placental insufficiency. After reaching a maximum of about 1 L at 37 weeks of gestation, amniotic fluid volume decreases gradually. The decrease in amniotic fluid may result in cord compression, fetal hypoxia, and a higher incidence of cesarean delivery for fetal heart rate (FHR) abnormalities. Intrapartum amnioinfusion, the installation of fluid into the amniotic cavity, significantly improves neonatal outcome and lessens the rate of cesarean section in the presence of oligohydramnios.[40]

Fetal macrosomia——increases the risk of cesarean delivery for dystocia (abnormal or difficult childbirth) and increases the risk of birth trauma during vaginal delivery as a result of shoulder dystocia (when the anterior shoulder of the infant cannot pass below the mother's hip bone or requires significant manipulation to pass the pubic symphysis), resulting in brachial plexus palsy.

Meconium passage in utero is common after 42 weeks of gestation. It is associated with fetal hypoxia.. Aspiration of meconium may lead to obstruction of the respiratory passages and interference with surfactant function. For this reason, current recommendations include tracheal intubation of the limp, cyanotic newborn to remove meconium from below the vocal cords. A recent adequately powered randomized trial of amnioinfusion to prevent infant death or meconium aspiration failed to demonstrate any benefit to this intervention.[41] As a result, the American College of Obstetricians and Gynecologists recommends against routine ammnioinfusion to prevent meconium aspiration syndrome.[42]

Placental insufficiency is another hazard to the fetus. When the placenta "ages," it fails to provide the fetus with substantial nutritional requirements. This may result in fetal intrauterine growth restriction. In labor, poor beat-to-beat variability, late decelerations, and bradycardia may be signs of fetal compromise as a result of placental insufficiency.

To decrease fetal risk of adverse outcome, two strategies are widely used: antenatal surveillance and induction of labor. There is a lack of evidence that antenatal testing improves neonatal outcome. However, it became standard practice because of its universal acceptance. Because of the lack of evidence, it is not clear when to start antenatal surveillance. There are wide variations of practice regarding what method of testing to use (see Antenatal Assessment later in this chapter) and how often to perform testing. Furthermore, it is unclear whether labor induction results in a better outcome when compared with antenatal surveillance. The American College of Obstetricians and Gynecologists recommends labor induction for pregnancies at 41 weeks or more when the cervix is favorable. When the cervix is unfavorable, cervical ripening followed by labor induction and fetal antenatal surveillance are acceptable options.[43]

Labor induction can be achieved with various medications when the cervix is favorable for induction. Intravenous infusion of **oxytocin,** a hormone secreted from the posterior pituitary that stimulates uterine contractions and milk letdown, is most commonly used. Oxytocin is started at a rate of 1 or 2 mU/min and increased periodically until an adequate pattern of uterine contractions is achieved. Possible side effects include water retention with long use of high doses (usually more than 20 mU/min). This can result in hyponatremia with seizures and coma in the mother. Oxytocin also causes hypotension when administered rapidly as an intravenous bolus. Uterine rupture and amniotic fluid embolism have been cited with oxytocin use.

When the cervix is unfavorable for induction, its texture, dilation, and effacement can be improved by several modalities. Mechanical methods include placement of a Foley catheter balloon or osmotic dilator (**Laminaria tents**) into the cervical canal. Laminaria tents are thought to act by absorbing water from the cervix, rendering it softer, resulting in dilation and effacement, a process referred to as cervical ripening. Pharmacological agents have also been used for cervical ripening. Prostaglandin E_2 cervical gel (Prepidil) and vaginal insert (Cervidil) are widely used. They act by causing dissolution of collagen fibers in the cervix. The most common side effects include maternal fever, nausea, vomiting, and diarrhea. Misoprostol (Cytotec) is a prostaglandin E_1 analog that is approved by the Food and Drug Administration for the prevention of ulcers that occur during long-term treatment with nonsteroidal antiinflammatory drugs. Because of its uterotonic effect, it has been increasingly used for cervical ripening and labor induction. Its popularity stems from its effectiveness, low cost, and stability at room temperature.[44] Safety concerns have been raised in view of reports of uterine rupture occurring after misoprostol induction in patients with previous uterine scars[45] and in multiparous patients.[46]

ANTENATAL ASSESSMENT

To ascertain the pregnancy at risk for an adverse outcome, one must begin with a thorough history and physical examination. Technological advances have made it possible to make many assessments of fetal condition. Both invasive and noninvasive methods of evaluating fetal structure and function are used with regularity. It is possible to view fetal anatomy, measure fetal biochemical and genetic status, assess fetal biophysical status, evaluate uteroplacental function, and determine the ability of the fetus and placenta to function during the normal stresses of labor. Depending on the characteristics of any given pregnancy, most perinatal centers are capable of performing detailed antepartum assessment.

Ultrasound

One of the most widely used methods of noninvasive assessment of the fetus is ultrasonography (see Figure 3-2). Using ultra-high-frequency sound waves and transabdominal or transvaginal transducers to obtain real-time images, the clinician can diagnose multifetal pregnancy and evaluate fetal anatomy, growth, and position. One can also localize the placenta within the uterus, measure amniotic fluid volume, estimate fetal growth over time, and assess fetal biophysical status. In addition, Doppler flow studies measure blood flow to fetal organs. **Doppler ultrasonography** measures the shifts in frequency in the emitted ultrasound waves and their echoes, making it possible to measure the velocities of moving objects. This measurement permits early identification of fetuses at risk, enabling opportune delivery or transport to sophisticated perinatal centers. Ultrasonography is also invaluable for guiding the physician while performing amniocentesis, umbilical blood sampling, and other invasive procedures.

Three-dimensional ultrasound imaging has been introduced to the obstetrics field. It offers better visualization of fetal organs (especially the face, heart, and spine) than the conventional two-dimensional ultrasound imaging Outcome studies are under way, accompanied by an increase in the use of three-dimensional ultrasound imaging among obstetricians and maternal–fetal specialists.[47]

Amniocentesis

The most commonly performed invasive procedure to assess fetal condition is amniocentesis. In this procedure, under sterile conditions a needle is inserted through the skin and uterine wall to obtain a sample of fluid from the amniotic sac (Figure 3-3) Depending on the reason for performing the procedure, the concentration of many substances in the fluid can be measured. For example, as the fetal lung matures, pulmonary surfactant is secreted from the fetal lung into the amniotic fluid, where its concentration can be measured. Fetal cells isolated from amniotic fluid can be used to assess for fetal chromosomal abnormalities (e.g., trisomy 21), fetal enzyme deficiencies (e.g., Tay-Sachs), and certain discrete genetic mutations (e.g., sickle cell disease).

Nonstress Test and Contraction Stress Test

Fetal well-being is highly dependent on placental function. Placental function is commonly assessed by monitoring

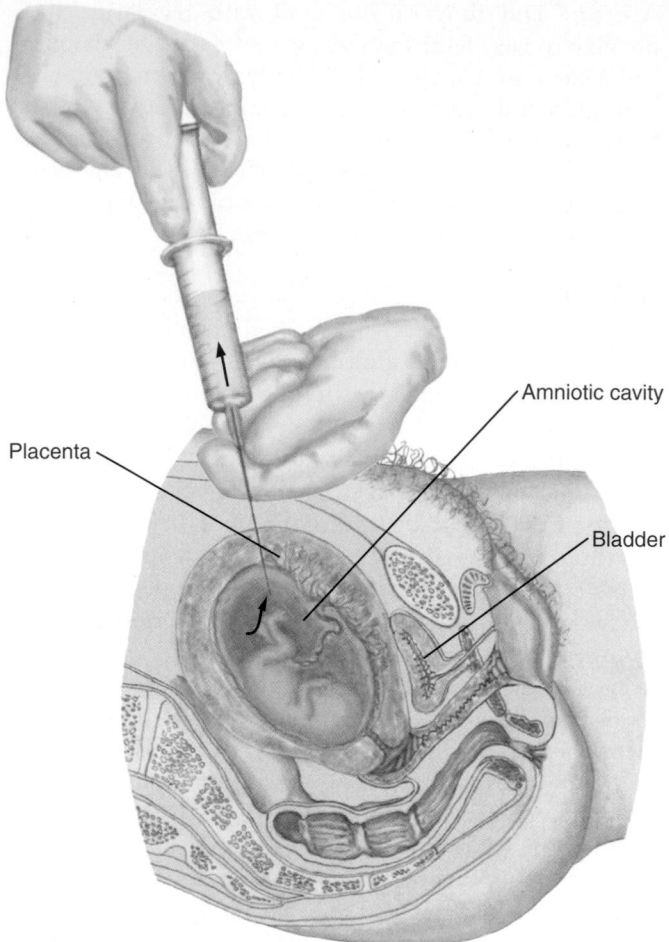

Placenta

Amniotic cavity

Bladder

FIGURE 3-3 In amniocentesis, a needle is inserted through the expectant mother's abdomen to aspirate fluid from the amniotic sac. The fluid can then be tested to detect chromosomal abnormalities in fetal cells or other problems and to determine fetal lung maturity. (From McKinney E, James S, Murray S, Nelson K, Ashwill J. *Maternal-child nursing*, ed 4, WB Saunders: Philadelphia, 2012.)

the fetal heart rate response when the fetus moves spontaneously **(nonstress test [NST])** or in reaction to induced uterine contractions **(contraction stress test [CST])**. For both tests, the FHR is monitored continuously. In the normally oxygenated fetus (as with a child or adult), cardiac output rises to support physical activity. This rise in cardiac output can be mediated by an increase in either heart rate or stroke volume. In the fetus, cardiac output rises by increasing the heart rate.

A reactive NST (Figure 3-4) requires at least two accelerations in fetal heart rate, each of at least 15 beats per minute and lasting at least 15 seconds, associated with maternal perception of fetal movement over a period of 20 minutes. A reactive NST is highly correlated with normal uteroplacental function. If no change in maternal clinical status transpires, this result predicts normal fetal survival when this test is performed within 1 week of delivery.[48]

The CST is conducted by continuously monitoring the FHR while uterine contractions are stimulated by intravenous infusion into the mother of a dilute solution of oxytocin. In a normal pregnancy, fetal Po_2 (partial pressure of oxygen) decreases with each uterine contraction and then rapidly returns to normal. A fetal Po_2 drop below 12 mm Hg, resulting in slowing of the FHR, indicates uteroplacental insufficiency. This slowing of the FHR in response to uterine contractions is called a late deceleration. A negative CST is one in which no late decelerations of the FHR develop with a frequency of three contractions, each lasting 40 to 60 seconds, per 10 minutes. A positive CST is diagnosed when late decelerations follow at least 50% of contractions. A suspicious CST is one in which late decelerations are inconsistent (follow less than 50% of contractions). Assuming no change in maternal clinical status, a negative CST predicts fetal survival if performed within 1 week of delivery. An abnormal CST must prompt further evaluation or delivery.

Fetal Biophysical Profile

The fetal **biophysical profile (BPP)** (Table 3-3) assesses placental function and fetal well-being.[49] The BPP has been likened to the Apgar score (a quick method to assess the health of a newborn baby, based on the scoring of five factors [see Chapter 4]). In producing a BPP, five determinants of fetal status are assessed and given a score of 0 to 2. Four are assessed by ultrasonography. They include fetal breathing, fetal tone, fetal gross body movement, and amniotic fluid volume. The fifth determinant is the NST. A BPP score of 8 to 10 is considered normal and reassuring; a score of 6 is equivocal and is generally repeated within 24 hours; BPP scores of 0 to 4 are clearly abnormal, are associated with poor perinatal outcomes, and require careful evaluation and usually immediate delivery.[50]

Mode of Delivery

Most deliveries occur spontaneously by the vaginal route. Typically, infants born vaginally are delivered head first (vertex presentation). However, there are times when assisted vaginal delivery (with forceps or vacuum) or abdominal delivery (cesarean) is needed. Breech presentation (legs or buttocks first) occurs in 3% to 4% of all births.

Breech Presentation

The breech position creates a situation in which there is greater potential for complications at the time of delivery. Predisposing factors for breech presentation include multiparity, previous breech delivery, uterine anomalies, fetal anomalies, multiple gestation, and polyhydramnios. The Term Breech Trial Collaborative Group conducted a multicenter randomized controlled trial of planned cesarean versus planned vaginal delivery for breech presentation at term. It concluded that planned cesarean

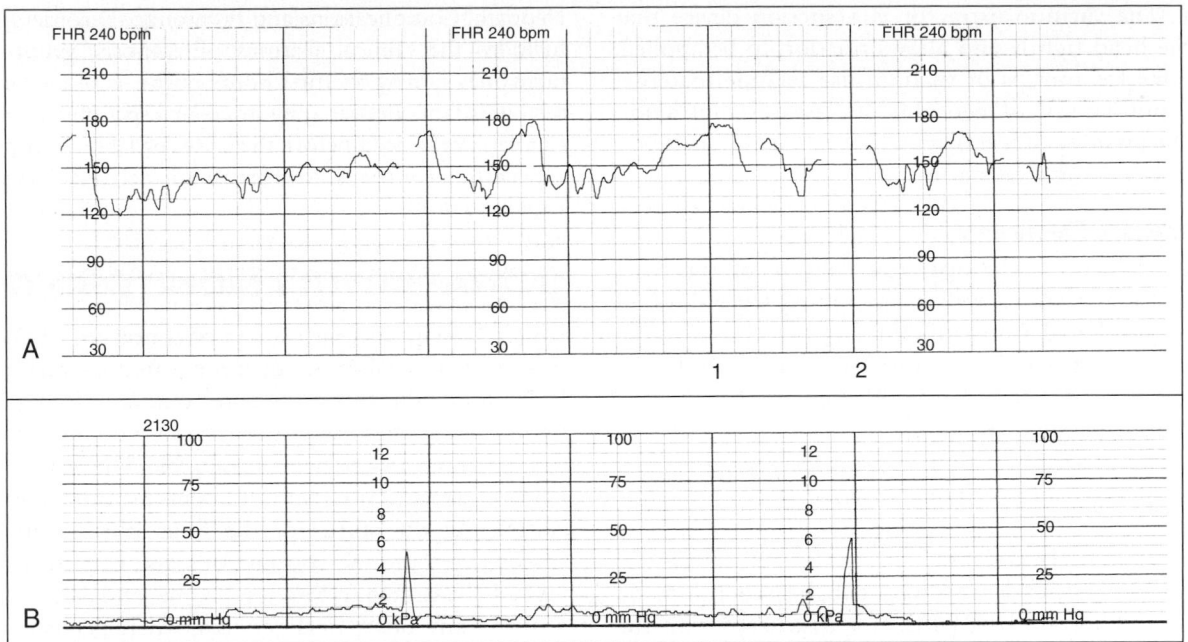

FIGURE 3-4 A nonstress test recording, produced with a cardiotocograph. **A,** The fetal heart rate (FHR) is recorded with an ultrasound probe as changes in beats per minute (bpm) over time. **B,** Uterine contractions (UC) are recorded with a pressure transducer as changes in pressure (mm Hg) over time. In this case the nonstress test is *reactive,* indicating normal uteroplacental function.

TABLE 3-3

Biophysical Profile Scoring

Biophysical Variable	Normal (Score = 2)	Abnormal (Score = 0)
Fetal breathing movements	At least one episode of FBM, lasting at least 30 sec, in 30 min	No FBM or no episode lasting >30 sec in 30 min
Gross body movements	At least three discrete body/limb movements (episodes of active continuous movement, considered as a single movement) in 30 min	Two or fewer episodes of body/limb movements in 30 min
Fetal tone	At least one episode of active extension with return to flexion of fetal limb or trunk; opening and closing of hand considered normal tone	Either slow extension with return to partial flexion movement of limb in full extension or absent fetal movement
Reactive FHR	At least two episodes of FHR acceleration of >15 bpm and lasting at least 15 sec associated with fetal movement in 20 min	Fewer than two episodes of acceleration of FHR or acceleration of <15 bpm in 40 min
Qualitative AFV	At least one pocket of AF that measures at least 1 cm in two perpendicular planes	Either no AF pockets or a pocket <1 cm in two perpendicular planes

AF, Amniotic fluid; AFV, amniotic fluid volume; bpm, beats per minute; FBM, fetal breathing movements; FHR, fetal heart rate.
Modified from Manning FA et al: Fetal biophysical profile score and the nonstress test: a comparative trial, *Obstet Gynecol* 1984;64:326.

delivery is preferred because of less risk for perinatal mortality or serious morbidity and no increase in serious maternal complications.[51] Two small randomized controlled trials published earlier did not find planned cesarean delivery of substantial benefit to the fetus.[52, 53] At present, the American College of Obstetricians and Gynecologists recommends that patients with persistent breech presentation at term in a singleton gestation should have a planned cesarean delivery. This recommendation does not apply to patients who present with breech presentation in labor and with imminent delivery.[54] Transverse lie, in which the fetus is oriented transversely inside the uterus, is another malpresentation that requires cesarean delivery.

Assisted Vaginal Delivery

Obstetrical forceps is an instrument used to cradle and guide the fetal head while applying traction to expedite delivery. The vacuum extractor is a suction device that holds the head tightly and allows traction to be applied. Indications for forceps or vacuum use include maternal cardiac, pulmonary, or neurological disease (contraindicating the pushing process); maternal exhaustion in labor; and nonreassuring fetal status.

Cesarean Delivery

Cesarean delivery is the operative delivery of the fetus through the abdominal wall. It accounted for 33% of all births in the United States in 2011.[55]

Major indications for cesarean delivery include the following:
- Previous cesarean delivery
- Failure to progress in labor
- Malpresentation (breech or transverse)
- Placenta previa
- Nonreassuring fetal status

Although cesarean delivery might be the least traumatic method of delivery of the fetus, it is associated with the following:
- An increased risk of significant maternal blood loss
- Anesthesia complications
- Intraoperative bladder or bowel injuries
- Postoperative wound infection
- **Endomyometritis**
- Thromboembolic events

Transient Tachypnea of the Newborn/ Type II Respiratory Distress Syndrome

The syndrome of transient tachypnea of the newborn (wet lung or type II respiratory distress syndrome [see Chapter 22,

Neonatal Complications and Pulmonary Disorders]), which includes the clinical features of cyanosis, grunting, and tachypnea during the first hours of life, is more commonly seen in infants delivered by cesarean, especially if that cesarean was performed before the onset of labor. The preferred explanation for the clinical features is delayed absorption of fetal lung fluid.[56]

INTRAPARTUM MONITORING

Evidence suggests that the use of continuous FHR monitoring during labor in uncomplicated pregnancies has little to no impact on neonatal outcome.[57] Despite this finding, its use has become routine in the United States. Its utility in high-risk patients is valuable. The response of the FHR to uterine contractions does provide information concerning the status of the fetus during labor. FHR responses to uterine contractions and their likely etiologies are illustrated in Figures 3-5, 3-6, and 3-7.

On many obstetrical services, when persistent severe variable or late decelerations of the FHR are diagnosed, fetal scalp blood is obtained via transvaginal fetal scalp puncture, and blood gas measurements can be obtained. Scalp blood pH greater than 7.25 is considered reassuring; values of 7.15 or less signal high risk of fetal acidemia. Many clinicians believe that scalp blood gas assessment in the face of an abnormal FHR pattern more precisely defines the fetus at risk and can thus prevent unnecessary forceps and cesarean deliveries.

An alternative to scalp blood gas assessment is fetal scalp stimulation. Using the underlying rationale of the NST, transvaginal stimulation of the fetal scalp to

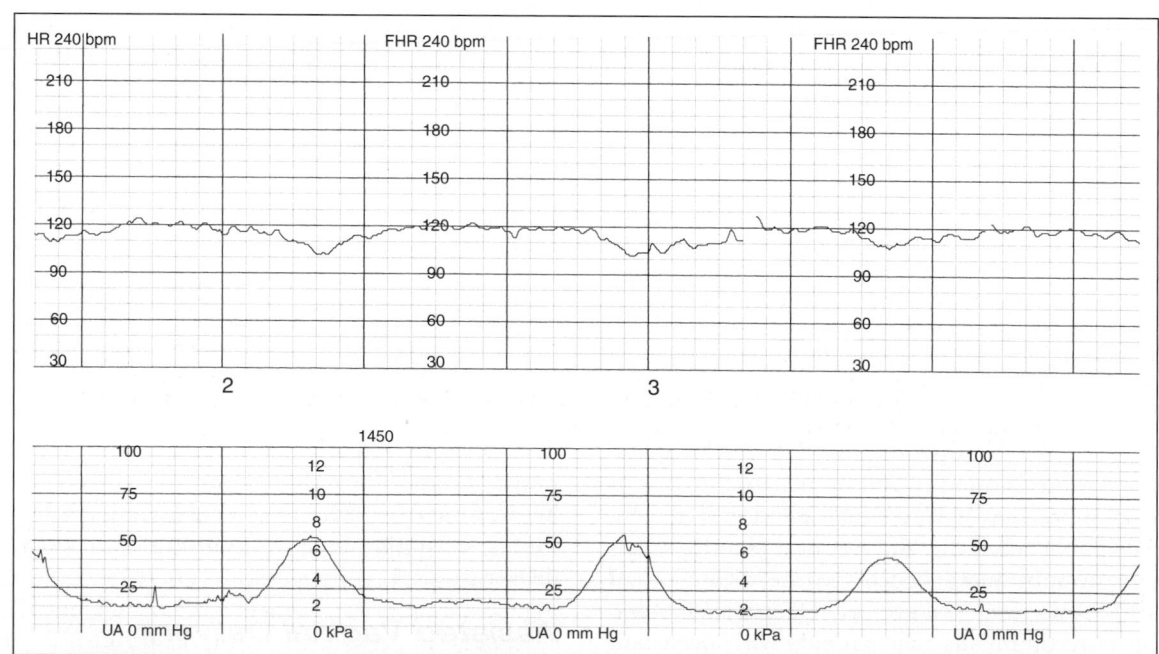

FIGURE 3-5   Early decelerations (coinciding with uterine contraction) usually are due to fetal head compression and pose little threat to the fetus.

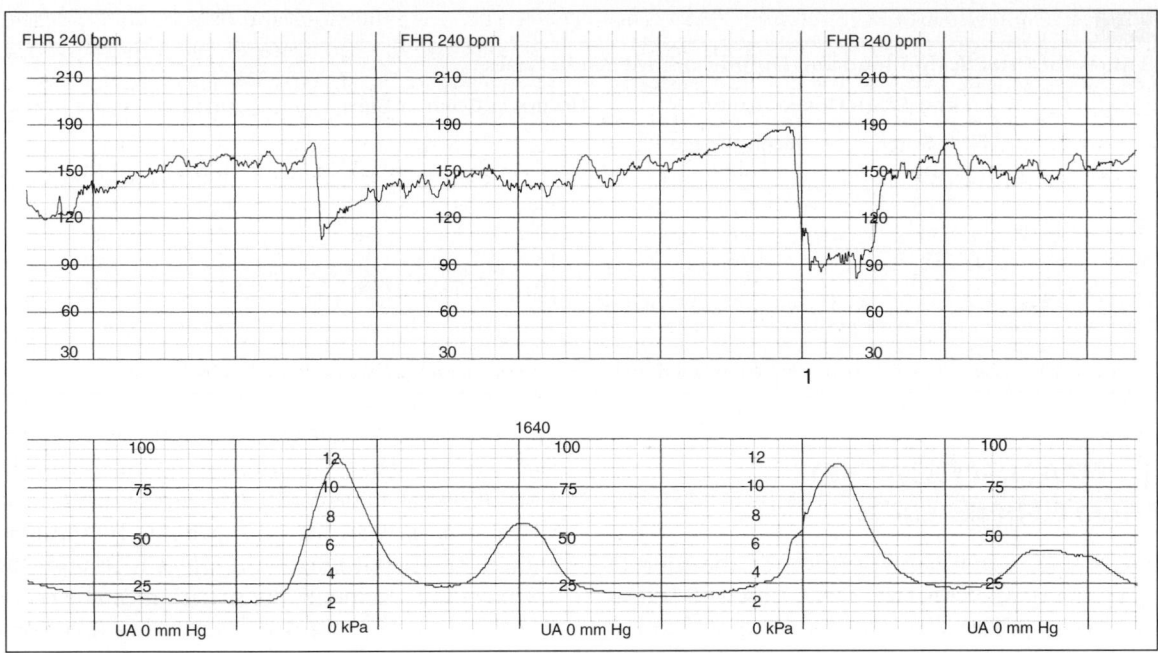

FIGURE 3-6 Variable decelerations are the most common. They are due to cord compression and have different configurations. Repetitive severe variable decelerations are associated with increased risk of fetal hypoxia.

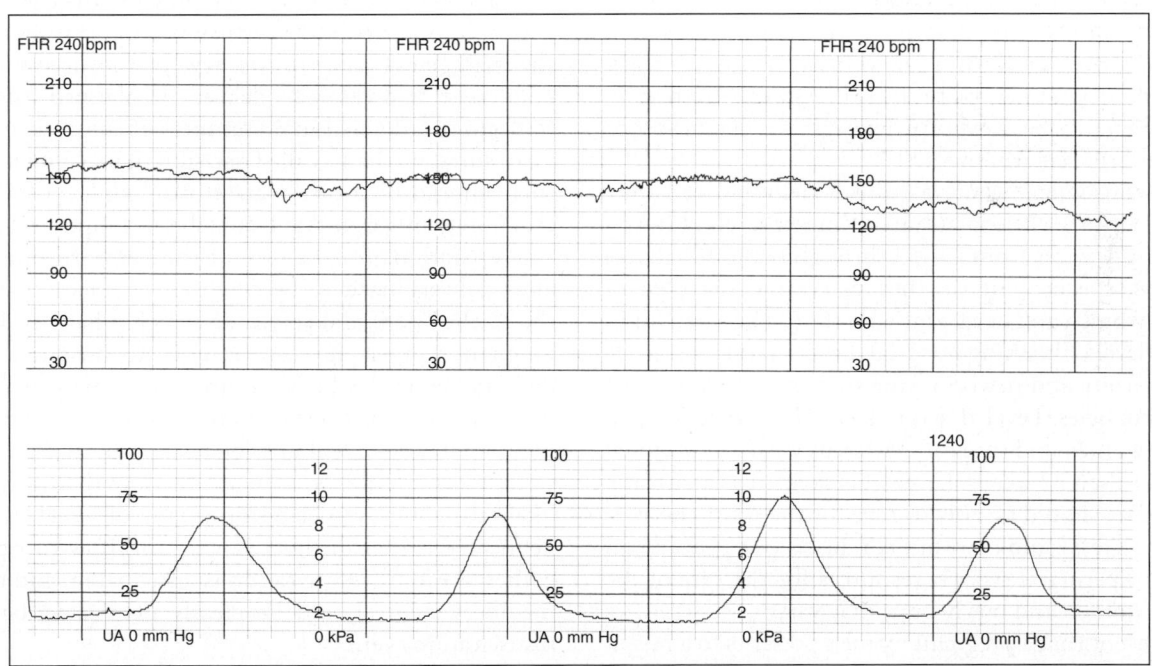

FIGURE 3-7 Late decelerations are due to uteroplacental insufficiency. They usually begin at the peak of the contraction and are associated with fetal distress.

induce fetal movement results in acceleration of the fetal heart rate and reassures the clinician that the fetus is not hypoxemic or acidemic.[58] Table 3-4 lists normal values for fetal scalp blood and umbilical cord blood gases.

Fetal oxygenation as determined by fetal pulse oximetry has been studied for intrapartum fetal assessment. A randomized controlled trial of intrapartum fetal pulse oximetry revealed a decrease in the number of cesarean deliveries performed for nonreassuring fetal heart tracing. The fetal pulse oximetry did not change the overall cesarean delivery rate.[59] More randomized controlled trials comparing fetal pulse oximetry with conventional fetal surveillance techniques are under way.

TABLE 3-4

Normal Values for Fetal Scalp Blood and Umbilical Cord Blood Gases

	FETAL SCALP DURING LABOR		UMBILICAL CORD AT BIRTH		ARTERIAL SAMPLE AFTER BIRTH		
	First-Stage Labor	Second-Stage Labor	Umbilical Artery	Umbilical Vein	5-10 Min	30 Min	60 Min
pH	7.33	7.29	7.24	7.32	7.21	7.30	7.33
P_{CO_2} (mm Hg)	44	46	49	38	46	38	36
P_{O_2} (mm Hg)	22	16	16	27	50	54	63
Bicarbonate (mEq/L)	20	17	19	20	17	18	19

P_{CO_2}, Carbon dioxide pressure; P_{O_2}, oxygen pressure.
Data from Beard RW, Nathanielsz PW: *Fetal physiology and medicine.* New York: Marcel Dekker, 1984; and Koch G, Wendel H. Adjustment of arterial blood gases and acid–base balance in the normal newborn infant during the first week of life, *Biol Neonate* 1968;12:136.

FETAL TRANSITION TO EXTRAUTERINE LIFE

Appropriate evaluation and intervention at the time of delivery of a fetus/newborn is key to the successful transition from a pattern of fetal circulation to that of the newborn. The physiological changes include increased PaO_2, decreased pulmonary vascular resistance, increased systemic vascular resistance, and closure of the foramen ovale and ductus arteriosus. These adaptations to extrauterine life occur immediately after delivery or in the first several hours after birth. The majority of newborns transition without intervention, but all newborns require a knowledgeable clinician to evaluate the success of the transition and intervene if the newborn displays maladaptation to the extrauterine environment.[60]

The environment where a baby is delivered can vary. The Guidelines for Perinatal Care delineate levels of hospital birthing services from Level I through Level III.[61] These levels have specific criteria that determine the type of pregnant women and newborns who should be cared for in a specific level of birthing hospital. Level I services provide basic maternity and newborn care to women with normal term pregnancies. Level II services care for moderately ill pregnant women and care for newborns with a gestational age greater than 32 weeks. Level III is defined as a birthing hospital that should be able to care for the most complex of maternal, fetal, and newborn conditions. Depending on the level of perinatal service, resources for the care of the pregnant women and newly born may vary.

In the event that a pregnant women presents to a hospital with a perinatal designation that does not meet the needs of her pregnancy or the fetus, intrauterine transport to a higher level of perinatal service should be accomplished if at all possible. These transfers may also occur after delivery. Many states have regionalized perinatal care systems that provide an organized approach to the transfer of pregnant women and newborns to higher levels of perinatal service as determined by level of illness and complexity and hospital resources.[61]

When a high-risk delivery occurs, whether planned or an emergency, key personnel, equipment, and supplies and medications, including blood products, need to be available. In most circumstances information from a woman's medical records can be obtained so there are baseline data regarding the patient. In trauma circumstances or when a pregnant patient is brought in unconscious or incapacitated, the situation can be very difficult. When a woman or fetus is deemed too unstable or labor has progressed too far to transfer the pregnant woman, preparation for delivery should occur. Maternal preparation should include intravenous access, fetal and contraction monitoring, 100% oxygen via non-rebreather mask, and side-lying position to take pressure off the vena cava and maximize placental perfusion. Importantly, the team that will assess and provide newborn resuscitation must be alerted. If a cesarean delivery is planned, the goal is to begin surgery within 30 minutes of the decision to perform surgery—the so-called decision to incision time. Thus there should be a care plan in place that ensures timely availability of surgical and anesthesia support staff.[62]

Preparations for the care of the newborn immediately after delivery need to be carefully planned regardless of the level of perinatal service in which a baby is delivered. Pregnant women are also brought to hospitals without delivery services, which requires that emergency departments be prepared to facilitate transition to extrauterine life for a newborn and provide resuscitation if necessary.

Systems should be in place for identifying newborns likely to require resuscitation (many of which have been delineated earlier in this chapter) and how to notify and gather a team if resuscitation is anticipated, and the team members roles should be clearly delineated before the resuscitation event.

At a minimum, staff should be familiar with the recommendations for newborn resuscitation and have the equipment and medications necessary for the assessment and resuscitation of a newborn. The most recent edition of the American Heart Association and American Academy of Pediatrics *Textbook of neonatal resuscitation* (NRP), sixth edition, provides an excellent in-depth source for the most recent standards for newborn resuscitation in hospitals.[63]

One of the biggest changes to accepted resuscitation standards for newborns in the sixth edition of NRP (2011) is the need for compressed air and pulse oximetry for all newborns requiring resuscitation. If ventilation is necessary, term infant ventilation is started with room air (21%) via positive pressure device and changes in oxygen concentration are made using clinical assessment and preductal pulse oximetry. Specific guidelines for preductal pulse oximetry readings in the first 10 minutes of life in term babies are published and should be used to guide resuscitation maneuvers and administration of oxygen.[64] Preterm infant resuscitation is started with oxygen, at a concentration of less than 100%, with changes in oxygen concentration being based on clinical assessment and pulse oximetry data.

Most newborns make a successful transition to extra-uterine life without intervention. The lower the gestational age of the newborn, the more likely he or she will require assistance. The transition needs to be observed by a skilled clinician. This can be done with the term infant placed on the mother's chest, skin to skin. Interventions are made in the event that the newborn is apneic or has gasping respirations, is bradycardic, or does not transition from cyanotic to pink within the excepted time frame. These interventions are completed on a newborn resuscitation table, which may be present in the delivery room or located in an adjacent newborn stabilization room.

Thermal management is critically important to a successful extrauterine transition. Efforts should be made to reduce heat loss as much as possible. There is a marked increase in glucose and oxygen consumption when a newly born infant is cold stressed. In an infant with a difficult transition, cold stress may precipitate the development of persistent pulmonary hypertension, a clinical situation in which pulmonary vascular resistance remains high, fetal shunts remain open, and blood flow to the newborn lung is minimal.[60]

In utero, a fetus may pass meconium. Meconium is the first stool a newborn passes and contains debris from amniotic fluid, vernix, and bowel exudate. If passed and the newly born infant is depressed (i.e., decreased heart rate, respiratory effort, or tone), the newborn should be intubated via the trachea and suctioned via a meconium aspirator.[65] If the newborn is further compromised, immediate implementation of addition resuscitation steps are mandated.

Based on the observers' assessment of the newborn's response, resuscitation continues. Infants who are apneic may be in primary or secondary apnea. The first maneuver is to clear the airway with either a bulb syringe or suction catheter. An apneic newborn needs to be immediately stimulated to breathe. The response to stimulation will indicate primary or secondary apnea. The newborn will begin to breathe if the apnea was primary. Secondary apnea is only resolved with the implementation of positive pressure ventilation.

If assistance with respiratory effort is needed, there are three currently accepted methods of providing positive pressure ventilation (PPV): the self-inflating bag, the flow-inflating bag, and the T-piece resuscitator.[63] The self-inflating bag does not require a compressed gas source to fill and can be used without a gas source; self-inflating bags do not provide positive end-expiratory pressure (PEEP) without attaching a PEEP valve. The flow inflating bag requires a gas source to distend it and can provide PEEP without an additional valve. The third device, the T-piece resuscitator requires the operator to preset a peak inspiratory pressure and PEEP before providing PPV.

The amount of pressure delivered by the self-inflating and flow-inflating bags is determined by the seal of the mask to the newborn's face and the squeeze the operator delivers when compressing the bag. The T-piece pressures are preset. The rate of ventilation recommended is 40 to 60 breaths per minute and is determined by how frequently the bag is squeezed, in the case of the self-inflating and flow-inflating bags. The rate when using the T-piece resuscitator is determined by depressing a valve on the tubing that attaches the T-piece device to the newborn mask. All devices used for newborn ventilation require safety features to avoid excessive pressure, which can result in lung injury and air leak. Recent literature suggests that the T-piece most reliably delivers ventilation at the prescribed pressures.[66]

Once ventilation is established, the newborn's response needs to be assessed. Chest rise and improvement in color should occur. A member of the team should have attached the pulse oximeter to the preductal (right hand or wrist) limb and be preparing to check an apical heart rate. Using these data, the need for further resuscitation efforts can be made. Decisions include the need to increase to FiO_2 and the need to perform chest compressions. Simultaneously another member of the team will prepare an advanced airway for placement and prepare for the administration of medications.[67]

Chest compressions should be provided if the newborn's heart rate is less than 60 beats per minute. A skilled team member should place an endotracheal tube at this juncture if one has not already been placed.

Medications should be prepared for administration if the heart rate remains below 60. Placement of an umbilical catheter is ideal for epinephrine administration. However, the first dose of epinephrine may be given via the endotracheal (ET) tube if the placement of the umbilical line delays prompt administration of the medication. Doses of epinephrine will vary based on the route of administration.[67]

Special thermal management strategies are necessary for preterm infants. These include the use of conductive heat–gaining mattresses and polyethelene wrap for infants 32 weeks of gestation or less.[68,69]

There is one situation where it is acceptable to allow a newborn's core temperature to drop to between 33°C and 34°C. Infants who have had a difficult transition and may have neonatal encephalopathy and meet specific criteria, the first one being a gestation of more than 36 weeks, may benefit from therapeutic hypothermia. This specific therapy is done in Level III perinatal centers and should not be undertaken without their guidance.[70,71]

The time of the initiation of resuscitation needs to be documented, along with frequent documentation of respiratory effort, heart rate, and oxygen saturations. If the baby does not improve or remains asystolic, decisions regarding additional strategies need to be made.[72]

Simulation of difficult deliveries and subsequent newborn resuscitations are helpful in identifying the level of staff's competence and the validity of the systems that support their efforts in these challenging situations. Knowledge of the equipment and the sequence of resuscitation needs to be evaluated, as well as the evidence of teamwork. Administrative support is necessary to ensure that the time and resources needed to complete simulation are available and issues identified during the scenarios are rectified.[73]

When a delivery is imminent, preparation is critical. All staff, equipment, and medications should be available and ready for use. Using the accepted sequence, resuscitation should proceed. After the resuscitation, the staff should debrief the experience and use challenges to improve performance in the future.[73]

CASE STUDY

Ms. S is a 19-year-old woman who is gravida 2, para 1 at 42 weeks and 1 day. Her pregnancy has been uncomplicated. She denies tobacco, alcohol, and drug use. Her pap smear is normal. She is O Positive Direct Antiglobulin test (DAT-), Rapid Plasma Reagin (RPR) non-reactive NR, gonorrhea negative, rubella immune (RI), GBS negative, HIV negative, HbSAg negative, with a normal 1-hour glucose challenge test. She was seen in the obstetrical clinic yesterday and had a BPP done. Results were reported to be within normal limits. A single comment was documented, stating a "slightly decreased volume of amniotic fluid."

She presents today to labor and delivery with regular, strong contractions. Her vaginal exam (VE) shows she is 4 cm dilated, 80% effaced, −2 station. The presenting fetal part is the head.

An epidural anesthetic is placed for pain control during labor. Two hours after admission her membranes spontaneously rupture and a small amount of green-tinged fluid appears. At this time her VE shows that she is 6 cm dilated, 90% effaced, 0 station. Dark green, thick meconium is present on the glove of the examiner. The fetal heart rate tracing shows that heart rate is 160 beats per minute with variability of 25 to 30 beats per minute, no decelerations.

Two hours later Ms. S is fully dilated, with variable decelerations on the fetal heart rate monitor. She is now pushing. The neonatal team is called to attend the delivery of this postmature fetus with meconium-stained amniotic fluid.

The team arrives before the delivery and prepares the resuscitation table for the birth of a term infant with potential for meconium aspiration. The neonatologist prepares the laryngoscope, endotracheal tubes, and meconium aspirator. The respiratory therapist prepares the blended gas source (air and oxygen), the T-piece resuscitator, and the self-inflating bag and mask. The registered nurse prepares the resuscitation table by turning on the heat and the pulse oximeter and prepares the pulse oximetry probe.

The baby is delivered limp, with decreased respiratory effort. The baby is placed on the warmer, immediately intubated, and a small amount of meconium is recovered from below the vocal cords. The team elects not to reintubate the baby and begins to clear the infant's airway further and stimulate the baby. At 1 minute the baby is noted to have a heart rate greater than 100 beats per minute, gasping respirations, limited tone, and no reflexes and remains cyanotic, with an Apgar score of 4. The pulse oximetry probe is placed preductally and SaO_2 reads 70%. The respiratory therapist notes the gasping respirations and begins to ventilate the baby with the T-piece resuscitator. The T-piece is set at 21%, peak inspiratory pressure (PI) of 25 cm H_2O and positive end-expiratory pressure (PEEP) of 5 cm H_2O with a rate of approximately 40 breaths per minute. Chest excursion is observed bilaterally with the delivery of the breaths. The nurse again checks the heart rate and it is noted to be more than 100 beats per minute. Breath sounds are equal.

The infant begins to breath spontaneously and cry under the mask, begins to flex limbs, and becomes less blue. The SaO_2 now reads 80% at 5 minutes. The ventilation is discontinued. The neonatologist assigns a 5-minute Apgar of 8, 1 off for color and 1 off for tone. Two minutes later the infant is well flexed and has a lusty cry. The pulse oximeter reads 89%. The baby is then wrapped in a blanket and is placed on her mother's chest. The staff remains to ensure that the infant continues to transition successfully.

1. How often does gestation exceed 42 weeks?
2. What are some of the potential risk factors associated with a postterm pregnancy?
3. Why do you think amniotic fluid volume may be decreasing?
4. Did the neonatal team adequately prepare for the birth of the infant?
5. What are your comments about their teamwork? How would you brief and debrief this clinical situation?
6. Are the newborn's recorded oxygen saturations as expected?

See Evolve Resources for answers.

KEY POINTS

- Identification of prepregnancy chronic diseases and careful continuous assessment for disorders specific to pregnancy are important in maximizing maternal and fetal outcome.
- Fetal and cervical ultrasound, Doppler, and continuous electronic fetal monitoring are tools that can inform the progress of the pregnancy and maternal and fetal well-being. These tools often are used to determine maternal management, medications, bed rest, and indicated preterm delivery.
- Preterm labor can often be predicted. Strategies to lengthen gestation and improve the newborn outcome should be initiated as soon as preterm delivery is anticipated.
- Postterm pregnancy can be associated with maternal and fetal morbidity. Careful attention to fetal size

and well-being should be implemented when a pregnancy becomes prolonged.
- Evidence-based strategies recently have been published regarding assisting newborns in the transition to extrauterine life. The use of titrated oxygen concentrations in response to the newborn's successful establishment of respiratory effort, vital signs, and preductal oxygen saturations are recommended.

ASSESSMENT QUESTIONS

See Evolve Resources for answers.

1. All of the following are criteria for diagnosis of severe preeclampsia except:
   A. Headache
   B. Diastolic blood pressure higher than 110 mm Hg
   C. Generalized edema
   D. Intrauterine growth restriction
2. Cesarean delivery is indicated for which one of the following maternal infections:
   A. Group B *Streptococcus*
   B. Hepatitis B
   C. Hepatitis C
   D. Anogenital herpes simplex virus
3. Polyhydramnios is associated with all of the following except:
   A. Gestational diabetes
   B. Anencephaly
   C. Twin–twin transfusion syndrome
   D. Use of prostaglandin synthase inhibitors
4. Late decelerations are usually caused by:
   A. Uteroplacental insufficiency
   B. Fetal anemia
   C. Umbilical cord compression
   D. Fetal head compression
5. The earliest sign of magnesium sulfate toxicity is:
   A. Hypotension and tachycardia
   B. Loss of deep tendon reflexes
   C. Respiratory depression
   D. Acute renal failure
6. When used for labor induction, misoprostol is contraindicated for patients with:
   A. Postterm pregnancy
   B. Preeclampsia
   C. Previous cesarean section
   D. Nulliparous pregnancy
7. All of the following are true about the use for induction of fetal lung maturity except:
   A. Corticosteroids are contraindicated for patients with premature rupture of membranes.
   B. Betamethasone and dexamethasone are the most commonly used corticosteroids.
   C. Corticosteroid use is associated with a decreased risk of fetal intracranial hemorrhage.
   D. Corticosteroid therapy reduces risk of RDS and other morbidities by 50%.

8. In preparing the delivery or operating room for the delivery of an infant expected to require resuscitation, all of the following should be prepared except:
   A. A warmed environment.
   B. A device that can only provide positive pressure ventilation at 100% oxygen.
   C. Staff skilled in assisting a newborn's transition to extrauterine life.
   D. A pulse oximeter for the newborn that is capable of accurate readings in low perfusion states.
9. Full-term newborn infants initially resuscitated with 21% FiO$_2$ may require an increase in the concentration of inspired oxygen. This determination should be made based on:
   A. The infant's skin color
   B. The infant's respiratory effort
   C. The postductal oxygen saturation (as measured by pulse oximeter)
   D. The preductal oxygen saturation (as measured by pulse oximeter)
10. Preterm infants require additional strategies to prevent hypothermia in the delivery room. These include:
   A. Polyethylene wrap for infants 28 weeks of gestation or less
   B. Conductive heat–gaining mattress for infants 32 weeks of gestation or less
   C. A and B
   D. None of the above

References

1. American Diabetes Association: Standards of medical care in diabetes—2011, *Diabetes Care* 34:S15, 2011.
2. Moretti ME, Rezvani M, Koren G: Safety of glyburide for gestational diabetes: a meta-analysis of pregnancy outcomes, *Ann Pharmacother* 42:483, 2008.
3. American College of Obstetricians and Gynecologists: *Prevention of early-onset group B streptococcal disease in newborns.* Committee Opinion 279. Washington, DC, 2002, American College of Obstetricians and Gynecologists.
4. Centers for Disease Control and Prevention: Sexually transmitted diseases guidelines, *MMWR* 59:1, 2010.
5. Hollier LM, Wendel GD: Third trimester antiviral prophylaxis for preventing maternal genital herpes simplex (HSV) recurrences and neonatal infection, *Cochrane Database Syst Rev* I: CD004946, 2008.
6. Centers for Disease Control and Prevention: Epidemiology of HIV/AIDS—United States, *MMWR* 55:589, 2006.
7. MacGregor SN: Human immunodeficiency virus infection in pregnancy, *Clin Perinatol* 18:33, 1997.
8. Connor EM, Sperling RS, Gelber R, et al: Reduction of maternal–infant transmission of HIV-1 with zidovudine treatment. Pediatric AIDS Clinical Trials Group Protocol 076 Study Group, *N Engl J Med* 331:1173, 1994.
9. European Mode of Delivery Collaboration: Elective caesarean section versus vaginal delivery in prevention of vertical HIV transmission: a randomized clinical trial, *Lancet* 353: 1035, 1999.
10. World Health Organization: *Hepatitis B.* WHO Fact Sheet No. 204. www.who.int/mediacentre/factsheets/fs204/en. Accessed February 18, 2013.

11. Bernstein HB: Maternal and perinatal infection—viral. In Gabbe SB, Niebyl JR, Simpson JL, Landon MB, Galan NL, Jauniaux, Driscoll DA ERM, editors: *Obstetrics: normal and problem pregnancies*, ed 6, New York, 2012, Churchill Livingstone, pp 1132.

12. Substance Abuse and Mental Health Service Administration: *Results from the 2010 National Survey on Drug Use and Health: Summary of national findings.* http://www.samhsa.gov/data/NSDUH/2k10MH_Findings/2k10MHResults.htm Accessed February 18, 2013.

13. Jones KJ, Smith DW, Ulleland CN, Streissguth P: Patterns of malformation in offspring of chronic alcoholic mothers, *Lancet* 1:1267, 1973.

14. Committee on Substance Abuse and Committee on Children with Disabilities: Fetal alcohol syndrome and fetal alcohol effects, *Pediatrics* 91:1004, 1993.

15. Hammoud AO, Bujold E, Sorokin Y, et al: Smoking in pregnancy revisited: findings from a large population-based study, *Am J Obstet Gynecol* 192:1856, 2005.

16. Harger JH, Hsing AW, Tuomala RE, et al: Risk factors for preterm premature rupture of membranes: a multicenter case control study, *Am J Obstet Gynecol* 163:130, 1990.

17. Ananth C, Smulian JC, Vintzileos AM: Incidence of placental abruption in relationship to cigarette smoking and hypertensive disorders in pregnancy: a meta-analysis of observational studies, *Obstet Gynecol* 93:622, 1999.

18. Taylor JA, Sanderson M: A reexamination of the risk factors for sudden infant death syndrome, *J Pediatr* 126:887, 1995.

19. Shiono PH, Klebanoff MA, Nugent RP, et al: The impact of cocaine and marijuana use on low birth weight and preterm birth: a multicenter study, *Am J Obstet Gynecol* 172:19, 1995.

20. American College of Obstetricians and Gynecologists: *Diagnosis and management of preeclampsia and eclampsia.* Practice Bulletin 33, Washington, DC, 2002, American College of Obstetricians and Gynecologists.

21. Cunningham FG, Leveno KJ, Bloom SL, Hauth JC, Rouse DJ, Spong CY, editors: *Williams obstetrics*, ed 23, New York, 2010, McGraw-Hill, p 709.

22. Sibai BM, El-Nazer A, Gonzalez-RuizAR: Severe preeclampsia-eclampsia in young primigravida women: subsequent pregnancy outcome and remote prognosis, *Am J Obstet Gynecol* 155:1011, 1986.

23. Rinehart BK, et al: Single umbilical artery is associated with an increased incidence of structural and chromosomal anomalies and growth restriction, *Am J Perinatol* 17:229, 2000.

24. Cunningham FG, Leveno KJ, Bloom SL, et al, editors: *Williams obstetrics,* ed 23, New York, 2003, McGraw-Hill, p 763.

25. Baron C, Morgan MA, Garite TJ: The impact of amniotic fluid volume assessed intrapartum on perinatal outcome, *Am J Obstet Gynecol* 173:167, 1995.

26. Mathew TJ, Mac Dorman MF: Infant mortality statistics from the 2008 period linked birth/infant death data set, *Natl Vital Stat Rep* 60(5), 2012.

27. Carr-Hill RA, Hall MH: The repetition of spontaneous preterm labor, *Br J Obstet Gynaecol* 92:921, 1985.

28. Lockwood CJ, et al: Fetal fibronectin in cervical and vaginal secretions as a predictor of preterm delivery, *N Engl J Med* 325:669, 1991.

29. Andersen HF: Use of fetal fibronectin in women at risk for preterm delivery, *Clin Obstet Gynecol* 43:746, 2000.

30. Pircon RA, et al: Controlled trial of hydration and bed rest versus bed rest alone in the evaluation of preterm uterine contractions, *Am J Obstet* Gynecol 161:775, 1989.

31. American College of Obstetricians and Gynecologists: *Management of preterm labor. Practice Bulletin 4.* Washington, DC, 2003, American College of Obstetricians and Gynecologists.

32. Haas DM, Caldwell DM, Kirkpatrick P, McIntosh JJ, Welton NJ: Tocolytic therapy for preterm delivery: systematic review and network meta-analytics, *Brit Med J* 345:E6226, 2012.

33. American College of Obstetricians and Gynecologists: *Antenatal corticosteroid therapy for fetal maturation.* Committee Opinion 402. Washington, DC, 2008, American College of Obstetricians and Gynecologists.

34. NIH Consensus Development Panel on the Effect of Corticosteroids for Fetal Maturation on Perinatal Outcomes. Effect of corticosteroids for fetal maturation on perinatal outcomes. *JAMA* 273:413, 1995.

35. Meis PJ, Klebanoff M., Thom, E et al: Prevention of recurrent preterm delivery by 17α-hydroxyprogesterone caproate, *N Engl J Med* 348:2379–2385, 2003.

36. Drakeley AJ, Roberts D, Alfirevic Z: Cervical stitch (cerclage) for preventing pregnancy loss in women, *Cochrane Database Syst Rev* 1:CD003253, 2003.

37. American College of Obstetricians and Gynecologists: *Cervical insufficiency. Practice Bulletin 48.* Washington, DC, 2003, American College of Obstetricians and Gynecologists.

38. Caughey AB, Stotland NE, Washington AE, Escobar GJ: Who is at risk for prolonged and post term pregnancy? *Am J Obstet Gynecol* 200:683, 2009.

39. Leddy MA, Powers ML, Schulkin J: The impact of maternal obesity on maternal and fetal health, *Rev Obstet Gynecol* 1(4):170, 2008.

40. Pitt C, et al: Prophylactic Amnioinfusion for intrapartum oligohydramnios: a meta-analysis of randomized controlled trials, *Obstet Gynecol* 95:861, 2000.

41. Fraser WD, Hofmeyr J, Jede R, et al: Amnioinfusion for the prevention of meconium aspiration syndrome. Amnioinfusion Trial Group, *N Engl J Med* 353:909, 2005.

42. American College of Obstetricians and Gynecologists: *Amnioinfusion does not prevent meconium aspiration syndrome.* Committee Opinion. Washington, DC, 2006, American College of Obstetricians and Gynecologists, pp 346.

43. American College of Obstetricians and Gynecologists: *Management of postterm pregnancy. Practice Bulletin 55.* Washington, DC, 2004, American College of Obstetricians and Gynecologists.

44. Wing DA, et al: Misoprostol: an effective agent for cervical ripening and labor induction, *Am J Obstet Gynecol* 172:4844, 1995.

45. Wing DA, Lovett K, Paul RH: Disruption of prior uterine incision following misoprostol for labor induction in women with previous cesarean delivery, *Obstet Gynecol* 91:828, 1998.

46. Khabbaz AY, et al: Rupture of an unscarred uterus with misoprostol induction: case report and review of the literature, *J Matern Fetal Med* 10:141, 2001.

47. Timor-Tritsch IE, Platt LD: Three-dimensional ultrasound experiences in obstetrics, *Curr Opin Obstet Gynecol* 14:569, 2002.

48. American College of Obstetricians and Gynecologists: *Intrapartum fetal heart rate monitoring: nomenclature, interpretation and general management principles. Practice Bulletin 106.* Washington, DC, 2009, American College of Obstetricians and Gynecologists.

49. Manning FA, et al: Fetal biophysical profile score and the non-stress test: a comparative trial, *Obstet Gynecol* 64:326, 1984.

50. Vintzileos AM, Campbell WA: Fetal biophysical scoring: current status, *Clin Perinatol* 16:661, 1989.

51. Hannah ME, et al: Planned caesarean section versus planned vaginal birth for breech presentation at term: a randomized multicentre trial, *Lancet* 356:1375, 2000.

52. Collea JV, Chein C, Quilligan EJ: The randomized management of term frank breech presentation: a study of 208 cases, *Am J Obstet Gynecol* 137:235, 1990.

53. Gimovsky ML, et al: Randomized management of the non-frank breech presentation at term: a preliminary report, *Am J Obstet Gynecol* 146:34, 1983.

54. American College of Obstetricians and Gynecologists: *Mode of term singleton breech delivery*. Committee Opinion 265. Washington, DC, 2001, American College of Obstetricians and Gynecologists.

55. Martin JA, Hamilton, BE, Ventura SJ, et al: Births: final data for 2010, *Natl Vital Stat Rep* 61:1, 2012.

56. Rozance PJ, Rosenberg AA: The neonate. In Gabbe SB, Niebyl JR, Simpson JL, et al, editors: *Obstetrics: normal and problem pregnancies*, ed 6, New York, 2012, Churchill Livingstone, p 485.

57. American College of Obstetricians and Gynecologists: *Intrapartum fetal heart rate monitoring. Practice Bulletin 62*. Washington, DC, 2005, American College of Obstetricians and Gynecologists.

58. Skupski DW, Rosenberg CR, Eglinton GS: Intrapartum fetal stimulation tests: a mete-analysis, *Obstet Gynecol* 99:129, 2002.

59. Kuhnert M, Schmidt S: Intrapartum management of non-reassuring fetal heart rate patterns: a randomized controlled trial of fetal pulse oximetry, *Am J Obstet Gynecol* 191:1989, 2004.

60. Blackburn ST, Loper, DL: The respiratory system. In Blackburn ST, Loper DL, editors: *Maternal, fetal and neonatal physiology: a clinical perspective*. Philadelphia, 1992, Saunders, p 692.

61. American Academy of Pediatrics, American College of Obstetricians and Gynecologists. Organization of perinatal healthcare. In Lockwood C, Lemons J, editors: *Guidelines for perinatal care*, Elk Grove Village, IL, 2012, AAP, p 6.

62. Crosby, WM, Cook, LJ: Unit 1: Is the mother sick? Is the fetus sick? In Kattwinkel J, Cook LJ, Hurt H, Nowacek GA, Short JG, editors: *Maternal and fetal evaluation and immediate newborn care*, Elk Grove Village, IL, 2007, AAP, p 16.

63. American Heart Association/American Academy of Pediatrics: Overview and principles of resuscitation. In Kattwinkel J, editor: *Neonatal resuscitation textbook plus*, Elk Grove Village, IL, 2011, AAP, p 1.

64. Mariani G, Dik PB, Ezquer A, et al: Pre-ductal and post-ductal O_2 saturations in healthy term neonates after birth, *J Pediatrics* 150:418, 2007.

65. Wiswell, TE, Gannon, CM, Jacob J, et al: Delivery room management of the apparently vigorous meconium stained neonate: results of the multicenter, international collaborative trial, *Pediatrics* 105(1 Pt 1):1, 2000.

66. Bennett S, Finer N, Rich W, Vaucher Y: A comparison of three neonatal resuscitation devices, *Resuscitation* 67:113, 2005.

67. Barber CA, Wycoff MH: Use and efficacy of endotracheal versus intravenous epinephrine during neonatal cardiopulmonary resuscitation in the delivery room, *Pediatrics* 118:1028, 2006.

68. Vohra S, Roberts, RS, Zhang, B, Janes, M, Schmidt, B: Heat loss prevention (HeLP) in the delivery room: a randomized controlled trial of polyethelene occlusive skin wrapping in very preterm infants, *J Pediatrics* 145:750, 2004.

69. Singh A, Duckett, J, Newton, T, Watkinson, M: Improving neonatal unit admission temperatures in preterm babies: exothermic mattresses, polythene bags, or a traditional approach? *J Perinatology* 30:45, 2010.

70. Gluckman PD, Wyatt JS, Azzopardi D, et al: Selective head cooling with mild systemic hypothermia after neonatal encephalopathy: multicentre randomised trial, *Lancet* 365:663, 2005.

71. Shankaran S, Laptook AR, Ehrenkranz RA, et al: Whole body hypothermia for neonates with hypoxic ischemic encephalopathy, *N Engl J Med* 353:1574, 2005.

72. Laptook AR, Shankaran S, Ambalavanan N, et al: Outcomes of term infants using apgar score at 10 minutes following hypoxic ischemic encephalopathy, *Pediatrics* 124:1619, 2009.

73. Edelson DR, Litzinger B, Arora V, et al: Improving inhospital cardiac arrest process and outcomes with performance debriefing, *Arch Intern Med* 168:1063, 2008.

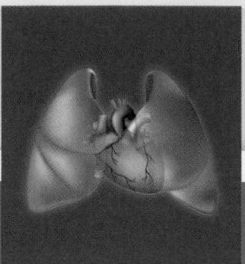

Chapter 4

Examination and Assessment of the Neonatal and Pediatric Patient

KRISTEN HOOD

LEARNING OBJECTIVES

After reading this chapter the reader will be able to:

1. List steps for initial stabilization of the newborn
2. Describe care to be given to infants born with meconium staining
3. Describe the Apgar scoring system and how and when it is performed on the newborn
4. List criteria for determining whether an infant is large for gestational age, appropriate for gestational age, or small for gestational age
5. List critical vital signs to be evaluated as part of the newborn's initial physical examination
6. Describe criteria for determining whether an infant is displaying apneic spells
7. Identify signs and symptoms of respiratory distress in the newborn
8. Describe the technique for rapid identification of a pneumothorax in a newborn
9. List the elements of a basic neurological examination in the newborn
10. Identify and use historical and physical findings to develop a differential diagnosis of a child's respiratory condition
11. Determine the severity of a child's respiratory condition
12. Communicate important historical and physical findings concerning a child's respiratory condition to the health care team in a timely manner

KEY TERMS

Acrocyanosis
Apgar score
Apnea
Ballard score
Bilateral choanal atresia
Bronchial fremitus
Chief complaint
Encephaloceles
Fontanels
Gastroschisis
Grunting
Head bobbing

Hygromas
Lanugo
Leukocytosis
Leukopenia
Kyphosis
Micrognathia
Microstomia
Mottling
Myelomeningoceles
Nasal flaring
Omphalocele
Pectus carinatum

Pectus excavatum
Periodic breathing
Prune belly syndrome
Scoliosis
Sternocleidomastoids
Stretor
Stridor
Subgaleal hemorrhage
Tactile fremitus
Transillumination
Vernix caseosa

The first few moments of an infant's life are the most critical. At this time the newborn must make the transition from intrauterine to extrauterine life. Most infants enter extrauterine life with crying and vigorous activity. However, of the approximately 4 million babies born in the United States each year, 7.3% are low birth weight, or 1500 to 2500 g, and 1.3% are very low birth weight, or less than 1500 g.[1] Adverse maternal and fetal conditions contribute to the need to initiate resuscitative efforts in approximately 6% to 10% of all deliveries, with extensive resuscitation required in less than 1%.[2]

Ideally, a detailed history of perinatal problems associated with an infant who may require resuscitation (Box 4-1) should be available.

STABILIZING THE NEONATE

Stabilizing the newborn starts with proper positioning followed by drying and warming. Immediately after delivery place the infant on a preheated radiant warmer (Figure 4-1), and position the infant with the neck slightly flexed. Placing a small roll under the shoulders often attains the correct position.

Drying and Warming

Preventing heat loss is critical when caring for a newborn, because cold stress increases oxygen consumption and impedes effective resuscitation. If possible, deliver the infant in a warm, draft-free area.[3] Heat loss can be greatly reduced by rapidly drying the infant's skin, immediately removing wet linens, and wrapping the infant in prewarmed blankets.[4]

Clearing the Airway

Suspect airway obstruction if the newborn's respiratory efforts are not effective. Immediately reposition the head and suction to clear the airway of potential obstruction. Use either a bulb syringe or a suction catheter clearing the mouth first and then the nose. To avert injury and atelectasis, as well as interference with the infant's ability to

---

| Box 4-1 | Perinatal Factors Associated with Increased Risk of Neonatal Depression |

ANTEPARTUM (FETOMATERNAL)

- Maternal diabetes
- Postterm status (born at greater than 42 weeks of gestation)
- Maternal infection (especially group B *Streptococcus* or herpes)
- Hemorrhage
- Substance abuse
- No prenatal care
- Age greater than 35 years
- Multifetal gestation
- Diminished fetal activity
- Maternal anemia or Rh isoimmunization
- Oligohydramnios or polyhydramnios
- Small fetus for maternal dates
- Previous fetal or neonatal death
- Immature pulmonary maturity studies
- Chronic or pregnancy-induced hypertension
- Preterm labor or premature rupture of membranes

- Other maternal illness (e.g., cardiovascular, thyroid, neurological)
- Drug therapy (e.g., magnesium, adrenergic blockers, lithium)
- Congenital abnormalities

INTRAPARTUM

- Maternal or fetal infection
- Prolapsed cord
- Prolonged labor
- Maternal sedation
- Operative or device-assisted delivery
- Meconium-stained delivery
- Prolonged rupture of membranes
- Breech or other abnormal presentation
- Indices of fetal distress (e.g., abnormal heart rate)

See Chapter 3, Antenatal Assessment and High-Risk Delivery.

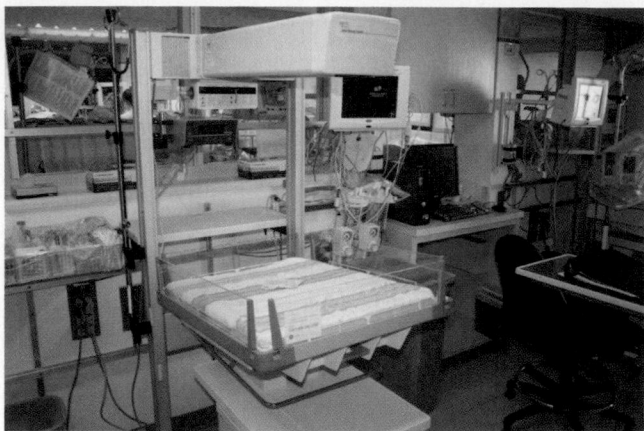

FIGURE 4-1   Radiant warmer. (From Price D, Gwin J. *Pediatric nursing: an introductory text,* ed 11. Philadelphia: Saunders, 2012.)

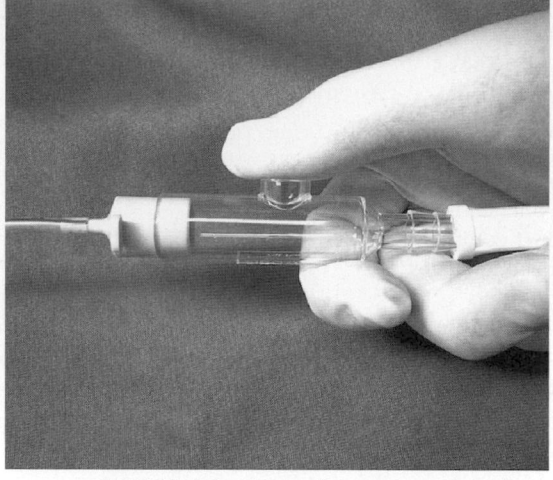

FIGURE 4-2   Meconium aspirator.

establish adequate ventilation, avoid excessive suctioning of clear fluid from the nasopharynx.[2]

Attempts to suction meconium from the pharynx or trachea before birth, during birth, or after birth increase the likelihood of severe aspiration pneumonia.[5] Some obstetricians orally and nasally suction meconium-stained infants after delivery of the head but before delivery of the shoulders. However, a large, multicenter, randomized trial showed no benefit from this practice.[6] Therefore, current recommendations for infants with meconium staining are the following:

· No intrapartum suctioning should occur.
· Infants who are vigorous at birth (i.e., strong respiratory effort, heart rate greater than 100 beats per minute, good muscle tone) should not receive tracheal suctioning.
· Infants who are not vigorous (i.e., no or poor respiratory effort, heart rate less than 100 beats per minute, poor muscle tone) may receive direct laryngotracheal suctioning.[5]

For direct laryngotracheal suctioning, intubate the infant and apply suction directly to the endotracheal tube with the help of a meconium aspirator (Figure 4-2). Constantly apply suction while removing the tube from the airway. Repeat the intubation and suctioning procedure until meconium is no longer visible in the airway or until resuscitation is required.

Providing Stimulation

If the newborn does not respond to the extrauterine environment with a strong cry, good respiratory effort, and the movement of all extremities, the infant requires stimulation. Flicking the bottoms of the feet, gently rubbing the back, and drying with a towel are all acceptable methods of stimulation. Slapping, shaking, spanking, and holding the newborn upside down are contraindicated and potentially dangerous to the infant.[7] In the delivery room the initial steps of warming, clearing the airway, and stimulation of the non–meconium-stained infant should occur within 30 seconds after birth.[5]

Apgar Score

Introduced in 1952 by Virginia Apgar, the **Apgar score** (Table 4-1) is an evaluation of newborns based on five factors: heart rate, respiratory effort, muscle tone, reflex irritability, and skin color.[8] Historically, proponents of the Apgar score have encouraged evaluation of newborns immediately after birth. It has also been used as a predictive index of neonatal mortality and neurological or developmental outcome and continues to be used as the best-established index of immediate postnatal health.[9] The Apgar score obtained 1 minute after delivery provides an immediate evaluation of the infant and an objective measure for evaluating future interventions. However, in the

TABLE 4-1

Apgar Scoring

Parameter	APGAR SCORE		
	0	1	2
Heart rate	None	<100 beats/min	>100 beats/min
Respiratory rate	None	Weak, irregular	Strong cry
Skin color	Pale blue	Body pink, extremities blue	Completely pink
Reflex irritability (response to stimulation)	No response	Grimace	Cry, cough, or sneeze
Muscle tone	Limp tone	Some flexion	Well flexed

delivery room resuscitation may be well under way at the 1-minute mark and should not be interrupted for Apgar scoring.

Scoring again at 5 minutes of age gives information about the infant's ability to recover from the stress of birth and adapt to extrauterine life. When the 5-minute Apgar score is less than 7, additional scores are usually obtained at 5-minute intervals until the score is greater than 7. Survival of the infant is unlikely if the score remains 0 after 10 minutes of resuscitation.[10]

The most important of the signs is heart rate, which indicates life or death. Failure of the heart rate to respond to resuscitation is an ominous prognostic sign.[9] Heart rate appears to be least affected by developmental maturity but may still be inadequate because of developmental difficulties in establishing cardiorespiratory function at birth.

In the immediate newborn period, skin color has the weakest correlation with the other four components of the Apgar score. Also, color does not reliably correlate with umbilical arterial pH, carbon dioxide pressure, and base excess.[11]

GESTATIONAL AGE AND SIZE ASSESSMENT

Ideally, gestational age assessment is performed before the neonate is 12 hours old, to allow the greatest reliability for infants less than 26 weeks of gestational age.[12-14] Evaluating gestational age requires consideration of several factors. The three main factors are as follows:

· Gestational duration based on the last menstrual cycle
· Prenatal ultrasound evaluation
· Postnatal findings based on physical and neurological examinations

Postnatal examinations for determining gestational age include the **Ballard score,** which is based on external physical findings, and neurological criteria. Often a gray-white cheeselike substance, called **vernix caseosa,** is present in the skin folds of a term infant. However, vernix is even more abundant on a preterm infant and suggests an earlier gestational age. The presence of **lanugo,** the fine hair that covers premature infants mostly over the shoulders, back, forehead, and cheeks, indicates an even younger gestational age (Figure 4-3).

Once gestational age is determined, weight, length, and head circumference are plotted on a standard newborn grid. Any infant whose birth weight is less than the tenth percentile for gestational age is small for gestational age; similarly, an infant whose birth weight is more than the ninetieth percentile is large for gestational age. When using intrauterine growth curves, it may be necessary to consider specific charts that are race and gender specific.[15] Along with prematurity, abnormal gestational age and size for gestational age are associated with many neonatal disease processes (Figure 4-4).

PHYSICAL EXAMINATION OF THE NEONATE

The physical examination of an adult is generally conducted in a rigid head-to-toe format. When examining an infant, however, the order of the examination is modified to establish critical information; for example, auscultation of the heart and lungs is done before the infant becomes agitated and begins to cry. However, the examiner must still completely examine the baby in an orderly and prioritized manner. As a general rule the following order works best, although this approach may require modification based on the clinical situation.

Vital Signs

Quickly assess the vital signs of the infant. Table 4-2 lists normal ranges for neonatal blood pressure. Absolute numbers are not as important as the relative ranges when considering the clinical situation. Heart rate of a neonate is often best assessed by listening with a stethoscope for the apical beat over the precordium. In the delivery room, lightly grasping the base of the umbilical cord and feeling the pulse can quickly estimate heart rate. As an example, the heart rate is normally 120 to 170 beats per minute. The heart rate of a term infant in deep sleep may decrease to 80 or 90 beats per minute. An infant undergoing a painful procedure or who is hungry may have a transient heart rate greater than 200 beats per minute. In comparison, a neonate older than 35 weeks of gestation has greater variability in heart rate than an infant born at 27 to 35 weeks of gestation. Presumably, in the younger infant, parasympathetic–sympathetic interaction and function are less developed.[16]

Normal values for temperature are 97.6 ± 1°F (axillary) and 99.6 ± 1°F (rectal); however, temperature on arrival in the nursery may be lower if the delivery room was cold or may be higher if the radiant warmer was operating at a higher temperature because of incorrect probe position or warmer malfunction.

Record the respiratory rate and blood pressure when determining vital signs.

General Inspection

Observing the infant's overall appearance is an important aspect of the physical examination. Ideally, examine the infant as he or she lies quietly and unclothed in a neutral thermal environment. Body position and symmetry, both at rest and during muscular activity, provide valuable information regarding possible birth trauma. For example, an infant who does not move his or her arms symmetrically could have a broken clavicle or an injury to the brachial plexus (Figure 4-5).

The infant's skin is an indicator of intravascular volume, perfusion status, or both. Both perfusion and underlying skin color affect the appearance of the skin. Capillary refill time should be less than 3 seconds. Assess refill by

Neuromuscular maturity

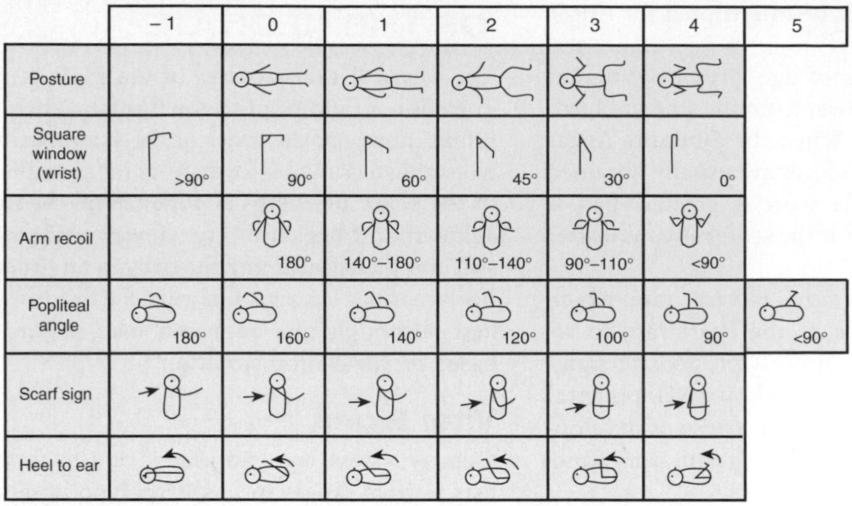

	−1	0	1	2	3	4	5
Posture							
Square window (wrist)	>90°	90°	60°	45°	30°	0°	
Arm recoil		180°	140°–180°	110°–140°	90°–110°	<90°	
Popliteal angle	180°	160°	140°	120°	100°	90°	<90°
Scarf sign							
Heel to ear							

Physical maturity

Skin	Sticky Friable Transparent	Gelatinous red, translucent	Smooth pink, visible veins	Superficial peeling &/or rash, few veins	Cracking pale areas, rare veins	Parchment, deep cracking, no vessels	Leathery, cracked, wrinkled
Lanugo	None	Sparse	Abundant	Thinning	Bald areas	Mostly bald	
Plantar surface	Heel-toe 40-50 mm: −1 <40 mm: −2	>50 mm no crease	Faint red marks	Anterior transverse crease only	Creases anterior 2/3	Creases over entire sole	
Breast	Imperceptible	Barely perceptible	Flat areola, no bud	Stippled areola, 1-2 mm bud	Raised areola, 3-4 mm bud	Full areola, 5-10 mm bud	
Eye/ear	Lids fused loosely: −1 tightly: −2	Lids open; pinna flat, stays folded	Sl. curved pinna; soft, slow recoil	Well-curved pinna; soft but ready recoil	Formed & firm; instant recoil	Thick cartilage; ear stiff	
Genitals (male)	Scrotum flat, smooth	Scrotum empty, faint rugae	Testes in upper canal, rare rugae	Testes descending, few rugae	Testes down, good rugae	Testes pendulous, deep rugae	
Genitals (female)	Clitoris prominent, labia flat	Prominent clitoris, small labia minora	Prominent clitoris, enlarging minora	Majora & minora equally prominent	Majora large, minora small	Majora cover clitoris & minora	

Maturity rating

score	weeks
−10	20
−5	22
0	24
5	26
10	28
15	30
20	32
25	34
30	36
35	38
40	40
45	42
50	44

FIGURE 4-3   New Ballard score.

pressing the sole of the infant's foot or the palm of its hand with a finger. Perfusion should be good and skin color pink. Some infants have blue hands and feet with decreased perfusion, or acrocyanosis, in the immediate postnatal period. True cyanosis is associated with blue or dusky mucous membranes and circumoral area.

Observing skin and color often provides diagnostic clues. *Mottling* refers to irregular areas of dusky skin alternating with areas of pale skin. An extremely pale or mottled infant suggests hypotension or anemia. A ruddy, reddish blue appearance is often associated with a high hematocrit value or polycythemia and neonatal hyperviscosity syndrome (hematocrit > 65%).[17] The yellow color associated with mild to moderate jaundice is common among newborns after the first day of life. Jaundice on the

first day of life, however, is always an indication for immediate evaluation.[18]

An infant exposed to meconium-stained amniotic fluid in utero for more than a few hours often presents with yellow-green staining of the skin, nails, and umbilical cord. Irregular areas of pale blue-black pigmentation over the sacrum and buttocks (Mongolian spots; Figure 4-6) are commonly seen on black and Asian infants. These spots are often confused with bruising (Table 4-3).

Respiratory Function

The normal newborn respiratory rate is 40 to 60 breaths per minute but may vary depending on multiple factors. Watch the infant's respiratory effort closely and note irregular respirations. Respiratory rates that exceed

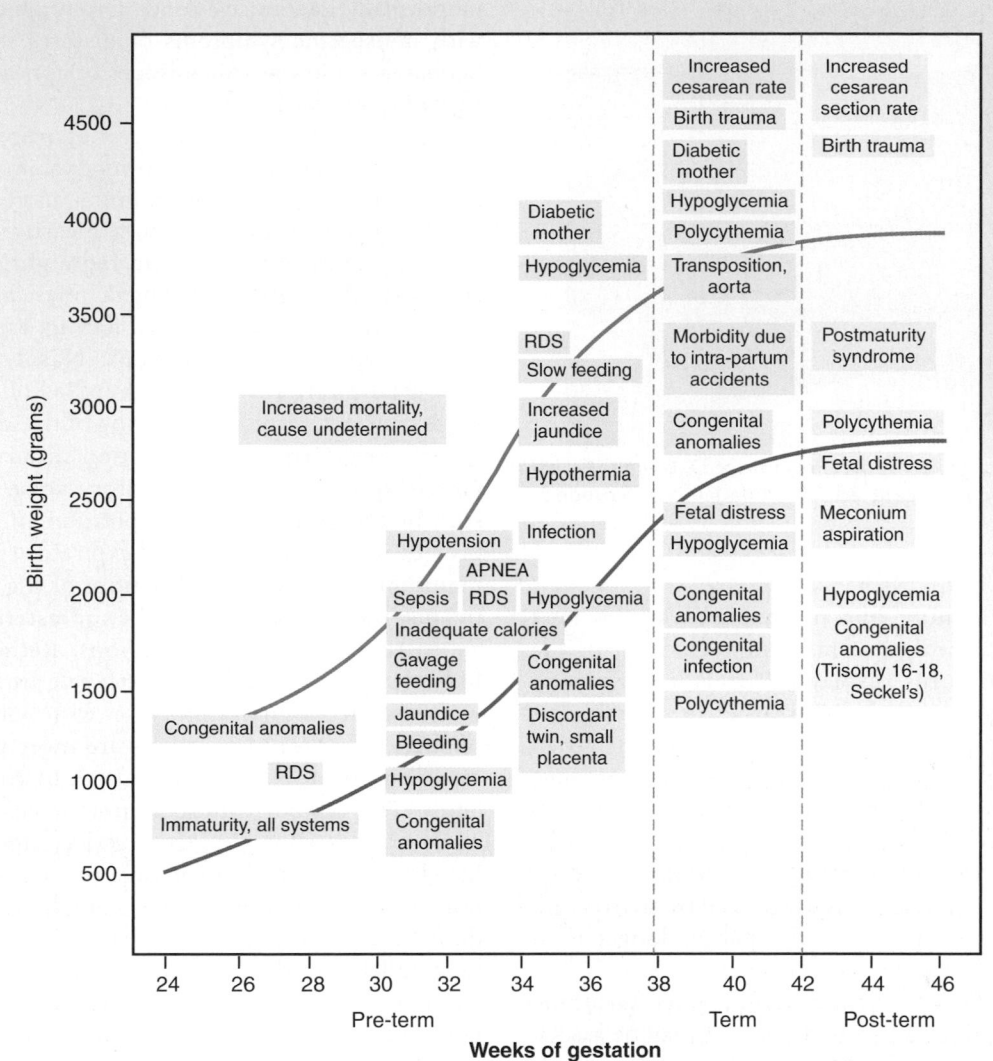

FIGURE 4-4 Weeks of gestation.

TABLE 4-2		
Normal Values for Vital Signs in the Neonatal Patient		
Birth Weight (g)	**Systolic/Diastolic Blood Pressure (mm Hg)***	**Mean Blood Pressure (mm Hg)**
>600	45/20	25
>1000	48/25	35
>2000	50/30	40
>3000	50/35	45
>4000	65/40	50
Newborn older than 12 hr	75/50	60
Respiratory rate (30-60 breaths/min)		
Heart rate (120-170 beats/min)		

*From Versmold HT et al. Aortic blood pressure ranges during the first 12 hours of life in infants with birth weight 610 to 4220 grams, *Pediatrics* 1981;67:607.

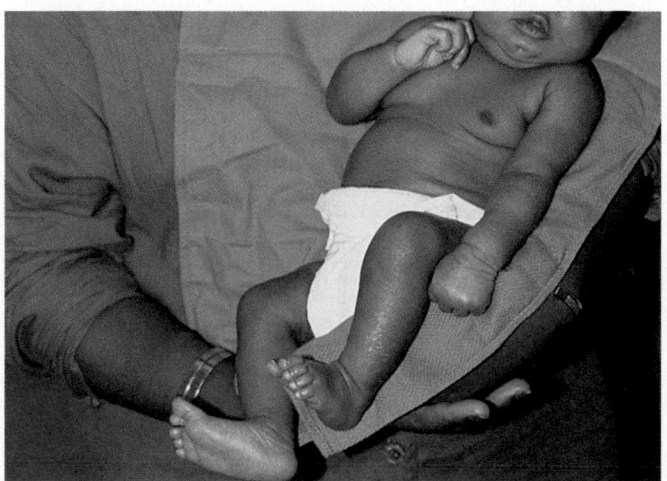

FIGURE 4-5 Left-sided brachial plexus. (From Hockenberry M, Wilson D. *Wong's essentials of pediatric nursing*, ed 8. St. Louis: Mosby, 2013.)

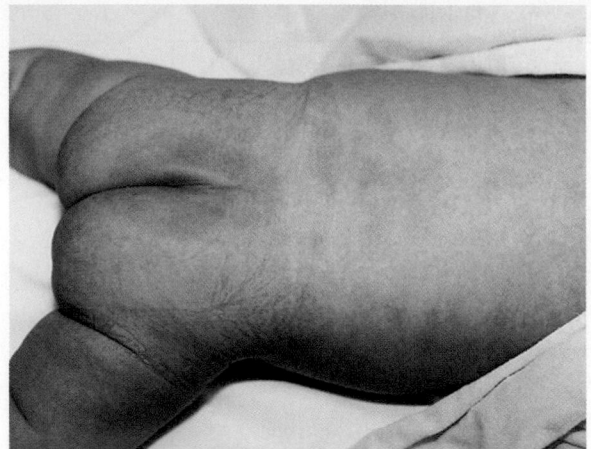

FIGURE 4-6   Mongolian spot. (From Price D, Gwin J. *Pediatric nursing: an introductory text,* ed 11. Philadelphia: Saunders, 2012.)

60 breaths per minute but normalize over the next several hours may indicate transient tachypnea of the newborn. All newborns display an irregular breathing pattern. The neonate normally breathes in the range of 70 to 80 breaths per minute for 10 to 20 seconds, slows to a rate of 20 or 30 breaths per minute for a short time, and then breathes at a faster rate again. The average respiratory rate over several minutes is 40 to 60 breaths per minute. **Periodic breathing,** a common finding among premature infants, is characterized by an irregular pattern of intermittent respiratory pauses longer than 5 seconds.

Apnea is a pathological condition in which breathing ceases for longer than 20 seconds. Apnea may be associated with cyanosis, bradycardia, pallor, and hypotonia (abnormally low muscle tone). Often apnea is associated with nonspecific symptoms of diseases seen with many neonatal conditions. All episodes of apnea must be investigated to establish the cause.[19]

It is important to note signs of respiratory distress (Table 4-4). The Silverman scoring system considers multiple factors to quantify an infant's distress (Figure 4-7). Although not always used as a measure of respiratory distress, the Silverman system highlights important respiratory observations during a physical examination. Signs of distress include nasal flaring, expiratory grunting, tachypnea, and retractions. **Nasal flaring** occurs during inspiration when the muscles of the nasal passages contract, resulting in flaring of the alae nasi, widening of the nostrils, and reduction in airway resistance. **Grunting** is an audible expiratory noise caused by closure of the glottis during expiration in an attempt to provide increased positive end-expiratory pressure and to maintain lung volume. Retractions of the chest wall during inspiration may occur in the suprasternal, substernal, subcostal, and intercostal regions. Retractions usually indicate reduced lung compliance but are also associated with obstructive airway processes with normal lung compliance. Chest wall retractions are more prominent and easily observed in the neonate than in an older child or adult. The newborn musculature is relatively thin and weak, and the thoracic cage is very compliant. The flexible chest wall and thoracic cage of the newborn exhibit noticeable retractions as lung compliance worsens. Abdominal and thoracic respiratory muscles normally move in parallel. Paradoxical respirations represent thoracic and abdominal respiratory efforts that are not synchronous. This "see-saw" effect often indicates severe respiratory distress.

TABLE 4-3

Common Dermal Findings in the Neonatal Patient

Finding	Description	Condition
Jaundice	Yellowish skin	Hyperbilirubinemia
True cyanosis	Centrally blue or dusky skin	Hypoxia
Acrocyanosis	Bluish hands and feet	Cold stress, ↓ circulation; normal for first few hours
Petechiae	Pinpoint hemorrhagic areas	Birth trauma, thrombocytopenia
Telangiectatic nevi	"Stork bites": red, flat areas	Capillary dilation, benign
Subcutaneous fat necrosis	Discrete firm masses in subcutaneous tissue	Trauma
Lanugo	Fine hair	More noticeable in preterm infants, benign
Sclerema	Hardening of skin	Septicemia, shock, cold stress
Ruddy complexion	Deep reddish skin	Polycythemia or high hematocrit value
Ecchymoses	Bruising of various sizes	Birth trauma, disseminated intravascular coagulation
Mongolian spots	Irregular areas of pale blue over sacrum and buttocks	Benign, common in black and Asian infants
Strawberry hemangiomas	Bright red, flat spots 1-3 mm in diameter	Benign, usually resolve spontaneously
Milia	White papules <1 mm on forehead, chin, and nose	Distended sebaceous glands that disappear later
Erythema toxicum	Whitish pink papular rash	Cause unknown
Pallor	Pale or white skin	Blood loss or hypovolemia
Vernix caseosa	Whitish gray, cheeselike substance	More abundant on preterm infants
Mottled skin	Uneven color, blotchy	Decreased perfusion

TABLE 4-4

Signs of Respiratory Distress in the Neonatal Patient

	Apnea	Tachypnea	Refractions	Grunting	Nasal Flaring	Stridor	Cyanosis	Breath Sounds	Other Findings
Respiratory distress syndrome		++	++	++	++		+	Decreased, rales	Premature infants, infants of diabetic mothers
Pneumothorax		++	+	+	+		+	Decreased, asymmetrical	Asymmetry of the chest, PMI shifted
Pneumonia	+	++	++	++	++		+	Rales and rhonchi	
Upper airway obstruction	+	±		++		++			Gasping or labored breathing
Diaphragmatic hernia		++		+	++		++	Bowel sounds in chest	Scaphoid abdomen, often associated with pneumothorax
Meconium aspiration	+	++	++	+	+		+	Decreased	Hyperexpansion of chest, atelectasis, pneumothorax
Transient tachypnea		++	+	+	+			Fine rales	Resolves in <24 hr
Apnea of prematurity	+++		±				±	Normal	Bradycardia

PMI, Point of maximal cardiac impulse.

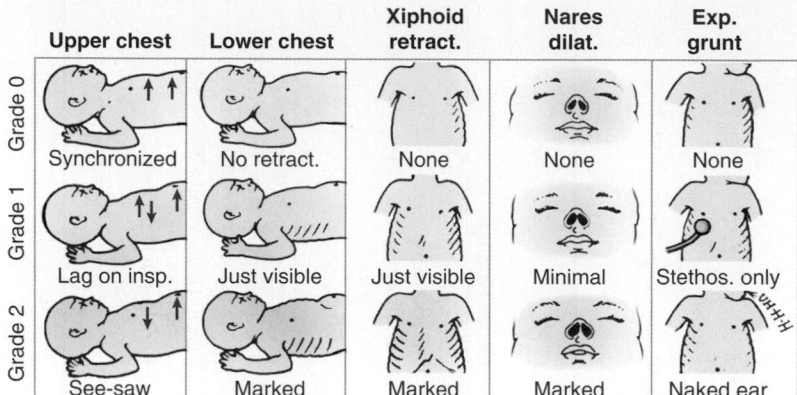

FIGURE 4-7   Silverman score.

Auscultation of the newborn can sometimes prove difficult. The newborn chest is small, and sounds easily transmit from one lung region to another. Abdominal sounds may even transmit to the lungs, although bowel sounds heard from the chest in place of absent breath sounds may indicate a diaphragmatic hernia (see Chapter 23 Surgical Disorders in Childhood That Affect Respiratory Care). Localizing auscultation findings in a preterm infant is often difficult or impossible with single-head stethoscopes. Auscultation with a double-head stethoscope has proved useful in some situations.[20] Comparison of the breath sounds from the right and left sides helps distinguish asymmetries. Asymmetrical sounds may indicate unilateral disease such as pneumothorax or a malpositioned endotracheal tube. Diminished breath sounds, wheezes, and stridor can occur in neonates. See Auscultation later in this chapter for a detailed discussion of pediatric breath sounds.

Chest and Cardiovascular System

The circumference of a newborn's chest is equivalent to the head circumference. Inspection of the chest may reveal malformations such as **pectus carinatum** (protruding xiphisternum or xiphoid process, also called pigeon chest) or **pectus excavatum** (funnel chest). Bulging or asymmetry of the chest wall usually indicates important pathological conditions.

The point of maximal cardiac impulse (PMI) is the position on the chest wall at which the cardiac impulse can be maximally seen. The PMI is usually seen in newborns because of the relatively thin and flexible chest wall. Typically, the PMI is relatively close to the sternal border because of the predominance of the right ventricle in the fetal period. A mediastinal shift caused by a pneumothorax will move the PMI away from the affected side of the chest.

With suspected pneumothorax, perform **transillumination** of the chest wall, using a high-energy flashlight or fiberoptic device in a darkened room. Place the light source on the chest wall of the suspected side. A large pneumothorax will reveal an excessively pink and illuminated, usually irregular area of light, or "glowing" area, through the chest wall when compared with the contralateral side.

Heart rate variations from 120 to 170 beats per minute may be normal depending on gestational age, as discussed earlier. The rapid rate and rhythm of heart sounds make them difficult to determine. Neonates have a high incidence of arrhythmias in the first few days of life. From 1% to 5% of all newborns exhibit some disturbance in heart rate or rhythm.[21] Many demonstrate "dropped beats," which on evaluation are premature atrial contractions. These episodes are usually benign, but any newborn with an irregular rhythm should have an electrocardiogram performed to assess the arrhythmia.

Cardiac murmurs are described as a soft to loud, harsh sound similar to a forcible exhalation with the mouth open. Many heart murmurs are transient and not associated with anomalies.

The heart size, shape, and thoracic positioning on chest X-ray film are often helpful in assessing infants with congenital heart disease.

Palpating the pulses of the quiet infant often provides important diagnostic information. Weak pulses suggest low cardiac output states such as shock and hypoplastic left-sided heart syndrome. Bounding pulses are seen in infants with patent ductus arteriosus and left-to-right shunt. The bounding characteristic of the pulse results from rapid runoff of the blood into the low-resistance pulmonary circulation. This lowers the systolic blood pressure and produces a wider pulse pressure. Brachial and femoral pulses should be equal in intensity and felt simultaneously. A delayed or weak femoral pulse can indicate coarctation of the aorta.

The range of normal blood pressures at various weights has been well established (see Table 4-2). In the absence of data, calculate an adequate mean blood pressure (MBP) as follows:

Adequate MBP = Gestational age (weeks) + 5

For example, an infant of 24 weeks of gestation should have an MBP of approximately 29 mm Hg, and a term newborn, 40 weeks of gestation, should have an MBP of approximately 45 mm Hg.

A pulse oximeter can provide valuable information in the evaluation of the cardiovascular system. Because the sensor of the pulse oximeter is applied to a distal extremity, the oximeter will display a low pulse rate and perfusion signal as peripheral pulses and perfusion decrease. The cause of this poor perfusion must be determined. However, if the oximeter suggests decreased perfusion while central blood pressure remains normal, the cause may be volume depletion with compensatory peripheral vasoconstriction. In addition, placing pulse oximeters on preductal and postductal sites allows for assessing right-to-left ductal level shunting, as seen with persistent pulmonary hypertension of the newborn. In this case the right arm, or preductal site, will have a higher saturation, while the postductal site, or left arm and lower extremities, will have a lower saturation because of venous admixture occurring postductally.

Abdomen

Successful abdominal examination requires a calm and quiet infant. Observe the contour of the abdomen and determine whether it is scaphoid (sunken anterior wall), flat, or distended. Distention is a significant finding characterized by tightly drawn skin through which engorged subcutaneous vessels can easily be seen. More noticeable abnormalities of the abdomen include **prune-belly syndrome,** which is a congenital lack of abdominal musculature; **omphalocele,** a protrusion of the membranous sac that encloses abdominal contents through an opening in the abdominal wall into the umbilical cord; and **gastroschisis,** a defect in the abdominal wall lateral to the midline with protrusion of the intestines (Figure 4-8).[22]

When examining the abdomen, auscultate and palpate over all four quadrants. Bowel sounds are usually heard over the entire abdomen, generally described as a "tinkling" or "rumbling." Because bowel sounds are not continuous, it may take several seconds to hear them.

Decreases or increases in the amount or changes in the characteristics of bowel sounds may indicate a pathological abdominal condition.

The umbilical cord is yellowish white with three blood vessels. The two small and thick-walled arteries and one large and thin-walled vein are easily visible at the end of a freshly cut cord. Wharton's jelly surrounds the vessels. A single umbilical artery suggests congenital anomalies, especially those of the urinary tract. The presence of meconium in the amniotic fluid causes a greenish yellow staining of the umbilical cord. The umbilical cord of an infant who is large for gestational age and born to a diabetic mother is often large and fat. Conversely, infants with intrauterine growth retardation often have thin cords with little Wharton's jelly. With an umbilical hernia the intestinal muscles do not close around the umbilicus, and the intestines protrude into this weakened tissue. Such a defect may require surgery or may resolve without intervention as the muscles become stronger.

Head and Neck

The head is usually the presenting part and often shows evidence of bruising and molding as a result of pressures exerted during the birth process. Molding of the skull with overlapping cranial bones is common. In term infants the molding should resolve within a few days. The **fontanels** are the nonossified areas between the cranial bones that make up the skull. The fontanels and suture lines should be soft and should not bulge. Craniotabes are soft skull areas that can be compressed like a ping-pong ball and may be a normal finding, especially in premature infants.

Any evidence of edema under the scalp should be examined carefully, especially in infants having vacuum or forceps-assisted delivery. Rarely edema is attributed to a **subgaleal hemorrhage,** tearing of the emissary veins, where edema from blood loss can extend from the eyes to the nape of the neck. Blood loss may occur fairly rapidly

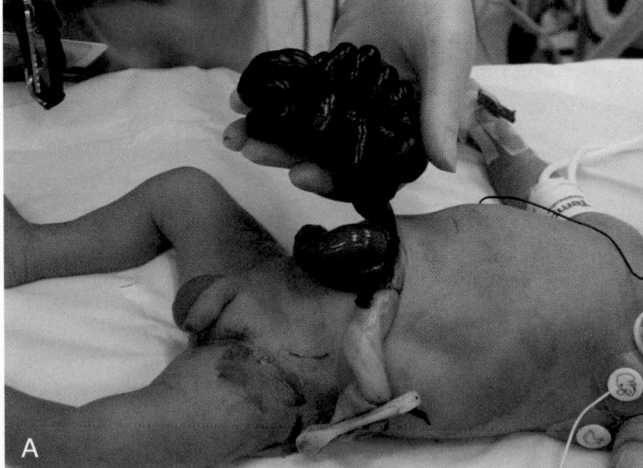
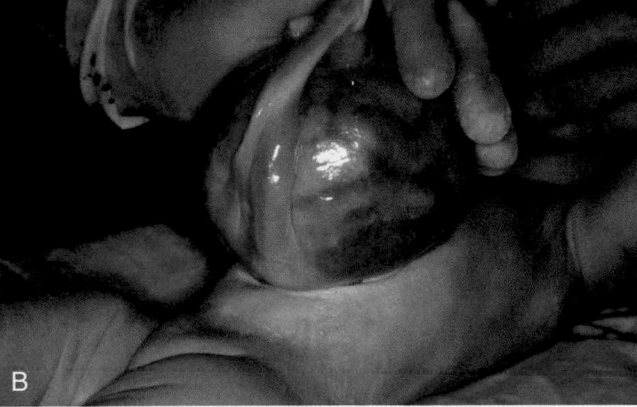

FIGURE 4-8   A, Gastroschisis. **B,** Omphalocele. (From Price D, Gwin J. *Pediatric nursing: an introductory text,* ed 11, Philadelphia: Saunders, 2012.)

after delivery and be sufficient to cause hypovolemic shock.[23,24]

More than 150,000 children are born with notable birth defects and syndromes in the United States each year.[25] Congenital anomalies are the leading cause of infant mortality in the postneonatal period. Unusual facies may suggest a number of distinct dysmorphic genetic syndromes. *Smith's Recognizable Patterns of Human Malformation* is an invaluable resource in the evaluation of infants with an unusual facies.[26] It also provides standard measurements for the newborn. Facial paralysis or an asymmetrical facies is often noticed in the otherwise normal-appearing infant. Facial paralysis may be readily apparent only when the infant cries.

The eyes are often swollen and edematous from the birth process. After resolution of the swelling, assess the eyes for excessive spacing and any unusual slant. Apply antibiotic ointment or silver nitrate to the eyes after delivery to prevent infection. In infants older than 28 weeks of gestation, the pupils should be round and regular and should react to light. Examine the ears for placement and deformation. Deformed, posteriorly rotated, or low-set ears are associated with various genetic anomalies. Consider ears low set when the upper insertion of the ear is below the level of a line drawn through the corner of the orbits of the eyes.

Newborns breathe preferentially through the nose; therefore alternately occlude each side and listen to breath sounds to assess the patency of each nostril. If the infant appears to be breathing comfortably, many nurseries no longer attempt to pass catheters because nasal trauma, obstruction, and edema are serious risks. An oral airway or endotracheal tube is often required if **bilateral choanal atresia,** the incomplete opening into the nasopharynx as a result of membranous or bony structures, is present. Abnormalities of the mouth, lips, and oral cavity are seen in many infants. **Microstomia,** small mouth, is commonly seen in infants with the chromosomal defect trisomy 18, whereas midfacial clefts, cleft lip and palate, are commonly seen with trisomy 13. Pierre Robin syndrome is characterized by a cleft palate, posteriorly displaced tongue, and **micrognathia,** a small lower jaw.[27]

Examination of the oral cavity and pharynx for less obvious palatal clefts, mucous cysts, Epstein's pearls, or natal teeth can be performed with a flashlight or laryngoscope blade light. Examine the neck for obvious shortening, vertebral anomalies, or limitations in movement. A variety of cysts, **hygromas** (sacs of fluid resulting from a blockage in the lymphatic system), sinuses, and masses may be present laterally or at the midline. Large neck lesions may apply pressure to the trachea and impair breathing.

The clavicles are often broken during the delivery of large infants with shoulder dystocia (difficult delivery as a result of the fact that the anterior shoulder of the infant cannot pass below the mother's hip bone) or in breech deliveries. Commonly the injury is noted when the infant refuses to move the affected shoulder. The break is usually easily palpable as an area of crepitus overlying the bone. Therapy is usually not necessary for fractured clavicles in the newborn because they heal without intervention.

Musculoskeletal System, Spine, and Extremities

The intrauterine environment often affects the extremities and musculoskeletal system. Many limb and other deformations in the fetus result from intrinsic (fetal) or extrinsic (uterine) factors.

Extra digits may be familial or may be associated with a number of syndromes. They can be present on hands or feet or both. The digits can vary from fully formed and articulated to simple skin tags.

Joint contractures or abnormal positioning of one or more limbs may result from a fetal problem or intrauterine compression. Clubfoot, talipes equinovarus, is a typical example.[28,29] An isolated joint-extremity malformation suggests extrinsic factors, whereas multiple deformations are more often seen with primary fetal neurological or muscular diseases.

The symmetry and bony structure of the spine are easily examined in the newborn. Suspend the infant in a prone position with one hand, then visually and digitally evaluate the structures. Many infants have a small indentation (sacral dimple) near the end of the spine. If the bottom of the dimple is easily seen without associated bony defects, no further evaluation is required. However, if the defect cannot be fully visualized or if there are bony defects, associated tufts of hair, or drainage of clear fluid, further evaluation is required. A few infants have the congenital malformations collectively called spina bifida (Figure 4-9). These defects result from failure of the embryonic neural tube to form correctly in the third to fifth week of gestation. The defects usually involve bone, skin, the covering of the central nervous system (meninges), and nerve tissue. Defects that occur over the spine are called **myelomeningoceles** (Figure 4-10), and those involving the brain are called **encephaloceles.**

It is important to evaluate the hips of all infants even if there is no evidence of asymmetry or other bone, joint,

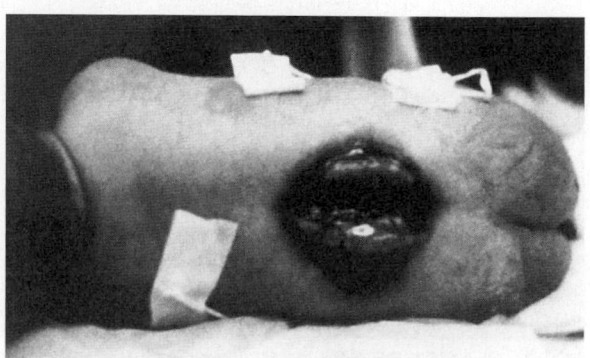

FIGURE 4-9 Infant with spina bifada.

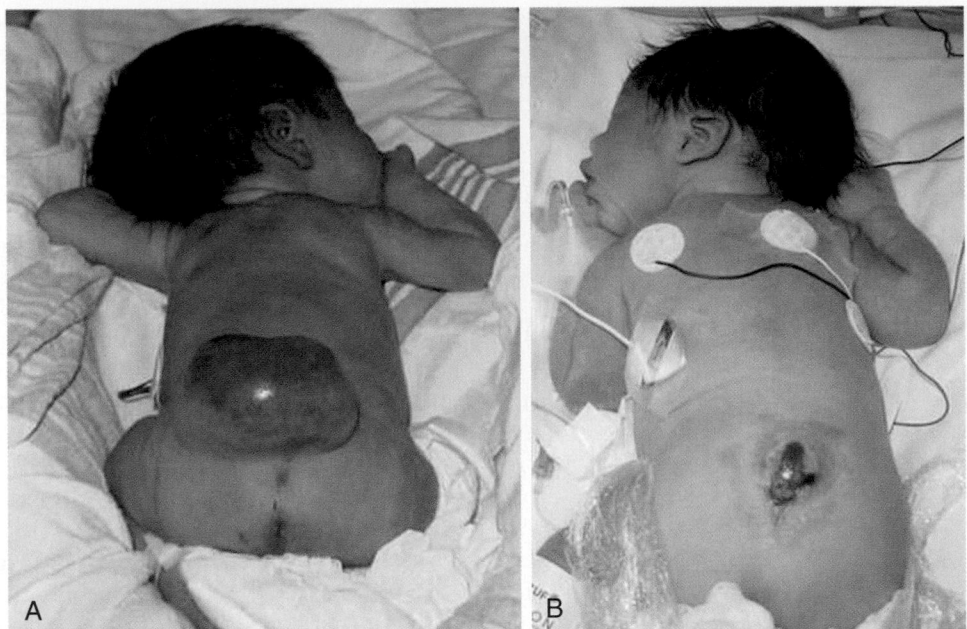

FIGURE 4-10   **A,** Myelomeningocele with intact sac. **B,** Myelomeningocele with ruptured sac. (From Hockenberry M, Wilson D. *Wong's essentials of pediatric nursing,* ed 8. St. Louis: Mosby, 2013.)

or muscular problems. Stabilize the pelvis on a flat surface while the joint is flexed and abducted to the surface. A telescoping feeling or the presence of a "clunk" suggests congenital laxity or dislocation of the hip.[29] Often, several days must pass before the hips of infants born in the breech position can be appropriately evaluated.

Cry

After the examiner has obtained some newborn experience, it is impressive how much information something as simple as a baby's cry can provide. A loud and vigorous cry is usually a sign of a healthy infant. A moaning, weak, or faint cry suggests illness. Often, an infant with respiratory distress syndrome strains with a grunting cry. An infant with a piercing, high-pitched cry often has a neurological injury, drug withdrawal, or increased intracranial pressure. Hoarse crying can be associated with laryngeal edema, as in recently extubated infants. However, a hoarse cry may also be heard with congenital hypothyroidism, cretinism, or hypocalcemia with laryngospasm. Perhaps the most distinctive cry is associated with a deletion of the short arm of the fifth chromosome. The catlike cry of these infants gives the syndrome the name *cri du chat,* French for "cry of the cat."

NEUROLOGICAL ASSESSMENT

The general neurological state of the infant is assessed during much of the physical examination. Note whether the infant responds appropriately to his or her surroundings or is lethargic or overly irritable. It is also important to determine whether the infant moves all extremities and

whether the movements are symmetrical and smooth or jittery and jerky. Infants with evidence of difficult delivery may manifest signs of extremity weakness associated with trauma to the brachial plexus.

Pick up the neonate under the arms to assess muscle tone in the term infant. A normal infant will suspend well. An infant with decreased tone will noodle through the hands. Infants with normal tone will maintain their extremities in a flexed position at rest.

A number of reflexes are present in the newborn. Everyone has observed the grasp reflex, in which the newborn infant grasps a finger placed in the palm of the hand. A similar downward curving of the toes occurs if a finger is pressed against the sole of the foot; this is referred to as the plantar grasp reflex. The startle reaction to sound or touch is similar to the Moro reflex (Figure 4-11), which occurs when the head is allowed to fall back slightly. The normal term infant's extremities will extend rapidly with open hands. The neonate will then slowly flex them back toward the body. Infants will respond to a bright light by shutting their eyelids tight. They will often turn toward unique sounds or sights and may focus on objects, especially faces. Suspending the infant and touching the top of the foot against a surface can demonstrate the stepping reflex: The infant should lift the leg and then place it flat on the surface.[30]

PEDIATRIC PATIENT HISTORY

Unlike neonatal patients, children present with previous history, and despite numerous advances in laboratory testing, the ability to obtain a pediatric history remains

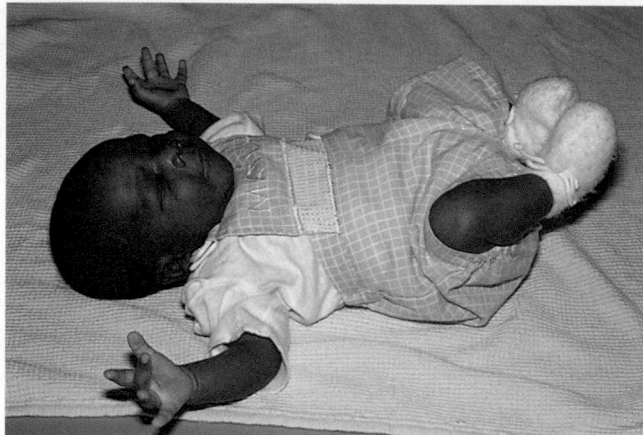

FIGURE 4-11   Moro reflex. (From Price D, Gwin J. *Pediatric nursing: an introductory text,* ed 11. Philadelphia: Saunders, 2012.)

essential to the practice of pediatric respiratory care. In most encounters of children with respiratory conditions, the history provides the necessary information to formulate a differential diagnosis and suggest additional evaluation and management. Thus the respiratory therapist (RT) should spend considerable effort enhancing history-taking skills.

The history for a new patient can be divided into the following categories:
· Chief complaint or primary concern
· History of the present illness (HPI)
· Medical history (MH)
· Review of symptoms (ROS)
· Family history
· Social and environmental histories

Chief Complaint

The **chief complaint** consists of the reason the child presents for health care. The chief complaint may simply be a symptom or sign observed by the child or caregivers and in need of further evaluation, as in the case of a new patient who presents for the evaluation of cough or chest pain. The chief complaint may also be a specific established diagnosis, as in the case of a child admitted to the hospital for treatment of acute asthma or a pulmonary exacerbation of cystic fibrosis (CF). For a new patient, the initial step is to establish the chief complaint or primary concern. Additional information in the form of a medical history is then sought to further elucidate and clarify historical findings that point to either a specific diagnosis or set of diagnoses (differential diagnosis) that then leads to further evaluation (e.g., physical examination, laboratory testing).

New Patient History

For a new patient, the medical history consists of specific components including the HPI, MH, ROS, family history, and social and environmental histories (Box 4-2). Important components of the HPI include duration, intensity or severity, and improvement or deterioration of symptoms.

Knowledge of the following may help point to a specific disease or narrow the differential diagnosis:
· Triggers of symptoms
· Aggravating or alleviating factors
· Medications that have previously or are currently being used and whether or not these medications have been helpful
· Chronicity
· Recurrence or seasonality of symptoms

Review of current medications, including nonprescription and alternative medications, dosing, and when and how taken, as well as what the medications are taken for, may provide useful information.

Where the child lives, adult visitors from areas of endemic tuberculosis, and recent travel history may also suggest unsuspected exposures or diseases.

Follow-up or Established Patient History

For a follow-up or established patient, the medical history is not usually focused on developing differential diagnoses or establishing a specific diagnosis but rather on determining current lung health and whether there have been any changes since the last visit. In this situation, the medical history consists of an interim history and review of key components of the MH, ROS, and social and environmental histories (Box 4-3). Questions are directed to determining whether there were any interim respiratory infections or exposures and whether these triggered exacerbation of the primary disease.[31] Exposure to environmental tobacco smoke should be asked about specifically.[32] If an exacerbation of the primary disease occurs, did this exacerbation lead to a clinic visit, emergency room visit, or hospitalization or were the caregivers able to manage the exacerbation at home? Information concerning the presence or absence of allergic, nasal, respiratory, or gastrointestinal symptoms is sought. If symptoms are present, are they better or worse than at the previous visit? Are new symptoms present and are these related to the primary disease? Quality-of-life issues should be explored. Missing school, inability to participate in normal daily and physical activities, or the caregiver(s) missing work because of an increase in the child's respiratory symptoms suggests that disease management is less than optimal. Review of current medications, including nonprescription and alternative medications; dosing; when and how taken; what the medications are taken for; and whether or not there have been changes in medications, dosing, or both since the previous visit also yields important information. Adherence with and understanding of the treatment plan should be explored. Changes in school and family situations; exposure to environmental tobacco smoke, allergens, and airway irritants; and recent travel or exposure to sick adults may also yield clues to changes in status of the primary disease. If an explanation of worsening or less than optimal control of the primary disease is not forthcoming, then the RT should take a more detailed history similar to the initial medical history.

Box 4-2	New Patient History

CHIEF COMPLAINT OR PRIMARY REASON FOR VISIT
- History of present illness
- Duration
- Intensity or severity
- Improvement or deterioration
- Triggers
- Aggravating or alleviating factors
- Medications (past and current)
- Chronicity
- Seasonality

MEDICAL HISTORY
- Perinatal history
- Acute care and emergency room visits
- Hospitalizations and surgeries
- Immunizations
- Previous evaluations

REVIEW OF SYMPTOMS
- Family history
- Social and environmental histories

Important components of the medical history that may contribute to establishing a diagnosis include the following:
- History of prematurity
- Birth weight
- Need for and duration of oxygen therapy, assisted ventilation, or both in the neonatal period
- Previous emergency room visits, hospitalizations, or both for respiratory disturbances (including intensive care unit admissions and any need for assisted ventilation)
- Previous surgeries
- Immunization history

Results of previous evaluations may also provide important diagnostic clues.

The ROS attempts to identify symptoms that were not identified in the HPI and that may be related or contribute to the child's underlying respiratory condition. A systematic review of symptoms in the following categories may suggest contributions of atopic diseases, gastroesophageal reflux, and immunodeficiency, as well as thoracic cage, neurological, and neuromuscular disorders, to the presenting pulmonary complaint:
- Allergic
- Dermatological
- Developmental
- Gastrointestinal
- Immunological
- Otolaryngological
- Musculoskeletal
- Neurological
- Neuromuscular

The family history may also provide valuable information. Important conditions in the biological parents, siblings, and other close relatives to ask about include the following:
- Presence or absence of asthma
- Chronic or seasonal bronchitis
- Atopic diseases
- Recurrent pneumonia
- CF
- Immunodeficiency
- Infertile males (may suggest CF)
- Tuberculosis
- Hemoptysis
- Early childhood serious illnesses or deaths
- Congenital heart disease
- Dextrocardia (heart situated on the right side of the body)
- α_1-Antiprotease deficiency

Important components of the social and environmental histories include the following:
- Who the child lives with
- Who assists the child with medications and therapies
- Level of adherence to medications and therapies
- Occupations of the caregivers
- Housing conditions
- Environmental tobacco smoke exposure
- Personal smoking
- Presence of visible mold
- Pets in the home
- Other significant exposures
- Use of day care
- School grades and performance
- Participation in and any difficulties with extracurricular activities

Box 4-3	Follow-up or Established Patient History

CHIEF COMPLAINT OR PREVIOUS DIAGNOSIS OR PROBLEM
Interim History
- Respiratory infections
- Exacerbations of primary disease
- Triggers and/or exposures
- Quality of life
- Medications

Review of Key Components
- Medical history
- Review of symptoms
- Social and environmental histories

PULMONARY EXAMINATION

The RT should also be proficient at performing a pediatric pulmonary examination. The setting in which an examination occurs determines the pace of the examination as well as the information gained. A child with respiratory distress may require rapid physical assessment and immediate institution of therapy. A crying child is almost impossible to examine. Efforts should be made to perform an examination in a calm, expeditious, and professional manner as well as in such a manner as not to upset the child. Examination of the small child in the caregiver's lap may be particularly helpful in allaying the child's fears and keeping the child calm. In general, the pulmonary examination includes inspection, palpation, percussion,

Box 4-4	Pulmonary Examination

- Inspection
- Vital signs
- Heart rate
- Respiratory rate
- Temperature
- Blood pressure
- Oxygen saturation
- Respiratory distress
- Tachypnea
- Breathlessness
- Head bobbing
- Grunting
- Nasal flaring
- Retractions
- Chest wall
- Shape
- Muscle mass and strength
- Adipose tissue
- Palpation
- Neck
- Masses or adenopathy

- Trachea
- Chest
- Fremitus
- Motion with deep breathing
- Percussion
- Hyperresonance
- Dullness
- Auscultation
- Grunting
- Stridor
- Stertor
- Breath sounds
- Symmetry
- Intensity
- Location: lobes and segments
- Phases: inspiration, expiration, or both
- Adventitious sounds
- Crackles: fine or coarse
- Wheezes: low or high pitched
- Monophonic or polyphonic

and auscultation (Box 4-4) and begins at the initiation of contact with the child. All components of the pulmonary examination yield valuable information, and the impulse to primarily or only use one's stethoscope should be avoided. Establishing a specific examination routine is helpful in assisting in completion of all the evaluation components and in increasing one's comfort and expertise in physical assessment of the child with respiratory disease.

Inspection

Inspection begins at the bedside with review of the child's vital signs and first contact with the child and caregiver. Vital signs of importance to the RT include heart rate, respiratory rate, temperature, blood pressure, and, if available, pulse oximetry. Initial inspection is directed to determining whether the child is in respiratory distress. A child in respiratory distress may display both nonpulmonary and pulmonary signs. Nonpulmonary signs of respiratory distress include anxiety, fussiness, irritability, depressed level of consciousness or responsiveness, and tachycardia. Pulmonary signs include tachypnea, breathlessness, head bobbing, grunting, nasal flaring, retractions, oxygen saturation less than 90%, and cyanosis. A child in severe respiratory distress requires rapid assessment and immediate institution of appropriate therapy. Inspection of the chest wall is done to evaluate for chronic obstructive lung, neuromuscular, and musculoskeletal diseases. Inspection for respiratory distress and of the chest wall is best done with the child's upper torso unclothed.

The respiratory rate can be a sensitive indicator of the severity of underlying lung disease.[31-33] Normal respiratory rates vary on the basis of age and activity level (Table 4-5). In general, the respiratory rate is best determined when the

TABLE 4-5						
Normal Respiratory Rates in Sleeping and Awake Pediatric Patients						
	SLEEPING BREATHS PER MINUTE			AWAKE BREATHS PER MINUTE		
Age	Number Studied	Mean	Range	Number Studied	Mean	Range
6-12 mo	6	27	22-31	3	64	58-75
1-2 yr	6	19	17-23	4	35	30-40
2-4 yr	16	19	16-25	15	31	23-42
4-6 yr	23	18	14-23	22	26	19-36
6-8 yr	27	17	13-23	28	23	15-30
8-10 yr	19	18	14-23	19	21	15-31
10-12 yr	11	16	13-19	17	21	15-28
12-14 yr	6	16	15-18	7	22	18-26

From Iliff A, Lee VA. Pulse rate, respiratory rate, and body temperature of children between two months and eighteen years of age, *Child Dev* 1952;23:237.

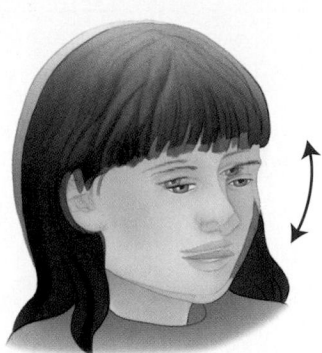

FIGURE 4-12   Head bobbing.

child is asleep or resting quietly.[34,35] In the ill-appearing child, the presence of fever may be a confounding factor that results in tachypnea proportional to the degree of fever and the appearance of respiratory distress. In the child with no underlying lung disease, relief of fever should result in resolution of tachypnea and apparent respiratory distress.

Head bobbing, nasal flaring, and grunting are common signs of respiratory distress in infants and young children and are compensatory mechanisms to decrease the work of breathing. **Head bobbing** occurs when the **sternocleidomastoids** (neck muscles that serve to flex and rotate the head), in an attempt to overcome decreased lung compliance, increased airway resistance, or both, contract during inspiration, pulling the head down and the clavicles and rib cage up (Figure 4-12). This results in the head bobbing forward in synchrony with each inspiration. Nasal flaring and grunting can be present in the pediatric patient as well. The presence of one or more of these signs typically indicates significant airway obstruction or lung disease.

Suprasternal, intercostal, and subcostal/substernal retractions and asynchronous chest and abdominal wall motion are common signs of respiratory distress in both younger and older children and may be due to significant airway obstruction, lung disease, or both. Retractions result from the pulling in of the skin between and below the ribs, above the sternum in the suprasternal notch, or both, because of significant airway obstruction and lung disease (Figures 4-13, 4-14, and 4-15). Suprasternal retractions are also referred to as "tracheal tugging." In most circumstances, a direct correlation exists between the degree of retractions and the severity of respiratory distress. Infants, young children, and children with muscle weakness may develop paradoxical inward motion of the chest wall and concomitant outward movement of the abdominal wall (i.e., asynchrony of chest and abdominal wall, or "see-sawing" motion) with increasing degrees of respiratory distress. As discussed earlier, in neonates, infants, and young children this see-sawing motion occurs because of their compliant rib cage, whereas in older children with muscle disease it occurs because of weakness of the abdominal wall musculature.

Inspection of the chest wall may reveal increased anteroposterior diameter, abnormal shape, muscular weakness, or obesity. Chest wall inspection should include anterior, posterior, and lateral examination. Chronic obstructive lung diseases such as severe asthma, advanced CF, and severe bronchopulmonary dysplasia may be associated with increased anteroposterior diameter of the chest as a result of increased air trapping. The chest wall may be abnormally shaped, such as in pectus carinatum ("pigeon breast"), pectus excavatum ("sunken chest"), **kyphosis** ("hunchback" appearance), and **scoliosis** (abnormal "sideways" spinal curvature). The chest wall may also be bell shaped or have obvious rib abnormalities. Muscular weakness may result in decreased chest wall muscle mass; poor head control; or obvious weakness of the trunk, extremities, or both. Obesity may cause excessive deposition of adipose tissue around the neck, chest, and abdomen. Abnormal chest wall shape, muscular weakness, and obesity can result in significant restrictive lung dysfunction.

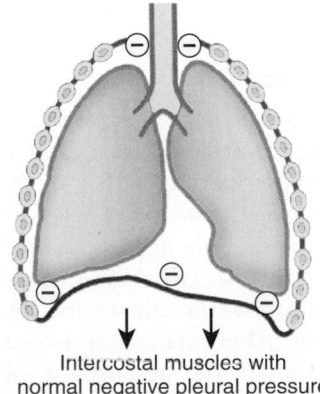

Intercostal muscles with normal negative pleural pressure during inhalation

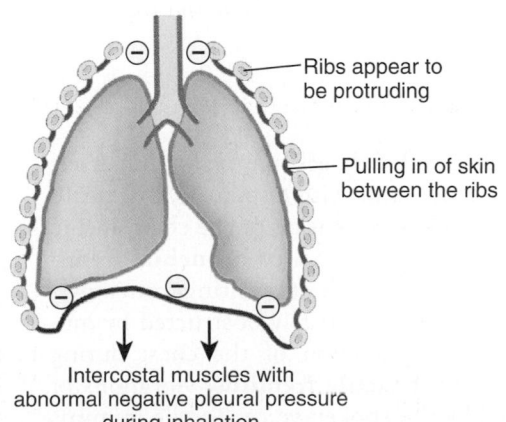

Ribs appear to be protruding

Pulling in of skin between the ribs

Intercostal muscles with abnormal negative pleural pressure during inhalation

FIGURE 4-13   Intercostal retractions. Soft tissue between the ribs is pulled inward (retracted) because of the extremely high negative pleural pressure.

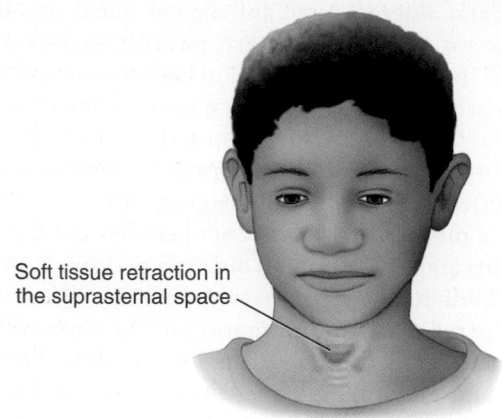

Soft tissue retraction in
the suprasternal space

FIGURE 4-14 Suprasternal retractions. Soft tissue in the suprasternal space is retracted because of high negative pressure, most often caused by the patient's attempt to breathe against an airway obstruction.

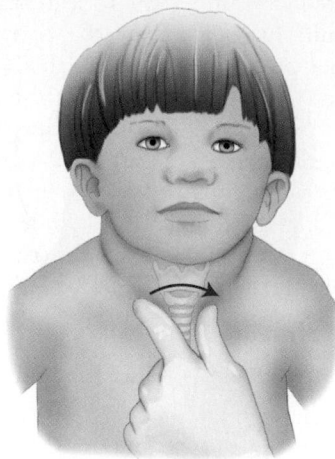

FIGURE 4-16 Technique for determining tracheal position in the older child.

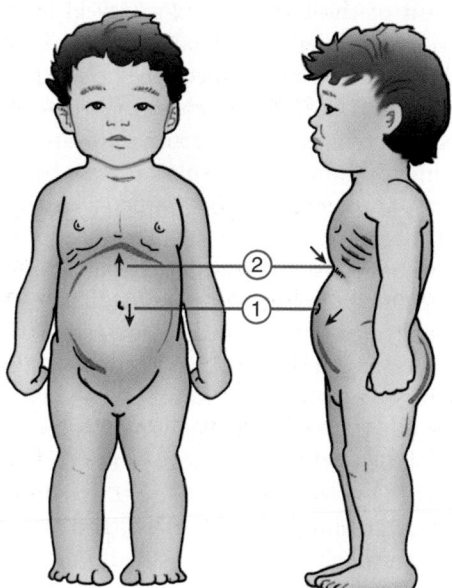

FIGURE 4-15 Subcostal/substernal retractions. Airway obstruction results in a pulling inward of the lower costal margins. The abdomen is protruding (*1*), and there is a sunken substernal notch (*2*). See-saw movement of the chest and stomach is also present.

Palpation

Palpation of the chest wall and neck may be helpful in the physical examination of a child with respiratory disease. In infants and young children, palpation of the chest during quiet breathing may elicit rhonchal or **bronchial fremitus,** which are vibrations of the chest resulting from movement of air through airways partially obstructed by mucus. In an older child, palpation of the chest during normal speech may elicit **tactile fremitus,** vibrations of the chest produced by the spoken voice. Tactile fremitus may be increased over areas of the chest wall corresponding to underlying pulmonary consolidation. In an older

child, assessment of chest wall excursion can be accomplished by placement of the examiner's hands on both sides of the thoracic spine, with thumbs toward the spine, and observing the motion of the hands and patient's ribs during deep inspiration. Palpation of the anterior neck may be helpful in determining whether the trachea is in the midline (Figure 4-16) and whether there are masses or adenopathy compressing the trachea.

Percussion

Percussion of the chest wall may be helpful in the physical examination of an older child but is typically unrewarding in the examination of an infant or younger child. Chest percussion is performed by tapping the finger of one hand with a finger of the other hand over corresponding areas of the patient's chest, usually while the patient is sitting upright. A relatively high-pitched percussion note, or hyperresonance, suggests focal or generalized air trapping or pneumothorax. A relatively dull percussion note indicates atelectasis, consolidation, or pleural effusion. In the case of pleural effusion, changes in the level of the dull percussion note over time can be used to assess worsening or improvement.

Auscultation

Auscultation involves listening to the sounds of the heart, lungs, and gastrointestinal tract, sometimes with the ears alone but more generally with a stethoscope. Breathing is normally quiet, so that noises heard without the stethoscope or audible noises during "quiet" breathing are always abnormal. Grunting was previously discussed Other audible noises include stridor, stertor, and occasionally wheezing. Abnormal chest noises, or adventitious sounds, heard with the stethoscope include crackles and wheezes.[38-40] Stridor and wheezes are sometimes further described as monophonic sounds. Wheezes may also be described as polyphonic sounds. Monophonic sounds are usually associated with upper and central airway disorders and sound similarly throughout the chest. Polyphonic sounds are usually associated with small airway disorders and sound different in different parts of the chest. Auscultation with the stethoscope should be done while the child is calm and quiet. Intensity and symmetry of breath sounds as well as duration of inspiration and expiration should be noted. Prolonged inspiration suggests extrathoracic (larynx and upper trachea) airway obstruction, whereas prolonged expiration suggests intrathoracic (lower trachea, mainstem bronchi, and smaller bronchi) airway obstruction.

Stridor is a high-pitched, monophonic, audible noise that may occur during inspiration or expiration or may be biphasic.[40,41] Inspiratory stridor suggests extrathoracic airway obstruction, such as occurs in laryngomalacia, subglottic stenosis, and croup. Expiratory stridor suggests intrathoracic central airway obstruction, such as occurs in mass or vascular compression of the trachea, tracheomalacia, and bronchomalacia. Biphasic stridor typically indicates a more severe degree of laryngeal or central airway obstruction and may be associated with signs of respiratory distress. To distinguish stridor from wheezing, place the head of the stethoscope over the neck area. If the sound is louder over the neck than over the chest, then it is most likely the result of stridor rather than wheezing. **Stertor** is a low-pitched, wet sound similar to snoring and suggests nasopharyngeal, oropharyngeal, and/or hypopharyngeal airway obstruction, such as occurs in adenotonsillar hypertrophy.[42,43] Audible wheezing may occur in asthma or in intrathoracic central airway obstruction, typically indicates a more severe degree of obstruction, and may be associated with signs of respiratory distress.

The classification of adventitious sounds is confusing. Most modern terminology primarily uses the term *wheezes* for continuous sounds and *crackles* for discontinuous sounds.[38-40] Continuous sounds typically last for at least 250 msec, whereas discontinuous sounds last for less than 20 msec.[38] Wheezes can be further described as inspiratory, expiratory, monophonic, polyphonic, high pitched, or low pitched. Polyphonic high-pitched wheezes typically occur in asthma, and as airway obstruction worsens, wheezes tend to progress from end-expiratory, to expiratory, to both expiratory and inspiratory sounds. The term *rhonchus* (plural, *rhonchi*) has also been used to describe a low-pitched wheeze and suggests movement of air through large airways partially obstructed by mucus. Crackles can be further described as inspiratory, expiratory, fine, and coarse. Fine crackles are less loud crackles with high-frequency components and short duration and are usually associated with distal small airway or alveolar diseases such as pneumonia or pulmonary edema. Coarse crackles are louder crackles with lower frequency and longer duration and are usually associated with medium or large airway disease such as bronchitis.[44] Where in the chest adventitious sounds are heard is also important to note and may suggest an etiology. Unilateral wheezes or wheezes heard over a specific segment or lobe suggest foreign body airway obstruction. Fine crackles heard over a specific segment or lobe suggest localized pneumonia.

NONPULMONARY EXAMINATION

In addition to examining the chest, a general examination should be done, including assessment of growth (weight, weight percentile, height, and height percentile) and examination of several other areas of the body, including the eyes, ears, nose, throat, heart, abdomen, skin, and extremities, for clues to underlying or contributing conditions (Box 4-5). Descriptions of many of the pathological findings that may be found during a pediatric examination are outside the scope of this chapter, and the interested reader

---

Box 4-5	Nonpulmonary Examination: Findings Possibly Associated with Pulmonary Disease

GENERAL
- Poor growth (weight, height, or both less than the fifth percentile for age)
- Developmental delay
- Neurological abnormalities or cerebral palsy
- Muscle weakness or atrophy
- Adenopathy

EARS, EYES, NOSE, THROAT
- Serous otitis media
- Conjunctivitis
- Allergic shiners
- Morgan-Dennie lines
- Nasal crease
- Nasal secretions
- Edematous, pale nasal mucosa
- Tonsillar hypertrophy
- Posterior pharyngeal mucus (postnasal drip)

HEART
- Abnormal rhythm
- Murmurs or gallop
- Prominent second heart sound

ABDOMEN
- Distention
- Hepatosplenomegaly

SKIN
- Atopic dermatitis
- Urticaria
- Poor circulation
- Hemangiomas, telangiectasias
- Cyanosis

EXTREMITIES
- Digital clubbing
- Edema
- Arthritis

is referred to other sources. Conditions potentially associated with respiratory disease that can be detected during a general examination include significant poor growth, developmental delay, neurological abnormalities or cerebral palsy, muscle weakness or atrophy, and adenopathy. Poor growth, manifested by weight, height, or both weight and height less than the fifth percentile for age, suggests a potentially serious chronic condition. Developmental delay, neurological abnormalities, and muscle weakness or atrophy may result in ineffective cough, dysphagia with pulmonary aspiration, chest wall deformities, or restrictive lung dysfunction. Adenopathy may suggest immunodeficiency or an oncological process.

Examination of the ears, eyes, nose, and throat, although usually performed by a physician, is part of the pulmonary examination and may reveal findings associated with a respiratory disease. Allergic disorders are suggested by the findings of serous otitis media; conjunctivitis; allergic shiners; Morgan-Dennie lines; nasal crease; nasal secretions; edematous, pale nasal mucosa; and posterior pharyngeal mucus (postnasal drip). Obstructive sleep apnea is suggested by severe tonsillar hypertrophy.

Cardiac dysfunction may contribute to or be the result of pulmonary dysfunction. Findings of an abnormal rhythm, murmur, gallop, or prominent second (pulmonic) heart sound during cardiac examination suggest cardiac dysfunction and should be noted.

Evaluation of the abdomen may reveal distention or hepatosplenomegaly that can be associated with CF or may result in impaired diaphragmatic excursion with resultant restrictive lung dysfunction.

Inspection of the skin may reveal evidence of an allergic disorder, such as atopic dermatitis or urticaria; cardiac dysfunction, such as poor circulation or cyanosis; severe hypoxemia, such as cyanosis; or lesions that suggest more generalized diseases with a pulmonary component, such as hemangiomas (a benign tumor of blood vessel endothelial cells that may obstruct large airways or, if in the lung, result in right-to-left shunting of blood, causing hypoxemia) or telangiectasias (small dilated blood vessel malformations that if multiple or present in the nose may suggest hereditary hemorrhagic telangiectasia).

Inspection of the extremities may reveal evidence of cardiac dysfunction or hypoproteinemia, such as edema; immunological disease, such as arthritis; or both. The finding of digital clubbing (Figure 4-17) in a child with any respiratory condition should strongly suggest chronic, potentially severe and life-threatening diseases such as CF, interstitial lung disorders, or other serious lung disorders. Although digital clubbing may be familial, it is also found in cyanotic congenital cardiac disease, infective endocarditis, cirrhosis, inflammatory bowel disease, and other infectious, neoplastic, inflammatory, and vascular disorders.[46] Thus, the finding of digital clubbing should always lead to additional laboratory evaluation.

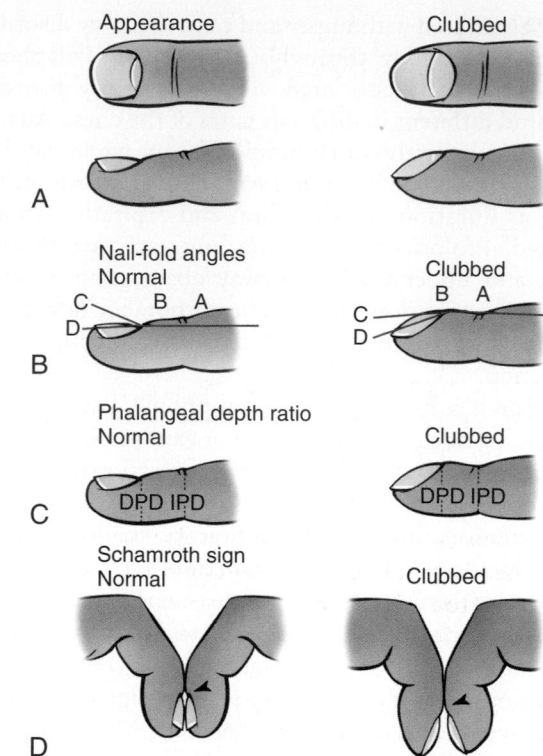

FIGURE 4-17 **A,** Normal finger, viewed from above and in profile, and the changes occurring in established clubbing, viewed from above and in profile. **B,** The finger on the left demonstrates normal profile (*ABC*) and normal hyponychial (*ABD*) nail-fold angles of 169 and 183 degrees, respectively. The clubbed finger on the right shows increased profile and hyponychial nail-fold angles of 191 and 203 degrees, respectively. **C,** Distal phalangeal finger depth (*DPD*)/interphalangeal finger depth (*IPD*) represents the phalangeal depth ratio. In normal fingers, the *IPD* is greater than the *DPD*. In clubbing, this relationship is reversed. **D,** Schamroth sign: in the absence of clubbing, opposition of the index fingers nail-to-nail creates a diamond-shaped window (*arrowhead*). In clubbed fingers, the loss of the profile angle because of an increase in tissue at the nail bed causes obliteration of this space (*arrowhead*).

LABORATORY ASSESSMENT

Routine laboratory studies play a limited but important role in the immediate newborn period. Most laboratory abnormalities seen in the first 24 hours of life result from sepsis, abnormally high or low levels of red blood cells, red blood cell isoimmunization, or temporary derangement in the regulation of glucose metabolism.

The white blood cell (WBC) count of the newborn is usually significantly higher than pediatric or adult values. **Leukopenia,** WBCs less than 3500/mm^3, and **leukocytosis,** WBCs greater than 25,000/mm^3, suggest infection. WBCs greater than 25,000/mm^3, however, are not unusual in the immediate newborn period. Similarly, the absolute number of platelets is associated with fetal/neonatal infection. A platelet count of less than 150,000 cells/mm^3 is abnormally low and is usually seen with acute or chronic infections.

TABLE 4-6

Laboratory Values in the Neonatal Patient

Age	Hgb	Hct	WBCs	Platelets
	(g/dl)	(%)	(×1000 cells/mm³)	(×1000 cells/mm³)
28 wk of gestation	14.5	45	—	275
32 wk of gestation	15	47	—	290
Term newborn	16.5	51	18.1	310
1-3 days	18.5	56	18.9	300

Hgb, Hemoglobin; Hct, hematocrit; WBCs, white blood cells.
Data from Oski FA, Naiman JL. *Hematological problems in the newborn infant.* Philadelphia: WB Saunders, 1981.

The newborn infant tends to have increased hemoglobin and hematocrit levels at birth. The fetus requires extra hemoglobin to maintain appropriate oxygen transport in the relatively low oxygen pressure of the fetal environment. The newborn's hematocrit is affected by many factors, including gestational age, the presence of placental abnormalities, the speed and mode of delivery, and the length of time after delivery that the infant remains attached to the placenta (with or without cord stripping by the obstetrician). Table 4-6 lists the range of normal values for newborns.

After completion of the history and physical examination of a pediatric patient, laboratory testing may be required for further diagnostic evaluation, objective quantification of disease severity, assessment of previous management, or longitudinal follow-up (Box 4-6). Typically, diagnostic laboratory evaluation proceeds from noninvasive to invasive studies in a stepwise progression. Noninvasive diagnostic studies that may be considered for a child with a respiratory condition include chest radiography, pulmonary function testing (spirometry, lung volume determinations, Dlco [diffusing capacity of the lungs for carbon monoxide], bronchial challenge testing [exercise, cold air, and methacholine]), exercise desaturation testing, sweat chloride analysis, complete blood cell count, serum immunoglobulins (IgG, IgA, IgM, and IgE), blood gas analysis (arterial, venous, and capillary), allergy skin testing, tuberculosis skin testing, sputum cultures (bacterial, fungal, mycobacterial, and viral), barium esophagography, chest computed tomography, chest magnetic resonance imaging, overnight polysomnography, and so on. Invasive diagnostic studies that may be considered include a 24-hour pH probe study, rigid or flexible bronchoscopy, lung biopsy (bronchoscopically directed, thoracoscopic, and open), and others. Studies used to quantitate disease severity, to assess previous management, or for longitudinal follow-up include pulmonary function testing (spirometry, lung volume determinations, Dlco, bronchial challenge testing [exercise, cold air, and methacholine]), exercise desaturation testing, sputum cultures (bacterial, fungal, mycobacterial, and viral), chest radiography, chest computed tomography, and others. Although pulse oximetry may be considered a laboratory evaluation in some clinical settings, because of its widespread availability it should be considered a vital sign.[47]

THE HEALTH CARE TEAM

Because of the complexity and severity of their respiratory disease and/or contributing disorders, many children with respiratory conditions require evaluation and management by a health care team, including the following:

- Physicians
- Nurses
- RTs
- Speech pathologists
- Physical and occupational therapists

Box 4-6 | Laboratory Evaluation

- Diagnostic
- Noninvasive
- Chest radiography
- Pulmonary function testing (spirometry, lung volume determinations, Dlco, and bronchial challenge testing [exercise, cold air, and methacholine])
- Exercise desaturation testing
- Sweat chloride analysis
- Complete blood cell count
- Serum immunoglobulins (IgG, IgA, IgM, and IgE)
- Blood gas analysis (ABG, VBG, and CBG)
- Allergy skin testing
- Tuberculosis skin testing
- Sputum cultures (bacterial, fungal, mycobacterial, and viral)
- Barium esophagography
- Chest computed tomography
- Chest magnetic resonance imaging
- Overnight polysomnography
- Invasive
- 24-Hour pH probe study
- Rigid or flexible bronchoscopy
- Lung biopsy (bronchoscopically directed, thoracoscopic, and open)
- Assessment of disease severity, management, and follow-up
- Pulmonary function testing (spirometry, lung volume determinations, Dlco, and bronchial challenge testing [exercise, cold air, and methacholine])
- Exercise desaturation testing
- Sputum cultures (bacterial, fungal, mycobacterial, and viral)
- Chest radiography
- Chest computed tomography

ABG, Arterial blood gas; CBG, capillary blood gas; Dlco, diffusing capacity of the lungs for carbon monoxide; VBG, venous blood gas.

The RT has unique opportunities during airway clearance, delivery of inhaled medications, or pulmonary function testing to contribute to the care of children with respiratory conditions by obtaining additional history and observing physical findings and then communicating these observations to the appropriate member of the health care team. Because children with respiratory conditions often have multiple encounters with the RT, the RT can make repeated observations of technique for delivery of inhaled medications and airway clearance and give encouragement to the child and caregiver for good technique or report any need for changes in technique to the appropriate member of the health care team. During the health care team's decision-making process regarding further evaluation and management, such information provided by an observant and caring RT often proves invaluable.

CLINICAL HIGHLIGHT

A 6-year-old girl is brought by her mother to the pulmonary office because of recurrent pneumonia. This establishes the chief complaint. With only this information the RT faces an extensive differential diagnosis that might include CF, immunocompromise, aspiration, chronic infection, and asthma. Further questioning reveals that the child has had at least one episode of pneumonia in each of the last 4 years, usually in the winter months. Her symptoms during the acute illness include cough, fever, and dyspnea. Only one of the pneumonias resulted in hospitalization. The patient recovered completely between episodes.

At this point the RT needs to pursue additional history. The girl's growth has been good, and she does not have frequent gastrointestinal symptoms or greasy bowel movements, making CF less likely. Her mother is healthy and has no acquired immunodeficiency syndrome (AIDS) risk factors, making AIDS less likely. Each of the pneumonia episodes started with a common cold, often accompanied by wheezing. The patient has had occasional coughing when exposed to irritating smells such as cigarette smoke and cold air. During one emergency department visit, she received a nebulized medication, which greatly relieved her respiratory distress. These findings suggest that her primary disease might be asthma (Box 4-7).

The child has had no recognized exposure to tuberculosis and no foreign body aspiration history. She denies swallowing difficulty, frequent emesis (vomiting), or heartburn. She has had a red itchy rash in the elbow and knee regions in the past that her mother thinks is eczema. The patient has not had welts or hives (i.e., urticaria). The associated atopic history also points to asthma as the underlying explanation for the pneumonias.

Family History

The family history may also reveal valuable clues. In the case of this 6-year-old girl, her older brother was diagnosed with asthma as a young child; there was no recognized CF, infertile males, dextrocardia, immunodeficiency, or α_1-antiprotease deficiency. This further supports asthma as a potential cause of her recurrent pneumonia.

Box 4-7	History Taking in the Pediatric Patient with Asthma

MANIFESTATIONS
- Cough
- Wheeze
- Dyspnea
- Chest pain

AGGRAVATING FACTORS
- Upper respiratory tract infections
- Exercise or activity
- Allergens or exposures
- Irritants
- Emotions

ALLEVIATING FACTORS
- Bronchodilators
- Avoidance of aggravating factors

FAILED MEDICATION TRIALS
- Antibiotics
- Decongestants
- Humidification
- Other

ASSOCIATED CONDITIONS (REVIEW OF SYMPTOMS)
- General: poor growth, activity intolerance
- Allergy/atopy: conjunctivitis, rhinitis, eczema, urticaria
- Gastrointestinal: dysphagia, dyspepsia, emesis, steatorrhea
- Pulmonary: recurrent pneumonia, foreign body aspiration
- Ear, nose, and throat: mouth breathing, snoring
- Exposure to infections: pertussis, tuberculosis, bronchiolitis, influenza, common cold

FAMILY HISTORY
- Allergic/atopic diseases: asthma, rhinitis, eczema, urticaria, food allergy
- Cystic fibrosis
- Infertile males (history of male infertility might suggest CF and need for further diagnostic testing)
- α_1-Antiprotease deficiency
- Dextrocardia
- Immunodeficiency states

ENVIRONMENTAL EXPOSURES
- Pets (cats, dogs, ferrets, hamsters, gerbils, birds, etc.)
- Tobacco smoke
- Visible household mold
- Areas of indoor dampness or water damage

CLINICAL HIGHLIGHT

A 6-year-old patient with asthma was undergoing pulmonary function testing during a follow-up asthma clinic visit. She reported to the pulmonary nurse that her asthma had been under worse control over the past 2 months, especially during exercise and at night. The attending physician was prepared to prescribe a short course of oral prednisone and double the baseline dose of the inhaled corticosteroid. During administration of the inhaled bronchodilator as part of the pulmonary function test, the RT noticed that the metered-dose inhaler technique was quite poor (despite prior demonstration of correct technique). Further questioning identified that the spacing device prescribed to improve aerosol deposition had been "lost" several weeks ago. Neither the patient nor her family realized the significance of this loss. After discovering this, the RT told the asthma team about her concerns that neither the inhaled steroids nor the bronchodilators were likely to be optimally deposited in the lower airways. Rather than increase the patient's exposure to corticosteroids, inhaler technique was reviewed and another spacing device was prescribed. Both the patient and her mother were reeducated about the importance of adherence and the proper technique for use of a metered-dose inhaler and spacing device.

In this example, the RT's participation with the health care team helped avoid unnecessary additional medications.

CLINICAL HIGHLIGHT

A 28-month-old boy is admitted to the hospital for respiratory distress and pneumonia. During the initial assessment, the RT noted that the child is somewhat thin and anxious but sitting quietly in his mother's arms. The child's pulse is 140 beats per minute, respiratory rate is 52 breaths per minute, room air oxygen saturation is 91%, and he has mild intercostal retractions. Auscultation reveals diffuse fine crackles. The child does not have clubbing. The RT appropriately places the child on low-flow nasal cannula oxygen. Further history reveals that the boy has had recurrent cough since he was several months of age, several bouts of pneumonia, and recently has developed a productive cough and lost 3 pounds. The RT communicates these findings to the child's physician and asks if the child could have a chronic respiratory illness such as cystic fibrosis. After initiating appropriate immediate therapy, the physician obtains a sweat chloride analysis that is positive and refers the child to a nearby cystic fibrosis center for further evaluation and management.

In this example, the RT's brief assessment and recognition that the child not only had an acute respiratory illness but also a probable chronic pulmonary disease led to communication with the child's physician. This communication resulted in further diagnostic testing, leading to a diagnosis and referral to more specialized care.

KEY POINTS

- Initial stabilization of the newborn minimally involves the following:
  Drying and warming the infant
  Opening and clearing the infant's airway if indicated
  Stimulating the infant to breathe
- Direct laryngotracheal suctioning should occur in the nonvigorous (i.e., no or poor respiratory effort, heart rate < 100, or poor muscle tone) meconium-stained newborn.
- Apgar score is an evaluation of newborns based on five factors: heart rate, respiratory effort, muscle tone, reflex irritability, and skin color. Apgar scoring is performed at 1 minute and 5 minutes after birth. Additional scoring may be indicated when the 5-minute Apgar is less than 7.
- Small-for-gestational-age infants have a birth weight less than the tenth percentile for gestational age. An infant whose birth weight is more than the ninetieth percentile is large for gestational age.
- Critical vital signs for initial assessment of the newborn include the following:
  Heart rate (120-170 beats per minute)
  Respiratory rate (40-60 breaths per minute)
  Blood pressure
  Temperature $97.6 \pm 1°F$ (axillary) and $99.6 \pm 1°F$ (rectal)
- Periodic breathing is normal in the neonate. Apnea is diagnosed by a 20-second cessation of respiration.
- Grunting, nasal flaring, and retractions indicate respiratory distress in the normal newborn. The Silverman score provides an objective measure of newborn respiratory distress.
- Transillumination of the neonatal chest wall with a high-energy light source can rapidly diagnose a pneumonthorax. A pneumothorax will "light up" brighter than normal lung tissue.
- Neurological examination of the newborn involves observing the infant's response to the environment (bright lights and sounds), muscle tone, and presence of various reflexes (e.g., grasp, plantar grasp, Moro, and stepping reflexes).
- Examination of a pediatric patient may occur in the lap of a caregiver. A crying child is difficult to examine.
- Head bobbing is sign of respiratory distress in the small child or infant.
- Respiratory rate varies in the pediatric patient with activity level but is still a sensitive indicator of the severity of underlying lung disease.

ASSESSMENT QUESTIONS

See Evolve Resources for answers.

1. What is the proper procedure to implement for an infant known to have experienced meconium aspiration before birth?
   A. The obstetrician should suction the mouth, nose, and pharynx after delivery of the head, but before delivery of the shoulders.
   B. Intubate immediately and aspirate the trachea, using a meconium aspirator regardless of whether the infant is vigorous.
   C. Treat the infant exactly as if meconium was not present.
   D. Intubate and suction only if the infant is not vigorous; otherwise, follow the normal resuscitation procedures.

2. Appropriate stimulation of a newborn includes which of the following:
   A. Flicking the bottoms of the feet
   B. Gently shaking the shoulders
   C. Drying with a warm towel
   D. Gently rubbing the back
   E. A and B
   F. A, C, and D

3. The Apgar score includes which of the following criteria:
   A. Color
   B. Evaluation of the Moro reflex
   C. Heart rate
   D. Reflex irritability
   E. A and B
   F. A, C, and D
   G. C and D

4. The best indicator of an infant's overall cardiopulmonary status immediately after birth is
   A. Heart rate
   B. Apgar score
   C. Color
   D. Respiratory effort

5. The ideal time to assess the gestational age of a newborn is
   A. Within the first 30 minutes after birth
   B. Within the first hour of life
   C. Within the first 12 hours of life
   D. Within the first 24 hours of life

6. Ideally, gestational age is evaluated on the basis of
   A. The gestational duration since the mother's last menstrual cycle
   B. Prenatal ultrasound evaluations
   C. The Ballard scoring system
   D. All of the above

7. Apnea is a pathological condition in which breathing ceases for a period of _____ seconds or longer.
   A. 10
   B. 20
   C. 45
   D. 60

8. Signs of respiratory distress in a newborn include which of the following:
   A. Vesicular breath sounds
   B. Grunting
   C. Nasal flaring
   D. B and C
   E. A and B

9. The umbilical cord normally has _____ artery(ies) and _____ vein(s).
   A. 1 and 1
   B. 2 and 2
   C. 1 and 2
   D. 2 and 1

10. An 8 month old presents with head bobbing. The following is true about head bobbing:
    A. It usually suggests a brainstem lesion.
    B. It is a voluntary action that can be stopped on command.
    C. It usually suggests respiratory distress, airway obstruction, or decreased lung compliance.
    D. It is unrelated to cardiopulmonary disease.

11. Palpation of a patient's chest produces a vibration of the chest wall during quiet breathing. This suggests partial obstruction of the large airways by mucus. The name of this sign is:
    A. Fine crackles
    B. Rhonchal or bronchial fremitus
    C. Clubbing
    D. Pectus carinatum
    E. Stridor

12. An infant produces an audible noise that appears to be stridor. The following is true about stridor:
    A. It is a high-pitched, monophonic, audible noise.
    B. It may occur during inspiration or expiration or may be biphasic.
    C. Patients with laryngomalacia or subglottic stenosis may have inspiratory stridor.
    D. Patients with a double aortic arch compressing the trachea, or tracheomalacia, may have expiratory stridor.
    E. All of the above.

13. A teenager has a temperature of 38.5°C, a respiratory rate of 28 breaths per minute, increased thoracic anteroposterior diameter, minimal subcostal retractions, and fine and coarse crackles heard over the right and left upper lobes. Further evaluation reveals mild digital clubbing of the fingers. This child probably has the following underlying disease:
    A. Asthma
    B. Gastroesophageal reflux
    C. Bilateral bronchomalacia
    D. Cystic fibrosis
    E. Acute respiratory distress syndrome

14. In the emergency room, the respiratory therapist is asked to give a 2 year old in respiratory distress an albuterol treatment. Pretreatment assessment reveals a mildly uncomfortable afebrile child with a respiratory rate of 36 breaths per minute, mild subcostal retractions, and expiratory wheezes best heard over the right middle and lower lobes. Posttreatment assessment is unchanged except that the respiratory rate is now 32 breaths per minute. A brief history reveals that coughing began abruptly several days ago and wheezing was noted this morning. The family has no history of atopic disease (allergic rhinitis, allergic conjunctivitis, asthma, or atopic dermatitis). This child was previously healthy with no history of chest disease. The respiratory therapist speaks with the attending physician and suggests that the child most likely has the following disorder/disease:
    A. Pneumonia
    B. Cystic fibrosis
    C. Foreign body aspiration
    D. Laryngeal cleft
    E. Double outlet right ventricle

References

1. Bernstein S, Heimler R, Sasidharan P: Approaching the management of the neonatal intensive care unit graduate through history and physical assessment, *Pediatr Clin North Am* 45:97, 1998.
2. Wolkoff L, Davis J: Delivery room resuscitation of the newborn, *Clin Perinatol* 26:641, 1999.
3. Chahine A, Ricketts R: Resuscitation of the surgical neonate, *Clin Perinatol* 26:693, 1999.
4. Kattwinkel J, Niermeyer S, Nadkami V, et al: An advisory statement from the pediatric working group of the international liaison committee on resuscitation, *Pediatrics* 103:E56, 1999.
5. Kattwinkel J, Perlman JM, Aziz K, et al: Neonatal resuscitation: 2010. American heart association (AHA) guidelines for cardiopulmonary resuscitation (CPR) and emergency cardiovascular care (ECC), *Pediatrics* 126:E1400–1413, 2010.
6. Vain NE, Szyld EF, Prudent LM, et al: Oropharyngeal and nasopharyngeal suctioning of meconium-stained neonates before delivery of their shoulders: multicentre, randomized controlled trial, *Lancet* 364:597, 2004.
7. Nadkarni V, Hazinski MF, Zideman D: Pediatric resuscitation: an advisory statement from the pediatric working group of the international liaison committee on resuscitation, *Circulation* 95 2185, 1997.
8. Juretschke L: Apgar scoring: its use and meaning for today's newborn, *Neonatal Network* 19:17, 2000.
9. Weinberger B, Anwar M, Hegyi T, et al: Antecedents and neonatal consequences of low Apgar scores in preterm newborns: a population study, *Arch Pediatr Adolesc Med* 154:294, 2000.
10. Jain L, Ferre C, Vidyasagar D, et al: Cardiopulmonary resuscitation of apparently stillborn infants: survival and long-term outcome, *J Pediatr* 118:778, 1991.
11. Catlin E, Carpenter MW, Brann IV BS, et al: The Apgar score revisited: influence of gestational age, *J Pediatr* 109:865, 1986.
12. Donovan E, Tyson J, Ehrenkranz R, et al: Inaccuracy of Ballard scores before 28 weeks' gestation, *J Pediatr* 135:147, 1999.
13. Sanders M, Allen M, Alexander GR, et al: Gestational age assessment in preterm neonates weighing less than 1500. grams, *Pediatrics* 88:542, 1991.
14. Ballard JL, Khoury JC, Wedig KL, et al: New Ballard score to include extremely premature infants, *J Pediatr* 199:417, 1991.
15. Thomas P, Peabody J, Turnier V, et al: A new look at intrauterine growth and the impact of race, altitude, and gender, *Pediatrics* 106:e21, 2000.
16. Dunster K: Physiologic variability in the perinatal period, *Clin Perinatol* 26:801, 1999.
17. Rosenkrantz T: Polycythemia and hyperviscosity in the newborn, *Semin Thromb Hemost* 29:515, 2003.
18. Bhutani V, Gourley G, Adler S, et al: Noninvasive measurement of total serum bilirubin in a multiracial predischarge newborn population to assess the risk of severe hyperbilirubinemia, *Pediatrics* 106:e17, 2000.
19. Rigatto H, Brady JP: Periodic breathing and apnea in preterm infants: hypoxia as a primary event, *Pediatrics* 50:219, 1972.
20. Ackerman NB, Bell RE, DeLemos RA: Differential pulmonary auscultation in neonates, *Clin Pediatr* 21:566, 1982.
21. Page J, Hosking M: An approach to the neonate with sudden dysrhythmia: diagnosis, mechanisms, and management, *Neonatal Network* 16:7, 1997.
22. Blakelock RT, Harding JE, Kolbe A, et al: Gastroschisis: can the mortality be avoided? *Pediatr Surg Int* 12:276, 1997.
23. Furdon S, Clark D: Differentiating scalp swelling in the newborn, *Adv Neonatal Care* 1:22, 2001.
24. Davis DJ: Neonatal subgaleal hemorrhage: diagnosis and management, *Can Med Assoc J* 164:1452, 2001.
25. Bodurtha J: Assessment of the newborn with dysmorphic features, *Neonatal Network* 18:27, 1999.
26. Jones KL: *Smith's recognizable patterns of human malformation*, ed 4, Philadelphia, 1988, WB Saunders.
27. Dennison WM: The Pierre Robin syndrome, *Pediatrics* 36:336, 1965.
28. Hashimoto BE, Filly RA, Callen PW: Sonographic diagnosis of clubfoot in utero, *J Ultrasound Med* 5:81, 1986.
29. Fernach S: Common orthopedic problems of the newborn, *Nurs Clin North Am* 33:583, 1998.
30. Majnemer A, Brownstein A, Kadanoff R, et al: A comparison of neurobehavioral performance of healthy term and low risk pre-term infants at term, *Dev Med Child Neurol* 34:417, 1992.
31. Glezen WP, Greenberg SB, Atmar RL, et al: Impact of respiratory virus infections on persons with chronic underlying conditions, *JAMA* 283:499, 2000.
32. DiFranza JR, Aligne CA, Weitzman M: Prenatal and postnatal environmental tobacco smoke exposure and children's health, *Pediatrics* 113:1007, 2004.
33. Morley CJ, Thorton AJ, Fowler MA, et al: Respiratory rate and severity of illness in babies under 6 months old, *Arch Dis Child* 65:834, 1990.
34. Harari M, Spooner V, Meisner S, et al: Clinical signs of pneumonia in children, *Lancet* 338:928, 1991.
35. Margolis P, Gadomski A: Does this infant have pneumonia? *JAMA* 279:308, 1998.
36. Iliff A, Lee VA: Pulse rate, respiratory rate, and body temperature of children between two months and eighteen years of age, *Child Dev* 4:237, 1952.
37. Rusconi F, Castagneto M, Porta N, et al: Reference values for respiratory rate in the first three years of life, *Pediatrics* 94:350, 1994.
38. Loudon R, Murphy RL: State of the art: lung sounds, *Am Rev Respir Dis* 130:663, 1984.
39. Mikami R, Murao M, Cugell D, et al: International symposium on lung sounds, *Chest* 92:342, 1987.
40. Cugell DW: Lung sound nomenclature, *Am Rev Respir Dis* 136:1016, 1987.
41. Eavey RD: A sound workup for evaluating airway obstructions, *Contemp Pediatrics* 3:78, 1986.
42. Tan HK, Holinger LD: How to evaluate and manage stridor in children, *J Respir Dis* 15:245, 1994.
43. Cotton RT, Reilly JS: Stridor and airway obstruction. In CD Bluestone, SE Stool, MD Scheetz, editors: *Pediatric otolaryngology*, Philadelphia, 1990, WB Saunders, pp 1098–1111.
44. Piirila P, Sovijarvi AR: Crackles: recording, analysis and clinical significance, *Eur Respir J* 8:2139, 1995.
45. Zitell BJ, Davis HW: *Atlas of pediatric physical diagnosis*, Philadelphia, 2002, WB Saunders.
46. Myers KA, Farquhar DR: Does this patient have clubbing? *JAMA* 286:341, 2001.
47. Mower WR, Sachs C, Nicklin EL, et al: Pulse oximetry as a fifth pediatric vital sign, *Pediatrics* 99:681, 1997.

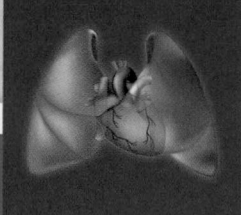

Chapter 5

Pulmonary Function Testing and Bedside Pulmonary Mechanics

KATRINA M. HYNES, CARL D. MOTTRAM

OUTLINE

LEARNING OBJECTIVES

After reading this chapter the reader will be able to:

1. Define the terminology and various abbreviations used in describing specific aspects of interpreting pulmonary function tests
2. Identify specific techniques used to elicit acceptable and repeatable results in children when performing pulmonary function tests
3. Describe the special challenges specific to neonates, infants, and children when performing pulmonary function tests or assessing respiratory function
4. Appraise the standard and alternative instrumentation techniques available for pulmonary function testing of the newborn and the child
5. Differentiate among the infant, child, and adult chest wall and pulmonary mechanics that affect correct interpretation of the pulmonary function data
6. Compare the various techniques available for measuring airway function in both infants and children

7. Compare the various techniques available for measuring lung volumes in both infants and children
8. Explain the methods used to challenge, or provoke, the airways to assess more subtle lung function abnormalities or airway reactivity, and their role in developing a treatment
9. Recognize the cut point for an abnormal exhaled nitric oxide test
10. Distinguish the difference between resistance and reactance measured during impulse oscillometry testing
11. Describe the various tests and techniques used at the bedside to assess pulmonary function and lung mechanics in the spontaneously breathing and mechanically ventilated patient

Airway resistance
"All-age" reference equations
Body plethysmography
Bronchial provocation
Cardiopulmonary exercise testing
  (CPET)
Diffusing capacity
Dynamic lung compliance

Exhaled nitric oxide
Functional residual capacity
Hug technique
Impulse oscillometry
Lung compliance
Pulmonary mechanics
Rapid shallow breathing index
Reactance

Respiratory inductance
  plethysmography
Specific conductance
Spirometry
Tension time index
Thoracic gas volume
Transpulmonary pressure
Work of breathing

INTRODUCTION

Pulmonary function testing (PFT) is an objective measurement of the respiratory system under various conditions of normal, disease, and stress states. Pulmonary function measurements can be used as a primary diagnostic tool or to frequently monitor disease progression by comparing previous or subsequent assessments.[1,2] PFT results corroborate a diagnosis suspected from the other components of the pulmonary assessment, primarily the patient history and physical examination. The American Thoracic Society and European Respiratory Society (ATS-ERS) publishes standards and guidelines for testing system performance characteristics, quality control, and test methodology in adults, adolescents, and preschool-aged children.[3] The pulmonary function laboratory equipment quality control program needs to follow these recommendations to ensure accurate test results regardless of the size and age of the subject being tested.

Assessing whether a specific measurement is "normal" may be complex because of the wide range of variability in normal children. Recent reference equations have been published for spirometry, diffusing capacity, and other variables that help to define lung function in young subjects. The **"all-age" reference equations** published in 2012 by the European Respiratory Society Global Lung Initiative taskforce define normal values for common spirometry indices down to 3 years of age.[4] PFT measurements remain an integral component in evaluation and lengthy follow-up of children with pulmonary dysfunction over time. PFT measurements evaluate the degree of illness and quantitatively determine the efficacy of various therapeutic interventions.

Laboratory testing includes measurement of lung compliance, assessment of airway caliber, lung volumes, gas exchange, and airway inflammation.[5,6] These tests can be performed in a laboratory setting or at the bedside and may include maneuvers that require active or passive participation by the subject.

Bedside pulmonary function studies apply PFT systems in the intensive care unit at the bedside to aid in mechanical ventilator management. Mechanical ventilators now provide the opportunity to measure and display airway graphics of pressure, flow, and volume on the ventilator screen. This provides real-time displays and is useful when assessing the interaction between the ventilator and the patient. These measurements are used to optimize ventilator support and to reduce the potential complications of positive-pressure ventilation. Because of the differences in purpose, test conditions, and clinical application, these types of studies at the bedside are differentiated from standard laboratory PFT studies.

DEFINITIONS

The terminology used to describe tests that are included in specific orders may vary across institutions. "Complete pulmonary function testing" may denote an extensive testing protocol at one institution or a more select group of tests at another. Similar variations exist for "lung function survey" and "pulmonary screening." Therefore, clinicians need to be familiar with the specific testing protocols within their institution.

In this chapter, the term **spirometry** represents flow-volume or volume–time measurements of basic lung function parameters. Spirometric measurements include forced vital capacity (FVC), forced expiratory volume in 1 second (FEV_1), the ratio of FEV_1 to FVC (FEV_1/FVC), forced expiratory flow at 25% to 75% of vital capacity (FEF_{25-75}), and forced expiratory flow at 50% of vital capacity (FEF_{50}). Lung volumes describe the measurements of **thoracic gas volume,** functional residual capacity (FRC), residual volume (RV), total lung capacity (TLC), and the ratio of RV to TLC (RV/TLC). Consider other measurements, such as carbon monoxide diffusing capacity, resistance or conductance, compliance, and maximal voluntary ventilation as separate tests. Sophisticated and seldom used tests are not addressed in this chapter, and more extensive texts for additional information are available. [1,2,9-12]

Bedside PFT refers to those tests often performed at the bedside, typically in the intensive care unit, including tidal volume (V_T), vital capacity (VC), minute ventilation ($\dot{V}_E$), peak expiratory flow rate (PEFR), and respiratory muscle strength measurements of maximal inspiratory pressure (MIP) and maximal expiratory pressures (MEP). **Pulmonary mechanics** are the interaction of forces and physical principles that determine the characteristics of gas movement into and out of the lungs. Elasticity of the lung and chest wall, resistance to flow through the airways, and the action of the respiratory muscles (diaphragm, intercostal muscles, and accessory muscles) are measurable forces affecting ventilation.

MECHANICS OF BREATHING IN NEWBORNS

With the first breaths of extrauterine life, a newborn must replace the in utero lung fluid with air. Surface tension forces in the fluid-filled lung require high negative pressures within the chest to establish normal air volume in the lungs. Newborns, particularly those born prematurely with respiratory distress syndrome, have low lung compliance. More pressure, or energy, is required to provide the normal amount of air volume brought into the baby's lungs with each breath. Because the newborn's ribs are mostly cartilage, the chest wall is flexible. With significant lung disease, the infant's chest wall may actually be more compliant than the lungs, causing retractions, in which the ribs and sternum distort inward during inspiration instead of expanding the lungs. The lung-thorax mechanical relationship is less of the traditional "bag in a box" analogy and more like a "bag in a bag."

The combination of **lung compliance** (C) and airway resistance (Raw) is the major force opposing inspiration, whereas elastic recoil is the force responsible for passive normal exhalation. When measured under static conditions (i.e., no gas flow into or out of the lungs), C is an assessment of the elasticity (compliance) of the total respiratory system (Crs).[13]

Lung Inflation and Transpulmonary Pressure

For both spontaneous and mechanically assisted breaths, the change in pressure within the airways is the driving force for gas movement into and out of the lungs. During spontaneous inspiration, moving the diaphragm and other muscles of ventilation expands the chest volume, which creates subatmospheric pressure in the thorax. During mechanically assisted breathing the ventilator applies positive pressure to the airways. Expiration is usually considered passive, but in fact the elastic recoil of the lungs and chest wall that causes gas movement out of the lungs requires energy.

Pulmonary mechanics are calculated by determining the change in pressure across the lung simultaneously with flow and volume measurements. During mechanically assisted ventilation, pressure in the airway is measured at the endotracheal tube. Gas flow and airway pressure are measured with a sealed face mask for spontaneous breathing studies. Pleural pressure may be approximated with a catheter placed in the esophagus.[13-15] The catheter is connected to a pressure transducer and either is filled with fluid or has an air-filled balloon at its tip.

Transpulmonary pressure is the pressure exerted on the lungs for gas movement; it is the difference between pleural and airway pressure. Pleural pressure measurements may not always be performed in assessing pulmonary mechanics for ventilator–patient management. In general, under these circumstances it is assumed that the pressure in the large airways equalizes to the distal airways in the lungs. In this case the compliance measurements are actually of the respiratory system, including the chest wall, rather than of the lungs alone.

NEONATAL PULMONARY FUNCTION TESTING IN THE LABORATORY

A laboratory offering PFT for infants must be prepared to meet the special needs of these patients.[12] Commercially available equipment typically uses the most technically advanced flow sensors and analyzers and may be expensive for a pulmonary laboratory to purchase. Before pursuing this type of testing, the laboratory should thoroughly evaluate its expectations, goals, and resources available to perform quality testing.[2]

Routine infant and adolescent PFTs require certain technical obstacles be overcome. The use of computers and precision electronics surmounts many of these challenges, which include high respiratory rates, the need for low dead space in the airway connection, and accurate measurements of very small gas volumes. Current instrumentation employs rapid-response gas flow sensors that are easily calibrated, remain stable, and are accurate in a measurement range that extends to the gas volumes of the smallest newborns.[1,16] A more complete discussion of equipment characteristics can be found in other sources.[2]

In infant testing, the subject may need to be lightly sedated in the laboratory for 2 to 3 hours to complete a full set of studies. Sedation carries some risk, and testing should not be viewed as routine. In a study by Heinstein et al., the NPO guidelines from the hospital sedation policy allowed infants younger than 6 months to receive formula and solids for up to 6 hours, breast milk for up to 4 hours, and clear liquids for up to 2 hours before sedation. Children who are 6 months or older may receive solids and liquids for up to 6 hours and clear liquids for up to 2 hours before sedation.[17]

Some drugs may alter pulmonary mechanics or the normal characteristics of breathing. Chloral hydrate is preferred by many laboratories and can be administered as an oral solution or rectally. The recommended dosage ranges from 50 to 90 mg/kg with a maximum dosage of 1 g given. Although normally a safe sedative for this purpose, using chloral hydrate when oxygen saturations are reduced increases the risk of respiratory distress. The infant should be continuously monitored from the time of drug administration until discharge.[17]

A face mask is required when testing neonates and infants. To ensure accurate testing, minimize both mask resistance and mask dead space volume during the measurement. Exercise caution, using a face mask can cause trigeminal nerve stimulation and induce vagal reflexes that may alter the pattern of heart or respiratory rhythm. A physician, emergency supplies, and equipment for infant resuscitation must be readily available in the laboratory area.

Plethysmography (Baby Box)

The principle of **body plethysmography** is similar to that of the gas concentration techniques.[18] In a closed system the product of pressure and volume is constant (Boyle's law). When performing pulmonary function testing in infants, the child is sedated and placed in the supine position. A tight-fitting mask with a small dead space volume is placed over the infant's nose and mouth. Putty is placed around the edges to create an airtight seal (Figure 5-1, *B*). Rapidly moving valves may make airway occlusions at end inspiration or end expiration for determination of thoracic gas volume (TGV) and airway resistance. The infant does not pant; however, tidal breaths may be shallow. Therefore the pressure transducers and flow sensors must be critically precise and accurate. In addition, the infant body box is relatively small and

temperature changes can drastically alter these measurements. Therefore the temperature in the box must be controlled and the air vented.

Signal-to-noise ratios are particularly critical in an infant plethysmograph. Although the child is motionless, safety features must permit rapid access to the box and the baby. The breathing apparatus should be easily removable in case the child is in distress or vomits. The advantage of plethysmography in infants is that it accurately measures TGV, the total gas in the thorax, and thus FRC may be determined. FRC is the easiest volume for the subject to reproduce consistently. Because the infant is not capable of performing a voluntary maximal inspiration nor expiration, residual volume and TLC cannot be obtained in the traditional manner. However, if the infant pulmonary function system is capable of performing raised volumes and forced thoracic compressions, then a full set of fractional lung volumes can be estimated.[2]

Functional residual capacity (FRC) is the resting volume of the lung at end expiration.[5] The chest wall of newborns is very compliant, and supine FRC values are lower than adult values—approximately 20% of total lung capacity. Preterm infants with respiratory distress syndrome have an abnormally low FRC because of alveolar collapse. The low FRC value results in low lung volume, low compliance, and increased work of breathing to achieve adequate tidal volume. Figure 5-2 shows tidal volume–pressure loops at various FRC levels. Note that the slope of compliance is best, and thus work of breathing is least, at a normal FRC. Some infants maintain a dynamic FRC at this level by incorporating breathing strategies that limit the expiratory flow rate, such as expiratory grunting and increased postinspiratory diaphragmatic muscle tone. Neonates with severe respiratory distress syndrome need positive airway pressure during expiration to establish a normal FRC.

Several methods may be used to determine FRC. Systems using helium dilution and nitrogen washout techniques are basically scaled-down versions of adult systems. The helium dilution technique uses a closed-circuit

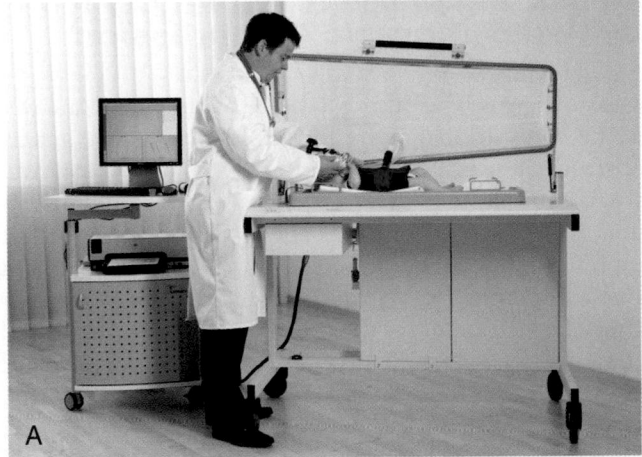

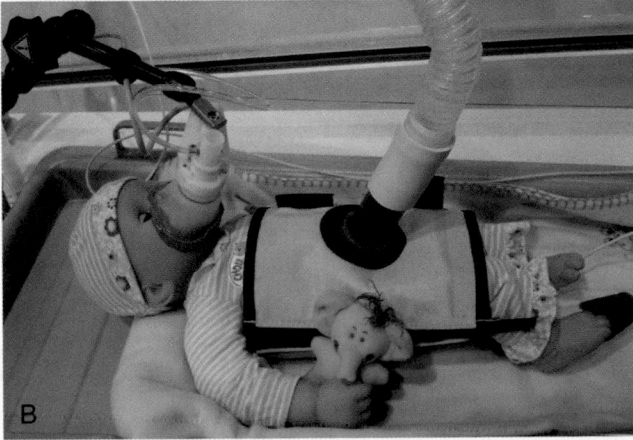

FIGURE 5-1 **A,** Positioning a patient in a "baby box" plethysmograph. **B,** Close-up of sedated baby with face mask, putty to form a seal, and pneumatic belt to perform the "hug technique."

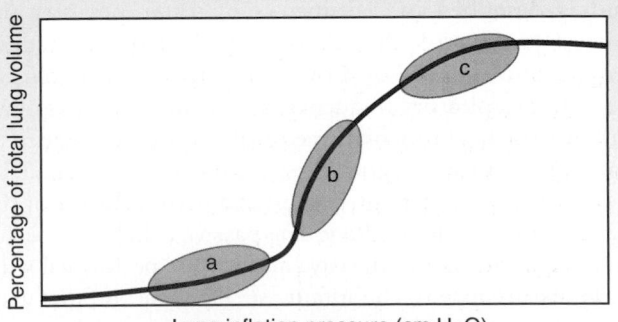

FIGURE 5-2 Volume–pressure loops of tidal breathing at various levels of functional residual capacity (FRC). **A,** Low FRC; **B,** normal FRC; **C,** elevated FRC.

system. Applying petroleum jelly to the edges of a disposable mask is helpful to ensure an airtight seal with no leaks on the infant's face. The infant breathes the helium–oxygen mixture while connected to a spirometer, until the helium concentration equilibrates between the circuit and lungs. The reduction in measured helium concentration in the circuit is equated to the FRC. The helium dilution method may be used for very sick infants with a fraction of inspired oxygen as high as 0.95.[6]

The nitrogen washout method also uses a sealed face mask. The infant breathes 100% oxygen in an open circuit, which displaces nitrogen in the lungs. The circuit must have no gas leaks. The system measures the volume of nitrogen washed out of the lungs. This method cannot measure the FRC if the infant's fraction of inspired oxygen is greater than 0.65.[19] Atelectasis may result from washout of poorly ventilated and partially obstructed areas of the lung.

The helium dilution and nitrogen washout techniques are described in further detail in the pediatric pulmonary function section of this chapter.

Measuring Static Compliance and Airway Resistance

Static compliance (Crs) describes the elastic properties of the total respiratory system. Crs is measured during no airflow, using the passive exhalation occlusion technique, and assesses elasticity of the respiratory system.[6,18,20] Volume and pressure are measured with a pneumotachometer at two points of a passive resting exhalation. The airway is momentarily occluded at end inspiration by a shutter placed between the face mask and the pneumotachometer to stimulate the Hering-Breuer reflex. The occlusion creates an apneic pause and relaxes the respiratory muscles. Pressure is measured during the occlusion, and passive exhaled volume is measured after the shutter opens. Crs is calculated by dividing the total passive expiratory volume by the corresponding pressure change at the airway opening.

Airway resistance (Raw) reflects the nonelastic airway and tissue forces resisting gas flow. Raw is calculated from the ratio of airway occlusion pressure to expiratory flow and is described in centimeters of water per liter per second (cm H_2O/L/s). Raw is dependent on the radius, length, and number of airways and varies with volume, flow, and respiratory frequency. The small diameters of an infant's tracheobronchial tree result in high resistance to gas flow. Airway irregularities; partial blocks caused by mucus, tumor, or foreign bodies; and partial closure of the glottis can also elevate Raw. The passive exhalation occlusion technique is noninvasive and can be performed with little disturbance to the infant.[21,22] However, infants with severe lung disease have an increased respiratory drive, and it may not be possible to induce a Hering-Breuer response.[6]

Raw measurements may be derived from body plethysmograph data, using a modified infant incubator as the enclosure. Because a pulmonary plethysmograph measures lung volumes, FRC and TLC measurements are acquired along with Raw.

Another method of determining Raw is to generate random noise signals at high frequencies at the mouth while the infant is breathing normal tidal breaths through a mouthpiece or mask. This technique is known as forced oscillation and is described later in this chapter. Similar to the plethysmograph, the forced oscillation technique may also be another method used to determine thoracic gas volume measurements. This technique is tolerated well by the infant with minimal discomfort.

Crs and Raw measurements may be useful in the following patients:

- Those receiving diuretics for chronic lung disease such as bronchopulmonary dysplasia
- Patients undergoing high-frequency ventilation
- Those with meconium aspiration syndrome
- Subsequent to extracorporeal membrane oxygenation
- Patients with respiratory syncytial virus infections and pneumonias
- Patients with diaphragmatic hernia
- Patients receiving aerosolized bronchodilator therapy

Measuring Maximal Expiratory Flow by Rapid Thoracic Compression Technique

Measuring gas flow during a forced expiratory maneuver is the conventional procedure used to evaluate airway obstruction in a cooperative infant. A relatively noninvasive technique to generate a partial expiratory flow volume (PEFV) curve in infants allows the measurement of expiratory flows during a forced maneuver in infants and small children.[3,6,18] A rapid thoracic compression or "hug" is delivered to the sleeping infant's chest and abdomen with an inflatable jacket to produce a forced expiration (Figure 5-1, *B*). A pneumotachometer with a sealed face mask measures exhaled gas flow. The flow at the end-expiratory point of a normal resting tidal breath (FRC) is measured on the PEFV curve. This flow value, the maximal expiratory flow at FRC, is reported as liters per second (Figure 5-3). Multiple tests at various jacket inflation pressures are conducted for a "best test" assessment.

The maximal expiratory flow test can demonstrate flow limitation in airway disease and is valuable for evaluating the response to bronchodilator therapy in infants.[23] PEFV studies are often performed before and after aerosolized bronchodilator therapy. An increase in maximal expiratory flow at FRC by at least 20% demonstrates a positive response to bronchodilator therapy. A significant number of infants with chronic lung disease have a negative bronchodilator response.[24]

Problems with the "**hug technique**" occur infrequently in experienced hands. The clinician must avoid collapsing the upper airway as a result of hyperextending the neck,

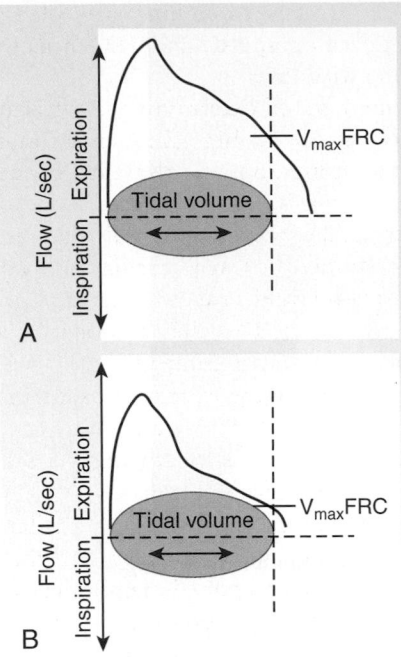

FIGURE 5-3 Partial expiratory flow–volume (PEFV) curves with identification of maximal expiratory flow at FRC (VmaxFRC), demonstrating a normal resting tidal breath and one with flow limitation. **A,** Normal; **B,** Abnormal (flow limited).

resulting in forced airflow limitation solely because of positioning. Other types of upper airway impedance may also affect the accuracy of the intrathoracic flow rates, and reflex glottis closure may complicate testing.[6]

Thoracoabdominal Motion Analysis by Respiratory Inductance Plethysmography

Respiratory inductance plethysmography (RIP) is a method used to indirectly measure tidal breathing over a wide age range, including infants. Compliant elastic bands are wrapped around the abdomen and chest of the infant. These bands are used to analyze thoracoabdominal motion in addition to the degree to which chest and abdominal excursions are out of phase (asynchronous). Thoracoabdominal asynchrony (TAA) should increase with increased respiratory resistance (upper or lower airways, lung tissue), decreased lung compliance (CL) (parenchymal disease), and increased chest wall compliance (floppy rib cage, neuromuscular disease). RIP can be calibrated to measure VT or uncalibrated so that the chest and abdominal signal reflect the timing and direction of volume change but not absolute volume changes. Because body movement and nonsinusoidal breathing can make accurate measurements challenging, data collection should occur during natural, quiet breathing, which most often occurs during sleep in infants. Although there are multiple limitations to take into consideration and a limited number of studies, RIP may be a useful screening tool in overall respiratory system function in infants.[3]

PEDIATRIC PULMONARY FUNCTION TESTING IN THE LABORATORY

Pediatric Testing

The greatest obstacle to obtaining satisfactory pulmonary function measurements in children lies in enlisting their cooperation and effort. Clinicians who work predominantly with children develop their own unique systems for making children comfortable and eliciting an appropriate testing effort. Conversely, pulmonary function laboratories that have limited experience with children often do not obtain satisfactory cooperation, and therefore the test results are inconclusive and the information may not be useful.

Several key factors are common to successful approaches in performing PFT on children. The testing environment or laboratory should have a warm and friendly atmosphere with pediatric-oriented pictures and toys. Each portion of the testing procedure should be carefully explained at an age-appropriate level, and the child's participation should be elicited in a playful rather than challenging fashion. For children undergoing their first PFT procedure, several efforts may be required before a satisfactory test is achieved. There is no substitute for patience and tolerance in this setting. Satisfactory performance can generally be achieved in the 5- or 6-year-old child, but some 8-, 9-, and 10-year-old children continue to have difficulty. Although uncommon, 3-year-old children may be able to do well, and good results have been reported more commonly among 4-year-old children. If the child is unable to perform satisfactorily at the first session, repeated attempts at subsequent visits should be encouraged, because most children learn quickly and often do much better at the next opportunity.

Spirometry

Spirometry is a common test performed in the pediatric subject and requires active participation and cooperation to elicit acceptable and repeatable results. Spirometers are categorized into two general types: volume and flow. Volume spirometers collect the expired air and divide the subject's expiratory time to derive flow. These spirometers are large because they are required to measure up to 8 L of air.[25] Flow-based spirometers use a pneumotachometer, or some other flow-sensing device, to measure flow, which in turn is multiplied by the subject's expiratory time to calculate volume. Flow spirometers are more common because they are inherently smaller than a volume spirometer and can easily be integrated into a variety of testing systems. An assortment of flow-based spirometers are available, including handheld devices, standalone systems integrated with a computer or laptop, and spirometers that are a component of a complex testing system that might include a body plethysmograph.

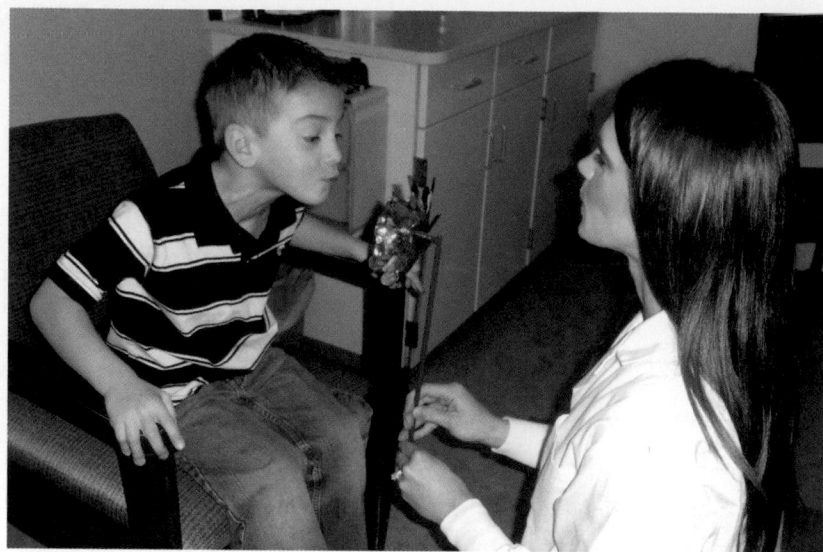

FIGURE 5-4   A child practices blowing out using a pinwheel before spirometry testing.

The FVC maneuver performed during spirometry is composed of three major components: the deep breath, the initial blast, and exhaling until empty. The latter two, however, are inconsequential if the subject does not take a deep breath. Demonstrating test performance before testing can greatly enhance the success rate of getting results that represent the subject's true lung function. The practitioner can use visual aids to help the child understand the test expectations. In Figure 5-4, the child uses a pinwheel to practice the technique needed for spirometry testing. This fun, interactive method demonstrates to the young subject the need for both a quick initial blast out and also to sustain "the blow" to keep the pinwheel spinning as long as possible. Some spirometers are integrated with computers and have software with interactive incentive screens. These screens, through a variety of methods (e.g., blowing out candles on a cake), give feedback to the young child to blast hard and fast and keep blowing until completely empty.

Following are the ATS-ERS acceptability criteria for a maneuver:

Free from artifact
· Cough during the first second of exhalation
· Glottis closure that influences the measurement
· Early termination or cutoff
· Effort that is not maximal throughout
· Leak
· Obstructed mouthpiece

Good start
· Extrapolated volume 5% of FVC or 0.15 L, whichever is greater

Satisfactory exhalation
· Duration of 6 seconds (3 seconds for children younger than 10 years old) or
· A plateau in the volume–time curve

The maneuver is considered "usable" if there is no cough in the first second and/or glottis closure that influence the measurement.[25] Usable maneuvers typically underestimate the subject's vital capacity, so usable variables would include peak flow, $FEV_{0.5}$, and FEV_1.

The traditional volume–time spirogram (Figure 5-5) is used to calculate timed flows such as FEV_1 and FEF_{25-75} and measure the FVC. It is also used to assess the end-of-test criteria of reaching a plateau.

Flow–Volume Loop

The flow–volume loop and its specific measurements are shown in Figure 5-6. The flow-volume curve is useful in identifying the quality of the maneuver, and its shape can be characteristic of a specific disease process. One advantage to the flow–volume representation is its clear depiction of whether subjects exhale to RV or whether they terminate their effort prematurely (Figure 5-7). "Early termination" is assessed by how gradual flow approaches zero and the duration of the exhalation effort displayed on the volume–time graph. An example of early termination is glottis closure which can be common in young subjects (Figure 5-8, *B*). Other acceptability indicators, such as cough in the first second (Figure 5-8, *A*) and excessive back extrapolation volume (Figure 5-8, *C*), are easily identified by the effect on the F-V curve. In addition, the shape of a flow–volume loop may also be of value in determining extrathoracic and intrathoracic sources of airway obstruction. Flow–volume loops that demonstrate fixed airway obstruction show a plateau on both inspiratory and expiratory phases of the loop (Figure 5-9, *A*). Flow limitation on the inspiratory portion of the loop is characteristic of an extrathoracic obstruction (Figure 5-9, *B*). This is common in children with vocal cord dysfunction (VCD). Flow limitation on the expiratory part of the loop demonstrates an

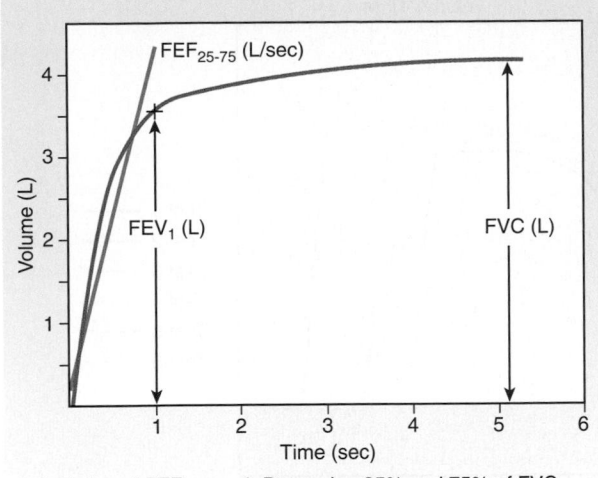

Calculation of FEF$_{25-75}$: 1. Determine 25% and 75% of FVC
2. Slope of line through 25% and 75% =
$$\frac{(V_{75}) - (V_{25})}{(T_{75}) - (T_{25})} \text{ (L/sec)}$$

FIGURE 5-5 A normal standard volume–time spirometry graph depicting the forced vital capacity (*FVC*), forced expiratory volume in 1 second (*FEV$_1$*), and forced expiratory flow between 25% and 75% of vital capacity (*FEF$_{25-75}$*).

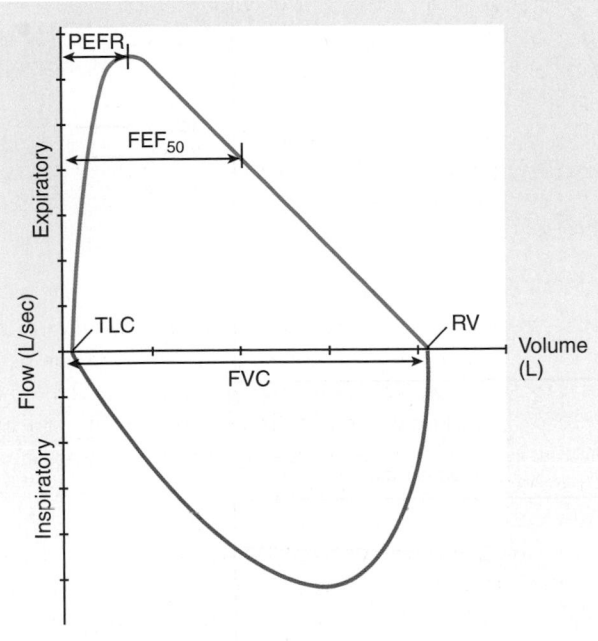

FIGURE 5-6 Normal flow–volume loop showing both the expiratory and inspiratory loops. The usual flow rates are identified. Note that no forced expiratory volume in 1 second (*FEV$_1$*) is evident because there is no time axis. *FEF$_{50}$*, Forced expiratory flow at 50% of vital capacity; *FVC*, forced vital capacity; *PEFR*, peak expiratory flow rate; *RV*, residual volume; *TLC*, total lung capacity.

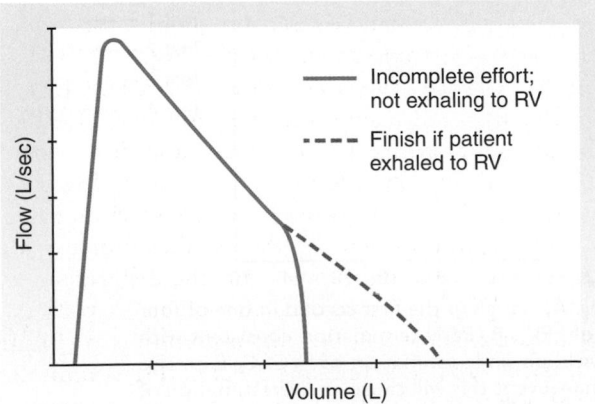

FIGURE 5-7 This expiratory flow–volume loop demonstrates the patient's failure to exhale completely to residual volume (*RV*). This will artificially decrease FVC and increase FEF$_{50}$.

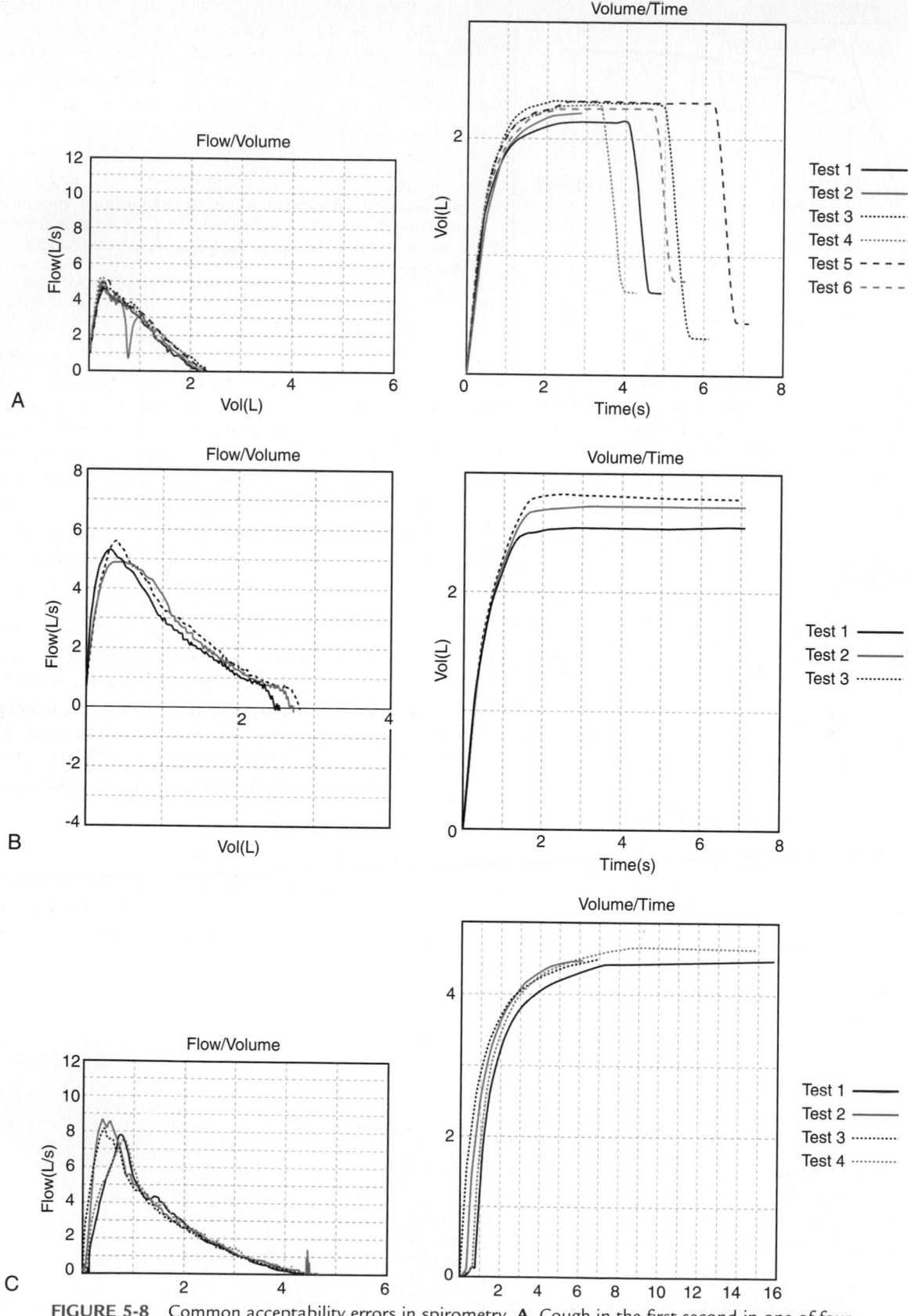

FIGURE 5-8 Common acceptability errors in spirometry. **A,** Cough in the first second in one of four maneuvers; this will interfere with proper measurement of FEV₁. **B,** Early termination consistent with glottis closure in all three maneuvers; this will typically yield an underestimation of FVC. **C,** Excessive back extrapolation volume in two of the four performed maneuvers; this will cause an overestimation of FEV₁ in the affected maneuvers.

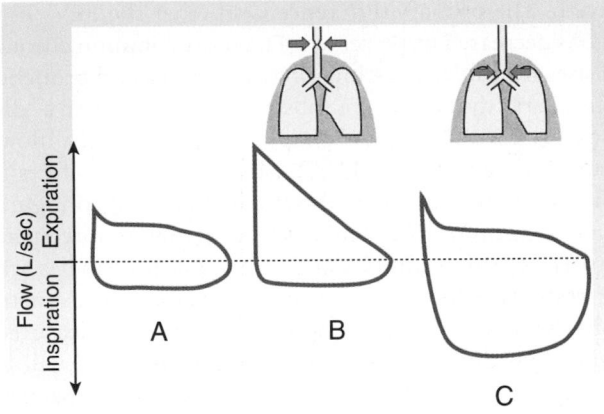

FIGURE 5-9 Flow–volume loops showing various forms of airway obstruction. **A,** Fixed obstruction; **B,** variable extrathoracic obstruction; **C,** variable intrathoracic obstruction. An easy mnemonic is *What's in is out, out is in.* In other words, if it affects the expiratory loop, it is inside the chest (variable intrathoracic), and if it affects the inspiratory loop, it is outside the chest (variable extrathoracic).

intrathoracic obstruction (Figure 5-9, C). A simple mnemonic for determining variable obstruction: "What's in is out, what's out is in." In other words, a variable inspiratory obstruction affects the expiratory portion of the F-V curve and a variable expiratory obstruction affects the inspiratory portion of the F-V curve.[2]

Some obstructions may also show a flutter, or irregular flow pattern, on either portion of the loop; this may be secondary to redundant tissue of the upper airway.

Forced Vital Capacity, Forced Expiratory Volume, and the Ratio

The most common measurements from spirometry include the FVC, FEV_1, and FEV_1/FVC ratio. These measurements are reproducible for many disease states in adult patients, such as chronic obstructive pulmonary disease. Physiologists were concerned, however, that the FVC and FEV_1 might be relatively preserved despite the presence of moderately severe small airway disease, and thus significant lung disease might be missed by using only these measurements. Because small airways less than 2 mm in diameter contribute only a small part of the total lung resistance, 20% or less, these tiny airways have been described as the "silent zone" of the lung. In an effort to measure their function more independently, without the large airway functions obscuring the measurements, the "maximal mid-expiratory flow rates" are calculated.[9] In current terminology, this is the FEF_{25-75} or the FEF_{50}.

Forced Expiratory Flow at 25% to 75% and at 50% of Vital Capacity

Although the FEF_{25-75} and FEF_{50} have been supported as reflecting the function of smaller airways, their measurement

is considerably more variable than that of the FEV_1 or FVC.[5,12,25] This decreases their usefulness in distinguishing normal from abnormal and requires a considerably larger change to be considered physiologically significant, as opposed to just the normal variability found from one measurement to another.[3] In addition, if the child does not fully exhale to residual volume, FEF_{25-75} may be artificially elevated because of reduced vital capacity.

Reference Values and Relevant Change

To interpret the test results, the laboratory needs to select a reference set and know the variability and clinically significant change for the most common spirometric and lung volume measurements in children (Table 5-1). The ERS Global Lung Initiative (GLI) has established the "all-age" reference set down to the age of 3 and should be considered the preferred reference equations in this age range.[4] Furthermore, the interpreter should be aware of the effects associated with changes in vital capacity and expiratory time on mid-flow variables (e.g., FEF_{25-75}) as they interpret these variables. Many childhood lung diseases, such as asthma and cystic fibrosis, have their roots in the distal airways; thus variables that are more sensitive, although more variable, may enhance the overall interpretation of the test. An abnormality isolated to the measurement of FEF_{25-75} or FEF_{50} is uncommon but more likely in children than adults. Therefore, most pediatric PFT centers pay careful attention to this variable as an early indicator of obstructive disease. Figure 5-10 demonstrates the potential importance of these measurements in a child with asthma.

Spirometry Values

Spirometry values are commonly used to determine whether a disease has a restrictive or obstructive pattern. Table 5-2 demonstrates the expected changes with each

TABLE 5-1		
Pulmonary Function Measurements in Children		
	Variability	Important Change
Measurement	(%)	(%)
FVC	5-7	>10
FEV_1	8	>15
FEV_1/FVC	—	—
FEF_{25-75}	15	>30
FEF_{50}	15	>30
TLC	7	>10
RV	7	>10
RV/TLC	7	—

FEF_{25-75}, Forced expiratory flow at 25% to 75% of vital capacity; *FEF_{50},* forced expiratory flow at 50% of vital capacity; *FEV_1,* forced expiratory volume in 1 second; *FVC,* forced vital capacity; *RV,* residual volume; *TLC,* total lung capacity.

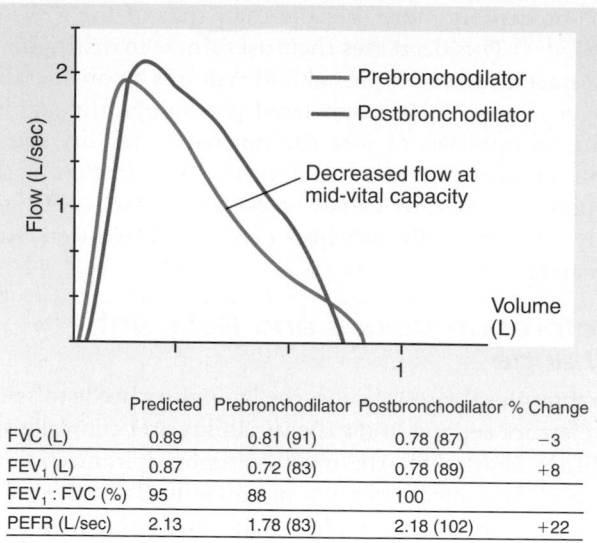

	Predicted	Prebronchodilator	Postbronchodilator	% Change
FVC (L)	0.89	0.81 (91)	0.78 (87)	−3
FEV$_1$ (L)	0.87	0.72 (83)	0.78 (89)	+8
FEV$_1$: FVC (%)	95	88	100	
PEFR (L/sec)	2.13	1.78 (83)	2.18 (102)	+22
FEF$_{50}$ (L/sec)	1.66	0.90 (54)	1.53 (92)	+70

FIGURE 5-10 Prebronchodilator and postbronchodilator expiratory loops produced by a 5-year-old patient with asthma. The prebronchodilator curve is slightly concave with respect to the volume axis, which is not evident on the postbronchodilator curve. The FEF$_{50}$ is the only prebronchodilator measurement below the expected normal range of variability; it increased by 70% after bronchodilator therapy. *FEF$_{50}$,* Forced expiratory flow at 50% of vital capacity; *FEV$_1$,* forced expiratory volume in 1 second; *FVC,* forced vital capacity; *PEFR,* peak expiratory flow rate.

TABLE 5-2

Characterization of Obstructive and Restrictive Patterns in Pulmonary Function Testing

Measurement	Obstructive	Restrictive
FVC	Normal or decreased	Decreased
FEV$_1$	Decreased	Decreased
FEV$_1$/FVC	Decreased	Normal or increased
TLC	Normal or increased	Decreased
RV	Increased	Normal or decreased
RV/TLC	Increased	Normal or increased

FEV$_1$, Forced expiratory volume in 1 second; *FVC,* forced vital capacity; *RV,* residual volume; *TLC,* total lung capacity.

---

pattern. The primary difference is whether the FEV$_1$/FVC ratio is decreased or preserved. The most common chronic diseases in children—asthma, cystic fibrosis, and bronchopulmonary dysplasia—are obstructive. Obstructive diseases produce a concave shape or scoop to the flow-volume curve (Figure 5-11, *C*). Most restrictive defects in children are related to an abnormal chest wall configuration or neuromuscular weakness rather than to interstitial fibrosis, as seen in adults. Caution must be used in describing restrictive lung disease on the basis of spirometry alone, because complete lung volumes are not measured. If the child did not take a deep breath, the FVC will be artificially decreased and mimic the restrictive pattern. Therefore, if restrictive lung disease is a concern, consider performing one of the lung volume studies described in the next section. The restrictive pattern is typically characterized by preserved flows with a reduction in the volume. This produces a visual pattern that has been described as a "witch's hat" (Figure 5-11, *B*).[2]

Diffusing Capacity

The **diffusing capacity** of the lung (D$_{LCO}$) assesses the functionality of the alveolar–capillary interface. A reduction in the D$_{LCO}$ might indicate problems with perfusion of the pulmonary capillary bed, bleeding within the lung, or thickening of the alveolar–capillary membrane. Abnormalities in D$_{LCO}$ may reflect pathological changes in the lung and are often correlated with outcome.[26] Indications for testing in the pediatric population that may produce a reduced D$_{LCO}$ include pulmonary fibrosis (primary disease or secondary to radiation treatment or chemotherapy), immunological disorders (scleroderma, systemic lupus erythematosus), bronchiolitis obliterans, pulmonary edema, and hematological disorders. An abnormally high D$_{LCO}$ may be seen in pediatric patients with acute hemorrhagenous bleeds, such as pulmonary vasculitis.[2] The single-breath D$_{LCO}$ procedure requires subjects to hold their breath for 8 to 12 seconds, which may be challenging for the very young. In addition, traditional testing routines require minimal washout (500 ml) and sample analysis

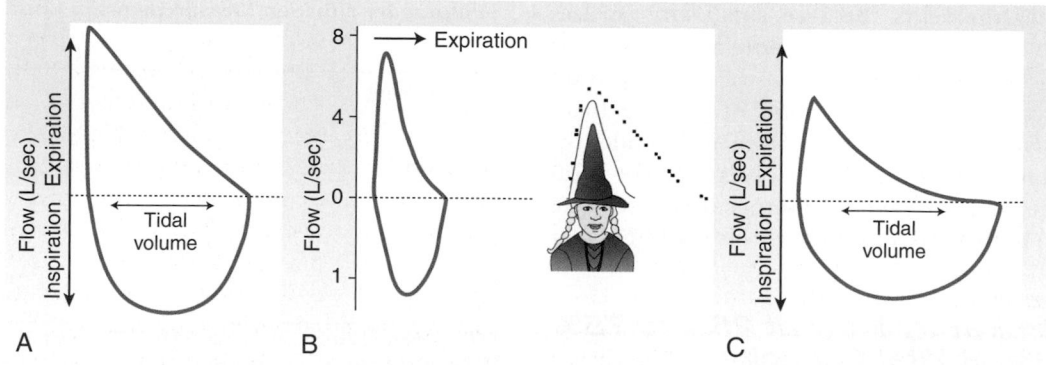

FIGURE 5-11 Patterns in flow–volume loops. **A,** Normal; **B,** restrictive (also known for its characteristic "witch's hat" shape); **C,** obstructive (concave).

volumes (500 ml), which may eliminate some children from testing.[27] Some DLCO systems have rapid analyzer technology that lets the technologist identify when dead space has been cleared and allows testing in subjects with a vital capacity less than 1 L. DLCO has been successfully performed on young children; however, as with all pulmonary function testing, it depends on the subject's maturation rather than their age. Reference values have been established in the pediatric subjects.[28] Kim and colleagues published regression equations in healthy Caucasian children ages 5 to 19.[29]

Lung Volumes

In contrast to the relative simplicity of spirometry, lung volume measurements are somewhat more involved and more difficult to perform. They include FRC, RV, TLC, RV/TLC ratio, and TGV. With the child sitting, the same techniques described earlier are used to measure lung volumes. These methods include helium dilution, nitrogen washout, and body plethysmography.[29,30-32]

Helium Dilution Method

The helium dilution method of calculating FRC measures only the gas that is in direct communication with the central airways. Helium dilution is described as the closed circuit technique as the subject rebreathes within a closed system (typically a bag). This uses the principle that the concentration of a gas in one volume is proportional to the concentration of that same gas in another volume, provided there is no production or consumption of the measured gas. Therefore, knowing the concentration of the gas inside the lungs and outside, as well as knowing the external volume, allows calculation of the lung volume. The volume of gas in the lung at end expiration (FRC) mixes and equilibrates with a known amount and concentration of helium (usually 5% to 10%) in a closed breathing circuit. The challenge for the young child is keeping a tight seal on the mouthpiece during the test because any leak will make the results invalid. The child breathes on the test system until helium equilibration is achieved. Helium equilibration is considered to be complete when the change in helium concentration is 0.02% for 30 seconds.[30] Testing time is typically less than 3 minutes but can last up to 10 minutes in a subject with severe airway obstruction.

Nitrogen Washout Method

The nitrogen washout method of calculating FRC also measures only the gas that is in direct communication with the central airways. Nitrogen washout is described as the open circuit technique because the subject's air is measured and expelled from the system. The child breathes 100% oxygen for up to 7 minutes via a mouthpiece, which displaces nitrogen in the lungs. The circuit must have no gas leaks. The system measures the volume of nitrogen washed out of the lungs. On the basis of the starting alveolar concentration of nitrogen, the computer uses a regression equation to calculate the volume of air in the lungs at end expiration, which is the FRC.[2]

Plethysmography

Body plethysmography requires that the patient sit in an airtight acrylic glass box, commonly called a body box. There are three types of body plethysmographs: volume, flow, and pressure. Most of the currently available body boxes are the latter, which uses a constant-volume, pressure-variable technique (Figure 5-12, *A*).[31] During constant-volume body plethysmography, the child voluntarily pants against a closed shutter (Figure 5-12, *B*). Using Boyle's law, the change in pressure against the closed shutter attached to a pneumotachometer is used to calculate a volume measurement, the TGV. TGV is measured at a known FRC value rather than on the basis of assumed values. TLC, the inspiratory capacity, is obtained by spirometry and added to the FRC. To calculate the RV, the expiratory reserve volume is subtracted from the FRC (Figure 5-13). In addition to measuring lung volumes, body plethysmography measures resistance and **specific conductance**.

Several potential errors are common when children perform these tests. If they are uncomfortable and anxious, pediatric patients may breathe at a slightly higher lung volume. If they are unable to start spirometry at TLC or exhale to RV, the values of inspiratory capacity and expiratory reserve volume will be incorrect. Therefore it is important to demonstrate the maneuver and make the child completely comfortable and relaxed.

Lung volume measurements are most useful in revealing restrictive lung diseases, in which they are decreased. It is critical to determine whether the lung volumes are smaller than expected because of a musculoskeletal problem (e.g., scoliosis and kyphosis), muscle weakness (e.g., Duchenne's muscular dystrophy and spinal muscular atrophy), or lung parenchymal disease (e.g., idiopathic pulmonary fibrosis). If it can be established that the patient's FVC as measured by spirometry correlates well with the TLC as measured on the basis of lung volumes, spirometry may be sufficient for most patients' follow-up.

In addition to lung volumes, measuring maximal inspiratory and expiratory pressures helps assess overall respiratory muscle strength and augments volume measurements when assessing patients with muscle weakness.

Airway Resistance. The body plethysmograph also allows the measurement of airway resistance (Raw) and the volume-associated parameters of specific airway resistance (sRaw) and conductance (sGaw). Raw is the pressure difference per unit flow as gas flows into or out of the lungs. The reciprocal of airway resistance (1/Raw) is conductance (Gaw). If obtained during lung volumes, the derivation of sRaw and sGaw can be calculated. Because some patients have changes in sGaw without changes in FEV_1 or FVC after a bronchodilator, and such changes are thought to be

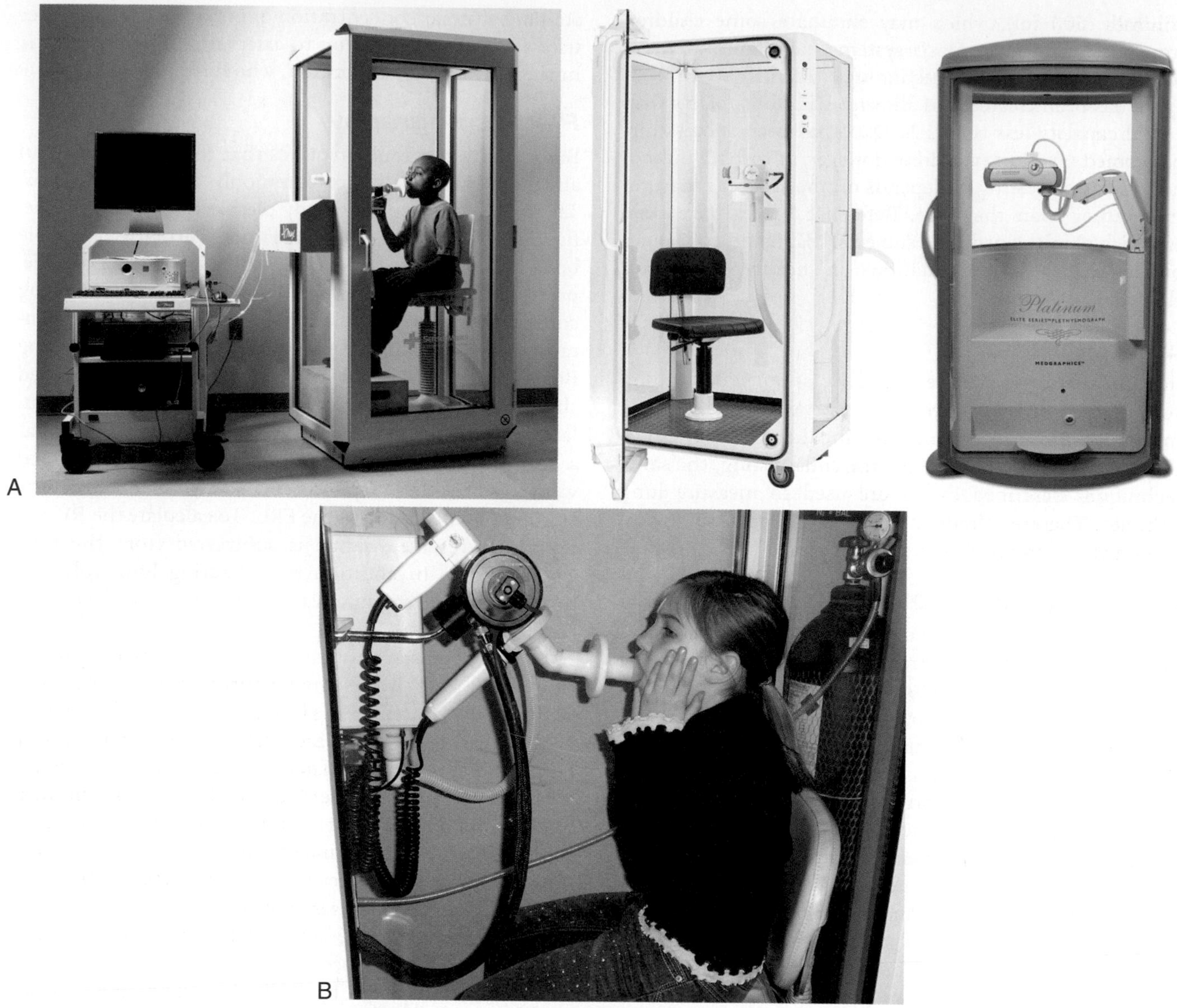

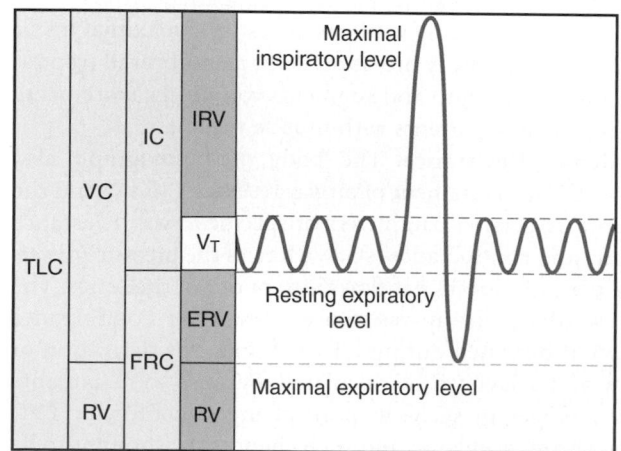

FIGURE 5-12 **A,** Three different vendor body plethysmographs. (Courtesy CareFusion, nSpire, and MGC Diagnostics.) **B,** Child supporting cheeks, panting, while performing lung volumes using a body box.

FIGURE 5-13 Graphic display of a simple spirogram depicting the subdivisions of lung volumes and capacities. *TLC,* total lung capacity; *VC,* vital capacity; *RV,* residual volume; *IC,* inspiratory capacity; *FRC,* functional residual capacity; *IRV,* inspiratory reserve volume; *ERV,* expiratory reserve volume; *VT,* tidal volume.

clinically significant, measuring bronchodilator response by sGaw may be more sensitive than relying on spirometry indices only, although a change of 35% to 40% is required. The measurement may also be helpful in pediatric subjects who cannot perform acceptable spirometry. Reference values have been published in children for ages 3 to 10 years.[33]

Impulse Oscillometry

Impulse oscillometry (IOS), also referred to as the forced oscillation technique (FOT), is a method to evaluate airway caliber using a miniature loudspeaker to produce oscillations within the airway (Figure 5-14, *A*). The pressure oscillations generated are of two types: those in phase with airflow, termed resistance (Rrs), and those "out of phase" with airflow, termed **reactance** (Xrs). Impulse oscillometry is a simple test that does not require the active cooperation of the child, and studies have shown IOS can be performed successfully in 3- to 6-year-olds with asthma.[34] Typical measured frequencies include 5, 10, 15, and 20 hertz (Hz), and reference equations have been published in children.[34] Current guidelines state that technologists/therapists can achieve competency after 10 to 15 supervised tests where they learn to recognize patient and technical problems that can occur during testing.[3] For this procedure the child should be seated, wear a nose clip, and firmly support the cheeks and mouth floor. The child is then instructed to breathe calmly and avoid obstructing the mouthpiece with his or her tongue. We have found that practice tests and sometimes distracters, such as a movie, can assist in achieving quiet tidal breathing in the young subject (Figure 5-14, *B*). The data acquisition should cover several breathing cycles, typically lasting 10 to 20 seconds. IOS can be used to assess bronchodilator with cut points ranging from a 10% to 30% decrease in Rrs5.

Response to methacholine using IOS has been described. In one study an Rrs5 increase of 45% compared with the baseline showed the optimal combination of sensitivity and specificity (0.72 and 0.73, respectively).[35]

CLINICAL HIGHLIGHT

Impulse Oscillometry

The patient is a 4-year-old girl with a history of coughing and wheezing. Current height is 109.4 cm; weight is 20 kg. Currently she is taking the following medications:

- Albuterol 0.083 % nebulized solution, 3 ml by inhalation every 4 hours as needed
- Flovent HFA 44 mcg/actuation aerosol, 2 puffs by inhalation two times a day

Her impulse oscillometry results were as follows:

Airway Reactivity	Baseline	Post-bronchodilator	Percent Change
R5Hz (kPa/L/sec)	1.28	0.87	−32%

Bronchial Provocation (Challenge) Testing

Challenge testing, also known as **bronchial provocation**, may be used in documenting bronchial hyperreactivity.[2,6,36-38] This can help solidify the diagnosis of hyperreactive airway disease, or asthma, in a patient whose symptoms may not be typical of asthma. Alternatively, for the patient who has symptoms that might mimic asthma, the lack of bronchial oversensitivity may help initiate the search for an alternative explanation. Bronchoprovocation tests are classified as direct or indirect, based on their mechanism of action. Common agents such as histamine and

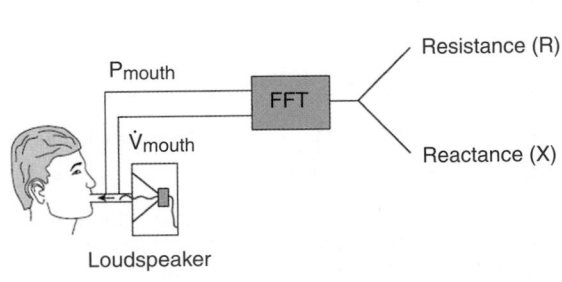

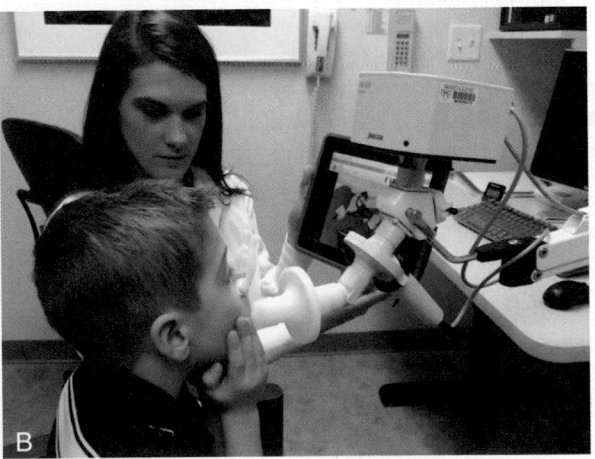

FIGURE 5-14 Components of the impulse oscillometry apparatus. **A,** A loudspeaker generates flow signals consisting of many pulsations. These pulsations are delivered to the mouth while mouth pressure (*P*) and flow (*V*) are measured. The computer then calculates resistance (*R*) and reactance (*X*). **B,** A 5-year-old boy performing IOS. Patient is using a nose clip, supporting the cheeks, and making a tight seal with the lips at the mouthpiece of the IOS apparatus. The therapist uses a movie as a distracter during the test procedure so the young boy breathes calming throughout the data acquisition period.

methacholine act directly on the smooth muscle cells of the airways to cause bronchoconstriction and airway hyperresponsiveness (AHR). Indirect bronchoprovocation tests, such as mannitol and adenosine monophosphate (AMP), act through inducing the release of bronchoconstricting mediators. Another indirect test such as hyperventilation, either at rest or during exercise, results in heat and water loss from the airway, which provokes a bronchospasm in susceptible patients.

Methacholine and mannitol are two very common inhalation challenge agents that have well-described protocols.[2] In methacholine testing, a test is considered positive if the FEV$_1$ falls more than 20% from baseline.[3,37,38] The concentration of the challenge drug is used as a marker of the degree of bronchial reactivity and is called the PD20, the provocative dose that produces a 20% fall in FEV$_1$. For example, a patient with highly reactive asthma may have a fall in FEV$_1$ of 20% with a methacholine concentration of 0.25 mg/ml. A patient with mild asthma may experience a 20% fall in the FEV$_1$ at 10 mg/ml. In mannitol testing a 15% decline in FEV$_1$ is considered a positive response.

Antigen inhalation is infrequently used as a challenge because of the difficulty in quantifying the dose of antigen to administer. Furthermore, antigen inhalation carries the risk of a late-phase reaction 6 to 8 hours after the challenge, at which time the patient is unlikely to be near a medical facility for therapeutic intervention.

Many laboratories have used exercise as a challenge. Unfortunately, because the primary driving forces for bronchoconstriction appear to be lack of humidity and low air temperature, an exercise challenge in the typically temperature-controlled pulmonary function laboratory may not be provocative. This has led some investigators to use hyperventilation while having the patient breathe cold air, without exercise, as the provocation test.

The Clinical Highlight on page 78 shows a positive methacholine challenge test in a 7-year-old girl evaluated for a chronic cough. This positive study led to therapy for asthma and ultimately resolved her cough. Interestingly, her previous spirometric measurements were normal and showed no improvement after bronchodilator therapy. The responses to exercise and cold air are measured by the duration of the challenge as well as the work performed during the exercise test. If other test parameters are used, such as the peak expiratory flow rate or specific Raw, different critical levels of positivity are used.

Cardiopulmonary Exercise Test

Cardiopulmonary exercise testing (CPET) is performed in the pediatric age group to evaluate symptoms that only occur during exercise or as a more general assessment of the subject's exercise tolerance in specific disease states.[2] The American Heart Association (AHA) has published guidelines on CPET in the pediatric age group and lists the common reasons for testing.[39] Box 5-1 expands on the AHA reasons to include specific disease states that might necessitate evaluation using CPET.

Current technology and testing devices easily adapt to the young subject. Cycle ergometers typically used in pediatric testing can be modified to varying body sizes using saddle height, crank-shaft length, and handlebar adjustments (Figure 5-15). This allows testing in subjects as young as 5 years of age. Ventilatory and metabolic responses to exercise can be assessed using small, close-proximity pneumotachometers, which can be positioned using mouthpieces or mask adaptations. Traditional measurements of electrocardiogram and blood pressure responses can be correlated to responses in oxygen consumption (V$_{O_2}$), minute ventilation (V$_E$), and other metabolic derivatives to evaluate exercise tolerance, ventilatory limitation, and inappropriate breathing strategies. The physiological responses to exercise are well defined in the pediatric age group but are beyond the scope of this chapter.[2] The Clinical Highlight on page 80 demonstrates the

---

CLINICAL HIGHLIGHT

Positive Methacholine Challenge in a 7-Year-Old Girl with Chronic Cough*

METHACHOLINE		PULMONARY FUNCTION		
Concentration (mg/ml)	Cumulative Dose (mg/ml)	FVC (L)	FEV$_1$ (L)	Percent Change in FEV$_1$
Saline	0	1.51 (83% predicted)	1.4 (82% predicted)	—
Methacholine				
0.025	0.125	1.51	1.38	−1%
0.25	1.375	1.64	1.53	+9%
2.5	13.875	1.54	1.39	−1%
10	63.875	1.33	1.07	−24%
Albuterol	—	1.41	1.26	−10%

FEV$_1$, Forced expiratory volume in 1 second; *FVC*, forced vital capacity.

*In a methacholine challenge test, the patient first breathes aerosolized saline (as a baseline), followed by a breathing test. The subject then takes five breaths of methacholine at a low concentration, followed by another breathing test. The process continues with increasing concentrations of methacholine until there is a 20% change in lung function or the maximal amount of methacholine has been inhaled. Albuterol, a bronchodilator, is then administered to help open the airways.

Box 5-1	Common Reasons for Pediatric Exercise Testing and Specific Clinical Applications

Evaluate specific signs and symptoms induced by exercise
Assess or identify abnormal responses to exercise
Assess efficacy of specific medical or surgical treatments
Assess functional capacity for athletic and vocational activities
Evaluate prognosis
Establish baseline data for rehabilitation

SPECIFIC CLINICAL APPLICATIONS
- Cardiac disorders
  - Aortic stenosis
  - Cardiomyopathy
  - Tetralogy of Fallot, Ebstein's anomaly
  - Coarctation of the aorta
  - Prolonged QT syndrome
- Pulmonary
  - Asthma
  - Cystic fibrosis
  - Chest wall (e.g., pectus excavatum)
  - Vocal cord dysfunction
- Others
  - Obesity
  - Neuromuscular disease
  - Exercise-induced syncope (e.g., postural orthostatic tachycardia syndrome [POTS])

Adapted from Paridon SM, Alpert BS, Boas SR, et al. Clinical stress testing in the pediatric age group: a statement from the American Heart Association Council on Cardiovascular Disease in the Young, Committee on Atherosclerosis Hypertension, and Obesity in Youth. *Circulation* 2006;113:1905-1920.

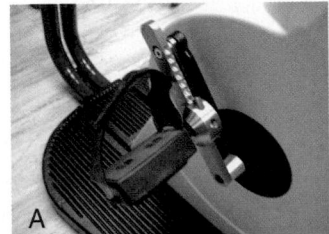
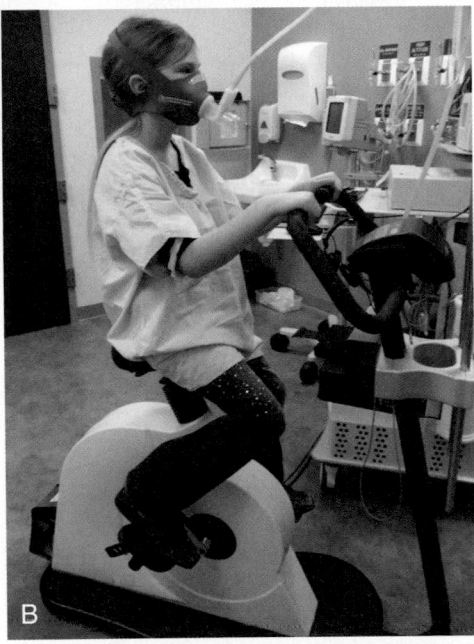

FIGURE 5-15   A, A cycle ergometer with adjustable pedal crank shafts to test smaller size patients. **B,** An 8-year-old child on a cycle ergometer with a face mask interface to a pneumotachometer to measure exhaled air.

use of the test in evaluating a teenage subject with symptoms during exercise.

The subject exercised on a cycle ergometer to a maximal workload of 160 watts. This appeared to be a maximal exercise test based on heart rate criterion. The subject has normal exercise tolerance with a maximum oxygen consumption ($\dot{V}O_2$max) of 83% predicted. The heart rate and blood pressure response were within the normal range, and the electrocardiogram did not show any signs of arrhythmia or ischemic changes. Minute ventilation increased to 74 L/min. There was no evidence of ventilatory limitation ($\dot{V}E$/maximum voluntary ventilation), although she used an inappropriate breathing strategy

with small tidal volumes (VT/FVC 33%) and higher breathing frequencies to increase her minute ventilation. Gas exchange assessed using pulse oximetry was normal (SpO_2 98%). Flow-volume loops obtained during CPET also demonstrated an improper breathing strategy, with the subject moving up in lung volumes during exercise and also showing evidence of variable extrathoracic obstruction (truncation and up-sloping inspiratory curve) suggestive of vocal cord dysfunction (VCD). The subject did exhibit audible stridor at peak exercise. The interpretation was that she had normal exercise tolerance with evidence of VCD and inappropriate breathing strategy.

CLINICAL HIGHLIGHT

The patient is a 14-year-old girl. She is an athlete who participates in cross-country running and figure skating.

History of present illness includes a 1-year history of dyspnea. The patient reports that "I can't catch my breath" with activity. She had been treated empirically with albuterol but still complained of her symptoms.

- Medications: Albuterol 2 puffs before activity
  Current evaluation included the following:
- Methacholine challenge: negative
- Exhaled nitric oxide: 10 ppb

A cardiopulmonary exercise test was ordered to further evaluate her symptoms, which occur with exercise.

CPET Results

Exercise		Rest	Maximum	Predicted	Percent Predicted
Workload	watts		160	190	84
Time	min:sec		12.3		
SpO$_2$	%	98	98		
VO$_2$	L/min	0.384	1.945	2.331	83
VO$_2$/kg	ml/kg		32		
R		0.75	1.00		
Cardiac Function					
Heart rate	bpm	58	191	199	96
Blood pressure (cuff)	mmHg	100/64	146/60	170/88	86/68
Oxygen pulse	VO$_2$/HR	7	10	11	91
Ventilation					
Minute ventilation	L/min	11.9	74.2	160.0	46
Respiratory rate	per min	10	45		
Tidal volume	L	0.367	1.650		
VT/FVC	%		33	45-50	

HR, Heart rate; *SpO$_2$*, oxygen saturation by pulse oximetry; *VO$_2$*, oxygen consumption; *VT/FVC*, tidal volume/forced vital capacity ratio.

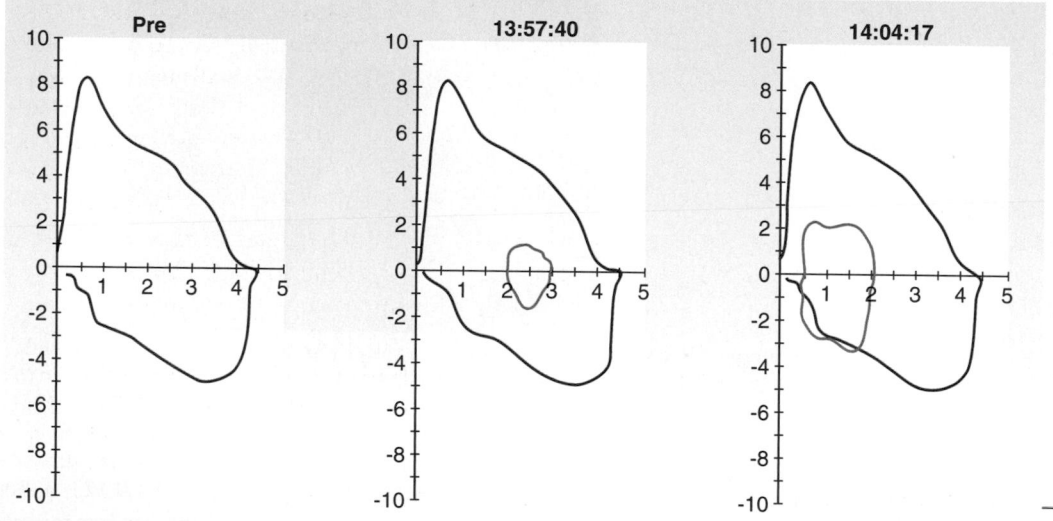

Exhaled Nitric Oxide

Exhaled nitric oxide (ENO) is a biomarker of airway inflammation and is a simple and noninvasive test for diagnosing and monitoring asthma in children. The fraction of nitric oxide (FENO) can be measured with either a chemiluminescent or electrochemical analyzer and is reported in parts per billion (ppb). Analyzers can be integrated with data acquisition software, which allows for incentive programs to help the child maintain the required flow, pressure, and duration of each maneuver (Figure 5-16). The child should refrain from eating or drinking (except water) for 2 hours before testing. "Because spirometric maneuvers have been shown to transiently reduce exhaled NO levels, it is recommended that ENO analysis be performed before spirometry."[40] According to current interpretation guidelines, a value greater than 35 ppb in children can be used to indicate that eosinophilic inflammation is present; in

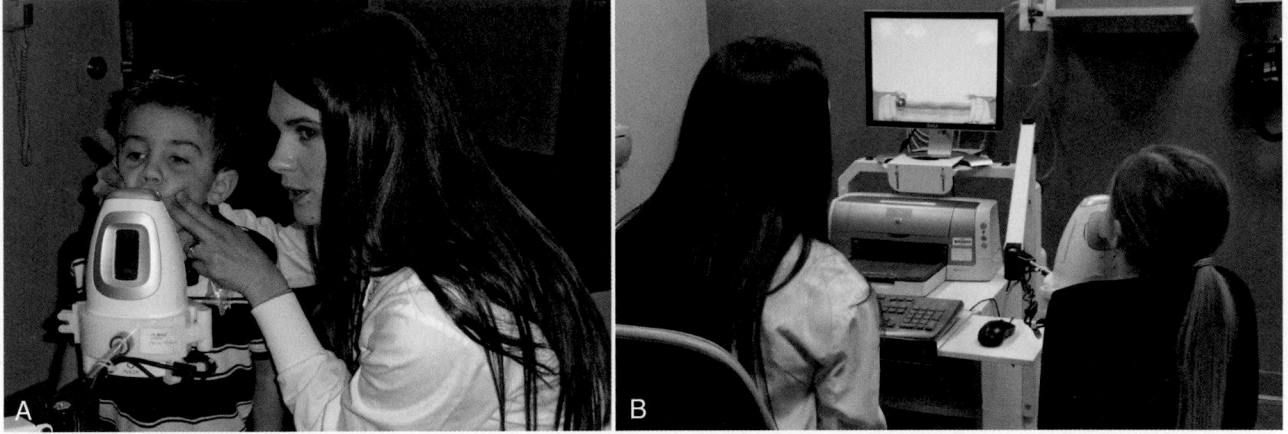

FIGURE 5-16   A, Therapist actively assisting a 5-year-old boy in successfully performing an exhaled nitric oxide test. **B,** Therapist passively coaching an 8-year-old girl using an incentive program.

symptomatic patients, there is a high likelihood the child will respond to inhaled corticosteroids.[41]

MEASURING PULMONARY MECHANICS AT THE BEDSIDE

Tidal Volume

Tidal volume (VT) is the gas volume (in milliliters) inhaled and exhaled during each resting breath. Often VT is indexed to body weight and reported as milliliters per kilogram (ml/kg). Some PFT systems report inspired and expired VT values separately, whereas some combine the two values. Infants in a neonatal intensive care unit may not normally inhale the same volume as they exhale for any given breath. This is visible in flow–volume (F–V) and pressure–volume (P–V) loops that are not closed. Typically, an average of at least 10 resting breaths is a better method of reporting VT. Infants receiving positive-pressure ventilation may have a gas leak around the uncuffed endotracheal tube. In this case, it is more accurate to report expired VT. Some PFT systems report leakage as a percentage of exhaled to inhaled VT, which is helpful in determining the delivered effective tidal volume. A system used for ventilator patient management should report VT values for spontaneous and ventilator-delivered breaths separately.[42]

Respiratory Frequency

Most PFT systems report respiratory frequency, or rate, as breaths per minute. If the child or infant is intubated and receiving mechanical ventilation, the system should report spontaneous and ventilator breaths separately. Often, increased respiratory frequency is one of the first signs of reduced compliance, increased resistance, or fatigue.

Minute Ventilation

Minute ventilation is the volume of gas inspired and expired each minute by the infant or child. It is reported as liters per minute (L/min) or as liters per minute per kilogram (L/min/kg) of body weight and is the product of VT and respiratory frequency. Viewing spontaneous and ventilator-delivered breathing separately or as a fraction of the total minute volume indicates the mechanical contribution of ventilation. This is helpful in assessing progress in weaning of a patient from assisted mechanical ventilation.

Rapid Shallow Breathing Index

The **rapid shallow breathing index** (RSBI) is a value that integrates two variables to determine the efficiency of tidal breathing. The RSBI is the ratio of spontaneous respiratory rate to VT: Divide the respiratory rate by VT (in liters) to calculate the index. A calculated value less than 100 to 105 is predictive of a successful extubation in adults.[43,44] The RSBI has less predictive value when applied to children and infants.[45-47] Factors such as age, endotracheal tube size, agitation, sedation, and duration of mechanical ventilation all contribute to the success of extubation and the usefulness of the RSBI as a pediatric weaning tool. The RSBI can be a useful tool in evaluating relative increases or decreases in work of breathing and monitoring an infant before and after extubation. For infants and pediatrics, normalize the RSBI equation for body size by dividing the VT by weight. The resulting unit of measure becomes breaths per milliliter per kilogram and allows easier comparison among the various measurements.[43,46,48] Because of the range of normal respiratory rates and tidal volumes, no single RSBI value will predict extubation success in the pediatric population.

Inspiratory and Expiratory Times

PFT systems measure inspiratory and expiratory times (TI and TE) by gas flow. The reported values will be different from the set, or duty cycle, times of a mechanical ventilator. Some systems also calculate the inspiratory-to-expiratory

TI/TE ratio or inspiratory time percent (TI/TTOTAL) from measured time.

Lung Compliance

At the bedside, compliance (C) is measured by the same technique as in the PFT laboratory. When making bedside measurements, it is important to know the compliance test conditions to interpret the meaning of the reported value. *Specific lung compliance* describes compliance when it is measured at a known level of total lung volume. When measuring compliance under static conditions by airway occlusion, compliance is similar to the value derived in the laboratory and assesses Crs. **Dynamic lung compliance** (Cdyn) is measured during resting tidal breathing and is affected by Raw.

There are some limitations to Cdyn measurement. This value reflects true compliance only when measuring transpulmonary pressure during spontaneous breathing with an esophageal catheter. Most centers do not routinely place an esophageal catheter for ventilator management studies. Instead, if the graph demonstrates that gas flow reaches zero at the end of inspiration and expiration, it is assumed that pressure has equalized from the proximal airway to the lungs. Compliance varies at different points of total lung volume, which is usually unknown during dynamic testing.

Airway Resistance

During bedside testing, the best evaluation of Raw also uses transpulmonary pressure measurements. A high Raw value is visualized on the P–V loop, described later, as a bowing out of the curve from the line of idealized compliance, or slope of the curve. The presence of an endotracheal tube with a small inner diameter is an airway obstruction causing Raw to be high. Changes in mechanical ventilator settings greatly affect Raw values, as do airway impairments such as secretions, bronchospasm, and edema. Bedside measurements of Raw usually preclude techniques used in the laboratory and are derived from the passive occlusion technique.

Time Constants

Respiratory time constants, tau (τ), are the mathematical product of compliance and resistance expressed as seconds, because all the units of pressure and volume measurement cancel out except time. A time constant is an interval over which a given change occurs, as a percentage of total change. Three time constants are required to reach 95% of inflation or exhalation. TI, or inflation time, and TE should be at least three times the respiratory time constants for optimal inspiration or expiration to occur.[49]

Pressure, Flow, and Volume over Time

Most infant PFT systems graphically display measured airway (or transpulmonary) pressure, inspired and expired gas flow rates, and VT on appropriate scales over a horizontal time axis on screen as the data are collected by the computer. This type of graphic display is also a component of most neonatal mechanical ventilators. Figure 5-17 shows a scalar tracing of pressure, flow, and volume over time. Pressure (Figure 5-17, *top tracing*) is either transpulmonary pressure or airway pressure measured at the endotracheal tube connection with the ventilator circuit. Gas flow at the airway (Figure 5-17, *middle tracing*) shows the inspiratory flow rate as a downward deflection and the expiratory flow rate as an upward deflection, with the center line being zero flow. VT (Figure 5-17, *bottom tracing*) portrays inspiration as upward, with a return to the baseline as volume is exhaled. The vertical dashed lines delineate the change from inspiration to expiration for each breath. Breaths are numbered from left to right; 1, 2, 4, and 5 are mechanically ventilated. Breath 3 is a spontaneous breath, with a lower VT than the ventilator-delivered breaths.

Flow–Volume Loops

During bedside testing, F–V loops are typically generated during tidal breathing.[32,50] The peak of expiratory flow

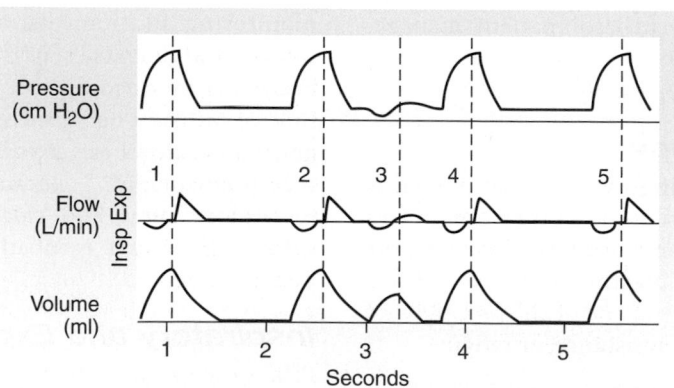

FIGURE 5-17 Tracing of pressure, flow, and volume over time (in seconds). *Exp,* Expiration; *Insp,* inspiration.

normally occurs within the first one third of expiratory volume. F–V loops that show decreased flow with relatively normal volume indicate an obstructive process in the airways; loops with decreased volume and normal flow suggest a restrictive disorder.

Pressure–Volume Loops

Graphically displaying a tidal breath with pressure change (airway or transpulmonary) on the horizontal axis and volume on the vertical axis also forms a loop. Spontaneous breathing is evidenced by a negative pressure change, and mechanical ventilator breaths display pressure in the positive direction. If the action of inhalation had only the elastic forces of lung tissue to overcome, the P–V graph would not be a loop but rather a straight line between the beginning and end points of inspiration (the dashed line in Figure 5-18). The P–V loop bows out from that line of pure compliance, mostly because of pressure needed for gas flow through narrow, resistive airways. The loop meets the line of ideal compliance at the end points of a tidal breath, where gas flow is zero. The slope of the line, and of the loop as a whole, depends on compliance. The more compliant the lung, meaning less pressure needed for normal VT, the more vertical the P–V loop appears.

Lung Overdistension

Ventilator-induced lung injury and pulmonary barotrauma are major complications of positive-pressure ventilation in all patient populations. Applying excessive distending airway pressures results in a characteristic distortion in the appearance of the normal P–V loop (Figure 5-19). To visualize this, imagine blowing up a balloon. At first it is necessary to blow hard (i.e., apply a large amount of pressure) to get any volume into the balloon. It then seems easier to push additional volume into the balloon as it expands. Finally, as the balloon reaches its expansion limit—that is, starts to overdistend—it again becomes more difficult to blow up. In other words, the compliance of the balloon or lung changes with total volume.

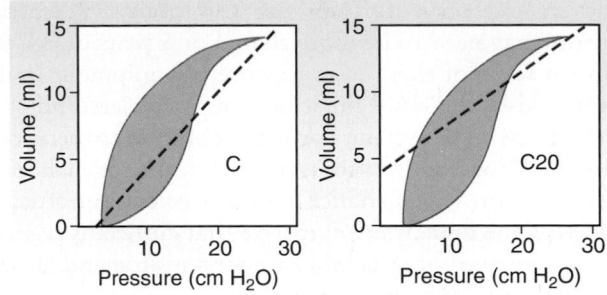

FIGURE 5-19 Pressure–volume loops demonstrating overdistention. Note the "penguin" or "bird's beak" appearance in the shape of the loops. These loops demonstrate idealized slopes (*dashed lines*) for change in compliance for the entire breath (*C*) and change in compliance in the last 20% of inspiratory pressure (*C20*). The C20:C ratio identifies lung overdistention.

Applying additional pressure to an overdistended lung produces little or no increase in delivered volume and is hazardous to the patient. Lung overdistention is quantified by comparing compliance change in the last 20% of inspiratory pressure (C20) with compliance change for the entire breath (C), in the ratio C20/C (see Figure 5-19). A C20/C value less than 0.8 indicates lung overdistention during mechanical ventilation. Gas exchange can be improved in mechanically ventilated neonates with lung overdistention by reducing peak inspiratory pressure.[51]

Work of Breathing

The calculated **work of breathing** is determined as the integral of esophageal pressure for a given tidal volume and reflects the amount of energy required by the patient to breathe. Work of breathing is usually indexed to body weight, reported as grams-centimeters per kilogram (g-cm/kg) or as joules per liter (J/L). Work of breathing measurements has proven particularly useful when evaluating new ventilator techniques and response to various therapies.

Other Bedside Tests

Other common pulmonary function measurements performed at the bedside are vital capacity, peak expiratory flow rate, and maximal inspiratory pressure, often referred to as negative inspiratory force (NIF). These measurements require a respirometer or pneumotachometer, a peak flow meter, and an NIF meter. The values are helpful in a variety of clinical situations, including weaning from mechanical ventilation, evaluating neuromuscular disorders such as myasthenia gravis or muscular dystrophy, and evaluating treatment for reactive airways.

Each of these measurements depends on patient cooperation and effort, which makes it challenging with

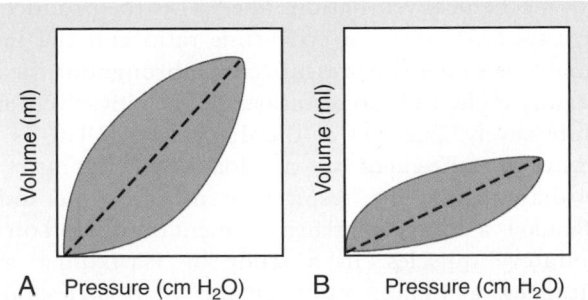

FIGURE 5-18 Pressure–volume loops demonstrating normal and decreased lung compliance. **A,** Normal lung compliance; **B,** decreased lung compliance.

children and prevents their use for infants. Pediatric patients may need to be more than 4 or 5 years of age to perform some of these tests because of equipment limitations. Also, the child must be able to understand the instructions and use the correct technique to perform the tests. Thoroughly explain the technique for each maneuver and provide a chance for practice before actually collecting the data. It is imperative that clinicians record their impression of the child's understanding and effort with the actual measurements.

Vital Capacity

VC is the maximal amount of gas that can be expired after a full inspiration. The patient inhales to TLC and then exhales completely through a respirometer or other measuring device. VC values are effort dependent, and the child must cooperate completely when asked to perform the maneuver. Incomplete effort will result in an artificially low value, which may lead to misdiagnosis. Forced vital capacity differs from VC in that during the FVC maneuver the patient exhales as forcefully and rapidly as possible after a maximal inspiration. FVC is usually the same as a slow VC, except in patients who experience airway collapse with rapid, forceful expiration.

Peak Expiratory Flow Rate

PEFR is the maximal achievable flow during a rapid, forced expiration. The PEFR is used primarily to monitor patients with hyperreactive airways. It is generally measured with handheld devices that sense flow against a turbine, through a variable orifice, or against a spring-loaded diaphragm. With increasing flow rates, an indicator advances linearly on a scale that reveals the PEFR, usually as liters per minute. Note that the PEFR on the F–V loop measures the same function as the peak flow meter, air flow in the large airways, but reported as liters per second. The PEFR measurement made during the recording of an F–V loop is an actual measurement of air flow. Because the handheld peak flow meter measures only the inertia from the initial blast of air, the value is not identical to the value reported during an F–V loop measurement.

Portable peak flow meters are used extensively in the study and management of patients with asthma. A significant decrease in the individual's baseline PEFR may indicate worsening asthma and the need for therapeutic interventions. In addition, measuring PEFR before and after bronchodilator administration evaluates the effectiveness of the therapy.[52]

Portable hand held models are inexpensive and easy to use at home, at school, or in an office. When using hand held peak flow meters, care must be taken to avoid partial occlusion of the flow exit orifice during exhalation. Partial occlusion decreases the amount of flow required to raise the flow indicator, resulting in overestimation of PEFR. This measurement can also be erroneously high if the patient uses a "spitting" action during exhalation.[6,53]

Maximal Inspiratory Pressure

Maximal inspiratory pressure, also called negative inspiratory force, is the maximal negative pressure, expressed as centimeters of water, generated during inspiration against an occlusion. Connect the patient's airway to an inspiratory pressure gauge with an adapter that allows occlusion of the airway during inspiration. Instruct the patient to exhale and then occlude the airway while the patient inhales with maximal effort, which results in measuring the maximal negative pressure.

MIP is an important measure to help differentiate weakness from other causes of restrictive lung disease. It can be an important differentiating point for children and young adults with various neuromuscular diseases. These patients usually have a combination of scoliosis and muscle weakness, both of which might contribute to reduced lung volumes. Measuring MIP helps in determining how much reduction might be caused by weakness. Because many neuromuscular diseases are progressive, MIP helps to document this progression. MIP may also indicate the patient's physical ability to take a deep breath and is often measured when weaning a patient from mechanical ventilation is being considered.

Complex Bedside Measurements

Automated and computer monitors allow the measurement of more complex breathing variables at the bedside. Usually these measurements are useful for weaning a child from mechanical ventilation, but they may also be helpful when evaluating the pulmonary status of a neuromuscular patient.

An example of such a measurement is the P0.1, pronounced "P one hundred." It is similar to MIP but measures the negative pressure generated in the first 100 msec. P0.1 appears to be more indicative of the ability to sustain respiratory drive and predict successful extubation or weaning from mechanical ventilation.

Another such measure is the **tension time index (TTI)**, which may assist in predicting successful weaning from mechanical ventilation. The TTI is the product of the inspiratory time-to-cycle time ratio and the integrated area under the pressure curve throughout the respiratory cycle. TTI can be measured both invasively and noninvasively. The TTI of the diaphragm (TTdi) is an invasive measurement of the load capacity ratio of the diaphragm. The respiratory muscle time index (TTmus) is a noninvasive measurement of the load on all respiratory muscles. In a study by Harikumar and colleagues, a TTmus value greater than 0.18 and a TTdi value greater than 0.15 had sensitivities and specificities of 100% in predicting extubation failure. Invasive and noninvasive measurements of TTI may provide accurate prediction of extubation outcome in mechanically ventilated children.[54]

KEY POINTS

- Pulmonary function testing is a vital part of the diagnosis and management of many respiratory diseases in both the intensive care unit and outpatient laboratory.
- Obtaining reliable pulmonary function data from infants and pediatric subjects may be challenging but provides extremely valuable insight into their respiratory mechanics.
- Traditional diagnostic tools such as spirometry, lung volume measurement techniques (e.g., plethysmography and dilution methods), diffusing capacity, and provocation tests are used in assessing lung function.
- A multitude of other diagnostic test modalities (e.g., impulse oscillometry, exhaled nitric oxide, CPET, etc.) may be used to identify and manage the care of infant and pediatric patients.
- Understanding the physiological principles of the tests and their specific application across a variety of clinical arenas is a useful skill set of the neonatal and pediatric practitioner.
- The continued advancement of pulmonary diagnostic technology and their application by skilled clinicians has dramatically enhanced the reliability and accuracy of pulmonary function testing in these age groups.

ASSESSMENT QUESTIONS

See Evolve Resources for answers.

1. When interpreting pulmonary function test results in children, assessing whether values are "normal" is complicated by:
   A. Applying the process of obligatory miniaturization
   B. The wide range of variability in normal children
   C. Lack of predicted normal values
   D. A and C
   E. B and C

2. Why do inspiratory retractions distort the ribs and sternum inward during distressed breathing in a premature newborn?
   A. Negative inspiratory pressures exceed transpulmonary pressure.
   B. The chest wall is compliant and does not expand the lungs.
   C. The specific conductance of the lungs is higher than the recoil of the chest wall.
   D. Time constant differences result in a lag between lung expansion and chest wall movement.
   E. None of the above.

3. Airway resistance (Raw) reflects the nonelastic airway and tissue forces resisting gas flow. How is Raw calculated?
   A. By dividing the peak ventilating pressures by the peak flow rate
   B. Using a modified Fick equation for gas flow
   C. From the ratio of airway occlusion pressure to expiratory flow
   D. Using a tonometer and paramagnetic analyzer
   E. By dividing the ratio of upper airway flow by lower airway compliance

4. Which of the following are possible tests that may be used to determine lung volume in an infant?
   I. Functional residual volume
   II. Helium dilution
   III. Plethysmography
   IV. Thoracic gas volume
   V. Nitrogen washout
   A. II, III, and V
   B. I, III, and V
   C. II and IV
   D. III and IV
   E. IV and V

5. What is the difference between pleural pressure and airway pressure?
   A. End-expiratory pressure
   B. Hyperinflation pressure
   C. PD20
   D. Isovolume pressure
   E. Transpulmonary pressure

6. Which of the following are considered a complication of using a face mask during infant pulmonary function tests?
   I. Trigeminal nerve damage
   II. Vagal reflex stimulation
   III. Increased lung compliance
   IV. Increased dead space volume
   V. Recurrent pharyngeal nerve damage
   A. I, II, and IV
   B. I, III, and IV
   C. II and IV
   D. II, III, and V
   E. III, IV, and V

7. What is one advantage to using a flow–volume loop instead of volume–time spirometry?
   A. A flow–volume loop is not dependent on patient cooperation or effort.
   B. Volume–time spirometry causes early fatigue in children.
   C. Flow–volume measurements are easier to record.
   D. A flow–volume loop displays early termination of the exhalation effort.
   E. Time–volume displays are not real time measurements.

8. How are spirometric values affected if a child fails to begin exhalation at 100% of total lung capacity?
   A. Reported tidal volume value is higher than the actual value.
   B. Reported FEF_{50} value is higher than the actual value.
   C. Reported FVC value is lower than the actual value.
   D. Reported PEFR value is higher than the actual value.
   E. All values are reported accurately.

9. Measuring flow from airways less than 2 mm in diameter is determined by evaluating:
   A. The maximal midexpiratory flow rates
   B. The forced expiratory flow at 25% to 75% of exhalation
   C. The forced expiratory flow at 50% of exhalation
   D. B and C
   E. A, B, and C

10. When using a handheld peak flow meter, a 6-year-old patient with asthma partially occludes the exit orifice of the meter. On the basis of the flow meter results, the physician may:

   A. Erroneously prescribe the wrong medication dose because the value reported is lower than the actual value

   B. Prescribe the correct medication dose because there is no effect on the actual value

   C. Not prescribe medication because the value reported is higher than the actual value

   D. Prescribe a medication dose that is proportionate to the erroneous reduction in peak flow

   E. None of the above

References

1. Majaesic CM: Clinical correlations and pulmonary function at 8 years of age after severe neonatal respiratory failure, *Pediatr Pulmonol* 42:8290, 2007.

2. Mottram CD: *Ruppel's manual of pulmonary function testing*, ed 10, St. Louis, 2012, Elsevier.

3. Beydon N, Davis SD, Lombardi E, et al: An official American Thoracic Society/European Respiratory Society statement: pulmonary function testing in preschool children, *Am J Respir Crit Care Med* 175:1304, 2007.

4. Quanjer PH, Stanojevic S, Cole TJ, the ERS Global Lung Function Initiative, et al: Multi-ethnic reference values for spirometry for the 3–95-yr age range: the global lung function 2012. equations, *Eur Respir J* 40:1324–1343, 2012.

5. Miller MR, Crapo R, Hankinson J, et al: An official American Thoracic Society/European Respiratory Society statement: general considerations for lung function testing, *Eur Respir J* 26:153, 2005.

6. Davis S, Johnson R, Flucke R, Kisling J, Myers T: American association for respiratory care clinical practice guideline: infant/toddler pulmonary function tests, *Respir Care* 53(7): 929–945, Revised & Updated July 2008.

7. Hanrahan JP, Tager IB, Castile RG, et al: Pulmonary function measures in healthy infants, *Am Rev Respir Dis* 141:1127, 1990.

8. Rosenfeld M, Pepe M, Longton G, et al: Effect of choice of reference equation on analysis of pulmonary function in cystic fibrosis patients, *Pediatr Pulmonol* 31:227, 2001.

9. Hyatt RE: Expiratory flow limitation, *J Appl Physiol* 55:1, 1983.

10. Castile R: Novel techniques for assessing infant and pediatric lung function and structure, *Pediatr Infect Dis J* 23:S246–S253, 2004.

11. Seed L, Wilson D, Coates AL: Children should not be treated like little adults in the PFT lab, *Respir Care* 57(1):61–71, 2012.

12. Blonshine SB: Pediatric pulmonary function testing, *Respir Care Clin North Am* 6:27, 2000.

13. Bhutani VK, Sivieri EM: Pulmonary function and graphics. In Goldsmith JP, editor: *Assisted ventilation of the neonate*, ed 4, Philadelphia, 2003, WB Saunders, pp 293–309.

14. Talmor D, et al: Esophageal and transpulmonary pressures in acute respiratory failure, *Crit Care Med* 34:1389, 2006.

15. Saslow JG, et al: Work of breathing using high-flow nasal cannula in preterm infants, *J Perinatol* 26:476, 2006.

16. Frey U, et al: Specifications for equipment used for infant pulmonary function testing: ERS/ATS Task Force on Standards for Infant Respiratory Function Testing, European Respiratory Society/American Thoracic Society, *Eur Respir J* 16:731, 2000.

17. Heistein LC, Ramaciotti C, Scott WA, Coursey M, Sheeran PW, Lemler MS: Chloral hydrate sedation for pediatric echocardiography: physiologic responses, adverse events, and risk factors, *Pediatrics* 117:434, 2006.

18. Stocks J, Godfrey S, Beardsmore C, et al. European Respiratory Society/American Thoracic Society: Plethysmographic measurements of lung volume and airway resistance: ERS/ATS task force on standards for infant respiratory function testing, *Eur Respir J* 17:302, 2001.

19. Tepper RS, Asdell S: Comparison of helium dilution and nitrogen washout measurements of functional residual capacity in infants and very young children, *Pediatr Pulmonol* 13:250, 1992.

20. Brar G, et al: Respiratory mechanics in very low birth weight infants during continuous versus intermittent gavage feeds, *Pediatr Pulmonol* 32:442, 2001.

21. Katier N, et al: Passive respiratory mechanics measured during natural sleep in healthy term neonates and infants up to 8 weeks of life, *Pediatr Pulmonol* 41:1058, 2006.

22. Katier N, et al: Feasibility and variability of neonatal and infant lung function measurement using the single occlusion technique, *Chest* 128:1822, 2005.

23. Maynard RC, et al: Partial forced expiratory flow (PFEF) measurements in premature infants at discharge, *Pediatr Res* 29:324, 1991.

24. Becker MA, Donn SM: Real-time pulmonary graphic monitoring, *Clin Perinatol* 34:1, 2007.

25. Miller MR, Hankinson J, Brusasco V, ATS/ERS Task Force, et al: Standardisation of spirometry, *Eur Respir J* 26:319–338, 2005.

26. Ginsberg JP, Aplenc R, McDonough J, et al: Pre-transplant lung function is predictive of survival following pediatric bone marrow transplantation, *Pediatr Blood Cancer* 54:454–460, 2010.

27. Macintyre N, Crapo RO, Viegi G, et al: Standardisation of the single-breath determination of carbon monoxide uptake in the lung, *Eur Respir J* 26:720–735, 2005.

28. Koopman M, Zanen P, Kruitwagen CL, et al: Reference values for paediatric pulmonary function testing: the Utrecht dataset, *Respir Med* 105:15–23, 2011.

29. Kim YJ, Hall GL, Christoph K, et al: Pulmonary diffusing capacity in healthy Caucasian children, *Pediatr Pulmonol* 47:469–475, 2012.

30. Gappa M, et al: Lung function tests in neonates and infants with chronic lung disease: lung and chest-wall mechanics, *Pediatr Pulmonol* 41:291, 2006.

31. Wanger J, et al: Standardization of the measurement of lung volumes, *Eur Respir J* 26:511, 2005.

32. Pfaff JK, Morgan WJ: Pulmonary function in infants and children, *Pediatr Clin North Am* 41:401, 1994.

33. Kirkby J, Stanojevic S, Welsh L, et al: Reference equations for specific airway resistance in children: the Asthma UK initiative, *Eur Respir J* 36:622–629, 2010.

34. Nowowiejska B, Tomalak W, Radlin J, Siergiejko G, Latawiec W, Kaczmarski M: Transient reference values for impulse oscillometry for children aged 3–18 years, *Ped Pulmonol* 43:1193–1197, 2008.

35. Schulze J, Smith H, Fuchs J, et al: Methacholine challenge in young children as evaluated by spirometry and impulse oscillometry, *Respir Med* 106:e627–e634, 2012.

36. Godfrey S, et al: Timing and nature of wheezing at the endpoint of a bronchial challenge in preschool children, *Pediatr Pulmonol* 39:262, 2005.

37. Wanger J, Blonshine S, Foss C, Mottram C, Ruppel G: AARC Guideline: Methacholine challenge testing, *Respir Care* 46(5):523–530, Revised & Updated 2001.

38. Crapo RO, Casaburi R, Coates AL, et al: Guidelines for methacholine and exercise challenge testing—1999. This official statement of the American Thoracic Society was adopted by the ATS Board of Directors, July 1999, *Am J Respir Crit Care Med* 161:309, 2000.

39. Paridon SM, Alpert BS, Boas SR, et al: Clinical stress testing in the pediatric age group: a statement from the American Heart Association Council on Cardiovascular Disease in the Young, Committee on Atherosclerosis Hypertension, and Obesity in Youth, *Circulation* 113:1905–1920, 2006.

40. American Thoracic Society/European Respiratory Society: ATS/ERS recommendations for standardized procedures for the online and offline measurement of exhaled lower respiratory nitric oxide and nasal nitric oxide, *Am J Respir Crit Care Med* 171:912–930, 2005.

41. Dweik RA, Boggs PB, Erzurum SC, et al: An official ATS clinical practice guideline: interpretation of exhaled nitric oxide levels (FENO) for clinical applications, *Am J Respir Crit Care Med* 184:602–615, 2011.

42. Mammel MC, et al: Effect of spontaneous and mechanical breathing on dynamic lung mechanics in hyaline membrane disease, *Pediatr Pulmonol* 8:222, 1990.

43. Berg KM, Lang GR, Salciccioli JD, et al: The rapid shallow breathing index as a predictor of failure of noninvasive ventilation for patients with acute respiratory failure, *Respir Care* 57(10):1584, 2012.

44. Vassilakopoulos T, Spyros Z, Roussos C: The tension–time index and the frequency/tidal volume ratio are the major pathophysiologic determinants of weaning failure and success, *Am J Respir Crit Care Med* 158:378, 1998.

45. Chatila V, et al: The unassisted respiratory rate–tidal volume ratio accurately predicts weaning outcome, *Am J Med* 101:61, 1996.

46. Venkataraman ST, Khan N, Brown A: Validation of predictors of extubation success and failure in mechanically ventilated infants and children, *Crit Care Med* 28:2991, 2000.

47. Farias JA, et al: Weaning from mechanical ventilation in pediatric intensive care patients, *Intensive Care Med* 24:1070, 1998.

48. Thiagarajan RR, et al: Predictors of successful extubation in children, *Am J Respir Crit Care Med* 160:1562, 1999.

49. Kamlin COF, Davis PG: Long versus short inspiratory times in neonates receiving mechanical ventilation, *Cochrane Database Syst Rev* 18(4):CD004503, 2004.

50. Lucangelo U, Bernabe F, Blanch L: Respiratory mechanics derived from signals in the ventilator circuit, *Respir Care* 50:55, 2005.

51. Kuschel C: Ventilation graphics and respiratory function monitoring, *Newborn Serv Clin Guideline* http://www.adhb.govt.nz/newborn/teachingresources/ventilation/RespiratoryFunctionMonitoringAndGraphics.htm June 2003.

52. Slieker MG, van der Ent CK: The diagnostic and screening capacities of peak expiratory flow measurements in the assessment of airway obstruction and bronchodilator response in children with asthma, *Monaldi Arch Chest Dis* 59:155, 2003.

53. Nair SJ, Daigle KL, DeCuir P, Lapin CD, Schramm CM: The influence of pulmonary function testing on the management of asthma in children, *J Pediatr* 147:797–801, 2005.

54. Harikumar G, Egberongbe Y, Nadel S, et al: Tension-time index as a predictor of extubation outcome in ventilated children, *Am J Respir Crit Care Med* 180(10):982–988, 2009.

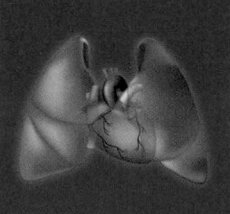

Radiographic Assessment

NINA KOWALCZYK

LEARNING OBJECTIVES

After reading this chapter the reader will be able to:

1. Recognize differences in radiographic positions/projections that affect the appearance of the visualized anatomy
2. Identify normal chest structures
3. Examine the chest radiograph for proper placement of endotracheal tubes and vascular catheters
4. Identify the pathologies most commonly visualized on soft tissue images of the neck
5. List the most common causes that lead to radiographic evaluation of the newborn chest
6. Describe how atelectasis affects the individual lobes of each lung
7. Describe the radiographic appearance of cystic fibrosis
8. List the complications of chest trauma, and identify the placement of support devices

KEY TERMS

Air bronchogram
Atelectasis
Barium swallow
Bronchiectasis
Computed tomography
Croup
Dysphasia
Epiglottitis
Esophogram
Hila
Horizontal fissure

Mass effect
Major fissure
Mediastinum
Minor fissure
Oblique fissure
Patent ductus arteriosus
Picture archiving and
  communication system (PACS)
Pneumatocele
Pneumomediastinum

Pneumothorax
Position
Projection
Pulmonary interstitial emphysema
Retropharyngeal cellulitis
Silhouette sign
Spine sign
Tracheoesophageal fistula
Tracheomalacia
Vascular ring

Radiographic assessment of the chest and airway is often critical in patient evaluation by the respiratory care practitioner: the position of lines and tubes can be accurately determined; visualized lung fields on the radiographs can be correlated with the physical examination; and airways can be assessed for patency and abnormalities.

RADIOGRAPHIC IMAGING

Conventional chest radiographs may be obtained with a mobile radiographic unit at the patient's bedside or by using stationary radiographic equipment in the radiology department. To ensure the highest quality images, radiographic examinations should be performed on stationary radiographic units whenever possible. Mobile radiographs should only be obtained when it is not safe or feasible to transport the patient to the radiology department. Mobile radiography is most commonly used when imaging neonates and patients in critical care units. Digital radiography has largely replaced film/screen imaging, so radiographs are increasingly being viewed on monitors within the patient unit or by accessing images on a computer via a **picture-archiving and communication system** or PACS (an electronic network to manage digital images).

Patient **position** and the radiographic **projection** are critical conditions to consider when evaluating a radiographic image. *Position* refers to the arrangement of the patient's body (e.g., erect, supine, recumbent), and *projection* refers to the path of the x-ray beam (e.g., posteroanterior [PA], meaning entering through the body's posterior surface and exiting the anterior surface). The standard projections for chest radiography are the erect PA and left lateral obtained on full inspiration.[1] The PA and anteroposterior (AP) projections demonstrate chest anatomy in relation to right and left sides of the body. With the addition of the lateral projection, most commonly a left lateral, the anatomical structures can also be visualized from anterior to posterior. This allows the anatomical structure to be examined three-dimensionally. When imaged with stationary radiographic equipment within the radiology department, a PA projection is obtained with the patient in an upright position with his or her chest against the radiographic imaging device. The x-ray tube is placed behind the patient's back with the x-ray beam projected through the patient in a posterior-to-anterior path. An upright left lateral projection of the chest is also obtained with the patient's arms raised above his or her head to avoid superimposition of the arms within the lung apices. The x-ray beam is projected through the patient in a right side to left side path. These positions place the heart close to the image receptor and prevent engorgement of the heart and great vessels. However, when the radiograph is performed at the patient's bedside with mobile radiographic equipment, the image receptor is placed behind the patient's back and the x-ray tube is placed in front of the patient's chest. This obtains a frontal view in the AP projection, with the beam passing from anterior to posterior. Whenever possible, mobile chest radiographs are obtained with the patient's head raised, but in some cases, such as in neonates, the image must be obtained with the patient lying flat on his or her back. An AP projection causes magnification of structures such as the heart because it places the anatomy further from the image receptor. When the chest radiograph is obtained with the patient in a supine position, the abdominal organs rise, the lungs cannot be fully distended, and the heart appears enlarged. Therefore knowledge of how the frontal view is obtained (anteroposterior vs. posteroanterior) is useful in evaluating heart size.

Although most chest radiographs are performed with PA and left lateral projections, other projections may contribute additional information. The lateral decubitus position is a frontal projection performed with the patient lying on either the right side (right lateral decubitus) or on the left side (left lateral decubitus). The down side can be evaluated for presence of fluid, such as a mobile pleural effusion, and the up side will demonstrate free air, such as in the case of a **pneumothorax** (air in the pleural cavity). Decubitus chest radiographs may also be used if a foreign body is lodged in a bronchus, causing air trapping. The down-side lung normally loses volume but may remain expanded when a foreign body obstructs airflow out of the bronchus.

As mentioned earlier, chest radiography is usually performed on full inspiration. Forced expiratory images are used in assessing the presence of a pneumothorax and to evaluate for foreign body aspiration in small children. When assessing foreign body aspiration in very young patients, the radiographer may gently add pressure to the abdomen during expiration. If an obstruction is present, the affected lung will not decrease in size but remains normal to hyperexpanded (Figure 6-1). In older and cooperative children the radiographer will have the patient inspire and expire without assistance while the radiographs are obtained. Oblique views are usually rotated 45 degrees from the frontal position. They are typically used in the evaluation of rib fractures and to better evaluate the entire heart border.

Although the thoracic trachea and mainstem bronchi are demonstrated on chest radiographs, soft tissue AP and lateral projections of the neck allow evaluation of the extrathoracic airway. These images may show **mass effect** on the airway from a retropharyngeal abscess or can show distortion of the tracheal caliber caused by croup and subglottic stenosis.

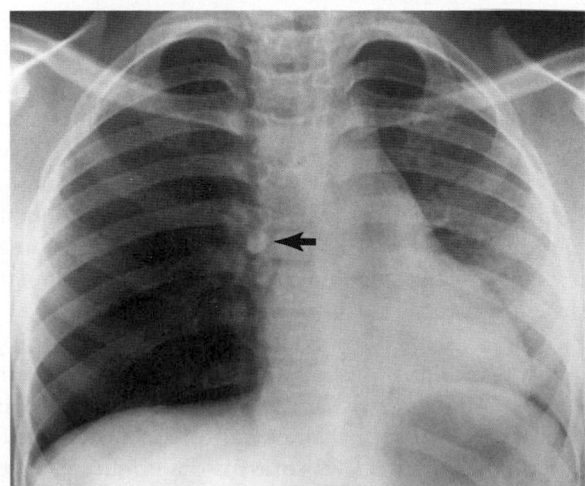

FIGURE 6-1 Expiratory frontal chest radiograph shows normal decrease in left lung volume. Tooth (*arrow*) obstructs the right mainstem bronchus and causes air trapping in the right lung.

Real-time imaging of the airway by fluoroscopy will show the dynamic collapse of tracheal walls known as **tracheomalacia.** If a **barium swallow,** also known as an **esophogram,** is performed as well, the presence of a **vascular ring** (in which the trachea and esophagus are encircled by connected segments of the aortic arch and its branches) or **tracheoesophageal fistula** (an abnormal connection between the trachea and the esophagus) can be excluded. Swallowing studies are performed with the assistance of a speech therapist, using various consistencies of barium-impregnated food to determine which the patient is unlikely to aspirate.

Computed tomography (CT) creates sectional images of the chest that can be viewed in multiple imaging planes: transverse, sagittal, and coronal. Volumetric CT offers the advantage of imaging the entire chest with one breath hold, which allows better evaluation of the chest, especially the diaphragm area. However, the radiation dose associated with CT is much higher than the radiation dose received from a conventional chest radiograph. Therefore, the use of CT in imaging pediatric patients is limited. CT of the chest is the method of choice for evaluation of pulmonary adenopathy. Standard radiographs are only about 50% sensitive to chest disease, typically displaying advanced pathologic conditions.[1] CT of the neck is also appropriate in older children with a palpable neck mass, whereas ultrasound of the neck is preferable in patients under the age of 14 years because it does not expose the child to ionizing radiation. However, if the mass is located in the retropharyngeal area, an enhanced CT of the neck is appropriate for pediatric patients of all ages.[2]

NORMAL CHEST ANATOMY

The normal structures that are visualized on a chest radiograph are distinguishable because of differences in the absorption of the x-ray beam by the organs and tissues within the thoracic cavity. Bone and metallic orthopedic hardware appear bright white because of greater x-ray absorption and less exposure of the image receptor. In contrast, air has little beam absorption, and therefore well-expanded lungs appear relatively black. Soft tissue organs and fluid usually appear as shades of gray in between the white bones and black lungs. However, incorrect exposure of the image receptor may alter the normal gray scale. Digital radiographic images are automatically rescaled to allow proper image contrast and brightness, and the image can be manipulated by the clinician after it is processed.

By using specialized tools available for adjusting images on a PACS monitor or computer, the image may be manipulated to enhance visualization of the lung detail and to clarify the presence of abnormal collections of free air. Adjusting the window level controls the brightness of the image on the monitor, and adjusting the window width changes the gray scale on the monitor. This is helpful in evaluating the soft tissue structures within the chest and neck. The zoom features are particularly useful to help magnify specific areas on the radiographic image. Inversion of the image sometimes will clarify the tip position of small catheters. Because of the complexity of image retrieval and portrayal with a PACS, instruction is usually provided to the clinicians by the PACS administrators from the radiology department.

A chest radiograph is a two-dimensional representation of a three-dimensional object. When an x-ray beam passes through the chest, the densities of all the structures it encounters are summated. Thus a flat object such as platelike **atelectasis** (collapse of all or part of the lung) may add little to the opacity of the chest in one projection but may appear opaque when viewed on edge in another projection. Pulmonary vessels appear as white dots when viewed in cross section but are fainter when viewed as tubes.

Differences in tissue density allow the viewer to discriminate between different structures. The heart, which is composed of soft tissue of muscle density, is clearly demarcated by a distinct edge from the adjacent air-filled lung. However, if the lung becomes denser from loss of air, as in atelectasis, or if the alveoli become filled with pus, as in pneumonia, the sharp edge between the heart and the lung is no longer apparent. The sign caused when two normal structures lose their distinct edge and blend imperceptibly is widely known as the **silhouette sign** (Figure 6-2).

The normal structures that the respiratory care practitioner must evaluate on all chest radiographs are the heart, lungs, and airways (Figure 6-3). Other structures that may be important in a specific patient include the diaphragm, soft tissues, bones, and organs in the upper abdomen. Although the heart is centrally located within the chest, it lays in an oblique plane; thus the left ventricle normally projects into the left hemithorax. As mentioned earlier, it is important to remember that the heart size may be magnified by anteroposterior projection as well as decreased lung expansion. Pulmonary bronchi, arteries, and veins form confluent areas on either side of the heart called the right and left pulmonary **hila.** Enlargement of the hila may be caused by increased caliber of the pulmonary vessels or enlarged lymph nodes. The side of the aortic arch should also be noted. Normally the aortic arch is on the left and causes a prominent bulge of the superior mediastinum and a mild indentation on the trachea.

The **mediastinum** is composed of the heart, aorta, main pulmonary artery and proximal branches, origins of the great vessels from the aorta, the superior vena cava, and the thymus. Thymic tissue is usually prominent in the neonate and becomes less apparent with age because of regression of the thymus and growth of surrounding structures. Because it is an anterior mediastinal structure, the thymus in the small child fills the anterior clear space normally seen on the lateral projection of a teenager or adult. On the AP or PA projection it may only cause widening of the superior mediastinum. When the thymus projects away from the mediastinum, typically into the right

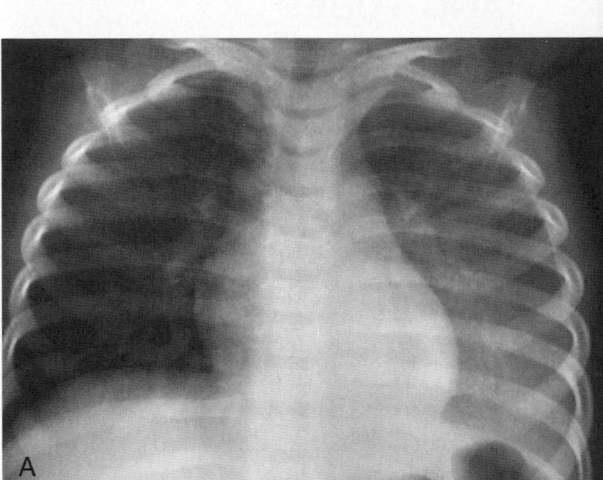
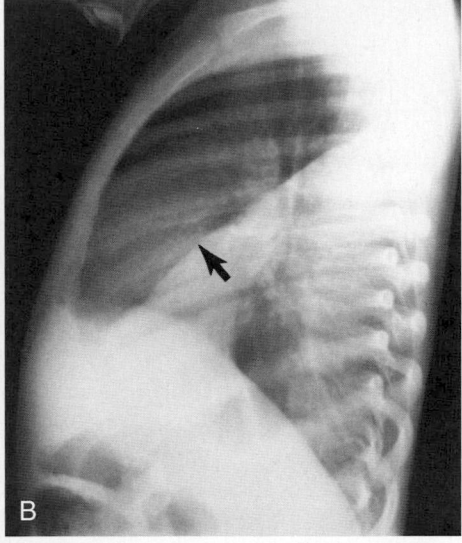

FIGURE 6-2   A, Left lower lobe pneumonia abuts the diaphragm, leading to nonvisualization of the normal edge of the diaphragm. The cardiac border is demarcated because the *lingula* (a segment of the upper lobe of the left lung) is normally aerated. **B,** Only the right hemidiaphragm is visualized because the left is obscured by the left lower lobe pneumonia. Major fissure appears as an edge (*arrow*).

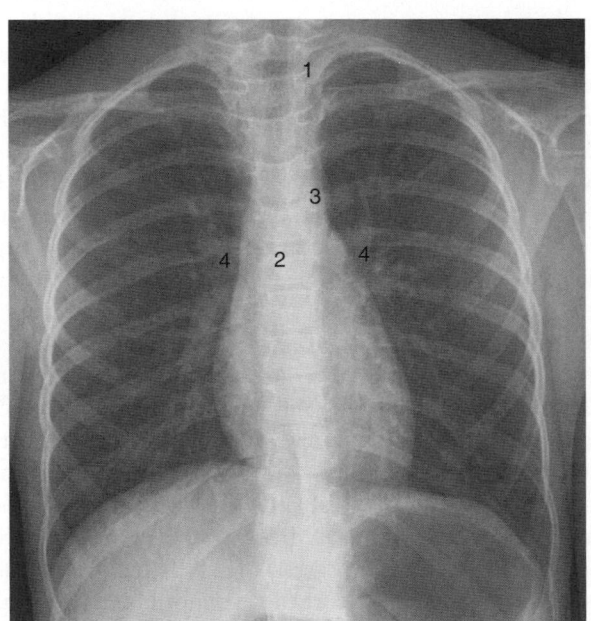

FIGURE 6-3   Normal frontal view of the chest demonstrating the thoracic inlet (*1*), *carina* (the point at which the trachea splits into the two mainstem bronchi) (*2*), the aortic arch (*3*), and pulmonary hila (*4*).

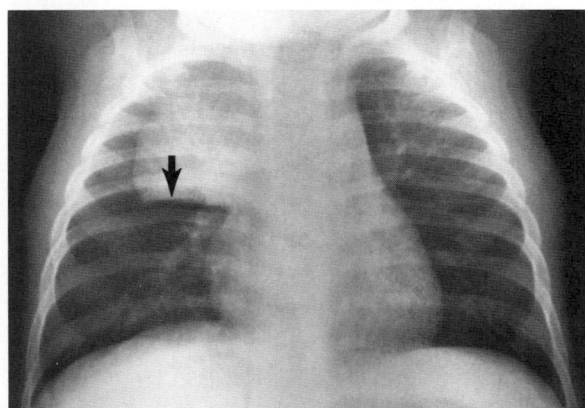

FIGURE 6-4   Normal thymus abuts the minor fissure (*arrow*) and has a curved lateral margin.

lingula of the left upper lobe may be thought of as corresponding to the right middle lobe, at least in location. A frontal view of the chest primarily demonstrates the upper and middles lobes of the lungs. Separating the upper and lower lobes, the **major fissures** (also called **oblique fissures**) extend diagonally on the lateral projection in an anteroinferior-to-posterosuperior plane. Fluid in the fissures increases their visibility. The posterior lobes are visualized on the lateral projection of the chest. The **minor fissure** (also called the **horizontal fissure**) separates the middle lobe from the right upper lobe. It is horizontal in orientation on both frontal and lateral projections and terminates at the major fissure on lateral projection.

Lung density is greatly affected by the degree of inspiration. Poor inspiration will cause crowding of pulmonary vessels and airways, leading to an overall increase in lung

upper lung, it appears as a "sail" with a sharp inferior margin. The lateral margins often have a characteristic wavy contour (Figure 6-4). Unlike a pathological mass such as lymphoma, the normal thymus does not exert mass effect on the trachea.

The right lung is divided into three lobes and the left lung into two lobes. Both lungs have upper and lower lobes, but the right lung also has a middle lobe. The

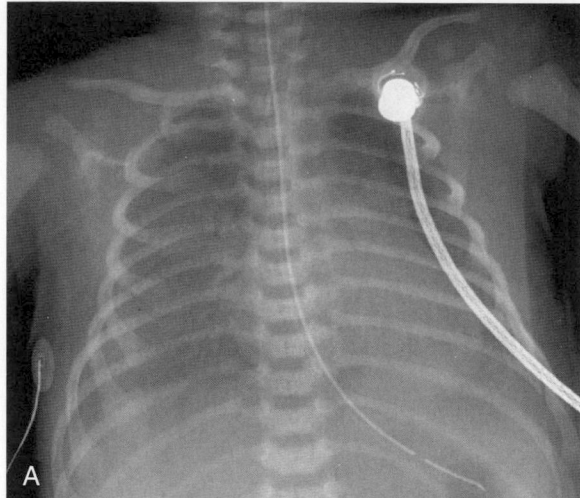

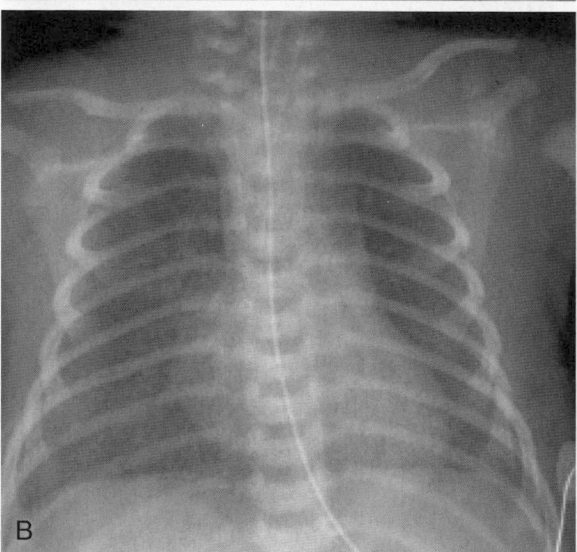

FIGURE 6-5 A, Infant with respiratory distress syndrome on lower ventilator setting. **B,** Same infant on higher ventilator setting.

density. When comparing the present chest radiograph with a prior image, the depth of inspiration should be taken into account and excluded as a cause of the change in appearance of both the lungs and size of the heart (Figure 6-5). When viewing infant and pediatric radiographs, body rotation may be difficult to avoid. Evaluating thoracic symmetry helps when interpreting the loss of lung volume or increased density in the rotated patient.

Evaluation of the trachea and mainstem bronchi should include the caliber as well as evidence of abnormal displacement or distortion by an adjacent mass. Truncation of a mainstem bronchus is often a sign of a mucous plug when the lung is collapsed. Although the right hemidiaphragm is usually slightly higher than the left because of the underlying liver, the position of the diaphragm may indicate hemidiaphragm paralysis or abdominal pathology. Congenital fusion anomalies may be seen in the neonatal rib cage, and rib fractures may contribute to difficult ventilation in a trauma patient.

POSITIONING OF LINES AND TUBES

Chest radiography is considered the "gold standard" in assessing endotracheal tube placement. The frontal chest radiograph can readily be used to assess the proper placement of the endotracheal (ET) tube, which should be positioned in the midtracheal region between the inferior clavicular border and the carina.[3,4] If the tip is located above the clavicular border, the ET tube is too shallow. If the tube is at the carina or in one of the mainstem bronchi, overaeration of one lung and atelectasis of the opposite lung may result. The position of the head, especially in a neonate, may result in a significant change in position of the endotracheal tube tip: the tip will advance toward the carina when the head is flexed.

If a chest radiograph is obtained for suspected esophageal intubation, the stomach, small bowel, and esophagus will be distended with air while the lungs will be underinflated. Although usually not necessary, a lateral projection would demonstrate the endotracheal tube in the more posterior esophagus. The lateral projection may be more useful for showing adequate tracheal positioning and length in long-term placement of a tracheostomy tube.

A chest tube is inserted through the chest wall between the ribs to allow drainage of air (e.g., pneumothorax) or fluid (e.g., pleural effusion or hemothorax) from the thoracic cavity. Those placed lower on the chest wall are usually for fluid drainage; those placed higher are usually for air removal. Proper insertion of a central venous pressure line (CVP) places the tip of the catheter in the distal superior vena cava just above the right atrium. A pulmonary artery catheter is a multilumen catheter that serves to evaluate cardiac function. The pulmonary artery catheter measures pulmonary wedge pressure, reflecting left atrial pressure, and it is positioned in the pulmonary artery. Access catheters such as a Hickman catheter or a Port-a-Cath are usually inserted via the subclavian vein. Hickman catheters are open to the outside of the body with the tip of the catheter placed in the superior vena cava. Port access devices are placed under the skin, just below the clavicle.[1] The positions of vascular catheters should also be evaluated and repositioned if necessary. If the tip of the catheter is in the right atrium, arrhythmia may result. Pneumothorax and new ipsilateral pleural effusion could result from error in catheter placement.

AIRWAY OBSTRUCTION

The adenoids are posterior to the nasopharynx on the lateral neck radiograph. The palatine tonsils are best seen between the oropharynx and nasopharynx. Enlargement of these normal lymphoid structures are a major cause of sleep-related apnea. An acute infection can also cause adenoidal and tonsillar enlargement, leading to airway obstruction (Figure 6-6).

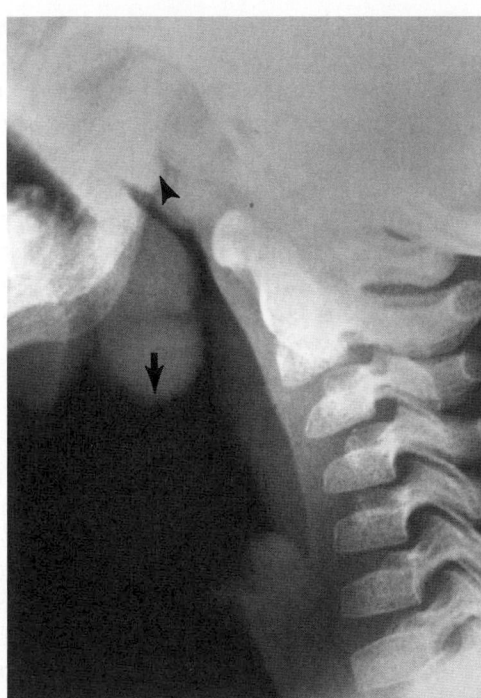

FIGURE 6-6 Enlarged tonsils (*arrow*) appear to hang down into the hypopharynx. The nasopharynx (*arrowhead*) is narrowed from enlarged adenoids located posterior and superior.

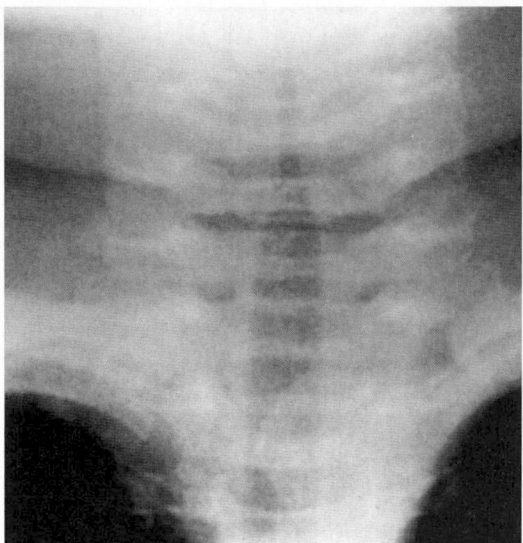

FIGURE 6-7 "Steepling" of the subglottic airway is caused by croup.

Croup (laryngotracheobronchitis) is the most common cause of upper airway obstruction in children, with a peak incidence in infants and children 6 months to 5 years of age.[5] Most cases are virally induced (parainfluenza) and cause inspiratory stridor with a barking cough. Frontal and lateral neck radiographs may show the characteristic subglottic narrowing below the vocal cords with loss of the normal "shouldering" of the airway and resultant "church steeple" appearance. The hypopharynx usually appears overdistended (Figure 6-7).

Whereas croup usually improves within a few days of supportive therapy, **epiglottitis** is a life-threatening disease causing acute inspiratory stridor, fever, and **dysphasia** (speech impairment). The usual pathogen is *Haemophilus influenzae*, with the risk of infection now greatly reduced by immunization programs. The diagnosis should be made by physical examination or by direct visualization through a scope. If a lateral radiograph of the neck is obtained, the epiglottis is enlarged (referred to as the thumb sign), and the aryepiglottic folds are thickened, with overdistention of the hypopharynx. The radiograph is performed upright in the position most comfortable for the patient to breathe. Because safety of the child is of primary concern, the radiograph should be performed portably in the emergency department, where intubation can be performed quickly if necessary (Figure 6-8).

Retropharyngeal cellulitis and abscess are usually preceded by an upper respiratory infection, often with cervical adenopathy (enlargement of the cervical lymph nodes). Spread of infection along lymph channels leads to

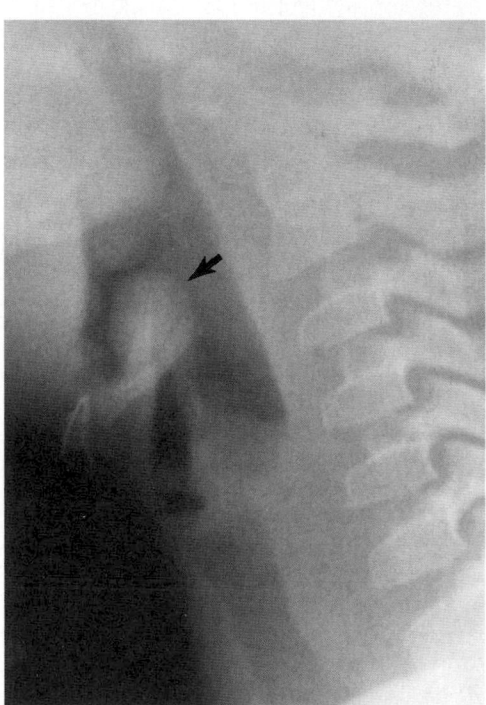

FIGURE 6-8 Enlarged epiglottis (*arrow*) appears as a "thumb" projecting into the airway.

enlargement of the retropharyngeal (prevertebral) soft tissues on the lateral neck radiograph with forward displacement and bowing of the airway (Figure 6-9). As discussed earlier, CT is the imaging modality of choice for distinguishing cellulitis from an abscess, which will appear as a walled-off fluid collection needing surgical drainage.

On occasion the child being evaluated for stridor has aspirated a foreign body, such as a peanut, into the bronchus and the airway is blocked, or the child has ingested an

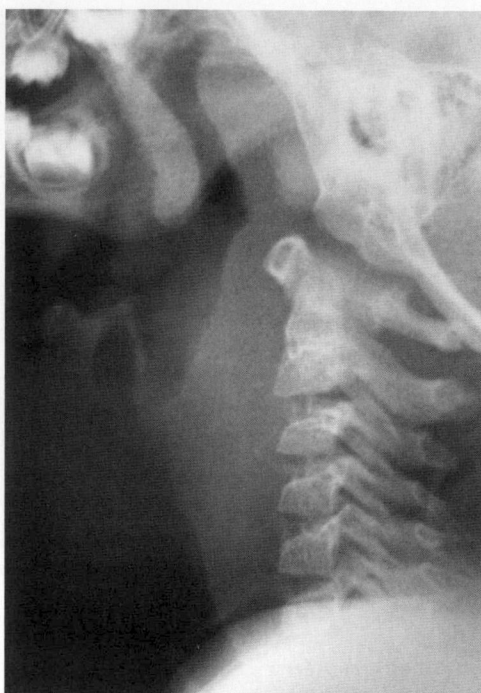

FIGURE 6-9   Hypopharynx and trachea are displaced away from the cervical spine by a retropharyngeal abscess.

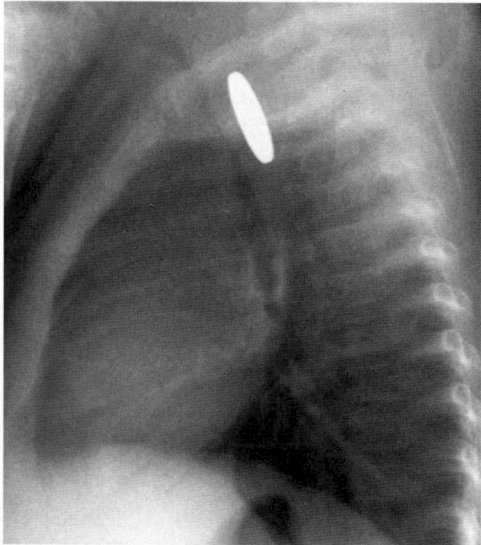

FIGURE 6-10   Edema from a coin in the upper esophagus causes marked narrowing of the adjacent trachea. The child presented with stridor and difficulty with swallowing.

object such as a coin into the esophagus, causing compression of the trachea. If the child is suspected of ingesting a coin or other object, a lateral radiograph of the neck and frontal views of the chest and abdomen are usually obtained to locate the object (Figure 6-10). Nonradiopaque objects that are aspirated may be difficult to see unless outlined by air in the trachea or bronchi. Forced expiratory chest radiographs are most useful in demonstrating the air trapping that may result when a foreign body is aspirated

into a bronchus. In some instances, decubitus radiographs or fluoroscopy may be warranted.

Tracheomalacia is diagnosed when the thoracic trachea abnormally collapses during expiration, leading to an expiratory wheeze. Although this may be seen in premature infants, other associations include tracheoesophageal fistula and vascular rings. The abnormal collapse may be easily demonstrated by airway fluoroscopy, which may be combined with a barium swallow to exclude a fistula or ring.[6,7]

RESPIRATORY DISTRESS IN THE NEWBORN

The various causes and conditions that can result in respiratory distress in the newborn may be combined under the mnemonic *CHAMPS* (Box 6-1).

One of the most common causes of respiratory distress in the newborn is transient tachypnea of the newborn. Conditions that decrease the thoracic squeeze to clear the lungs of fluid at delivery include cesarean section, mild or moderate prematurity, maternal diabetes, and precipitous delivery. The radiographic findings usually show mild vascular congestion with pulmonary edema and small pleural effusions. The chest radiograph clears rapidly by 24 hours and is usually normal by 48 to 72 hours of age with conservative treatment.

Respiratory distress syndrome (RDS), or hyaline membrane disease, occurs in premature infants, particularly those under 36 weeks of gestation. It is caused by a deficiency in pulmonary surfactant and deficiency in alveolar surface area for gas exchange in the immature lungs.[3] By lowering the surface tension in the alveoli, surfactant prevents atelectasis. When surfactant is deficient, the chest radiograph shows the characteristic pattern of low lung volumes with a ground-glass or granular pattern of alveolar collapse surrounding **air bronchograms** (air-filled bronchus against surrounding opacified alveoli, indicating alveolar disease) (Figure 6-11).

Artificial surfactant given through the endotracheal tube may lead to rapid improvement demonstrated radiographically, but it may also lead to asymmetrical patterns of aeration if distributed unevenly. Gradual improvement over 1 week occurs with mild or moderate cases of RDS, but severe disease usually results in the chronic lung changes of bronchopulmonary dysplasia. This chronic

Box 6-1	Respiratory Distress in the Newborn

C: Cardiac, congenital anomalies
H: Hyaline membrane disease
A: Airway
M: Meconium aspiration
P: Pneumonia
S: Surgical lesions

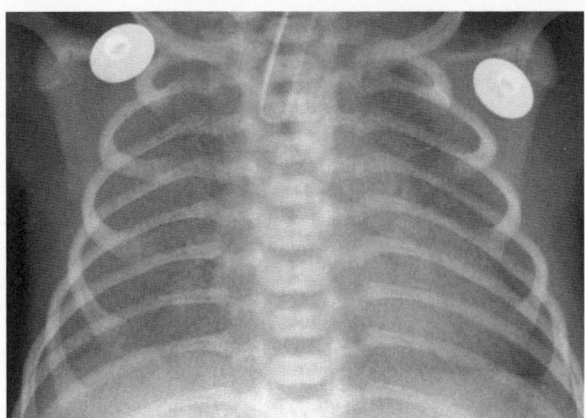

FIGURE 6-11   Even after intubation, the lungs are hypoinflated and have a granular pattern with faint air bronchograms in this infant with respiratory distress syndrome.

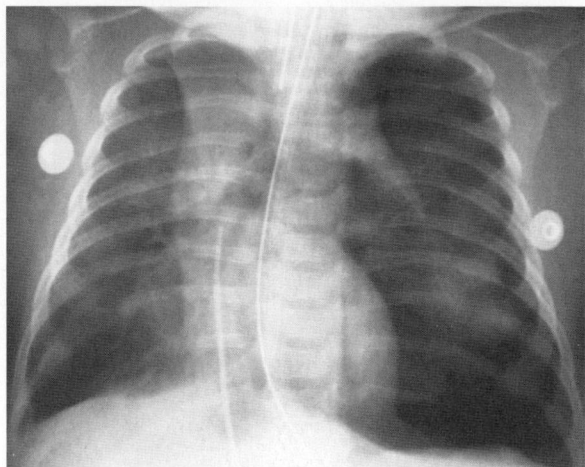

FIGURE 6-13   Pneumomediastinum elevates the left lobe of the thymus to produce a "spinnaker sail" in this child, who also has a large left pneumothorax.

disease is characterized by coarse, linear areas of scarring or atelectasis interspersed with areas of air trapping as well as shifting atelectasis. Both RDS and bronchopulmonary dysplasia may produce a variety of air leaks related to mechanical ventilation, including pneumothorax, **pneumomediastinum,** and **pulmonary interstitial emphysema.**

Pneumothoraces are the most common air leaks and are caused when air dissects in the pleural space surrounding the lung. On an AP supine chest radiograph, air is usually seen lateral to the lung but may be subpulmonic (between the lung and diaphragm) or medial (next to the heart), in the latter case mimicking a pneumomediastinum (Figure 6-12). If the hemithorax appears hyperlucent or the lateral costophrenic margin is too clearly visualized, a decubitus view or cross-table lateral view (patient supine with x-ray beam parallel to the table and passing through the patient from one side to the other side) may be helpful to exclude a pneumothorax. An upright, PA chest radiograph is preferred in older children in whom the pneumothorax accumulates above the lung apex.

When air dissects into the mediastinal tissues, it is called a pneumomediastinum. This air elevates the thymus, producing a "spinnaker sail" appearance, and may dissect under the heart, leading to a continuous diaphragm appearance (Figure 6-13). A lateral decubitus image may cause a medial pneumothorax to shift to the elevated lateral pleural space, which distinguishes it from a pneumomediastinum. Air in a pneumopericardium surrounds only the heart and does not extend around other mediastinal structures such as the aorta. Neither a medial pneumothorax nor a pneumopericardium will elevate the thymus.

Pulmonary interstitial emphysema results from air dissecting within the interstitium of the lung. This condition appears as a diffuse pattern of random, small radiolucent bubbles combined with an irregular network of branching radiolucencies. Distribution is variable from entire lung to lobar to segmental. Interestingly, the pattern of involvement may shift from one lobe of one lung to another lobe in the other lung (Figure 6-14).

The radiographic appearance of RDS can also be complicated by the superimposition of a **patent ductus arteriosus** (in the newborn, a failure of the connection between the aorta and the pulmonary artery to close) or hemorrhage. The appearance of pleural effusions with increased heart size and edema several days after birth suggests patent ductus arteriosus. Whiteout of a lung or lobe without volume loss may result from pulmonary hemorrhage.

Although meconium staining of amniotic fluid occurs in 12% of deliveries, only 2% of these newborns develop meconium aspiration syndrome. Predisposing factors are postmaturity, intrauterine stress, and small size for gestational age. The aspirated meconium produced by the bowel plugs bronchi and produces a chemical pneumonitis. The chest radiograph is characterized by coarse, patchy

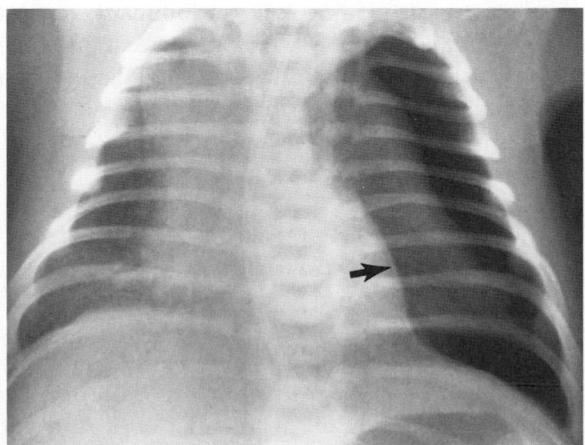

FIGURE 6-12   Large left pneumothorax appears black and outlines the partially collapsed left lung and left cardiac border (*arrow*).

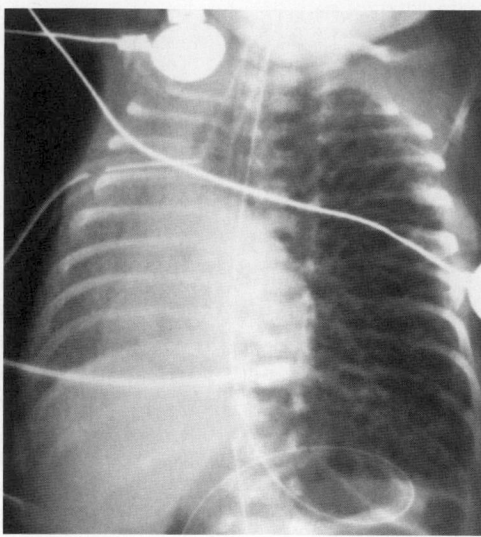

FIGURE 6-14 Massive pulmonary interstitial emphysema throughout the left lung causes shift of the mediastinum to the right and downward displacement of the left hemidiaphragm.

opacities secondary to atelectasis from bronchial obstruction alternating with areas of hyperinflation (Figure 6-15). The severity of the radiographic abnormalities does not always correlate with the clinical severity of the disease. Likewise, an infant with relatively mild radiographic findings may be worse clinically because of persistent pulmonary hypertension. Pneumothoraces and pneumomediastinum develop in about 25% of infants with meconium aspiration syndrome. Resolution of the radiographic findings may take several weeks.

Although a variety of organisms may cause neonatal pneumonia, the most common is group B *Streptococcus,* which is usually acquired by the fetus before birth. Premature rupture of the membranes and maternal infection are predisposing factors. The radiographic findings are variable and may mimic other disease entities. For example,

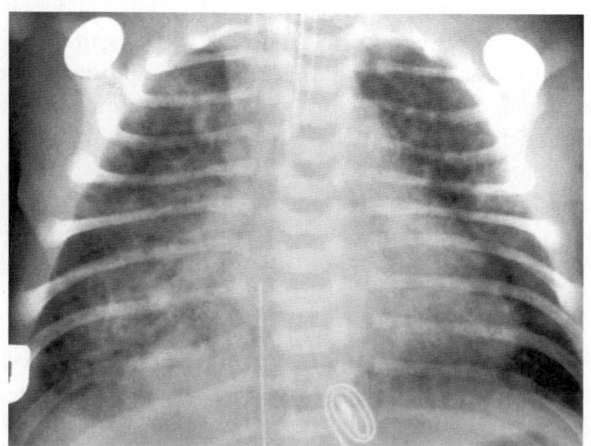

FIGURE 6-15 Meconium aspiration appears as a coarse, asymmetrical pattern. Enlargement of the heart may be secondary to fluid overload in this infant.

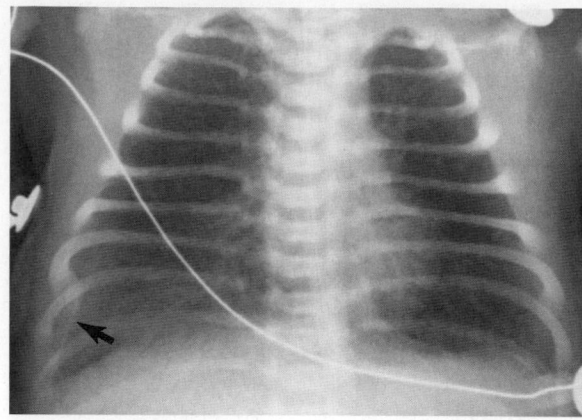

FIGURE 6-16 Group B streptococcal pneumonia presents in this infant with hyperinflation, small right pleural effusion (*arrow*), and hazy infiltrative pattern.

pneumonia may have a pattern resembling RDS; however, the presence of pleural effusions is rare in RDS but common in neonatal pneumonia (Figure 6-16). Treatment is usually begun on the basis of the clinical assumption of pneumonia, with the radiographs used to monitor progress of the disease.[8]

Two surgical entities that may cause a cystic appearance in the lung are congenital diaphragmatic hernia and cystic adenomatoid malformation. In congenital diaphragmatic hernia, bowel herniates through the defect in the diaphragm, leading to a "cystic" appearance as the loops fill with air. If the stomach herniates as well, placement of a nasogastric tube may confirm the diagnosis. Because the bowel is in the chest, the abdomen will appear scaphoid (concave). Most of the hernias occur on the left. Patient outcome depends on the degree of pulmonary hypoplasia caused by compression of the developing lung tissue (Figure 6-17).

Cystic adenomatoid malformation is a derangement in normal pulmonary tissue development, leading to cysts ranging from millimeters to several centimeters in size. Initially the cysts are fluid filled but become air filled over the first day or two of life. A large dominant cyst could mimic congenital lobar overinflation, whereas cysts appearing to fill one lung could mimic congenital diaphragmatic hernia. The presence of a normal amount of bowel in the abdomen would make a hernia unlikely.[7]

ATELECTASIS

Atelectasis is caused by an absence of air in the lung parenchyma from myriad causes, including bronchial obstruction or extrinsic compression. Most atelectasis is subsegmental in extent and appears as discoid or platelike opacities, often radiating from the hila or located just above the diaphragm. Segments, lobes, and entire lungs may be collapsed, or atelectatic. This loss of volume may shift fissures toward the area of atelectasis, cause a

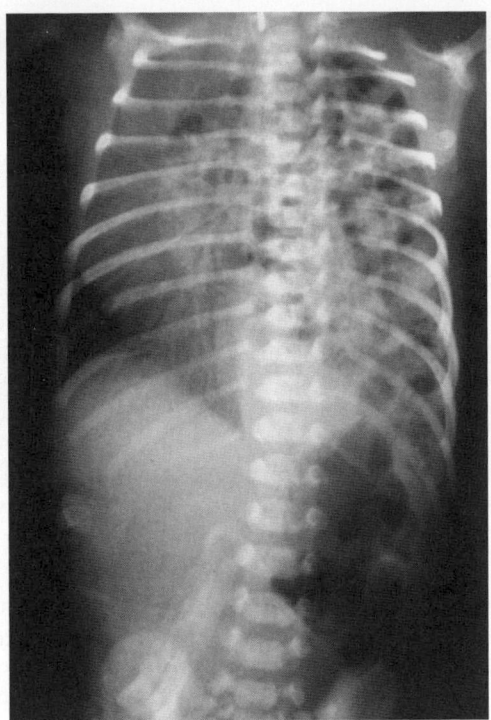

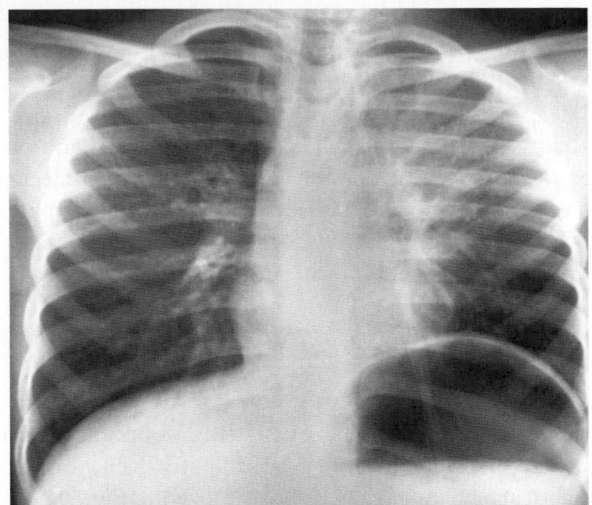

FIGURE 6-18   Left upper lobe collapse causes elevation of the left hemidiaphragm and crowding of the left ribs from volume loss. The cardiac and superior mediastinal borders are indistinct because of the "silhouette sign," whereas the diaphragm remains demarcated by the aerated left lower lobe.

FIGURE 6-17   Multiple "cysts" in the left hemithorax are air-filled loops of bowel that herniated through a defect in the left hemidiaphragm. The abdomen is scaphoid from decreased bowel content.

mediastinal shift toward the affected side, and elevate the ipsilateral diaphragm. Crowding of the pulmonary vascular and interstitial markings in the affected region will occur. The other lung or adjacent lobes may become more lucent secondary to hyperexpansion.

When atelectasis occurs in the right upper lobe, the minor fissure and posterior half of the major fissure shift upward. The collapsed right upper lobe appears as a triangular wedge of opacity adjacent to the superior mediastinum on the frontal radiograph and as a triangular wedge at the apex in the lateral radiograph. Because no minor fissure is present on the left, collapse of the left upper lobe appears different from the right, with the major fissure shifting in an anterior direction. The collapsed left upper lobe on frontal projection appears as opacity in the upper two thirds of the lung that obscures superior mediastinal and left cardiac borders and lacks a sharply defined border with the aerated lower lobe (Figure 6-18). In lateral projection the left upper lobe collapses adjacent to the anterior chest wall, with the major fissure defining the edge against the lower lobe. Isolated lingular atelectasis obscures the left cardiac border.

Right middle lobe collapse is commonly seen in children with asthma and causes the major and minor fissures to approximate. The resultant triangular wedge or platelike opacity is most diagnostic in lateral projection and extends from the hilum to the anterior chest wall (Figure 6-19). It is less defined in frontal projection and may appear as a vague loss of the right-sided cardiac border.

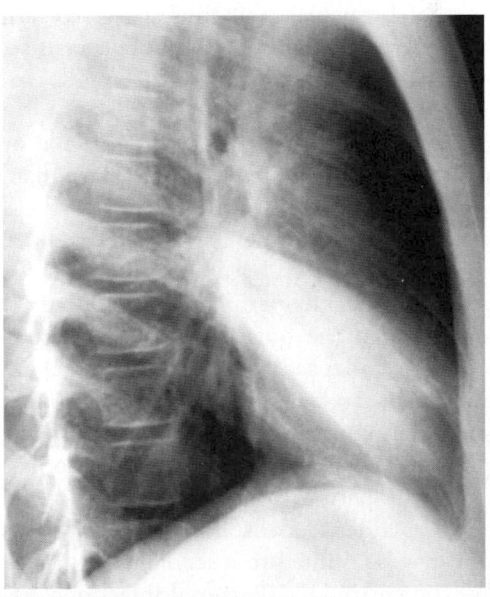

FIGURE 6-19   Collapsed right middle lobe appears as a triangular wedge of increased density extending anteriorly and inferiorly toward the anterior chest wall and diaphragm.

Both right and left lower lobe atelectasis cause downward and posterior displacement of the major fissure. The lower lobe collapses toward the posterior aspect of the diaphragm on the lateral view and retrocardiac adjacent to the spine on the frontal view. The sharp border of the adjacent diaphragm becomes obscured in both projections. In the lateral radiograph the normally more lucent-appearing lower thoracic vertebral bodies appear denser than normal because the x-ray beam must penetrate through the adjacent collapsed lower lobe. This increased density of the lower thoracic vertebral bodies has been termed the **spine sign.** Left lower lobe collapse is commonly seen in postoperative patients, especially those having undergone cardiothoracic surgery.

The previously described silhouette sign is useful in localizing suspected atelectasis. The right cardiac border loses its sharp definition with right middle lobe atelectasis, whereas the left border is associated with lingular pathology. The diaphragmatic border is lost when atelectasis or other pathology occurs in the adjacent lower lobe.[9]

PNEUMONIA

Viruses are the most common cause of pneumonia in children, especially in the outpatient population. Many bacterial pneumonias are superimposed over viral infections but may also be seen in hospitalized patients. Fungal and less common infections should be suspected in the immunocompromised patient.

Infections may involve primarily the airways, mainly the peripheral airspaces, or a combination of both. Bronchiolitis in the younger child and bronchitis in the older child are viral infections of the airways leading to a radiographic appearance of bronchial wall thickening. Hyperinflation of the lungs as well as linear areas of atelectasis secondary to airway plugging by mucus are often associated with airway inflammation.

Patchy areas of poorly defined parenchymal opacification characterize bronchopneumonia. The inflammation in the airways extends outward to involve the adjacent air spaces. The opacities may be caused by the air space inflammation as well as by atelectasis from associated mucous plugging of the peripheral airways. Air bronchograms occur when the open airways are surrounded by consolidated or collapsed air spaces. Both viral and bacterial pneumonias can cause a bronchopneumonia pattern. Although it may mimic other pulmonary diseases, *Mycoplasma* presents typically as a bronchopneumonia.

Filling of the peripheral air spaces with an infectious exudate causes a dense, consolidated appearance. The involvement may be limited to a segment of lung or spread to involve the entire lobe. Bacterial infections are usually the cause of consolidated, or lobar, pneumonia.

Pneumonia may be associated with hilar adenopathy and pleural effusions. When the pleura becomes infected, the resulting empyema may need to be surgically drained. Although decubitus radiographs may be able to differentiate an uncomplicated mobile pleural effusion from loculated fluid or thickening, both ultrasound and CT can be used to better characterize the pleural fluid. Pulmonary abscesses are rare complications, but **pneumatoceles** (thin-walled, air-filled cavities in the lungs) may occur after staphylococcal pneumonia. Round pneumonias are usually of pneumococcal origin (Figure 6-20).[9-12]

The American College of Radiology (ACR) has developed appropriateness criteria for imaging pediatric patients who

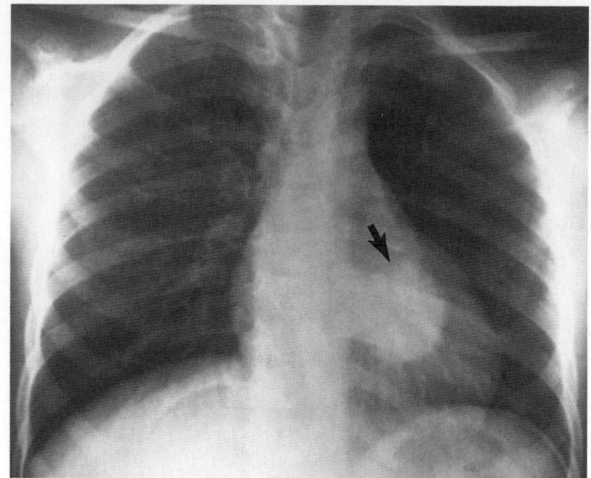

FIGURE 6-20   Round pneumonia (*arrow*) in the left lower lobe simulates a mass.

present with a fever with an unknown source.[2] Although the source of a fever may be determined medically through patient evaluation, history, and laboratory tests, chest radiographs are considered appropriate in the acute evaluation of infants and children with a fever without a source, especially if the patient displays chest symptoms. Chest radiographs may also be appropriate for evaluation in a pediatric patient who does not have chest symptoms but does have a fever, oxygen saturation of 95% or lower, and a white blood cell count of $20,000/mm^3$ or more.[2]

ASTHMA

Asthma is caused by recurrent bronchospasm of the large intrathoracic airways, leading to wheezing and labored breathing. Chest radiographs are usually obtained to exclude the presence of pneumonia causing the acute episode. Typical findings are hyperinflation and bronchial wall thickening. Mucous plugging of the airways may lead to atelectasis and focal air trapping. Atelectasis is the usual cause of a focal opacity in the lung. Pneumomediastinum occurs in a small percentage of children evaluated for an acute asthma attack and is a cause of acute chest pain.[11-14]

CYSTIC FIBROSIS

Cystic fibrosis is a genetic disorder affecting the function of exocrine glands, causing increased viscosity of the respiratory mucus. This mucus is difficult to clear from the airways, leading to obstruction and promotion of bacterial infection. Cystic fibrosis involves many organs in addition to the respiratory system. In the respiratory system, evidence suggests that the lungs are histologically normal at birth. Pulmonary damage is initiated by gradually increasing secretions from the hypertrophy of bronchial

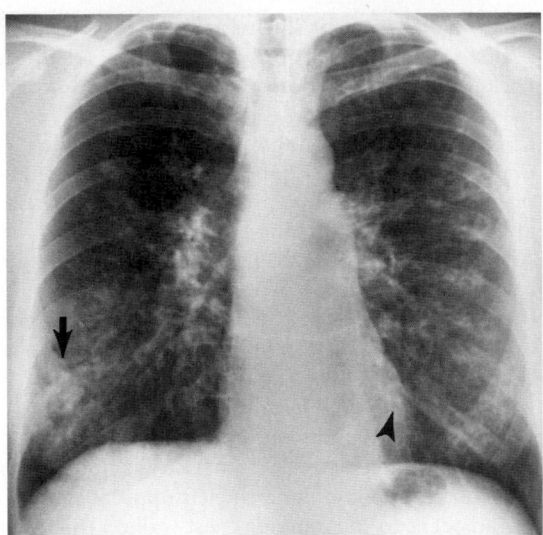

FIGURE 6-21 Coarse interstitial markings, hyperinflation, bronchiectasis, mucous plugging (*arrow*), atelectasis (*arrowhead*), and enlarged pulmonary hila are all demonstrated in this child with cystic fibrosis.

glands, leading to obstruction of the bronchial system. The resultant plugging promotes staphylococcal infection, followed by more tissue damage, as well as atelectasis (collapse of lung tissue) and emphysema.[4] Early childhood radiographs may show nonspecific findings of airway disease with peribronchial thickening, atelectasis, and air trapping. These early changes are similar to the chest radiographs of a patient with asthma. As the disease progresses, fingerlike mucoid impaction of the airways may be demonstrated along with abnormal dilation of the airways, called bronchiectasis, lobar atelectasis, scarring, pulmonary artery and right ventricular enlargement, and overinflation of the lung and chest wall. Recurrent infections are common. Striking hyperinflation is seen in older patients, often with enlarged hila from pulmonary hypertension (Figure 6-21).[13]

ACUTE RESPIRATORY DISTRESS SYNDROME

Although originally described in adults, acute respiratory distress syndrome may occur in children as well. These patients present initially with either sepsis, pneumonia, near drowning, inhalation injury, aspiration, or trauma. The acute lung insult can lead to increased capillary permeability, pulmonary edema, surfactant inactivation, alveolar filling, and reduced lung compliance. This leads to profound hypoxemia and acute respiratory distress syndrome. The disease passes through stages of acute lung injury, exudative alveolitis, fibroproliferative repair, and finally recovery if the patient survives. The mortality rate is high. Pneumothoraces and pneumomediastinum are common complications (Figure 6-22).[15]

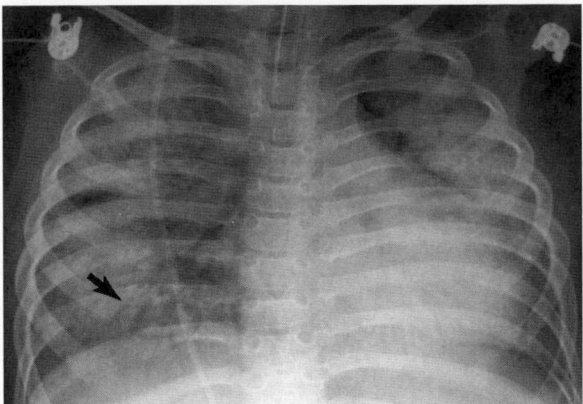

FIGURE 6-22 Pneumonia was the precipitating precursor to acute respiratory distress syndrome, with densely consolidated lungs and air bronchograms (*arrow*).

CHEST TRAUMA

When an injured child is evaluated in the emergency department, initial radiographs to screen for trauma usually include an AP projection of the chest. Lines and tubes inserted at the accident site or on arrival in the emergency department should be assessed for position and effectiveness. A right mainstem intubation may lead to collapse of the left lung. The position of a chest tube may not be optimal for evacuating a pneumothorax, and the nasogastric tube may need to be advanced into the stomach.

Consolidation in the patient with blunt trauma may result from pulmonary contusion with hemorrhage into the air spaces. Aspiration leading to patchy consolidation in the upper lobes should be considered in the patient with loss of consciousness. Laceration of the lung may lead to cysts in the parenchyma as well as a pneumothorax. The rib cage should be evaluated for fractures, especially adjacent to an area of lung injury. Multiple contiguous rib fractures may result in a flail chest (three or more rib fractures resulting in paradoxical motion of the chest wall with respiration) with associated ventilation difficulties (Figure 6-23).

Widening of the superior mediastinum suggests hemorrhage, which could be venous or related to aortic injury. Traumatic aortic rupture is rare in children as opposed to adults. Small children have prominent thymic tissue, so this should be excluded as the cause of mediastinal widening. Tracheal and bronchial fractures are rare but cause massive air leaks. Enlargement of the cardiac silhouette from a traumatic pericardial effusion is rare.

When significant chest injury is suspected clinically or demonstrated on chest radiographs, CT scans of the chest more clearly demonstrate the extent of the injury than conventional radiographs. These are often rapidly performed in conjunction with imaging of the abdomen. Lung and mediastinal injury as well as placement of chest tubes can be further clarified. More injury is often shown

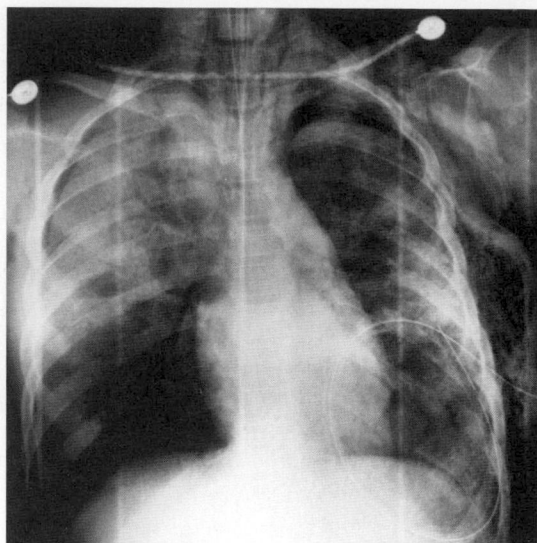

FIGURE 6-23   Trauma to the chest resulted in extensive bilateral air leaks and densely consolidated pulmonary contusions. Multiple rib fractures are present.

by CT scans than was suspected on chest radiographs. Not uncommonly, small pneumothoraces are found by CT that cannot be seen even in retrospect on conventional radiographs. CT angiography of the chest has supplanted catheter aortography for exclusion of aortic injury. The need for CT is usually made clear after assessment of the previously obtained chest radiographs. Although CT scanning of the chest may provide additional information, routine scanning in children is discouraged because of the added radiation dose.[13-15]

KEY POINTS

- *Position* refers to the arrangement of the patient's body and *projection* refers to the path of the x-ray beam.
- The PA and AP projection demonstrates chest anatomy in relation to right and left sides of the body. The lateral projection demonstrates the anatomical structures from anterior to posterior. The lateral decubitus position is a frontal projection performed with the patient lying on either the right or left side.
- The normal structures that are visualized on a chest radiograph are distinguishable because of differences in the absorption of the x-ray beam. Bone and metallic orthopedic hardware appear white, well-expanded lungs appear relatively black, and soft tissue organs and fluid usually appear as shades of gray.
- The endotracheal tube should be located between the thoracic inlet and the carina. The tip of the CVP catheter should be in the distal superior vena cava just above the right atrium. The pulmonary artery catheter should be positioned in the pulmonary artery.

- Common reasons for soft-tissue neck radiographic evaluation include croup and epiglottitis. CT of the neck is useful in the evaluation of retropharyngeal masses and abnormalities.
- Chest radiography is appropriate in neonates to evaluate for a fever without a source, RDS, pneumonias, congenital diaphragmatic hernias, and cystic adenomatoid malformation.
- Atelectasis may affect segments, lobes, or the entire lung. The collapsed right upper lobe appears as a triangular wedge of opacity adjacent to the superior mediastinum in the frontal radiograph and as a triangular wedge at the apex in the lateral radiograph. The collapsed left upper lobe appears as opacity in the upper two thirds of the lung, obscuring the superior mediastinal and left cardiac borders on the frontal projection and the left upper lobe collapsing adjacent to the anterior chest wall on the lateral projection. Right middle lobe collapse is best visualized on the lateral projection as a triangular wedge or platelike opacity extending from the hilum to the anterior chest wall. Both right and left lower lobe atelectasis cause downward and posterior displacement of the major fissure.
- The radiographic appearance of cystic fibrosis in early childhood demonstrates nonspecific findings of airway disease with peribronchial thickening, atelectasis, and air trapping. As the disease progresses, fingerlike mucoid impaction of the airways may be demonstrated along with bronchiectasis, lobar atelectasis, scarring, pulmonary artery and right ventricular enlargement, and overinflation of the lung and chest wall.
- Chest trauma resulting in pulmonary contusion often is demonstrated radiographically as consolidation from hemorrhage into the air spaces. Aspiration pneumonia is demonstrated as patchy consolidation in the upper lobes should be considered in the patient with loss of consciousness. Laceration of the lung may lead to pneumothorax, atelectasis, and cyst formation within the lung parenchyma. Multiple contiguous rib fractures may result in a flail chest with associated ventilation difficulties.

ASSESSMENT QUESTIONS

See Evolve Resources for answers.

1. A mother states that she found her 18-month-old child choking near an open can of peanuts. Which set of chest radiographs would most likely suggest airway obstruction?
   A. Frontal and bilateral oblique
   B. Frontal inspiratory and frontal forced expiratory
   C. Frontal and lateral
   D. Frontal and left-side down lateral decubitus

2. The normal thymus has a characteristic appearance with which of the following radiographic findings?
   I. Displacement of the trachea to the opposite side of the mediastinum
   II. Appearance of a sail
   III. Wavy margins
       A. I and II only
       B. I and III only
       C. II and III only
       D. I, II, and III

3. A pneumothorax is suspected on the left in a child's portable radiograph from the intensive care unit. Which of the following may better image and confirm a suspected pneumothorax?
   I. Cross-table lateral
   II. Upright frontal
   III. Left-side down decubitus
   IV. Right-side down decubitus
       A. I, II, and III only
       B. I, II, and IV only
       C. I, III, and IV only
       D. II, III, and IV only

4. Subglottic edema causing a "church steeple" appearance of the trachea on the frontal neck radiograph is characteristic of which infection?
   A. Retropharyngeal abscess
   B. Epiglottitis
   C. Adenoiditis
   D. Croup

5. Before intubation, the chest radiograph of a premature newborn reveals low lung volumes and diffuse ground-glass opacification of the lungs. These radiographic findings are most characteristic of
   A. Meconium aspiration
   B. Respiratory distress syndrome
   C. Bronchopulmonary dysplasia
   D. Transient tachypnea of the newborn

6. The initial chest radiograph of a neonate in severe respiratory distress and having a scaphoid abdomen reveals multiple round air-filled structures in the left side of the chest, displacing the mediastinum to the right. The most likely etiology is:
   A. Congenital adenomatoid malformation
   B. Pulmonary interstitial emphysema
   C. Congenital diaphragmatic hernia
   D. Staphylococcal pneumonia

7. Left lower lobe collapse (atelectasis) is associated with which of the following radiographic findings?
   I. Loss of the left-side heart border
   II. Loss of the left hemidiaphragm border
   III. Increased retrocardiac density
   IV. "Spine sign"
       A. I, II, and III only
       B. I, II, and IV only
       C. I, III, and IV only
       D. II, III, and IV only

8. Pneumatoceles are occasionally seen as a complication of which of the following infections?
   A. Mycoplasmal
   B. Viral
   C. Streptococcal
   D. Staphylococcal

9. Which of the following is a hallmark of cystic fibrosis and is *not* also seen with asthma?
   A. Hyperinflation
   B. Atelectasis
   C. Bronchiectasis
   D. Airway disease

10. CT scans of the chest in a pediatric trauma patient are not routinely obtained because of
    A. The high radiation dose
    B. The time necessary to complete the scan
    C. A contraindication to the use of IV contrast agents
    D. The additional costs associated with CT imaging

References

1. Kowalczyk N: *Radiographic pathology for technologists*, ed 6, St. Louis, 2013, Mosby/Elsevier.
2. American College of Radiology Appropriateness criteria: *Pediatric Imaging*. http://www.acr.org/Quality-Safety/Appropriateness-Criteria/Diagnostic/Pediatric-Imaging. Accessed January 17, 2013.
3. Harris EA, Arheart KL, Penning DH: Endotracheal tube malposition within the pediatric population: a common event despite clinical evidence of correct placement, *Can J Anesth* 55(10):685–690, 2008.
4. Peterson J, Johnson N, Deakins K, Wilson-Costello D, Jelvsek JE, Chatburn R: Accuracy of the 7-8-9 rule for endotracheal tube placement in the neonate, *J Perinatology* 26:333–336, 2006.
5. McCance KL, Heuther SE, Brashers VL, Rote NS: *Pathophysiology: the biologic basis for disease in adults and children*, ed 6, St. Louis, 2010, Mosby/Elsevier.
6. Strife JL: Upper airway and tracheal obstruction in infants and children, *Radiol Clin North Am* 26:309, 1988.
7. Griscom NT: Diseases of the trachea, bronchi and smaller airways, *Radiol Clin North Am* 31:605, 1993.
8. Newman B, Bowen AD, Sang OK: A practical approach to the newborn chest, *Curr Probl Diagn Radiol* 19:41, 1990.
9. Newman B, Sang OK: Abnormal pulmonary aeration in infants and children, *Radiol Clin North Am* 26:323, 1988.
10. Paré JA, Fraser R: *Synopsis of diseases of the chest*, Philadelphia, 1983, WB Saunders.
11. Eggli KD, Newman B: Nodules, masses, and pseudomasses in the pediatric lung, *Radiol Clin North Am* 31:651, 1993.
12. Hedlund GL, Kirks DR: Emergency radiology of the pediatric chest, *Curr Probl Diagn Radiol* 19:133, 1990.
13. Kirks DR: Practical pediatric imaging: *Diagnostic radiology of infants and children*, ed 3, Philadelphia, 1998, Lippincott-Raven.
14. Hilton SV, Edwards DK: *Practical pediatric radiology*, Philadelphia, 1994, WB Saunders.
15. Kuhn JP, Slovis JP, Haller JO, Caffey J, eds. *Caffey's pediatric diagnostic imaging*, ed 10, Mosby, 2004, Philadelphia.

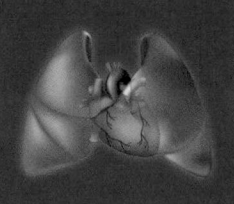

Chapter **7**

Pediatric Flexible Bronchoscopy

PETER M. LUCKETT, DANIELLE CORRIGAN

LEARNING OBJECTIVES

After reading this chapter the reader will be able to:

1. Identify common indications for bronchoscopy in infants and children and the differences between rigid and flexible bronchoscopy
2. Prepare equipment and the patient for a flexible bronchoscopy procedure
3. Monitor a patient during a flexible bronchoscopy, including what complications to watch for during and after the procedure
4. Clean and disinfect bronchoscopes after procedures

KEY TERMS

Bronchiectasis
Bronchoalveolar lavage
Bronchomalacia
Conscious sedation
Flexible fiberoptic bronchoscopy

High-level disinfection
Laryngeal web
Laryngomalacia
Papillomatosis
Rigid bronchoscopy

Stridor
Tracheomalacia
Vocal cord dysfunction

Flexible fiberoptic bronchoscopy was first introduced for clinical practice in 1968, with the invention of flexible scopes containing fiberoptic bundles to illuminate and visualize the airways.

The procedure was initially performed in adults because of the relatively large size of the fiberscopes. The development of smaller bronchoscopes in the late 1970s led to the widespread use of this procedure in children.[1] Pediatric flexible bronchoscopy is now performed by many medical specialists, including pediatric pulmonologists, otolaryngologists, surgeons, anesthesiologists, and pediatric intensivists. It is done in a variety of settings, including bronchoscopy suites, operating suites, intensive care units, and procedure rooms.[2-5] Since the 1990s the direct visual inspection of the pediatric airways with or without **bronchoalveolar lavage** has been a major tool in the assessment of the child with respiratory disease.

INDICATIONS

Flexible bronchoscopy is indicated when (1) information valuable to the management of a patient cannot be obtained by less invasive techniques or (2) therapeutic interventions need to be directly administered to the airway (Box 7-1). As with any invasive procedure, the potential benefits to be gained in any given patient must be weighed against the risks of the procedure, even the most minor risk.

Diagnostic Bronchoscopy

For diagnostic purposes, persistent or recurrent respiratory symptoms are the most common indication for flexible bronchoscopy. These symptoms may include stridor, an abnormal voice, wheeze, cough, and recurrent or persistent abnormalities on chest radiography.

Stridor

Stridor is a high-pitched wheeze produced by turbulent airflow through a partially obstructed airway. It can be

Box 7-1	Indications for Flexible Bronchoscopy

DIAGNOSTIC
Airway Anatomy Evaluation
- Fistulas
- Hemangiomas or tumors
- Stenoses or strictures
- Tracheal bronchus
- Tracheostomy evaluation
- Vascular rings
- Congenital anomalies

Bronchoalveolar Lavage and Biopsy
Cytopathology
- Lipid-laden macrophages
- Hemosiderin-stained macrophages
- Malignant cells

Microbiology
- Bacteria
- Fungi
- *Pneumocystis*
- *Mycobacterium tuberculosis*
- Viruses

Foreign Body Aspiration
Functional Airway Evaluation
- Laryngomalacia, tracheomalacia, bronchomalacia
- Vocal cord dysfunction or paralysis
- Persistent hoarseness

Inhalation Injury
- Hemoptysis
- Recurrent pneumonia

THERAPEUTIC
- Atelectasis
- Endotracheal intubation
- Foreign body aspiration
- Laser therapy

inspiratory, expiratory, or biphasic. Inspiratory stridor associated with extrathoracic lesions is the most common. Expiratory stridor or mixed expiratory/inspiratory stridor is typically associated with intrathoracic lesions. Because stridor always has an anatomical basis, visual inspection of the airway is usually required for definitive diagnosis. It is the most common indication for diagnostic flexible bronchoscopy in infants. The possible causes of recurrent or persistent stridor include laryngeal pathology, subglottic stenosis, mass or tumor, extrinsic compression of the tracheobronchial tree, and vocal cord paralysis. **Vocal cord dysfunction** (VCD), an uncontrolled adduction of the vocal cords, is seen in older children and adolescents.

Stridor often varies in intensity depending on the extent of a child's activity or agitation, which increases the child's minute ventilation. This increase in airflow results in louder stridor. Thus stridor is a dynamic process in children, and flexible bronchoscopy is ideally suited for its evaluation. Because flexible bronchoscopy can be performed on a sedated but spontaneously breathing patient, the dynamics of the airways are preserved without disruption by general anesthesia, positive-pressure ventilation, or the oral approach of rigid bronchoscopy. Of all indications of diagnostic pediatric flexible bronchoscopy, stridor receives the highest diagnostic yield for the procedure, identifying specific lesions in more than 80% of patients.[6,7]

The most common cause of inspiratory stridor in neonates is **laryngomalacia,** the inward collapse of the softer than normal cartilage of the upper airway over the airway opening during inspiration. It is a congenital condition that is usually not serious. The exact cause is not known. Laryngomalacia will resolve 90% of the time by 12 to 18 months. The condition occurs in three patterns:
- The prolapse of one or both arytenoids into the supraglottic space during inspiration
- The lateral infolding across the airway of a soft epiglottis that is more omega shaped than crescent shaped in a young infant
- The anteroposterior bending of a soft epiglottis across the supraglottic space

Other laryngeal lesions that can produce stridor include unilateral or bilateral vocal cord paralysis from congenital lesions, birth trauma, or recurrent laryngeal nerve injury after thoracic surgery; laryngeal **papillomatosis;** and **laryngeal webs.** Inspiratory or biphasic stridor may also arise from subglottic lesions, such as congenital or acquired subglottic stenosis, subglottic edema resulting from infection or chronic acid aspiration, or subglottic hemangiomas.

Tracheomalacia, caused by a congenital or acquired weakness in tracheal cartilaginous support, may cause inspiratory stridor but is more often associated with biphasic or expiratory stridor. Tracheomalacia may be seen in up to one third of patients with laryngomalacia. It is also present when a tracheoesophageal fistula or vascular ring deforms the tracheal cartilage, and it may develop with long-standing tracheal inflammation, as seen in infants with bronchopulmonary dysplasia. If the weakness in support extends into the mainstem bronchi, the condition is termed **bronchomalacia.**

Additional causes of expiratory stridor include extrinsic tracheal or bronchial obstruction from vascular rings or slings, anomalous arteries, congenital heart disease, hilar adenopathy, and mediastinal mass lesions.

Wheeze

Recurrent wheezing, a continuous, coarse, whistling sound, is another common respiratory symptom in the pediatric population. Wheezing usually results from a more distal site of airway obstruction than stridor. The most common cause of recurrent wheezing in children is asthma, and most patients with asthma do not require bronchoscopy as part of their evaluation. Exceptions include asthmatics with recurrent or persistent atelectasis (lung collapse, often of the right middle lobe) or asthmatics with gastroesophageal reflux who may have chronic aspiration. A flexible bronchoscopic evaluation is often indicated to investigate other causes of wheezing, particularly when the wheezing is unilateral, is present at birth or at a young age, or is refractory to asthma medications. Nonasthmatic causes of wheezing include anatomical abnormalities of the airway (e.g., bronchomalacia, stenosis, and extrinsic compression of the left mainstem bronchus from a dilated heart), anomalies of the great vessels (vascular ring), recurrent aspiration, and foreign body aspiration. Vocal cord dysfunction may masquerade as asthma.

Cough

Some disorders may produce chronic cough in addition to wheezing, and bronchoscopy is often indicated because of chronic refractory cough. This indication is particularly strong when there is radiographic indication of **bronchiectasis**—that is, chronic dilation of the bronchi and bronchioles associated with secondary infection in an area of lung. There is little role for bronchoscopy in evaluating the cough that accompanies common childhood conditions such as upper and uncomplicated lower respiratory tract infections, sinusitis, postnasal drip syndrome, asthma, and exposure to environmental irritants. On the other hand, bronchoscopy should be considered to evaluate the possibilities of gastroesophageal reflux or aspiration, anatomical abnormalities of airways or large vessels, and any occult endobronchial lesions or foreign bodies, as well as to obtain culture specimens from children not responding to therapy.

Radiographic Abnormalities

Flexible bronchoscopy is indicated in the evaluation of a number of radiographic abnormalities in children, including recurrent or persistent atelectasis or infiltrate, localized pulmonary consolidation or hyperinflation, recurrent pneumonia, and focal atelectasis. Often, airway anatomical anomalies, mucous plugs, or unsuspected foreign body aspiration may be found. Children with lobar atelectasis or consolidation who have failed medical management may benefit from direct instillation of mucolytic agents and removal of mucous plugs via flexible bronchoscopy. Biopsies may also be obtained through the larger flexible bronchoscopes. These may include mucosal biopsies for the evaluation of ciliary motion and ultrastructure, as well as transbronchial biopsies for the diagnosis of certain pulmonary conditions, especially rejection or infection in lung transplant patients.

Foreign Body Aspiration

The flexible bronchoscope may be used to rule out the presence of a foreign body in the lower airways of children in whom the diagnosis is not strongly suspected. If a foreign body is discovered, the flexible bronchoscope can be used to evaluate the rest of the airways to look for the presence of a second foreign body. However, when the presence of a foreign body is confirmed or highly suspected either by radiographic evaluation or by history, the preferred approach is to identify and remove the foreign body by rigid bronchoscopy. Although some authors believe that the flexible bronchoscope can be used for the therapeutic purpose of foreign body removal, rigid bronchoscopy is a better and safer approach in children. It allows better ventilation of the patient under general anesthesia and facilitates safer delivery of large foreign bodies through the subglottic area and the larynx compared with the flexible bronchoscope.

Hemoptysis

Flexible bronchoscopy is sometimes indicated in selected pediatric patients with hemoptysis who need visual inspection of the airways for localization of their bleeding site. It can be useful for therapeutic purposes as well, by removal of blood clots and placement of single-lumen or double-lumen endotracheal tubes and balloon catheters to tamponade (i.e., to exert direct pressure on) a bleeding site in the airway. In situations with massive hemoptysis or brisk bleeding, however, the flexible bronchoscope is usually inadequate because of its limited visualization and suction capabilities compared with the rigid bronchoscope.

Inhalation Injury

In patients with acute inhalation of a toxic or heated gas, flexible bronchoscopic evaluation of the upper and lower airways can be helpful in judging the extent of injury and determining the therapy and level of respiratory support needed. The decision for elective intubation with the assistance of bronchoscopy may be made if significant laryngeal edema is visualized.

Therapeutic Bronchoscopy

The flexible bronchoscope is an excellent therapeutic tool. It is useful in placing an endotracheal tube in difficult intubation cases. The direct instillation of medications such as N-acetylcysteine (Mucomyst), dilute sodium bicarbonate, or recombinant human deoxyribonuclease I (DNase) can help dislodge retained secretions or viscous mucous plugs before bronchoscopic suctioning. The flexible bronchoscope has also been used to administer surfactant in patients with acute respiratory distress syndrome. Laser surgery of airway lesions can be done through a flexible bronchoscope, but a rigid scope allows for mechanical as well as laser resection and for better control of bleeding complications.

Flexible Nasopharyngoscopy

The flexible bronchoscope may also be used for examination of the nasophaynx. However, the flexible nasopharyngoscope is more convenient for this purpose. The procedure is performed on an awake patient with only local anesthesia. In a tertiary center it is customary for our ear, nose, and throat (ENT) colleagues to perform this examination. This type of examination might be performed in the pulmonary function laboratory by a pulmonologists in the context of a VCD evaluation. This technique is useful to examine the upper airway for foreign bodies, polypoid disease, mass lesions, adenoidal anatomy, and septal anatomy and to obtain a dynamic view of palatal, laryngeal, and vocal cord function. Examination of the airway below the vocal cords is reserved for the flexible bronchoscope.

CONTRAINDICATIONS

Flexible bronchoscopy has been shown to be a safe procedure, even when performed on ill pediatric patients. However, certain conditions can place a patient at risk for complications (Box 7-2). Although there are no absolute contraindications for flexible bronchoscopy, there are conditions where the risk may be too great. If it is determined by a trained specialist that the possible benefit of bronchoscopy outweighs the risks, and appropriate equipment and personnel are available, then the procedure may be performed.

Flexible bronchoscopy often causes hypoxemia, most often as a result of occlusion of the airway by the bronchoscope during the procedure, and hypoventilation or apnea from sedation. Pulse oximetry and cardiac and respiratory tracings should be continuously monitored during and after the procedure. Supplemental oxygen should be provided to maintain oxygen saturation, optimally above 95%. If the patient is already hypoxemic, flexible bronchoscopy can further worsen the hypoxemia and place the patient at serious risk. Flexible bronchoscopy through an LMA may improve the safety of the procedure. Patients with impending respiratory failure may be electively intubated before the bronchoscopy, in anticipation of worsening ventilation and oxygenation during and after the procedure.

Elective flexible bronchoscopy should not be performed in the patient who has cardiovascular instability, uncontrolled asthma, coagulopathy, pulmonary hypertension, severe upper airway obstruction, or superior vena cava obstruction until these conditions are stabilized. It should be performed selectively and with great caution in patients with acute laryngotracheitis because of the risks of sudden laryngospasm during the procedure and additional postprocedural airway edema that may severely compromise an already swollen airway. The bronchoscope should never be inserted forcefully past any area of airway narrowing, to avoid further injury and compromise to that site. As noted earlier, the strong suspicion of foreign body aspiration is a relative contraindication to flexible bronchoscopy and an indication for rigid bronchoscopy.

EQUIPMENT

Flexible Bronchoscope

The flexible bronchoscope may be divided into three sections: (1) the insertion tube, (2) the control head and eyepiece, and (3) the light source connector.

Insertion Tube

The insertion tube is the flexible portion of the bronchoscope that is inserted into the patient's airways. These tubes have the same working length of 55 cm, but they vary in outer diameter from less than 2 mm to 6.3 mm. The instruments most often used in pediatric patients are 2.2-mm-diameter scopes for neonates, 2.8- to 3.7-mm scopes for older children, and 4.7- to 4.9-mm scopes for adolescents (Figure 7-1). The composition of the tubes varies somewhat according to the diameter. All scopes contain one or two fiberoptic bundles for light transmission from the light source to the airway, as well as one

Box 7-2	Contraindications to Flexible Bronchoscopy

CONDITIONS IN WHICH RISK IS LIKELY TO BE TOO GREAT
- Inability to oxygenate the patient adequately
- Cardiovascular instability
  - Hypotension
  - Malignant arrhythmias
  - Myocardial infarction

CONDITIONS IN WHICH RISK IS MORE LIKELY TO BE MANAGEABLE
- Severe bleeding diatheses/coagulopathy
- Hypercapnia with acidosis
- Hypoxemia
- Severe pulmonary hypertension
- Severe upper airway obstruction
- Superior vena cava obstruction
- Uncooperative patient
- Uncontrolled asthma
- Uremia

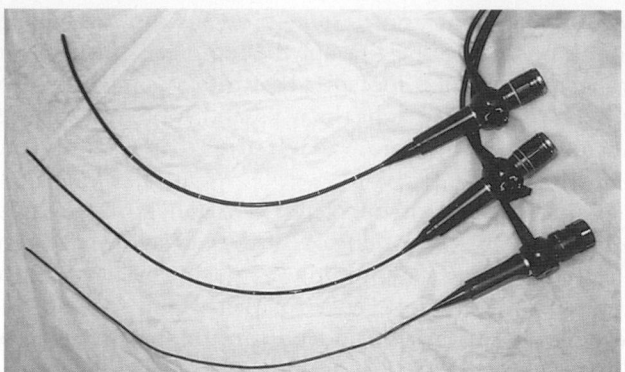

FIGURE 7-1 Three different sizes of pediatric flexible bronchoscopes. *Top to bottom*: 4.5-, 3.6-, and 2.2-mm outer diameter. Note that all scopes have similar working tube lengths.

fiberoptic cable for transmission of the airway image from the tip of the scope to the eyepiece. These fiberoptic bundles consist of thousands of tiny (8-μm) glass fibers that are coated with a highly reflective glass material. These fibers transmit light and images by internal reflections at the core–coating interface. This arrangement of highly reflective, minute glass fibers accounts for the bronchoscope's flexibility and high image quality. However, it also imparts substantial fragility to the instrument. Efforts to miniaturize charge-coupled devices (CCDs) have led to the development of bronchoscopes with tiny CCDs in their tips that record an image and then transport it electronically to the recording device. The CCD bronchoscopes provide larger and clearer images, free of the dots characteristic of fiberoptic images. Unfortunately, CCD video chips small enough to be used in pediatric flexible bronchoscopes (3.5 mm or smaller) are not yet available.

The insertion tubes of the thinnest bronchoscopes, less than 2.2 mm in diameter, contain only light and image bundles. They are nondirectable because they lack the cables necessary to direct the distal section of the scope. Appropriately, they have been nicknamed "spaghetti scopes," and their use is limited to visualization of an airway via insertion down an endotracheal tube.

Larger, flexible bronchoscopes have two control cables aligned 180 degrees from each other that connect a hinged bending section at the distal tip of the tube to a control lever at the head of the scope. These cables allow the operator to flex and extend the distal tip of the bronchoscope in order to direct the passage of the scope through the airways. The 2.2-mm scopes have this directable capability, but they lack the third major component of the insertion tube, a suction channel. The larger scopes contain suction channels, varying in diameter from 1.2 mm in the 2.8- to 3.7-mm scopes to 3.2 mm in the 4.5-mm scopes. These suction channels allow for the suction of airway secretions, the instillation of lavage fluids or medications into the airway, and the passage of brushes and biopsy forceps for obtaining airway cytology and pathology specimens.

The channel, direction cables, and fiberoptic bundles are enmeshed in a woven metal sheath and then enclosed in a nonlatex flexible plastic membrane.

Control Head and Eyepiece

The control head directs the insertion tube and use of the bronchoscope and transmits its images to the operator. Transmission is accomplished with an eyepiece and focusing ring. The operator may look through the eyepiece directly at the distal image. Alternatively, a camera attached to the eyepiece and displayed on a video monitor during the procedure records the image. On directable bronchoscopes, the control head contains an angulation lever, which regulates the cables attached to the bending tip of the scope. On the larger scopes there is also a channel port attached or in addition to a button that activates suction through the suction channel. Syringes attach to the port for airway lavage, and instruments may be passed through the port for the collection of airway specimens. A suction adapter extends at a right angle from the head of the bronchoscope and attaches to tubing connected to the suction source.

Light Source Connector

The control head is also attached to a cable. The other end of the cable contains the light source connector for the transmission of light from a source to the fiberoptic cables in the insertion tube. The light source houses a bright halogen or xenon lamp, which provides adequate illumination via the fiberoptic cables.

Video Recording Equipment

Video recording has proven to be invaluable in flexible bronchoscopy procedures. Video allows the bronchoscopist to review the findings after the procedure, identifying or clarifying lesions missed during the actual procedure and at other times allowing for consultation with medical or surgical colleagues. Video of the recorded procedure may also be shown to the patient and family when discussing the patient's condition and treatment plan. The video also provides a record of the findings that may be used for comparison with past or future bronchoscopies.

PREPARATION

To perform an efficient and safe procedure the practitioner needs to fully prepare the bronchoscopy area, the equipment, medications, the patient, and the personnel who will participate in the procedure.

Equipment and Supplies

The proper selection and preparation of equipment are important to ensure a safe and effective procedure. The preparation of this equipment and certain medications is usually the responsibility of the respiratory therapist who will assist in the procedure.

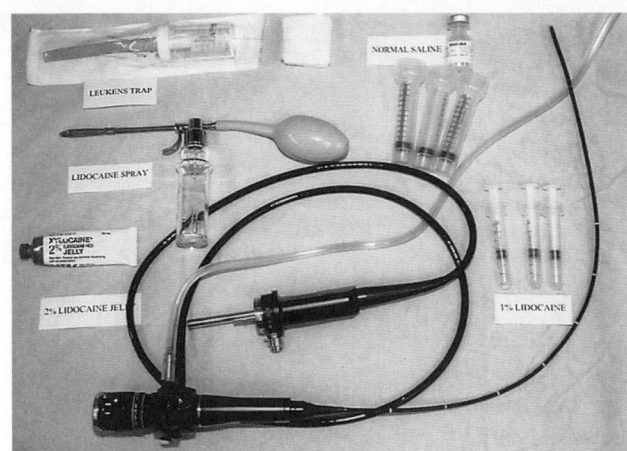

FIGURE 7-2 Necessary equipment for basic pediatric flexible bronchoscopy includes bronchoscope, attached suction tube, 2% lidocaine jelly, lidocaine spray, three 1-ml aliquots of 1% lidocaine solution, Lukens trap, gauze pads, and three to five 10-ml aliquots of normal saline for bronchoalveolar lavage. These items are placed on a clean drape on top of a portable bronchoscopy cart.

The light source, video recorder, and monitor are usually maintained on a portable bronchoscope cart. Equipment, such as 1% to 2% lidocaine spray, 2% lidocaine jelly, syringes containing aliquots of 1% to 2% lidocaine, a Lukens trap, 10-ml normal saline aliquots for lavage, and clean gauzes, may be placed on top of the cart for easy access (Figure 7-2). A cardiac monitor, pulse oximeter, noninvasive blood pressure monitor, and emergency resuscitation cart should also be placed at the bedside. Appropriately sized resuscitation bag and mask, laryngoscopes and endotracheal tubes, and resuscitation medications must be readily available. Wall suction and oxygen should be connected and turned on for prompt access if needed. Two sources of wall suction should be used: one connected to the bronchoscope to clear the field of vision and to obtain specimens, and the other connected to a suction catheter or Yankauer suction tip for use if the patient has excessive oropharyngeal secretions or vomits during the procedure. On certain occasions, special equipment or medications may be needed, such as a swivel adapter for an endotracheal tube, positive end-expiratory pressure (PEEP) valves, tracheostomy tubes, wire brushes for cytology, transbronchial needle catheters, sodium bicarbonate, N-acetylcysteine, and DNase (Box 7-3).

During the procedure, all pediatric patients will require some type of sedation. The most common approach is **conscious sedation** following the guidelines of the American Academy of Pediatrics (1992). For administration of conscious sedation, the presence of a trained clinician to attend to the sedation alone is required. Intravenous drugs are preferable to intramuscular medications because of their quicker onset, shorter duration, and titratable dosage for optimal effects. Although various sedative agents are available, the combination of a benzodiazepine

(e.g., midazolam) and a narcotic (e.g., fentanyl or morphine) is widely accepted. In addition to sedative effects, the narcotic provides analgesic and antitussive effects, and the benzodiazepine offers anxiolytic effects and antegrade amnesia. The most common side effect of this combination is respiratory depression. On occasion, benzodiazepines can induce cardiovascular depression, and narcotics can elicit muscular rigidity and impaired liver and kidney functions. Fortunately, if these complications occur, specific reversal agents, naloxone (0.01 mg/kg per dose) and flumazenil (0.2 mg/kg per dose) can be given to restore the patient's respiratory status. These antagonists, along with atropine and epinephrine for adverse cardiac events, should be immediately available.

Additional medications that should be available include aerosolized albuterol to treat any bronchospasm that may develop, aerosolized epinephrine for airway edema, and diphenhydramine and a corticosteroid to treat any potential anaphylactic reaction to the sedating medications. The presence of an anesthesiologist to manage the sedation and monitoring of the patient is increasingly common.

Patient

Patient preparation includes a thorough history and physical examination before the procedure. Any radiographic studies should be reviewed. Information regarding the child's current health status and drug allergies must be obtained. Elective bronchoscopic procedures should be postponed if the patient has a reversible condition or acute illness that may increase the risk for complications from the sedation or the procedure itself. After a thorough description of the procedure to the parents and to the patient, if the child is able to understand, written informed consent must be obtained. One of the major risks of flexible bronchoscopy is aspiration of gastric contents. Infants younger than 6 months should not take anything by mouth for 3 to 4 hours before the procedure, older infants and toddlers for 4 to 6 hours, and older children 8 hours, to ensure an empty stomach.

Flexible laryngoscopy may be performed in infants and cooperative older children with only topical anesthesia because it causes no more trauma than nasopharyngeal suctioning and can be equally brief when done by an experienced operator. When the bronchoscope is to be passed below the glottis, intravenous access is recommended.

For psychological support and patient comfort, parents should be allowed to stay with the patient as long as possible before starting the procedure. However, they should not overstimulate the patient, especially when conscious sedation is used. The importance of a calm, nonstimulating atmosphere in the bronchoscopy area cannot be overstated. This may be achieved by low-level lighting, calm and quiet actions by the bronchoscopist and support personnel, and a smooth prebronchoscopy routine. Premedication with a benzodiazepine 30 to 60 minutes before the

Box 7-3	Equipment and Supplies for Pediatric Flexible Bronchoscopy

Bronchoscope with light source
Endotracheal tube swivel adapter
Water-soluble lubricant
Monitoring equipment
• Cardiac monitor with electrode patches
• Pulse oximeter with probes
• Respiratory monitor
• Sphygmomanometer
• Stethoscope
Oxygen and aerosol equipment
• Aerosol mask
• Cannula with nasal prongs clipped
• Flow meter
• Nebulizer
• Oxygen mask with nose cut out
• Oxygen source
• Oxygen tubing with connectors
Specimen collection equipment
• Biopsy forceps
• Channel brush
• Fixative
• Glass slides
• Lukens trap
• Retrieval baskets and cages
• Syringes with nonbacteriostatic saline for bronchoalveolar lavage
• Transport media
Suction equipment
• Sterile gloves
• Suction canisters
• Suction catheters
• Suction tubing
• Tonsil-tip or Yankauer-type suction catheter
• Vacuum suction source
Intravenous equipment
• Isotonic saline
• Intravenous infusion sets
• Syringes with flush solution
Medications
• Topical anesthetics
  • Lidocaine solution (1% to 2%)
  • Lidocaine viscous (2%)

• Sedatives
  • Diazepam
  • Fentanyl
  • Meperidine
  • Midazolam
  • Morphine
• Aerosols
  • Albuterol
  • Racemic epinephrine
• Emergency drugs
  • Atropine
  • Bicarbonate
  • Epinephrine (1:1000)
  • Flumazenil
  • Furosemide
  • Intravenous corticosteroids
  • Naloxone
  • Phenobarbital
  • Succinylcholine
Resuscitation equipment
• Bite block
• Endotracheal tubes
• Laryngoscope with blades
• Oral airways
• Resuscitation bag with oxygen tubing attached
• Stylets
Extra batteries for laryngoscope
Extra lightbulbs
Facemasks
Video camera with recording equipment
Bronchoscopist and assistant equipment
• Eye protectors
• Gloves
• Gown
• Mask
• Scissors

procedure can help the patient relax before starting the procedure.

Personnel

Typically the flexible bronchoscopy team includes a bronchoscopist, a nurse, a respiratory therapist, and the clinician providing conscious sedation. All team members should be informed of the patient's diagnosis, indication for bronchoscopy, allergies, and biological risks to the patient and team members. In addition, the team should be fully informed of the planned procedures and any difficulties that may arise. Everyone should wear a clean protective gown, gloves, mask, and eye protection. All body

fluids, including bronchoalveolar lavage specimens, should be handled carefully using universal precautions.

Personnel safety is increased by identifying patients with potentially transmissible pathogens, such as hepatitis viruses, human immunodeficiency virus, and *Mycobacterium tuberculosis*. Approved high-efficiency particulate air (HEPA) filter masks should be worn for all procedures involving patients with suspected *M. tuberculosis* infection, and the procedure should be performed in a room that meets ventilation requirements for tuberculosis. Patients with, or at risk of having, tuberculosis should be kept in a respiratory isolation room before and after the procedure.

PROCEDURE

Most pediatric flexible bronchoscopies are performed with the patient in a supine position on a bed. The height of the bed should be adjusted to the bronchoscopist's comfort level. When the patient and bronchoscopy team are ready and all preparations are completed, a "time-out" procedure is performed according to institutional policy and the selected sedation is initiated. Appropriate sedation will decrease the patient's anxiety, discomfort, and unwanted physiological effects. Nevertheless, many younger patients may need a gentle restraining system even when sedated.

Conscious Sedation

Several different conscious sedation regimens have been used safely and successfully for pediatric flexible bronchoscopy. As noted earlier, one of the most widely accepted is a combination of a benzodiazepine (e.g., midazolam) and a narcotic (e.g., fentanyl or meperidine) given intravenously. The usual pediatric dose of intravenous midazolam ranges from 0.05 to 0.1 mg/kg to a maximal total dose of 0.4 to 0.6 mg/kg (or 6-10 mg). Typically, sedation is begun with a small dose (0.05-0.1 mg/kg) and is then titrated upward every 5 minutes to achieve the optimal sedative effect. The same approach is also used for intravenous fentanyl, 1 to 2 µg/kg to a maximal total dose of 5 to 10 µg/kg, starting with a 1-µg/kg dose and titrating upward every 5 minutes. Some bronchoscopists prefer a stronger sedative, such as intravenous ketamine (1 mg/kg per dose) or intravenous propofol (1-2 mg/kg per dose).[5]

Other combinations of drugs are given intramuscularly and include meperidine, promethazine, and chlorpromazine and the combination of droperidol, promethazine, and chlorpromazine. The disadvantages of intramuscular sedation include the inability to titrate the optimal dose of the medications and the lack of intravenous access in case of an emergency. However, the intramuscular approach is sometimes justified for short procedures in stable children with difficult intravenous access. Intranasal midazolam has also been shown to induce adequate sedation for pediatric patients undergoing endoscopic procedures or imaging studies.[8] The usual dose of intranasal midazolam ranges from 0.2 to 0.5 mg/kg. Regardless of the method, optimal sedation is achieved when the child is sleepy and has minimal reaction to noxious stimuli, while still maintaining adequate ventilation and protective airway reflexes. In patients who are at increased risk for cardiopulmonary compromise during conscious sedation, general anesthesia may be preferred.

Topical Anesthesia

Conscious sedation is augmented by application of the local anesthetic agent, 1% to 2% lidocaine, to the nasal cavity, posterior pharynx, vocal cords, and tracheobronchial tree. Another technique is to pretreat the subject with a lidocaine aerosol (4-8 mg/kg) given by nebulizer.[9] Lidocaine 2% jelly may also be applied to the nares with a cotton-tipped applicator or small syringe. With small infants, care should be taken that the total lidocaine dose does not exceed the maximal therapeutic range of 3 to 4 mg/kg. Toxic lidocaine levels have been reported with topical airway administration.

Patient Monitoring

Continuous cardiac, respiratory, and oximetry monitoring must be performed during and after the procedure. During the procedure the patient should be closely monitored for cardiac and respiratory rates and tracings, blood pressure, oxygen saturation, clinical airway obstruction, chest wall movement, peripheral perfusion, and cyanosis. Ideally, oxygen saturation should be maintained above 95% at all times, with supplemental oxygen delivered to the patient if necessary.

Technique

When the bronchoscope is balanced on the left hand, the left thumb controls the angulation lever on the control head and the right thumb and index finger direct the insertion tube at the naris (for right-handed operators). Routes for bronchoscopic approaches include nasal, oral, and endotracheal tube; tracheostomy tube; and LMA.

The most common route for nonintubated pediatric patients is the transnasal approach. The flexible bronchoscope is lubricated with lidocaine jelly or another sterile water–based lubricant and then inserted through a nostril into the nasopharyngeal area. A topical decongestant (e.g., phenylephrine) may be administered to the nasal mucosa first to facilitate passage of the scope past edematous tissue and to reduce the risk of bleeding. The nasopharyngeal and laryngeal anatomy is visualized. The vocal cords are assessed for movement and then anesthetized with lidocaine sprayed through a suction channel of the bronchoscope. Adequate laryngeal anesthesia is critical to avoid sudden laryngospasm. The bronchoscope is then passed through the vocal cords into the tracheobronchial tree. Another dose of 1% to 2% lidocaine is usually applied to the carina to minimize the cough reflex. The tracheobronchial anatomy is then examined.

If bronchoalveolar lavage is performed, the bronchoscopist wedges the bronchoscope in the selected segmental or subsegmental bronchi, and normal saline is instilled in three to five aliquots of up to 1 ml/kg per aliquot. The saline is then suctioned back through the suction channel. Typically, one third to one half of the instilled volume is recovered with suctioning. A specimen is usually collected in a Lukens trap and sent for microbiology or pathology studies. Ideally, if a specimen is collected for microbiological evaluation, suction should not be applied until the bronchoscope is inside the trachea to minimize contamination of the channel with nasopharyngeal secretions. In some cases, a protected catheter may be introduced through the working channel and used to obtain a clean specimen when a larger bronchoscope is in use. In special cases, consultation with the microbiologist or pathologist beforehand ensures that the specimen is large enough for the requested study and is handled and sent appropriately.

During the bronchoscopy the respiratory therapist is often responsible for connecting and disconnecting suction, attaching normal saline syringes and traps for lavage, and giving certain transbronchoscopic medications. The therapist and assisting nurse may divide responsibility for monitoring the patient's oxygenation and respiratory status, stabilizing the patient's head and upper airway, and comforting the patient. Because the bronchoscopist is focused on the procedure, the therapist and nurse are responsible for detecting and promptly notifying the bronchoscopist of any untoward patient occurrence. In most instances, the licensed independent practitioner providing conscious sedation will provide this function. The respiratory therapist is also responsible for assisting in emergency respiratory management, such as maintaining patency of the patient's airway, suctioning oropharyngeal secretions, handling emergency equipment, and giving certain respiratory medications.

A PEEP-Keep is used when performing flexible bronchoscopy in a patient through an endotracheal tube or LMA. In a patient who is being mechanically ventilated, the risk of further compromise to the patient's respiratory condition is higher with a partially occluded endotracheal tube. Special considerations should be made for maximizing the patient's ventilation and oxygenation and compensating for air leaks and increased resistance that may occur. In this situation the respiratory therapist or anesthesiologist is responsible for ventilator adjustment and stabilization of the endotracheal tube. It is often necessary to remove the patient from the ventilator to provide ventilation by bag-valve mask (Ambu bag) during the procedure.

POSTPROCEDURAL MONITORING AND COMPLICATIONS

Monitoring of the patient must continue after the procedure until the patient has fully awakened or has returned to preprocedural baseline status. Children, particularly anxious toddlers, often require large doses of medications, with the level of sedation increasing after the procedure, when the agents are still active and the child is no longer stimulated by the procedure. It is essential to continue to monitor the adequacy of the patient's oxygenation, ventilation, and airway patency until the sedation has completely resolved. Breath sounds should be monitored for the development of any stridor or wheezing after the procedure. To prevent aspiration, oral fluids are withheld until the patient is fully awake and the topical laryngeal

anesthesia has worn off, usually about 1 hour after administering the topical anesthetic.

In general, flexible bronchoscopy is a safe and well-tolerated procedure in pediatric patients, especially when it is performed by an experienced bronchoscopy team that employs careful monitoring and takes appropriate precautions. Patient risk factors for adverse events include upper airway pathology, preprocedure hypoxemia, and weight less than 10 kg. The most common complications include transient cough, respiratory depression, hypoxemia, hypercapnia, and bronchospasm during the procedure.[10] Cough is almost universally seen during and after the procedure, but it is usually self-limited and resolves within 24 hours. Minor epistaxis is common and does not require therapy. Respiratory depression is usually associated with oversedation and sometimes requires reversal agents. Any bronchospasm is relieved promptly in most patients by bronchodilator aerosol treatments.

A less common but potentially more serious complication is laryngospasm. This problem can be avoided by application of topical lidocaine to the vocal cords. If laryngospasm occurs, the bronchoscope must be withdrawn immediately and airway resuscitation initiated. These measures include jaw thrust, suction of secretions, and mask ventilation. Rarely, laryngospasm may become life threatening and require paralysis and endotracheal intubation.

Up to 20% of patients may have fever after bronchoalveolar lavage, but pneumonia is uncommon.[10] Subglottic edema is the most common complication of rigid bronchoscopy but is very unusual with flexible bronchoscopy. Other more serious complications, including arrhythmias, pulmonary hemorrhage, and pneumothorax, are seldom encountered during pediatric flexible bronchoscopy. Deaths are extremely rare, with no bronchoscopy-related mortality reported in more than 3500 pediatric flexible bronchoscopy procedures.[10,11]

EQUIPMENT MAINTENANCE

Because the bronchoscope and its accessories are extremely fragile and expensive, special attention must be taken during cleaning and maintenance procedures. Proper care can increase the life span of the equipment, decrease repair and replacement costs, and reduce the potential risk of cross-contamination. Handling requires the avoidance of any excessive angulation or twisting of the scope, actions that can damage the quartz fiber bundles. Inadequate disinfection of a bronchoscope can result in serious adverse outcomes to a patient. The organisms most often responsible for cross-contamination between bronchoscopies are *Mycobacterium* and *Pseudomonas* spp.

The flexible bronchoscope should be cleaned immediately after each procedure. Soak the instrument in enzymatic detergent for at least 5 to 10 minutes. Dried secretions or blood will prevent penetration of the disinfecting agent.

Therefore the exterior surface should be wiped or gently scrubbed with a soft cloth or brush. The suction port should be irrigated and flushed with detergent solution and then scrubbed with a short, thick brush. The suction channel should be scrubbed with a long, thin brush, and afterward the brush should be examined for retained blood or mucus. It may be necessary to run the brush through the channel a number of times until it is clear of debris. If the suction valve is not disposable, it should be disassembled and flushed thoroughly with a cleaning solution. Because flexible bronchoscopy is not a sterile procedure, cleaning a bronchoscope does not require routine sterilization and high-level disinfection has been considered satisfactory. **High-level disinfection** is a cleaning method that inactivates all viruses, fungi, and vegetative microorganisms but not necessarily all bacterial spores. The most common agent used is 2% alkaline glutaraldehyde. Immersion in glutaraldehyde for 20 minutes can destroy virtually all pathogens surviving on a well-cleaned bronchoscope.[12]

Because of increasing concern about more virulent and resistant microorganisms, many centers are adopting routine sterilization of their bronchoscopes. Two highly effective methods against all types of microorganisms are ethylene oxide gas sterilization and peracetic acid submersion. Ethylene oxide is noncorrosive and able to penetrate all portions of the bronchoscope without requiring high pressures. However, a venting cap must be placed to equalize the pressure between the interior and the exterior of the bronchoscope. The major disadvantage of ethylene oxide sterilization is that it is time-consuming, taking at least 12 to 16 hours to complete the process. An alternative method is the STERIS system (Figure 7-3), an automated, microprocessor-controlled device using a sterilant concentrate, peracetic acid, as the active biocidal agent. This chemical sterilization process requires only 25 minutes. Once the disinfection or sterilization process is completed, the bronchoscope is rinsed with tap water

and may be wiped with alcohol before storage in a dry, clean cabinet.

COMPARISON WITH RIGID BRONCHOSCOPY

Rigid bronchoscopy is most often performed in the operating room by surgeons or otolaryngologists, with general anesthesia administered to the patient by an anesthesiologist. This rigid bronchoscope has some advantages over flexible bronchoscopy, including its relatively large internal diameter, improved anatomical definition, the ability to provide ventilation during the procedure, and the ability to use larger instruments. It is particularly useful in removal of a foreign body or when laser therapy is required. Relative disadvantages of rigid bronchoscopy include the inability to allow inspection of distal airways, the inability to assess the dynamic and natural state of the airways, and the complications associated with general anesthesia. Thus the risks and benefits of each procedure must be carefully considered for each patient before choosing the bronchoscopic method. The two procedures may be coordinated and performed sequentially in the operating room for different diagnostic and therapeutic purposes in select patients.

CASE STUDY

You are called to the bedside of a 4-year-old girl in the intensive care unit (ICU). The patient was born 24 weeks premature and has a history of bronchopulmonary dysplasia requiring tracheostomy and ventilator support; she was admitted for respiratory distress. At home she is on a tracheostomy heat moisture exchanger (HME) during the day and ventilator support at night. Over the past several days she has been unable to come off her ventilator during the day because of lower saturation requiring increased FiO_2 and higher PEEP and peak inspiratory pressure (PIP). She has also been spiking high fevers, and her chest x-ray examination shows worsening areas of atelectasis and collapse. The ICU has requested a flexible bronchoscopy to further evaluate her airway. While examining the airway, you encounter what appears to be a foreign object in the left mainstem bronchus.

What is your next action? (NOTE: More than one answer may be acceptable.)

See Evolve Resources for answers.

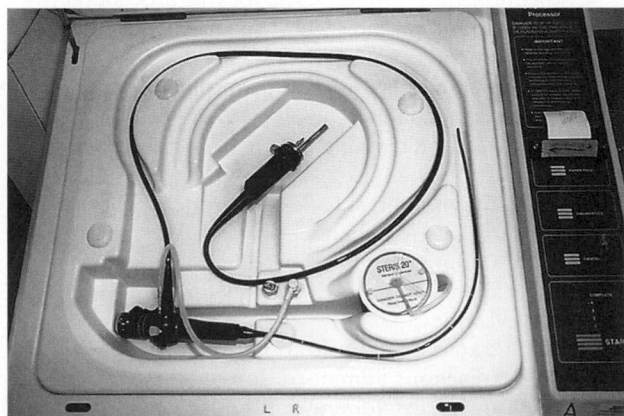

FIGURE 7-3 Correct placement of flexible bronchoscope in STERIS cleaning apparatus, used for chemical sterilization of the instrument.

KEY POINTS

- Flexible bronchoscopy allows for the examination of the lower airway and collection of diagnostic specimens, including cultures and biopsy material. Therapeutic intervention may also be possible. Rigid bronchoscopy is indicated when the information obtained will be of higher quality or when the safety of the procedure is enhanced.

- The performance of safe and efficient bronchoscopy requires adequate preparation. All equipment should be readily available on a cart. All medications should be drawn up beforehand. The light sources and video equipment should be tested. The patient should be prepared; a child life service is very helpful in this regard. The consent must be signed and placed in the chart. The child should have nothing by mouth, following institutional guidelines for conscious sedation or general anesthesia. A time-out procedure should always be performed.

- Close monitoring of the patient is critical for safe performance of bronchoscopy. In most cases the heart rate, respiratory rate, and saturation will be continuously monitored. Blood pressure will be measured frequently according to directives related to conscious sedation policies. Frequent inspection and auscultation of breathing should be performed. Ideally, saturation should be maintained above 95% and supplemental oxygen should be used when necessary. During conscious sedation a licensed independent practitioner should be available to monitor the patient. Common complications include cough, transient hypoxia, respiratory depression, and wheezing. Complications should be anticipated, and sufficient personnel and resources to manage them must be available.

- The safe use of the equipment requires reliable and consistent cleaning between procedures. The bronchoscope must be soaked in enzymatic solution sufficiently long enough to loosen biological material. The bronchoscope should be scrubbed with detergent, and the suction and working channels should be meticulously cleaned with a scrub brush. High-level disinfection or gas sterilization is then performed. An institutional cleaning protocol should be used to ensure consistency of performance.

ASSESSMENT QUESTIONS

See Evolve Resources for answers.

1. Flexible bronchoscopy is commonly performed in all the following settings *except*:
   A. Operating rooms
   B. Bronchoscopy suites
   C. Pulmonary clinic rooms
   D. Intensive care units
   E. Procedure rooms
2. The most common diagnostic indication for flexible bronchoscopy in infants is:
   A. Stridor
   B. Wheezing
   C. Hoarse voice
   D. Persistent atelectasis
   E. Difficult intubation

3. Which of the following disorders may cause *only* inspiratory stridor?
   A. Vocal cord dysfunction
   B. Laryngomalacia
   C. Vascular ring
   D. Cardiomegaly
   E. Bronchial foreign body
4. Airway dynamics can be disrupted by:
   A. General anesthesia
   B. Conscious sedation
   C. Topical lidocaine
   D. Intranasal midazolam
   E. Sleep
5. Flexible bronchoscopy is indicated in the evaluation of wheezing in all the following settings *except*:
   A. Wheezing that is unilateral
   B. Wheezing that has been present since birth
   C. Wheezing that is refractory to asthma therapy
   D. Wheezing that is triggered by viral infections
   E. Wheezing associated with persistent atelectasis
6. Bronchoalveolar lavage may be performed to look for:
   A. Infection
   B. Malignancy
   C. Bleeding
   D. Aspiration
   E. All of the above
7. The only absolute contraindication to flexible bronchoscopy is when:
   A. The diagnosis could be obtained by open lung biopsy
   B. The patient is hypoxemic
   C. The patient requires intubation and mechanical ventilation
   D. The patient is febrile with acute pneumonia
   E. The risks of bronchoscopy outweigh the potential benefits of the procedure
8. A 3-year-old child is intubated with a 4.5-mm endotracheal tube and is mechanically ventilated for severe pneumonia. The respiratory therapist is asked to set up a bronchoscope for bronchoalveolar lavage to obtain microbiology specimens. What is the most appropriate scope for this procedure?
   A. 1.8-mm nondirectable "spaghetti" bronchoscope
   B. 2.2-mm directable flexible bronchoscope without suction channel
   C. 2.7-mm directable flexible bronchoscope with suction channel
   D. 4.5-mm directable flexible bronchoscope with large suction channel
   E. 4.0-mm rigid bronchoscope
9. Topical anesthesia of the airway may be achieved by:
   A. Intranasal administration of midazolam
   B. Intravenous administration of fentanyl
   C. Intravenous administration of midazolam
   D. Airway instillation or nebulization of lidocaine
   E. Airway instillation or nebulization of a topical corticosteroid

10. During a bronchoscopy, the respiratory therapist may do each of the following *except*:
- **A.** Connect and disconnect suction and specimen traps
- **B.** Administer supplemental oxygen as needed
- **C.** Administer saline lavages or transbronchoscopic medications
- **D.** Administer conscious sedation medications
- **E.** Assist in emergency airway management

11. The most common complication after flexible bronchoscopy is:
- **A.** Cough
- **B.** Wheezing
- **C.** Hemoptysis
- **D.** Fever
- **E.** Pneumothorax

12. Acceptable cleaning and decontamination of a flexible bronchoscope include all the following *except*:
- **A.** Washing the exterior and channel of the scope with a detergent solution
- **B.** Immersion in 70% ethanol solution
- **C.** Immersion in 2% alkaline glutaraldehyde solution
- **D.** Ethylene oxide gas sterilization
- **E.** Immersion in peracetic acid

References

1. Wood RE: Spelunking in the pediatric airways: explorations with the flexible fiberoptic bronchoscope, *Pediatr Clin North Am* 31:785, 1984.
2. Wang KP, Mehta AC, editors: *Flexible bronchoscopy*, Cambridge, MA, 1995, Blackwell Science.
3. Brutinel WM, Cortese DA: Fiberoptic bronchoscopy. In Burton GG, Hodgkin JE, Ward JJ, editors: *Respiratory care: a guide to clinical practice*, ed 4, Philadelphia, 1997, Lippincott, pp 281-294.
4. Hollinger LD, Lusk RP, Green CG, editors: *Pediatric laryngology and bronchoesophagology*, Philadelphia, 1997, Lippincott-Raven.
5. Midulla F, de Blic J, Barbato A, et al: 2003 ERS Task Force: flexible endoscopy of paediatric airways, *Eur Respir J* 22:698, 2003.
6. Barbato A, de Blic J, Barbato A: Use of the pediatric bronchoscope, flexible and rigid, in 51 European centers, *Eur Respir J* 10:1761, 1997.
7. Godfrey S, Avital A, Maayan C: Yield from flexible bronchoscopy in children, *Pediatr Pulmonol* 23:261, 1997.
8. Fishbein M, Lugo RA, Woodland J: Evaluation of intranasal midazolam in children, undergoing esophagogastroduodenoscopy, *J Pediatr Gastroenterol Nutr* 25:261, 1997.
9. Gjonaj ST, Lowenthal DB, Dozor AJ: Nebulized lidocaine administered to infants and children undergoing flexible bronchoscopy, *Chest* 112:1665, 1997.
10. de Blic J, Marchac V, Scheinmann P: Complications of flexible bronchoscopy in children; prospective study of 1,328 procedures, *Eur Respir J* 20:1271, 2002.
11. Nussbaum E: Pediatric fiberoptic bronchoscopy, *Clin Pediatr* 34:430, 1995.
12. Woodcock A, Campbell I, Collins JV: Bronchoscopy and infection control, *Lancet* 2:270, 1989.
13. Committee on Drugs, American Academy of Pediatrics: Guidelines for the elective use of conscious sedation, deep sedation, and general anesthesia in pediatric patients, *Pediatrics* 89:1110-1115, 1992.

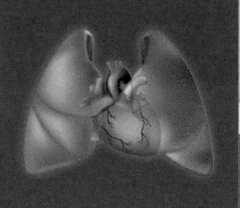

Chapter **8**

Invasive Blood Gas Analysis and Cardiovascular Monitoring

MICHAEL DAVIS

LEARNING OBJECTIVES

After reading this chapter the reader will be able to:

1. Describe indications for obtaining blood gas samples
2. Identify common anatomical sampling sites used to obtain blood gases
3. Describe potential patient and caregiver complications associated with blood gas sampling
4. Interpret a complete hemodynamic profile of a patient
5. Illustrate the progression of blood pressure waveforms seen during the proper placement of a pulmonary artery catheter

6. Describe invasive, semi-invasive, and noninvasive techniques for monitoring cardiac output and index in children
7. Discuss various measurements that can be used to determine the adequacy of cellular oxygenation
8. Identify variables that can shift the oxygen dissociation curve

KEY TERMS

Arterial blood gas
Capillary blood gas
Carboxyhemoglobin

Cardiac index
Cardiac output
Central venous catheter

Central venous oxygen saturation
Central venous pressure
Cutdown method

Blood gases are considered the most effective test for evaluating the efficiency of gas exchange and cardiopulmonary interaction. Evaluating an infant or child with respiratory impairment requires the analysis of blood gases in umbilical, arterial, capillary, or mixed venous blood samples. To interpret these blood gas values correctly, the clinician must understand acid–base balance and gas exchange and be able to recognize normal and abnormal blood gas values. The techniques of blood gas sampling can affect the results. This chapter reviews the procedures, indications, complications, and contraindications for each technique. It also reviews various clinical techniques that are used to monitor and evaluate cardiac performance, response to therapeutic interventions, and severity/progression of disease processes in pediatrics. It is beyond the scope of this chapter to describe noninvasive methods to measure gas exchange. Chapter 9, Noninvasive Monitoring in Neonatal and Pediatric Care, provides a complete overview of these concepts.

BLOOD GAS SAMPLING

Blood gas sampling may occur from arterial (ABG), venous (VBG), or capillary (CBG) sites. Blood gas analysis (BGA) is indicated when an accurate measurement of acid–base balance or pulmonary gas exchange is required.[1] This analysis may be needed for a variety of reasons (Box 8-1).[2] Figure 8-1

shows the various anatomical sites that provide access for percutaneous arterial puncture and catheterization; Figures 8-2 and 8-3 show recommended sites for capillary puncture. **Venous blood gas** sampling can occur at any site approved for venipuncture for routine purposes.

Pain Control

Blood gas sampling can be a painful procedure, but the resulting information is often a vital part of patient management. Because painful procedures do not always evoke vigorous pain responses in critically ill newborns, many believe that such newborns are not being affected by pain.[3] However, infants probably have a higher sensitivity to painful procedures than older age groups.[4,5] For infants more than 4 months of age and for children, anesthetic cream or a lidocaine injection may be used to control the pain felt during a blood gas procedure.[6] For nonintubated infants and premature newborns, a pacifier dipped in 24% sucrose is effective in helping to ameliorate the effects of pain. If the newborn is intubated, the sucrose can be administered as drops on the tongue or palate from an oral medication syringe.[7] Depending on the type and duration of procedure, more potent short-acting analgesic or anesthetic agents may be appropriate.[8]

Arterial Sampling Sites

Figure 8-1 illustrates potential sites for arterial puncture or catheterization in infants or children. Arterial sampling sites provide the most accurate blood gas results. The brachial and femoral sites are usually avoided because both feed large distal networks and neither has collateral circulation. Also, the brachial pulse is difficult to palpate in infants and small children because of the naturally large fat pad located in that area of the arm. Injury to the brachial nerve can also result in serious complications. Only a highly skilled clinician should perform a brachial artery puncture if necessary.

In a child, the femoral artery is reserved for an emergency, and then only as a last resort. In the neonate or infant, the femoral artery lies close to the femoral vein, nerve, and hip joint, and because of their proximity, damage inflicted on any one of these structures by femoral puncture is likely to cause severe complications and is thus not indicated for this population.[9]

The preferred site in both neonatal and pediatric populations is the radial artery. The radial artery provides good

---

Box 8-1	Indications for Blood Gas Analysis

- To evaluate ventilation ($Paco_2$, $Pvco_2$, $Pcco_2$)
- To evaluate acid–base balance (pH, $Paco_2$, $Pvco_2$, $Pcco_2$)
- To evaluate oxygenation (Pao_2, oxyhemoglobin)
- To evaluate the oxygen-carrying capacity (Pao_2, oxyhemoglobin, hemoglobin, dyshemoglobin)
- To evaluate intrapulmonary shunt
- To quantify response to therapy
- Supplemental oxygen
- Mechanical ventilation
- To assist in diagnosis
- To monitor the severity or progress of a disease
- To assess early goal-directed therapy (EGDT) in patients with sepsis, septic shock, and after major surgery ($Scvo_2$)
- To assess inadequacy of circulatory response

Paco_2, Partial pressure of carbon dioxide in arterial blood; *Pao_2*, partial pressure of oxygen in arterial blood.

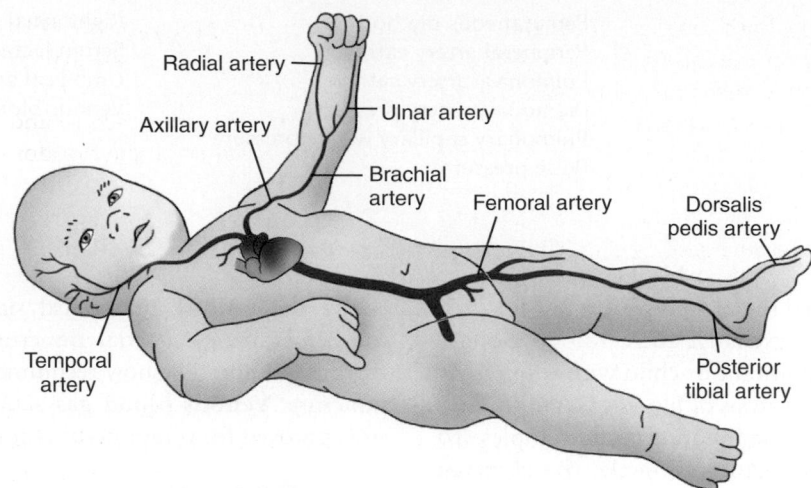

FIGURE 8-1 Arterial sites that may be used for peripheral artery puncture in infants and children.

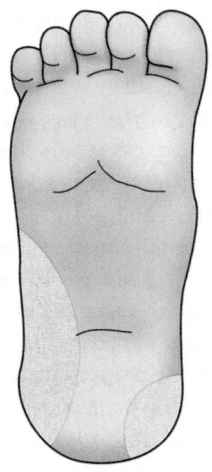

FIGURE 8-2 Recommended puncture sites (*shaded areas*) in infant's heel to obtain capillary blood for analysis.

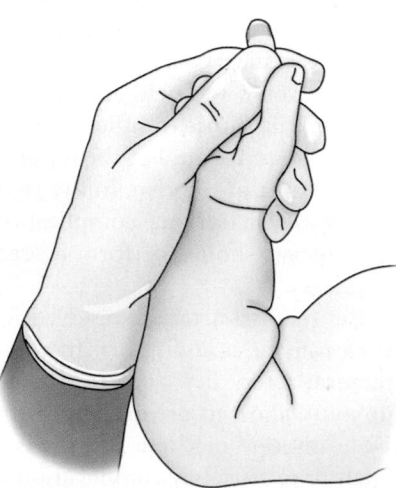

FIGURE 8-3 Technique for grasping the finger for a capillary puncture, with recommended site for puncture indicated (*shaded area*).

access as well as collateral circulation to the hand by the ulnar artery. There are usually no nerves or veins directly adjacent to the radial artery, and the patient's wrist is easier to manipulate than other body parts. The bone and firm ligaments of the wrist make it easy to palpate, stabilize, and compress the radial artery.[1,7] A **modified Allen's test** (described in the next section) is performed to ensure collateral circulation around the radial artery and to avoid complications. The ulnar artery should be avoided because it runs adjacent to the ulnar nerve.

The dorsalis pedis or posterior tibial artery is considered if the radial artery shows signs of poor collateral circulation. In addition, the temporal artery provides an alternative site for the premature or newborn infant. Access is generally good because two branches are close to the scalp. In most premature and neonatal patients, the temporal artery branches are larger than the radial artery.

Modified Allen's Test

The modified Allen's test is used to verify the presence of collateral circulation to the hand and should be performed to confirm whether poor circulation exists before puncturing the radial, posterior tibial, or dorsalis pedis artery. To assess blood flow to the hand, hold the child's wrist with both hands, thumbs on top. Ask the child to make a tight fist, and then occlude the radial and ulnar arteries by pressing down on them with the thumbs, one on each artery. Keeping both arteries occluded, ask the child to unclench the fist and note whether the palm is blanched, which indicates impaired blood flow. Then remove the pressure from the ulnar artery. The palm will become pink within 5 seconds if the ulnar artery is patent and able to provide collateral circulation.[7]

The passive method for performing the modified Allen's test, used on an infant or child who cannot follow commands, is performed by gently squeezing or elevating the hand while occluding both arteries. Once the ulnar artery is released, the results are interpreted as previously described.[1] Allen's test can also be used to verify collateral circulation when using one of the arteries of the foot as a puncture site, by elevating the foot and compressing the dorsalis pedis and posterior tibial arteries. Collateral circulation is confirmed by releasing pressure from the artery that will not be punctured and assessing the nail beds and sole of the foot for return of blood flow.[1,7]

ARTERIAL PUNCTURE

When infrequent sampling is required, **arterial blood gas** samples are obtained by arterial puncture. This procedure involves percutaneously puncturing one of the aforementioned peripheral artery sites. Obtaining a blood gas sample from an infant or child is generally more difficult than in an adult and requires more patience, skill, and time. However, an experienced clinician using proper technique can quickly obtain a sample that yields accurate results. Two individuals are helpful when performing an arterial puncture on a child who is too young to understand the need for the test but strong enough to react to the procedure. On a small infant or neonate, a transilluminating light placed behind the wrist may help visualize the location of the radial artery.[1,7]

Procedure

Performing a successful arterial puncture requires knowledge of the anatomy involved and proficient technical skills. Collect the equipment required for the arterial puncture (Box 8-2). Use the following sequence of technical steps as a guideline for performing the puncture.[1,7]

1. Wash hands and adhere to universal precautions for bloodborne pathogens, using proper-fitting examination gloves, along with eye and splash protection.[2,9-11]
2. Palpate the pulse at various sites (see Figure 8-1) to determine the best site for testing.
3. Perform the modified Allen's test if appropriate for the artery being sampled.
4. Use an assistant to help restrain the child and immobilize the limb if required.

Box 8-2	Equipment for Arterial Puncture and Blood Gas Collection

- 1-ml preheparinized* tuberculin syringe
- 25-gauge needle *or* preheparinized* 25-gauge butterfly needle infusion kit
- Correctly fitting examination gloves
- Povidone-iodine and alcohol wipes
- Sterile gauze
- Needle-capping and protection device
- Eye and splash shield
- Patient label

*Use dry heparin or expel liquid heparin from the syringe and needle hub or butterfly set before starting the procedure.

5. Scrub the puncture site with an approved antiseptic swab and allow to air dry, or use a sterile gauze pad. Do not blow on the site to dry it.
6. Palpate the artery again, and position the index and middle finger of the nondominant hand to stabilize the artery.
7. Maintain a clean field around the syringe and syringe kit while opening it. Prepare the kit for use, and heparinize the syringe if required. Remember to expel the heparin completely from the barrel of the syringe and hub of the needle.
8. Insert the needle of the syringe or butterfly catheter into the artery at a 35- to 45-degree angle with the bevel up, and advance it gently. Enter the artery from the direction opposite, or against, the blood flow. A flash in the hub of the syringe or butterfly catheter verifies that the needle penetrated the artery and is located in the lumen. In the small pediatric patient it is quite easy to pass through the artery with the needle. If a good pulse is palpated and no blood return occurs after the needle is inserted, pull the needle back incrementally and continue to watch for a flash of blood. If resistance is met when inserting the needle, slowly withdraw it immediately and change direction because it has most likely touched the bone.
9. Obtain the required amount of blood. Because the arterial pressure is usually high enough, manual aspiration is not required. If manual aspiration is required, however, the barrel of the syringe is withdrawn slowly. When using a butterfly catheter, attach the syringe to the catheter and slowly aspirate the correct amount of blood into the syringe. Maintain the sample amount as close to the technically feasible minimal volume as possible.[2,7]
10. After obtaining the sample, withdraw the needle and immediately apply firm pressure to the puncture site with a sterile gauze pad for at least 5 minutes. Apply pressure for a longer period if the patient has a coagulopathy or is receiving anticoagulation therapy (e.g., heparin). Avoid using pressure dressings. Patients should not apply the pressure because they may not press hard or long enough.
11. While holding the site, gently remove air bubbles from the sample. If using a butterfly catheter, remove it from the syringe.
12. Continue compressing the site, and seal the syringe with a one-handed safety cover device to prevent exposure of the sample to air. Gently roll the syringe between the hands or fingers to mix the heparin with the specimen.[3]
13. Immediately apply the proper patient label to the specimen according to institutional policy.
14. For accurate results, analyze the sample immediately, or analyze room temperature samples within 10 to 15 minutes after they are drawn. Samples placed on ice should be analyzed within 1 hour.[12]

Contraindications

The major contraindication to an arterial puncture is lack of collateral circulation. Punctures should not be performed at sites where the extremity has previously blanched, which may result from arterial obstruction or spasm. Punctures should not be performed through a site distal to or through a surgical shunt, as in a dialysis patient. If a limb is infected or shows evidence of peripheral vascular disease, an alternative site should be selected.[10]

Complications

Hematoma formation is the most common complication during arterial puncture and is seen more often in brachial than in radial artery punctures. Complications can be minimized by immediately applying adequate pressure to the puncture site after the needle is withdrawn. As with any invasive procedure, infection is a possible complication but is relatively low with aseptic technique. Scarring, laceration of the artery, and hematoma formation are more likely to occur with repeated puncture of an artery.[8] Alternating puncture sites decreases this risk. Other complications associated with arterial punctures in infants and children include nerve damage, bleeding, obstruction of the artery by clots or spasms, trauma to the artery, and pain.

Because the median nerve is close to the brachial artery, the nerve may be punctured as well during the procedure, which will cause intense pain down the arm. Because the posterior tibial artery and nerve are also close to one another, special care should also be taken to avoid nerve damage during puncture of this artery. Although the femoral artery is much easier to puncture, complications in infants tend to occur more often, including thrombosis, nerve damage, and necrosis of the head of the femoral bone.[7]

Although gloves are worn and universal precautions applied during all arterial punctures, needle sticks remain a risk to the clinician and are the most common source of transmission of bloodborne pathogens to health care workers.[2,8,9,13] Most of these complications are avoided by having only thoroughly trained and highly skilled clinicians perform a puncture.

CLINICAL HIGHLIGHT

Arterial complications are more severe than most capillary and venous complications. Special care should be taken to rule out contraindications to arterial puncture. Collateral circulation should also be verified via active or passive modified Allen's test before arterial puncture.

CAPILLARY BLOOD GAS SAMPLES

Capillary blood gas sampling provides a common alternative to ABG analysis in the infant or child. Punctures for capillary samples are less invasive than arterial punctures, are easier and quicker to perform, and can be used when there is no arterial catheter for drawing ABG samples.[13,14] Drawing a CBG sample is usually less painful, but local anesthetic application helps alleviate pain associated with the procedure.[6,7,15]

In general, a CBG sample correlates best with arterial pH and carbon dioxide tension ($PaCO_2$) values. Correlation of capillary samples with arterial samples varies depending on the parameters measured.[10,16,17] When a capillary sample site is adequately "arterialized" and puncture and sampling procedures are performed correctly, the pH and carbon dioxide partial pressure (PCO_2) of capillary samples can accurately reflect those of arterial samples. Often, capillary PO_2 is lower than arterial values; however, given a clinically acceptable difference between capillary PO_2 and PaO_2, the capillary PO_2 may trend with increases and decreases in arterial values.[11,16] Although some studies have shown a significant correlation between capillary PO_2 and PaO_2, the use of capillary PO_2 to determine oxygenation is currently not recommended.[2] The accuracy of capillary blood gas values is severely attenuated by the presence of hypotension, hypothermia, hypovolemia, and lack of perfusion.[12] Conversely, correlation of capillary and arterial blood gas values improves with hypoxemia, as venous and arterial PO_2 converge. Special consideration should be given to patients with circulatory defects. Decreased venous return, secondary to cor pulmonale or decreased cardiac output, leads to venous congestion and peripheral pooling, which may result in an increase in PCO_2. Conversely, increased blood flow may result in decreased capillary PCO_2.[13]

Although capillary punctures are less invasive, it is necessary to obtain an arterial sample at some point to ensure correlation and accuracy regardless of the specific marker being evaluated. Using noninvasive monitors such as pulse oximeters or transcutaneous oxygen/carbon dioxide monitors to evaluate oxygenation and ventilation when arterial samples are not obtained is an effective way to eliminate the need for frequent CBGs.[12] However, many factors that lead to inaccurate CBG sampling may also affect the accuracy of monitoring (see Chapter 9, Noninvasive Monitoring in Neonatal and Pediatric Care).[1]

Puncture Sites

The least hazardous puncture site for infants is the posterolateral foot, just anterior to the heel (Figure 8-2).[1,11] The posterior heel curvature and back of the heel must be avoided because the lancet could puncture the bone and result in calcaneous osteomyelitis. Do not perform a capillary puncture on the medial aspect of the heel, which is the location of the posterior tibial artery. For children and some infants, use the palmar or fleshy surface of the distal aspects of the fingers (middle or ring) and toes (Figure 8-3).[10,11,13] The earlobes are a secondary site for puncture in children. In general, avoid punctures on the fingers and toes of neonates because of the higher risk of nerve damage in this area.[11,13] Previous puncture sites or inflamed areas with an apparent or possible infection should not be used. As previously discussed, extremities with localized swelling or edema should be avoided because of the effect of extracellular or interstitial fluid on sample accuracy. Cyanotic areas should also be avoided.[13]

Procedure

Successful capillary puncture is not complicated, but it does require proficient technical skill. Collect the equipment required (Box 8-3), and use the following sequence of steps as a guide to collect a CBG sample.[1,7,11]

1. Select a puncture site and warm the area for 5 to 10 minutes. Use a warm (greater than 37° C but less than 42 to 45° C) wet cloth or disposable warming pack, and apply with caution.[1,7]

2. Give a 12% to 24% sucrose solution pacifier 2 minutes before the procedure, or apply an anesthetic cream or subcutaneous injection for pain control.[3,5-7]

3. Wash hands and adhere to universal precautions for bloodborne pathogens, using proper-fitting examination gloves, along with splash protection.[8,9]

4. Remove the warming device. Clean the site with an antiseptic, and dry with a sterile gauze pad; alcohol will hemolyze the blood.

5. Immobilize the area by properly grasping the hand or foot (see Figures 8-3 and 8-4) and stabilize the area by anchoring the hand or foot on a hard surface. Use an assistant to help restrain a child, and immobilize the limb if required. Restrain infants by swaddling them in a blanket.[7]

6. Finger or toe stick: Hold the digit (patient's finger or toe) with the thumb and forefinger, supporting the digit behind or close to the nail (see Figure 8-3). Keep fingertips well away from the puncture site.

7. Heel stick: Consider using venipuncture or a digit first, because either may be less painful and require less resampling.[3-7] Hold the heel gently but firmly. Wrap the forefinger around the infant's upper heel and ankle while holding the arch of the foot with the thumb (see Figure 8-4).

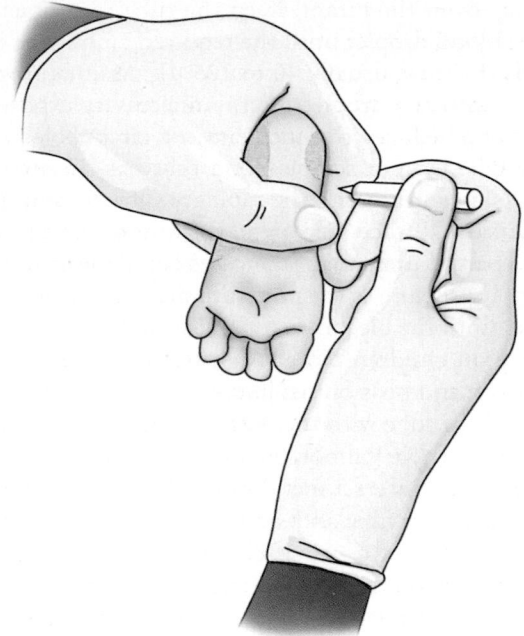

FIGURE 8-4   Technique for stabilizing the heel for a capillary puncture.

8. Position the lancet.
    a. For a finger or toe stick, hold the lancet at a 10- to 20-degree angle to the longitudinal axis of the phalangeal bone. Do not direct it into the bone.
    b. For a heel stick, hold the lancet between the thumb and index finger of the opposite hand, perpendicular to the puncture site.

9. Poke the point of the lancet into the skin with one continuous, deliberate motion. Correct depth depends on the infant, but 1 to 2 mm is generally sufficient to produce a free-flowing drop of blood.[7,16,17] Use a mechanical puncture when available because most produce consistent results with less need for resampling.[7,15] Avoid superficial punctures and the need to repeat the puncture. Do not slice, dig, or make multiple punctures.[1,6,7,16] Ease thumb pressure after the lancet is removed.

10. Wipe away the first drop of blood, which may be contaminated with intracellular, interstitial, or lymphatic fluids, with a dry sterile gauze pad.

11. Apply moderate pressure to the heel or digit, without massaging or squeezing, until a free-flowing drop of blood appears. Squeezing or "milking" the sample may cause red blood cell hemolysis, especially in newborns, because their hematocrit levels are higher and their red blood cells more fragile. Squeezing also results in bruising and contamination of the specimen with lymphatic and venous drainage.

12. Collect the blood by placing the tip of the capillary tube into the blood droplet without touching the puncture wound. Hold the capillary tube angled horizontally, or slightly downward, with the colored ring

Box 8-3	Equipment for Capillary Puncture and Blood Gas Collection

- Warming device or warm damp cloth
- Lancet and mechanical puncture device
- Lancet disposal system
- Correctly fitting examination gloves
- Alcohol wipes
- Sterile gauze
- Adhesive bandage
- Eye and splash shield
- Preheparinized capillary tubes
- Metal "flea," magnet, and capillary tube caps (if required)
- Patient label

away from the infant. Keep the tube in contact with the blood droplet until the required amount of blood fills the tube, usually 40 to 125 μl.[7] Maintaining contact with the droplet limits unnecessary exposure to air and reduces the incidence of air bubbles in the sample. Do not scrape blood that has smeared onto the skin surface into the capillary tube. Scraping from the skin surface increases exposure to air and alters the partial pressure of the gases being measured.[1,7,9]

13. Apply pressure to the puncture site with a sterile gauze pad until the bleeding stops. Use an adhesive bandage only on children old enough not to place it in their mouth and possibly aspirate it.

14. Label the tube with the proper patient information.

15. If the sample cannot be analyzed immediately after collection, insert a metal mixing bead (or "flea") into the capillary tube and seal it. Mix the sample by running a magnet gently back and forth along the tube, and place the sample on ice; this decreases the incidence of sample clotting. Remove the metal flea before analyzing the blood.

Contraindications

CBG sampling should not be performed when accurate assessment of oxygenation or ABG values is necessary. CBGs should not be used for routine blood gas monitoring when less painful or noninvasive measurements provide results that are more accurate.

Capillary puncture is contraindicated in neonates less than 24 hours old. A newborn has a low systemic output, and vasoconstriction tends to be maximal during this stage secondary to a decrease in environmental temperature and an increase in circulating catecholamines.[11,16,18,19] CBG sampling is not recommended in a patient with decreased peripheral blood flow, especially in the case of hypotension.[11,16,20] CBG sampling may be difficult to perform on a patient with polycythemia (hematocrit greater than 65%) because of the short clotting time. Do not use areas that are edematous, inflamed, or infected, or other areas previously mentioned. Avoid heel samples from ambulatory children who have formed calluses on the soles of their feet.[7,21]

Complications

Serious complications may result in medical management if capillary results do not accurately reflect the patient's condition. Consider potential errors in correlation with arterial values before deciding on a clinical course of action based on CBG values.[9,11,20]

Although capillary puncture is a relatively safe procedure, complications have been observed. Burns have been reported secondary to heel warming, but using a prepackaged warming kit that does not require an external heat source minimizes this problem. Other complications include infection, scarring, calcaneous osteomyelitis, calcifications, nerve damage, arterial laceration, bruising, cellulitis,

hematoma, and bleeding.[1,10,11] Some of these complications may seem benign at first but lead to developmental delays in such milestones as grasping and walking.

CLINICAL HIGHLIGHT

CBG samples are more vulnerable to inaccuracies caused by sampling technique and site selection than ABGs and VBGs. Special care must be taken during CBG sampling and analysis.

ARTERIAL CATHETERS

For frequent blood gas sampling, an **umbilical artery catheter** (UAC) in the newborn and a **peripheral artery catheter** or arterial line in the older infant or child is used for critically ill patients (Figure 8-5). Arterial catheters provide access for arterial blood pressure analysis and ABG sampling. UACs and arterial catheters also allow blood pressure monitoring in patients who are hemodynamically unstable.

Umbilical Artery Catheterization

In the infant the umbilicus typically provides ready access to two arteries. Facing the child, the two umbilical arteries are located at about the 5 and 7 o'clock positions. Prompt catheterization is essential in neonates because these vessels will undergo arterial spasm in the presence of increased arterial oxygen, making cannulation difficult if not impossible.[7]

It should be noted that some congenital anomalies may be associated with an umbilicus with a single artery.

Two positions are typically used to place the tip of the UAC. In the **high position** the catheter overlies the sixth through eighth thoracic vertebrae (T6 to T8); this position avoids major tributaries of the aorta because it is below the ductus arteriosus and above the celiac access. The **low position** is usually at the third to fourth lumbar (L3 to L4) space, between the renal artery and aortic intersection and above the takeoff of the inferior mesenteric artery. The UAC is placed to avoid the large tributaries supplied by these vessels to minimize trauma and hemodynamic disturbances of vital organs.[22]

The choice of high or low catheter placement is empiric. Hospitals tend to favor one site or the other; both are associated with their own set of complications related to hypoglycemia, hypotension, vasospasm, and embolic disturbances of organs distal to the catheter tip. A meta-analysis and literature reviews demonstrate a small advantage when using the high position over the low position.[23]

The starting point for how far a catheter should be inserted is determined by first measuring the distance from the umbilicus to the shoulder. This measurement is then looked up on a *nomogram* (a diagram allowing computation of a function) to determine the correct catheter insertion distance.[24-28]

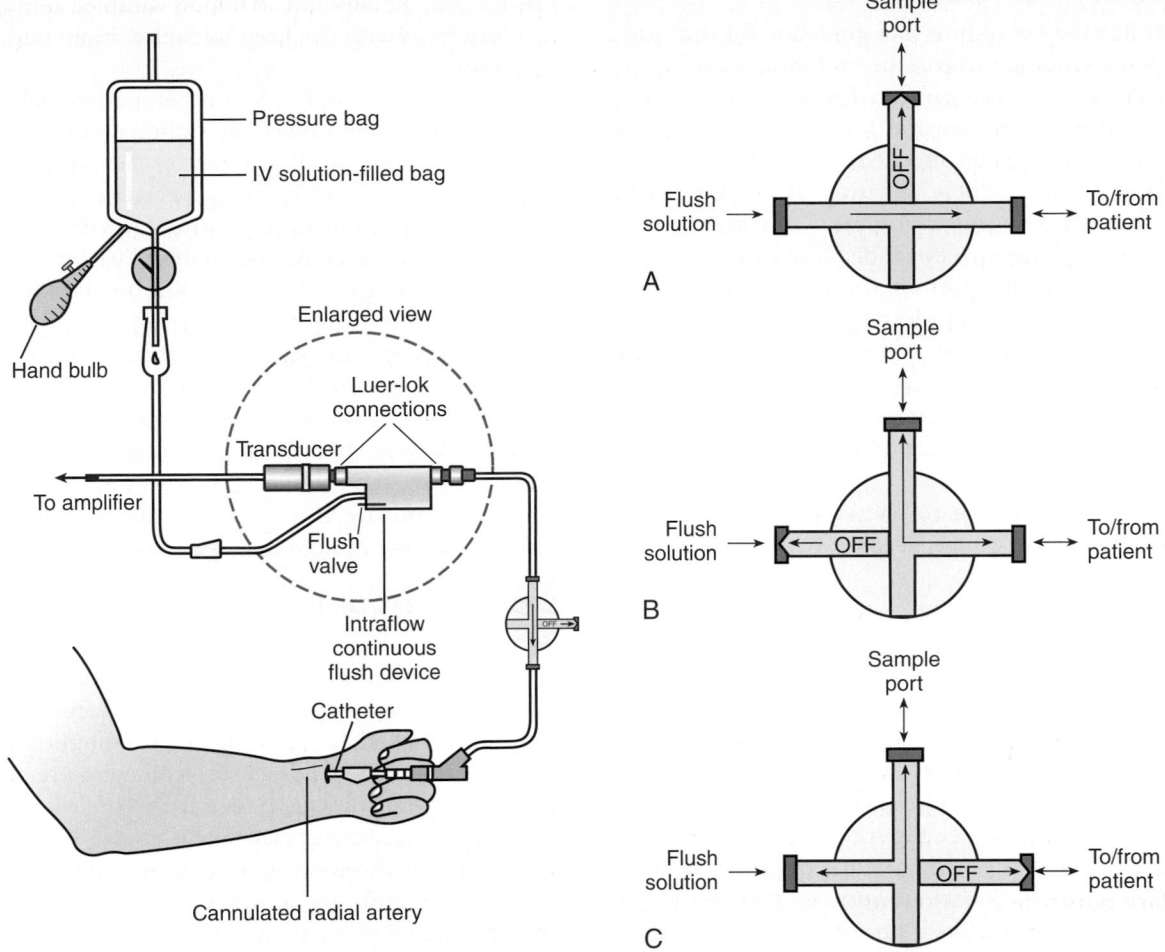

FIGURE 8-5 An indwelling arterial line and continuous infusion/flush system used to monitor blood pressure and obtain blood gas samples. Exploded view shows a three-way stopcock system. **A,** Normal position with stopcock off to sampling port allows continuous monitoring of blood pressure and flushing of the line if using a (pigtail) flush system. **B,** Position to draw blood or inject flush solution to the patient with stopcock turned off to flush solution. **C,** Position to flush sample port with stopcock off to patient. All ports are closed at all intermediary positions.

Using sterile technique, insert the catheter into one of the arteries. The artery that is less tortuous upon initial insertion will be easier to cannulate. Direct the tip toward the ipsilateral groin. The catheter is advanced with a gentle downward pressure, using a rotating motion to allow the catheter to seek the arterial lumen. Advance to a distance one third the infant's body length plus 1 cm for the high position. Patency is confirmed by the ease of blood flow. Connect the UAC to a prepared fluid pressure–transducing system (see Figure 8-5).[7,18]

The catheter is secured by suturing it into the umbilical artery, and taping it to the abdomen. Chest and abdominal radiographs help to confirm placement. A UAC may remain in place for several days to weeks as indicated by patient need.[1,18,24]

Peripheral Artery Catheterization

The clinician must rely on peripheral arterial catheterization in the pediatric patient. An arterial line is also used for blood gas monitoring in an infant or a newborn without umbilical artery access.

Arterial line placement is accomplished by using either a percutaneous method (through the skin) or a cutdown method (a small surgical stoma that allows direct visualization and cannulation of the isolated vessels). As previously noted, the most commonly used site is the radial artery; the posterior tibial and dorsalis pedis arteries are occasionally used. Other monitoring sites, such as the brachial artery, superficial temporal artery, and femoral artery, are rarely used because of the increased risk of complications. Arterial catheter sizes range from 22 to 24 gauge for a neonate and from 20 to 22 gauge for a pediatric patient.[24]

Before placing an arterial catheter, the modified Allen's test previously described can be performed to observe collateral blood flow to the hand or foot being punctured.[1,7] When performing a radial artery puncture in small children and infants, the use of a transilluminating light to locate the radial artery is helpful.[28]

Procedure for Sampling

Use the following procedure as a guideline for drawing a blood sample from an arterial or umbilical artery catheter.[1,28] Both catheters are connected to a heparinized normal saline continuous infusion/flush source and blood pressure–monitoring transducer (see Figure 8-5).

1. Wash hands and adhere to universal precautions for bloodborne pathogens, using proper-fitting examination gloves, along with eye and splash protection.[8,9]

2. Uncap the locking port of the three-way stopcock. Apply appropriate antibacterial solution to the stopcock port or rubber infusion port, depending on institutional procedures, and allow to dry.[1] Because multiple syringes are required, maintain a clean field around the site and a place to set the syringes that are not in use.

3. Attach a 3-ml syringe to the stopcock, or attach a syringe with a 25-gauge needle to the infusion port (see Figure 8-5, *A*).

4. Turn the stopcock off to continuous infusion/flush line, aspirate 1.25 to 2 ml of blood diluted with the infusion fluid, and remove the syringe. Do not discard this sample, and keep the tip sterile because it must be reinfused after the blood sample is acquired.

5. Close the stopcock by making a one-quarter turn between the syringe and the line to the continuous infusion/flush line (see Figure 8-5, *B*).

6. Attach a sterile preheparinized syringe to the port. Switch the stopcock back one-quarter turn toward the continuous infusion/flush line to the off position.

7. Aspirate 0.25 to 1 ml of blood into the sampling syringe, depending on the volume required by the blood gas analyzer.

8. Close the stopcock by making a one-quarter turn back toward the syringe, and remove the sample (see Figure 8-5, *A*).

9. Reattach the syringe with the aspirated infusion volume, and switch the stopcock toward the infusion line (see Figure 8-5, *B*) to the off position and toward the sampling syringe to the on position. Slowly reinfuse the solution from the syringe.

10. Repeat the procedure for turning the stopcock off to the continuous infusion/flush line, remove the syringe, and attach a syringe prefilled with flush solution.

11. Open the stopcock back to the flush syringe, and infuse 0.5 to 1.5 ml of solution to flush blood from the line. Turn the stopcock off to the sampling port, and remove the flush syringe. Return the stopcock cap to its position.

12. If using a flush device (pigtail) instead of a flush syringe then turn the stopcock off to the patient (see Figure 8-5, *C*) and open to the continuous infusion/flush line, then flush solution through the sample port and then turn stopcock off to the sample port to flush blood through the line to the patient.

13. Record the amount of blood sampled and flush solution infused to keep accurate input and output records.

14. Immediately apply the proper patient label to the specimen according to institutional policy.

15. For accurate results, analyze the sample immediately, or analyze room-temperature samples within 10 to 15 minutes after they are drawn. Samples placed on ice should be analyzed within 1 hour.[10]

When infusing or reinfusing solution into the umbilical or arterial line, tapping the syringe while holding it upward releases bubbles to the surface, where they can be expelled before attaching the syringe to the stopcock. When infusing, keep the syringe in a perpendicular position to allow air bubbles to rise toward the plunger. If bubbles form, tap them so they rise toward the plunger. Continue infusing the solution, but do not infuse air bubbles into the arterial line.

Complications

As with any invasive method of monitoring, peripheral artery catheterization carries an increased risk of infection.[24,25] The risk is greater when a catheter has been in place for longer than 72 hours. Some complications associated with the use of arterial catheters are related to thrombotic phenomena, either at the site of the catheter tip or distal to catheter placement.

The risk of thrombosis tends to depend on the size of the catheter and the duration of placement. Children younger than 5 years are at greater risk. Once significant perfusion or thrombotic problems are identified, remove the catheter as soon as possible, and manage the affected extremity to improve perfusion.

The circulating blood volume in a neonate is approximately 85 to 90 ml/kg; it is 70 to 75 ml/kg in children.[26] Therefore it is important to record and limit the amount of blood drawn from these patients. Hemorrhage may occur during insertion, from frequent or excessive blood sampling and if the catheter tubing is inadvertently disconnected. Blood transfusions are given to replace the blood volume lost as a result of these factors. Pallor, decreased pulses, and poor capillary refill are all signs of ischemia. Injection of even a small amount of air into the arterial system can result in rapid and devastating air embolism to the brain.

UAC complications may also include intraventricular hemorrhage, altered mesenteric blood flow, and necrotizing enterocolitis.[24,29] These and other complications, such as misplacement into the iliac artery or infarction of various organ systems, including the kidney, liver, and spinal cord,[30,31] may result in life-threatening or prolonged severe disability.

Measurements

The placement of arterial catheters allows direct measurement of arterial blood pressure values: the systolic and diastolic pressures. Monitoring arterial pressure waveforms helps to determine the patency of the arterial line and the quality of the pulse pressure and to calculate the **mean arterial pressure** (MAP). The arterial line monitor calculates MAP internally. However, use the following formula to obtain an indirect measurement of MAP with a sphygmomanometer:

$$MAP = \frac{[(2 = diastolic) + systolic]}{3}$$

MAP is often used as an indication of left ventricular afterload, thus representing the resistance against which the left ventricle must pump. The **pulse pressure** is the difference between the systolic and the diastolic blood pressure. A decreasing pulse pressure may indicate hypovolemia, and an increasing pulse pressure may indicate a restoration of normal volume status.

CONTINUOUS INVASIVE BLOOD GAS MONITORING

In-line continuous infant blood gas monitors can be used as an alternative strategy for patients requiring frequent blood gas analysis. These devices are specifically designed for small patients with low blood volumes and volume restriction. The monitor is placed directly in-line with an arterial or umbilical catheter (Figure 8-6). Using a closed loop system, it obtains a 1.5-ml sample of arterial blood, measures the blood gases via an in-line microelectrochemical sensor, and reinfuses the blood back into the patient. Clinical trials using in-line monitors in neonates found

that this method provided frequent, reliable results in a short amount of time, while substantially reducing the amount of blood loss and less exposure to health care providers.[32] Other continuous monitors are currently undergoing Phase I testing but are not currently available for clinical use.[33,34]

CENTRAL VENOUS CATHETERS

Indications for a **central venous catheter** are as follows:
· Cardiovascular instability
· Intravascular volume disturbances (e.g., extreme dehydration, hemorrhage, increased intracranial pressure, renal failure, and diabetic ketoacidosis)
· Administration of drugs, fluids, or nutritional support to the central circulation
· The need for **central venous pressure** (CVP) monitoring[35]
· Central venous catheterization is also indicated when other peripheral access sites have been exhausted. Placing a CVP line allows measurement of right atrial pressure (RAP) to assist in the following:
  · Managing fluid volume
  · Infusing fluid volumes larger than a peripheral intravenous catheter can accommodate
  · Administering total parenteral nutrition, and providing a secure long-term venous site in a chronically ill child[32,36,37]

Monitoring Sites

Techniques for central line placement in infants and children vary according to the patient's age and condition. *Monitoring sites* for central venous catheterization are locations where a peripheral vein can be cannulated by either the percutaneous or the cutdown method and the catheter can be advanced to a central location in the vena cava. The percutaneous technique is relatively safe and easy, with many potential sites.

The **cutdown method,** or surgical cannulation, reduces the risk of trauma to the vein and adjacent tissue. Cutdown also provides additional sites for patients with poor peripheral perfusion or lack of percutaneous sites. Cutdown locations include the internal and external jugular veins, common facial vein, brachial vessels, saphenous vein, and femoral veins. The cutdown technique requires experience to avoid surgical complications such as bleeding, inadvertent interruption of arterial flow, and dissection through vital structures such as muscles and nerves.

Common vessels used for percutaneous approaches are the external and internal jugular veins (the right is preferred over the left vein), subclavian vein, brachial veins, and saphenous vessels.[38,39]

The umbilicus offers a unique site in the newborn because the umbilical vein is available for placement of a central catheter.[36]

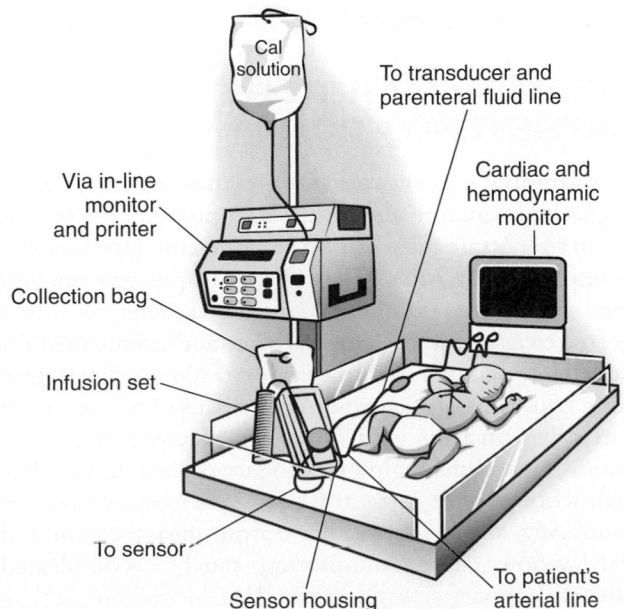

FIGURE 8-6 An ex vivo in-line continuous blood gas monitor designed for use in critically ill newborn infants.

Cal solution
To transducer and parenteral fluid line
Via in-line monitor and printer
Cardiac and hemodynamic monitor
Collection bag
Infusion set
To sensor
Sensor housing
To patient's arterial line

Procedure

Placement of the catheter is performed under sterile conditions with the child sedated and in accordance with the recommendations for pain control.[6] The site is usually anesthetized with lidocaine before the catheter is placed in the vein. Advance the catheter until an RAP waveform appears on the monitor. Connect a flush line and pressure transducer as with any indwelling catheter used for pressure monitoring. Confirm catheter placement with a chest radiograph.

Complications

The major complication of venous catheter use in general is catheter-related *sepsis*, especially when the catheter is in place longer than 72 hours.[32] Fungal sepsis is especially significant in the neonatal population.[40,41] In older children the additional complication of *pulmonary embolism* is significant.[42] Embolism appears to be a largely unrecognized clinical entity in the neonate.

The percutaneous approach may be difficult in patients with poor peripheral perfusion and in those with chronic disease who require many venous catheters. The cutdown method requires a higher degree of skill and training than the percutaneous approach to avoid complications. Cardiac arrhythmias may occur if the catheter tip slips into the right ventricle. Inadvertent placement of the catheter tip in the left atrium is possible if the patient has a patent foramen ovale or atrial septal defect. Perforation of the trachea is rare but has occurred with insertion into the jugular vein. Saphenous and femoral vein sites tend to be at higher risk for thrombosis. Air embolus may occur during insertion and when tubing is disconnected.[42]

Catheterization should be discontinued at the first sign of inflammation or when the patient's condition no longer requires its use. Percutaneous sites should be rotated on a regular basis. Any vein may be safely reused after 4 to 7 days.

Measurements

The placement of a central venous catheter allows measurement of the **right atrial pressure,** which represents the filling pressure of the right atrium. Systemic venous return, intravascular volume, tricuspid valve performance, myocardial function, and right ventricular pressure all affect the RAP. Normal values for RAP range from 2 to 7 cm H_2O but must be interpreted cautiously, because filling pressures vary with changes in thoracic and intrapleural pressure, such as during mechanical ventilation. The value of the RAP measurement is useful in monitoring trends and after changes in therapy.

Central venous oxygen saturation can be used to provide information about the peripheral extraction, delivery, and consumption of oxygen. Central venous oxygen saturation can be sampled from a truly "central" location ($ScvO_2$) or from a mixed venous source (SvO_2). Venous oximetry aids in the monitoring and implementation of early goal-directed therapies (EGDT) for patients with septic shock; it may also help reduce morbidity and mortality of patients undergoing major and/or traumatic surgery.[43-46] Blood samples taken from the right atrium may be similar to mixed venous samples; however, the "gold standard" for measuring mixed venous oxygenation is obtained by using a pulmonary artery catheter. This approach demands caution because catheter tip placement may be influenced by venous return from one portion of the body rather than the whole body. Of note, the presence of a high gradient between central venous PCO_2 ($PcvO_2$) and arterial PCO_2 can be indicative of poor circulatory response in the settings of severe hemorrhagic shock, poor cardiac output, cardiopulmonary resuscitation, and post-cardiopulmonary bypass.[47-51]

CLINICAL HIGHLIGHT

Central line infections are a major concern when sampling from this type of line. Please take extra precautions and sample as infrequently as possible.

Decreased CVP values usually indicate hypovolemia. Reduced CVP values occur during fluid imbalance, hemorrhage, extreme vasodilation, and shock. Increased CVP values may result from the following:

- Hypervolemia, as with sudden fluid shifts or volume overload
- Interference with the right ventricle's ability to pump blood, such as tricuspid valve regurgitation or stenosis, right ventricular failure or infarction, increased pulmonary vascular resistance, or cardiac tamponade
- Increased systemic vasoconstriction
- Left ventricular failure[38]

PULMONARY ARTERY CATHETERIZATION

The **pulmonary artery catheter** provides important physiological information about the cardiopulmonary vascular system (not attainable with other catheters), intravascular volume status, and the effects of various pharmacological therapies.[52] The pulmonary artery catheter is often referred to as a "Swan-Ganz" catheter and is indicated for critically ill patients with respiratory failure or profound shock requiring vasoactive drugs. It is used to assess left ventricular function, guide fluid management, and aid in diagnosing and managing pulmonary disease and cardiac dysfunction. Direct intracardiac and pulmonary pressure monitoring, along with cardiac output measurement and mixed venous oxygen monitoring, can be accomplished with a pulmonary artery catheter.[53,54]

Pulmonary artery catheters are used less often in pediatrics and are generally reserved for the sickest of patients.

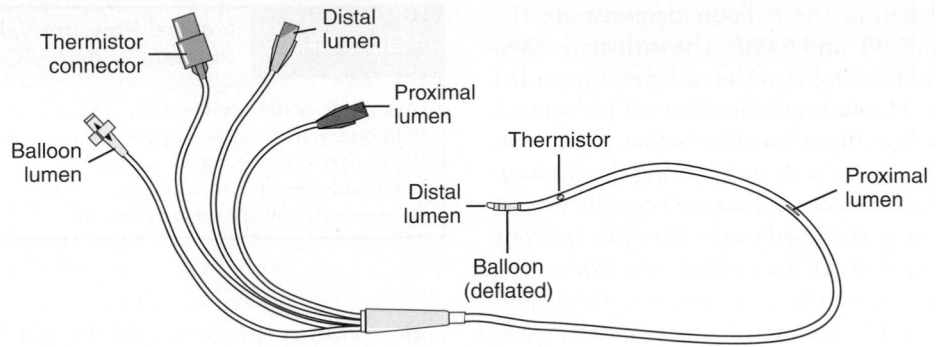

FIGURE 8-7   Conventional pulmonary artery (Swan-Ganz) thermodilution catheter.

The standard use of pulmonary artery catheters is divergent and its implementation varies from hospital to hospital. An analysis of risk versus benefit should be considered before using pulmonary artery catheters.

Pulmonary artery catheters contain quadruple lumens and come in 5-Fr (for patients less than 18 kg) and 7-Fr outer diameters. They are marked in 10-cm increments along the outside, and a balloon is fastened 1 to 2 mm from the tip. A four-lumen catheter has the following ports (Figure 8-7):

· Proximal port for placement in the right atrium—this port terminates in an opening at the tip of the catheter and is used to measure RAP.

· Distal port for placement in the pulmonary artery—this lumen terminates in an opening at the tip of the catheter and lies in the pulmonary artery. It is used to measure **pulmonary artery pressure** (PAP) and **pulmonary capillary wedge pressure** (PCWP) and to sample mixed venous blood.

· Port for inflation of the balloon at the catheter tip—when inflated, the balloon should surround but not cover the tip of the catheter.

· Port for the temperature-measuring thermistor—this port connects to the cardiac output monitor. The thermistor wires transmit the temperature of the blood flowing over them to the cardiac output monitor.[55]

Procedure

If tolerable, the patient is placed in the Trendelenburg position to prevent air embolism and to enhance neck vein filling. The catheter is primed with intravenous flush solution, and the integrity of the balloon is evaluated by injecting air into it. The catheter is placed in a large vessel, using a cutdown or percutaneous approach, and advanced until an RAP tracing appears on the monitor. The balloon is inflated with air and floated through the tricuspid valve into the right ventricle. The catheter is advanced into the pulmonary artery and then into a wedged position, where the catheter occludes the artery. As the catheter is advanced, characteristic waveforms are observed for each heart and vessel location, which assists with placement (Figures 8-8 and 8-9). Once the catheter is wedged, the balloon is deflated and the pulmonary artery waveform is confirmed on the monitor.

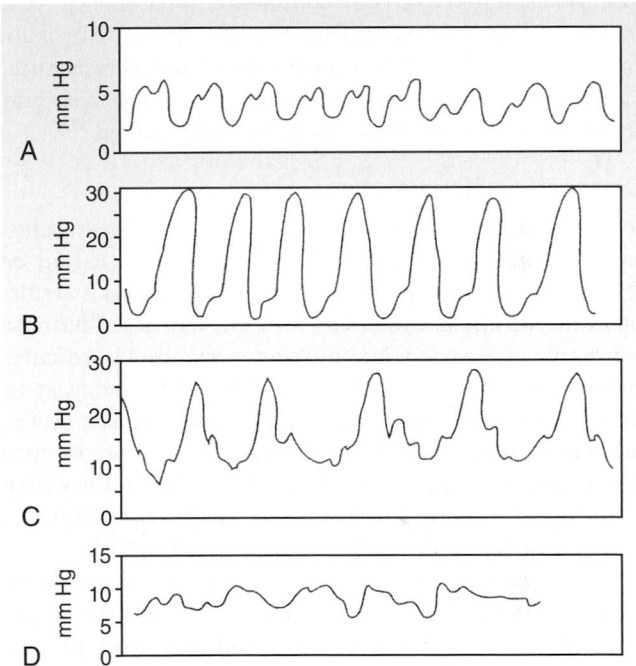

FIGURE 8-8   Examples of pressure waveform patterns at various locations in and around the heart. **A,** Central venous pressure; **B,** right ventricular pressure; **C,** pulmonary artery pressure; **D,** pulmonary capillary wedge pressure.

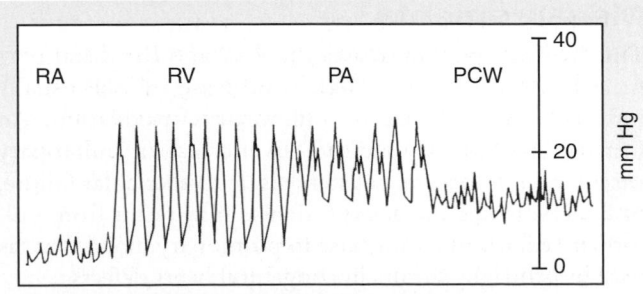

FIGURE 8-9   Pressure waveforms as the catheter travels through the right atrium (*RA*), right ventricle (*RV*), and pulmonary artery (*PA*), becoming wedged (pulmonary capillary wedge pressure [*PCWP*]).

Inflating and deflating the balloon demonstrate the ability to acquire a PCWP and a PAP. The catheter is then sutured in place, and the length of the catheter is recorded at the insertion site. The catheter should never be inserted to a length greater than that measured before placement. This avoids complications, such as knotting or unintentional wedging of the catheter without balloon inflation. A chest radiograph can be obtained immediately to rule out a pneumothorax and to verify the catheter's position.

Continuous monitoring of the catheter waveforms and pressures is necessary. On the monitor, the catheter position is maintained to produce a PAP waveform, except for those brief intervals when PCWP readings are obtained. To obtain a PCWP reading, a syringe is attached to the balloon port and aspirated to ensure complete emptying of the balloon, which avoids overinflation and rupture. Normally when inflating the balloon there is some initial resistance. If there is no resistance, the integrity of the balloon should be evaluated and inflation should be discontinued.[38,56]

Complications

At insertion, complications include bleeding, pneumothorax, tricuspid or pulmonic valve damage, right atrium or right ventricle perforation, and cardiac arrhythmias resulting from the catheter traversing the right ventricle. The most commonly observed arrhythmias are premature ventricular contractions and ventricular tachycardia. Overinflation of the balloon may result in rupture of the pulmonary artery, pulmonic valve obstruction, and air embolization. Pulmonary infarction may occur if the catheter is left in the wedge position for extended periods. The major complications remain catheter-induced thrombosis and sepsis.[56-64]

Positive-pressure ventilation affects PCWP measurements. Erroneous measurements may result from changes in baseline during the inspiratory and expiratory phases. Other sources of measurement error are failure to zero-set or calibrate the transducer properly, misalignment of the transducer with the tip of the catheter in the pulmonary artery, and dampening of the waveform secondary to thrombus formation.[25] Accurate hemodynamic values can be difficult to obtain in children with intracardiac shunts and tricuspid regurgitation.

Measurements

The proximal port measures the RAP and the distal port measures the PAP (Box 8-4). A decrease in PAP usually indicates hypovolemia or pulmonary vasodilation. An increase in PAP may indicate an increase in pulmonary vascular resistance, mitral stenosis, left ventricular failure, or hypervolemia. Increased PAP also may result from pulmonary edema or an increase in pulmonary blood flow, as with left-to-right shunts in congenital heart defects.

The PCWP reflects downstream pressures in the left side of the heart under conditions of absent flow in the pulmonary capillary bed. Variations in airway pressures, such as during mechanical ventilation, with positive

Box 8-4	Normal Pressure Values from Pulmonary Artery Catheters	
Mean right atrial pressure	2-7 mm Hg
Pulmonary artery systolic pressure	15-30 mm Hg
Pulmonary artery diastolic pressure	5-15 mm Hg
Mean pulmonary artery pressure	10-20 mm Hg
Pulmonary capillary wedge pressure	5-15 mm Hg

end-expiratory pressure (PEEP), can influence PCWP. The degree to which ventilation affects the relationship between PCWP and left atrial pressure depends on lung compliance. Under normal conditions, only 50% of the alveolar pressure is transmitted to the intrapleural space. Patients with low lung compliance, and hence low lung volumes, experience a negligible effect from variations in positive pressure on the PCWP. Higher compliance results in larger lung volumes and higher alveolar pressures. Therefore, higher intrapleural pressure is transmitted to the adjacent cardiovascular structures. PCWP should be measured at end expiration and without PEEP if tolerated by the patient. Measuring the PCWP with PEEP to establish trends in changes in clinical conditions is common. If not caused by PEEP, increased PCWP usually indicates left ventricular failure, hypervolemia, or intravascular fluid overload. Pulmonary artery catheters can have an additional fiberoptic lumen that provides continuous measurement of Svo_2 from the pulmonary artery.[55,58]

Cardiac Output

Cardiac output is the single most important hemodynamic measurement used to evaluate cardiac function and to determine the therapeutic effects of various treatments in critically ill pediatric patients. Cardiac output is the amount of blood ejected from the heart over the course of 1 minute. It is the product of stroke volume and heart rate. At birth, a newborn's cardiac output is approximately 0.6 L/min and increases to 6 L/min in an adolescent male.[29] Cardiac output is referenced to the body surface area as the **cardiac index.** The cardiac index is normally 3 to 4.5 L/min/m² throughout childhood.[29] Traditionally, cardiac output measurements use the thermodilution technique. Measurements are derived from injecting a known volume of liquid at a set temperature, 22 to 24° C, or iced, 0 to 4° C, into the right atrium through the right atrial port of the catheter. The solution is injected with a rapid and constant motion. The exact temperature and amount of liquid are entered into the cardiac output computer. As the liquid mixes with the blood and passes through the right ventricle into the pulmonary artery, the thermistor measures the rate of change in blood temperature from the value entered into the computer. The computer calculates the rate at which the blood warms the liquid, which is proportional to blood flow, and yields cardiac output.

By using the cardiac output and pressure measurements from the pulmonary and peripheral artery catheters, clinicians can construct a complete hemodynamic profile of a patient (Table 8-1).[25,57,61]

The injectate volume used with pediatric patients is smaller than that used with adults. However, it is important to limit excessive fluid administration by reducing the number of tests being done.

Pulmonary artery catheters are now available that do not require a cold injectate bolus to determine the cardiac output. Thermodilution is applied by using a thermal element on the catheter that warms up the surrounding blood, making it a warm bolus with a known temperature. Cardiac output is calculated, as the area under the curve, on the basis of the temperature change of the blood bolus as measured by a downstream thermistor.

Pulse contour analysis offers a minimally invasive technique that uses measurements obtained from arterial and central venous catheters to continuously calculate cardiac output. This method analyzes variations in the arterial pressure waveform during ventilation to determine stroke volume and hence cardiac index.[62] In addition, this method integrates a thermal dilution technique, using a central venous catheter, for initial and periodic system calibrations.

Pulse contour analysis has been shown to be an effective way to measure cardiac index in pediatric patients without using a pulmonary artery catheter or subjecting small patients to excessive fluid boluses.[63]

NONINVASIVE MEASUREMENT OF CARDIAC OUTPUT AND PERFUSION

Because of the inherent risks and limitations associated with pulmonary artery catheters, trends favoring noninvasive techniques to accurately measure cardiac output and tissue perfusion have resulted in new technologies.

A noninvasive cardiac output monitor that uses partial rebreathing of CO_2 to determine cardiac output via the Fick principle can now be used in mechanically ventilated children. A study has shown that this method correlates well with simultaneous cardiac output measurements obtained from a pulmonary artery catheter in patients with a body surface area of at least 0.6 m^2 and a tidal volume of at least 300 ml.[62] The values derived from these methods are not interchangeable and measurements from a pulmonary arterial catheter may be more sensitive. Nonetheless, the noninvasive method may be suitable for detecting large changes in cardiac output.[65]

Signal extraction pulse oximetry, which uses signal extraction software to analyze the plethysmographic waveform to determine pulsatile strength, is now being used to provide continuous noninvasive measurements of peripheral perfusion.[60] The perfusion index (PI) is the ratio of the pulsatile blood flow to the nonpulsatile or static blood in peripheral tissue.[64] The (PI) has been used as an objective parameter to evaluate perfusion and determine severity of illness in critically ill neonates.[66] The pulse variability index (PVI) continuously detects the cyclic changes of the perfusion index signal caused by variations in the intrathoracic pressure during a complete respiratory cycle. The PVI value has been shown to reliably predict fluid responsiveness in mechanically ventilated patients.[67]

PATIENT INFORMATION

It is important to monitor and record several parameters when taking a blood gas sample. Documenting the specific puncture or sample site and whether it is arterial, venous, mixed venous, or capillary is essential. The caregiver should also record the date and time at which the sample was taken, along with the patient's respiratory variables. Important respiratory variables include respiratory frequency, temperature, fraction of inspired oxygen (FiO_2), and specific oxygen device used. If the patient is mechanically ventilated, include the type of ventilator, mode of ventilation, tidal volume, peak inflation pressure, PEEP, and other relevant settings. Note the patient's position (e.g., upright in an infant seat), activity level (e.g., whether crying or breath holding), clinical appearance, and other signs of respiratory distress. Be sure to document any adverse reactions, along with the corrective action taken.

FREQUENCY

The clinical status of the patient, rather than an arbitrarily set time or frequency, should dictate the need for arterial and capillary punctures.[2,11,13] It is also important to understand that an infant, especially a premature neonate, has a much smaller quantity of blood. Frequent

---

TABLE 8-1

Normal Ranges of Derived Hemodynamic Parameters

Parameter	Formula	Range
Cardiac index	CO/BSA	3-4.5 L/min/m^2
Stroke volume	CO/HR	50-80 ml/beat
Stroke volume index	SV/BSA	30-65 ml/beat/m^2
Systemic vascular resistance	MAP – LAP/CO	11-18 mm Hg/L/min
Pulmonary vascular resistance	PAP – PCWP/CO	1.5-3 mm Hg/L/min
Shunt fraction	$(Cc_{O_2} - Ca_{O_2})/$ $(Cc_{O_2} - C\bar{V}_{O_2})$	Less than 5%

BSA, Body surface area; *Ca*$_{O_2}$, arterial oxygen content; *Cc*$_{O_2}$, pulmonary end-capillary oxygen content; *CO*, cardiac output; *C$\bar{V}$*$_{O_2}$, mixed venous oxygen content; *HR*, heart rate; *LAP*, left atrial pressure; *MAP*, mean arterial pressure; *PAP*, pulmonary artery pressure; *PCWP*, pulmonary capillary wedge pressure; *SV*, stroke volume.

TABLE 8-2

Approximate Normal Range of Arterial Blood Gas Values

Parameter	ELBW (<1000 g) Premature Infant	VLBW (<1500 g) Premature Infant to Late-Term Infant	Term Infant to Toddler	Child to Adult
	(<28 wk of GA)	(28-40 wk of GA)	(Up to 2 yr)	(>2 yr)
pH	≥7.25 (≥7.20)*	≥7.25 (≥7.20)*	7.3-7.4	7.35-7.45
Arterial carbon dioxide tension (PaCO$_2$, mm Hg)	45-55 (60)	45-55 (60)	30-40	35-45
Arterial oxygen tension (PaO$_2$, mm Hg)	45-65	50-70	80-100	80-100
Bicarbonate (HCO$_3^-$) (mEq/L)	15-18	18-20	20-22	22-24

ELBW, Extremely low birth weight; *GA*, gestational age; *VLBW*, very low birth weight.
*Values in parentheses may be accepted for certain lung protection ventilator strategies.
Modified from Pagtakhan RD, Pasterkamp H. Intensive care for respiratory disorders. In Chernick V, editor: *Kendig's disorders of the respiratory tract in children*, ed 5. Philadelphia: WB Saunders, 1990:205–224; and Durand DJ, Philips P, Boloker J: Blood gases: technical aspects and interpretation. In Goldsmith JP, Karotkin EH, editors: *Assisted ventilation of the neonate*, ed 4. Philadelphia: WB Saunders/Elsevier Science, 2003.

blood sampling results in hypovolemia and anemia in these patients. During mechanical ventilation, wait 10 minutes after changing the FiO$_2$ in a patient without chronic pulmonary disease to take an ABG sample.[68] Samples should not be drawn until 20 to 30 minutes after changing the FiO$_2$ of a spontaneously breathing patient without chronic pulmonary disease. Patients with chronic pulmonary disease should not have samples drawn for at least 30 minutes after an FiO$_2$ change.[2,13]

BLOOD GAS INTERPRETATION

Although a thorough discussion of blood gas interpretation is beyond the scope of this chapter, using the blood gas result requires some explanation of acid–base balance and gas exchange. *Gas exchange* refers to the exchange of oxygen and carbon dioxide between air and blood and then between blood and tissue. Proper gas exchange depends on many factors, such as blood flow, cardiac output, metabolic rate, diffusion, shunting, and gas concentration of the inspired air. An abnormality in any of these factors will result in a change in blood gas values and possibly an increase in the work of the cardiopulmonary system. Usually, only three values are measured during blood gas analysis: pH, PCO$_2$, and PO$_2$. Bicarbonate (HCO$_3^-$) and oxygen saturation are also usually calculated using the Henderson-Hasselbach equation, temperature, blood pH and the oxyhemoglobin dissociation curve. On occasion, other non–blood gas values may be measured simultaneously, depending on the analyzer in use at the time.

Typically, interpretation of blood gas values involves acid–base interpretation, to evaluate the pH and PCO$_2$ values, and evaluation of oxygenation, or PO$_2$, separately. Normal PaO$_2$ and PaCO$_2$ values reflect normal gas exchange, whereas an abnormality in gas exchange results in abnormal values. Normal values can vary considerably, based on patient age. Some mechanical ventilator strategies that use a lung-protective strategy have redefined normal ranges in acid–base status, especially in premature infants. Recognizing normal and abnormal values helps to understand more completely, and to interpret, blood gas values (Table 8-2).

Acid–Base Balance

Assessing acid–base balance is accomplished by evaluating the pH, PaCO$_2$, and HCO$_3^-$ values for acidosis or alkalosis and the degree of compensation present (Table 8-3). PaCO$_2$ is directly proportional to the adequacy of alveolar ventilation.

TABLE 8-3

Laboratory Values for Acid–Base Disturbances

Disease	pH	PaCO$_2$	HCO$_3^-$
Metabolic acidosis			
Uncompensated	↓	N	↓
Partially compensated	↓	↓	↓
Compensated	N	↓	↓
Metabolic alkalosis			
Uncompensated	↑	N	↑
Partially compensated	↑	↑	↑
Compensated	N	↑	↑
Respiratory acidosis			
Uncompensated	↓	↑	N
Partially compensated	↓	↑	↑
Compensated	N	↑	↑
Respiratory alkalosis			
Uncompensated	↑	↓	N
Partially compensated	↑	↓	↓
Uncompensated	N	↓	↓
Mixed acidosis	↓	↑	↓
Mixed alkalosis	↑	↓	↑

HCO$_3^-$, Bicarbonate; *N*, normal; *PaCO$_2$*, arterial carbon dioxide tension.
*Compensation of metabolic alkalosis by hypoventilation is limited by the physiological response to hypoxic hypoxia caused by the elevated PaCO$_2$.

Thus acid–base abnormalities are classified as primarily respiratory or metabolic. The amount to which the pH is balanced by the metabolic or respiratory processes determines the degree of compensation. Boxes 8-5 to 8-8 list common causes of metabolic acidosis/alkalosis and respiratory acidosis/alkalosis.

Box 8-5	Causes of Metabolic Acidosis

Diarrhea
Small bowel, biliary, or pancreatic tube or fistula drainage
Parenteral nutrition
Ingestion of chloride-containing compounds
• Calcium chloride
• Magnesium chloride
• Ammonium chloride
• Hydrochloric acid
Renal tubular acidosis
Renal failure
Carbonic anhydrase deficiency
Lactic acidosis
• Tissue hypoxia
• Sepsis
• Neonatal cold stress
Ketoacidosis
• Diabetes mellitus
• Starvation
Ingestion of toxins
• Salicylate poisoning
• Methanol poisoning
• Ethylene glycol poisoning
• Prolonged use of paraldehyde
Inborn errors of metabolism

Modified from Brewer ED. Disorders of acid–base balance. *Pediatr Clin North Am* 1990;37:429.

Box 8-6	Causes of Metabolic Alkalosis

Vomiting
Nasogastric suctioning
Congenital chloride-wasting diarrhea
Dehydration
Drugs
• Diuretics
• Steroids
• Sodium bicarbonate
Cushing syndrome
Bartter syndrome
Hypokalemia
Hypochloremia
Chewing tobacco
Massive blood transfusion
Infants with cystic fibrosis fed regular formula or breast milk (low in sodium)

Modified from Brewer ED. Disorders of acid–base balance. *Pediatr Clin North Am* 1990;37:429.

Box 8-7	Causes of Respiratory Acidosis

LUNG DISEASE
Upper airway obstruction
• Laryngotracheobronchitis (croup)
• Epiglottitis
• Foreign body
Small airway obstruction
• Asthma
• Bronchiolitis
Chronic obstructive pulmonary disease
• Cystic fibrosis
• Bronchopulmonary dysplasia
• Bronchiectasis
Pneumonia
Pulmonary edema
Respiratory distress syndrome
Aspiration
• Meconium
• Foreign body
Pulmonary hypoplasia
IMPAIRED LUNG MOTION
Pleural effusion
Pneumothorax
Thoracic cage abnormalities
• Flail chest
• Scoliosis
• Osteogenesis imperfecta
• Thoracic dystrophy
APNEA
NEUROMUSCULAR DISORDERS
Brainstem/spinal cord injury or tumor
Paralysis of diaphragm
Drug overdose/oversedation
Muscular dystrophy
Guillain-Barré syndrome
Myasthenia gravis
Poliomyelitis
OTHER
Botulism
Extreme obesity

Modified from Brewer ED. Disorders of acid–base balance. *Pediatr Clin North Am* 1990;37:429.

Oxygenation

The arterial partial pressure of oxygen (PaO_2) reflects exchange of oxygen, or oxygenation. Oxygen moves into the airway and the alveolus, at which point a pressure gradient causes it to diffuse across the alveolar–capillary membrane into the pulmonary capillary blood. It is then carried in the blood to the tissues in two forms: (1) dissolved in plasma and (2) bound to hemoglobin. Although the amount of oxygen dissolved in plasma is small, it is critical because it determines the pressure gradients among the inspired air, the blood, and the tissues. Hemoglobin carries the majority of the oxygen as oxyhemoglobin.

Box 8-8	Causes of Respiratory Alkalosis

Anxiety
Fever
Sepsis
Hypoxemia
• Pneumonia
• Atelectasis
• Pulmonary emboli
• Congestive heart failure
• Asthma
Central nervous system disorders
• Head injury
• Brain tumor
• Infection
• Cerebrovascular accident
• High altitude
Liver failure
Reye's syndrome
Hyperthyroidism
Salicylate poisoning
Mechanical ventilation

Modified from Brewer ED. Disorders of acid–base balance. *Pediatr Clin North Am* 1990;37:429.

The amount of oxygen bound to hemoglobin is expressed as *arterial oxygen* saturation (SaO_2) or % O_2 Hb saturation. The oxyhemoglobin dissociation curve illustrates the relationship between PaO_2 and SaO_2 regarding the loading and unloading of oxygen by the hemoglobin molecule (Figure 8-10). The sigmoid shape of the curve shows that the hemoglobin loads and unloads oxygen

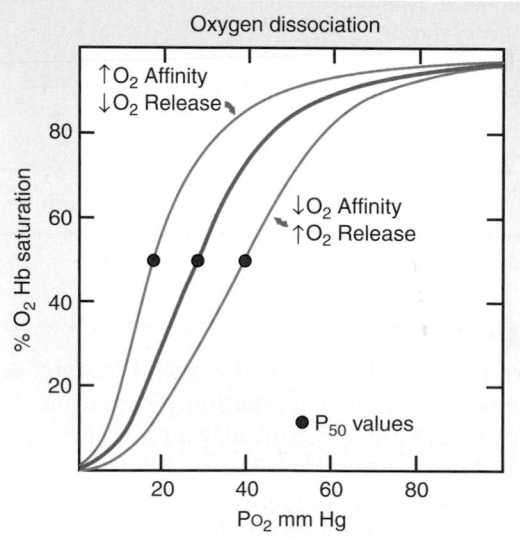

FIGURE 8-10 Oxyhemoglobin dissociation curve, illustrating the P_{50} value (PO_2 at 50% saturation) with the effects of right and left shifts of the curve. As the curve shifts to the right, the oxygen affinity of hemoglobin decreases, more oxygen is released at a given PO_2, and the P_{50} value increases. When the curve shifts to the left, there is increased oxygen affinity, less oxygen is released at a given PO_2, and the P_{50} value decreases.

differently at various PaO_2s. The PaO_2 at which the SaO_2 is 50% saturated is known as the P_{50} value. Under normal conditions, the P_{50} is approximately 26.5 mm Hg; however, this value can change depending on conditions that cause shifts in the oxyhemoglobin dissociation curve. The oxyhemoglobin dissociation curve is affected by several factors and may shift left or right (Table 8-4). A shift to the *right* results in a decrease in oxygen affinity, decrease in oxyhemoglobin, and increase the unloading of oxygen at the cellular level. A shift to the *left* increases oxygen affinity, increases oxyhemoglobin, and decreases the unloading of oxygen at the cellular level.

The oxygen content of the blood, expressed as a percentage, is the sum of the oxygen dissolved in the plasma and the oxygen in combination with hemoglobin (Hb, g/dl). Oxygen content accurately reflects the amount of oxygen in the blood, as follows:

$$O_2 \text{ content} = (Hb \times 1.34 \times SaO_2) + (PaO_2 \times 0.003)$$

Oxygen delivery, expressed as milliliters per minute, is the product of the O_2 content of the arterial blood and the cardiac output (Figure 8-11). Oxygen delivery reflects the total oxygen available at the cellular level in 1 minute as follows:

$$O_2 \text{ delivery} = O_2 \text{ content} \times \text{cardiac output} \times 10$$

Normal oxygen delivery ranges from 133 to 200 ml/min in newborns and from 200 to 400 ml/minute during infancy, and 460 to 1200 ml/min during childhood.[29]

Determining **serum lactate** in a blood sample provides important information about oxygenation. Lactic acid is commonly the byproduct of anaerobic metabolism, which results from hypoxia at the cellular level. Higher lactate levels are indicative of decreased O_2 delivery. Normal values for serum lactate typically range from 0.7 to 1.3 mmol/L.[69] A serum lactate concentration of 4.8 mmol/L and greater has been associated with increases in morbidity and mortality in children.[70]

TABLE 8-4	
Factors That May Shift Oxyhemoglobin Dissociation Curve	
Increased Affinity (Shift to Left)	**Decreased Affinity (Shift to Right)**
Increased pH	Decreased pH
Decreased PCO_2	Increased PCO_2
Decreased temperature	Increased temperature
Decreased 2,3-DPG	Increased 2,3-DPG
Fetal hemoglobin	
Carboxyhemoglobin	
Methemoglobin	

2,3-DPG, 2,3-diphosphoglycerate; *PCO_2*, partial pressure (tension) of carbon dioxide.

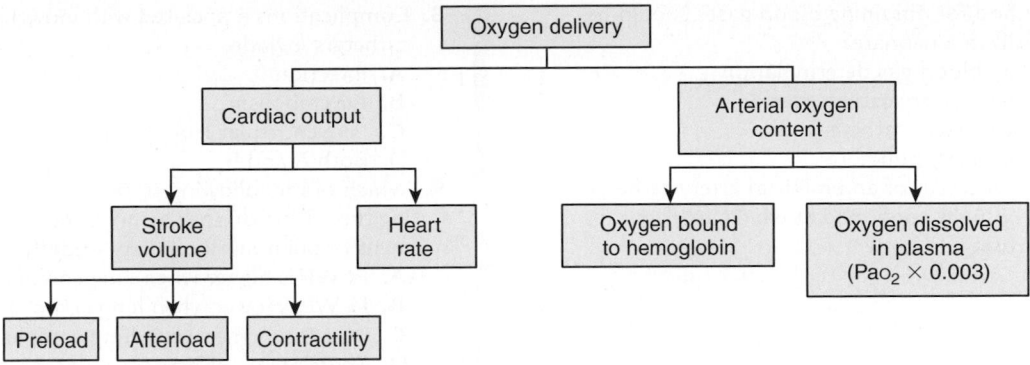

FIGURE 8-11 Components of oxygen delivery.

ABNORMAL HEMOGLOBIN

Abnormal hemoglobin may also have an effect on the capacity of hemoglobin to combine with oxygen. The following hemoglobins are sometimes encountered in the infant and pediatric population. **Fetal hemoglobin** accounts for approximately 85% of the hemoglobin in the full-term infant. It causes a shift to the left of the oxyhemoglobin dissociation curve and consequently an increased affinity of hemoglobin for oxygen. In utero, this compensates for the low fetal PaO_2 and causes more oxygen to be picked up in the placenta. At about 6 months to 1 year of age, all fetal hemoglobin should be converted to normal hemoglobin.

Methemoglobin forms when hemoglobin is oxidized to the ferric state. It causes the oxyhemoglobin dissociation curve to shift to the left, resulting in a decrease in hemoglobin's ability to combine with oxygen. Nitrate-containing molecules in medications and therapeutic gases may cause methemoglobinemia.

Carboxyhemoglobin forms when carbon monoxide combines with hemoglobin, which reduces the amount of oxygen that can attach to the hemoglobin. In carbon monoxide poisoning the patient has reduced oxygen content even though the PaO_2 may be normal (see Chapter 31, Pediatric Trauma). A left-shifted oxyhemoglobin dissociation curve compounds the tissue hypoxia further.

- Patient or caregiver complications may arise from blood gas sampling. Patient complications commonly include minor hematomas but may be as severe as neurovascular injury or infection. Caregiver complications are commonly related to inadvertent needle sticks. Universal precautions should always be applied during blood gas sampling and analysis.
- Indwelling catheters can provide valuable hemodynamic data. Arterial catheters can be used to monitor mean arterial pressure; central venous catheters can be used to evaluate RAP, CVP, and $ScvO_2$.
- Pulmonary artery catheters illustrate pressure waveforms from the venous, right atrial, right ventricular, and pulmonary artery regions. These catheters can also be used to monitor cardiac output and PCWP. Cardiac output can be determined noninvasively using rebreathing techniques and the Fick principle.
- Cellular oxygenation can be evaluated arterially (PaO_2, SaO_2), in conjunction with cardiac output measurements), in conjunction with cardiac output measurements (total oxygen delivery), or via venous values ($ScvO_2$, SvO_2). Serum lactate is also an indicator of cellular oxygenation, as lactic acid is a common byproduct of anaerobic metabolism.
- Functional understanding of the oxyhemoglobin dissociation curve is necessary to evaluate oxygenation, as this curve illustrates the oxygen affinity of hemoglobin at various PaO_2s. A shift of the curve to the right indicates an increase in this affinity; a shift to the left indicates a decrease in this affinity.

KEY POINTS

- Blood gas samples should be used to evaluate the efficiency of gas exchange, acid–base homeostasis, and cardiopulmonary interaction.
- Blood gas samples may be obtained from arterial, capillary, or venous sources. When selecting an arterial sampling site, those with adequate collateral circulation are preferred. The posterolateral foot is the least hazardous site for capillary puncture. For frequent sampling, indwelling catheters may be placed in either peripherally or centrally located vessels.

ASSESSMENT QUESTIONS

See Evolve Resources for answers.

1. The most accurate way to detect changes in oxygenation in the blood is by obtaining the following:
   A. Capillary blood gas
   B. Mixed venous blood gas
   C. Arterial blood gas
   D. Pulse oximetry

2. What method for obtaining blood gases should be tried initially in a neonate?
   A. Capillary blood gas determination
   B. Pulmonary artery catheterization
   C. Umbilical artery catheterization
   D. Femoral artery puncture

3. The high placement of an umbilical artery catheter should be visually confirmed at which anatomical landmark using an X-ray?
   A. T6-T8
   B. T3-T4
   C. L1-L2
   D. T1-T3

4. The most important advantage of continuous in-line blood gas sampling compared with umbilical blood gas sampling in neonates is:
   A. Lower risk of infection
   B. Lower incidence of clot formation
   C. Decreased amount of blood wasted
   D. The advantage of also being able to measure the cardiac index

5. The cardiac index is calculated by the following equation:
   A. $CaO_2/SpO_2 \times 100$
   B. Stroke volume/cardiac output
   C. $CaO_2 \times CO$
   D. Cardiac output/BSA

6. Common factors that can reduce pulmonary vascular resistance include:
   A. Hypoxemia and acidosis
   B. High mean airway pressure
   C. Fluid resuscitation
   D. Nitric oxide

7. Which of the following measurements requires a pulmonary (Swan-Ganz) artery catheter?
   A. Pulse variability index
   B. Pulse contour analysis
   C. Partial CO_2 rebreathing, using the Fick method
   D. Pulmonary capillary wedge pressure

8. Complications associated with indwelling vascular catheters include:
   A. Infection
   B. Air embolism
   C. Periventricular leukomalacia
   D. Both A and B

9. Which of the following statement(s) is correct regarding the effects of positive pressure on the measurement of pulmonary capillary wedge pressure?
   A. PCWP is higher when lung compliance is low.
   B. PCWP is lower when lung compliance is high.
   C. PCWP is higher when lung compliance is high.
   D. There are no effects from positive pressure on PCWP.

10. Oxygen delivery is composed of all of the following, except:
    A. Cardiac index
    B. Cardiac output
    C. Hemoglobin
    D. CaO_2
    E. A and C
    F. A, C, and D

11. Venous oximetry is helpful in reducing morbidity and mortality in the setting(s) of:
    A. Septic shock
    B. Major surgery
    C. Inhalation injury
    D. A and B

References

1. Czervinske MP: Arterial blood gas analysis and other cardiopulmonary monitoring. In Koff PB, Neu J, editors: *Neonatal and pediatric emergency care*, St. Louis, 1988, Mosby.
2. AARC clinical practice guideline: In-vitro pH and blood gas analysis and hemoximetry. American Association for Respiratory Care, *Respir Care* 46:498, 2001.
3. Johnston CC, Stevens BJ, Franck LS, Jack A, Stremler R, Platt R: Factors explaining lack of response to heel stick in preterm newborns, *J Obstet Gynecol Neonatal Nurs* 28(6): 587–594, 1999.
4. Anand KJ: Clinical importance of pain and stress in preterm neonates, *Biol Neonate* 73(1):1–9, 1998.
5. Johnston CC, Stevens BJ, Yang F, Horton L: Differential response to pain by very premature neonates, *Pain* 61(3):471–479, 1995.
6. Stevens B, Yamada J, Ohlsson A: Sucrose for analgesia in newborn infants undergoing painful procedures, *Cochrane Database Syst Rev* (3):CD001069, 2004.
7. Lefrak L, Burch K, Caravantes R, et al: Sucrose analgesia: identifying potentially better practices, *Pediatrics* 118 (Suppl 2):S197–S202, 2006.
8. Anand KJ: Consensus statement for the prevention and management of pain in the newborn, *Arch Pediatr Adolesc Med* 155(2):173–180, 2001.
9. National Committee for Clinical Laboratory Standards (Clinical and Laboratory Standards Institute): *Procedures for the collection of arterial blood specimens*, ed 4, NCCLS document no. H11-A3, Wayne, PA, 2004, Clinical and Laboratory Standards Institute.
10. Centers for Disease Control: Update: universal precautions for prevention of transmission of human immunodeficiency virus, hepatitis B virus, and other bloodborne pathogens in health-care settings, *MMWR Morb Mortal Wkly Rep* 37(24): 377–382, 387–388, 1988.
11. Occupational Safety and Health Administration: *Final rule: Occupational exposure to bloodborne pathogens*, Washinton, DC, 12/12/2008, OSHA.
12. Escalante-Kanashiro R, Tantalean-Da-Fieno J: Capillary blood gases in a pediatric intensive care unit, *Crit Care Med* 28(1):224–226, 2000.
13. American Association for Respiratory Care. AARC clinical practice guideline. Capillary blood gas sampling for neonatal and pediatric patients, *Respir Care* 39(12):1180–1183, 1994.
14. McLain BI, Evans J, Dear PR: Comparison of capillary and arterial blood gas measurements in neonates, *Arch Dis Child* 63(7 Spec No):743–747, 1988.
15. Johnson KJ, Cress GA, Connolly NW, Burmeister LF, Widness JA: Neonatal laboratory blood sampling: comparison of results from arterial catheters with those from an automated capillary device, *Neonatal Netw* 19(1):27–34, 2000.

16. Courtney SE, Weber KR, Breakie LA, et al: Capillary blood gases in the neonate. A reassessment and review of the literature, *Am J Dis Child* 144(2):168–172, 1990.

17. Yildizdas D, Yapicioglu H, Yilmaz HL, Sertdemir Y: Correlation of simultaneously obtained capillary, venous, and arterial blood gases of patients in a paediatric intensive care unit, *Arch Dis Child* 89(2):176–180, 2004.

18. Koch G: Comparison of carbon dioxide tension, Ph and standard bicarbonate in capillary blood and in arterial blood with special respect to relations in patients with impaired cardiovascular and pulmonary function and during exercise, *Scand J Clin Lab Invest* 17:223–229, 1965.

19. Cousineau J, Anctil S, Carceller A, Gonthier M, Delvin EE: Neonate capillary blood gas reference values, *Clin Biochem* 38(10):905–907, 2005.

20. Ueta I, Jacobs BR: Capillary and arterial blood gases in hemorrhagic shock: a comparative study, *Pediatr Crit Care Med* 3(4):375–377, 2002.

21. Sell EJ, Hansen RC, Struck-Pierce S: Calcified nodules on the heel: a complication of neonatal intensive care, *J Pediatr* 96 (3 Pt 1):473–475, 1980.

22. Symansky MR, Fox HA: Umbilical vessel catheterization: indications, management, and evaluation of the technique, *J Pediatr* 80(5):820–826, 1972.

23. Barrington KJ: Umbilical artery catheters in the newborn: effects of position of the catheter tip, *Cochrane Database Syst Rev* (2):CD000505, 2000.

24. Cole FS, Todres ID, Shannon DC: Technique for percutaneous cannulation of the radial artery in the newborn infant, *J Pediatr* 92(1):105–107, 1978.

25. Eshali H, Ringertz S, Nystrom S, Faxelius G: Septicaemia with coagulase negative staphylococci in a neonatal intensive care unit. Risk factors for infection, and antimicrobial susceptibility of the bacterial strains, *Acta Paediatr Scand Suppl* 360:127–134, 1989.

26. Hazinski MF: Hemodynamic monitoring of children. In Daily EK, Schroeder JS, editors: *Techniques in bedside hemodynamic monitoring*, ed 5, St. Louis, 1994, Mosby, pp 275–341.

27. MacDonald MG: Umbilical artery catheterization. In Avery GB, Fletcher MA, MacDonald MG, editors: *Neonatology: pathophysiology and management of the newborn*, Philadelphia, 1999, Lippincott Williams & Wilkins, pp 1338.

28. Tibby SM, Murdoch IA: Monitoring cardiac function in intensive care, *Arch Dis Child* 88(1):46–52, 2003.

29. Lott JW, Conner GK, Phillips JB: Umbilical artery catheter blood sampling alters cerebral blood flow velocity in preterm infants, *J Perinatol* 16(5):341–345, 1996.

30. Brown MS, Phibbs RH: Spinal cord injury in newborns from use of umbilical artery catheters: report of two cases and a review of the literature, *J Perinatol* 8(2):105–110, 1988.

31. Cumming WA, Burchfield DJ: Accidental catheterization of internal iliac artery branches: a serious complication of umbilical artery catheterization, *J Perinatol* 14(4):304–309, 1994.

32. Widness JA, Kulhavy JC, Johnson KJ, et al: Clinical performance of an in-line point-of-care monitor in neonates, *Pediatrics* 106(3):497–504, 2000.

33. Jin W, Wu L, Song Y, et al: Continuous intra-arterial blood pH monitoring by a fiber-optic fluorosensor, *IEEE Trans Biomed Eng* 58(5):1232–1238, 2011.

34. Jin W, Jiang J, Song Y, Bai C: Real-time monitoring of blood carbon dioxide tension by fluorosensor, *Respir Physiol Neurobiol* 180(1):141–146, 2012.

35. Duck S: Neonatal intravenous therapy, *J Intraven Nurs* 20(3):121–128, 1997.

36. Hamilton H, Fermo K: Assessment of patients requiring i.v. therapy via a central venous route, *Br J Nurs* 7(8):451–454, 456–460, 1998.

37. Chiang VW, Baskin MN: Uses and complications of central venous catheters inserted in a pediatric emergency department, *Pediatr Emerg Care* 16(4):230–232, 2000.

38. Jordan W: Arterial catheters. In Blumer JL, editor: *A practical guide to pediatric intensive care*, St. Louis, 1990, Mosby, pp 825.

39. MacDonald MG: Umbilical vein catheterization. In Avery GB, Fletcher MA, MacDonald MG, editors: *Neonatology: pathophysiology and management of the newborn*, Philadelphia, 1999, Lippincott Williams & Wilkins, p 148.

40. Trotter CW: Percutaneous central venous catheter-related sepsis in the neonate: an analysis of the literature from 1990 to 1994, *Neonatal Netw* 15(3):15–28, 1996.

41. Green C, Yohannan MD: Umbilical arterial and venous catheters: placement, use, and complications, *Neonatal Netw* 17(6):23–28, 1998.

42. Wynsma LA: Negative outcomes of intravascular therapy in infants and children, *AACN Clin Issues* 9(1):49–63, 1998.

43. Blasco V, Leone M, Textoris J, Visintini P, Albanese J, Martin C: [Venous oximetry: physiology and therapeutic implications], *Ann Fr Anesth Reanim* 27(1):74–82, 2008.

44. Christensen M: Mixed venous oxygen saturation monitoring revisited: thoughts for critical care nursing practice, *Aust Crit Care* 25(2):78–90, 2012.

45. Marx G, Reinhart K: Venous oximetry, *Curr Opin Crit Care* 12(3):263–268, 2006.

46. Walkey AJ, Farber HW, O'Donnell C, Cabral H, Eagan JS, Philippides GJ: The accuracy of the central venous blood gas for acid-base monitoring, *J Intensive Care Med* 25(2):104–110, 2010.

47. Futier E, Robin E, Jabaudon M, et al: Central venous O_2 saturation and venous-to-arterial CO_2 difference as complementary tools for goal-directed therapy during high-risk surgery, *Crit Care* 14(5):R193, 2010.

48. Idris AH, Staples ED, O'Brien DJ, et al: Effect of ventilation on acid-base balance and oxygenation in low blood-flow states, *Crit Care Med* 22(11):1827–1834, 1994.

49. Steedman DJ, Robertson CE: Acid base changes in arterial and central venous blood during cardiopulmonary resuscitation, *Arch Emerg Med* 9(2):169–176, 1992.

50. Utoh J, Moriyama S, Goto H, et al: [Arterial-venous carbon dioxide tension difference after hypothermic cardiopulmonary bypass], *Nihon Kyobu Geka Gakkai Zasshi* 45(5):679–681, 1997.

51. Weil MH, Tang W, Noc M: Acid-base balance during cardiopulmonary resuscitation, *Crit Care Med* 21(9 Suppl):S323–S324, 1993.

52. Osgood CF, Watson MH, Slaughter MS, MacIntyre NR: Hemodynamic monitoring in respiratory care, *Respir Care* 29(1):25–34, 1984.

53. Katz RW, Pollack MM, Weibley RE: Pulmonary artery catheterization in pediatric intensive care, *Adv Pediatr* 30:169–190, 1983.

54. Abou-Khalil B, Scalea TM, Trooskin SZ, Henry SM, Hitchcock R: Hemodynamic responses to shock in young trauma patients: need for invasive monitoring, *Crit Care Med* 22(4):633–639, 1994.

55. Marini JJ: Obtaining meaningful data from the Swan-Ganz catheter, *Respir Care* 30:572, 1985.

56. Pollack MM, Reed TP, Holbrook PR, Fields AI: Bedside pulmonary artery catheterization in pediatrics, *J Pediatr* 96(2):274–276, 1980.

57. Moodie DS, Feldt RH, Kaye MP, Strelow DA, van der Hagen LJ: Measurement of cardiac output by thermodilution: development of accurate measurements at flows applicable to the pediatric patient, *J Surg Res* 25(4):305–311, 1978.

58. White KM: Completing the hemodynamic picture: Svo2, *Heart Lung* 14(3):272–280, 1985.

59. WH P: Invasive measurements in the PICU. In Fuhrman BP, editor: *Pediatric critical care*, St. Louis, 1998, Mosby, pp 70–86.

60. Goldman JM, Petterson MT, Kopotic RJ, Barker SJ: Masimo signal extraction pulse oximetry, *J Clin Monit Comput* 16(7):475–483, 2000.

61. Koppl J: Hemodynamic monitoring using a PiCCO in a ten month old infant suffering from serious burn injury, *Bratisl Lek Listy* 108:359, 2000.

62. Levy RJ, Chiavacci RM, Nicolson SC, et al: An evaluation of a noninvasive cardiac output measurement using partial carbon dioxide rebreathing in children, *Anesth Analg* 99(6):1642–1647, 2004.

63. Fakler U, Pauli C, Balling G, et al: Cardiac index monitoring by pulse contour analysis and thermodilution after pediatric cardiac surgery, *J Thorac Cardiovasc Surg* 133(1):224–228, 2007.

64. Masimo Corporation: *Clinical applications of perfusion index.* http://www.masimo.com/pdf/whitepaper/LAB3410F.pdf. Retrieved August 2008.

65. Kotake Y, Yamada T, Nagata H, Suzuki T, Takeda J: Can mixed venous hemoglobin oxygen saturation be estimated using a NICO monitor? *Anesth Analg* 109(1):119–123, 2009.

66. De Felice C, Latini G, Vacca P, Kopotic RJ: The pulse oximeter perfusion index as a predictor for high illness severity in neonates, *Eur J Pediatr* 161(10):561–562, 2002.

67. Cannesson M, Slieker J, Desebbe O, et al: The ability of a novel algorithm for automatic estimation of the respiratory variations in arterial pulse pressure to monitor fluid responsiveness in the operating room, *Anesth Analg* 106(4):1195–1200, 2008.

68. Hess D, Good C, Didyoung R, et al: The validity of assessing arterial blood gases 10 minutes after an FIO_2 change in mechanically ventilated patients without chronic pulmonary disease, *Respir Care* 30:1037, 1985.

69. Vincent JL: Lactate and biochemical indexes of oxygenation. In Tobin MJ, editor: *Principles and practices of intensive care monitoring*, New York, 1998, McGraw-Hill, pp 369–375.

70. Basaran M, Sever K, Kafali E, et al: Serum lactate level has prognostic significance after pediatric cardiac surgery, *J Cardiothorac Vasc Anesth* 20(1):43–47, 2006.

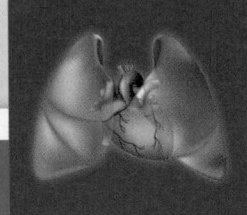

Chapter 9

Noninvasive Monitoring in Neonatal and Pediatric Care

CRAIG D. SMALLWOOD

LEARNING OBJECTIVES

After reading this chapter the reader will be able to:

1. Describe the fundamental monitoring methods used to assess heart rate, respiratory rate, and blood pressure
2. Recognize the principles of operation of pulse oximetry
3. Describe proper placement of a pulse oximeter probe
4. Describe the difference between end-tidal CO_2 monitoring and volumetric capnography
5. Explain the physiological phenomenon responsible for a gradient between end-tidal and arterial CO_2 measurements
6. Interpret specific abnormalities associated with capnograms
7. Explain the importance of proper transcutaneous site selection and application
8. List two problems associated with transcutaneous monitoring
9. State the objective of indirect calorimetry
10. Identify limitations of indirect calorimetry

KEY TERMS

Alveolar volume
Calorimetry
Capnography
Carbon dioxide production (Vco_2)
Carboxyhemoglobin
CO_2 elimination
Dead-space volume
Deoxyhemoglobin
Direct calorimetry

Electrocardiography
End-tidal CO_2
Energy expenditure
Indirect calorimetery
Infrared spectrometry
Mainstream capnography
Oxygen consumption (Vo_2)
Oxyhemoglobin
Postductal oxygen saturation

Preductal oxygen saturation
$P_{TC}O_2$
$P_{TC}CO_2$
Pulse oximetry
Resting energy expenditure
Sidestream capnography
Transcutaneous monitor
Volumetric capnography

Monitoring of the neonatal and pediatric patient is essential during each phase of the disease process (from the outpatient clinic to emergency room to the intensive care unit). Close monitoring of physiological function can provide clinicians with information that helps guide decision making. Appropriate monitoring (including proper application, use, and interpretation of data) can delineate the need for clinical interventions and the effect of those interventions over time. Respiratory-related illness is a leading reason for hospital admission in pediatrics and is therefore critical. Technologies have evolved over the last few decades to enhance the accuracy of measurements, eliminate the propensity for human error and bias, and readily display information dynamically and as a trend. These efforts have led to a number of specific devices that the respiratory therapist must learn to master to provide the best care possible, which can prove to be lifesaving.[1]

FUNDAMENTAL MONITORING

Heart rate, respiratory rate, and blood pressure are three of the four vital signs that can be noninvasively monitored and are readily available in a variety of clinical settings. Because these were discussed in Chapter 4, here we give only a brief summary of essentials for patients who are continuously monitored, such as in the intensive care unit.

Electrocardiography

Electrocardiography (ECG) is used to measure and display the heart rate and rhythm by measuring body surface electric potentials generated by the heart. It is easy to perform, noninvasive, and has been used for many years. Typically, ECG monitoring uses a set of three electrodes, which are placed on the upper left (LA), upper right (RA), and lower left (LL) portions of patient's thorax. Most lead manufacturers color code the leads to assist with appropriate placement: LA is black, RA is white, LL is red. A simple mnemonic to ensure proper placement of the electrodes is *White on the right, smoke over fire. White* refers to the white lead, *smoke* refers to the black lead, and *fire* refers to the red lead. Electrodes are available in different sizes to be applied according to patient size. The electrodes are typically plugged into the bedside monitor so that data (heart rate and waveform) can be displayed at the bed side and transmitted to a central telemetry console for remote monitoring. Continuous monitoring and interpretation of the ECG can ensure adequate heart rate and detect potentially life-threatening changes in rate and rhythm (such as severe bradycardia or ventricular fibrillation). A normal ECG waveform will have several distinct features, including depolarization and repolarization of the atria and ventricles. The most prominent feature is the QRS complex, which results from ventricular contraction. However, limitations of the technology, included inaccurate measurements caused by motion artifact, for instance, should be considered when interpreting results. Additionally, infant electrocardiographs present extra challenges caused by rapidly changing hemodynamics. A full-term infant will have a different ECG than a premature baby (34 weeks of gestation or less). In addition, the ECG of a normal infant will undergo changes during the baby's first few weeks of life. Not until a child is approximately 3 years of age will the ECG start to resemble that of an adult, although still with considerable differences.[2]

Impedance Respiratory Rate

Using the same electrodes as those employed during ECG monitoring, respiratory rate (RR) and impedance tracing can be measured and displayed on a bedside monitor and telemetry console for continuous monitoring and assessment. The monitor works by injecting a small alternating current into the patient, which is not felt by the patient and is monitored by one of the other electrodes. Because body tissue and air impede the flow of electricity, it is possible to detect RR based on changes in impedance. It is important to note that impedance RR monitors do not measure respirations (gas exchange) but simply chest excursions. In some cases, children may exhibit ineffective breathing movements (in which case the thorax could change shape) without actually inhaling or exhaling a breath. Although rare, in this case the impedance monitor would not provide an accurate reflection of respiratory rate. A more accurate monitor of respiration is end-tidal CO_2, which will be discussed later. However, for most patients, impedance RR equals the number of respirations; therefore it is widely monitored and used throughout the hospital.

Noninvasive Blood Pressure

Blood pressure (BP) is another of the four vital signs and is an essential metric of physiological health in the intensive care unit. Although not a direct measure of cardiac output, BP may be used, with caution, as a surrogate for cardiac output (along with proper assessment of HR, perfusion, etc.). It is therefore a physiological variable, and increases and decreases in BP can be life threatening, requiring immediate intervention. Additionally, in mechanically ventilated children, increases in intrathoracic pressure (by increasing positive end-expiratory pressure, for example) can reduce venous return, resulting in decreased BP. Close BP monitoring is therefore necessary for mechanically ventilated children, particularly the most severely ill. Although BP can be determined by using an indwelling arterial catheter, the procedure is invasive and increases the risk for infection. Noninvasive BP monitoring can provide periodic monitoring for those patients who do not require such intensive monitoring. Generally, a noninvasive BP is determined by using a cuff affixed to an upper extremity. In larger patients, generally the cuff is placed around the bicep, but for small children or infants, a cuff can be placed around a leg. Although this measure can be determined manually, most ICUs have an automated system that is integrated into the bedside monitor. Unlike manual determination of systolic and diastolic blood pressure by auscultation of Korotkoff sounds, an automated system uses a sensitive transducer to measure simultaneously the total pressure in the cuff as well as oscillations that result from the pulsating blood vessel. The systolic and diastolic blood pressures are recognized by the changes in oscillation intensity. Often, monitors can calculate BP at clinician-determined intervals (anywhere from minutes to hours) and display the results as needed. Care should be taken to ensure proper placement of the cuff or results will not reflect the patient's true BP. As mentioned previously, noninvasive BP by cuff cannot be monitoring continuously and may not be sufficient for some acutely ill children. In mechanically ventilated children, increases in intrathoracic pressure (by increasing positive end expiratory pressure for example) can reduce venous return, resulting in decreased BP.

PULSE OXIMETRY

Oxygenation monitoring is essential in the neonatal and pediatric patients, particularly those who are critically ill, such as during supported ventilation. *Hypoxemia,* reduced blood oxygen content, can lead to tissue and end organ damage, brain and developmental delays, and death. Conversely, *hyperoxemia,* elevated blood oxygen content, can cause retinopathy of prematurity in neonates, and long-term exposure to elevated concentrations of oxygen can cause chronic changes in pulmonary tissue or even fibrosis. Skilled caregivers cannot always detect hypoxemia by visual assessment when oxygen saturation levels drop below 80%. **Pulse oximetry** provides a means of monitoring oxygenation level trends over time or in response to therapeutic interventions. Pulse oximetry is simple to use, accurate (when applied correctly), and poses minimal discomfort to the patient. Despite limited scientific evidence showing improved outcomes with pulse oximetry, it is widely used to continuously monitor patients throughout the hospital, in clinic, and at home.[3]

Principles of Operation

Oxygen is carried in the blood in two forms: bound and dissolved. Approximately 98% of the oxygen found in arterial blood is bound to hemoglobin, whereas the remaining 2% is dissolved in the plasma.[3] The hemoglobin binds with oxygen in the pulmonary circulation and is then released at the tissue level for use. The saturated concentration of oxygen in the artery (SaO_2) is related to that which is dissolved in the plasma (PaO_2). This relationship and its modified response to pH, CO_2, and other factors is described by the **oxyhemoglobin** dissociation curve. Pulse oximeters measure the relative concentration of oxyhemoglobin to total hemoglobin in pulsatile arterial blood (SpO_2).[3]

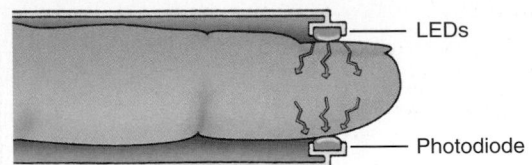

FIGURE 9-1 Proper alignment of light-emitting diodes (LEDs) opposite the photodiode in a sensor applied to a patient's finger.

A pulse oximeter sensor has two light-emitting diodes (LEDs) that function as light sources and a photodiode that measures the amount of light from the LEDs (Figure 9-1). One LED emits red light, and the other diode emits infrared light. The sensor is placed over a translucent part of the body (finger, toe, earlobe, etc.). As the light from the diodes passes through the blood and tissue, some of the light from both the red and the infrared diodes is absorbed by oxyhemoglobin. The photodiode then measures the amount of light that passes through the body without being absorbed. Because oxyhemoglobin (hemoglobin bound with oxygen) and **deoxyhemoglobin** (hemoglobin not bound with oxygen) absorb significantly different amounts of light, the proportion of oxyhemoglobin (expressed as a percentage) is determined (Figure 9-2). To measure arterial blood, the sensor detects pulsatile blood as it enters the tissue.

Application

Pulse oximeters do not require calibration at the bedside because they are precalibrated during the manufacturing process and the calibration is built in to the device's algorithm. The wavelength of the sensor diodes is checked and then coded into a calibration resistor. The instrument decodes the resistor each time it is turned on, at periodic intervals during use, or when a new sensor is used.

Various sensors are available for different clinical settings. The disposable bandage type for wrapping around a finger or toe is used most often for neonates and larger children (Figure 9-3). Application of the sensor is crucial to the quality of readings from the pulse oximeter. The sensor should be placed over a vascular area with the diodes and the photodiode directly opposite each other and in good contact with the skin. The sensors should be placed firmly to avoid falling off or motion artifact, but care should be taken to avoid overtightening and compromising local circulation.[4] The sensor sites should be changed routinely and the monitoring sites assessed for tissue injury. Finger and ear clips are also available for larger patients. Care must be taken with the clip type of sensors because the clinician has limited control of the spring tension and the pressure created on the extremity.

The gold standard for blood oxygen measurement is the arterial blood gas. However, this requires an arterial sample be obtained using a needle and syringe or indwelling

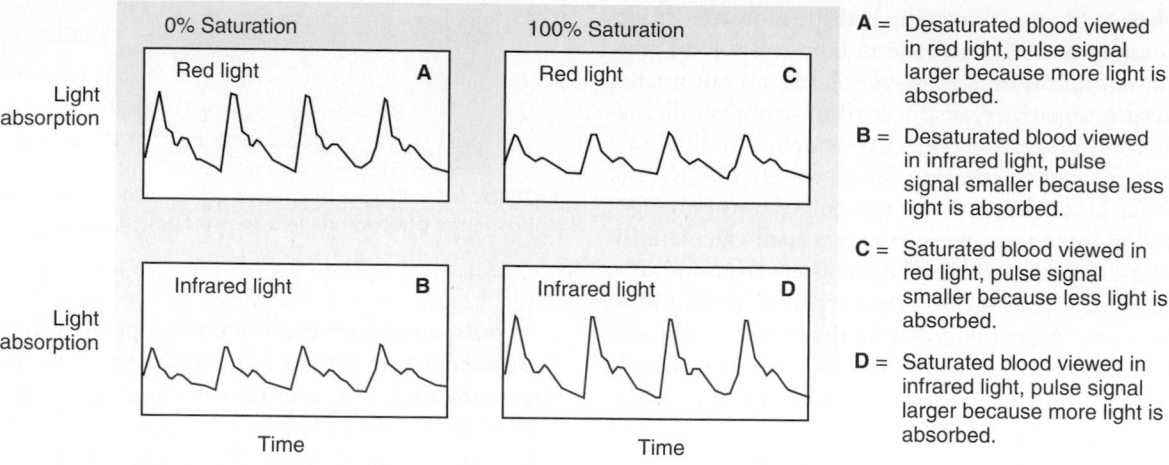

FIGURE 9-2   Differences in light absorption between deoxygenated hemoglobin (0% saturation) and oxygenated hemoglobin (100% saturation) during pulsatile signals.

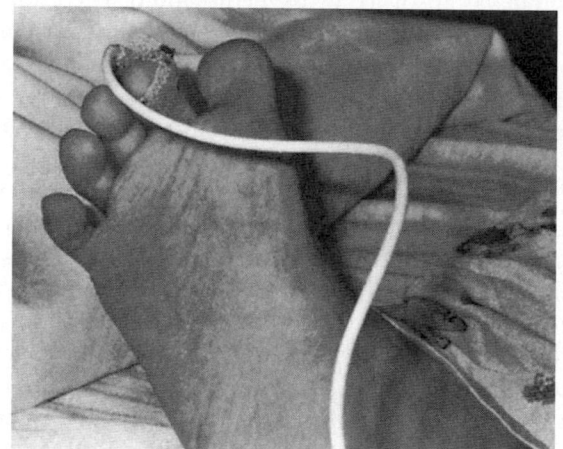

FIGURE 9-3   Pulse oximeter probe attached to a child's toe.

catheter. Needles sticks can be traumatic for some children, and the pain associated with it can increase agitation, thus increasing respiratory and heart rates, which may unintentionally affect gas exchange, rendering the arterial blood gas biased and limited in usefulness. Conversely, pulse oximetry is noninvasive, comfortable, and therefore routinely used to assess oxygenation in the neonatal and pediatric population.[4]

In the premature infant, site selection is crucial. In cardiac circulation, you will recall that the ductus arteriosus provides a communication between the aorta and the pulmonary artery during fetal circulation. The failure of the duct to close after birth results in a left to right shunt, referred to as a patent ductus arteriosus (PDA). Three arterial vessels take off from the aorta. The first diverts blood to the right arm and head, before the PDA (preductal). The remaining vessels occur postductal and therefore contain some proportion of deoxygenated blood resulting from shunting of deoxygenated pulmonary blood into the arterial circulation. **Preductal oxygen saturation** reflects an

infant's blood occurring before the ductus arteriosus and before it has a chance to be mixed with deoxygenated blood. A **postductal oxygen saturation** is a measurement taken after the ductus arteriosus and has been mixed with deoxygenated blood from the pulmonary circulation. Therefore, sensor placement on right arm or head will reflect preductal values and the left arm and the lower parts of the body will reflect postductal oxygen saturation values. In some premature infants, pre- and postductal oxygen saturations are simultaneous monitored. The difference between pre- and postductal oxygen saturation can reflect the degree of shunting, response to related therapies and need for intervention. This phenomenon can be observed using a transcutaneous monitor as well, which is discussed later in this chapter.

Limitations

Pulse oximetry was originally developed by anesthesiologists for use in the operating room. Unlike the operating room, however, patients can be awake, alert, and active. This introduces motion artifact that adversely, albeit temporarily, affect the accuracy of pulse oximetry.[5] Artifact typically manifests in two ways. First, the device may continue to read SpO_2 but underestimate the true concentration of oxyhemoglobin, potentially setting off a lower alarm limit. Second, if the artifact obscures the pulse, the "loss of pulse" alarm could be triggered, indicating the device is not able to pick up any information. Furthermore, electrical noise and changes in ambient light (e.g., fluorescent) can produce artifacts that affect pulse oximeters; however, with improved technology, this is less of a problem than in the past. Accuracy of arterial oxygen saturation measurement is reduced at levels below 80%. However, the clinical relevance of this is limited because saturations less than 80% indicate a medical emergency for most children. When using a finger probe, some nail polishes can negatively affect SpO_2 accuracy, causing displayed values to be falsely low. Acrylic nails do not appear to interfere with pulse oximetry readings.[3] It is important to note that impaired peripheral perfusion (perfusion to where the sensor is placed) can affect the SpO_2. Conditions such as low cardiac output, vasoconstriction, vasoactive therapy, and hypothermia can adversely affect the accuracy of pulse oximetry, and therefore care should be taken in these circumstances when interpreting results.[4]

Some studies have questioned the correlation of pulse oximeters and arterial blood gases in the neonate.[6] Neonatal patients with hyperbilirubinemia or anemia and those receiving hyperalimentation, total parenteral nutrition (TPN), or inotropic infusions may not yield ideal correlation with arterial blood gases. The sensitivity of pulse oximetry to detect the presence and degree of hyperoxia may be limited in the neonatal patient. If the oximeter is reading an SpO_2 of 100%, the arterial oxygen tension (PaO_2) could be between 90 and 250 mm Hg. However, many neonatal intensive care units target an SpO_2 below a certain threshold to reduce the risk of retinopathy of prematurity in premature babies. Proper site selection, understanding the principles of operation, and routinely assessing the patient to correlate the SpO_2 with other physiological data should help to minimize these limitations and ensure that the pulse oximeter remains a valuable clinical tool.[3-7]

Another important limitation concerns other gases that can be combined with hemoglobin, such as carbon monoxide (yielding **carboxyhemoglobin**). Most pulse oximeters cannot differentiate between oxyhemoglobin and carboxyhemoglobin. Therefore, in subjects with suspected carbon monoxide inhalation, a pulse oximeter will yield a percentage of hemoglobin with bound gases, not specifically those bound with oxygen. Caution should be exercised when interpreting pulse oximetry data in patients with suspected inhalation injury.

Recent technological advancements in pulse oximtery, such as signal extraction technology (SET), and noninvasive hemoglobin and oxygen content measurements, may prove to benefit patients with enhanced monitoring. SET pulse oximetry combines the traditional method based on red and infrared pulse oximeter signals with advanced techniques allowing signal "noise" produced by venous blood movement during motion to be filtered out, producing more accurate measurements of the arterial oxygenation of patients who are moving or with poor tissue perfusion. Noninvasive hemoglobin and oxygen content can be measured using dedicated pulse oximtery devices and specialized sensors. Some studies have shown that this provides an accurate measurement of hemoglobin in most subjects.[9] However, more research is needed to assess the accuracy and agreement of measurements in critically ill infants and children, particularly because these patients may have reduced peripheral perfusion that could adversely affect hemoglobin measurements during pulse oximetry.

CAPNOGRAPHY

Capnography is the measurement and representation of exhaled carbon dioxide. Capnography uses a noninvasive airway adapter or specialized nasal cannula as well as a dedicated monitoring device to measure the exhaled partial pressure of CO_2 (PCO_2) and also the total volume of exhaled CO_2 per unit of time. This technique is especially useful during mechanical ventilation because it can provide clinicians with important information about ventilation (such as changes in hemodynamics, confirmation of endotracheal tube placement, and response to changes in therapy, as well as others).[10] **End-tidal CO_2** refers to the partial pressure of CO_2 and the end of an exhalation ($PetCO_2$) and is commonly displayed in the unit mm Hg. **Volumetric capnography** refers to the simultaneous measurement of gas flow and CO_2 concentrations such that volumetric CO_2 values can be numerically and graphically displayed. Volumetric carbon dioxide elimination (VCO_2) is typically measured in milliliters per minute (ml/min).

Principles of Operation

The most common methods used to continuously measure carbon dioxide concentration in an exhaled gas employ **infrared spectroscopy** and mass spectrometry. Infrared spectrometry is based on the fact that infrared light is strongly absorbed by carbon dioxide. Mass spectrometry uses an electronic beam that ionizes gases. The resulting particles are then deflected emitting a specific wavelength by which the concentration of the gas can be determined. Infrared spectrometry allows for real-time, continuous measurement and display of PCO_2 with a delay time of about 0.25 second. Mass spectrometry is also accurate but has a delay time of 0.1 to 80 seconds. In addition, it is expensive, is not as portable, and is therefore rarely used at the bedside.[11]

Gases from an exhaled breath can reach the sample chamber in one of two ways. **Mainstream capnography** is used primarily during mechanical ventialtion, with placement at the proximal end of an endotracheal tube (Figure 9-4). This method employs infrared spectrometers. **Sidestream capnography** analyzers continuously aspirate a sample of gas through a small tube to the analyzer and can be used during mechanical ventilation and spontaneous breathing. Bedside sidestream monitors also primarily use infrared spectroscopy, although some do employ mass spectrometry. However, the narrow tubing can become occluded with mucus or water, causing inaccuracies. In addition, infants with small tidal volumes can contaminate the sample line with fresh gases. It is important to choose the correct adapter given a patient's size and gas flows. An infant CO_2 adapter has a small internal diameter and therefore small dead space (which reduces the amount of added mechanical dead space) but increases the airway resistance. If an infant CO_2 adapter is used on a larger child, airway resistance is elevated, which

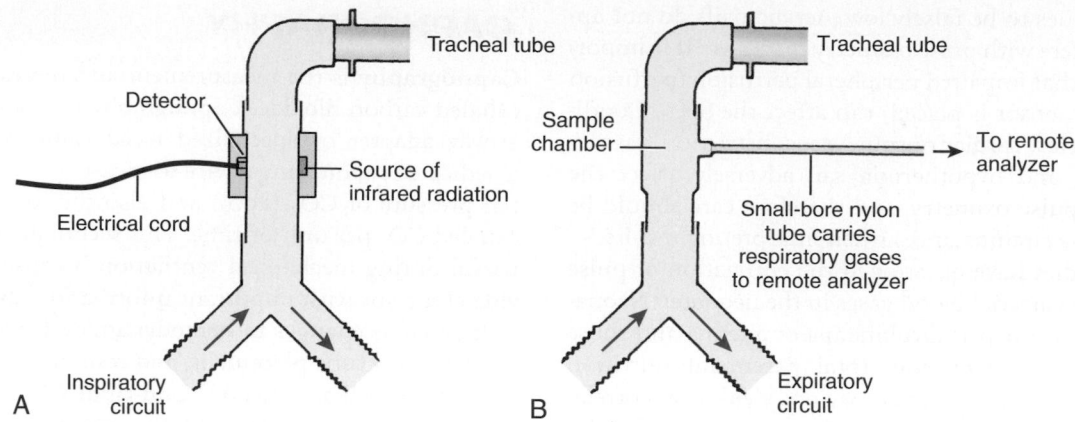

FIGURE 9-4   Location of mainstream airway adapter (**A**) and sidestream adapter (**B**) in patient's airway.

could cause significant discomfort for the patient and limit ventilation. On the other hand, if an adult sensor is placed on a small infant, the proportion of added mechanical dead space to the breathing circuit could cause rebreathing of CO_2, impeding appropriate ventilation. It is therefore important to follow manufacturer's recommendations for sensor selection.

$PetCO_2$ can be used as a surrogate for the arterial partial pressure of CO_2 ($PaCO_2$) within physiological limits. Normally, $PetCO_2$ is 2 to 5 mm Hg below $PaCO_2$. The reason for this is the proportion of dead-space ventilation. At the alveolar level, $PaCO_2$ will equal the partial pressure of CO_2 in the alveolar gas ($PACO_2$) as diffusion occurs across the alveolar capillary membrane. Recall that each breath contains a portion that is not involved in gas exchange, referred to as the **dead-space volume** (such as that in the endotracheal tube and conducting airways). **Alveolar volume** is that which is involved in gas exchange as it comes into direct contact with capillaries for O_2 and CO_2 exchange. In healthy infants and children, dead space accounts for around 30% to 40% of ventilation. This means that for a tidal volume of 100 ml, we would expect 30 ml to not be involved in gas exchange and therefore not contain CO_2. Let us assume that $PaCO_2$ and consequently $PACO_2$ contain 40 mm Hg. In this example, 70 ml contains 40 mm Hg of CO_2 and 30 ml contains 0 mm Hg. As these gases are mixed and exhaled, the alveolar gas is "diluted" by dead space and the $PetCO_2$ concentration may be around 35 mm Hg. It is essential that the clinician has a firm understanding of this physiological phenomenon because changes in dead space will affect the gradient between $PetCO_2$ and $PaCO_2$; increased dead space will increase the gradient and reduced dead space will reduce the gradient. $PetCO_2$ monitoring has also been used to help ensure the adequacy of chest compressions during cardiopulmonary resuscitation and to confirm proper placement of endotracheal tubes after intubation.

If $PetCO_2$ is thought of as the concentration of CO_2 in an exhaled breath, VCO_2 is thought of as the flow of CO_2

out of the patient (**CO_2 elimination**). Some CO_2 monitors, and often those that are integrated into the mechanical ventilator, provide simultaneous PCO_2 and flow data. A plot of PCO_2 and volume can therefore be plotted. The PCO_2–volume plot enables the estimation of airway dead-space volume, alveolar volume, CO_2 elimination, and alveolar minute ventilation (Figure 9-5). CO_2 elimination is normally 2 to 3 ml/kg/min in adults. However, typical values seen in children are greater when normalized to body weight. Newborn infants can range approximately 5 to 7 ml/kg/min and older children anywhere from 3 to 5 ml/kg/min.[12] Monitoring CO_2 elimination may help guide decision making and response to ventilator titration in mechanically ventilated children.[10]

Limitations

Although both methods for PCO_2 monitoring require the placement of an airway adapter proximal to the patient's breathing circuit, mainstream capnography adapters tend to be a bit more bulky because the sensors used to measure PCO_2 are located at the airway. In small infants, the added weight of the mainstream sensor can be a concern. In some cases it may not be used because of this, but in most cases can be used safely with careful attention to sensor placement and endotracheal tube securement. As discussed earlier, inappropriate sensor selection can have a detrimental effect on ventilation with each method. Water condensation and secretions can also build up to the point that they occlude either the sensor window in mainstream analyzers or the samples line in sidestream analyzers. Frequent assessment of the sensor, sensor replacement, and appropriate secretion and humidification management will ensure that PCO_2 is measured continuously without protracted interruptions.

Interpretation of Capnogram

Trending $ETCO_2$ will give the bedside clinician a good sense of the adequacy of ventilation for the patient. An increase in $ETCO_2$ from previous levels might indicate hypoventilation.

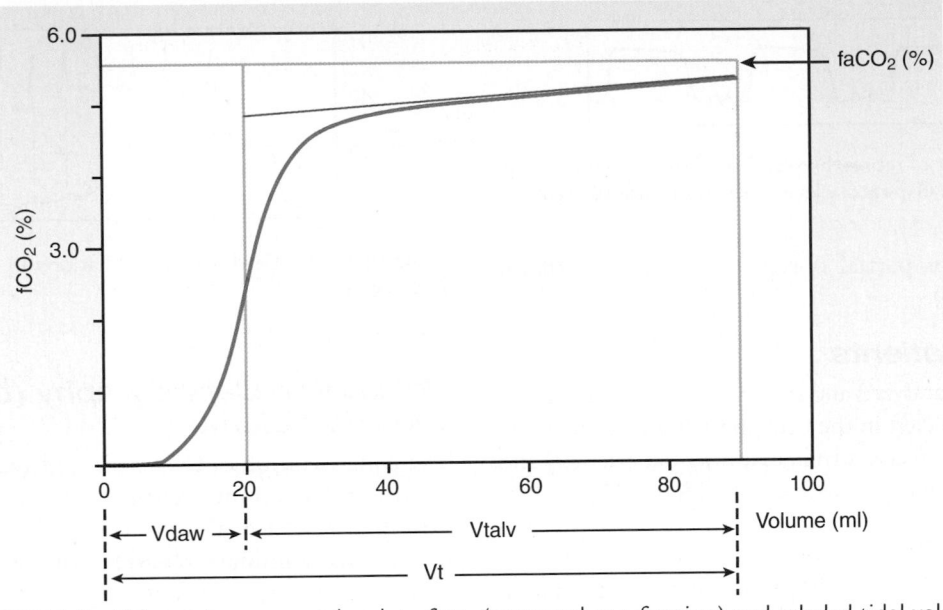

FIGURE 9-5 Volumetric capnography plot of CO_2 (expressed as a fraction) and exhaled tidal volume showing airway dead space, alveolar volume, and dead-space volume.

The possibility of decreased tidal volume or respiratory rate should be investigated. A decrease in $ETCO_2$ from previous levels might indicate hyperventilation. Interpretation of the capnogram (waveform display of the exhaled carbon dioxide) can also help the clinician detect other ventilatory abnormalities.

The normal capnogram can be divided into four phases (Figure 9-6):

Phase A-B: The inspiratory phase, during which the sensor detects no carbon dioxide

Phase B-C: The initial expiratory phase, during which carbon dioxide rapidly increases as the alveoli begin to empty

Phase C-D: The completion of expiration as the alveoli empties (alveolar plateau) and shows a slight increase in carbon dioxide

Phase D-E: The beginning of inspiration as the waveform returns to zero

Detection of Ventilation Problems

The clinician can use the capnogram to detect important ventilation problems in neonatal and pediatric patients.

Endotracheal Tube in Esophagus

A normal capnogram provides evidence that the endotracheal tube is in the proper position and that alveolar ventilation is occurring. When the endotracheal tube is placed incorrectly in the esophagus, no carbon dioxide will be detected or only small transient capnograms will be present.

Rebreathing

Rebreathing is characterized by an elevation in the A-B phase of the capnogram, with a corresponding increase in $ETCO_2$. It indicates the rebreathing of previously exhaled carbon dioxide. Rebreathing can be caused by allowing an insufficient expiratory time or by inadequate inspiratory flow (Figure 9-7).

Obstructed Airway

Obstruction of the expiratory flow of gas will be noted as a change in the slope of the B-C phase of the capnogram. The B-C phase may diminish without a plateau. Obstruction can be caused by a foreign body in the upper airway, increased secretions in the airways, the patient having

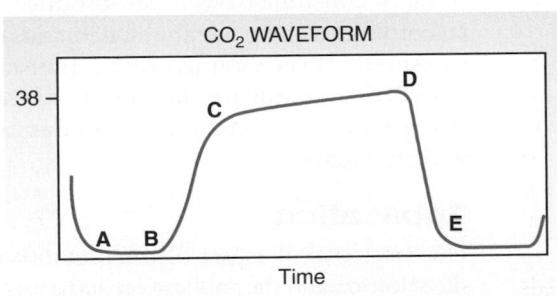

A–B: Exhalation of CO_2 free gas from dead space.

B–C: Combination of dead space and alveolar gas.

C–D: Exhalation of mostly alveolar gas (alveolar plateau).

D: "End-tidal" point—CO_2 exhalation at maximum point.

D–E: Inhalation of CO_2 free gas.

FIGURE 9-6 Normal capnogram.

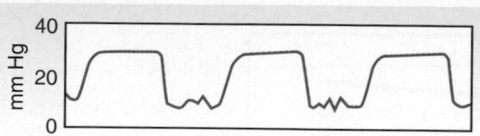

FIGURE 9-7 Effect of rebreathing carbon dioxide on the capnogram. Note that the inspiratory level does not return to zero.

bronchospasms, or partial obstruction of the ventilator circuit (Figure 9-8).

Paralyzed Patients

Patients who are paralyzed and receiving mechanical ventilation may develop a cleft in the C-D phase of the capnogram. The cleft may indicate a return in diaphragmatic activity and the need for additional paralytic agents (Figure 9-9).

Pneumothorax

A stair-stepping of the D-E phase of the capnogram, caused by unequal and incomplete emptying of the lungs, and a failure to return to baseline may suggest a pneumothorax (Figure 9-10).

Cardiogenic Oscillations

Cardiogenic oscillations may be seen in patients with long expiratory times and slow respiratory rates. The oscillations will be seen in the D-E phase of the capnogram and occur as the heart contracts and moves the lungs, causing gas flow (Figure 9-11).

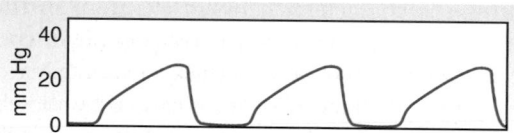

FIGURE 9-8 Capnogram with sloping alveolar plateau representative of airway obstruction.

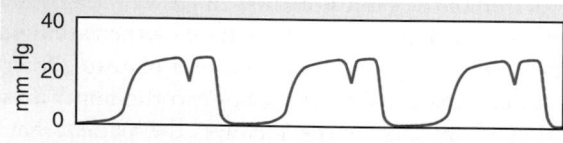

FIGURE 9-9 Curare cleft in the alveolar plateau.

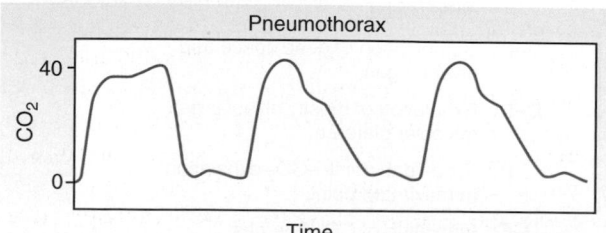

FIGURE 9-10 Stair effect on the descending limb of the capnogram indicating a potential pneumothorax.

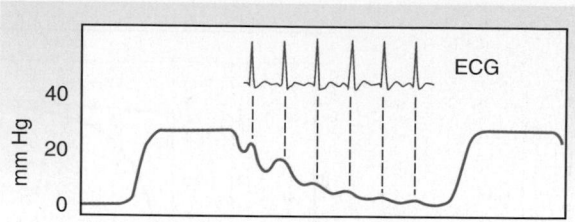

FIGURE 9-11 Cardiogenic oscillations in synchrony with the ECG signal.

Volumetric Capnography (the Carbon Dioxide–Volume Plot)

The concentration of CO_2 is plotted against exhaled tidal volume to determine relevant ventilation data such as airway dead space, alveolar tidal volume, and extrapolation of CO_2 elimination and alveolar minute ventilation.

TRANSCUTANEOUS MONITORING

In the hands of an experienced and trained clinician, a well-maintained and properly calibrated **transcutaneous monitor** will provide accurate information regarding the pediatric patient's oxygenation status.[13] Transcutaneous measurement of the partial pressure of oxygen (**P_{TcO_2}**) and carbon dioxide tension (**P_{TcCO_2}**) provides continuous information about the body's ability to deliver oxygen to the tissues and to remove carbon dioxide. Because the sensor is placed on surface tissue, it is important to note that measurements may not reflect arterial blood gas tensions but rather that of the underlying tissue. When hemodynamic conditions are stable, transcutaneous measurements correlate well with arterial values, but this correlation does not necessarily mean that the measured values will be identical.

Principles of Operation

Transcutaneous measurements of P_{O_2} and P_{CO_2} require a heating element, built in to the sensor, that elevates the temperature in the underlying tissue. Increasing the skin's temperature increases capillary blood flow to the tissues, making it more permeable to gas diffusion. The tissue under which the sensor is placed will continue to consume oxygen and produces carbon dioxide (according to their metabolic demands). Consequently, measured values obtained with a transcutaneous monitor will differ from arterial values.[14,15] Generally, the P_{O_2} is slightly lower than in the arteries, and the P_{CO_2} is slightly higher.

Application

The most critical aspect of transcutaneous monitoring is site selection and the application of the sensor (Figure 9-12). The site should be a highly vascular area such as the earlobe,

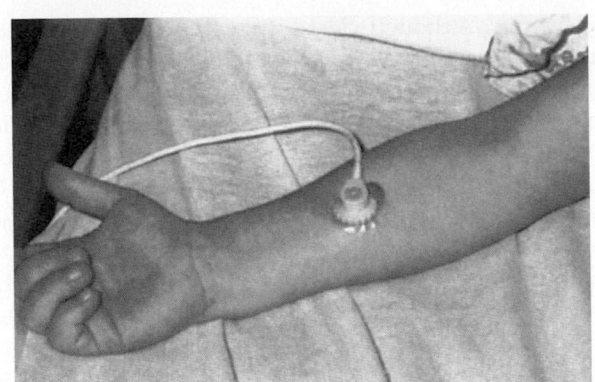

FIGURE 9-12 Transcutaneous oxygen monitor electrode placed on a child's arm.

upper chest, abdomen, or thighs or the lower back if the patient is supine; bony areas and those with limited perfusion, such as over the spine, should be avoided.

Selecting a sensor temperature is important to proper operation.[16] The temperature range is usually 41° to 44° C. Heating of the sensor requires that the site be changed on a routine basis to prevent thermal injuries. The frequency of site changes ranges from 4 to 12 hours (depending on the device and sensor temperature) but can be reduced if necessary.

Meticulously following the manufacturer's membrane changing procedure and calibration instructions will result in the most accurate readings. Once the machine has been prepared and the site selected, the skin must be cleaned to wipe away dead skin, oils, and medications. The accuracy of the sensor is improved by using 1 or 2 drops of contact gel or even normal saline or sterile water. This liquid-to-liquid medium makes the diffusion of gases more efficient. The sensor is then attached to the skin with a fixation ring (or earlobe clip). This ring must form a good seal between the sensor and skin, eliminating air bubbles.

Limitations

Transcutaneous monitoring provides a noninvasive, simple means of continuously monitoring ventilation. However, it can be labor intensive, involving sensor preparation, frequent site and membrane changes, and calibration.[15] Additionally, because transcutaneous monitors require the tissue to be heated, a period of time (usually just a few minutes) exists immediately after application during which no values can be measured. Once the tissue has been appropriately heated, values can be displayed. For long-term monitoring this is generally not a concern; however, in emergency situations requiring immediate action, a transcutaneous monitor may not be ideal. A transcutaneous monitor is limited in its usefulness during cardiopulmonary resuscitation and airway obstruction or apnea detection.

Changes in perfusion can adversely affect the accuracy of transcutaneous measurements. The skin reacts to cold, shock, and certain drugs by contracting the superficial blood vessels, opening larger, deeper arterioles to achieve a shunting effect. Capillary blood flow is reduced upon exposure to cold temperatures in order to reduce the loss of body heat. Shock and certain medications can also divert blood from capillaries to the central circulation. In all cases of reduced capillary perfusion, the capillary blood, which is measured using a transcutaneous monitor, may reflect measurements associated with venous blood, with a considerably lower P_{O_2} and higher P_{CO_2} (compared with values obtained with good capillary perfusion).[15] If a patient has poor skin integrity, transcutaneous monitoring may also be contraindicated.

Some sensors combine oxygen saturation (S_{O_2}) and transcutaneous carbon dioxide measurements in a single ear sensor. The sensor is heated to 42° C to maximize capillary blood flow. The location of the sensor on the ear may decrease motion artifact because less head movement occurs in neonates. This type of sensor reduces the number of wires attached to the patient's chest, enabling a clearer view for chest X-ray examinations. When end-tidal carbon dioxide measurements are not possible, or are found to be limited in some way (e.g., in newborns with large air leaks or those requiring high-frequency ventilation), a transcutaneous sensor may be optimal.

CALORIMETRY

Appropriate nutrition in children is associated with reduced risk of hospital mortality.[17] However, ensuring that nutritional requirements are correctly met for critically ill neonatal and pediatric patients can be difficult. By correctly assessing nutritional needs and tracking adequate intake, outcomes may be improved. **Calorimetry** is the measurement of gas exchange and the determination of **energy expenditure** (where energy expenditure is the amount of energy burned by a patient per unit of time, typically expressed in kilocalories per day [kcal/day]). *Gas exchange* refers to the volume of oxygen that is consumed by the patient (**oxygen consumption [V_{O_2}]**) and the volume of carbon dioxide that is produced by the patient (**carbon dioxide production [V_{CO_2}]**). **Resting energy expenditure** (REE) is generally defined as the amount of energy required in a 24-hour period during which the body is performing minimal activity (typically expressed as kcal/day). The determination of a patient's REE, appropriate energy prescription, and intake can reduce the risk of overfeeding and underfeeding. A neonate's energy expenditure, when expressed per unit of body weight, is higher at birth compared with other times in life.[21] Equations are available that relate a child's gender, age, height, and weight into an estimation of energy expenditure. An example that is commonly used in neonates and pediatric patients is the Schofield equation (Table 9-1).[18] However, formulas are known to be inaccurate in many children, particularly those requiring mechanical ventilation.[19] Therefore, determination of REE through measurement of V_{O_2} and V_{CO_2} is often required.[20]

TABLE 9-1

The Schofield Equation

Age	Males	Females
<3 y	0.167W + 15.174H – 617.6	16.252W + 10.232H – 413.5
3-10 y	19.59W + 1.303H + 414.9	16.969W + 1.618H + 371.2
10-18 y	16.25W + 1.372H + 515.5	8.365W + 4.65H + 200.0
18-30 y	15.057W – 0.1H + 705.8	13.623W + 2.83H + 98.2

H, Ht. in cm; W, wt. in kg.
From Schofield WN. Predicting basal metabolic, new and review of previous work. *Hum Nutr Clin Nutr* 39(C Suppl 1):5-41, 1985.

Two methods exist for measuring calorimetry: direct and indirect. **Direct calorimetry** extrapolates energy expenditure by measuring heat produced and lost from the body, whereas **indirect calorimetry** combines measurements of V_{O_2} and V_{CO_2} into an equation to calculate energy expenditure. Most energy expenditure reports contain results for V_{O_2}, V_{CO_2}, REE, and respiratory quotient (which is V_{CO_2}/V_{O_2} and can be used to determine substrate utilization). For critically ill, mechanically ventilated patients, V_{O_2} will be approximately 4.5 to 6.3 ml/min/kg for newborns and infants, 2.7-4.5 ml/min/kg for older children and 1.6-2.4 ml/kg/min for large teenagers and adults.

Principles of Operation

Direct calorimeters are bulky, expensive, and not suitable for critically ill infants and children. Indirect calorimeters, on the other hand, can be transported to the patient's bedside. Open- and closed-circuit designs are available on indirect calorimeters. Although closed-circuit indirect calorimeters may sometimes be, open-circuit devices are much more common. The open-circuit indirect calorimeter measures the volume of consumed oxygen and eliminated carbon dioxide (V_{O_2} and V_{CO_2}, respectively). To accomplish this, inspiratory and expiratory gas concentrations are measured with an O_2 sensor (typically a galvanic cell) and CO_2 sensor (typically a nondispersive infrared sensor similar to that used in ET_{CO_2} monitors, albeit with greatly improved accuracy) and a highly accurate flow sensor. All sensors must be precisely calibrated before usage. The system can be set up to take measurements during mechanical ventilation and during spontaneous breathing. During mechanical ventilation some systems use a sensor placed at the airway (similar to an end-tidal CO_2 sensor), whereas others require multiple connections: inspiratory gas concentration sample, expiratory gas concentration sample, and flow sensor placed at the ventilator exhaust (Figure 9-13). Alternatively, a spontaneously breathing child requires a canopy placed over the child's head (or on top of the infant if the patient is small enough) connected to the indirect calorimeter, which draws exhaled gases into a sample line for volume and gas concentration analysis (Figure 9-14). The difference between inspired and expired gas fractions are multiplied by the volume measurement to yield V_{O_2} and V_{CO_2}. The modified Weir equation uses the V_{O_2} and V_{CO_2} data to yield energy expenditure:

$$Energy\ expenditure = [3.941(V_{O_2}) + 1.106(V_{CO_2})] \times 1440$$

where V_{O_2} and V_{CO_2} are measured in L/min.[21] Fluctuations in energy expenditure can occur over time and can be greatly affected by temperature, pain or agitation, activity

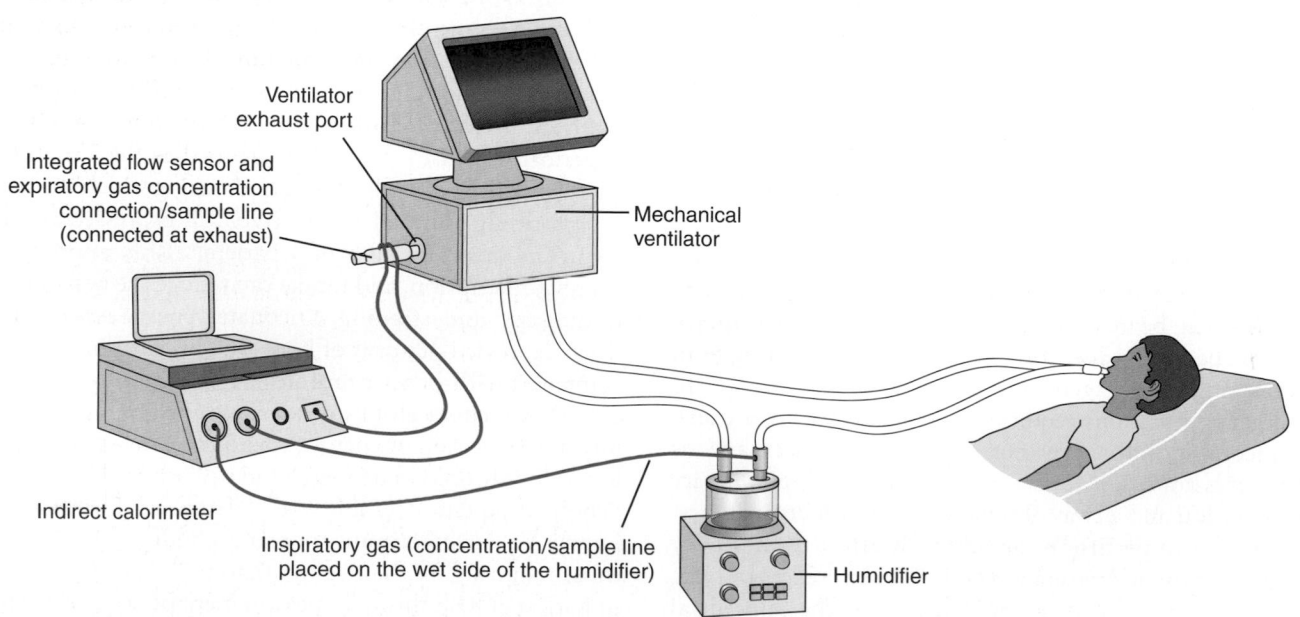

FIGURE 9-13 Typical setup of an indirect calorimeter used during mechanical ventilation.

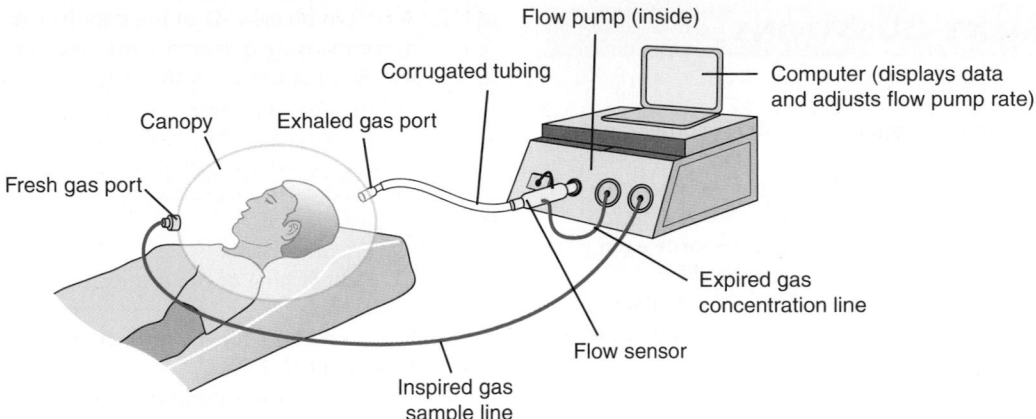

FIGURE 9-14   Typical setup of an indirect calorimeter for measurement of energy expenditure of the spontaneously breathing child or infant.

level, changes in disease state, and ventilator parameters. It is important to gather data with minimal fluctuations in gas exchange. Therefore, for indirect calorimetry results to be valid and used to adjust nutrient intake, measurements must reflect a steady-state period. Often, a metabolic test lasts 30 minutes. The on-board algorithm (of the indirect calorimeter) looks for periods when minimal fluctuations in Vo_2, Vco_2, RQ, and other parameters are observed. The steady-state results are shown on the display.

Limitations

Direct calorimetry is cost prohibitive, equilibration and measurement are time consuming, and few exist in the United States. Indirect calorimetry is not without its limitations: Devices can be costly, dedicated and well-trained personnel are required, and measurement errors can be introduced during certain conditions. Conditions that preclude the use of indirect calorimetry include uncuffed endotracheal tubes, cuff or ventilator circuit leaks greater than 10% to 15%, Fio_2 greater than 50%, need for high-frequency ventilation or extracorporeal membrane oxygenation, and active chest tube leakage. As previously mentioned, certain patient conditions, such as unstable hemodynamics and agitation, may also limit the utility of indirect calorimetry because these conditions may not reflect the patient's typical energy expenditure.[22] However, with proper understanding of the appropriate calibration, application, and interpretation of indirect calorimetry data, it can be a valuable tool to aid clinicians in determining proper nutritional support of the critically ill neonatal or pediatric patient.[23]

- Pulse oximetry uses a sensor that includes light-emitting diodes and photodiode sensor that measure the relative concentration of oxyhemoglobin to total hemoglobin in pulsatile arterial blood and displays the result as a percentage.
- Pulse oximeter sensors should be placed in a vascular area such as the finger or earlobe, with the diodes and the photodiode directly opposite each other and in good contact with the skin.
- *End-tidal CO₂ monitoring* refers to the measurement of CO_2 plotted against time and displays the partial pressure of CO_2 at end exhalation. *Volumetric capnography* refers to a plot of CO_2 and volume and typically provides a measure of carbon dioxide elimination, alveolar minute ventilation, and airway dead space.
- The gradient between end-tidal and arterial CO_2 measurements reflects dead-space ventilation and is normally between 0 and 5 mm Hg.
- Abnormalities that can be detected with capnograms include (but are not limited to) rebreathing exhaled gases, airway obstruction, and possible pneumothorax.
- Transcutaneous sensor placement is important to enhance accuracy and reduce risk of burns. Sensors should be placed in highly vascular area such as the earlobe, upper chest, abdomen, or thighs or the lower back if the patient is supine; bony areas and those with limited perfusion, such as over the spine, should be avoided.
- Potential problems that can adversely affect the accuracy of transcutaneous monitoring include improper site selection, not following manufacturer's guidelines, and changes in peripheral perfusion.
- Indirect calorimetry seeks to measure the amount of energy that is used by a patient and help guide clinicians in determining optimal nutrition intake.
- Indirect calorimetry may not be reliable in those children who require oxygen concentrations greater than 60%, during mechanical ventilation, who have an endotracheal tube leak greater than 10%, those requiring noninvasive or high-frequency ventilation, and those in whom steady state is not achieved.

KEY POINTS

- Fundamental monitoring methods to measure and assess heart rate, respiratory rate, and blood pressure include electrocardiography, impedance monitoring, and periodic cuff assessment, respectively.

ASSESSMENT QUESTIONS

See Evolve Resources for answers.

1. Which of the following demonstrates incorrect application of the pulse oximeter sensor?
   A. Tight placement over a bony area
   B. Placement over a vascular area
   C. Diodes and photodiode directly opposite each other and in good contact with the skin
   D. Firm placement to help avoid motion artifact

2. The following choices are all disadvantages of a pulse oximeter except:
   A. Ease of use
   B. Artifact
   C. Poor tissue perfusion
   D. Hypothermia

3. Which of the following measurements are obtained via transcutaneous monitoring in the neonatal and pediatric population?
   A. Hemoglobin
   B. pH, bicarbonate ion
   C. P_{O_2}, P_{CO_2}
   D. Oxygen saturation

4. Which of the following is *not* a disadvantages of transcutaneous monitoring?
   A. Use is labor intensive because of required frequent site and membrane changes and calibration requirements.
   B. Good correlation requires good peripheral blood perfusion.
   C. Use requires the patient to be paralyzed and sedated.

5. Trending $ETCO_2$ via capnometry enables the clinician to have a good sense of the adequacy of _____ for the patient.
   A. Oxygenation
   B. Ventilation
   C. Perfusion
   D. Saturation

6. The normal capnogram can be divided into four phases. Phase B-C, as illustrated below, is indicative of which phase?

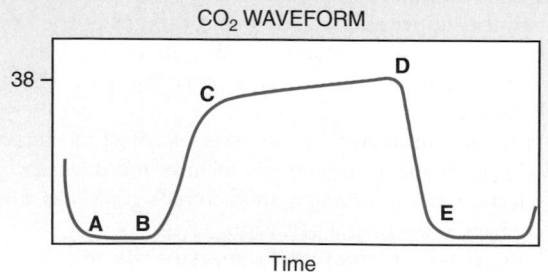

CO$_2$ WAVEFORM

   A. The completion of expiration as the alveoli empty (alveolar plateau)
   B. The initial expiratory phase, during which carbon dioxide rapidly increases as the alveoli begin to empty
   C. The inspiratory phase, during which the sensor detects no carbon dioxide
   D. The beginning of inspiration as the waveform returns to zero

7. A cleft in phase C-D of the capnogram in the figure accompanying question 7 may indicate:
   A. An obstruction in the airway, possibly caused by a foreign body in the upper airway, increased secretions in the airways, bronchospasms, or partial obstruction of the ventilator circuit
   B. Medication used to paralyze the infant is wearing off
   C. Pneumothorax
   D. Rebreathing of the previously exhaled carbon dioxide

8. What accounts for the difference between Pa_{CO_2} and end-tidal CO_2?
   A. Inadequate respiratory rate
   B. Dead-space ventilation
   C. Spontaneous ventilation
   D. Postductal oxygen concentration

9. What is the normal gradient between Pa_{CO_2} and end-tidal CO_2 (Pa_{CO_2} minus end-tidal CO_2)?
   A. -2 to -5 mm Hg
   B. 8 to 10 mm Hg
   C. 10 to 15 mm Hg
   D. 0 to 5 mm Hg

10. Indirect calorimetry requires which of the following to calculate energy expenditure?
    A. Oxygen saturation and end-tidal carbon dioxide
    B. Oxygen consumption and respiratory rate
    C. Oxygen consumption and carbon dioxide elimination
    D. Transcutaneous oxygen and carbon dioxide concentration

References

1. Folke M, Cernerud L, Ekström M, et al: Critical review of non-invasive respiratory monitoring in medical care, *Med Biol Eng Comput* 41:377, 2003.
2. Tipple M: Interpretation of electrocardiograms in infants and children, *Images Paediatr Cardiol* 1:3, 1999.
3. Jubran A: Pulse oximetry, *Crit Care* 3: R11, 1999.
4. Pulse Oximetry FORUM: The FORUM offers recommendations on best practices in pediatric pulse oximetry, *American Association for Respiratory Care Times* Apr:36-44, 2000.
5. Barker SJ, Shah NK: The effects of motion on the performance of pulse oximeters in volunteers, *Anesthesiology* 86:101, 1997.
6. Gibson LY: Pulse oximeter in the neonatal ICU: a correlational analysis, *Pediatr Nurs* 22:511, 1996.
7. Tallon RW: Oximetry: state of the art, *Nurs Manage* 27:43, 1996.
8. Trivedi NS, Ghouri AF, Lae E, Shah NK, et al: Pulse oximeter performance during desaturation and resaturation: a comparison of seven models, *J Clin Anesth* 9:184, 1997.
9. Dewhirst BE, Naguib A, Winch P, et al: Accuracy of noninvasive and continuous hemoglobin measurement by pulse co-oximetry during preoperative phlebotomy, *J Intensive Care Med* 2013. [Epub ahead of print].
10. Walsh BK, Crotwell DN, Restrepo RD, et al: Capnography/capnometry during mechanical ventilation: 2011, *Respir Care* 56:503, 2011.
11. Stock MC: Nonivasive carbon dioxide monitoring, *Crit Care Clin* 4:511, 1988.

12. Lindahl SG, Offord KP, Johannesson GP, et al: Carbon dioxide elimination in anaesthetized children, *Can J Anaesth* 36:113, 1989.

13. Dullenkopf A, Bernardo SD, Berger F, et al: Evaluation of a new combined $SpO_2/PtcCO_2$ sensor in anaesthetized paediatric patients, *Paediatr Anaesth* 13:777, 2003.

14. Bernet-Buettiker V, Ugarte MJ, Frey B, et al: Evaluation of a new combined transcutaneous measurement of PCO_2/pulse oximetry oxygen saturation ear sensor in newborn patients, *Pediatrics* 115:e64, 2005.

15. Tobias JD, Meyer DJ: Noninvasive monitoring of carbon dioxide during respiratory failure in toddlers and infants: end-tidal versus transcutaneous carbon dioxide, *Anesth Analg* 85:55, 1997.

16. Kocher S, Rohling R, Tschupp A: Performance of a digital PCO_2/SpO_2 ear sensor, *J Clin Monit Comput* 18: 75, 2004.

17. Mehta NM, Bechard LJ, Cahill N, et al: Nutritional practices and their relationship to clinical outcomes in critically ill children—an international multicenter cohort study, *Crit Care Med* 40:2204, 2012.

18. Schofield WN: Predicting basal metabolic rate, new standards and review of previous work, *Hum Nutr Clin Nutr* 39(Suppl 1):5, 1985.

19. Coss-Bu JA, Jefferson LS, Walding D, et al: Resting energy expenditure in children in a pediatric intensive care unit: comparison of Harris-Benedict and Talbot predictions with indirect calorimetry values, *Am J Clin Nutr* 67:74, 1998.

20. Mehta NM, Compher C, et al: A.S.P.E.N. Clinical guidelines: nutrition support of the critically ill child, *JPEN J Parenter Enteral Nutr* 33:260, 2009.

21. Weir JB: New methods for calculating metabolic rate with special reference to protein metabolism, *Nutrition* 6:213, 1990.

22. Flancbaum L, Choban PS, Sambucco S, et al: Comparison of indirect calorimetry, the Fick method, and prediction equations in estimating the energy requirements of critically ill patients, *Am J Clin Nutr* 69:461, 1999.

23. Mehta NM, Bechard LJ, Dolan M, et al: Energy imbalance and the risk of overfeeding in critically ill children, *Pediatr Crit Care Med* 12:398, 2011.

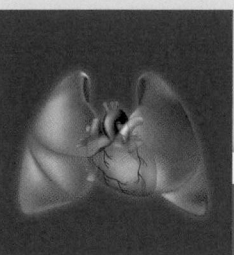

Chapter 10

Oxygen Administration

BRIAN WALSH

LEARNING OBJECTIVES

After reading this chapter the reader will be able to:

1. Discuss causes, clinical signs and symptoms, and evidence of hypoxemia
2. Identify adverse physiological effects and equipment-related complications associated with oxygen administration to neonates, infants, and children
3. Differentiate between variable-performance and fixed-performance oxygen delivery systems and provide examples of each
4. Discuss the indications and contraindications for use of oxygen delivery devices in the neonatal and pediatric populations
5. Describe the methods used to apply devices to deliver oxygen to neonates, infants, and children

KEY TERMS

Humidified high-flow nasal oxygen
Hypoxemia
Hypoxia

Nasal cannula
Oxygen hood
Oxygen therapy

Venturi mask
Simple oxygen mask

In 1774 Joseph Priestley was credited with discovering the colorless, odorless, tasteless gas that Antoine Lavoisier 1 year later named oxygen.[1] Nearly 150 years would pass before the Finnish pediatrician Arvo Ylppö recommended the intragastric administration of this gas to infants.[2] It was not until 1934 that Dr. Julius Hess, chief of pediatrics at the Michael Reese Hospital in Chicago, created the first inhaled oxygen delivery device for a premature infant. His "oxygen box," which consisted of a metal hood with a small window, was the first oxygen chamber used within an incubator.[3] Although the device was criticized both for making it difficult to view the infant and for its inability to maintain high oxygen concentrations, it led the way in the

development of oxygen administration devices for premature infants and children.[4] Further development and use of these delivery devices has resulted in significant health care benefits, including a reduction in mortality. Today the administration of oxygen by inhalation continues to play an essential role in the survival of infants and children.

The goal of oxygen administration is to achieve adequate tissue oxygenation. The system used to provide supplemental oxygen must be appropriate to the patient's size, gestational and postnatal age, and clinical condition. Selection of the oxygen delivery device and flow rate is targeted to meet the specific physiological needs and therapeutic goals of each patient.[5] Unfortunately, adverse reactions from the therapeutic use of oxygen are well documented in neonatal and pediatric patients. Therefore it is imperative that **oxygen therapy** be provided at accurate and safe levels with the lowest possible fractional concentration of inspired oxygen (FiO_2).

INDICATIONS

Documented or Suspected Hypoxemia

A need to correct **hypoxemia** (low oxygen content in the blood) is the most common indication for oxygen therapy.[6] Left untreated, hypoxemia progresses to **hypoxia** (low tissue oxygen) and possibly anoxia (absent tissue oxygen), which, if severe enough, leads to metabolic abnormalities and the development of acidosis.

Hypoxemia occurs as a result of decreased alveolar ventilation, decreased inspired oxygen, poor ventilation–perfusion relationships, intrapulmonary or cardiac shunting, diffusion defects, or short red blood cell transit times. In conditions such as anemia or carbon monoxide poisoning, the oxygen-carrying capacity of the blood is reduced despite the presence of normal arterial oxygen tension (PaO_2). Bradycardia, cardiac failure, hypotension, and hypothermia leave the circulatory system unable to provide adequate tissue oxygen. In rare cases, such as cyanide poisoning, the tissue is unable to accept and use oxygen, despite adequate oxygen delivery.[7] The documentation of hypoxemia through arterial blood gas sampling or pulse oximetry provides the most definitive evidence of actual or impending tissue hypoxia.

Administration of oxygen is also appropriate if hypoxia is strongly suspected on clinical grounds. However, substantiation of either the PaO_2 or the percentage of oxygen saturation (SpO_2) is required within an appropriate period after administration.[6,7] In emergency situations, such as severe respiratory distress, shock, or cardiopulmonary arrest, oxygen therapy is never withheld even if laboratory test results are unavailable.

Evidence of Hypoxemia
Measurement of Oxygen Tension and Saturation

In children a PaO_2 less than 80 mm Hg and an SpO_2 less than 95% usually indicate hypoxemia. However, generally agreed on practice is to only treat SpO_2 less than 90% or a PaO_2 less than 60 mm Hg. Because fetal hemoglobin has a much greater affinity for oxygen, the oxygen dissociation curve is shifted to the left, allowing a higher saturation for any given PaO_2. The normal immediate postnatal PaO_2 of 50 to 60 mm Hg corresponds closely with an SpO_2 of 85% to 90%. For this reason, it is generally agreed that a PaO_2 less than 50 mm Hg and an SpO_2 less than 88% in the newborn indicate hypoxemia and necessitate initiation of oxygen therapy. The PaO_2 and the SpO_2 are the principal clinical indicators used to begin, monitor, adjust, and terminate oxygen administration.

Clinical Signs and Symptoms

In the infant and child the earliest clinical manifestations of hypoxia are tachycardia and tachypnea. Worsening hypoxia results in decreased ventilation, apnea, and bradycardia. This is especially true in both the neonate and the term infant. Other physical signs of hypoxia include grunting, nasal flaring, retractions, paradoxical breathing, cyanosis, irritability, and increased restlessness.[8] Often the neonate or infant becomes lethargic and flaccid, with arms and legs extended in a "frog leg" position.

The presence of cyanosis has often been used to determine inadequate oxygenation. Although this clinical sign is somewhat useful in the pediatric and adult patient, its presence in infants is often a late sign of severe hypoxia. Peripheral cyanosis (acrocyanosis) is the bluish discoloration of the skin or extremities. It occurs when a decrease in body temperature results in poor peripheral circulation or vasoconstriction. Central cyanosis involves the warm and well-perfused areas of the tongue and mucous membranes. It does not occur until reduced hemoglobin reaches 4 to 6 g/dl in arterial blood. In the child and adult the reduced hemoglobin concentration at which cyanosis occurs corresponds to a PaO_2 of approximately 50 to 60 mm Hg and an SpO_2 of 85% to 90%. In the infant, the stronger affinity of fetal hemoglobin for oxygen results in the PaO_2 falling to a significantly lower level before reduced hemoglobin is present at 5 g/dl in arterial blood. In fact, by the time central cyanosis is present in the infant, oxygen delivery to the tissues is grossly insufficient. For this reason central cyanosis is considered an unreliable indicator of the degree of tissue hypoxia. The clinical impression of cyanosis in the infant must be confirmed by arterial blood gas analysis or pulse oximetry.

COMPLICATIONS

Complications of therapeutic oxygen administration are separated into two categories: adverse physiological effects and equipment-related complications. Adverse reactions that result directly from using a specific oxygen delivery device are discussed in later sections describing that device. Although potential risks are present whenever oxygen is administered, the consequences of hypoxia are more severe.

In certain chronic lung disorders, including cystic fibrosis and bronchopulmonary dysplasia, the normal response to ventilation is blunted because of chronic carbon dioxide retention. Abrupt and excessive increases in supplemental oxygen decrease the respiratory drive and result in hypoventilation and respiratory acidosis that may lead to respiratory arrest.[9] The goal of oxygen therapy in patients with this degree of chronic lung disease is to correct the hypoxemia without decreasing the pH. Supplemental oxygen should be initiated at a low FiO_2 and increased on the basis of the results of PaO_2 or SpO_2 monitoring.

The role of oxygen in the development of retinopathy of prematurity (ROP) is controversial. It is believed to cause constriction of retinal and cerebral vessels in neonates and infants, which can lead to ischemia, varying degrees of retinal scarring, and retinal detachment. Formerly referred to as "retrolental fibroplasia," ROP may resolve spontaneously or result in permanent visual impairment, including blindness. In the 1940s and 1950s when oxygen was administered to premature infants without blood gas monitoring, ROP reached epidemic proportions.[10,11] Many other factors, in addition to oxygen, appear to correlate with the development of ROP, including gestational age, intraventricular hemorrhage, sepsis, and low birth weight.[12]

Much has been described in the literature regarding the role of supplemental oxygen in the development of ROP.[13-16] The altered regulation of vascular endothelial growth factor (VEGF) has been suggested as one of the factors in the pathogenesis of ROP.[17,18] It thus is possible that repeated cycles of hyperoxia and/or hypoxia favor the progression of ROP.[19,20] It is possible that time outside the targeted oxygen saturation range is evidence in preterm infants that combines these two factors, hyperoxia and hypoxia, and ROP.

Current practice supports oxygen therapy targeting SpO_2 levels at 88% to 95% and maintaining a PaO_2 value of 50 to 80 mm Hg in infants weighing less than 1500 g. Studies that have examined the relationship between hospital policies concerning SpO_2 limits and the survival and ophthalmic and developmental outcome of premature infants who have received supplemental oxygen have concluded that vigilance concerning oxygen management, without adversely affecting death and disability, was in some part responsible for the current decline in severe ROP.[21-24] But despite the knowledge that hyperoxia (high levels of oxygen in the blood) can be detrimental to the premature infant, there remains a challenge in establishing limits for the rational use of supplemental oxygen in the extremely premature infant. The optimal range of oxygenation that can balance the risks of mortality, ROP blindness, chronic lung disease, and brain damage continues to be studied.[25] A recent randomized trial of a lower target range of oxygenation (85%-89%) compared with a higher range (91%-95%) found that death before discharge occurred more often in the lower-oxygen-saturation group (19.9% vs. 16.2%), whereas severe retinopathy among survivors occurred less often in this group (8.6% vs. 17.9%).

High concentrations of oxygen have been linked to atelectasis, pulmonary vasodilation, and pulmonary fibrosis. In the face of high oxygen levels, the alveolar oxygen tension (SpO_2) may increase and the alveolar nitrogen decrease, resulting in absorption atelectasis. As the nitrogen is replaced by oxygen, the blood rapidly absorbs the oxygen,

gas volume decreases, and atelectasis develops. High FiO_2 levels may also result in pulmonary vasodilation. As the pulmonary vasculature dilates and alveolar volumes decrease, areas of ventilation–perfusion mismatch occur with increased intrapulmonary shunting and worsening of arterial oxygen delivery. In patients with a hypoplastic left ventricle or a single ventricle, the increased PaO_2 that occurs with oxygen therapy has been reported to compromise the balance between pulmonary and systemic blood flow.[26] There are also reports of pulmonary fibrosis occurring after oxygen administration to patients with Paraquat poisoning and to those receiving the chemotherapeutic agent bleomycin.[27,28]

OXYGEN ADMINISTRATION

Many of the devices used to deliver supplemental oxygen to neonatal and pediatric patients are simply smaller versions of the adult devices. They are similarly classified in the same manner as either variable-performance oxygen delivery systems (low-flow and reservoir systems) or fixed-performance oxygen delivery systems (high-flow systems).[5]

Variable-performance oxygen delivery systems include devices that are not capable of meeting the patient's inspiratory demand and therefore provide a fractional concentration of delivered oxygen (FdO_2) that varies with the patient's rate and depth of ventilation and the flow rate of the gas. These devices include low-flow nasal cannulas, nasopharyngeal catheters, tracheostomy oxygen adapters, simple oxygen masks, partial-rebreathing masks, and non-rebreathing masks.

Fixed-performance oxygen delivery systems include devices that can meet or exceed the patient's inspiratory demand and thereby provide an accurate FdO_2 that is not affected by changes in the ventilatory pattern. These devices include high-flow nasal cannulas, air-entrainment masks, air-entrainment nebulizer systems, and oxygen blender systems. The last category of oxygen delivery devices includes enclosure systems that provide some means of controlling oxygen concentration, temperature, and humidity. These devices include oxygen hoods, oxygen tents, and closed incubators.[5]

Variable-Performance Oxygen Delivery Systems
Nasal Cannula
The **nasal cannula** consists of flexible small-bore tubing ending in two soft prongs that are about 1 cm in length (Figure 10-1). Oxygen flows from the cannula into the patient's nasopharynx, which acts as an anatomical reservoir. For many years, the cannula was used only in pediatric and adult patients. It was not until the 1980s that it was proposed for use in infants as well.[29] Today its ease of administration makes it the preferred and most commonly used device for oxygen delivery to neonates, infants,

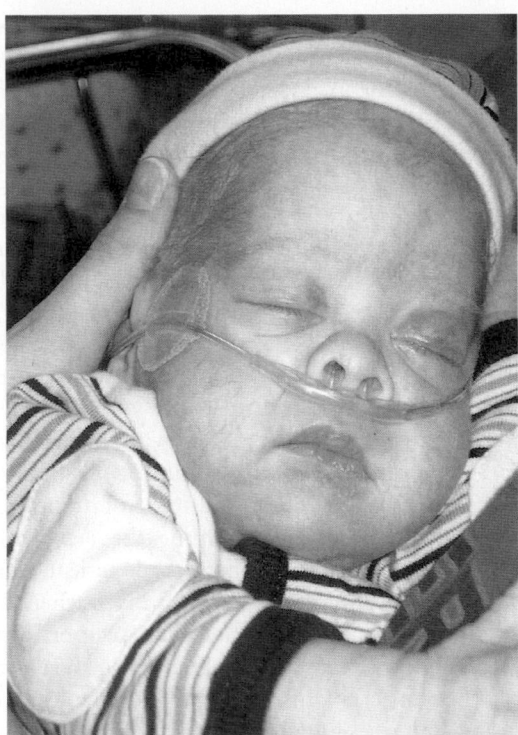

FIGURE 10-1 Infant with a neonatal nasal cannula.

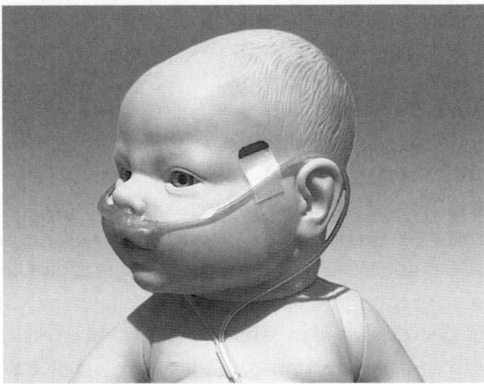

FIGURE 10-2 NeoHold cannula/tubing holder. The 4-cm-long strip attaches to the skin with hydrocolloid while the flap on top positions and secures the tubing in place. The clear flap allows visualization of the tubing.

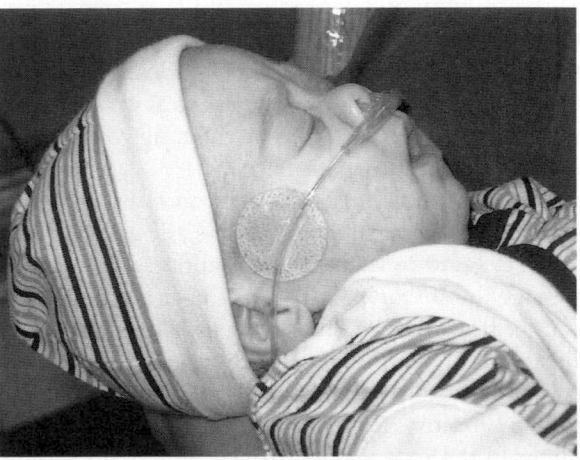

FIGURE 10-3 Tender Grip skin fixation pad. A round base of microporous tape is applied to the infant's skin. The flap on top of the base is designed to position and secure the tubing in place.

and children. As with the nasopharyngeal catheter, the cannula is designed to provide low oxygen concentrations from approximately 24% to 45%, with the FiO_2 varying with the patient's inspiratory flow.[30,31]

Indications and Contraindications. Caregivers are able to feed and provide for the patient without interrupting the delivery of oxygen. When compared with an oxygen hood, the nasal cannula allows the patient greater mobility, which may increase interactions with the patient's caregivers and environment.[32] Nasal cannulas are contraindicated in patients with nasal obstruction, such as facial trauma and choanal atresia.[5]

Application. Select the appropriate size cannula and insert the prongs into the patient's nares, making sure that the nares are not completely occluded. Wrap the lightweight tubing around the ears, and hold it under the chin with an adjustable plastic notch. In the very small or active infant, secure the cannula to the face to prevent dislodgment and position the tubing past the ears, securing it behind the head, instead of under the chin, to prevent airway obstruction. Oxygen is delivered from a flow meter and bubble humidifier through the small-bore oxygen tubing.

When adhesive tape is used to secure the cannula to the fragile skin of the neonatal patient, epidermal stripping can result each time the tape is moved to readjust the tubing. Skin irritation can also occur from a local allergic reaction to polyvinyl chloride.[5] Popular alternatives to using adhesive tape or stoma adhesive are the NeoHold cannula/tubing holder (Neotech Products, Valencia, CA) (Figure 10-2) and the Tender Grip skin fixation system

(Salter Labs, Arvin, CA) (Figure 10-3). These commercially available devices consist of a latex-free base with an adhesive backing of tinted microporous tape that is applied to the skin, usually on the patient's cheek. On top of this base is a clear tab with an adhesive backing. The tab folds over the cannula tubing and secures the cannula in place (cannula lies between the base and the tab). To reposition the cannula simply peel back the tab, adjust the tubing, and reapply the tab. The microporous tape allows the skin to breathe and the tab makes it easy to adjust the cannula without irritating the skin. The devices usually adhere to the skin for 1 to 3 weeks, staying in place even during baths.

Blenders and Low-Flow Flow Meters. Two methods of providing oxygen at low flows through a nasal cannula are common in neonatal and pediatric units. The first method entails connecting the cannula to a flow meter attached to an air–oxygen blender. The second method consists of simply connecting the cannula to a low-flow flow meter attached to a 100% oxygen source.

Oxygen blenders set at specific oxygen concentrations can be used to regulate the FiO_2 to infants receiving oxygen with nasal cannulas. Using this method, adjust both the oxygen concentration and the flow rate of the gas to achieve the appropriate FdO_2. With a cannula connected to the flow meter on the blender, set the oxygen concentration at 100% and the flow rate at the lowest possible flow. Many protocols begin the flow rate at 1 L/min. Adjust the flow rate, decreasing it in small increments until reaching the flow necessary to maintain adequate SpO_2 levels. Continue weaning by decreasing the flow rate until reaching the minimal flow setting of the flow meter. Proceed with weaning by decreasing the oxygen concentration setting on the blender to maintain adequate SpO_2 levels, or until oxygen is no longer required. Although some centers lower the oxygen concentration first, a lower flow rate may maximize the stability of delivered oxygen over time, as well as minimize the degree of change in FiO_2 during the weaning process.[33,34] Tables have been constructed to estimate hypopharyngeal oxygen concentrations at various settings, but reproducibility is affected by the range of infant sizes and variable breathing patterns.[34-36]

Because hypopharyngeal oxygen concentrations tend to be more stable when using lower flows, the use of a low-flow flow meter helps to optimize continuous oxygen administration in the infant population. Depending on the flow meter, the flow rates range from 0.1 to 3.0 L/min, with some adjustable in increments of less than 0.125 L/min.[5] Using this method, connect the cannula to a low-flow flow meter receiving 100% oxygen. Set an appropriate flow rate, as determined by the SpO_2, and wean the oxygen by decreasing the flow rate in small increments of 0.1 to 0.2 L/min. Continue weaning in small increments until the minimal desired SpO_2 is reached or until oxygen is no longer required.

Inspired Oxygen Determination. In the infant and child, FiO_2 provided with a nasal cannula is controlled primarily by varying the flow rate of the gas or the oxygen concentration of the blender. At low flow rates, FiO_2 also varies with the patient's minute ventilation and the relative duration of inspiration and expiration.[34] FiO_2 may decrease as a result of room-air entrainment that occurs during the patient's inspiration. In the small or premature infant, inspiratory flow rates are quite small and result in less room-air entrainment during inspiration. On the other hand, sedated infants may have decreased minute ventilation, resulting in an increase in the actual FiO_2.[37] The FiO_2 are higher in infants receiving oxygen via nasal cannula than in adults and can exceed potentially toxic levels.[38] Several studies have documented high FiO_2 when supplemental oxygen is supplied to neonates via nasal cannula, ranging from 22% to 95% on various flows of 100% oxygen.[33,35,39]

Oxygen delivered by nasal cannula is measured in liters per minute (L/min) rather than FiO_2. Translating a flow rate into an approximate FiO_2 is helpful in gauging the degree of respiratory compromise and comparing oxygen conditions in clinical studies. Tables and equations are available for this purpose and in fact were distributed in the multicenter Supplemental Therapeutic Oxygen for Prethreshold Retinopathy of Prematurity (STOP-ROP) study on the safety of oxygen use and the progression of ROP.[21,34] Although potentially it provides a more rational basis for oxygen prescription through a nasal cannula, the calculation and subsequent documentation of the effective FiO_2 are rarely implemented in clinical practice. Perhaps this is because the calculations are too cumbersome to undertake during routine clinical care.[32]

Because the concentration of oxygen inhaled into the lungs varies according to respiratory rate, tidal volume, inspiratory flow, and other factors such as ratio of mouth to nose breathing, it is difficult to determine the FiO_2 with certainty.[34,40,41] When compared with the adult patient, an infant can experience a substantial difference in FiO_2 when there is just a fraction of a change in the flow rate. An approximation of FiO_2 at low flows can be determined using the regression equation (Box 10-1).[33] This equation incorporates minute ventilation, but it does not account for changes in respiratory pattern and is more accurate for infants weighing less than 1500 g. Use such an equation only as a comparative estimate, and do not rely on it as an accurate determination of breath-to-breath FiO_2. During most routine clinical situations, approximating the FiO_2 from cannula flow is unnecessary. However, when weaning a patient from a cannula, the clinician can determine the measure of improvement by monitoring the incremental decreases in oxygen flow rate.

Hazards and Complications. Depending on the type of nasal cannula, the flow rate, and the infant's anatomy, an increase in exhaled resistance can result in substantial inadvertent positive expiratory airway pressure (PEP) being delivered to an infant's airway.[5,42] This occurs when using either the blender or the low-flow flow meter to deliver supplemental oxygen. Significant PEP tends to occur more often when the cannula has large-diameter prong tips and when flow rates are set above 2 L/min in smaller infants and toddlers.[39,42-45] PEP that impedes venous return may precipitate intraventricular hemorrhage in neonates and can be detrimental to an infant with obstructive

Box 10-1	Regression Equation for Estimating Nasal Cannula FiO_2 at Low Flow Rates

Approximate $FiO_2 =$
$$(O_2 \text{ flow} \times 0.79)[(0.21 \times V_E)/(V_E \times 100)]$$

This equation is most predictive with an assumed tidal volume of 5.5 ml/kg for infants less than 1500 g.

FiO_2, Fractional concentration of inspired oxygen; *O_2 flow,* expressed as milliliters per minute; *V_E* (minute ventilation) = tidal volume × respiratory rate.

pulmonary disease.[38] It also carries the potential risk of pneumothorax, pulmonary interstitial emphysema, and pneumopericardium. Although the amount and certainty of PEP may not be determined, keep in mind the possibility of such complications when improvement in response to nasal oxygen is less than expected.

Although the nasal cannula is relatively comfortable, lightweight, and easy to apply, the prongs are difficult to keep in the nares of active infants, often becoming displaced and resulting in loss of oxygen delivery.[46] Prongs that are too large can occlude the nares and increase the patient's work of breathing. An improperly sized cannula can cause irritation. Excessive flows may result in drying of the nasal mucosa as well as mucosal irritation. It is recommended that maximal flow be limited to 2 L/min in infants and newborns.[5] There is a slight risk of airway obstruction caused by mucus, especially in the low-birth-weight infant. Therefore it is important to inspect and clean the nostrils daily.[47] Keep the nose clean and free of mucus by gently cleaning the nostril areas with a soft, moist cloth, being careful to avoid causing irritation and swelling of the nasal mucosa. Also, monitor the skin around the patient's ears and face for irritation as well as proper fit and placement of the cannula and tubing.

Disadvantages to using a nasal cannula to deliver oxygen include the instability of oxygen administration in transitions between oral and nasal breathing and the lack of precise knowledge concerning the delivered oxygen concentration. Unknown FiO$_2$ values may contribute to inconsistent weaning practices that could potentially result in unnecessary days of supplemental oxygen, delays in hospital discharge, and high costs of care.[32]

Simple Oxygen Mask

The **simple oxygen mask** is a lightweight plastic reservoir designed to fit over the patient's nose and mouth and is secured by an elastic strap around the patient's head (Figure 10-4). Open ports on both sides of the mask allow exhalation and also allow the patient to draw in room air during inspiration. FiO$_2$ varies with the patient's inspiratory flow and the oxygen flow into the mask.[48] Room air is entrained through the exhalation ports in the mask if the patient's inspiratory flow rate exceeds the oxygen flow rate. Flow rates from 6 to 10 L/min provide a variable FiO$_2$ of 0.35 to 0.5; however, there are no data concerning newborns and infants to predict the effective FiO$_2$.[49]

Indications and Contraindications. Administration of oxygen with a simple mask is reserved for infants and children who need moderate concentrations of supplemental oxygen for short periods. Such situations include medical transport, emergency stabilization and postanesthesia recovery and during medical procedures. The oxygen concentrations may be higher in patients with small tidal volumes, and therefore simple masks are not suitable for infants and small children who require low or precise concentrations of oxygen.[5,6]

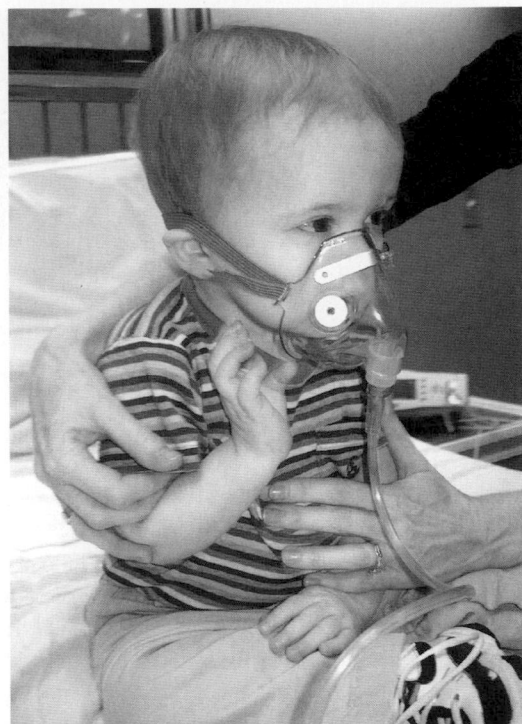

FIGURE 10-4 Infant with a simple oxygen mask.

Application. The mask is secured around the patient's head by a strap, and oxygen is delivered to the mask from a flow meter and bubble humidifier through small-bore tubing. The cone shape of the simple mask may act as a reservoir for accumulated exhaled carbon dioxide if a minimal flow of gas is not maintained. In older children and adults, 6 L/min is the recommended minimal flow rate to flush accumulated carbon dioxide.

Hazards and Complications. Because this mask is strapped to the face, infants and small children often refuse to keep the mask on. In addition, the confinement of the mask interferes with speech, eating, and breast- or bottle-feeding and may increase the risk for aspiration of vomitus. The elastic strap is often uncomfortable and can cause skin irritation with prolonged use.

Reservoir Masks

A reservoir mask consists of a soft, lightweight mask with a plastic reservoir bag attached to its front (Figure 10-5). Oxygen source gas flows directly into the neck of the mask and is directed into the bag during exhalation. When the patient inhales, high concentrations of oxygen can be delivered from the bag through the mask. Currently, there are two types of reservoir masks: partial-rebreathing and nonrebreathing masks.

If functioning properly, reservoir masks have the advantage of providing high concentrations of oxygen. However, the tight fit necessary to achieve optimal performance makes the masks impractical for long-term therapy. As with the simple oxygen mask, the elastic straps may cause the reservoir masks to be uncomfortable, confining, and

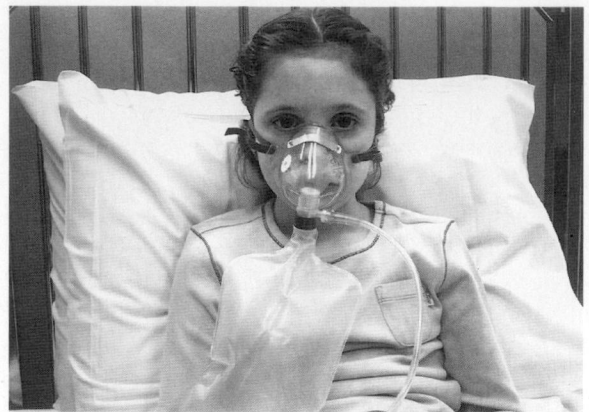

FIGURE 10-5 Pediatric patient with a partial-rebreathing mask, a type of reservoir mask.

not well tolerated by infants and children. The use of reservoir masks is limited to short-term situations requiring high FiO$_2$ administration or specific gas mixture therapy. Reservoir masks are not recommended for use in the neonatal population.[5]

Partial-Rebreathing Mask. The partial-rebreathing mask is similar to a simple oxygen mask but contains a reservoir bag at the base of the mask. It is designed to conserve oxygen by receiving 100% oxygen along with a small portion of the patient's exhaled volume (approximately equal to the volume of the patient's anatomical dead space). The oxygen concentration of the exhaled gases combined with the supply of fresh oxygen permits the use of oxygen flows lower than those necessary for other devices, potentially conserving oxygen use. The remaining portion of the patient's exhaled volume is vented through open exhalation ports located on the sides of the mask.

Fit the mask securely to the patient's face to minimize the amount of room air entrained during inspiration. Adjust the oxygen flow rate to a level sufficient to keep the bag partially inflated during inspiration; usually 6 to 15 L/min is sufficient. If the reservoir bag becomes totally deflated when the patient inspires, increase the flow rate. When there is an adequate seal around the mask and an appropriate flow rate is maintained, an FiO$_2$ of up to 0.6 is delivered to the patient.[5,48] However, this FiO$_2$, as in other variable performance devices, is also influenced by the patient's ventilatory pattern.

Nonrebreathing Mask. The nonrebreathing mask is similar in design to the partial-rebreathing mask but in addition has one-way valves that function to keep the patient from rebreathing any exhaled gas.[48] A one-way valve located between the face mask and the reservoir bag allows 100% source gas to enter the mask during inspiration, but unlike the partial-rebreathing mask, it prevents any of the patient's exhaled gas from entering the bag. Instead of entering the reservoir bag, the exhaled gas is directed through one-way leaflet valves located over the exhalation ports on the sides of the mask. The leaflet

valves also ensure minimal dilution from the entrainment of room air.

The nonrebreathing mask is designed to provide a higher FiO$_2$ than the simple and partial-rebreathing masks and the nasal delivery devices.[30] If there is an adequate seal around the mask and the flow rate is sufficient to keep the bag partially inflated during inspiration, oxygen concentrations can conceivably reach greater than 90%. Because it is designed to provide almost 100% source gas, the nonrebreathing mask is the recommended device to deliver specific gas mixtures, as in helium–oxygen therapy, or specific concentrations from a blender.[6,49]

Fixed-Performance Oxygen Delivery Systems
Air-Entrainment Mask

Air-entrainment masks, or **Venturi masks,** are examples of high-flow systems that provide the patient's entire inspiratory requirements while delivering predetermined, precise oxygen concentrations (Figure 10-6). This is accomplished by providing a total flow of gas that exceeds the patient's ventilatory demands, thus eliminating dilution of the oxygen concentration with room air, as occurs in low-flow devices.

The performance of the mask is based on principles described by Bernoulli.[50] As 100% oxygen under pressure flows through a small jet orifice entering the mask, the velocity increases, creating viscous shearing forces. As a result, room air is entrained through open ports located at the base of a reservoir tube attached to the front of the

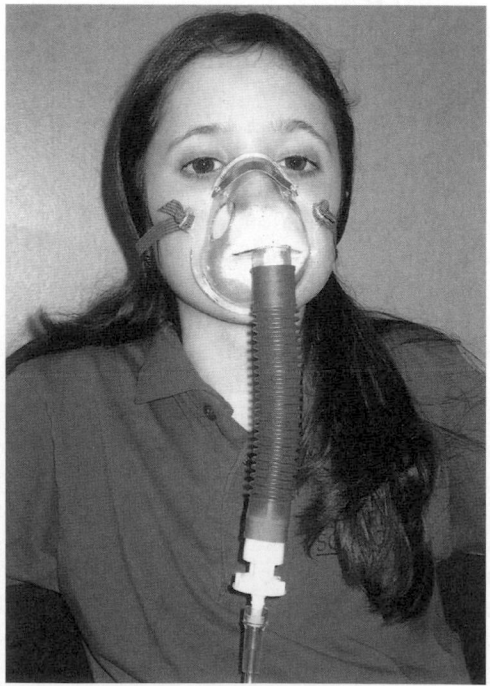

FIGURE 10-6 Pediatric patient with an air-entrainment mask.

mask. By varying either the diameter of the jet orifice or the size of the entrainment ports, the amount of room air entrained can be proportionally changed, resulting in higher total flows and specific concentrations delivered to the patient's proximal airway.

Indications and Contraindications. The air-entrainment mask is indicated for patients who require a controlled FiO_2 at either low or moderate levels. The commercially available masks are capable of providing oxygen concentrations ranging from 24% to 50%. In the hypoxic child with increased respiratory rates and tidal volumes, the air-entrainment mask is the preferred oxygen delivery system because it is capable of maintaining total flows in excess of the patient's inspiratory flow rate. For pediatric patients with chronic carbon dioxide retention who have the potential to hypoventilate with increased oxygen concentrations, the air-entrainment mask is ideal because it maintains a constant FiO_2 even at low concentrations.

Application. An air-entrainment mask is designed to fit over the patient's nose and mouth and contains a short corrugated hose with a jet orifice that is connected to oxygen supply tubing. Because the high total flows produced by this system can be quite drying, humidification is provided with a bubble-diffusion humidifier. At the lower concentrations of 24% and 28%, oxygen flow through the small, restricted orifice creates excessive backpressure in the humidifier. For these levels of oxygen concentration, an alternative method may be used in which a bland aerosol is applied through a 22-mm cuplike collar attached to the base of the corrugated hose at the air-entrainment ports. This collar is often placed on the hose even when no aerosol is applied, simply to act as a shield to prevent the accidental occlusion of the air-entrainment ports with bed linens.

Hazards and Complications. Correct performance of the air-entrainment mask can be altered by resistance to the flow of gas that may occur distal to the restricted orifice. The resistance to flow at this particular point creates backpressure, resulting in less air entrainment. As a result, higher oxygen concentrations and lower total flows are delivered to the patient. If total flow decreases significantly, room air may be inhaled around and through the mask ports. This same phenomenon will occur if the entrainment ports are partially or completely obstructed. Also, at the 50% oxygen setting, total gas flow delivered by the device is less than that at the lower concentrations. Because of this, there is the potential for the patient with an increased inspiratory flow requirement to receive an oxygen concentration less than 50%.

Air-Entrainment Nebulizer

The gas-powered, large-volume or all-purpose nebulizer is another fixed-performance system that provides particulate water and contains an adjustable air-entrainment port that controls oxygen concentrations.[51] The addition of heat gives this type of system the advantage of providing

100% body humidity when clinically indicated. The nebulizer provides oxygen at fixed concentrations by adjusting the size of the air-entrainment port located at the top of the nebulizer lid. The small size of the nebulizer jet restricts maximal flow to 15 L/min from any 50-psi gas source.

Indications and Contraindications. Air-entrainment nebulizers are used when high levels of humidity or aerosol are desired. Patient application devices used with the nebulizers include a tracheostomy collar, face tent, and aerosol mask (Figure 10-7).[5]

Application. Each patient application device is attached to the nebulizer unit with 4 to 6 ft of large-bore corrugated tubing that allows high gas flows and maximal aerosol delivery to the patient. Both the aerosol mask and the face tent apparatus are indicated primarily for short-term administration of oxygen with high humidity, as in postextubation or postanesthesia hypoxemia.[52]

When used to deliver oxygen to the older patient with an artificial airway, the aerosol is heated and the temperature of the gas–aerosol mixture is monitored. A tracheostomy collar is recommended for use with a tracheostomy; however, if a precise FiO_2 is required, a T-piece device may ensure delivery of a more exact FiO_2 because of its close fit on the tracheostomy tube. Provided that the gas flow from the nebulizer exceeds the patient's inspiratory flow rate, room-air entrainment is limited and the delivered FiO_2 is stable.

An air-entrainment nebulizer used with a collar or T-piece is not appropriate for oxygen delivery to infants and young children with a tracheostomy. Instead, a heated humidifier is recommended along with an oxygen blender used to regulate the FiO_2. Using small-bore oxygen supply tubing attached to the flow meter on the blender, the oxygen is directed through the humidifier where large-bore corrugated tubing is connected to the tracheostomy collar.

Hazards and Complications. As with all masks used to deliver oxygen therapy to the infant or pediatric patient, the aerosol mask and face tent frequently provoke unnecessary

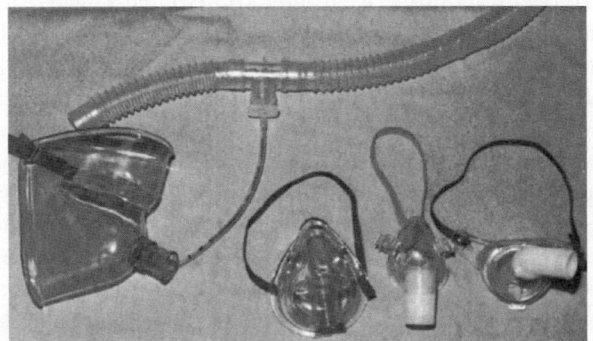

FIGURE 10-7 Various aerosol attachments. *Left to right*: Face tent, T-piece attached to an endotracheal tube, pediatric aerosol mask, infant aerosol mask, and tracheostomy mask (collar).

agitation and anxiety, especially in the treatment of postanesthesia hypoxemia. Infants and young children often find it difficult to keep the masks in place. Nebulizers are susceptible to bacterial contamination and require replacement according to hospital policy. Condensate in the aerosol tubing is considered infectious waste and should never be drained back into the nebulizer.[5] The condensate can completely obstruct gas flow or cause increased resistance to flow, which may increase the FiO_2 above the desired setting.

The weight of the T-piece and tubing assembly often creates torque on the endotracheal or tracheostomy tube, causing tracheal irritation and possible displacement. The tracheostomy collar may cause skin irritation around the patient's neck and condensate in the aerosol tubing may result in inadvertent tracheal lavage.[5]

A cool mist is not recommended for newborns because of the potential to induce cold stress.[53] If the gas flow from the oxygen source is cool and is directed toward the infant's face, stimulation of the trigeminal nerves may cause alterations in the respiratory pattern and lead to apnea.[54]

High-Flow Nasal Cannula

In the past the nasal cannula has always been classified as a low-flow, variable-performance oxygen delivery system, with recommendations that no more than 6 L/min gas flows be used with adults and that the maximal flow to newborn infants not exceed 2 L/min.[5,6,30] Flow limitations largely have been due to the airway cooling and drying that occur at higher flows. Using a bubble humidifier to humidify oxygen with a nasal cannula does not provide adequate humidification to premature infants and has been associated with decreased airway patency, nasal mucosal injury, and coagulase-negative staphylococcal sepsis in extremely low birth weight infants.[55-57] Although face masks can safely deliver oxygen at higher flows, these devices are confining and often poorly tolerated by infants and children.

Using a nasal cannula at high flows is still a relatively new means to deliver oxygen to infants and children. It has been used only a few years more in the adult population. However, studies with neonates through adults have been favorable, with data showing the heated, **humidified high-flow nasal cannula** (HHFNC) providing moderate-to-high FiO_2 values and possibly providing a cost-efficient alternative for patients who require this level of oxygen concentration.[58-60] One study indicated that when the oxygen is delivered through a HHFNC, adult patients with advanced obstructive airway disease experience an increase in oxygenation. The warm humidification may have likely contributed to the improvement of airway function by maximizing mucociliary clearance and preventing inflammatory reactions. Also, nasal breathing of warm, humidified gas tends to inhibit the bronchoconstrictor reflex, which in turn

prevents the increase in airway resistance that is often triggered by cold air.[61]

Washout of Nasopharyngeal Dead Space

Dead space has a significant and critical impact on the composition of inspiratory gas that reaches the lower, respiratory regions of the pulmonary system. When a breath begins, the first bolus of gas to be drawn into the lungs is the end-expiratory gas that was intended for exhalation. This phenomenon is the result of the anatomical dead space that must serve as a bidirectional conduit between nasal openings and the lung. Under normal conditions, this rebreathing of CO_2-rich and oxygen-depleted end-expiratory gas allows us to maintain an arterial CO_2 tension in the ideal range for our innate blood buffering system, as well as protect the lower respiratory tract form the supraphysiological partial pressure of oxygen found in atmospheric air. However, for a patient having trouble removing CO_2 or oxygenating the blood, elimination of anatomical dead space will improve breathing efficiency and therefore improve the composition of inspiratory gas within the lung.

Using HHFNC, gas flow rates that exceed inspiratory flow rates purge the nasopharyngeal cavity during the late expiratory phase and end-expiratory pause of respiration. This purging of anatomical dead space removes expiratory gas that is high in carbon dioxide concentrations and relatively depleted of oxygen. This creates an anatomical reservoir of the intended inspiratory gas mixture. Under these conditions, the subsequent breath is composed of less rebreathed expiratory gas and more delivered cannula gas. The new alveolar gas equilibrium supports alveolar ventilation (VA) with less minute ventilation (VE), and in this regard improves the efficiency of breathing.

Data from clinical studies on HHFNC confirm the reduction of dead space because of the immediate impact on ventilation rates.[62-65]

In the neonatal community, a number of clinical trials support the conclusion that dead-space washout provides a ventilation effect. Holleman-Duray and colleagues showed infants were able to be extubated to HHFNC from significantly greater ventilator rates (33 ± 8 vs. 28 ± 8 breaths per minute; $p < 0.05$) compared with other noninvasive support modes.[66] Additionally, a case report of a pediatric burn patient showed respiratory rate decreased immediately after initiation of HHFNC (63-38 breaths per minute), with a secondary sustained decrease in heart rate (175-144 beats per minute) after a short period of HHFNC.

Indications and Contraindications. Oxygen delivery with a high-flow nasal cannula is most often indicated for use in patients with hypoxemia who have not responded to oxygen administered with a low-flow nasal cannula. It may also be indicated for use in infants and children with lung disorders who require improved oxygenation or a reduction in work of breathing. The high-flow nasal cannula has also been recommended for infants in the management of apnea of prematurity.[43] As a less intrusive method to deliver high flows of oxygen, its use may reduce the potential risk of the iatrogenic injuries associated with nasal CPAP and mechanical ventilation.[67] Contraindications for use of the high-flow nasal cannula may include suspected or confirmed pneumothorax, severe upper airway obstruction, and absence of spontaneous ventilation.

Application. To provide optimal humidification, the high-flow nasal cannula must be used with a hydration system. The Vapotherm 2000i (Vapotherm, Stevensville, MD) system is credited with starting the high-flow therapy via nasal cannula. In 2004 it was approved by the U.S. Food and Drug Administration to humidify and deliver high-flow air or oxygen by nasal cannula and other patient interfaces. It is not approved, nor is it recommended for use, as a CPAP delivery system.[42-45] The Precision Flow (newest version of the Vapotherm system), through a novel humidification system, can provide oxygen flow at a relative humidity of 99.9% with a temperature setting of 37° C.[68] Oxygen is supplied to the unit from an air–oxygen blender. The flow rate of the gas is controlled by the flow meter on the blender. The oxygen travels through a vapor exchange cartridge, where it is separated from the water by a microporous membrane material with a pore size less than 0.01 μm.[69] The membrane allows water vapor to pass into the flow of gas, but the small pore size of the membrane prevents direct contact between the water source and the oxygen, effectively serving as a filter.[68] After it is warmed and humidified, the oxygen flows through a water-heated delivery tube that is connected to the nasal cannula. This tubing maintains the temperature of the gas and minimizes condensation in the cannula.

The Vapotherm system has cannulas available in six sizes:
· Premature
· Neonatal
· Infant
· Intermediate infant
· Pediatric
· Adult

It also has two vapor transfer cartridges: a low-flow cartridge that is used to deliver flows of 1 to 8 L/min and a high-flow cartridge that is used to deliver flows of 5 to 40 L/min. The temperature range is selectable from 33 to 43° C.*

---

*Note: Fisher & Paykel Healthcare (New Zealand) and Teleflex Incorporated (Research Triangle, NC) have heated, humidified high-flow nasal cannula systems with similar nasal cannula sizes, called Optiflow and Comfort Flo, respectively. Careful consideration needs to be taken because each device has unique features. Please refer to manuals of operations for specifics.

Select the cannula that is most appropriate for the size of the patient, making sure that the prongs do not occlude the patient's nares. Attach the high-flow nasal cannula to the patient in the same manner as one would a low-flow nasal cannula. Adjust the oxygen concentration with the blender and set the flow rate on the flow meter. Increase or decrease the flow in small increments. Assess the patient's breathing pattern, breath sounds, and vital signs. Also monitor the SpO_2 and chest radiographs to determine appropriate flow rates. The high-flow nasal cannula and the delivery tubing are single-patient disposables and are discarded after each patient's use.

Hazards and Complications. To a greater extent than with the low-flow nasal cannula, there is considerable concern as to the lack of knowledge of the exact amount of positive pressure generated. Although most studies present low levels of positive pressure in flow range commonly used, the development of gastric distention or lung overexpansion is a possibility if not carefully monitored.[64] A second concern is the level of FdO_2 that can be administered. An FdO_2 of more than 0.6 can be easily administered at higher flows. When needed, this ability is a blessing; however, it may disguise a progressive disease when mistakenly considered a low-flow, low-FdO_2 delivery device.

More data supporting the clinical efficacy of HHFNC are produced each year. Research continues to focus on when HHFNC transitions from simple heated and humidified oxygen therapy to respiratory support by dead-space reduction and the application of low-level positive pressure.

CLINICAL HIGHLIGHT

It is theorized that to improve ventilation efficiency with HHFNC the flow must be set to minimally exceed the expiratory flow rate of the patient. To provide additional low-level positive pressure with HHFNC, the flow must be set to exceed the inspiratory flow rate of the patient.

Exceeding expiratory flow rate (typically less than inspiratory flow rate) reduces dead space, increases oxygen delivery, and provides humidity. Exceeding inspiratory flow rates accomplishes deadspace washout and possibly provides some positive pressure expiratory pressure.

Table 10-1 represents estimated inspiratory flow rates of a wide patient population range. The assumptions in Table 10-1 are based on the notion that patients who are receiving HHFNC are in respiratory distress. Calculations are based on the highest known normal respiratory rate for each category, inspiratory time of 33%, and tidal volumes between 4-8 mL/Kg.

Oxygen Hood

The **oxygen hood** is a transparent enclosure constructed of clear plastic material in a cylinder or boxlike design

TABLE 10-1

Estimated Inspiratory Flow Rates of a Wide Patient Population Range

Weight (Kg)	Age	Low L/Kg/Min	Medium L/Kg/Min	High L/Kg/Min
<2.9	Neonate (Premature)	0.7	1.0	1.3
3.0-4.9	Neonate	0.6	0.9	1.2
5.0-9.9	<1 years	0.5	0.8	1.1
10-26.9	1-7 years	0.4	0.6	0.8
27-60.9	8-14 years	0.3	0.5	0.6
>61	>14 years	0.2	0.3	0.4

(Figure 10-8). Oxygen is administered through large-bore corrugated tubing attached to the back of the hood. The hood surrounds the infant's head, leaving the body accessible for nursing care. This design also allows the infant to be placed in a neutral thermal environment, such as an incubator, and still receive controlled oxygen concentrations. Variations in hood design allow access to the infant's head by removing the top lid or by opening large ports on the sides or top of the hood.

Indications and Contraindications. Hoods are indicated most often for neonates, infants, and small children who require supplemental oxygen with heated humidity. Hoods are used to provide a controlled FiO_2 and increased heated humidity to patients who are unable to tolerate other oxygen or humidification devices. An oxygen hood can also be used to perform an oxygen challenge (hyperoxia) test in a spontaneously breathing neonate. Oxygen concentration in a hood can be varied from 21% to 100% and is more stable than that provided by a tent.[5]

Application. Oxygen is delivered to the hood with heated humidification by means of an oxygen blender, dual air and oxygen flow meters, or a heated air-entrainment nebulizer. When using the heated air-entrainment nebulizer, power the nebulizer with compressed air, setting the oxygen concentration dial at 100% and bleeding oxygen into the nebulizer. In this way, oxygen concentrations are more easily regulated and noise levels are reduced.[70]

The oxygen blender system premixes oxygen concentrations and passes the blended gas through a heated humidifier before entering the hood. This allows more precise control over both oxygen concentration and temperature and virtually eliminates noise inside the hood. With dual air and oxygen flow meters, both air and oxygen are titrated through the heated humidifier and tubing into the hood and analyzed until accurate prescribed oxygen concentrations are obtained. Regardless of which system is used, oxygen is analyzed on a continuous basis to ensure accurate concentrations.

When high oxygen concentrations are used, a layering effect occurs inside the hood, with the highest oxygen concentrations settling toward the bottom. For this reason, place the oxygen analyzer sensor as close to the infant's head as possible. It is also important that an adequate flow of gas be delivered to wash out any carbon dioxide that may accumulate inside the hood. In general, flow rates should be greater than 7 L/min.[5] Flows of

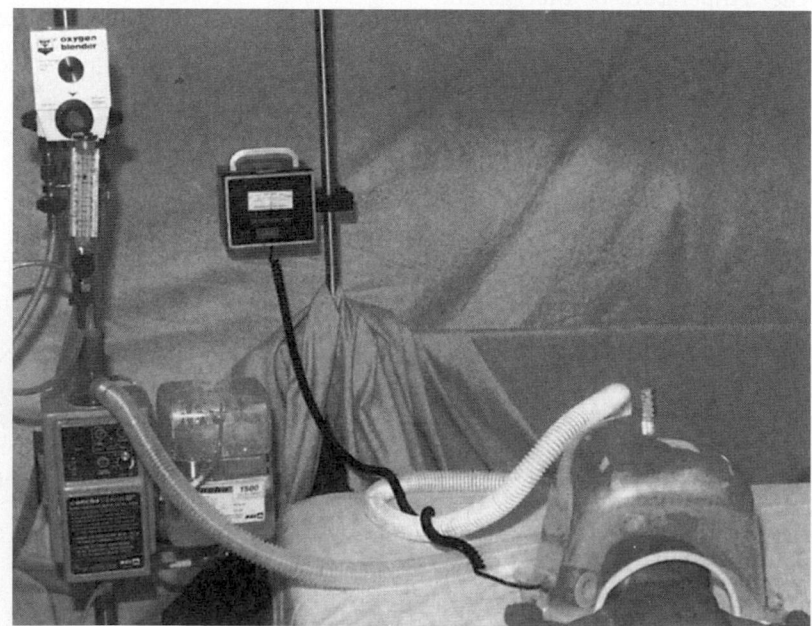

FIGURE 10-8 Infant oxygen hood with gas delivered through an oxygen blender system with heated humidification. The oxygen analyzer sensor is placed inside the hood close to the infant's head.

10 to 15 L/min are adequate for most infants and children.

It is important that adequate heat and humidity be maintained inside the hood. Administration of cool, dry gas induces cold stress in infants, resulting in increased oxygen consumption. Likewise, delivery of overheated gases induces apnea.[54] Temperature is maintained at or near body temperature with a thermometer placed inside the hood for continuous monitoring.

Oxygen hoods come in a variety of sizes to fit the very small neonate and very large infant. For patients too large for neonatal-size hoods, there are transparent enclosures in larger sizes called tent houses or huts (Figures 10-9 and 10-10). For optimal temperature, flow, and oxygen control, choosing the proper-sized hood is imperative.

Hazards and Complications. Limited mobility may be an issue with the oxygen hood if the infant requires oxygen for a prolonged period. Opening the hood decreases the oxygen concentration and can result in hypoxia. If the hood is opened for an extended period, such as during feeding and nursing procedures, it is appropriate to provide nasal oxygen with a cannula while the patient is eating or until the procedure is completed. Just as a loss of gas flow to the hood can result in hypoxia, hypercapnia, and even death, excessive oxygen concentrations can lead to irreversible complications. For these reasons, use an oxygen analyzer to continuously monitor the oxygen concentration in the hood, maintaining high and low alarms on the analyzer at all times. Although the oxygen hood is usually well tolerated, irritation to the infant's skin, especially around the neck, may occur because of pressure from an improperly sized hood or active movement of the patient. Cutaneous fungal infections have been associated with prolonged exposure to humidified oxygen in hoods.[71] High gas flow into the hood may produce noise levels that induce hearing impairment.[70]

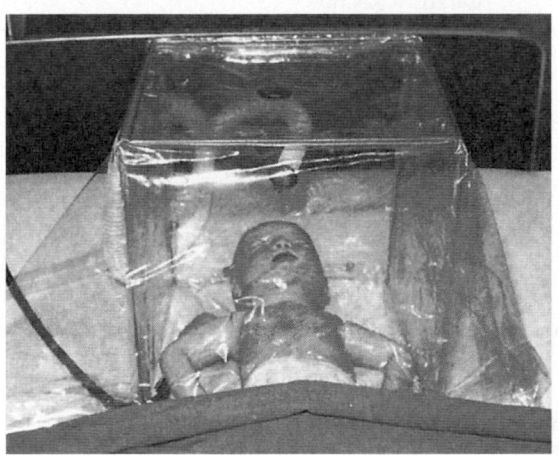

FIGURE 10-9 Tent house for oxygen administration to larger infants.

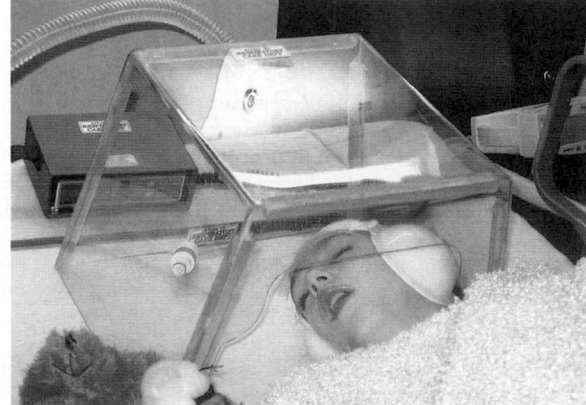

FIGURE 10-10 Older pediatric patient requiring low oxygen concentration after surgical repair of earlobes. Because use of a face mask or cannula would require straps or tubing placed around the patient's ears, a hood is used.

CASE STUDY

You are presented with providing oxygen therapy for a mildly hypoxic 12-year-old child with an SpO_2 of 86% to 88%. The child has been recently diagnosed with moderate persistent asthma. She is admitted for a moderate exacerbation. The patient is in moderate distress, tachypneic, with good air entry and prolonged expiratory wheezes. The last blood gas obtained from a referral hospital is only remarkable for a mild respiratory alkalosis. The physician asks you to initiate oxygen therapy with the device of your choice and to maintain the PaO_2 above 60 torr. Which of the following answers best describes the device you would choose and what noninvasive oxygen saturation range would you target?

   A. A nasal cannula and an SpO_2 of 92% to 95%
   B. A nasal cannula and an SpO_2 of 89% to 92%
   C. A venti-mask set at 28% to achieve an SpO_2 of 92% to 95%
   D. Do nothing because the patient's PaO_2 is already above 60

See Evolve Resources for answers.

KEY POINTS

- Oxygen is a drug and should be treated as one. Withholding oxygen can have detrimental effects, however continuing to provide oxygen therapy when it is no longer indicated can prolong hospitalization and increase the cost of care.
- Oxygen therapy is only one aspect of the oxygen delivery equation. One must ensure that oxygen content and

cardiac output are considered when assessing the effectiveness of oxygen therapy.

- Oxygen therapy device selection is vitally important. Care must be taken in the application process of such a wide patient population. Smaller pediatric patients are not small adults therefore assumed FiO_2 calculation cannot be assumed.

- Oxygen therapy has several physiologic effects that are similar to adults. However, there are several differences that if not carefully monitored can lead to blindness, poor perfusion (CHD patients), and/or brain injury.

- Abnormal breathing patterns such as apnea of prematurity, abnormal neurogenic breathing, or obstructive sleep apnea can make oxygen therapy more difficult to manage. Inappropriately providing oxygen therapy in the face of one of these abnormal breathing patterns will lead to larger swings in oxygen delivery. In some cases it may mask apnea.

ASSESSMENT QUESTIONS

See Evolve Resources for answers.

1. Bedside evaluation of the degree of hypoxemia may best be accomplished by which of the following?
   A. Auscultation
   B. Pulse oximetry
   C. Capillary blood gas analysis
   D. Capillary refill time

2. A 5-year-old patient with a history of asthma is admitted to the emergency department after complaining of chest tightness and wheezing. The pulse oximeter reading drops from 95% to 88%. Which of the following devices should be selected to deliver oxygen to this patient?
   A. Nasal cannula
   B. Oxygen hood
   C. Oxygen mist tent
   D. Nonrebreathing mask

3. What is the minimal flow rate that should be used to deliver oxygen through a hood to an infant?
   A. 5 L/min
   B. 6 L/min
   C. 10 L/min
   D. 15 L/min

4. The physician orders 32% oxygen for a 12-year-old patient with cystic fibrosis. Which of the following oxygen delivery devices would best ensure this oxygen concentration?
   A. Low-flow nasal cannula
   B. Simple mask
   C. Nonrebreathing mask
   D. Air-entrainment mask

5. A 9-year-old patient is admitted to the hospital after smoke inhalation. While receiving oxygen with a nonrebreathing mask, it is noted that the reservoir bag becomes totally deflated when the patient inspires. Which of the following actions should be taken?
   A. Increase the oxygen flow rate
   B. Decrease the oxygen flow rate
   C. Change to a nasal cannula
   D. Change to a partial rebreathing mask

6. A premature infant is receiving oxygen by nasal cannula at 1.5 L/min. The following capillary blood gas and pulse oximetry values are obtained:

pH	7.37
$PtcCO_2$	41 mm Hg
PCO_2	43 mm Hg
HCO_3	23 mEq/L
BE	−1 mEq/L
SpO_2	98%

   BE, Base excess in blood; HCO_3-, bicarbonate; $PtcCO_2$, partial pressure of carbon dioxide, determined transcutaneously; PCO_2, partial pressure of oxygen, determined transcutaneously; SpO_2, percentage of oxygen saturation.

   Which of the following should be recommended?
   A. Replace the nasal cannula with an oxygen hood
   B. Decrease the nasal cannula flow to 1 L/min
   C. Increase the nasal cannula flow to 2 L/min
   D. Discontinue the nasal cannula

7. What plausible ways does HHFNC improve oxygenation?
   A. Nasal pharyngeal CO_2 washout at flows that exceed expiratory gas flow
   B. Filling the nasal cavity with oxygen-enriched gas
   C. Positive pressure
   D. All of the above

8. What is a concern(s) when using a HHFNC?
   A. A lack of understanding of the actual fraction of oxygen delivered
   B. An increased risk of developing chronic lung disease
   C. A lack of knowledge concerning the actual amount of positive pressure applied to the patient's airways
   D. A and C

References

1. In: Partington JR, editor: *A short history of chemistry,* ed 3, New York, 1989, Dover, pp 110–152.
2. Saugstad OD: Oxygen toxicity in the neonatal period, *Acta Pediatr Scand* 79:881, 1990.
3. Hess JH: Oxygen unit for premature and very young infants, *Am J Dis Child* 47:916, 1934.
4. In: Baker JP, editor: *The machine in the nursery: premature technology and the origins of newborn intensive care,* Baltimore, 1996, Johns Hopkins University Press, p 152.
5. American Association for Respiratory Care: Clinical practice guideline: selection of an oxygen delivery device for neonatal and pediatric patients, *Respir Care* 47:707, Revised & Updated 2002.
6. American Association for Respiratory Care: Clinical practice guideline: oxygen therapy for adults in the acute care facility, *Respir Care* 47:717, Revised & Updated 2002.
7. Fulmer JD, Snider GL: American college of chest physicians/National heart, lung, and blood institute: National conference on oxygen therapy, *Chest* 1984;86:234. [concurrent publication in *Respir Care* 29:922, 1984].
8. Bonadio W: The history and physical assessments of the febrile infant, *Pediatr Clin North Am* 45:65, 1998.
9. Fisher AB: Oxygen therapy: side effects and toxicity, *Am Rev Respir Dis* 122:61, 1980.
10. Lanman JT, et al: Retrolental fibroplasia and oxygen therapy, *JAMA* 155:223, 1954.
11. Patz A: The role of oxygen in retrolental fibroplasia, *Pediatrics* 19:504, 1957.

12. George DS, et al: The latest on retinopathy of prematurity, *Maternal Child Nurs* 13:254, 1988.

13. Gaynon MW, Stevenson DK, Sunshine P, Fleisher BE, Landers MB: Supplemental oxygen may decrease progression of prethreshold disease to threshold retinopathy of prematurity, *J Perinatol* 17:434, 1997.

14. Phelps DL: Reduced severity of oxygen-induced retinopathy in kittens recovered in 28% oxygen, *Pediatr Res* 24:106, 1988.

15. Stuart MJ, Phelps DL, Setty BN: Changes in oxygen tension and effects on cyclooxygenase metabolites: III. Decrease of retinal prostacyclin in kittens exposed to hyperoxia, *Pediatrics* 82:367, 1988.

16. Kinsey VE, Arnold HJ, Kalina RE, et al: Pao_2 levels and retrolental fibroplasia: a report of the cooperative study, *Pediatrics* 60:655, 1977.

17. Pierce EA, Foley ED, Smith LE: Regulation of vascular endothelial growth factor by oxygen in a model of retinopathy of prematurity, *Arch Ophthalmol* 114:1219, 1996.

18. Robbins SG, Rajaratnam VS, Penn JS: Evidence for upregulation and redistribution of vascular endothelial growth factor (VEGF) receptors flt-1 and flk-1 in the oxygen-injured rat retina, *Growth Factors* 16:1, 1998.

19. Penn JS, Henry MM, Wall PT, Tolman BL: The range of Pao_2 variation determines the severity of oxygen-induced retinopathy in newborn rats, *Invest Ophthalmol Vis Sci* 36:2063, 1995.

20. Saito Y, Omoto T, Cho Y, et al: The progression of retinopathy of prematurity and fluctuation in blood gas tension, *Graefes Arch Clin Exp Ophthalmol* 231:151, 1993.

21. STOP-ROP Multicenter Study Group: Supplemental therapeutic oxygen for pre-threshold retinopathy of prematurity (STOP-ROP), a randomized, controlled, trial: primary outcomes, *Pediatrics* 105:295, 2000.

22. Tin W, et al: Pulse oximetry, severe retinopathy, and outcome at one year in babies of less than 28 weeks gestation, *Arch Dis Child Fetal Neonatal Ed* 84:F106, 2001.

23. Askie LM, et al: Oxygen-saturation targets and outcomes in extremely preterm infants, *N Engl J Med* 349:959, 2003.

24. Chow LC, et al: Can changes in clinical practice decrease the incidence of severe retinopathy of prematurity in very low birth weight infants? *Pediatrics* 111:339, 2003.

25. Silverman WA: A cautionary tale about supplemental oxygen: the albatross of neonatal medicine, *Pediatrics* 113:394, 2004.

26. El-Lessy HN: Pulmonary vascular control in hypoplastic left-heart syndrome: hypoxic- and hypercarbic-gas therapy, *Respir Care* 40:737, 1995.

27. Fairshter RD, et al: Paraquat poisoning: new aspects of therapy, *Q J Med* 45:551, 1976.

28. Ingrassia TS, et al: Oxygen-exacerbated bleomycin pulmonary toxicity, *Mayo Clin Proc* 66:173, 1991.

29. Kloor TH Jr, Carbajal D: Infant oxygen administration by modified nasal cannula, *Clin Pediatr* 23:447, 1984.

30. Leigh JM: Variation in performance of oxygen therapy devices, *Anaesthesia* 25:210, 1970.

31. Ooi R, et al: An evaluation of oxygen delivery using nasal prongs, *Anaesthesia* 47:591, 1992.

32. Walsh M, et al: Oxygen delivery through nasal cannulae to preterm infants: can practice be improved? *Pediatrics* 116:857, 2005.

33. Finer NN, et al: Low flow oxygen delivery via nasal cannula to neonates, *Pediatr Pulmonol* 21:48, 1996.

34. Benaron DA, Benitz WE: Maximizing the stability of oxygen delivered via nasal cannula, *Arch Pediatr Adolesc Med* 148:294, 1994.

35. Vain NE, et al: Regulation of oxygen concentration delivered to infants via nasal cannulas, *Am J Dis Child* 143:1458, 1989.

36. Stevens DP, et al: Hypopharyngeal O_2 concentration in infants breathing O_2 by nasal cannula [abstract], *Respir Care* 31:988, 1986.

37. Hammer J, et al: Effect of jaw-thrust and continuous positive airway pressure on tidal breathing in deeply sedated infants, *J Pediatr* 138:826, 2001.

38. Kuluz JW, et al: The fraction of inspired oxygen in infants receiving oxygen via nasal cannula often exceeds safe levels, *Respir Care* 46:897, 2001.

39. Fan LL, Voyles JB: Determination of inspired oxygen delivered by nasal cannula in infants with chronic lung disease, *J Pediatr* 103:923, 1983.

40. Miller MJ, et al: Oral breathing in newborn infants, *J Pediatr* 107:465, 1985.

41. Miller MJ, et al: Effect of maturation on oral breathing in sleeping premature infants, *J Pediatr* 109:515, 1986.

42. Locke RG, et al: Inadvertent administration of positive end-distending pressure during nasal cannula flow, *Pediatrics* 91:135, 1993.

43. Sreenan C, et al: High-flow nasal cannula in the management of apnea of prematurity: a comparison with conventional nasal continuous positive airway pressure, *Pediatrics* 107:1080, 2001.

44. Frey B, et al: Nasopharyngeal oxygen therapy produces positive end-expiratory pressure in infants, *Eur J Pediatr* 160:556, 2001.

45. Courtney SE, et al: Lung recruitment and breathing pattern during variable versus continuous flow nasal continuous positive airway pressure in premature infants: an evaluation of three devices, *Pediatrics* 107:304, 2001.

46. Thilo EH, et al: Home oxygen therapy in the newborn: costs and parental acceptance, *Am J Dis Child* 141:766, 1987.

47. Weber MW, et al: Comparison of nasal prongs and nasopharyngeal catheter for the delivery of oxygen in children with hypoxemia because of a lower respiratory tract infection, *J Pediatr* 127:378, 1995.

48. Cairo JM, Pilbeam SP: Administering medical gases: regulators, flowmeters, and controlling devices. In *Mosby's respiratory care equipment*, ed 7, St. Louis, 2004, Mosby, pp 71–72.

49. Redding JS, et al: Oxygen concentrations received from commonly used delivery systems, *South Med J* 71:169, 1978.

50. Scacci R: Air entrainment masks: jet mixing is how they work: the Bernoulli and Venturi principles are how they don't, *Respir Care* 24:928, 1979.

51. Cairo JM, Pilbeam SP: Humidity and aerosol therapy. In *Mosby's respiratory care equipment*, ed 7, St. Louis, 2004, Mosby, pp 73–74.

52. Amar D, et al: An alternative oxygen delivery system for infants and children in the post-anesthesia care unit, *Can J Anaesth* 38:49, 1991.

53. Scopes JW, Ahmed I: Ranges of critical temperatures in sick and premature newborn babies, *Arch Dis Child* 41:417, 1966.

54. Daily WJR, et al: Apnea in premature infants: monitoring, incidence, heart rate changes, and an effect of environmental temperature, *Pediatrics* 43:510, 1969.

55. Walsh B: Comparison of Vapotherm 2000i with a bubble humidifier for humidifying flow through an infant nasal cannula, *Respir Care* 48:1086, 2003.

56. Kopelman AE, Holbert D: Use of oxygen cannulas in extremely low birthweight infants is associated with mucosal trauma and bleeding and possibly with coagulase-negative staphylococcal sepsis, *J Perinatol* 23:94, 2003.

57. Kopelman AE: Airway obstruction in two extremely low birthweight infants treated with oxygen cannulas, *J Perinatol* 23:164, 2003.

58. Wettstein RB, et al: Delivered oxygen concentration using low-flow and high-flow nasal cannulas, *Respir Care* 50:604, 2005.

59. Wilkinson D, Andersen C, O'Donnell CP, De Paoli AG: High flow nasal cannula for respiratory support in preterm infants, *Cochrane Database Syst Rev* (5):CD006405, 2005. doi: 10.1002/14651858.CD006405.pub2.

60. Frizzola M, Miller TL, Rodriguez ME, Zhu Y, Rojas J, Hesek A, et al: High-flow nasal cannula: impact on oxygenation and ventilation in an acute lung injury model, *Pediatr Pulmonol* 46:67, 2011. doi: 10.1002/ppul.21326.

61. Chatila W, et al: The effects of high-flow versus low-flow oxygen on exercise in advanced obstructive airways disease, *Chest* 126:1108, 2004.

62. Byerly FL, Haithcock JA, Buchanan IB, Short KA, Cairns BA: Use of high flow nasal cannula on a pediatric burn patient with inhalation injury and post-extubation stridor, *Burns* 32:121, 2006. doi: S0305-4179(05)00150-6 [pii] 10.1016/j.burns.2005.05.003.

63. Calvano TP, Sill JM, Kemp KR, Chung KK: Use of a high-flow oxygen delivery system in a critically ill patient with dementia, *Respir Care* 53:1739, 2008.

64. Price AM, Plowright C, Makowski A, Misztal B: Using a high-flow respiratory system (Vapotherm) within a high dependency setting, *Nurs Crit Care* 13:298, 2008. doi: NCR299 [pii] 10.1111/j.1478-5153.2008.00299.x.

65. Roca O, Riera J, Torres F, Masclans JR: High-flow oxygen therapy in acute respiratory failure, *Respir Care* 55:408, 2010.

66. Holleman-Duray D, Kaupie D, Weiss MG: Heated humidified high-flow nasal cannula: use and a neonatal early extubation protocol, *J Perinatol* 27:776, 2007. doi: 7211. 25 [pii] 10.1038/sj.jp.7211825.

67. Juretschke R, Spoula R: High flow nasal cannula in the neonatal population, *Neonatal Intensive Care* 17:20, 2004.

68. Waugh JB, Lain DC: Evaluation of a new high flow gas humidification device [abstract], *Am J Respir Crit Care Med* 167:A996, 2003.

69. Vapotherm, Inc: *2000i operating instruction manual*, Stevensville, MD, 2000, Vapotherm, Inc.

70. Beckham RW, Mishoe SC: Sound levels inside incubators and oxygen hoods used with nebulizers and humidifiers, *Respir Care* 27:33, 1982.

71. Lanska MJ, et al: Cutaneous fungal infections associated with prolonged treatment in humidified oxygen hoods [letter], *Pediatr Dermatol* 4:346, 1987.

Chapter 11

Aerosols and Administration of Medication

JAMES B. FINK, ARZU ARI

OUTLINE

LEARNING OBJECTIVES

After reading this chapter the reader will be able to:

1. Describe impact of differences in patient size and age on aerosol delivery
2. Understand the basic mechanisms of operation of nebulizer, pressurized metered-dose inhalers, and dry powder inhalers

3. Select the best device for a pediatric patient for specific clinical applications
4. Initiate and modify aerosol therapy
5. Discuss the range of medications available for administration via aerosol

KEY TERMS

Aerosol
Aerosol therapy
Nebulizer

Pressurized metered-dose inhaler
Dry powder inhaler

Spacers
Valved holding chamber

Decades of research have established the scientific principles underlying the use of therapeutic aerosols. In general, the advantages of aerosol therapy include a smaller but targeted dose, lower cost, fewer side effects, efficacy comparable to or better than that observed with systemic administration of the drug, and usually a more rapid onset of action.[1] When inhaled drugs are delivered directly to the conducting airways, their systemic absorption is limited and systemic side effects are minimized, providing a high therapeutic index.[2] On the other hand, peptides and other macromolecules can be targeted to the terminal airways and alveoli for systemic administration across the pulmonary vascular bed. This is an exciting and evolving use for therapeutic aerosols.

The uses for aerosol devices vary widely, ranging from bronchodilation to insulin administration, and the range of uses for aerosol devices continues to increase. Nebulizers, pressurized metered-dose inhalers (pMDIs), and dry powder inhalers (DPIs) are often used as aerosol generators because they produce respirable particles with a mass median aerodynamic diameter (MMAD) of 0.5 to 5.0 μm.[3] Other types of nonpressurized metered-dose inhalers, such as nasal sprays, produce particles in the 10- to 100-μm range, too large for pulmonary delivery. Although pMDIs and DPIs are used chiefly to deliver bronchodilators and steroids, nebulizers can be used to administer antibiotics, mucoactive agents, and other drugs.[4] Given the appropriate formulation, even complex molecules can potentially be delivered by aerosol. The operating characteristics and limitations of aerosol-generating devices, how they are matched to the needs of specific patients, and how they are used largely determine the efficacy of aerosol therapy. This chapter reviews the key principles of how aerosols are generated, deposited, and administered in the neonatal and pediatric patient.

NEONATAL AND PEDIATRIC MEDICATION DELIVERY

Compared with adults, infants and children have smaller airway diameters, have higher and more irregular breathing rates, engage in nose breathing (which filters out large particles), and often have difficulty with mouthpiece administration. Cooperation and ability to perform aerosol inhalation techniques effectively vary with the child's age and developmental ability.

The size of the airways changes dramatically in the first years of life. Breathing patterns, flows, and volumes all change with growth and development. The resting respiratory rate decreases with age as tidal volume and minute ventilation increase. Tidal volume is approximately 7 ml/kg in the newborn, with a 300% increase in tidal volume in the first year. Inspiratory flow also increases with vital capacity. The low tidal volume, vital capacity, functional residual capacity, and short respiratory cycles of infants result in a low residence time for small particles, resulting in a further decrease in pulmonary deposition (Box 11-1).[5]

Box 11-1	Factors That Reduce Rate and Depth of Aerosol Particle Deposition in Neonatal and Pediatric Patients

- Large tongue in proportion to oral airway
- Nose breathing
- Narrow airway diameter
- Fewer and larger alveoli
- Fewer generations of airway
- More rapid respiratory rate
- Small tidal volume
- Inability to hold breath and coordinate inspiration
- High inspiratory flow rate during respiratory distress and crying

Direct information regarding inhaled particle mass, lung deposition, and regional distribution of aerosols is limited concerning neonates, infants, and young children. Nevertheless, the data suggest that aerosol delivery is substantially less efficient for this population. Pulmonary deposition of aerosol to neonates may be less than 1% of the nominal dose being nebulized, compared with 8% to 22% in an adult.[5]

This reduced efficiency may result in infants receiving weight-appropriate dosing compared with adults. For example, the deposition efficiency of 0.5% of a standard dose of albuterol sulfate (2500 μg) would result in a lung dose of 12.5 μg, or 6.25 μg/kg for a 2-kg infant, whereas a 70-kg adult with 10% deposition has a lung dose of 250 μg, equivalent to 3.6 μg/kg. In this example, the infant actually receives a similar but slightly greater dose per unit weight. To some extent, the reduced deposition of aerosolized bronchodilators results in safety and efficacy profiles for infants and children similar to those reported for adults. Extrapolation of data from Wildhaber and colleagues[6] (Figure 11-1) demonstrates that whereas deposition from a pMDI with nonelectrostatic valved holding chamber varies with child age, the amount of drug per kilogram of body weight is consistent across ages. This suggests that the same dose that is effective for an adult

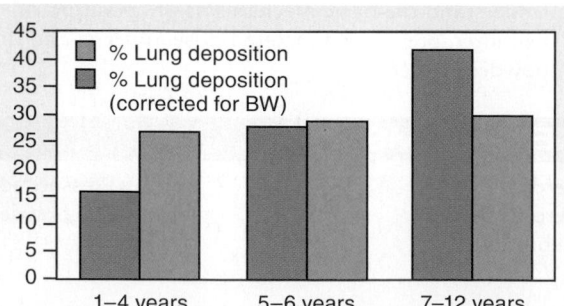

FIGURE 11-1 Although the percentage of drug deposited in the lung varies with age (*blue columns*), the percentage of lung deposition corrected for body weight (*orange columns*) is consistent across age groups.

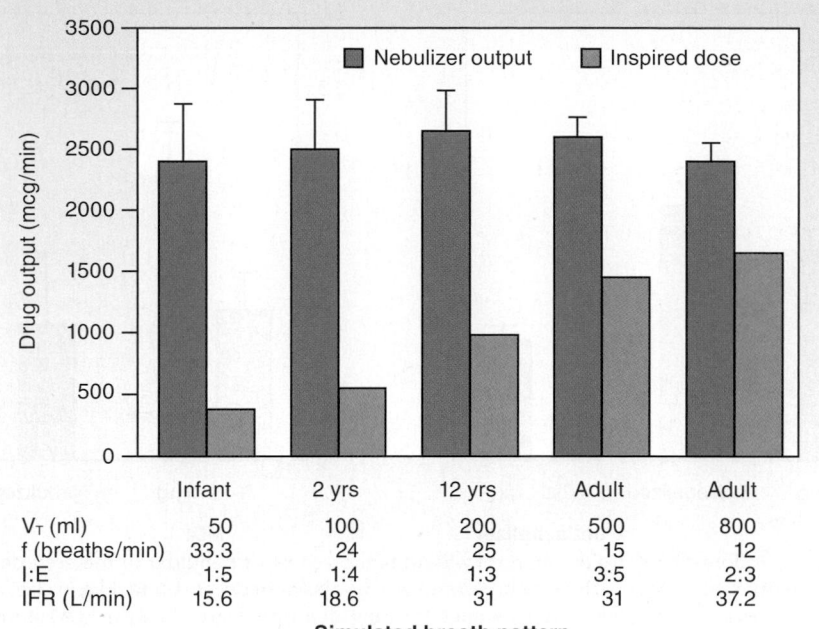

	Infant	2 yrs	12 yrs	Adult	Adult
V_T (ml)	50	100	200	500	800
f (breaths/min)	33.3	24	25	15	12
I:E	1:5	1:4	1:3	3:5	2:3
IFR (L/min)	15.6	18.6	31	31	37.2

Simulated breath pattern

FIGURE 11-2   Assessing nebulizer performance. *F,* Frequency; *I:E,* ratio of inspiratory to expiratory time; *IFR,* inspiratory flow rate; *V_T,* tidal volume.

will probably be safe in infants. In contrast, rationales to reduce drug doses for infants and small children have not been well substantiated in the literature.

Figure 11-2 illustrates the impact of changes in breathing patterns in the transition from infant to child to adult, with a lung simulator inhaling aerosolized drug from a continuous breath-enhanced nebulizer (PARI LC Star; PARI, Starnberg, Germany) producing a relatively consistent output.[7] The drug inhaled at the "mouth" of this in vitro model varies with the different simulated breath patterns, so that the infant and small child are apt to inhale less of the aerosol emitted from the nebulizer than the larger adult. Tidal volume, inspiratory-to-expiratory (I:E) ratio, and inspiratory flow rates are key to the ability to efficiently inhale output from a nebulizer. In infants less than 6 months of age, reduced inspiratory flow rates and broad I:E ratios result in less aerosol inhaled than by a larger child or adult.

These factors may decrease the rate and depth of aerosol deposition to the respiratory tract to as little as 0.1% to 1% of the medication dose placed in a nebulizer, or the dose emitted from a pMDI, regardless of whether the infant is breathing spontaneously or is intubated.[8]

AEROSOL ADMINISTRATION IN NONINTUBATED INFANTS AND CHILDREN

Limited studies are available that directly quantify deposition of aerosols in nonintubated infants and children.

Wildhaber and colleagues[9] studied children, 2 to 9 years of age, with stable asthma inhaling radiolabeled albuterol (salbutamol) from a nebulizer and a pMDI through a nonstatic holding chamber. Mean (absolute dose) total lung deposition expressed as a percentage of the nebulized dose was 5.4% (108 μg) in younger children (<4 years) and 11.1% (222 μg) in older children (>4 years). Mean (absolute dose) total lung deposition expressed as a percentage of the metered dose was 5.4% (21.6 μg) in younger children and 9.6% (38.4 μg) in older children. The authors reported equivalent percentages of total lung deposition of radiolabeled salbutamol aerosolized by either a nebulizer or a pMDI/holding chamber within each age group. However, the delivery rate per minute and the total dose of salbutamol deposited were significantly higher for the nebulizer.

Erzinger[10] studied 8 asymptomatic children between 18 months and 3 years of age with history of recurrent wheeze for the administration of radiolabeled salbutamol with either a vent-assisted nebulizer or a pMDI attached to a holding chamber. After the measurement of aerosol deposition with a gamma camera, they reported that lung deposition with a face mask leak was 0.2% and 0.3% with pMDI and nebulizer, respectively. Screaming children without a face mask leak had 0.6% lung deposition with pMDI and 1.4% with nebulizer. Lung deposition in children who were quietly breathing and without a face mask leak ranged from 4.8% to 8.2%.

DEPOSITION IN INTUBATED AND NONINTUBATED INFANTS

Fok and colleagues[8] measured radioaerosol deposition of Salbutamol by jet nebulizer and pMDIs with Valved Holding Chamber in ventilated and nonventilated infants (1-4 kg)

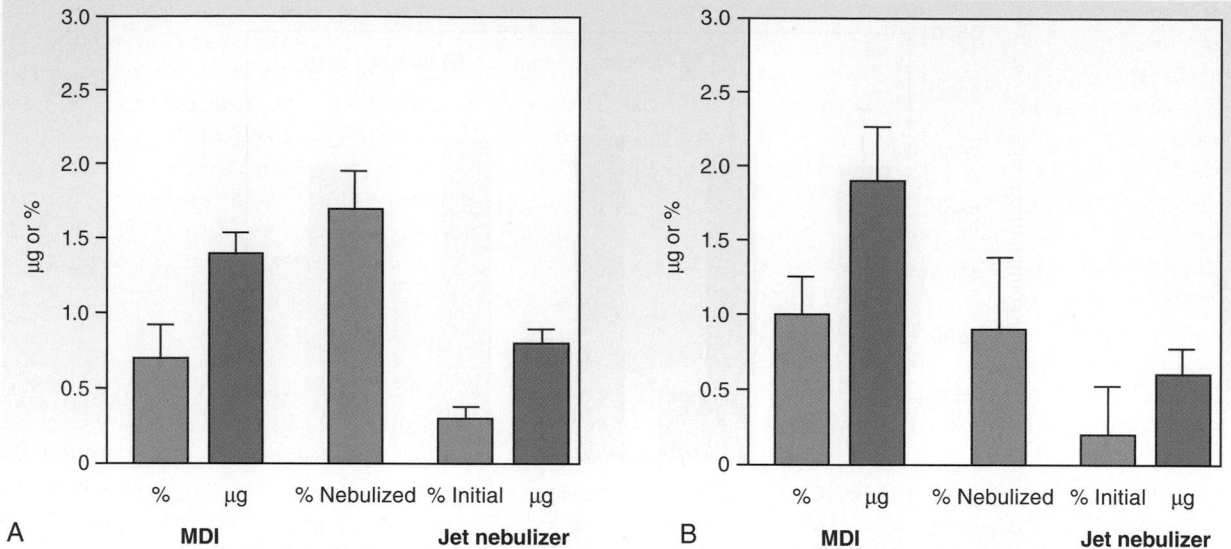

FIGURE 11-3   A dose of 200 μg of albuterol was administered by jet nebulizer or metered-dose inhaler (*MDI*) with chamber to infants with bronchopulmonary dysplasia, between 1 and 4 kg in size, and either ventilated or nonventilated. Mean (SEM) values for lung deposition are shown in (**A**) nonventilated infants (n = 13) and (**B**) ventilated infants (n = 10). Values are given as the percentage of the amount delivered to the infants and, for nebulizers, also as the percentage of the initial nebulizer dose. The absolute amount (μg) of salbutamol deposited in the lungs (*blue columns*) is given for reference.

with bronchopulmonary dysplasia, finding less than 1% of dose delivered to the lung in all cases (Figure 11-3). Delivery of aerosol was low for all delivery systems, and similar whether or not subjects were intubated, with considerable variability across patients. Lung deposition in the ventilated infants was similar to those obtained from previous in vitro, in vivo animal, and indirect human studies.

AEROSOL CHARACTERISTICS

Deposition of Particles

An **aerosol** is a group of particles that remain suspended in air for a relatively long time because of low terminal settling velocity. The terminal settling velocity of a particle is the velocity at which the particle will fall, because of gravity, through the air; it is related to the size and density of the particle.[9] Aerosols are also described by their geometric standard deviation (GSD), a measure of the particle size distribution. A monodisperse aerosol has a GSD less than 1.22, and a heterodisperse aerosol has a GSD greater than 1.22. Monodisperse aerosols are used for diagnostic and research purposes. Most therapeutic aerosols are heterodisperse, which means they contain a wider range of particle sizes. The greater the MMAD, the larger the median particle size, the greater the GSD, and the more heterodisperse is the aerosol. The particle size and size distribution of an aerosol are the major factors determining deposition efficiency and distribution in the lung.[11]

Gravitational sedimentation occurs when the aerosol particles lose inertia and settle onto the airway as a result of gravitational forces. The greater the mass of the particle,

the faster it settles, affecting particles with diameters of 0.5 μm or less. Breath holding for 4 to 10 seconds increases the residence time for particles in the lung, extending the time allowed for deposition through gravitational sedimentation, especially in the last six generations of the airway.[12] A breath hold can increase deposition of an aerosol by up to 10% and is associated with a shift of deposition from the central to peripheral airways. This marginal increase in deposition may explain why breath holding has not been demonstrated to significantly improve the clinical response to aerosolized medications. Breath holding after inhalation does not appear to influence the response to administration of a bronchodilator given by DPI to children with asthma.[13]

Inertial impaction is the primary mechanism for deposition of particles with diameters of 5 μm or greater and an important mechanism for particles as small as 2 μm in diameter. A particle traveling in a stream of gas that is diverted by a turn in the airway tends to continue on its initial path, impacting with and depositing on the surface of the airway. This tendency increases with the velocity and mass of the particle. The higher the inspiratory flow of gas, such as during crying, the greater the velocity and inertia of the particles, which increases the tendency for even smaller particles to impact and deposit in large airways. Common factors that increase the rate of inertial impaction of particles larger than 2 μm include turbulent flow, bifurcations, complex passageways, narrow or obstructed airways, and inspiratory flows greater than 30 L/min.

Diffusion, also known as brownian movement, is the primary mechanism for deposition of particles less than

3 μm in diameter in the airway. As gas reaches the more distal regions of the lung, gas flow ceases. Aerosol particles bounce against air molecules and each other and deposit on contact with the airway surfaces. Particle deposition in the particle size range of 0.5 to 3.0 μm is reported to be divided between the central and peripheral airways.[11]

Aerosol droplets in the respirable range (MMAD, 1.0 to 5.0 μm) have a better chance to deposit in the lower respiratory tract than larger or smaller particles.[11,12] For particles greater than 1.0 μm, the depth of penetration into the lung is inversely proportional to the size of the particles, whereas particles less than 1.0 μm are so small, light, and stable that a significant proportion entering the lung do not deposit and are exhaled. However, nanoparticles less than 0.1 μm have greater lung deposition than common medical aerosols; very large particles may be filtered out by impacting on surfaces en route and "rain out" before reaching the airway.

Translocation of Aerosols

To be effective as a therapeutic agent, an aerosol medication first must efficiently deposit in the airway and then must translocate across the mucous barrier, retaining bioactivity in this process. The optimal site of action depends on the agent administered. Bronchodilators and steroids need to reach the epithelium to be effective. Aerosolized antibiotics and mucolytics are most effective when dispersed in infected airway secretions at sites of maximal airway obstruction. Gene transfer therapy must not only access the epithelium through the mucous barrier but must then gain access to the submucous glands or basal progenitor cells of the epithelium.

Particle size, charge, and solubility, and the biophysical properties of secretions, all affect the ability of an aerosol to penetrate the mucous barrier. A consistent inverse relationship exists between molecular mass and particle diffusion through mucus, especially at molecular masses greater than 30 kD.[14] Turbulent flow and airway obstruction can affect the airway deposition pattern. Other factors limiting efficacy, especially of macromolecules, include binding to constituents of mucus, including mucin and DNA, and the breakdown of bioactive molecules by proteases and other enzymes. Translocation of macromolecules can be further compromised by the hypersecretion that accompanies inflammation and chronic pulmonary disease. These secretions can be a barrier to the penetration of any aerosol.[15,16]

The antibiotic diffusion barrier represented by mucin may be significant in vitro, particularly for nebulized antibiotics.[17] Some antibiotics bind to whole cystic fibrosis sputum, with the degree of binding dependent on the DNA concentration and the presence of acidic mucins.[18] Mucolytic agents might be able to increase diffusion and increase antibiotic levels in the sputum.[19] Similarly, treatment of the sputum-covered cells with recombinant human deoxyribonuclease at 50 μg/ml significantly improved gene transfer in patients with cystic fibrosis (CF).[20]

Factors promoting translocation include an effective surfactant layer and increased particle retention time. Discontinuity of mucus in the airway may assist deposition and translocation. The translocation of particles through the mucus layer is likely to depend partly on the presence of bronchial surfactant. In vitro experiments have shown that pulmonary surfactant promotes the displacement of some particles from air to the aqueous phase and that the extent of particle immersion depends on the surface tension of the surface-active film.[21,22]

Drug Dose Distribution

Dosing of aerosolized medication is an imprecise science. It is unclear how much, if any, drug is delivered to targeted areas of the lung with progressive disease states or during acute exacerbations. All the factors previously discussed decrease the rate and depth of aerosol deposition to the respiratory tract to as little as 0.5% of the medication dose placed in a nebulizer, regardless of whether the patient is breathing spontaneously or intubated. High flow increases aerosol impaction in larger airways, whereas lower inspiratory flow with high-resistance DPIs can reduce the amount of medication inhaled.

Humidity also influences medication delivery, especially for DPIs and in ventilator circuits. Droplets of solution may evaporate or grow, depending on the water content and temperature of the gas, and powder can clump or aggregate in high humidity. High ambient humidity can also result from a child exhaling into a DPI or from a DPI being brought into a warm indoor environment from the cold outdoors (or from inside a car on a very cold day), with condensation forming inside the device.[23]

Drug formulations dictate in part which aerosol options are available for medication delivery. Most solutions can be nebulized if the medication is soluble (corticosteroids are a notable exception), but the physical characteristics of the solution (or suspension) can affect particle size and nebulizer output. Furthermore, some macromolecules may not enter suspension well and can shatter into nonbioactive forms with the force of air required to generate an aerosol. Because of development costs, many aerosol medications are initially developed as nebulizer solutions and later reformulated for DPI or pMDI delivery.

Theoretically, if a particle can be milled to a respirable size while retaining bioactivity, it can be delivered by DPI or pMDI. However, development costs are greater for these devices than for nebulizer solutions. At present, DPI formulations are limited to only a few preparations. With more effective DPI devices being developed and the need to eliminate chlorofluorocarbon (CFC)–based propellants in accordance with the Montreal Protocol on Substances that Deplete the Ozone Layer (see http://www.unep.org/OZONE/pdfs/Montreal-Protocol2000.pdf), it is anticipated that a greater variety of DPI medications and devices will soon be commercially available. A greater variety of formulations are available for pMDIs, and more are being developed for the newer hydrofluoro-alkane (HFA)–based pMDIs.

AEROSOL DELIVERY

The most common methods of generating therapeutic aerosols are with **nebulizers** (jet pneumatic, ultrasonic [USN], and vibrating mesh [VMN]) and inhalers (pMDIs and DPIs). Older methods based on the spray "atomizer" or the addition of medications to room humidifiers are ineffective, and their use should be discouraged.

Pneumatic Nebulizers

Pneumatic nebulizers use the Bernoulli principle to drive a high-pressure gas through a restricted orifice and draw the fluid into the gas stream from a capillary tube immersed in the solution. Shearing of the fluid stream in the jet forms the aerosol stream that impacts against a baffle removing larger particles that may return to the reservoir.

An effective pneumatic nebulizer should deliver more than 50% of its total dose as aerosol in the respirable range in 10 minutes or less of nebulization time. Performance varies with diluent volume, operating flow, pressures, gas density, and manufacturer.[24] The amount of drug that is nebulized increases as the volume of diluent is increased. The residual volume of medicine that remains in commercial small-volume nebulizers (SVNs) varies from 0.5 to 2.0 ml depending on the specific device; thus increasing the fill volume allows a greater proportion of the active medication to be nebulized. For example, with a residual volume of 1 ml, a fill of 2 ml would leave only 50% of the nebulizer charge available for nebulization, whereas a fill of 4 ml would make 3 ml, or 75%, of the medication available for nebulization. No significant difference in clinical response has been shown with varying diluent volumes and flow rates.[25]

Droplet size and nebulization times are both inversely proportional to gas flow through the jet. Proper operating gas flow varies with each model of nebulizer, from 2 L/min (MiniHEART, Westmed Inc., Tucson, AZ) to 10 L/min (Misty Max, Cardinal Health, Dublin, OH). For any given nebulizer, the higher the flow to the nebulizer, the smaller the particle size generated and the shorter the time required to nebulize the full dose.[26,27] Nebulizers that produce smaller particle sizes by use of baffles such as one-way valves may have a lower total drug output per minute than the same nebulizer without baffling, requiring more time to deliver a standard dose of medication.

Gas density affects both aerosol generation and delivery of aerosol to the lungs, especially with low-density helium–oxygen mixtures. The lower the density of a carrier gas, the less turbulent the flow, which theoretically decreases aerosol impaction, allowing more aerosol to pass beyond an obstructed airway.[28] This is true with virtually any aerosol, with high-concentration heliox increasing aerosol delivery by as much as 50%. Heliox concentrations as low as 40% can improve aerosol delivery. When using heliox to drive a jet nebulizer, the aerosol output is much less than with air or oxygen, requiring double the flow to produce a comparable output of respirable aerosol per minute. Thus, although helium can increase the amount of aerosol reaching the lungs, it impairs the production of aerosol from jet nebulizers.[29]

Humidity and temperature affect the particle size and the concentration of drug remaining in the nebulizer. Evaporation of water and adiabatic expansion of gas can reduce the temperature of the aerosol to as much as 5°C below ambient temperature. Aerosol particles entrained into a warm and fully saturated gas stream increase in size. These particles can also stick together, further increasing the MMAD, and with a DPI this can severely compromise the output of respirable particles.

With three different fill volumes, albuterol delivery from a nebulizer was found to cease after the onset of inconsistent nebulization (sputtering).[30] Aerosol output declined by one half within 20 seconds of the onset of sputtering. The concentration of albuterol in the nebulizer cup increased significantly once the aerosol output declined, and further weight loss in the nebulizer was caused primarily by evaporation. The conclusion was that aerosolization past the point of initial jet nebulizer sputter is ineffective.

Nebulizer selection affects aerosol delivery. Only nebulizers that have been shown to work reliably under specific conditions, with specific medications, and with specific compressors should be used.[31] When used to treat small children or during mechanical ventilation, nebulizers producing aerosols with an MMAD of 0.5 to 3.0 μm are more likely to achieve greater deposition in the lower respiratory tract.[5]

Continuous aerosol generation wastes medication because the aerosol is produced throughout the respiratory cycle and is largely lost to the atmosphere (Figure 11-4, *A*). Patients with an I:E ratio of 1:3 lose a minimum of 75% of the aerosol generated to the atmosphere. If only 50% of the dose is available from the nebulizer as aerosol in the respiratory range and only 25% of that is inhaled by the patient, it is clear that less than 10% deposition is typically measured with nebulizer therapy.

A reservoir on the expiratory limb of the nebulizer conserves drug aerosol.[31] A simple approach is to place 6 inches of aerosol tubing on the expiratory side of the nebulizer T-tube device.

On the other hand, breath-enhanced nebulizers utilize a one-way inspiratory valve on the inlet of the nebulizer, and another on the mouthpiece or mask directing exhaled aerosol away from the nebulizer.[32,33] Theoretically, breath-enhanced nebulizers provide more aerosol when ambient air vents through the nebulizer during inhalation, and less aerosol is cleared from the device when when exhaled gas is routed out the expiratory one-way valve in the mouthpiece, Thus, breath-enhanced nebulizers may increase the inhaled dose by as much as 50% compared with continuous simple jet nebulizers (see Figure 11-4, *B*).

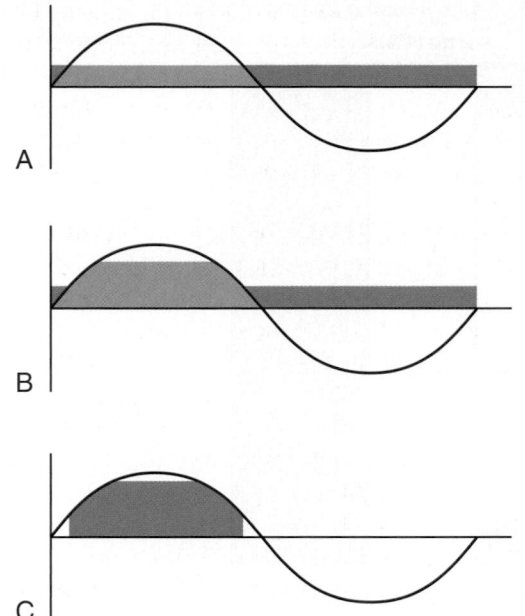

FIGURE 11-4 Aerosol generated and inhaled during nebulization therapy. **A,** Continuous nebulization; **B,** breath-enhanced nebulization; **C,** breath-actuated nebulization.

Several systems integrating a bag reservoir and one-way valves, such as the Piper (Piper Medical Products, Carmichael, CA) or Circulaire (Westmed, Tucson, AZ) systems collect aerosol in simple bag reservoirs during exhalation, allowing the small particles to remain in suspension for inhalation with the next breath while larger particles rain out in the bag or on the valves. The valves direct the aerosol from the reservoir to the patient and from the patient to the air, without exhaling back into the reservoir. These systems are also more efficient than simple jet nebulizers.

As another alternative to continuous nebulization, a three-way thumb control port, placed between the oxygen tubing and the gas inlet of the nebulizer, allows the patient to direct gas to the nebulizer only on inspiration. This improves efficiency by as much as threefold, but only if there is good hand–breath coordination. This increase of inhaled dose comes at the cost of longer administration time. An alternative to having the patient manually control when nebulization occurs, a mechanical or electronic design can automate breath actuation.[34]

Breath-actuated nebulization occurs by generating aerosol in synchrony with inspiration. Nebulizing only during inspiration is more efficient than continuous or vented systems (see Figure 11-4, C). Previous studies showed that breath-actuated nebulizers (BANs) produce smaller particles and more lung dose than continuous pneumatic nebulizers.[32,35-37] However, to nebulize the same total dose placed in the nebulizer, the breath-actuated system may take two to four times longer than the continuous nebulizer.[32] The AeroEclipse (Monaghan Medical, Plattsburgh, NY) is a purely mechanical pneumatic device that generates aerosol when the patient produces

sufficient inspiratory flow (approximately 20 LPM) during inspiration. On the other technical extreme, the I-Neb with adaptive aerosol delivery (AAD) systems (Philips Respironics, Murrysville, PA) and Akita (Activaero, Wohra, DE) use a microprocessor and pressure transducer to sense inspiratory efforts and regulate nebulization during the first half of or all of inspiration.

A number of in vitro studies have shown greater deposition in adults and large children with BANs. Lin et al[38] studied the influence of nebulizer type with different pediatric aerosol masks on drug deposition in a model of a spontaneously breathing small child. After modeling toddler breathing patterns, they demonstrated substantial reductions in inhaled dose with a mechanical BAN, rather than simple continuous nebulizers, despite the BAN appearing to be actuating with every inspiratory maneuver.[38] This suggests that the appearance of breath actuation in vivo with young children may not ensure superior aerosol delivery.

There is no randomized trial in the literature showing greater bronchodilator efficacy with breath-actuated nebulizers than with pneumatic nebulizers. In a recent clinical study by Sabato et al.,[36] it was reported that the admission rate with the breath-actuated nebulizer and pneumatic jet nebulizer were both 40%. Lin and Huang[37] compared a breath-actuated nebulizer with a constant-flow pneumatic nebulizer in the treatment of children with acute asthma and showed a change in pulse rate 5 minutes after the treatment. Although these studies provide us with valuable information about breath-actuated nebulizers, future research is warranted to understand the efficacy, safety, and satisfaction measures of breath-actuated nebulizers in the treatment of children.[39,40]

A typical dose of albuterol sulfate solution is 2.5 mg (2500 μg). If only 34% (850 μg) leaves the nebulizer and is inhaled by the patient, and some of that drug deposits in the upper airways (50 μg) and is exhaled (500 μg), it should not be surprising that 12% deposition of the nominal dose, typical of ambulatory adult patients, would be 300 μg (Figure 11-5). In small children and infants, deposition can be less than 1%, representing less than 25 μg delivered to the lung.

Gas pressure and flow affect particle size distribution and output. A nebulizer that produces an MMAD of 2.5 μm when driven by a gas source at 50 psi with a flow rate of 6 to 10 L/min may produce an MMAD greater than 8 μm when used with a home compressor (or ventilator) providing only 10 psi. Insufficient flow can result in negligible respirable nebulizer output. As a consequence, nebulizers used for home care should be matched to the compressor on the basis of data supplied by the manufacturer so that the specific combination of equipment will efficiently nebulize the desired medications prescribed. European standards require equipment manufacturers to demonstrate that their nebulizer and compressor combination can nebulize the appropriate fill volume of drug

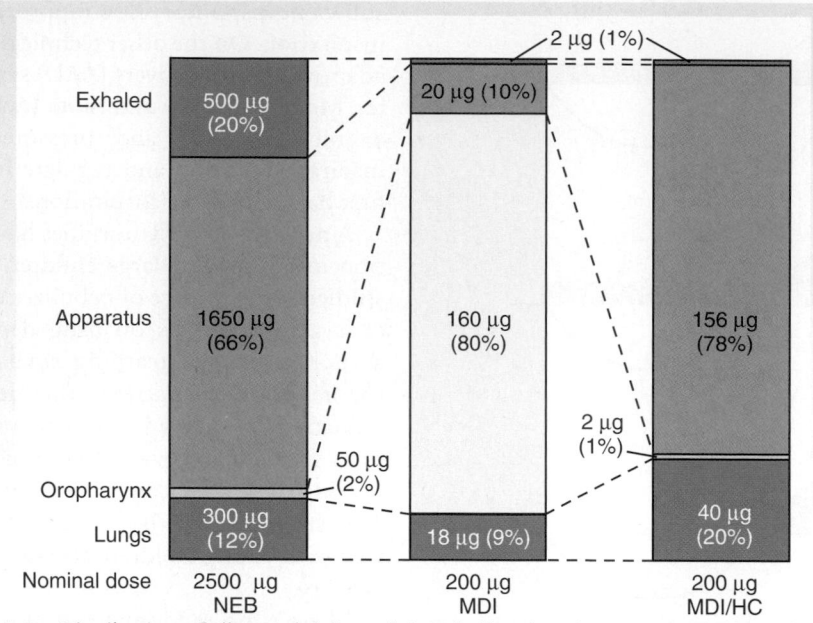

FIGURE 11-5 Distribution of albuterol delivered via nebulizer (*NEB*), pressurized metered-dose inhaler (*MDI*), and pressurized metered-dose inhaler with holding chamber (*MDI/HC*).

within 10 minutes, deliver more than 50% of the drug in the nebulizer as respirable particles, and identify all medications with which the nebulizer and compressor might reliably meet these two criteria.[41] Until such time that standards are required in the United States, clinicians should ascertain that patients are prescribed only systems that have been demonstrated to meet these criteria.

Repeated use of a nebulizer will not alter the MMAD, or output, as long as it is properly cleaned (rinsed and dried between treatments). Failure to clean the nebulizer properly results in degradation of performance, from clogging the jet (Venturi) nebulizer to increasing bacterial contamination, and buildup of electrostatic charge in the device.[42] The Centers for Disease Control and Prevention (CDC) recommend cleaning and disinfecting nebulizers or rinsing with sterile water between uses, and then air drying.[43] Storage of multidose solutions at room temperature and reuse of syringes to measure the solution represent the main sources of nebulizer microbial contamination.[44] Refrigerating the solution and disposing of syringes every 24 hours help to eliminate bacterial contamination.

Large-Volume Nebulizer

The large-volume pneumatic nebulizer (LVN) has a reservoir volume greater than 100 ml and can be used to administer an aerosol solution over a prolonged time. Indications for using an LVN to administer a bland solution (i.e., sterile water or saline) include the need to humidify medical gases when the upper airway is bypassed, control stridor with a cold aerosol, and induce sputum. Because nebulizers provide a route of transmission for pathogens, pass-over humidifiers and heater wire humidifiers are preferable.

LVNs work on the same principles as SVNs, except that the residual volume is greater and the effects of evaporation, changing the concentration of medication over time, are more profound.

Caution should be exercised when using LVNs with incubators or hoods because of the noise produced. The American Academy of Pediatrics recommends a sound level less than 58 dB to avoid hearing loss in patients in incubators and hoods. Many LVNs are designed to deliver controlled concentrations of oxygen and use a Venturi system to entrain air into the stream of gas administered to the patient. Standard entrainment nebulizers may deliver a fractional concentration of delivered oxygen approaching 1.00 but cannot provide a fractional concentration of inspired oxygen (FiO_2) greater than 0.40. High-flow nebulizers are designed to deliver high flow rates of oxygen, bringing the FiO_2 up to 0.60 to 0.80. Closed dilution and gas injection nebulizers provide high-flow access to the nebulizer from two gas sources, allowing gas to mix without compromising FiO_2.

Some LVNs are used for continuous medication delivery over a prolonged period. These nebulizers are also powered by a compressed gas source, and evidence indicates that continuous nebulization is safe, effective, and less time consuming compared with intermittent nebulization in the treatment of patients with asthma.[45-47] However, use of these nebulizers for a prolonged period results in changes in drug concentration over time. Therefore, empting and refilling the LVN every 5 hours are recommended.[48]

Small-Particle Aerosol Generator

The small-particle aerosol generator (SPAG; Valeant Pharmaceuticals International, Aliso Viejo, CA) is a jet

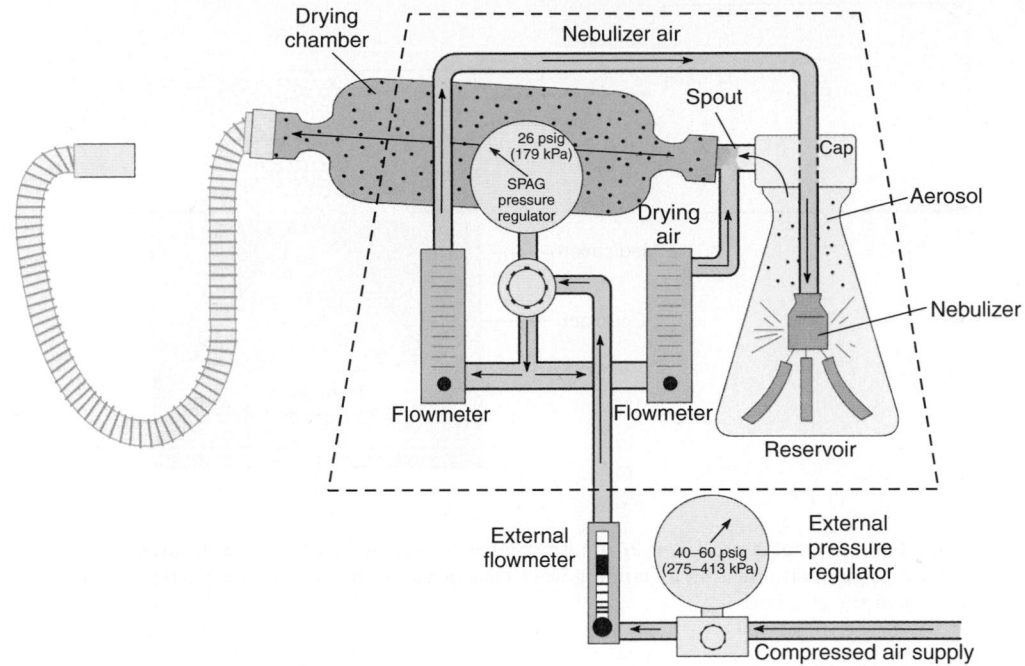

FIGURE 11-6 Diagram of small-particle aerosol generator (*SPAG*), which may be used with a hood, tent, mask, or ventilator. *psig,* Pounds-force per square inch gauge.

aerosol generator used to nebulize the antiviral agent ribavirin (Figure 11-6). The SPAG incorporates a secondary drying chamber that reduces the MMAD to 1.2 μm, with a GSD of 1.4 and relatively high output. The SPAG reduces the 50 psi of line pressure medical gas to 26 psi, which supplies gas to separate flow meters controlling flow to the nebulizer and the drying chamber. As the aerosol leaves the medication reservoir, it enters the long cylindrical drying chamber, where additional flow of dry gas reduces the size of the aerosol particles through evaporation. The nebulizer flow is adjusted to maximum, approximately 7 L/min, with a total flow from both flow meters equal to at least 15 L/min.

Ribavirin is an expensive antiviral agent that has been used to treat high-risk infants and children with severe respiratory syncytial viral infections. The effectiveness of ribavirin is poor, with few data to support its use for such a broad population. In addition, concerns about the secondhand exposure of health care workers to ribavirin have resulted in recommendations to avoid open-air administration, use specific room filtration techniques, and use personal protective equipment for staff and visitors.[49] Ribavirin tends to precipitate into a thick powder that forms on the surfaces of tubing and tents. Recommendations for ribavirin use are now limited to treatment of patients who have severe respiratory syncytial virus infection and require mechanical ventilation.[50] Risks of using ribavirin during mechanical ventilation include delivering excessive volume and pressure, so that care should be taken to place and frequently change filters in the expiratory limb of the circuit.[51]

Ultrasonic Nebulizers

The ultrasonic nebulizer (USN) uses a piezoelectric crystal vibrating at a high frequency (1.3 to 1.4 mHz) to create an aerosol. The crystal transducer converts electricity to sound waves, which creates motion and standing waves in the liquid immediately above the transducer, forming a geyser of droplets (Figure 11-7). USNs are capable of a broader range of aerosol output (0.5 to 7.0 ml/min) and higher aerosol densities than most conventional jet nebulizers. Particle size is affected by frequency, whereas output is affected by the amplitude of the signal. Particle size is inversely proportional to the frequency of vibrations. Frequency is device specific and is not user adjustable. For example, the DeVilbiss Porta-Sonic (DeVilbiss Healthcare, Somerset, PA) operates at a frequency of 2.25 MHz and produces a MMAD of 2.5 μm, and the DeVilbiss Pulmo-Sonic operates at 1.25 MHz and produces particles in the 4- to 6-μm range. Large-volume USNs, used mainly for bland aerosol therapy or sputum induction, incorporate air blowers to carry the mist to the patient. Low flow rates of gas through the nebulizer are associated with higher mist density. Unlike jet nebulizers, which cool through evaporation, USNs increase the temperature of the drug during use, which is associated with increased concentration; however, some medications may be denatured by the increased operating temperature.[52]

A number of small-volume USNs are available for aerosol drug delivery.[53] Unlike the larger reservoir USNs, these systems do not always use a water-filled couplant compartment; instead, medication is placed directly into the manifold on top of the transducer connected to a battery power

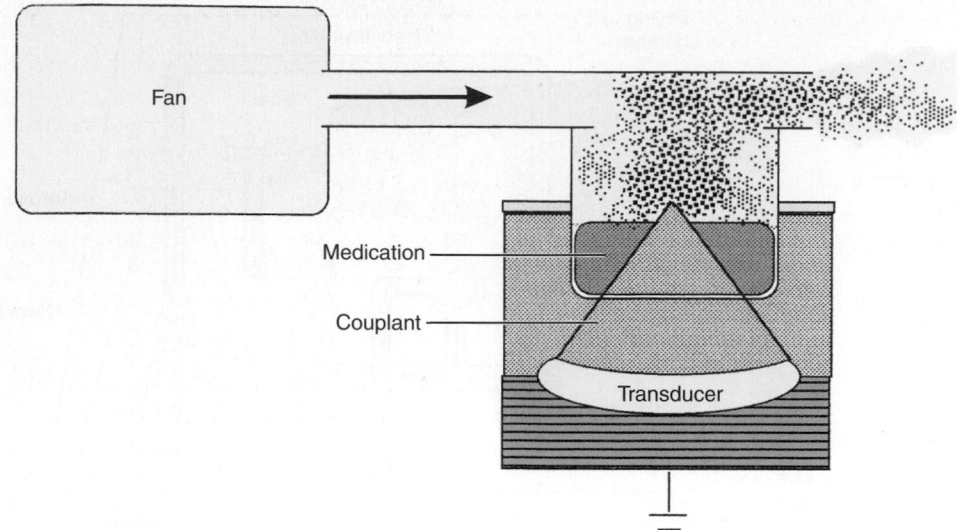

FIGURE 11-7   Aerosol is produced in an ultrasonic nebulizer by focusing sound waves, which disrupt the surface of the fluid, creating a standing wave that produces droplets. Flow from a fan pushes the aerosol out of the chamber.

source. The patient's inspiratory flow draws the aerosol from the nebulizer into the lungs. As the USN operates, the aerosol remains in the medication cup/chamber until a flow of gas draws the aerosol from the nebulizer. Thus, during exhalation, aerosol generated by the USN remains in the chamber, awaiting the next breath.

Small-volume USNs may have less residual drug volume than SVNs, reducing the need for a large quantity of diluent to ensure delivery of drugs. The contained portable power source provides convenience and mobility. These advantages of USNs may be outweighed by their high cost, however, which can be several orders of magnitude greater than that of pMDI therapy. USNs have been promoted for administration of a wide variety of formulations, ranging from bronchodilators to antiinflammatory agents and antibiotics.[54] In general, however, USNs have been shown to be less effective than other aerosol delivery devices.[55] This is particularly true with suspensions.

Several hazards, in addition to bacterial contamination, are associated with using a USN. The high-density aerosol from USNs has been associated with bronchospasm, increased airway resistance, and irritability in a substantial portion of the population. Overhydration may occur when using a USN for prolonged treatment of a neonate or small child or patients with renal insufficiency. The structure of the medication may be disrupted by acoustic power output rated greater than 50 W/cm^2.[56,57] Several ventilator manufacturers have provided USNs for administration of aerosols during mechanical ventilation. The advantage of the USN during ventilation is that no driving gas flow is added to the circuit, changing ventilator parameters and alarm settings.[58] Disadvantages may be the weight of the USN in the ventilator circuit, a tendency to heat up over time, and the potential for reduced therapeutic efficacy of medications.

Vibrating Mesh Nebulizers

Vibrating mesh nebulizers (VMNs) use electricity to stimulate a piezo element to vibrate a ceramic or metal disk, which in turn presses or pumps medication through multiple orifices. VMNs are of two types: Passive (static) mesh nebulizers use an ultrasonic horn to generate vibrations that produce aerosol to be inhaled by pushing medication through the static mesh, whereas active mesh nebulizers use a piezo ceramic element positioned surrounding a dome-shaped aperture plate containing 1000 to 4000 tapered apertures to vibrate the mesh at a frequency greater than 120 kHz, creating a micropumping action that makes liquid pass through the apertures and break up into fine droplets.[33] Particle size is dependent on the diameter of the orifices through which the medication passes, and VMNs can be manufactured to produce specific MMADs between 2 and 6 μm. VMNs typically operate at one tenth the frequency and consume less than one tenth the power of a USN, so medications are not heated or reconcentrated. This class of nebulizer can efficiently nebulize suspensions, with mean particle sizes that are smaller than the diameter of the apertures. These nebulizers are quite efficient, having residual drug volumes of medication ranging from 1 to 100 μL. Because the VMN does not add gas to the patient airway or ventilator circuit, greater aerosol concentrations can be reached than with jet nebulizers. VMNs produce the same size aerosol particles with air, oxygen, or helium. Handheld VMN nebulizers tend to be much more efficient than continuous jet nebulizers or USNs, with inhaled mass ranging from 25% to 55%. When used with mechanical ventilators, VMNs do not change volumes or flows.

Technique

The effectiveness of aerosol therapy with nebulizers can be optimized using the right technique. Box 11-2 describes

Box 11-2	Technique for Using Nebulizers

1. Assemble the tubing or cable, the nebulizer, and the mouthpiece or mask.
2. Place the prescribed amount of medication in the nebulizer's reservoir.
3. For a pneumatic nebulizer:
   - Connect the tubing to the flow meter or compressor.
   - Set the flow according to the manufacturer's recommendation (often 6-10 L/min).
4. For a vibrating mesh or small ultrasonic nebulizer:
   - Connect a clean nebulizer/medication reservoir to the mask or mouthpiece.
   - Attach the nebulizer/reservoir to the electronic controller.
   - Attach the nebulizer to a power source or make sure the device's battery has a sufficient charge.
5. Instruct the patient to sit in an upright position, as tolerated.
6. Apply the mouthpiece or mask and encourage the patient to breathe through the mouth. If an artificial airway is used, make sure the nebulizer is positioned appropriately and does not put undue pressure on the airway.
7. Encourage relaxed tidal breathing with low inspiratory flow rates and occasional deep breaths.
8. Operate the nebulizer in an upright position, 45 degrees from vertical.
9. Run the nebulizer until the onset of sputter or until aerosol is no longer produced.
10. At the conclusion of therapy, rinse, wash, disinfect, and air dry the nebulizer/reservoir or dispose of it.
11. Do not submerge the electronic controller or compressor in water or disinfectant.
12. Store the nebulizer in a clean, dry place.

Box 11-3	Cleaning and Disinfection of Nebulizers for Home Use[64]

After each use:
- Disassemble the nebulizer and mouthpiece or mask.
- Wash them in warm, soapy water.
- Rinse with tap water.
- Shake off the excess water.
- Place the parts on a clean, absorbent towel and allow them to air dry.
- Reassemble the nebulizer and store it in a clean, dry place.

Once a day:
- After washing the nebulizer and mouthpiece or mask, place them in a disinfectant solution to soak for 1 hour.
- Rinse with sterile or distilled water.
- Shake off the excess water and allow the parts to air dry.
- Reassemble the nebulizer and store it in a clean, dry place.

Some types of homemade disinfecting solutions:
- 1 oz quaternary ammonium compound (QAC) to 1 oz distilled water; discard weekly.
- 1 part vinegar (5% acetic acid) to 3 parts hot water; discard after each use.
- 1 teaspoon household chlorine bleach to 1 gallon of water; discard after use.

the optimal technique with each type of nebulizer used in the treatment of children with pulmonary diseases.

Care and Cleaning

In order to limit the transmission of airborne pathogens, cleaning and disinfection of nebulizers are essential. When pneumatic nebulizers are used at the hospital, they should be changed every 24 hours or at a frequency determined by the infection control team of the hospital.[33,43,59-63] Also, pneumatic nebulizers should be cleaned, rinsed with sterile water, and air dried after each treatment.[33,59,61,62] Box 11-3 describes cleaning and disinfection procedures of nebulizers for home use. Cleaning and disinfection procedures of vibrating mesh and ultrasonic nebulizers should be done based on the manufacturer's recommendations.[33,59]

Pressurized Metered-Dose Inhalers

The **pressurized metered-dose inhaler** (pMDI) is the most commonly prescribed device for aerosol delivery. pMDIs are used to administer bronchodilators, anticholinergics, and antiinflammatory agents. More drug formulations are available for administration by pMDIs than by any other nebulization system. Properly used, pMDIs are at least as effective as other nebulizers for drug delivery.[65] Therefore pMDIs are often the preferred method for delivering bronchodilators to spontaneously breathing, as well as intubated, ventilated patients.

A pMDI is a pressurized canister containing a drug in the form of a micronized powder or solution that is suspended with a mixture of propellants along with a surfactant or a dispersal agent (Figure 11-8).[5] Dispersing agents are present in concentrations equal to or greater than that of the medication. In some patients these agents may be associated with coughing and wheezing.[66] The bulk of the spray, up to 80% by weight, is composed of a propellant, typically a CFC such as Freon. Adverse reactions to CFCs are extremely rare.[67-69] More recently pMDIs have been developed to use more environmentally safe propellants such as HFA-134a. As HFA pMDIs are introduced, they represent newer technologies with potentially improved performance.

The output volume of the pMDI varies from 30 to 100 μl and contains 20 μg to 5 mg of drug. Lung deposition is estimated to be between 10% and 25% in adults, with high intersubject variability largely dependent on user technique. When proper technique is used, the pMDI delivers as much or more of the dose of medication to the lung than an SVN.

The pMDI canister contains a pressurized mixture containing propellants, surfactants, preservatives, and sometimes flavoring agents, with approximately 1% of the total

Metered-dose inhaler

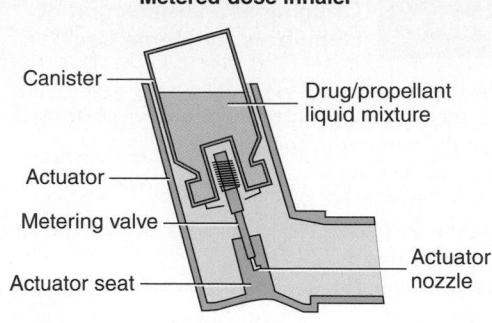

Metered-valve function

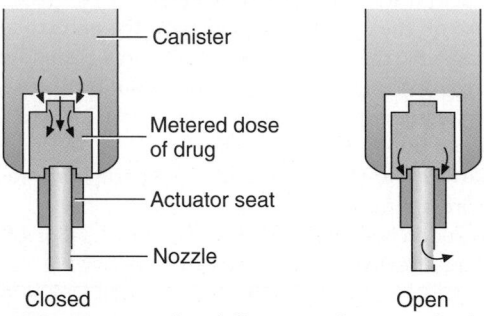

FIGURE 11-8 Cross-sectional diagrams of a pressurized metered-dose inhaler.

Box 11-4	Optimal Self-Administration Technique for Using Pressurized Metered-Dose Inhaler

- Warm pMDI canister to hand or body temperature.
- Shake the canister vigorously.
- Assemble the apparatus and uncap the mouthpiece.
- Ensure that no loose objects are in the device that could be aspirated or could obstruct outflow.
- Open the mouth wide.
- Keep the tongue from obstructing the mouthpiece.
- Hold the pMDI vertically with the outlet aimed at the mouth.
- Place the canister outlet between the lips, or position the pMDI 4 cm (two fingers) away from the mouth.*
- Breathe out normally.
- Begin to breathe in slowly (< 0.5 L/sec).
- Squeeze and actuate ("fire") the pMDI.
- Continue to inhale to total lung capacity.
- Hold breath for 4 to 10 seconds.
- Wait 30 seconds between inhalations (actuations).
- Disassemble the apparatus, and recap the mouthpiece.

pMDI, Pressurized metered-dose inhaler.
*Open-mouth technique is not recommended with ipratropium bromide.

---

contents being active drug. This mixture is released from the canister through a metering valve and stem that fits into an actuator boot, designed and tested by the manufacturer to work with the specific formulation. Small changes in actuator design can change the characteristics and output of the aerosol from a pMDI.

Up to 80% of the emitted dose from a pMDI impacts in the oropharynx. Actuation of a pMDI into a valved holding chamber decreases impaction losses by reducing the velocity of the aerosol jet,[5] allowing time for evaporation of the propellants and for the particles to "age" before impacting on a surface. The nominal dose of medication with a pMDI is much smaller than with a nebulizer. The quantity of albuterol exiting the actuator nozzle of a pMDI is 100 μg with each actuation, or 90 μg from the opening of the actuator boot; this is how pMDI aerosol actuations are characterized in the United States. Thus a dose of 2 to 4 actuations (200- to 400-μg nominal dose) is typically used. In ambulatory patients, 10% deposition may deliver a dose of 20 to 40 μg for an effective bronchodilator response.

Technique

Effective use of a pMDI is technique dependent. Up to two thirds of patients who use pMDIs and health professionals who prescribe pMDIs do not perform the procedure well enough to derive benefit from the medication.[70,71] Box 11-4 outlines the recommended steps for self-administering a bronchodilator with a pMDI.[72] Good patient instruction

can take 10 to 30 minutes and should include demonstration, return demonstration, practice, and confirmation of patient performance (demonstration placebo units should be available for this purpose). Repeated instruction with every visit improves performance.[73]

All pMDIs require priming, firing one to four actuations, before first use, and after the device has not been used for a prolonged period (1 to 4 days). The HFA pMDIs require less frequent priming than CFC devices (check the label for each specific device).

Problems with home use of pMDI devices include not only poor technique but also poor storage. The pMDI should always be stored with cap on, both to prevent foreign objects from entering the boot and to reduce humidity and microbial contamination.[73]

Each type of pMDI contains a specific number of actuations (between 60 and 400 actuations). After those doses have been administered the pMDI will continue to actuate, with or without medication emitted (tailing-off effect), placing the patient at risk of not receiving prescribed medication. Pressurized MDIs should always be discarded when empty to avoid administering propellant without medication. The suggestion that pMDIs can be tested for drug remaining by floating the canister in water has proven not to be accurate and to compromise performance of the pMDI.

It is more accurate for the patient or parent to note when the medication was started, the number of doses to be taken each day, and the number of doses in the canister, and from this information to calculate a discard date.

For example, if 200 actuations are in a canister (information always indicated on the canister label) and 4 "puffs" are taken per day, the canister should be discarded 50 days, or 7 weeks, after the start date. This discard date should be written on the canister label on the day the new canister is started. A more user-friendly alternative is to attach a dose counter to the pMDI. In the near future, the U.S. Food and Drug Administration will require new pMDIs to be manufactured with dose counters. Because pMDIs deposit up to 80% of their emitted dose in the oro- and hypopharynx, patients should "rinse and spit" to remove excess drug from the mouth and back of the throat.

Infants, young children up to age 3 years, and patients in acute distress may not be able to use a pMDI effectively. A "cold Freon effect" can occur when the aerosol plume reaches the back of the mouth and the patient stops inhaling. These problems can be corrected by using the proper pMDI accessory device (see the next section).

Accessory Devices

Various pMDI accessory devices have been developed to overcome the primary limitations of pMDI administration: hand–breath coordination problems, high oropharyngeal deposition, and difficulty in tracking doses. Accessory devices include flow-triggered pMDIs, spacers, valved holding chambers, and dose counters.

Flow-Triggered Device. The Maxair Autohaler (Graceway Pharmaceuticals, Bristol, TN) and Easyhaler (Orion Pharma, Espoo, Finland) are flow-triggered pMDIs designed to reduce the need for hand–breath coordination by firing in response to the patient's inspiratory effort.[74] To use the Autohaler, the patient cocks a lever on the top of the unit that spring-loads the canister against a vane mechanism. When the patient's inspiratory flow exceeds 30 L/min, the vane moves, allowing the canister to be pressed into the actuator, firing the pMDI. This device is available only with the β-agonist pirbuterol in the United States, but other formulations are in development. The Easyhaler has been introduced in Europe with several medications and may soon be available in North America. The flow required to actuate these devices may be too great for some children to generate, especially during acute exacerbations of disease.

Spacers and Holding Chambers. When properly designed, **spacers** and **valved holding chambers** do the following:
· Reduce oropharyngeal deposition of drug
· Relieve the bad taste of some medications by reducing oral deposition
· Eliminate the cold Freon effect
· Decrease aerosol MMAD
· Increase respirable particle mass
· Improve lower respiratory tract deposition
· Significantly improve therapeutic effects[55,72,75]

Spacers should be differentiated from valved holding chambers. A spacer device is a simple open-ended tube, chamber, or bag that has sufficiently large volume to provide space for the pMDI plume to expand by allowing the propellant to evaporate. To perform this function, a spacer device must have an internal volume greater than 100 ml and must provide a distance of 10 to 13 cm between the pMDI nozzle and the first wall or baffle. Smaller, inefficient spacers can reduce respiratory dose by 60% and offer no protection against poor coordination between actuation and breathing pattern. Spacers with internal volumes greater than 100 ml generally provide some protection against early firing of the pMDI, although exhaling immediately after the actuation clears most of the aerosol from the device, wasting the dose.

The valved holding chamber, usually 140 to 750 ml in volume, allows the plume from the pMDI to expand. It incorporates a one-way valve that permits the aerosol to be drawn from the chamber during inhalation only, diverting the exhaled gas to the atmosphere and not disturbing the remaining aerosol suspended in the chamber (Figure 11-9). Patients with small tidal volumes may empty the aerosol from the chamber with five to six breaths, except when there is a large dead space. A valved holding chamber can also incorporate a mask for use by an infant or child. These devices allow effective pMDI administration in a patient who is unable to use a mouthpiece because of size, age, coordination, or mental status.[76] With infants these masks should have minimal dead space, should be comfortable on the child's face, and should have a valved chamber that will open and close with the low inspiratory flow and volume generated by the patient. Box 11-5 describes the correct technique for using a pMDI with a holding chamber.

Valved holding chambers, which reduce the need to coordinate breathing with actuation, should be used with infants, small children, and any child taking steroids. In addition, the chambers reduce the pharyngeal dose of aerosol from the pMDI 10- to 15-fold over administration

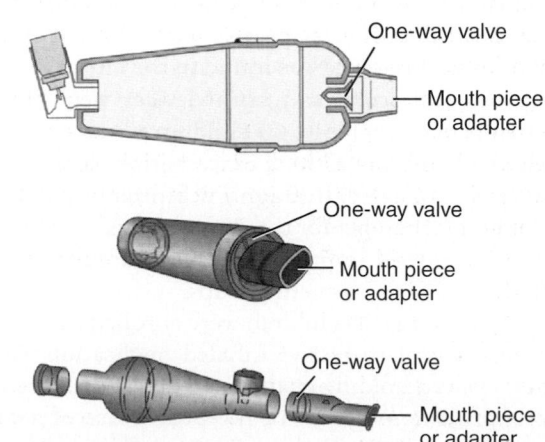

FIGURE 11-9 Metered-dose inhaler holding chambers are spacers with one-way valves that allow the chamber to be emptied only when the patient inhales, by preventing the exhaled gas from reentering the chamber.

Box 11-5	Optimal Technique for Using Pressurized Metered-Dose Inhaler with Valved Holding Chamber

- Warm the pMDI to hand or body temperature.
- Shake the canister vigorously, holding it vertically.
- Assemble the apparatus.
- Ensure that no loose objects are in the device that could be aspirated or could obstruct outflow.
- Place the holding chamber in the mouth (or place the mask completely over the nose and mouth), encouraging the patient to breathe through the mouth.
- Have the patient breathe normally, and actuate at the beginning of inspiration.
- For small children and infants, have them continue to breathe through the device for five or six breaths.
- For patients who can cooperate and clear the chamber with one breath, encourage larger breaths with breath holding.
- Allow 30 seconds between actuations.

pMDI, Pressurized metered-dose inhaler.

without a holding chamber. This decreases the total body dose from swallowed medications, which is an important consideration with steroid administration.[75,77,78] The high percentage of oropharyngeal drug deposition with steroid pMDIs can increase the risk of oral yeast infections (thrush). Rinsing the mouth after steroid use can reduce this problem, but most pMDI steroid aerosol impaction occurs deeper in the pharynx, which is not easily rinsed. For this reason, steroid MDIs should always be used in combination with a valved holding chamber.

Wheezing Infants

Valved holding chambers make pMDIs as reliable as SVNs for aerosol administration. In one study, 34 infants between 1 and 24 months of age and with acute asthma received two doses of terbutaline, 20 minutes apart, as either 2 mg/dose in 2.8 ml of 0.9% saline by nebulizer or as 0.5 mg/dose (5 puffs) by pMDI with a valved holding chamber.[79] No difference was found in the rate of improvement or clinical score, and both devices were reported equally effective. Similarly, 60 children 6 years of age or less who had an acute asthma exacerbation were randomized to receive albuterol through a nebulizer or pMDI with valved holding chamber for three treatments over 1 hour.[80] All patients showed improvement over baseline, with no difference between treatment groups.

In another study, 84 children were enrolled in the emergency department to receive inhaled medication with or without a valved holding chamber to determine whether a single brief demonstration of the proper use of a valved holding chamber would result in improved outcomes.[81] The valved holding chamber group reported significantly faster resolution of wheezing, fewer days of cough, and fewer missed days of school.

Evidence-based research does not support the belief that an SVN is better than a pMDI if the patient is not able to inhale with optimal technique. In fact, if unable to perform an optimal maneuver with a pMDI, the patient cannot perform an optimal maneuver with an SVN. Although optimal technique is always preferred, it is often difficult to attain with an infant, small child, or severely dyspneic patient. For such patients, an alternative may be to increase the pMDI or nebulizer dose (see later discussion).

Care and Cleaning

Particles containing drug settle and deposit within these devices, causing a whitish buildup on the inner chamber walls. This residual drug poses no risk to the patient but should be rinsed out periodically. After washing a plastic chamber or spacer with tap water, it is less effective for the next 10 to 15 puffs, until the static charge in the chamber (which attracts small particles) is once again reduced. Use of regular dish soap to wash the chamber reduces or eliminates this static charge. Metal and nonelectrostatic plastic spacers should be cleaned as recommended by their manufacturers.

Accessory devices either use the manufacturer-designed boot that comes with the pMDI or incorporate a "universal canister adapter" to fire the pMDI canister. Different formulations of pMDI drugs operate at different pressures, and devices have different orifice sizes in the boot specifically designed for use exclusively with the specific pMDI. Output characteristics of pMDIs will change when using an adapter with a different-size orifice; therefore spacers or holding chambers with universal canister adapters should be avoided. Devices that include the manufacturer's boot with the pMDI should be used when available.

Dry Powder Inhalers

Dry powder inhalers (DPIs) create aerosols by drawing air through a dose of dry powder medication. The powder contains micronized drug particles (MMAD less than 5 μm) with larger lactose or glucose particles (greater than 30 to 100 μm in diameter), or it contains micronized drug particles bound into loose aggregates.[82] Micronized particles adhere strongly to each other and to most surfaces. Addition of the larger particles of the carrier decreases cohesive forces in the micronized drug powder so that separation into individual respirable particles (disaggregation) occurs more readily. Thus the carrier particles aid the flow of the drug powder from the device. These carriers also act as "fillers" by adding bulk to the powder when the unit dose of a drug is small. Usually the drug particles are loosely bound to the carrier,[83] and they are stripped from the carrier by the energy provided by the patient's inhalation (Figure 11-10). The release of respirable particles of the drug requires inspiration at relatively high flow (30 to 120 L/min).[84,85] A high inspiratory flow results in

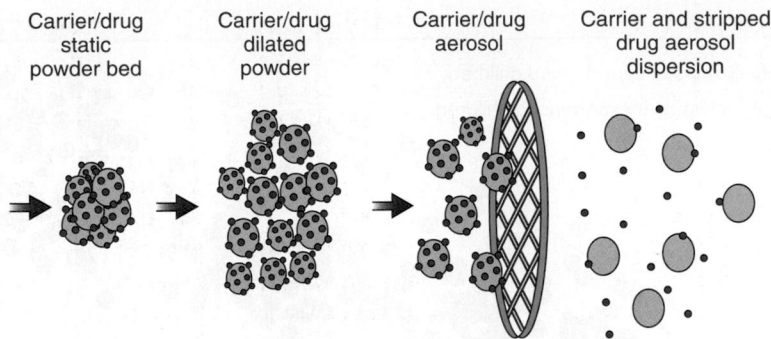

Carrier/drug static powder bed   Carrier/drug dilated powder   Carrier/drug aerosol   Carrier and stripped drug aerosol dispersion

FIGURE 11-10 As patient inhales through a dry powder inhaler, inspiratory flow disaggregates particles from the powder bed or capsule and is drawn through a screen that strips the small drug particles from the larger carrier particles, creating an aerosol dispersion.

pharyngeal impaction of the larger carrier particles that comprise the bulk of the aerosol and, as with pMDIs, results in up to 80% of the drug dose being deposited in the oro- and hypopharynx. Impaction of lactose carrier particles gives the patient the sensation of having inhaled a dose. Like with pMDIs, patients should rinse and spit after inhalation of steroid preparations from a DPI.

The internal geometry of the DPI device influences the resistance offered to inspiration and the inspiratory flow required to disaggregate and aerosolize the medication. Devices with higher resistance require a higher inspiratory flow to produce a dose. Inhalation through high-resistance DPIs may improve drug delivery to the lower respiratory tract compared with pMDIs as long as the patient can reliably generate the required flow rate.[67,86] High-resistance devices have not been shown to improve either deposition or bronchodilation compared with low-resistance DPIs. DPIs with multiple components require correct assembly of the apparatus and priming of the device to ensure aerosolization of the dry powder. Periodic brushing is needed to remove any residual powder accumulated within some DPIs.

DPIs produce aerosols in which most of the drug particles are in the respirable range, with distribution of particle sizes (GSD) differing significantly among various DPIs.[68] High ambient humidity produces clumping of the dry powder, creating larger particles that are not as effectively aerosolized.[69] Air with a high moisture content is less efficient at disaggregating particles of dry powder than dry air, such that high ambient humidity increases the size of drug particles in the aerosol and may reduce drug delivery to the lung. Newer DPI devices contain individual doses more protected from humidity. Humidity can accumulate once the device is opened, or if the DPI is stored with the cap off, or by condensation when the device is brought from a very cold environment into a warmer area.

Because the energy from the patient's inspiratory flow disperses the drug powder, the magnitude and duration of the patient's inspiratory effort influence aerosol generation from a DPI. Failure to perform inhalation at a sufficiently

fast inspiratory flow reduces the dose of the drug emitted from DPIs and increases the distribution of particle sizes within the aerosol with a variety of devices.[87,88] For example, the Advair Diskus (GlaxoSmithKline, London, UK) delivers approximately 90% of the labeled dose at an inspiratory flow ranging from 30 to 90 L/min, whereas the dose delivered by the high-resistance Pulmicort Turbuhaler (AstraZeneca, Lund, Sweden) is significantly lower at an inspiratory flow of 30 L/min compared with the dose delivered at 90 L/min. The variability between doses at different inspiratory flows is higher with the Turbuhaler.[89,90] Figure 11-11 shows the effect of two inspiratory flows (30 and 55 L/min) when using a pMDI, a breath-actuated MDI (Autohaler), a Rotahaler (previously GlaxoSmithKline) (DPI 1), a Turbuhaler (DPI 2), and a Diskhaler (GlaxoSmithKline) (DPI 3).[91] The peak inspiratory flow rate of children is limited and associated with age, making it unlikely that a child younger than 6 years could reliably empty a DPI requiring greater than 50 L/min (Figure 11-12).[91]

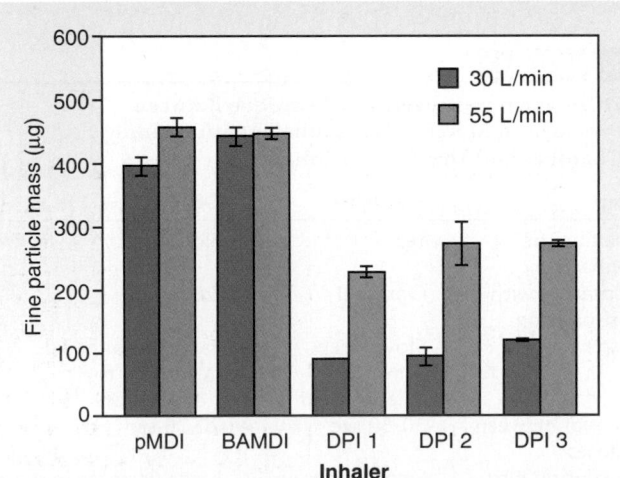

FIGURE 11-11 Fine particle mass delivered from a 100-µg target dose (±SD) as a function of flow rate. *pMDI,* Pressurized metered-dose inhaler; *BAMDI,* breath-actuated MDI (Autohaler); *DPI 1,* Rotahaler; *DPI 2,* Turbuhaler; *DPI 3,* Diskhaler.

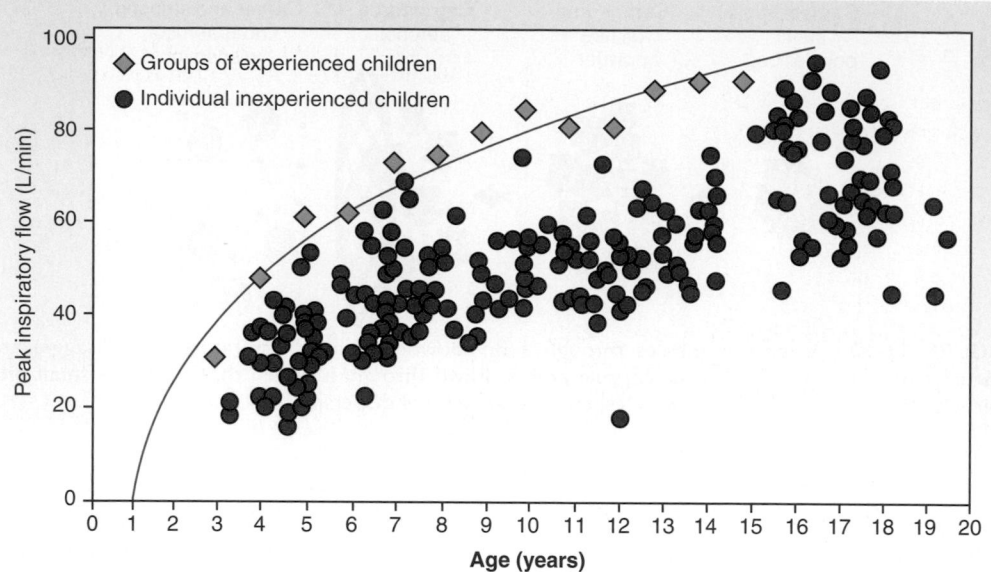

FIGURE 11-12   Peak inspiratory flows in individual inexperienced children and in groups of experienced children.

Technique

All commercially available DPIs are passive, requiring energy from the patient to disaggregate the powder from its carrier and container to form aerosol, and therefore are breath actuated, reducing the problem of coordinating inspiration with actuation. The technique of using DPIs differs in important respects from the technique employed to inhale drugs from a pMDI (Table 11-1). Although DPIs are easier to use than pMDIs, up to 25% of patients may use DPIs improperly.[91] DPIs are critically dependent on inspiratory airflow to generate the aerosol. The lower the inspiratory flow, the less drug is emitted by the device. Children younger than 6 years may not be able to generate

sufficient inspiratory flow for effective dosing with units requiring more than 60 LPM. Exhalation into a DPI may blow the powder from the container and into the device, away from the patient, reducing drug delivery. Moreover, the humidity in the exhaled air reduces subsequent aerosol generation from the DPI. Therefore patients must be instructed not to exhale into a DPI. Thus DPIs should be used with caution, if at all, in the very young or ill child, weak patients, elderly persons, and those with altered mental status. Patients may need repeated instruction before they can master the technique of using DPIs, and periodic assessment is necessary to ensure that patients continue to use an optimal technique.[91] Clinicians must also learn the correct technique of using DPIs to train their patients in the proper use of these devices. Box 11-6 outlines the basic steps in the use and care of DPIs.

Care and Cleaning

DPIs should be cleaned in accordance with the product label. Patients should be trained not to submerge DPIs in water, which will dramatically reduce available dose.[33]

DEVICE SELECTION AND COMPLIANCE

Whenever possible, patients should use only one type of aerosol-generating device for inhalation therapy. Each type requires a different technique, and repeated instruction is necessary to ensure that the patient uses a device appropriately. The use of different devices for inhalation can be confusing for patients and may decrease their compliance with therapy. This has been referred to as "device dementia."[73]

TABLE 11-1		
Differences in Inhalation Technique Between Pressurized Metered-Dose Inhaler with Holding Chamber and Dry Powder Inhaler		
Step	**pMDI/HC**	**DPI**
Shaking the inhaler	Yes	No
Actuation with inspiration	Optional	Essential
Inspiration	Slow, deep; improves deposition	Fast, prolonged; required for deposition
Interval between doses	30-60 sec	20-30 sec
Exhalation into device	Small decrease in dose	Large decrease in dose

DPI, Dry powder inhaler; *pMDI/HC,* pressurized metered-dose inhaler with holding chamber.

Box 11-6	Technique for Using Dry Powder Inhaler

Priming instructions: Before using a new DPI for the first time, check the manufacturer's instruction and prime the DPI. Steps for using the DPIs:

- Assemble the apparatus.
- Load dose based on the manufacturer's instruction.
- Exhale slowly to functional residual capacity.
- Exhale away from the mouthpiece.
- Seal lips around the mouthpiece.
- Inhale deeply and forcefully (>60 L/min). A breath-hold should be encouraged but is not essential.
- If more than one dose is required, repeat the previous steps.
- Monitor adverse effects.
- Replace the cover on the inhaler.
- Keep the inhaler clean and dry at all times (following manufacturer's instruction).
- Keep the device in a dry place at a controlled room temperature (i.e., 20° to 25° C [68° to 77° F]). Do not submerge in water.

TABLE 11-2

Comparison of Pressurized Metered-Dose Inhaler with Holding Chamber, Dry Powder Inhaler, and Nebulizer as Aerosol Delivery Device

Factor	pMDI/HC	DPI	Nebulizer
Performance			
Most aerosol particles <5 μm in size	+	+	±
High pulmonary deposition	+	±	±
Low mouth deposition	+	±	−
Reliability of dose	+	±	±
Influenced by humidity	−	+	−
Physical and chemical stability	+	+	+
Breath actuated	−	+	−
Risk of contamination	−	−	+
Convenience			
Lightweight, compact	+	+	−
Multiple doses	+	+	−
Dose indicator	−	+	−
Inexpensive	+	+	−
Easy and quick operation	±	±	−
Suitable for all ages	+	−	+
Suitable for multiple clinical situations	+	±	+

DPI, Dry powder inhaler; *pMDI/HC,* pressurized metered-dose inhaler with holding chamber.

At present, DPIs may be considered alternatives to pMDIs for patients who can generate inspiratory flow rates greater than 30 to 60 L/min but who are unable to use pMDIs effectively. DPIs are recommended for therapy for patients with stable asthma and chronic obstructive pulmonary disease but not for patients with acute bronchoconstriction or children younger than 6 years. Therefore one drawback of DPIs is that they do not substitute for pMDIs in all clinical situations. Moreover, dose adjustment may be needed when the same drug is administered by a DPI instead of a pMDI. Table 11-2 compares DPIs, pMDIs, and nebulizers. Deciding on the appropriate dose of inhaled corticosteroids may be a particularly vexing problem because it is difficult to determine bioequivalence with these agents. Further research is needed to determine equivalent doses when both the drug and the device used for inhalation therapy are altered.[92,93]

Selecting an Aerosol Device for Infants and Toddlers (Birth to 4 Years)

Children younger than 4 years of age may not be able to master specific breathing techniques and be unable to reliably use breath-actuated nebulizers, breath-actuated pMDIs, or DPIs, and such devices may not be appropriate for this patient population; therefore, administering aerosolized medications to infants should be done via a nebulizer or pMDI with VHC.[33,94,95]

Infants and small children, under the age of 4 years, may not be able to use a mouthpiece, requiring a mask for administration. Because some children may cry when a mask is applied, some clinicians have recommended the use of blow-by, that is, directing a stream of aerosol from a nebulizer toward the mouth and nose of an infant, often from up to 6 inches away. Just as crying greatly reduces lung delivery of aerosol[10,96,97] so does blow-by. Studies demonstrate that inhaled drugs should be given to infants when they are settled and breathing quietly because the administration of inhaled drugs to patients during sleep when infants have quite breathing results in greater inhaled dose.[98] However, it may be difficult to deliver aerosolized drugs to infants without waking them. An in vivo study showed that 69% of children woke up during aerosol therapy and 75% of them were distressed.[99] Multiple in vitro studies reported the importance of face mask seal during aerosol therapy[100,101] with both nebulizers and pMDIs with VHC. Several studies reported the importance of face mask seal[10,102-108] and showed differences in the efficiency to achieve a good face mask seal for the different face mask designs.[103,104,106-108] According to a recent in vitro study conducted by Mansour and Smaldone, aerosol delivery via blow-by can be a good alternative for uncooperative children if the breath-enhanced nebulizer is used for aerosol therapy as opposed to a standard jet nebulizer.[109] However, several studies indicated that aerosol delivery to children reduces as the distance between mask and face increases.[100,101,109] Therefore it is important to teach infants how to play with their mask and learn to tolerate it being placed on the face. This takes some time but with a little patience from the care provider, it can greatly enhance the efficacy of the aerosol therapy and the trauma to both patient and parent, as will comforting babies and providing other effective forms of distraction that will help optimize aerosol therapy in infants. If a face mask is not tolerated by the infant, use of a hood provides an option for administering inhaled medications via a nebulizer because it is better tolerated by some infants and preferred by parents. Some studies showed that the hood and face mask have comparable efficacy in infants and leads to a better therapeutic index with minimal deposition at the infant's eyes.[110-113] Another alternative to a face mask is the high-flow nasal cannula, where aerosol delivery at a lower flow appears to be as good or better than use of a tight-fitting mask. Although its *efficiency* has been reported by a few in vitro studies,[114,115] clinical studies are still needed in this area of research.

Selecting an Aerosol Device for Preschool Children (4-5 Years)

Nebulizers and pMDIs with VHC are suggested for use with preschool children.[33,94,116,117] Although the *efficiency* of both devices are similar, the shorter treatment time and portability of the pMDI with VHC makes it more desirable than the nebulizer. Once children reach age 5 years, their physical and cognitive abilities should be assessed to determine whether they can generate the sustained inspiratory flow rates required for specific devices. Children who can successfully master the more complex breathing techniques may be given breath-actuated pMDIs or DPIs. Although use of a mouthpiece is an option for preschool children, a face mask should be used until the child can comfortably use a mouthpiece.[94]

Selecting an Aerosol Device for Young Children (6-12 Years)

Young children can control their breathing. Their hand–breath coordination is usually good, and they can master complex inhalation techniques. Therefore, several aerosol devices, such as pMDI with or without VHC, DPI, and breath-actuated pMDI, can be used for this patient population.[94] The selection of an aerosol device should be based on patients' physical and cognitive abilities as well as their preference and acceptance.

EMERGENCY BRONCHODILATOR RESUSCITATION

When a patient comes to the emergency department with an acute exacerbation of asthma, the onset of the exacerbation is often 12 to 36 hours earlier. These children have often taken rescue medications without obtaining sufficient relief. They, and their parents, are anxious, uncomfortable, and exhausted. The goal is to provide relief as soon as possible and to decrease the work of breathing until antiinflammatory medications take effect. Administration of selective β_2-agonists and anticholinergics such as ipratropium (Atrovent) by aerosol is usually the first therapy given. Albuterol (salbutamol outside the United States) reaches 85% of bronchodilator effect in

the first 5 minutes after administration. The national asthma guidelines recommend albuterol administration with either 2.5 or 5.0 mg by jet nebulizer or 4 to 8 puffs of albuterol by pMDI with valved holding chamber at 20-minute intervals for the first hour.[118,119]

Inhaled short-acting bronchodilators are a mainstay of asthma treatment in the emergency room. Now the decision question is which aerosol device should be used for the delivery of inhaled bronchodilators to children in the emergency department. A few studies showed that the *efficacy* of pMDI/VHC is similar to the nebulizer for the treatment of acute asthma exacerbation in the emergency room.[120-129] A recent study also showed that use of a pMDI/VHC in the emergency room does not increase hospital admission and decreases not only length of inpatient stay but also cost per patient for children admitted to the hospital.[130] Despite the evidence, nebulizers are still commonly used for the treatment of acute exacerbation in the emergency room. The reasons for resistance to using pMDI/VHC in the emergency department include increased equipment costs, myths about the superiority of nebulization, concerns about its safety, increased workload, perceived resistance from patients/parents, interprofessional conflict, and lack of consensus about the benefits of pMDI/spacers among staff.[131-133] Overcoming all these barriers can be accomplished through the education programs tailored to physicians and health care professionals who will implement the change from nebulizers to pMDIs with spacers in the emergency room.[134]

Intermittent Versus Continuous Therapy

If the patient does not experience relief of symptoms with standard dosing, frequency of administration is often increased to hourly, or even every 15 to 20 minutes, in the emergency department. Treatments can be continued at this frequency until symptoms are relieved. The standard SVN treatment takes 10 to 15 minutes and requires that a clinician be at the bedside constantly. An alternative to intermittent treatments is continuous nebulization delivering at a controlled rate of medication over an extended period, with the patient monitored for rapid identification of increases in heart rate. Doses of albuterol between 7.5 and 15 mg/hr have been shown to be effective in treating acute exacerbation of asthma in adults and children.[135-138]

One strategy for continuous nebulization is to use an intravenous infusion pump to drip a premixed bronchodilator solution through a port into the reservoir of a standard SVN (operating at 6 to 8 L/min) or specialty nebulizer such as the MiniHEART nebulizer (Westmed) (operating at 2 L/min). More recently a VMN, the Aeroneb Solo (Aerogen, Dangan, Galway, Ireland), with a port for drip feed and continuous operation, has been introduced. Another solution is to use an LVN that produces an MMAD in the respirable range and that is known to deliver a consistent output of medication at a specific flow. Albuterol solution and normal saline are mixed in the reservoir, and the LVN is operated at a specific flow, identified by the manufacturer, to deliver the desired dose. Several LVNs are now commercially available for continuous administration of bronchodilators. The HEART high-output nebulizer (Westmed) has an output of approximately 30 ml/hr at a flow of 10 L/min for up to 6 or 8 hours. The HOPE nebulizer (B&B Medical Technologies, Loomis, CA) is a closed dilution nebulizer that allows drug output and oxygen or heliox administration. The medication can be delivered through an aerosol mouthpiece or mask or in-line with a ventilator circuit. For patients with moderately severe asthma, continuous therapy and intermittent therapy have similar effects with either low-dose or high-dose β-agonists. For patients with a severe asthma exacerbation, or forced expiratory volume in 1 second (FEV_1) less than 40% of predicted values, continuous therapy may work more rapidly.[138]

Although β_2-agonists are the first-line agents for acute exacerbation of asthma, data from both adults and children suggest that ipratropium bromide is synergistic with β-agonists for the therapy of acute asthma.[139-144] Combination bronchodilator therapy using albuterol and ipratropium in patients with severe asthma significantly reduced the percentage of patients hospitalized (Figure 11-13).[143] It is important to remember that poor relief of acute asthma with bronchodilators may signify a nonasthmatic cause of wheezing, such as foreign body aspiration or tracheitis. Infants with bronchiolitis respond poorly to bronchodilator medications, which are therefore not recommended for this condition.

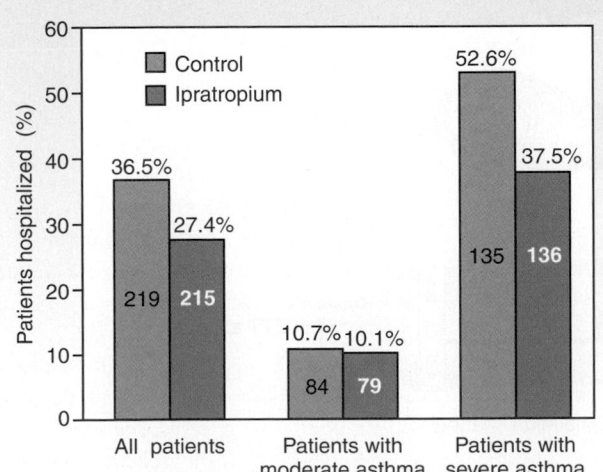

FIGURE 11-13 Rates of hospitalization of patients with asthma from the emergency department after treatment with albuterol (control) or with albuterol and ipratropium (ipratropium). Numbers in columns, number of children tested. In patients with moderate asthma, no difference was seen in hospitalization rate. In patients with severe asthma, the benefits of combined therapy were significant.

Undiluted Bronchodilator

A faster method of administering albuterol is achieved by placing undiluted medication into the nebulizer. Diluent is typically added to medication in the nebulizer to reduce the fraction of the dose that is trapped as residual volume. With undiluted administration, enough medication must be added to the nebulizer to exceed the residual volume of the nebulizer and to allow 1.0 to 2.0 ml of albuterol solution (5 to 10 mg) to be nebulized. Patients should be monitored closely during administration, and the treatment should be terminated if the patient has significant reduction of symptoms and begins to develop tremor or other side effect. Undiluted albuterol administered with specialty nebulizers achieves similar improvements in clinical status in less time. The osmolarity of undiluted medication may be a problem for some patients, especially children younger than 2 years old.

MECHANICAL VENTILATION

In the past the consensus was that the efficiency of aerosol delivery to the lower respiratory tract in mechanically ventilated patients was much lower than that in ambulatory patients. In 1- to 4-kg infants, Fok and colleagues[8] demonstrated less than 1% deposition with jet nebulizers and pMDIs with spacers during mechanical ventilation and spontaneous breathing.

Data suggest that this might be overly pessimistic, however, because a number of variables affect aerosol delivery during mechanical ventilation (Box 11-7).

Factors Affecting Aerosol Delivery
Ventilator–Patient Interface

The ventilator circuit is typically a closed system that is pressurized during operation, requiring the nebulizer or pMDI to be attached with connectors that maintain the integrity of the circuit during operation. The pMDI cannot be used with the actuator designed by the manufacturer, and use of a third-party actuator is required (Figure 11-14). The size, shape, and design of these actuators greatly affect respirable drug available to the patient and may vary with different pMDI formulations.[145]

Breath Configuration

During controlled mechanical ventilation (CMV), the pattern and rate of inspiratory gas flow and breathing differ from spontaneous respiration. Ambulatory adult patients under normal stable conditions tend to have sinusoidal inspiratory flow patterns of about 30 L/min, whereas ventilators may use square or decelerating waves with considerably higher flow. Also, the airways are pressurized on inhalation when using CMV, whereas spontaneous inspiration is generated by negative airway pressure drawing gas deep into the lungs. All these factors influence aerosol delivery to the lung.

| **Box 11-7** | Variables That Affect Aerosol Delivery and Deposition During Mechanical Ventilation |

VENTILATOR RELATED
Mode
Tidal volume
Respiratory frequency
Duty cycle
Inspiratory flow waveform
Trigger mechanism

DEVICE RELATED
Metered-dose inhaler
Type of spacer or adapter
Position of spacer in circuit
Timing of actuation
Nebulizer
Type of nebulizer
Fill volume
Gas flow
Cycling: inspiration versus continuous
Duration of nebulization
Position in circuit

CIRCUIT RELATED
Endotracheal tube
Inhaled gas humidity
Inhaled gas density

DRUG RELATED
Dose
Formulation
Aerosol particle size
Targeted site for delivery
Duration of action

PATIENT RELATED
Severity of airway obstruction
Mechanism of airway obstruction
Presence of dynamic hyperinflation
Patient–ventilator synchrony

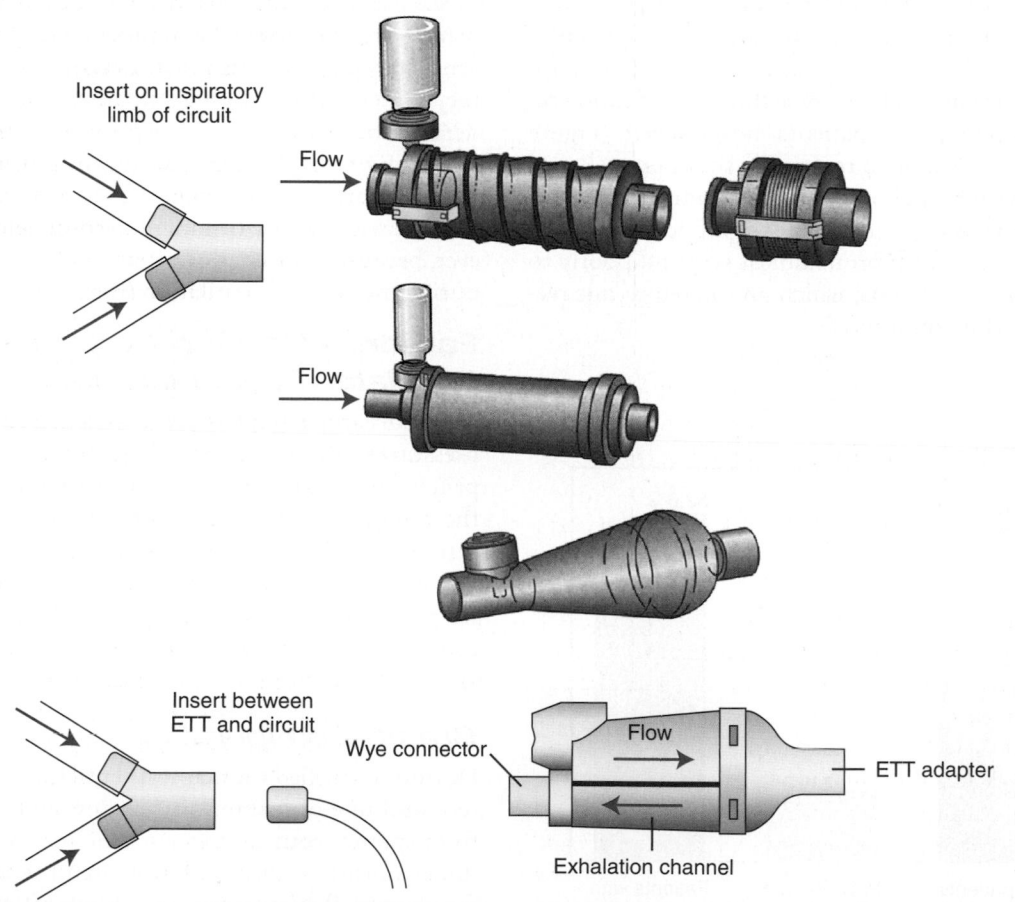

FIGURE 11-14   MDI holding chambers to use in-line with mechanical ventilator circuits or in intubated patients or those with tracheostomies.

Airway

In the mechanically ventilated patient, the conduit between the aerosol device and lower respiratory tract is narrower than the oropharynx and trachea. Although the endotracheal tube (ETT) is narrower than the trachea, its smooth interior surface may create a more laminar flow path than the structures of the glottis and larynx and may be less of a barrier to aerosol delivery than the ventilator circuit. In vitro studies demonstrate that three times more aerosol from the pMDI is delivered past the ETT during CMV under dry condition than deposits in the lung through an intact upper airway, raising some doubt that the ETT is the primary barrier to aerosol.[146]

Environment

Ventilator circuits are typically designed to provide heat and humidity for inspired gas to compensate for bypassing the normal airway. Humidity can increase particle size and reduce deposition during CMV, but no data suggest that this reduction is unique to the ventilated patient. The ambulatory patient receiving aerosol, from either an inhaler or nebulizer, in a hot, high-humidity climate may experience a similar reduction in delivered dose.

Response Assessment

The most common method by which to assess patient response to bronchodilator administration is through changes in expiratory flow. During mechanical ventilation, forced expiratory maneuvers are impractical, poorly reproducible, and rarely performed, requiring other, less sensitive methods such as monitoring pressure changes (peak and plateau) during ventilator-generated breaths (e.g., passive inspiration). Fok and colleagues demonstrated differences in the response in a rabbit model of ventilated infants and found that a pMDI was more effective than a jet nebulizer and that a USN was more effective than either (Figure 11-15).[147] Other changes in mechanics consistent with bronchodilator therapy include decreasing the pressure needed to deliver a set tidal volume during volume ventilation, decreasing the mean airway pressure (now continuously monitored electronically by most mechanical ventilators), and decreasing the requirement for supplemental oxygen. Flow–volume loops have been used to demonstrate bronchodilator response in infants, but unless the patient is sedated and paralyzed, respiratory efforts can provide misleading differences before and after bronchodilator administration. Chest auscultation to detect changes in wheezing is notoriously inaccurate and should never be used as the sole criterion for evaluating the effect of inhaled bronchodilators. For example, wheezing may become more prominent as severe bronchospasm is relaxed and the lungs begin to open up.

Nebulizer Placement

Placement of a continuous jet nebulizer 30 cm from the ETT is more efficient than placement between the patient

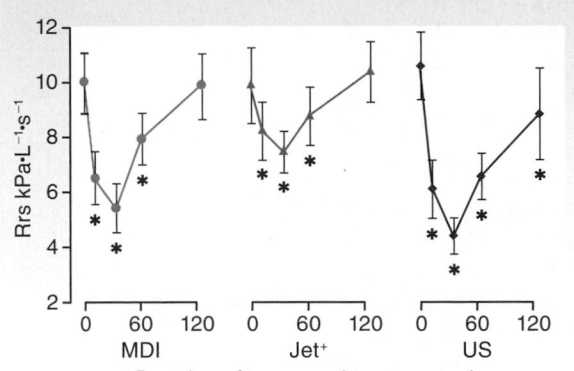

FIGURE 11-15 Measurements of respiratory system resistance (*Rrs*) before, and 15, 30, 60, and 120 min after, salbutamol treatment via a metered-dose inhaler (*MDI*), a jet nebulizer (Jet: Sidestream), and an ultrasonic nebulizer (*US*). *Posttreatment values were significantly lower than the pretreatment Rrs, $p < 0.0001$.

Y-device and the ETT because the inspiratory ventilator tubing acts as a spacer for the aerosol to accumulate between inspirations.[148] Addition of a spacer device between the nebulizer and ETT modestly increases aerosol delivery.[149] Placement of an ultrasonic or vibrating mesh nebulizer near the patient Y-device is more efficient than placement near the ventilator, unless bias flow exceeds 2 L/min. Operating the nebulizer only during inspiration is marginally more efficient for aerosol delivery compared with continuous aerosol generation.[148]

Ari et al. compared aerosol delivery from four types of generators (jet [JN], ultrasonic [USN], vibrating mesh [VMN] nebulizers, and pMDI) in three positions (between the ETT and Y, in the inspiratory limb near the Y, and proximal to the ventilator) during continuous mechanical ventilation with no bias or trigger flow.[150] When operated in the inspiratory limb near the Y, the pMDI, USN, and VMN delivered 16% to 17% of the dose distal to the ETT, whereas the jet nebulizer delivered 3.5% in a heated, humidified circuit. Moving the aerosol generator back toward the ventilator increased the jet nebulizer to 6%, but reduced efficiency of the other generators. In a similar experiment with 2 and 5 LPM of bias flow, both VMN and jet nebulizer were more efficient placed near the ventilator before the humidifier than in the inspiratory limb near the Y. This was demonstrated with both adult and pediatric circuits and parameters.[150,151] Figure 11-16 illustrates the experimental setup used by Ari et al. with jet nebulizer and vibrating mesh nebulizer; Figure 11-17 shows the effect of nebulizer type, placement, and bias flow on aerosol delivery in adult and pediatric lung models.[150]

Inhaler Adapters

Several types of commercial adapters are available to connect the pMDI canister to the ventilator circuit. Pressurized MDIs can be used with adapters that attach directly to

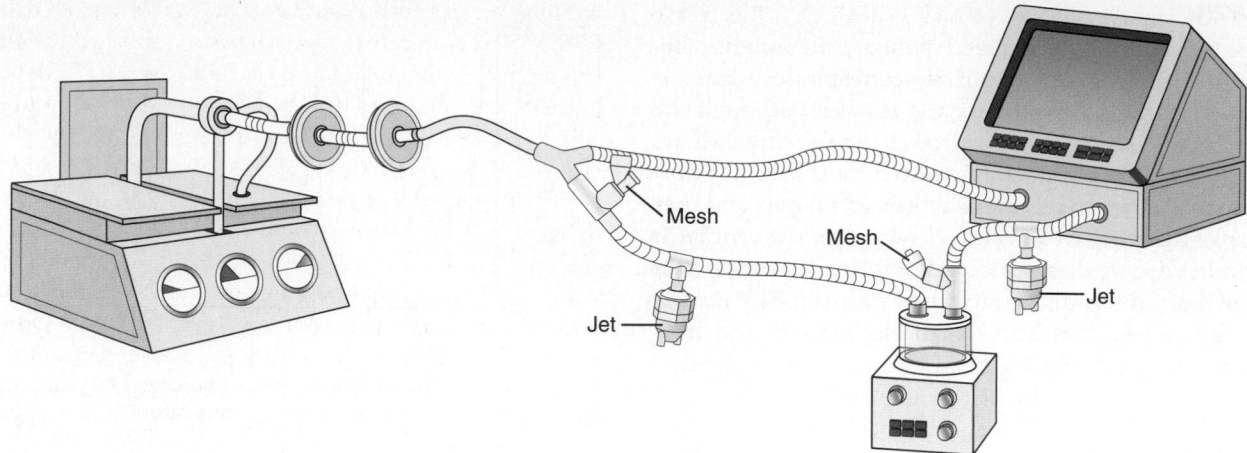

FIGURE 11-16 Experimental setup used with jet nebulizer (*above*) and vibrating mesh nebulizer (*below*) placed in two positions in an adult (22 mm ID) and pediatric (15 mm ID) ventilator circuits.

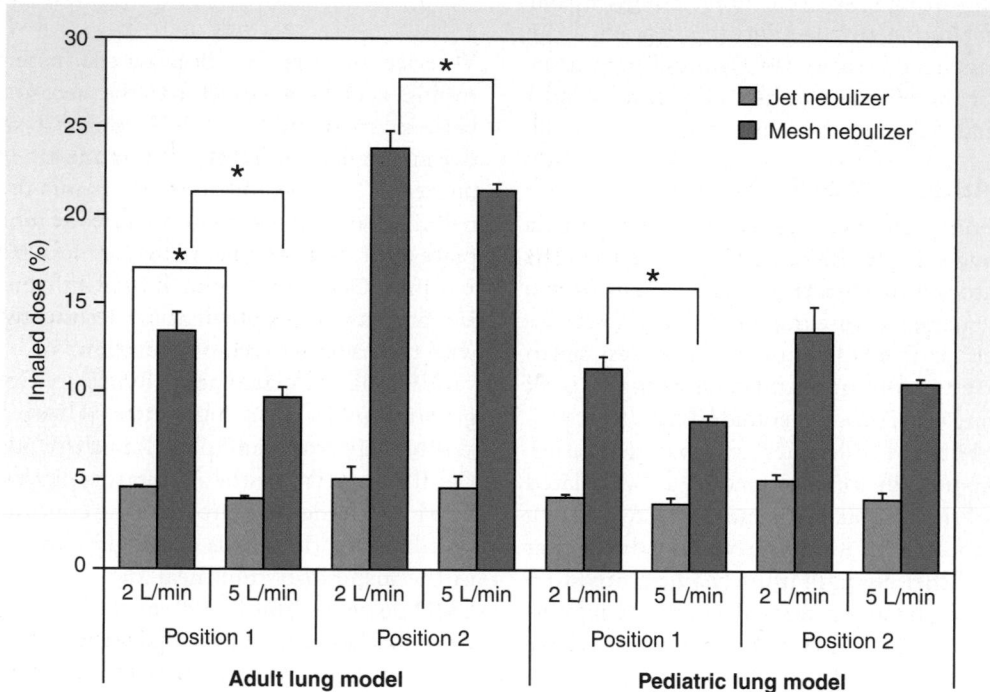

FIGURE 11-17 Effect of nebulizer type, placement, and bias flow on aerosol delivery from jet and mesh nebulizers in adult and pediatric lung models.

the ETT, with inline chamber or nonchamber adapters placed in the inspiratory limb of the ventilator circuit. In vitro and in vivo studies have shown that the combination of a pMDI and an accessory device with a chamber results in a four- to sixfold greater delivery of aerosol than pMDI actuation into a connector attached directly to the ETT or into an inline device that lacks a chamber.[76,148,149,152-154] When using the elbow adapter connected to the ETT, actuation of the pMDI out of synchrony with inspiratory airflow delivers little aerosol to the lower respiratory tract. This observation may explain the lack of therapeutic effect

with this type of adapter after administration of high doses (100 puffs, 1 mg of albuterol) of aerosol from a pMDI in some studies.[155]

Aerosol Particle Size

In mechanically ventilated patients the ventilator circuit and ETT act as baffles that trap particles with larger diameter en route to the bronchi, and hygroscopic particles might increase further in size in the ventilator circuit. Wide variability exists in the MMAD of aerosol particles produced by different brands of nebulizers. Nebulizers producing smaller aerosol particles (MMAD, <2 μm) are likely to produce greater deposition in the lower respiratory tract of ventilator-supported patients.[156]

Endotracheal Tube

Aerosol impaction in the ETT can reduce the efficiency of aerosol delivery in mechanically ventilated patients. The efficacy of aerosol delivery decreases when narrow ETTs are used in pediatric ventilator circuits.[156,157] The efficiency with which various nebulizers deliver aerosols beyond the ETT did not vary among tube sizes ranging in internal diameter from 7 to 9 mm.[152]

Heating and Humidification

Humidification of inhaled gas decreases aerosol deposition with pMDIs and nebulizers by approximately 40% using in vitro models, probably because of increased particle loss in the ventilator circuit.[76,156-158] More recently, evidence suggests that models that exhale humidity, more accurately simulating patient conditions, show little to no difference in delivered aerosol with passive or active humidity. This would eliminate any benefit of turning off active humidification before administration of aerosol. Absence of humidification may not pose problems during the brief period required to administer a bronchodilator with a pMDI; however, inhalation of dry gas for more than a few minutes can damage the airway.[76] In addition, the disconnection of the ventilator circuit required to bypass the humidifier interrupts ventilation and may increase the risk of ventilator-associated pneumonia. For routine bronchodilator treatment, we recommend using either a pMDI or a nebulizer with a humidified ventilator circuit.

Density of Inhaled Gas

High inspiratory flow with air or oxygen produces turbulence and increased aerosol impaction. Breathing less dense gas such as helium–oxygen improves aerosol deposition. Studies in ambulatory patients with airway obstruction reveal higher aerosol retention when breathing helium–oxygen compared with air.[159,160] Studies on the effects of helium–oxygen mixtures on aerosol deposition during mechanical ventilation demonstrated an up to 50% increase in deposition of albuterol from a pMDI or SVN during CMV of a simulated adult patient.[29]

Ventilator Mode and Settings

The ventilator mode and settings of tidal volume, flow, and respiratory rate influence the characteristics of the airflow used to deliver aerosol in mechanically ventilated patients. For optimal aerosol delivery, actuation of a pMDI into a spacer needs to be synchronized with the onset of inspiratory airflow. Actuation of a pMDI into a cylindrical spacer synchronized with inspiration results in approximately 30% greater efficiency of aerosol delivery compared with actuation during exhalation.[76] When using an elbow adapter, actuation of a pMDI that is not synchronized

with inspiratory airflow achieves negligible aerosol delivery to the lower respiratory tract. Aerosol can be delivered during assisted modes of ventilation, provided that the patient is breathing in synchrony with the ventilator. Albuterol deposition may be up to 23% higher during simulated spontaneous breaths than with controlled breaths of equivalent tidal volume.[158] For efficient aerosol delivery to the lower respiratory tract, the tidal volume of the ventilator-delivered breath must be larger than the volume of the ventilator tubing and ETT. Tidal volumes of 500 ml or greater in adults are associated with adequate aerosol delivery, but the higher pressures required to deliver larger tidal volumes can be detrimental to the lungs. For infants and small children, volumes that exceed the mechanical dead space of the circuit and airway help to optimize delivery.

Aerosol delivery directly correlates with longer inflation times.[156-158] Because nebulizers generate aerosol over several minutes, longer inspiratory times have a cumulative effect in improving aerosol delivery. However, pMDIs produce aerosol only over a portion of a single inspiration, and the mechanism by which longer inspiratory times increase aerosol delivery is unclear. Aerosol particles that deposit in the ventilator tubing may be swept off the walls and entrained by longer periods of inspiratory flow.

In addition, the diluent volume and the duration of treatment influence nebulizer efficiency.[155] Approximately 5% of the nominal dose of albuterol administered by a pMDI is exhaled in mechanically ventilated patients, whereas less than 1% is exhaled with the use of pMDIs in ambulatory patients.[29,161] The mean exhaled fraction (7%) with the use of nebulizers in mechanically ventilated patients is similar to that with MDIs, but considerable variability exists between patients (coefficient of variation, 74%).[162]

Technique of Aerosol Administration in Critical Care

Deposition of aerosol during mechanical ventilation varies with the type of aerosol generator used. During mechanical ventilation of adult patients under standard conditions (humidity on; I:E ratio, 1:2), 1% to 3% of the dose is delivered to the lungs.[163] Under similar conditions, a pMDI, with proper spacer and synchronized actuation, can deliver 11% of an emitted dose to the lungs. Both ultrasonic and vibrating mesh nebulizers may deliver 10% to 15% of a dose.[164,165]

In the infant, the deposition is considerably less (0.2% to 1.0%) with jet nebulizers and pMDIs, whereas the vibrating mesh nebulizer appears to be an order of magnitude more efficient (9% to 12.9%).[165]

In both adults and infants, the gas driving the jet nebulizer enters the ventilator circuit, with the potential for changing delivered volumes, pressures, and parameters; this can set off alarms. Because of the relatively low flow rates used in infant ventilator circuits, the addition of

2 to 6 L/min of gas can more than double the delivered volume. With other aerosol generators such as pMDIs and ultrasonic and vibrating mesh nebulizers, there is no substantial increase in gas volume and ventilator parameters remain consistent.

Specific techniques can improve the efficiency of every ventilator circuit. In vitro the best delivery with a jet nebulizer during CMV (15% to 35%) was accomplished with a nebulizer (e.g., AeroTech II; Biodex Medical Systems, Shirley, NY) that produces particles with an MMAD less than 2 μm, but it can take 35 minutes to administer a 3 ml dose of medication. This dose was nebulized into a dry ventilator circuit, with a duty cycle of 0.5 at inverse-ratio ventilation.[162] Admittedly, this approach might be difficult to tolerate for a patient requiring mechanical ventilation. A common nebulizer that generates particles with an MMAD of 3.5 μm takes half the time but may reduce the dose to the lung by up to 50%, reducing total deposition to 7.5%. Keeping the humidifier on during administration reduces delivery by another 40% (decreasing total deposition to 4%), and reducing the duty cycle to a normal 0.25 reduces deposition to 2%.[155]

Studies on the dose response to bronchodilators in mechanically ventilated patients have not been done in children and infants. This requires us to extrapolate data from adult ventilated patients, in whom bronchodilator effects were observed with the administration of a 3-ml unit dose containing 2.5 mg of albuterol with a jet nebulizer or 4 actuations (400 μg) with a pMDI.[166] The pMDI was administered to stable patients through a humidified ventilator circuit, with a chamber-style adapter placed in the inspiratory limb at the Y-piece. Actuations were synchronized to inspiration, with a pause of 20 to 30 seconds between actuations. Minimal therapeutic advantage was gained by administering higher doses, but the potential for side effects was increased.[165,166] In the routine clinical setting, higher doses of bronchodilators may be needed for patients with severe airway obstruction or if the technique of administration is not optimal. Because these results were observed with humidified ventilator circuits, we do not recommend bypassing the humidifier for routine bronchodilator therapy. In summary, when the technique of administration is carefully executed, most stable mechanically ventilated patients achieve near maximal bronchodilation after administration of 4 puffs of albuterol with a pMDI or 2.5 mg with a nebulizer. Dosing requirements for infants and small children during mechanical ventilation have not been established and should be titrated to effect. In this case, to a decrease in airway resistance or an increase in tachycardia or tremor. Some authors have recommended that flow–volume loops be monitored before and after bronchodilator administration to quantify changes in airway resistance. In patients who are not totally sedated, these loops can change with patient inspiratory efforts and may be misleading.

Single-dose ampoules of drug are preferred to multi-dose containers or bottles, which are more easily contaminated. Similarly, when the chamber spacer remains in the ventilator circuit between treatments, condensate collects inside. Using a heated wire circuit can reduce the formation of condensate within the spacer. Care must be taken to prevent the condensate in the spacer from being washed into the patient's respiratory tract when the spacer is pulled open during use. When a noncollapsible spacer chamber is used to actuate a pMDI, it should be removed from the ventilator circuit between treatments. No studies demonstrate contamination problems with administration of aerosol from a pMDI during CMV.

The administration of medication by pMDI to the mechanically ventilated neonate may not be well tolerated. Leaving a chamber device in-line is not practical because of the increased compressible volume incorporated into the ventilator circuit. Depending on the FiO_2 and the propellant gas volume, an inline pMDI actuation theoretically may result in the delivery of a hypoxic gas mixture to an infant receiving a tidal volume less than 100 ml. It is possible to deliver a pMDI aerosol medication to the intubated neonate, especially for medications available only in pMDI preparations. However, it may be preferable to hand ventilate the pMDI delivery of medication to the patient. If a chamber adapter is used, the infant must be removed from the circuit, the chamber placed in-line, and the infant reattached to the circuit before the pMDI is administered. The large dead space volume caused by placing a spacer or chamber at the end of the ETT must also be considered when administering pMDI medications to an infant.

BRONCHODILATOR ADMINISTRATION

Inhaler Versus Nebulizer

Nebulizers and pMDIs are equally effective in the treatment of airway obstruction in ambulatory children.[167] Similarly, nebulizers and pMDIs produce similar therapeutic effects in mechanically ventilated patients.

The use of pMDIs for routine bronchodilator therapy in ventilator-supported patients is preferred because of several problems associated with the use of jet nebulizers. The rate of aerosol production by nebulizers is highly variable, not only in nebulizers from different manufacturers but also in different batches of the same brand. Furthermore, the nature of the aerosol produced, especially the particle size, is also highly variable among different nebulizers. The issue is further complicated because the operating efficiency of a nebulizer changes with the pressure of the driving gas and with different fill volumes. Because the pressure of the gas supplied by a ventilator to drive the nebulizer during inspiration is lower than that supplied by a tank/air compressor unit, the efficiency of some nebulizers can be drastically decreased in a ventilator circuit. The gas flow driving the nebulizer produces additional airflow in the ventilator circuit, necessitating adjustment of tidal volume and inspiratory flow when the nebulizer is in use. When patients are unable to trigger the ventilator during assisted modes of mechanical ventilation because of the additional nebulizer gas flow, hypoventilation can result.[166] Therefore, before using a jet nebulizer to treat a ventilator-supported patient, it is imperative to characterize its efficiency in a ventilator circuit under the typical clinical conditions in which it will be used.

Box 11-8 outlines a modification of the technique of aerosol administration with jet nebulizers to mechanically ventilated patients. Box 11-9 provides another strategy for bronchodilator therapy using a pMDI.[5]

Care of Accessory Devices and Nebulizers

For intubated infants or children with increased work of breathing or poor I:E ratios and for those in whom intubation is imminent, a nebulizer or pMDI adapted to a resuscitation bag can be used. The same FiO_2 is used with the jet nebulizer and the resuscitation bag. Flow to the nebulizer should be optimal for the nebulizer used, and flow to the

---

Box 11-8	**Technique for Using Nebulizers to Treat Mechanically Ventilated Patients**

- Place drug solution in the nebulizer to the optimal fill volume (2-6 ml).*
- Place the nebulizer in the inspiratory line, about 30 cm from the patient's Y-piece.
- Ensure sufficient airflow (6-8 L/min) to operate the nebulizer.†
- Ensure adequate tidal volume (about 500 ml in adults, 7 mg/kg for infants and children). Attempt to use a duty cycle greater than 0.3, if possible.
- Adjust the minute volume, sensitivity trigger, and alarms to compensate for additional airflow through the nebulizer if required.
- Turn off flow-by or continuous-flow mode on the ventilator and remove the heat moisture exchanger (if present) from between the nebulizer and the patient.
- Observe the nebulizer for adequate aerosol generation throughout use.
- Disconnect the nebulizer when no more aerosol is being produced.
- Rinse with sterile water or air dry between uses. Store the nebulizer under aseptic conditions.
- Reconnect the ventilator circuit, and return to original ventilator and alarm settings. Confirm proper operation with no leaks in circuit.

*The volume of solution associated with maximal efficiency varies with different nebulizers and should be determined before using any nebulizer.
†The nebulizer may be operated continuously or only during inspiration; the latter method is more efficient for aerosol delivery. Some ventilators provide inspiratory gas flow to the nebulizer. Continuous gas flow from an external source can also be used to power the nebulizer.

Box 11-9	**Technique for Using Pressurized Metered-Dose Inhalers to Treat Mechanically Ventilated Patients**

1. Minimize the inspiratory flow rate during administration.
2. Aim for an inspiratory/expiratory ratio (excluding the inspiratory pause) greater than 0.3 of total breath duration.
3. Ensure that the ventilator breath is synchronized with the patient's inspiration.
4. Shake the pMDI vigorously.
5. Place the canister in the actuator of a cylindrical spacer situated in the inspiratory limb of the ventilator circuit.*
6. Actuate the pMDI to synchronize with precise onset of inspiration by the ventilator.†
7. Allow passive exhalation.
8. Repeat actuations after 20 to 30 seconds until total dose is delivered.‡

pMDI, Pressurized metered-dose inhaler.
*With pMDIs, it is preferable to use a spacer that remains in the ventilator circuit so that disconnection of the ventilator circuit can be avoided at the time of each bronchodilator treatment. Although bypassing the humidifier can increase aerosol delivery, it prolongs the time for each treatment and requires disconnection of the ventilator circuit.
†In ambulatory patients with the pMDI placed inside the mouth, actuation is recommended briefly after initiation of inspiratory airflow. In mechanically ventilated patients in whom a pMDI and spacer combination is used, actuation should be synchronized with onset of inspiration.
‡The manufacturer recommends repeating the dose after 1 minute. However, pMDI actuation within 20 to 30 seconds after the prior dose does not compromise drug delivery.

---

bag should be reduced to compensate for the flow from the nebulizer. When using a bag and mask to deliver medication, care must be taken to avoid gastric insufflation, pulmonary hyperinflation, and hyperventilation or hypoventilation. The mask is used to create a good seal, and attempts must be made to time the inflation with the inspiratory effort. Care must be taken to stabilize the ETT to prevent accidental extubation with the added weight of the equipment. The patient is ventilated using the same pressures and rate as with the mechanical ventilator. It is theoretically helpful to deliver an occasional sigh by providing a slight inspiratory hold at the peak inspiratory pressure, thereby enhancing the volume and depth of medication delivered while providing additional time for deposition to occur in the airways.

HOME CARE AND MONITORING COMPLIANCE

With most therapeutic aerosols being administered in the home, patient education and adherence with written medicine and action plans are critical. To improve compliance, aerosol therapy should be administered along with some easily remembered activity of daily living. For twice-daily administration, medications can be kept with the toothbrush and inhaled just before brushing teeth.

This approach also reduces aerosol corticosteroid deposition in the oral pharynx. It is always best to avoid the regular use of medication at school because the inconvenience can significantly reduce compliance and may embarrass some children. However, the availability of rescue medication at school (or day care or other caregiver's home) must be ensured. It helps to prepare written guidelines for medication use. Distribute these guidelines to all the places where the child stays, such as home, school, or the residence of each parent if divorced or separated.[78]

It is helpful, at least initially, to keep a diary of medication use. Lack of response to inhaled asthma medication can be related to a number of factors, including incorrect technique of inhalation; inhalation from depleted canisters of medications, thinking that they still contain active drug; not taking preventive medications as prescribed; change in the child's environment; or misdiagnosis. For example, children with aspirated foreign body, gastroesophageal reflux disease, or psychogenic wheeze will have a poor response to asthma therapy. Infants with tracheomalacia or bronchopulmonary dysplasia may even become much worse after inhaling a bronchodilator aerosol because of increased dynamic airway collapse.[79,169]

Standard nebulizers and pMDIs have no intrinsic mechanism for tracking use or compliance. The pMDI also has no mechanism to track how many doses remain in the canister. If accurately completed, medication diaries can help to track medication use and the use of rescue medications while monitoring prescription refill records.

Several aerosol delivery devices entering the market can directly track use and monitor compliance. These devices range from electronic models integrated with the nebulizer that track number of breaths taken, size of breaths, and duration and frequency of treatment, to simple counting devices attached to the pMDI actuator boot. More sophisticated devices allow monitoring of both pMDI use and expiratory maneuvers for later transmission to the care provider's office. Some newer DPI devices contain a built-in counter that advances each time a dose is loaded. These devices also give a visual signal when only a few doses remain in the device.

OTHER MEDICATIONS FOR AEROSOL DELIVERY

Antibiotics

Aerosol antibiotics can deliver high concentrations of antibiotics to the airway with low systemic bioavailability, thus reducing toxicity. This approach is of particular importance in patients with cystic fibrosis (CF), who often require courses of antibiotic therapy.[170] In a phase 3 registration study, 468 patients with CF were enrolled in a 6-month masked, placebo-controlled trial of preservative-free, nonpyrogenic tobramycin solution for inhalation (TOBI; Novartis, Emeryville, CA), alternating between 4-week courses of tobramycin and placebo. During treatment the patients received 300 mg of tobramycin in 5 ml of quarter-strength saline. The FEV_1 increased by more than 10% by the end of 6 months, with patients receiving tobramycin 26% less likely to be hospitalized and 36% less likely to require intravenous antipseudomonal antibiotics and a greater than 10-fold reduction in sputum bacterial density.[171] Follow-up studies in CF and non-CF bronchiectasis have generally been consistent with these earlier results.[172]

Other antibiotics are being prepared for aerosol delivery including colistin, gentamicin, ciprofloxacin, and aztreonam. As this chapter is being prepared, the latter has completed phase 3 trials in CF by Gilead Sciences (Foster City, CA) using a novel vibrating mesh aerosol delivery device (eFlow; PARI Pharma, Midlothian, VA). Although aerosolized antibiotics may find a role in the therapy of patients with severe bronchopulmonary dysplasia or those with chronic tracheostomies, the emergence of bacterial resistance to these antibiotics is a real risk and must be closely monitored.[173]

Mucoactive Agents

Sputum is expectorated mucus mixed with inflammatory cells, cellular debris, polymers of DNA and F-actin, as well as bacteria. Mucus is usually cleared by airflow and ciliary movement, and sputum is cleared by cough.[174] Dornase alfa (Pulmozyme; Genentech, South San Francisco, CA) was the first approved mucoactive agent for the treatment of CF.[9] Dornase alfa is safe and effective, even in patients with more severe pulmonary disease, defined as a forced vital capacity less than 40% of the predicted value.[175] Efficacy has not been demonstrated for the therapy of acute exacerbations of CF lung disease or for the treatment of other chronic airway diseases.[176] A small phase 1 study in non-CF bronchiectasis demonstrated no efficacy in non-CF bronchiectasis, and there was a suggestion that the use of dornase worsened disease in this adult population.[177] This may be due to the fact that secretions in bronchiectasis and chronic obstructive pulmonary disease are composed primarily of mucin and related proteins, thus constituting true mucous hypersecretion,[178] whereas in the CF airway there is significantly decreased mucin and mucus, the CF secretions being almost entirely neutrophil-derived pus.[179]

Other mucoactive agents under development include mucolytics such as Nacystelyn (N-acetylcysteinate lysine),[180] thymosin β4, and low-molecular-weight dextran[181]; mucokinetic agents such as surfactant; and P2Y2 chloride channel activators.[182] The use of hyperosmolar saline or mannitol to improve secretion clearance in CF is discussed in a following section (see Hyperosmolar Aerosols).

Surfactant

There is profound loss of surfactant in the inflamed airway with bronchitis or cystic fibrosis.[183] Randomized, masked, placebo-controlled studies demonstrate that surfactant aerosol improves pulmonary function and sputum transportability in patients with chronic bronchitis and that this effect is dose dependent with no significant side effects.[184] As a wetting and spreading agent, the surfactant also has the ability to increase the lower airway deposition of other aerosol medications, such as dornase alfa or gene therapy vectors, and may increase small particle translocation through the mucous layer.[21]

Hyperosmolar Aerosols

For many years, sputum induction by hyperosmolar saline inhalation has been used to obtain specimens for the diagnosis of pneumonia. In a pilot study, 58 patients with CF were randomly assigned to receive 10 ml of either 0.9% normal saline or 6% hypertonic saline twice daily by ultrasonic nebulization.[185] Spirometry was measured for 2 weeks during therapy and for 2 weeks after therapy. At 2 weeks there was a significant increase in the FEV_1 in the hypertonic saline group, with a return to baseline by 28 days. Despite pretreatment with 600 μg of inhaled albuterol, several patients had an acute decrease in FEV_1 after inhaling hypertonic saline. Similarly, hyperosmolar dry powder mannitol improves quality of life and pulmonary function in adult subjects with non-CF bronchiectasis and significantly improves the surface adhesivity and cough clearability of expectorated sputum.[186]

Subsequent studies, as reviewed in the *Cochrane Database of Systematic Reviews,* tend to confirm that the long-term use of inhaled hyperosmolar saline improves pulmonary function in patients with CF[187] and that inhaled hyperosmolar saline or mannitol is beneficial in non-CF bronchiectasis.[188] Although this therapy is readily available and inexpensive, it has been reported that hypertonic saline aerosol is not as effective as dornase alfa in the therapy of CF lung disease.[189]

Gene Transfer Therapy

Gene transfer therapy represents a novel use for aerosols. Efforts in this arena have centered largely on complementary (copy) DNA transfer of the normal CF transmembrane regulator (CFTR) gene to patients with CF. Gene transfer was first attempted by inserting the normal CFTR gene into a replication-defective adenovirus vector with bolus bronchoscopic delivery of the vector. An unanticipated host immune response to the vector led to reevaluation of this strategy.[190]

For gene transfer to be effective, the vector and its package must be nonimmunogenic, stable to shear forces during aerosolization, and safe to transfected cells. The vector should not increase cell turnover. It should either stably integrate into the progenitor (basal) cell genome or be safe and effective with repeated administration and should be able to reach the cellular target of relevance. Part of the difficulty with CF is that this cellular target has not been clearly identified as epithelial cell, goblet cell, submucous gland, or all of these. The amount of gene and vector and persistence in the airway must also be determined for each vector and delivery system.[191]

Viral vectors that have been studied include adenovirus, adeno-associated virus, and lentivirus. Adenovirus naturally targets the airway epithelium. Adeno-associated virus is a small organism that requires a "helper" virus to replicate. These viruses are capable of site-directed insertion into DNA, reducing the risk of insertional mutagenesis (initiating cancer by activation of an oncogene or inactivation of an oncogene suppressor). Gene therapy with adeno-associated virus appears to be especially promising.[192] Lentiviruses are retroviruses such as human immunodeficiency virus. They are able to transfect cells that are not terminally differentiated, such as the basal or airway progenitor cell, but insertional mutagenesis is a substantial risk.

The primary nonviral vectors studied to date have been cationic liposomes. These lipid capsules are able to form complexes with DNA and then enter cells. With the first generation of liposome vectors, the efficiency of gene transfer was poor; however, this has improved dramatically with newer systems.[193] The development of this technology will result in revolutionary aerosol generators.[194]

Aerosols for Systemic Administration

Aerosols can be targeted to different sites in the airway. Depending on the intrapulmonary behavior of each molecule, the aerosol mode of administration allows airway/secretion delivery, cellular delivery, or systemic delivery. Most medications are targeted to the airway epithelium, including the neuromuscular plexus (bronchodilators) and inflammatory cells (corticosteroids). Epithelial agents such as the P2Y2 ion channel activators are targeted directly to the ciliated epithelium. Mucolytics, proteases, and antibiotics are targeted to secretions in the airway rather than to the epithelial cells.

Small particles targeted to the alveolus can be effective for systemic delivery of macromolecules through the extensive pulmonary vascular bed. Insulin is likely to be the first such medication introduced for systemic administration through aerosol administration, but other peptides and macromolecules are under development. Considerations for systemic administration include cost, convenience, efficacy, and safety. The pulmonary behavior of an inhaled molecule is not predictable and must be studied individually.[195]

Insulin

Insulin was one of the first medications to be administered by aerosol. Because of the nebulizer and insulin formulation available at that time, absorption and efficacy were highly unpredictable. This has changed dramatically with the development of ultrafine particles and aerosol devices that can efficiently and reliably target the alveolar space.

With a rapid and smooth onset of action and elimination of the necessity for injections with their attendant risks and discomfort, inhaled insulin has great potential for clinical use. Intrapulmonary insulin administration to healthy subjects can induce significant hypoglycemia and a clinically relevant increase in serum insulin concentrations.[196] Once plasma glucose levels are normalized, postprandial glucose levels can be maintained below diabetic levels by delivering insulin into the lungs 5 minutes before ingestion of a meal.[197,198]

Studies have confirmed that inhaled insulin is safe and effective for the therapy of type 2 diabetes even when this is not controlled by diet[199,200] and that the addition of inhaled insulin or oral therapy with hypoglycemic agents improves glycemic control.[201]

With the success of inhaled insulin demonstrating the safe and effective systemic administration of complex peptides via the pulmonary bed, it is highly probable that we will see the development of other aerosol therapies that could revolutionize fields as diverse as endocrinology, critical care, immunology, and genetics.[202,203] Because the respiratory therapist will be at the front line for teaching and administering these novel therapies, this will greatly expand the role of the respiratory therapist in the future.

The use of therapeutic aerosol medications is evolving from a basis of optimizing the delivery of asthma medications to the airway to understanding how the extensive pulmonary vascular bed can be used for the systemic administration of a variety of macromolecules. Evolving and novel uses of therapeutic aerosols will require an understanding of aerosol generation, deposition, and translocation, as well as target organ physiology and pharmacology.

KEY POINTS

- Infants are obligate nose breathers up to 6 to 9 months.
- With growth, lung volumes increase, airways get larger, and respiratory rates decrease.
- Smaller airways filter out more aerosol, reducing lung doses compared with larger children and adults.
- From ages 3 to 13, pulmonary deposition increases but dose per kilogram is similar.
- Nebulizers vary in method of operation and delivered dose.
- Breath-actuated nebulizers can increase inhaled dose and dosing time by threefold compared with continuous nebulizers.
- Infants and toddlers may not be able to breath-actuate nebulizers.
- Jet and ultrasonic nebulizers have residual medication volumes of 0.5 to 1.4 ml.
- Nebulizers with medication cups that directly connect to vent circuit or mouthpiece are prone to contamination from drool and contaminated condensate.
- DPIs typically require high sustained inspiratory flows to disaggregate drug and may not be suitable for children younger than 5 years of age.
- No aerosol devices were specifically designed for infants and toddlers.

- DPI and pMDI alone are not suitable for children younger than 4 to 5 years.
- pMDI with VHC and nebulizers (continuous) are suitable for children younger than 4 years.
- Interface of aerosol device to patient is critical.
- Mask must be tightly fitted for optimal delivery with jet or pMDI.
- Blow-by has not been shown to be effective.
- Mask with jet nebulizer more than 2 cm from an infant's face is not effective.
- Agitated and crying infants do not receive much if any aerosol to lung.
- Nasal delivery of aerosol via high-flow nasal cannula may be a solution.
- As flow decreases, aerosol delivery increases in infants and small children.
- Heliox appears to improve aerosol delivery when inspiratory flow rates are higher.
- Very few inhaled medications have been approved based on studies in infants and small children, making administration to this population "off label."
- Caution should be exercised during administration of any aerosol to neonates and infants.
- New and developing medications are showing great promise for use with children.

ASSESSMENT QUESTIONS

See Evolve Resources for answers.

1. Which of the following is true when a standard unit dose is nebulized to patients of different sizes and ages?
   A. Smaller percentage of dose is delivered to bigger patients
   B. Larger percentage of dose is delivered to smaller patients
   C. Similar inhaled dose per kilogram of body weight
   D. Similar total inhaled dose
   E. No dose is delivered to infants

2. In infants between 1 and 4 kg, deposition of aerosol with a pMDI or jet nebulizer is:
   A. Similar whether intubated and mechanically ventilated or spontaneously breathing with a normal airway
   B. Less than 1% in all cases
   C. Slightly greater with a pMDI than with a jet nebulizer
   D. All of the above
   E. None of the above

3. What should the operator do when operating a jet nebulizer with a mixture of helium–oxygen?
   A. Provide the same total flow of gas to the nebulizer as with air or oxygen.
   B. Increase the flow of gas to the nebulizer by 2- or 3-fold.
   C. Reduce the flow of gas to the nebulizer by one half.
   D. Never use heliox to drive a nebulizer.
   E. Never use an air or oxygen flow meter.

4. Which of the following statements is true about the SPAG aerosol generator?
   A. It makes very small particles.
   B. It uses a secondary chamber to dry particles.
   C. It is used to administer ribavirin.
   D. It is often used with double containment systems.
   E. All of the above.

5. What is the most reliable way to determine how many actuations are left in a pMDI?
   A. Float the canister in water.
   B. Count the number of doses used.
   C. Actuate until it is empty.
   D. Use it for only 1 month.
   E. All of the above.

6. What limits use of DPIs for children less than 5 years of age?
   A. They are not big enough to generate sufficient inspiratory flow.
   B. They cannot use a mouthpiece.
   C. DPIs make them cough.
   D. They cannot coordinate actuation with inspiration.
   E. None of the above.

7. Which of the following statements is/are true about a large proportion of patients and their caregivers?
   A. They do not know how to properly use a DPI.
   B. They do not know how to properly use a pMDI.
   C. They do not know how to properly clean and assemble a nebulizer.
   D. They misuse their inhaler to the point of not benefiting from their medication.
   E. All of the above.

8. During bronchodilator administration in severe airway obstruction:
   A. An increased dose may be more effective than increased frequency.
   B. Undiluted bronchodilator may be substituted for diluted bronchodilator.
   C. Continuous nebulization may work better than intermittent nebulizations.
   D. Patients who do not respond to initial high doses are more often admitted to hospital.
   E. All of the above.

9. What is the most practical way to improve aerosol deposition during mechanical ventilation?
   A. Use a nebulizer with a small particle size.
   B. Use a ramp versus square-wave pattern.
   C. Minimize inspiratory flow rates.
   D. Use a pMDI instead of a nebulizer.
   E. All of the above.

10. Which drug was one of the first to be administered by aerosol?
    A. Mucolytics
    B. Antibiotics
    C. Gene therapy
    D. Surfactant
    E. Insulin

References

1. Newhouse M, Dolovich M: Control of asthma by aerosols, *N Engl J Med* 315:870, 1986.
2. Janson C: Plasma levels and effects of salbutamol after inhaled or i.v. administration in stable asthma, *Eur Repir J* 4:544, 1991.
3. Brain JD, Valberg PA: Deposition of aerosol in the respiratory tract, *Am Rev Resp Dis* 120:1325, 1979.
4. Gross NJ, Jenne J, Hess D: Bronchodilator therapy. In Tobin MJ, editor: *Principles and practice of mechanical ventilation*, New York, 1994, McGraw-Hill, pp 1077–1123.
5. Rubin B, Fink J: Aerosol therapy for children, *Respir Care Clin N Am* 7:100, 2001.
6. Wildhaber JH, Janssens HM, Pierart F, Dore ND, Devadason SG, LeSouef PN: High-percentage lung delivery in children from detergent-treated spacers, *Pediatr Pulmonol* 29:389, 2000.
7. Dolovich M: Assessing nebulizer performance, *Respir Care* 47:1290, 2002.
8. Fok TF, Monkman S, Dolovich M, et al: Efficiency of aerosol medication delivery from a metered dose inhaler versus jet nebulizer in infants with bronchopulmonary dysplasia, *Pediatr Pulmonol* 21:301, 1996.
9. Wildhaber JH, Dore ND, Wilson JM, Devadason SG, LeSouef PN: Inhalation therapy in asthma: nebulizer or pressurized metered-dose inhaler with holding chamber? In vivo comparison of lung deposition in children, *J Pediatr* 135:28, 1999.
10. Erzinger S, Schueepp KG, Brooks-Wildhaber J, Devadason SG, Wildhaber JH: Facemasks and aerosol delivery in vivo, *J Aerosol Med* 20:S78, 2007.
11. Fink J, Dhand R: Aerosol therapy: In Fink J, Hunt G, editors: *Clinical practice in respiratory care*, Philadelphia, 1998, Lippincott-Raven, pp 307–336.
12. Dolovich M: Physical principles underlying aerosol therapy, *J Aerosol Med* 2:171, 1989.
13. Pedersen S: Delivery systems in children: In Barnes P, Grunstein M, Leff A, Woolcock A, editors: *Asthma*, Philadelphia, 1997, Lippincott-Raven, pp 1925.
14. Desai M, Mutlu M, Vadgama P: A study of macro-molecular diffusion through native porcine mucus, *Experientia* 48:22, 1992.
15. Bolister N, Basker M, Hodges NA, Marriott C: The diffusion of beta-lactam antibiotics through mixed gels of cystic fibrosis-derived mucin and *Pseudomonas aeruginosa* alginate, *J Antimicrob Chemother* 27:285, 1991.
16. King M, Kelly S, Cosio M: Alteration of airway reactivity by mucus, *Respir Physiol* 62:47, 1985.
17. De Sanctis GT, Kelly SM, Saetta MP, et al: Hyporesponsiveness to aerosolized but not to infused methacholine in cigarette-smoking dogs, *Am Rev Respir Dis* 135:338, 1987.
18. Bataillon V, Lhermitte M, Lafitte JJ, Pommery J, Roussel P: The binding of amikacin to macromolecules from the sputum of patients suffering from respiratory diseases, *J Antimicrob Chemother* 29:499, 1992.
19. Taskar VS, Sharma RR, Goswami R, John PJ, Mahashur AA: Effect of bromhexeine on sputum amoxicillin levels in lower respiratory infections, *Respir Med* 86:157, 1992.
20. Stern M, Caplen NJ, Browning JE, et al: The effect of mucolytic agents on gene transfer across a CF sputum barrier in vitro, *Gene Ther* 5:91, 1998.
21. Schurch S, Gehr P, Im Hof V, Geiser M, Green F: Surfactant displaces particles toward the epithelium in airways and alveoli, *Respir Physiol* 80:17, 1990.
22. Kharasch VS, Sweeney TD, Fredberg J, et al: Pulmonary surfactant as a vehicle for intratracheal delivery of technetium

sulfur colloid and pentamidine in hamster lungs, *Am Rev Respir Dis* 144:909, 1991:

23. Newhouse M, Kennedy A: Rapid temperature change from 25°C to 15°C impairs powder deaggregation in Bricanyl Turbuhaler, *J Aerosol Med* 12:113, 1999.

24. Hess D, Fisher D, Williams P, Pooler S, Kacmarek RM: Medication nebulizer performance. Effects of diluent volume, nebulizer flow, and nebulizer brand, *Chest* 110:498, 1996.

25. Johnson M, Newman S, Bloom R, Talaee N, Clarke S: Delivery of albuterol and ipratropium bromide from two nebulizer systems in chronic stable asthma: efficacy and pulmonary deposition, *Chest* 96:6, 1989.

26. Hadfield JW, Windebank WJ, Bateman JR: Is driving gas flow rate clinically important for nebulizer therapy? *Br J Dis Chest* 80:50, 1986.

27. Douglas JG, Leslie MJ, Crompton GK, Grant IW: A comparative study of two doses of salbutamol nebulized at 4 and 8 litres per minute in patients with chronic asthma, *Br J Dis Chest* 80:55, 1986.

28. Hess DR, Acosta FL, Ritz RH, Kacmarek RM, Camargo CA, Jr: The effect of heliox on nebulizer function using a beta-agonist bronchodilator, *Chest* 115:184, 1999.

29. Goode ML, Fink JB, Dhand R, Tobin MJ: Improvement in aerosol delivery with helium-oxygen mixtures during mechanical ventilation, *Am J Respir Crit Care Med* 163:109, 2001.

30. Malone RA, Hollie MC, Glynn-Barnhart A, Nelson HS: Optimal duration of nebulized albuterol therapy, *Chest* 104:1114, 1993.

31. Thomas S, Lanford J, George R: Improving the efficiency of drug administration with jet nebulisers, *Lancet* 1:126, 1988.

32. Rau JL, Ari A, Restrepo RD: Performance comparison of nebulizer designs: constant-output, breath-enhanced, and dosimetric, *Respir Care* 49:174, 2004.

33. Ari A, Hess D, Myers TR, Rau JL: *A guide to aerosol delivery devices for respiratory therapists*, Dallas, 2009, American Association for Respiratory Care.

34. Newnham DM, Lipworth BJ: Nebuliser performance, pharmacokinetics, airways and systemic effects of salbutamol given via a novel nebuliser delivery system ("Ventstream"), *Thorax* 49:762, 1994.

35. Sangwan S, Condos R, Smaldone G: Lung deposition and respirable mass during wet nebulization, *J Aerosol Med* 16:379, 2003.

36. Sabato MK, Ward P, Hawk W, Gildengorin G, Asselin JM: Randomized controlled trial comparing a breath actuated nebulizer to a hospital's standard therapy to treat pediatric asthma in the emergency department, *Respir Care* 56:761, 2011.

37. Lin YZ, Huang FY: Comparison of breath-actuated and conventional constant-flow jet nebulizers in treating acute asthmatic children, *Acta Paediatr Taiwan* 45:73, 2004.

38. Lin HL, Wan GH, Chen YH, Fink JB, Liu WQ, Liu KY: Influence of nebulizer type with different pediatric aerosol masks on drug deposition in a model of a spontaneously breathing small child, *Respir Care* 57:1894, 2012.

39. Ari A, Fink JB: Effective bronchodilator resuscitation of children in the emergency room: device or interface? *Respir Care* 56:882, 2011.

40. Ari A, Fink JB: Breath-actuated nebulizer versus small-volume nebulizer: efficacy, safety, and satisfaction, *Respir Care* 57:1351, 2012.

41. The Nebuliser Project Group of the British Thoracic Society Standards of Care Committee: Current best practice for nebuliser treatment, *Thorax* 52:S4, 1997.

42. Standaert TA, Morlin GL, Williams-Warren J, et al: Effects of repetitive use and cleaning techniques of disposable jet nebulizers on aerosol generation, *Chest* 114:577, 1998.

43. Centers for Disease Control and Prevention: Guideline for prevention of nosocomial pneumonia, *Respir Care* 39:1191, 1994.

44. Oie S, Kamiya A: Bacterial contamination of aerosol solutions containing antibiotics, *Microbios* 82:109, 1995.

45. Kelly H, Keim K, McWilliams B: Comparison of two methods of delivering continuously nebulized albuterol, *Ann Pharmacotherapy* 37:23, 2003.

46. Papo MC, Frank J, Thompson AE: A prospective, randomized study of continuous versus intermittent nebulized albuterol for severe status asthmaticus in children, *Crit Care Med* 21:1479, 1993.

47. Khine H, Fuchs SM, Saville AL: Continuous vs intermittent nebulized albuterol for emergency management of asthma, *Acad Emerg Med* 3:1019, 1996.

48. Berlinski A, Willis JR, Leisenring T: In-vitro comparison of 4 large-volume nebulizers in 8 hours of continuous nebulization, *Respir Care* 55:1671, 2010.

49. Kacmarek R, Kratochvil J: Evaluation of a double-enclosure double-vacuum unit scavenging system for ribavirin administration, *Respir Care* 37:37, 1992.

50. Adderley RJ: Safety of ribavirin with mechanical ventilation, *Pediatr Infect Dis J* 9:S112, 1990.

51. Committee on Infectious Diseases, American Academy of Pediatrics: Reassessment of the indications for ribavirin therapy in respiratory syncytial virus infections, *Pediatrics* 97:137, 1996.

52. Phillips G, Millard F: The therapeutic use of ultrasonic nebulizers in acute asthma, *Respir Med* 88:387, 1994.

53. Summer W, Elston R, Tharpe L, Nelson S, Haponik EF: Aerosol bronchodilator delivery methods. Relative impact on pulmonary function and cost of respiratory care, *Arch Intern Med* 149:618, 1989.

54. Yuksel B, Greenough A: Comparison of the effects on lung function of two methods of bronchodilator administration, *Respir Med* 88:229, 1994.

55. Nakanishi AK, Lamb BM, Foster C, Rubin BK: Ultrasonic nebulization of albuterol is no more effective than jet nebulization for the treatment of acute asthma in children, *Chest* 111:1505, 1997.

56. Doershuk CF, Matthews LW, Gillespie CT, Lough MD, Spector S: Evaluation of jet-type and ultrasonic nebulizers in mist tent therapy for cystic fibrosis, *Pediatrics* 41:723, 1968.

57. Boucher RM, Kreuter J: The fundamentals of the ultrasonic atomization of medicated solutions, *Ann Allergy* 26:591, 1968.

58. Thomas SH, O'Doherty MJ, Page CJ, Treacher DF, Nunan TO: Delivery of ultrasonic nebulized aerosols to a lung model during mechanical ventilation, *Am Rev Resp Dis* 148:872, 1993.

59. Ari A, Restrepo RD: Aerosol delivery device selection for spontaneously breathing patients: 2012. *Respir Care* 57:613, 2012.

60. Boe J, Dennis JH, O'Driscoll BR, et al: European respiratory society guidelines on the use of nebulizers, *Eur Respir J* 18:228, 2001.

61. Tablan O, Anderson L, Besser R, Bridges C, Hajjeh R: Guidelines for Preventing Health Care–Associated Pneumonia. Recommendations of the CDC and the Healthcare Infection Control Practices Advisory Committee. *MMWR Recommendations & Reports,* 2004. http://www.cdc.gov/mmwr/preview/mmwrhtml/rr5303a1.htm. Accessed 19 January 2009.

62. Saiman L, Siegel J: Infection control recommendations for patients with cystic fibrosis: microbiology, important pathogens, and infection control practices to prevent patient-to-patient transmission, *Am J Infect Control* 31:S6, 2003.

63. O'Malley CA, VandenBranden SL, Zheng XT, Polito AM, McColley SA: A day in the life of a nebulizer: surveillance

for bacterial growth in nebulizer equipment of children with cystic fibrosis in the hospital setting, *Respir Care* 52:258, 2007.

64. Fink JB, Ari A: Humidity and aerosol therapy. *Mosby's respiratory care equipment*, 9th ed, St. Louis, 2013. Mosby-Elsevier.

65. Lin Y, Hsieh K: Metered dose inhaler and nebuliser in acute asthma, *Arch Dis Child* 72:214, 1995.

66. Newhouse M, Dolovich M: Aerosol therapy in children. In Chermick V, Mellins R, editors: *Basic mechanisms of pediatric respiratory disease: cellular and integrative*, Toronto, 1991, BC Decker.

67. Svartengren K, Lindestad P, Svartengren M, Philipson K, Bylin G, Camner P: Added external resistance reduces oropharyngeal deposition and increases lung deposition of aerosol particles in asthmatics, *Am J Respir Crit Care Med* 152:32, 1995.

68. Hill LS, Slater AL: A comparison of the performance of two modern multidose dry powder asthma inhalers, *Respir Med* 92:105, 1998.

69. Rajkumari N, Byron PR, Dalby RN: Testing of dry powder aerosol formulations in different environmental conditions, *Int J Pharm* 113:123, 1995.

70. Larsen JS, Hahn M, Ekholm B, Wick KA: Evaluation of conventional press-and-breathe metered-dose inhaler technique in 501 patients, *J Asthma* 31:193, 1994.

71. Guidry G, Brown W, Stogner S, George R: Incorrect use of metered dose inhalers by medical personnel, *Chest* 101:31, 1992.

72. Newman SP, Pavia D, Clarke SW: Simple instructions for using pressurized aerosol bronchodilators, *J R Soc Med* 73:776, 1980.

73. Fink JB, Rubin BK: Problems with inhaler use: a call for improved clinician and patient education, *Respir Care* 50:1360, 2005.

74. Hampson N, Mueller M: Reduction in patient timing errors using a breath-activated metered dose inhaler, *Chest* 106:462, 1994.

75. Toogood JH, Baskerville J, Jennings B, Lefcoe NM, Johansson SA: Use of spacers to facilitate inhaled corticosteroid treatment of asthma, *Am Rev Respir Dis* 129:723, 1984.

76. Diot P, Morra L, Smaldone GC: Albuterol delivery in a model of mechanical ventilation. Comparison of metered-dose inhaler and nebulizer efficiency, *Am J Respir Crit Care Med* 152:1391, 1995.

77. Salzman GA, Pyszczynski DR: Oropharyngeal candidiasis in patients treated with beclomethasone dipropionate delivered by metered-dose inhaler alone and with Aerochamber, *J Allergy Clin Immunol* 81:424, 1988.

78. Rubin BK: Pressurized metered-dose inhalers and holding chambers for inhaled glucocorticoid therapy in childhood asthma, *J Allergy Clin Immunol* 103:1224, 1999.

79. Closa RM, Ceballos JM, Gomez-Papi A, Galiana AS, Gutierrez C, Marti-Henneber C: Efficacy of bronchodilators administered by nebulizers versus spacer devices in infants with acute wheezing, *Pediatr Pulmonol* 26:344, 1998.

80. Williams JR, Bothner JP, Swanton RD: Delivery of albuterol in a pediatric emergency department, *Pediatr Emerg Care* 12:263, 1996.

81. Cunningham SJ, Crain EF: Reduction of morbidity in asthmatic children given a spacer device, *Chest* 106:753, 1994.

82. Ganderton D, The generation of respirable clouds from coarse powder aggregates, *J Biopharm Sci* 3:101, 1994.

83. Dolovich M: Measurement of the particle size and dosing characteristics of a radiolabelled albuterol sulphate lactose blend used in the SPIROS dry powder inhaler. In Dalby R, Byron PR, Farr S, editors: *Respiratory drug delivery*, Buffalo Grove, NY, 1996, Interpharm Press, pp 332–335.

84. Engel T, Heinig JH, Madsen F, Nikander K: Peak inspiratory flow and inspiratory vital capacity of patients with asthma measured with and without a new dry-powder inhaler device (Turbuhaler), *Eur Respir J* 3:1037, 1990.

85. Pedersen S, Hansen O, Fuglsang G: Influence of inspiratory flow rate upon the effect of a Turbuhaler, *Arch Dis Child* 65:308, 1990.

86. Thorsson L, Edsbacker S, Conradson TB: Lung deposition of budesonide from Turbuhaler is twice that from a pressurized metered-dose inhaler P-MDI, *Eur Respir J* 7:1839, 1994.

87. Hindle M, Byron PR: Dose emissions from marketed dry powder inhalers, *Int J Pharm* 116:169, 1992.

88. Gansslen M: Uber inhalation von insulin, *Klin Wochenschr* 4:71, 1925.

89. Bisgaard H, Klug B, Skamstrup K, Sumby B: Inspiratory flow rate through the discus/accuhaler inhaler and turbuhaler inhaler in children with asthma, *J Aerosol Med* 116:169, 1996.

90. Smith KJ, Chan HK, Brown KF: Influence of flow rate on aerosol particle size distributions from pressurized and breath-actuated inhalers, *J Aerosol Med* 11:231, 1998.

91. Pedersen S: Delivery options for inhaled therapy in children over the age of 6 years, *J Aerosol Med* 10:S41, 1997.

92. Fok TF, Lam K, Chan CK, et al: Aerosol delivery to nonventilated infants by metered dose inhaler: should a valved spacer be used? *Pediatr Pulmonol* 24:204, 1997.

93. Kesten S, Elias M, Cartier A, Chapman KR: Patient handling of a multidose dry powder inhalation device for albuterol, *Chest* 105:1077, 1994.

94. Ari A, Fink J: Guidelines to aerosol devices in infants, children and adults: which to choose, why and how to achieve effective aerosol therapy? *Expert Rev Respir Med* 5:561, 2011.

95. Everard ML: Guidelines for devices and choices, *J Aerosol Med* 14 Suppl 1:S59, 2001.

96. Everard ML: Trying to deliver aerosols to upset children is a thankless task, *Arch Dis Child* 82:428, 2000.

97. Iles R, Lister P, Edmunds AT: Crying significantly reduces absorption of aerosolised drug in infants, *Arch Dis Child* 81:163, 1999.

98. Janssens H, van der Wiel E, Verbraak A, de Jongste J, Merkus P, Tiddens H: Aerosol therapy and the fighting toddler: is administration during sleep an alternative? *J Aerosol Med* 16:395, 2003.

99. Esposito-Festen JE, Ijsselstjin H, Hop W, van Vliet F, de Jongste J, Tiddens H: Aerosol therapy by pMDI-spacer in sleeping young children: to do or not to do? *Chest* 130:487, 2006.

100. Lin HL, Restrepo RD, Gardenhire DS, Rau JL: Effect of face mask design on inhaled mass of nebulized albuterol, using a pediatric breathing model, *Respir Care* 52:1021, 2007.

101. Restrepo RD, Dickson SK, Rau JL, Gardenhire DS: An investigation of nebulized bronchodilator delivery using a pediatric lung model of spontaneous breathing, *Respir Care* 51:56, 2006.

102. Janssens H, Heijnen E, de Jong V, Holland W, de Jongste J, Tiddens H: Aerosol delivery from spacers in wheezy infants: a daily life study, *Eur Repir J* 16:850, 2000.

103. Smaldone GC, Berg E, Nikander K: Variation in pediatric aerosol delivery: importance of facemask, *J Aerosol Med* 18:354, 2005.

104. Smaldone GC: Assessing new technologies: patient-device interactions and deposition, *Respir Care* 50:1151, 2005.

105. Esposito-Festen JE, Ates B, van Vliet FJ, Verbraak AF, de Jongste JC, Tiddens HA: Effect of a facemask leak on aerosol delivery from a pMDI-spacer system, *J Aerosol Med* 17:1, 2004.

106. Amirav I, Newhouse MT: Aerosol therapy with valved holding chambers in young children: importance of the facemask seal, *Pediatrics* 108:389, 2001.

107. Esposito-Festen J, Ates B, van Vliet F, Hop W, Tiddens H: Aerosol delivery to young children by pMDI-spacer: is facemask design important? *Pediatr Allergy Immunol* 16:348, 2005.

108. Hayden J, Smith N, Woolf D, Barry P, O'Callaghan C: A randomised crossover trial of facemask efficacy, *Arch Dis Child* 89:72, 2004.

109. Mansour MM, Smaldone GC: Blow-by as potential therapy for uncooperative children: an in-vitro study, *Respir Care* 57:2004, 2012.

110. Amirav I, Balanov I, Gorenberg M, Groshar D, Luder AS: Nebuliser hood compared to mask in wheezy infants: aerosol therapy without tears! *Arch Dis Child* 88:719, 2003.

111. Kugelman A, Amirav I, Mor F, Riskin A, Bader D: Hood versus mask nebulization in infants with evolving bronchopulmonary dysplasia in the neonatal intensive care unit, *J Perinatol* 26:31, 2006.

112. Amirav I, Oron A, Tal G, et al: Aerosol delivery in respiratory syncytial virus bronchiolitis: hood or face mask? *J Pediatr* 147:627, 2005.

113. Amirav I, Shakked T, Broday DM, Katoshevski D: Numerical investigation of aerosol deposition at the eyes when using a hood inhaler for infants—a 3D simulation, *J Aerosol Med Pulm Drug Deliv* 21:207, 2008.

114. Ari A, Harwood R, Sheard M, Dailey P, Fink JB: In vitro comparison of heliox and oxygen in aerosol delivery using pediatric high flow nasal cannula, *Pediatr Pulmonol* 46:795, 2011:

115. Bhashyam AR, Wolf MT, Marcinkowski AL, et al: Aerosol delivery through nasal cannulas: an in vitro study, *J Aerosol Med Pulm Drug Deliv* 21:181, 2008.

116. Everard ML: Aerosol delivery to children, *Pediatr Ann* 35:630, 2006.

117. Everard ML: Inhalation therapy for infants, *Adv Drug Deliv Rev* 55:869, 2003.

118. National Asthma Education and Prevention Program: Expert Panel III. *Guidelines for the diagnosis and management of asthma.* Bethesda, MD, 2007, National Heart, Blood and Lung Institute.

119. Schuh S, Parkin P, Rajan A, et al: High- versus low-dose, frequently administered, nebulized albuterol in children with severe, acute asthma, *Pediatrics* 83:513, 1989.

120. Direkwatanachai C, Teeratakulpisarn J, Suntornlohanakul S, et al: Comparison of Salbutamol efficacy in children—via the metered-dose inhaler (MDI) with Volumatic spacer and via the dry powder inhaler, Easyhaler, with the nebulizer—in mild to moderate asthma exacerbation: a multicenter, randomized study, *Asian Pac J Allergy Immunol* 29:25, 2011.

121. Yilmaz O, Sogut A, Kose U, Sakinci O, Yuksel H: Influence of ambulatory inhaled treatment with different devices on the duration of acute asthma findings in children, *J Asthma* 46:191, 2009.

122. Mandelberg A, Tsehori S, Houri S, Gilad E, Morag B, Priel IE: Is nebulized aerosol treatment necessary in the pediatric emergency department? *Chest* 117:1309, 2000.

123. Ploin D, Chapuis FR, Stamm D, et al: High-dose albuterol by metered-dose inhaler plus a spacer device versus nebulization in preschool children with recurrent wheezing: a double-blind, randomized equivalence trial, *Pediatrics* 106:311, 2000.

124. Rubilar L, Castro-Rodriguez JA, Girardi G: Randomized trial of salbutamol via metered-dose inhaler with spacer versus nebulizer for acute wheezing in children less than 2 years of age, *Pediatr Pulmonol* 29:264, 2000.

125. Leversha AM, Campanella SG, Aickin RP, Asher MI: Costs and effectiveness of spacer versus nebuliser in young children with moderate and severe acute asthma (Structured abstract), *J Pediatrics* 4:497, 2000.

126. Deerojanawong J, Manuvakorn W, Prapphal N, Harnruthakorn C, Sritippayawan S, Samransamruaikit R: Randomized controlled trial of salbutamol aerosol therapy via metered dose inhaler-spacer vs jet nebulizer in young children with wheezing, *Pediatr Pulmonol* 39:466, 2005.

127. Delgado A, Chou KJ, Silver EJ, Crain EF: Nebulizers vs metered-dose inhalers with spacers for bronchodilator therapy to treat wheezing in children aged 2 to 24 months in a pediatric emergency department, *Arch Pediatr Adolesc Med* 157:76, 2003.

128. Sannier N, Timsit S, Cojocaru B, et al: [Metered-dose inhaler with spacer vs nebulization for severe and potentially severe acute asthma treatment in the pediatric emergency department], *Arch Pediatr* 13:238, 2006.

129. Chong Neto HJ, Chong-Silva DC, Marani DM, Kuroda F, Olandosky M, De Noronha L: Different inhaler devices in acute asthma attacks: a randomized, double-blind, placebo-controlled study (Structured abstract), *Jornal de Pediatria* 4:298, 2005.

130. Goh AE, Tang JP, Ling H, et al: Efficacy of metered-dose inhalers for children with acute asthma exacerbations, *Pediatr Pulmonol* 46:421, 2010.

131. Hurley KF, Sargeant J, Duffy J, Sketris I, Sinclair D, Ducharme J: Perceptual reasons for resistance to change in the emergency department use of holding chambers for children with asthma, *Ann Emerg Med* 51:70, 2008.

132. Osmond MH, Gazarian M, Henry RL, Clifford TJ, Tetzlaff J: Barriers to metered-dose inhaler/spacer use in Canadian pediatric emergency departments: a national survey, *Acad Emerg Med* 14:1106, 2007.

133. Scott SD, Osmond MH, O'Leary KA, Graham ID, Grimshaw J, Klassen T: Barriers and supports to implementation of MDI/spacer use in nine Canadian pediatric emergency departments: a qualitative study, *Implement Sci* 4:65, 2009.

134. Mecklin M, Paassilta M, Kainulainen H, Korppi M: Emergency treatment of obstructive bronchitis: change from nebulizers to metered dose inhalers with spacers, *Acta Paediatr* 100:1226, 2011.

135. Colacone A, Wolkove N, Stern E: Continuous nebulization of albuterol (salbutamol) in acute asthma, *Chest* 97:693, 1990.

136. Portnoy J, Aggarwal J: Continuous terbutaline nebulization for the treatment of severe exacerbations of asthma in children, *Ann Allergy* 60:368, 1988.

137. Rebuck AS, Chapman KR, Abboud R, et al: Nebulized anticholinergic and sympathomimetic treatment of asthma and chronic obstructive airways disease in the emergency room, *Am J Med* 82:59, 1987.

138. Amado M, OPortnoy J: A comparison of low and high doses of continuously nebulized terbutaline for treatment of severe exacerbations of asthma [abstract], *Ann Allergy* 60:165, 1988.

139. Rubin BK, Albers GM: Use of anticholinergic bronchodilation in children, *Am J Med* 100:49S, 1996.

140. Zorc JJ, Pusic MV, Ogborn CJ, Lebet R, Duggan AK: Ipratropium bromide added to asthma treatment in the pediatric emergency department, *Pediatrics* 103:748, 1999.

141. Lanes SF, Garrett JE, Wentworth CE 3rd, Fitzgerald JM, Karpel JP: The effect of adding ipratropium bromide to Salbutamol in the treatment of acute asthma: a pooled analysis of three trials, *Chest* 114:365, 1998.

142. Lin RY, Pesola GR, Bakalchuk L, et al: Superiority of ipratropium plus albuterol over albuterol alone in the emergency department management of adult asthma: a randomized clinical trial, *Ann Emerg Med* 31:208, 1998.

143. Qureshi F, Pestian J, Davis P, Zaritsky A: Effect of nebulized ipratropium on the hospitalization rates of children with asthma, *N Engl J Med* 339:1030, 1998.

144. Schuh S, Johnson DW, Callahan S, Canny G, Levison H: Efficacy of frequent nebulized ipratropium bromide added to frequent high-dose albuterol therapy in severe childhood asthma, *J Pediatr* 126:639, 1995.

145. Fink J, Tobin M, Dhand R: Bronchodilator therapy in mechanically ventilated patients, *Respir Care* 44:53, 1999.

146. Fink JB, Dhand R, Grychowski J, Fahey PJ, Tobin MJ: Reconciling in vitro and in vivo measurements of aerosol delivery from a metered-dose inhaler during mechanical ventilation and defining efficiency-enhancing factors, *Am J Respir Crit Care Med* 159:63, 1999.

147. Fok TF, Al-Essa M, Monkman S, et al: Pulmonary deposition of Salbutamol aerosol delivered by metered dose inhaler, jet nebulizer, and ultrasonic nebulizer in mechanically ventilated rabbits, *Pediatr Res* 42:721, 1997.

148. Hughes J, Saez J: Effects of nebulizer mode and position in a mechanical ventilator circuit on dose efficiency, *Respir Care* 32:1131, 1987.

149. Harvey C, O'Doherty M, Page C, Thomas S, Nunan T, Treacher D: Effect of a spacer on pulmonary aerosol deposition from a jet nebulizer during mechanical ventilation, *Thorax* 50:50, 1995.

150. Ari A, Areabi H, Fink JB: Evaluation of position of aerosol device in two different ventilator circuits during mechanical ventilation, *Respir Care* 55:837, 2010.

151. Ari A, Atalay OT, Harwood R, Sheard MM, Aljamhan EA, Fink JB: Influence of nebulizer type, position, and bias flow on aerosol drug delivery in simulated pediatric and adult lung models during mechanical ventilation, *Respir Care* 55:845, 2010.

152. Rau J, Harwood R, Groff J: Evaluation of a reservoir device for metered-dose bronchodilator delivery to intubated adults: an in-vitro study, *Chest* 102:924, 1992.

153. Bishop MJ, Larson RP, Buschman DL: Metered dose inhaler aerosol characteristics are affected by the endotracheal tube actuator/adapter used, *Anesthesiology* 73:1263, 1990.

154. Fuller HD, Dolovich MB, Turpie FH, Newhouse MT: Efficiency of bronchodilator aerosol delivery to the lungs from the metered dose inhaler in mechanically ventilated patients. A study comparing four different actuator devices, *Chest* 105:214, 1994.

155. Manthous C, Hall C, Schmidt G, Wood L: Metered-dose inhaler versus nebulized salbutamol in mechanically ventilated patients, *Am Rev Resp Dis* 148:1567, 1993.

156. O'Riordan TG, Greco MJ, Perry RJ, Smaldone GC: Nebulizer function during mechanical ventilation, *Am Rev Respir Dis* 145:1117, 1992.

157. Garner SS, Wiest DB, Bradley JW: Albuterol delivery by metered-dose inhaler with a pediatric mechanical ventilatory circuit model, *Pharmacotherapy* 14:210, 1994.

158. Fink J, Dhand R, Duarte A, Jenne J, Tobin M: Aerosol delivery from a metered-dose inhaler during mechanical ventilation. An in-vitro model, *Am J Respir Crit Care Med* 154:382, 1996.

159. Svartengren M, Anderson M, Philipson K, Camner P: Human lung deposition of particles suspended in air or in helium/oxygen mixture, *Exp Lung Res* 15:575, 1989.

160. Anderson M, Svartengren M, Bylin G, Philipson K, P. C: Deposition in asthmatics of particles inhaled in air or in helium-oxygen, *Am Rev Respir Dis* 147:524, 1993.

161. Moren F, Anderson J: Fraction of dose exhaled after administration of pressurized inhalation aerosols, *Int J Pharm* 6:295, 1980.

162. O'Riordan TG, Palmer LB, Smaldone GC: Aerosol deposition in mechanically ventilated patients. Optimizing nebulizer delivery, *Am J Respir Crit Care Med* 149:214, 1994.

163. Thomas SH, O'Doherty MJ, Fidler HM, Page CJ, Treacher DF, Nunan TO: Pulmonary deposition of a nebulised aerosol during mechanical ventilation, *Thorax* 48:154, 1993.

164. Dubus JC, Vecellio L, De Monte M, et al: Aerosol deposition in neonatal ventilation, *Pediatr Res* 58:10, 2005.

165. Fink J: Aerosol delivery to ventilated infants and pediatric patients, *Respir Care* 49:653, 2004.

166. Dhand R, Duarte A, Jubran A, et al: Dose response to bronchodilator delivered by metered-dose inhaler in ventilator supported patients, *Am J Respir Crit Care Med* 154:388, 1996.

167. Dolovich MB, Ahrens RC, Hess DR, et al: Device selection and outcomes of aerosol therapy: evidence-based guidelines: American College of Chest Physicians/American College of Asthma, Allergy, and Immunology, *Chest* 127:335, 2005.

168. Rubin BK, Newhouse M, Barnes P: *Conquering childhood asthma: an illustrated guide to the understanding and control of childhood asthma*, Hamilton, ON, 1998, BC Decker.

169. Rubin BK: Tracheomalacia as a cause of respiratory compromise in infants, *Clin Pulm Med* 6:195, 1999.

170. Rubin BK: Emerging therapies for cystic fibrosis lung disease, *Chest* 154:388, 1999.

171. Ramsey BW, Dorkin HL, Eisenberg JD, et al: Efficacy of aerosolized tobramycin in patients with cystic fibrosis, *N Engl J Med* 328:1740, 1993.

172. Sexauer W, Fiel S: Aerosolized antibiotics in cystic fibrosis, *Sem Respir Crit Care Med* 24:717, 2003.

173. Ryan G, Mukhopadhyay S, Singh M: Nebulised anti-pseudomonal antibiotics for cystic fibrosis, *Cochrane Database Syst Rev* 3:CD001021, 2003.

174. Rubin BK, van der Schans C: *Lung biology in health and disease*, Boca Raton, FL, 2004, CRC Press/Taylor & Francis.

175. McCoy K, Hamilton S, Johnson C: Effects of 12-week administration of dornase alfa in patients with advanced cystic fibrosis lung disease, *Chest* 110:889, 1996.

176. Wilmott RW, Amin RS, Colin AA, et al: Aerosolized recombinant human DNase in hospitalized cystic fibrosis patients with acute pulmonary exacerbations, *Am J Respir Crit Care Med* 53:1914, 1996.

177. O'Donnell AE, Barker AF, Ilowite JS, Fick RB: Treatment of idiopathic bronchiectasis with aerosolized recombinant human DNase I. rhDNase Study Group, *Chest* 113:1329, 1998.

178. Henke MO, Shah SA, Rubin BK: The role of airway secretions in COPD—clinical applications, *COPD* 2:377, 2005.

179. Henke MO, Renner A, Huber RM, Seeds MC, Rubin BK: MUC5AC and MUC5B mucins are decreased in cystic fibrosis airway secretions, *Am J Respir Cell Mol Biol* 31:86, 2004.

180. App EM, Baran D, Dab I, et al: Dose-finding and 24-h monitoring for efficacy and safety of aerosolized Nacystelyn in cystic fibrosis, *Eur Respir J* 19:294, 2002.

181. Feng W, Garrett H, Speert DP, King M: Improved clearability of cystic fibrosis sputum with dextran treatment in vitro, *Am J Respir Crit Care Med* 157:710, 1998.

182. Deterding R, Retsch-Bogart G, Milgram L, et al: Safety and tolerability of denufosol tetrasodium inhalation solution, a novel P2Y2 receptor agonist: results of a phase 1/phase 2 multicenter study in mild to moderate cystic fibrosis, *Pediatr Pulmonol* 39:339, 2005.

183. Griese M, Essl R, Schmidt R, et al: Sequential analysis of surfactant, lung function and inflammation in cystic fibrosis patients, *Respir Res* 6:133, 2005.

184. Anzueto A, Jubran A, Ohar JA, et al: Effects of aerosolized surfactant in patients with stable chronic bronchitis: a prospective randomized controlled trial, *JAMA* 278:1426, 1997.

185. Eng PA, Morton J, Douglass JA, Riedler J, Wilson J, Robertson CF: Short-term efficacy of ultrasonically nebulized hypertonic saline in cystic fibrosis, *Pediatr Pulmonol* 21:77, 1996.

186. Daviskas E, Anderson SD, Gomes K, et al: Inhaled mannitol for the treatment of mucociliary dysfunction in patients with bronchiectasis: effect on lung function, health status and sputum, *Respirology* 10:46, 2005.

187. Wark PA, McDonald V: Nebulised hypertonic saline for cystic fibrosis, *Cochrane Database Syst Rev* 1:CD001506, 2003.

188. Wills P, Greenstone M: Inhaled hyperosmolar agents for bronchiectasis, *Cochrane Database Syst Rev* 2:CD002996, 2006.

189. Suri R, Metcalfe C, Lees B, et al: Comparison of hypertonic saline and alternate-day or daily recombinant human deoxyribonuclease in children with cystic fibrosis: a randomised trial, *Lancet* 358:1316, 2001.

190. Knowles MR, Hohneker KW, Zhou Z, et al: A controlled study of adenoviral-vector-mediated gene transfer in the nasal epithelium of patients with cystic fibrosis, *N Engl J Med* 333:823, 1995.

191. Rochat T, Morris MA: Gene therapy for cystic fibrosis by means of aerosol, *J Aerosol Med* 15:229, 2002.

192. Moss RB, Rodman D, Spencer LT, et al: Repeated adeno-associated virus serotype 2 aerosol-mediated cystic fibrosis transmembrane regulator gene transfer to the lungs of patients with cystic fibrosis: a multicenter, double-blind, placebo-controlled trial, *Chest* 125:509, 2004.

193. Eastman SJ, Scheule RK: Cationic lipid: pDNA complexes for the treatment of cystic fibrosis, *Curr Opin Mol Ther* 1:186, 1999.

194. Flotte TR, Carter BJ: In vivo gene therapy with adeno-associated virus vectors for cystic fibrosis, *Adv Pharmacol* 40:85, 1997.

195. Mallet JP, Diot P, Lemarie E: Inhalation route for administration of systemic drugs, *Rev Mal Respir* 14:257, 1997.

196. Heinemann L, Traut T, Heise T: Time-action profile of inhaled insulin, *Diabet Med* 14:63, 1997.

197. Jendle JH, Karlberg BE: Intrapulmonary administration of insulin to healthy volunteers, *J Intern Med* 240:93, 1996.

198. Laube BL, Benedict GW, Dobs AS: The lung as an alternative route of delivery for insulin in controlling postprandial glucose levels in patients with diabetes, *Chest* 114:1734, 1998.

199. DeFronzo RA, Bergenstal RM, Cefalu WT, et al: Efficacy of inhaled insulin in patients with type 2 diabetes not controlled with diet and exercise: a 12-week, randomized, comparative trial, *Diabetes Care* 28:1922, 2005.

200. Dawson M, Wirtz D, Hanes J: Enhanced viscoelasticity of human cystic fibrotic sputum correlates with increasing microheterogeneity in particle transport, *J Biol Chem* 278:50393, 2003.

201. Rosenstock J, Zinman B, Murphy LJ, et al: Inhaled insulin improves glycemic control when substituted for or added to oral combination therapy in type 2 diabetes: a randomized, controlled trial, *Ann Intern Med* 143:549, 2005.

202. Laube BL: The expanding role of aerosols in systemic drug delivery, gene therapy, and vaccination, *Respir Care* 50:1161, 2005.

203. Edwards DA, Dunbar C: Bioengineering of therapeutic aerosols, *Annu Rev Biomed Eng* 4:93, 2002.

Chapter 12

Airway Clearance Techniques and Hyperinflation Therapy

BRIAN K. WALSH

LEARNING OBJECTIVES

After reading this chapter the reader will be able to:
1. Explain the indications and risks of airway clearance techniques
2. Apply the various techniques of airway clearance
3. Understand how to avoid complications associated with airway clearance techniques
4. Understand the role of hyperinflation therapy and its relationship to proper airway clearance

KEY TERMS

Airway clearance technique (ACT)
Cough

Hyperinflation therapy

Positive expiratory pressure (PEP) therapy

Traditional **airway clearance techniques (ACT)** are designed to remove secretions from the lungs and include postural drainage, percussion, chest wall vibration, and coughing. Newer techniques considered part of ACT are maneuvers to improve the efficacy of cough, such as the following:

· The forced expiration technique (FET)
· **Positive expiratory pressure (PEP) therapy**
· High-frequency chest compression (HFCC)
· Insufflator–exsufflator (e.g., Cough Assist)
· High-frequency chest wall oscillation with Cough Assist
· Intrapulmonary percussive ventilation
· Specialized breathing techniques, such as autogenic drainage (AD)

Because all these techniques share the same goal—removal of bronchial secretions—the term *bronchial drainage* is often employed to describe them collectively. This term may be preferable to *ACT* because it highlights the aims, rather than the means, of treatment. This chapter is devoted to describing and analyzing bronchial drainage techniques and how they should be applied to the infant or pediatric patient with lung disease or respiratory impairment.

HISTORY AND CURRENT STATUS OF AIRWAY CLEARANCE TECHNIQUES

Postural drainage was used as early as 1901 in the treatment of bronchiectasis.[1] In the 1960s and 1970s we saw an increase in the use of ACT.[2] It was introduced in many U.S. hospitals concurrent with a wave of mounting criticism of intermittent positive-pressure breathing (IPPB) therapy. Many institutions found that the routine use of IPPB was replaced with the routine use of ACT. Beginning in the late 1970s, experts in the field began to point to the lack of evidence to support the routine use of ACT in pulmonary disorders such as pneumonia and chronic bronchitis.[3] However, despite a steady stream of criticism, the use of ACT appears to have increased dramatically.[4-12] The clinician must evaluate the possible usefulness of airway clearance in the face of low-level evidence and intervene only when the benefit clearly outweighs the risk.

Traditional airway maintenance, airway clearance therapy, and principles of their application are similar for neonates, children, and adults. In the pediatric patient, distinct differences in physiology and pathology limit the application of adult derived airway clearance and maintenance modalities. One of the major obstacles in device research, particularly airway clearance or maintenance modality, is proper blinding and equipoise.

The lack of scientific rigor, among other issues, has led to a deficiency of high-level evidence. Yet airway maintenance and clearance therapy take a great deal of the clinician's time. Many clinicians feel that if the patient is producing secretions, we should do something about it. Although most studies have focused on the primary outcome of sputum production, it is not clear whether or not sputum volume is an appropriate indication or outcome of airway clearance. There is a perception that airway clearance may not help, but it won't hurt either. This attitude can lead to inappropriate orders and inadvertent complications. Many airway clearance techniques are not benign, particularly if they are not used as intended.

Physiological and Pathophysiological Considerations

Airway Clearance Mechanisms

Ciliary movement and **cough** are the two primary airway clearance mechanisms. Expulsion of mucus requires turbulent flow from the peripheral airway toward the trachea. The airway undergoes compression that creates moving choke points or stenosis that catch mucus and facilitate expiratory airflow propelling the mucus downstream[13] (Figure 12-1). This mechanism requires narrowing of the airway, but complete obstruction will inhibit this transfer. Children, particularly infants, are prone to complete airway obstruction that can lead to atelectasis and the elimination of expiratory flow. This result is particularly true in the heterotaxy population.

Infants and children have high chest wall compliance because they have less musculature, ossification, and stiffness of their rib cage than adults.[14] They also have a lower

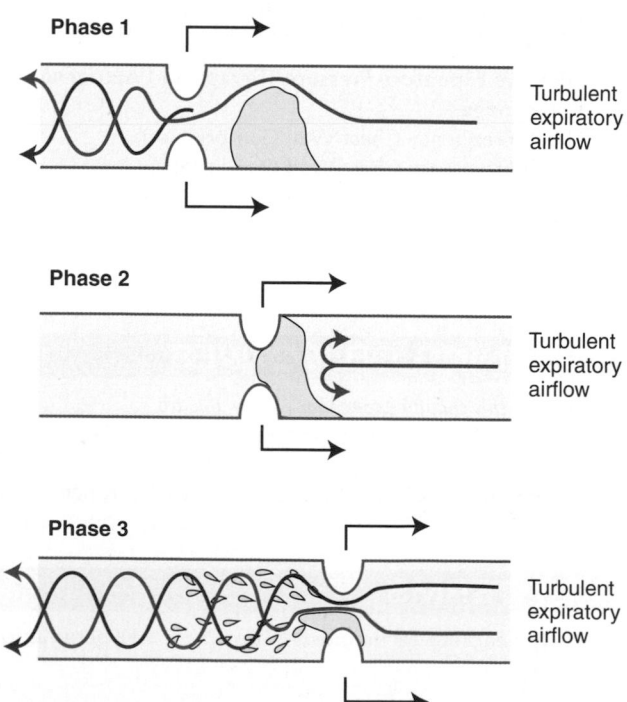

Phase 1

Turbulent expiratory airflow

Phase 2

Turbulent expiratory airflow

Phase 3

Turbulent expiratory airflow

FIGURE 12-1 Compression of the airways creates moving choke points or stenosis that facilitate mucus expulsion. Narrowing of the airway is required, but complete obstruction will inhibit this transfer.

pulmonary compliance and greater elasticity than adults, leading to a lower functional residual capacity (FRC) compared with their total lung capacity, which promotes premature airway closure.[15] The bronchus will collapse as pleural pressure exceeds intralumen airway pressure. This collapse is avoided by opposing forces that make up the rigidity of the airway structure, specifically smooth muscle in the peripheral airways and cartilage in the central airways. In infants, especially premature infants, the airway cartilage is less developed and more compliant than that of older children and adults.[16] This increased yielding leads to greater airway collapse at lower changes in pleural and airway pressure. Common neonatal disease states reduce pulmonary compliance and produce bronchial wall edema, enhancing the risk of airway collapse. The clinical picture of airway collapse often prompts ACT or bronchodilator orders. This airway collapse can be further exaggerated when chest percussion is performed or bronchodilators administered. Bronchodilators cause a decrease in smooth muscle tone, leading to increased collapsibility. This is why continuous positive airway pressure (CPAP) or PEP can be therapeutic in patients with airway collapse, because it tends to improve their FRC and establishes a fundamental airway clearance mechanism of producing air behind the secretions. Efforts to increase FRC can be valuable tools in your airway clearance arsenal.

Airway resistance is disproportionately high in children at baseline. Small changes in airway diameter such as caused by edema, secretions, a foreign body, or inflammation can lead to drastic changes in resistance. This decrease in airflow limits the child's ability to expel secretions and may contribute to the work of breathing. Furthermore, the upper airway, particularly the nose, can contribute up to 50% of the airway resistance, which is only compounded by nasal congestion.[17]

Interalveolar pores of Kohn and bronchiolar-alveolar canals of Lambert are compensatory mechanisms that contribute to the aeration of gas exchange units distal to obstructed airways in older children and adults (Figure 12-2).

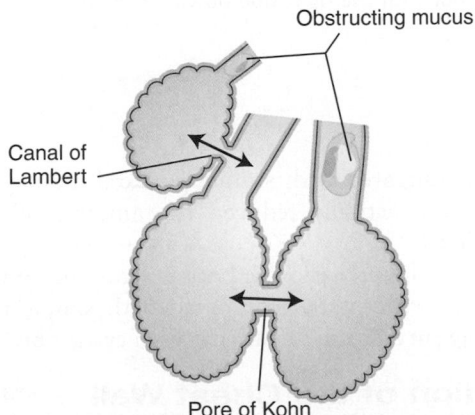

FIGURE 12-2 The location of collateral airways such as the interalveolar pores of Kohn and bronchiolar-alveolar canals of Lambert.

Yet these are missing in infants, in whom these collaterals are not well developed. This can hinder airway clearance and lead to large areas of atelectasis.

Traditional Airway Clearance Therapy Techniques

Traditional ACT has four components: (1) postural drainage, (2) percussion, (3) vibration of the chest wall, and (4) coughing.

Postural Drainage

Postural drainage attempts to use gravity to move secretions from peripheral airways to the larger bronchi, from which they are more easily expectorated. The patient is placed in various positions, each designed to drain specific segments of the lung, and may be supported by rolled towels, blankets, or pillows. Figures 12-3 and 12-4 illustrate postural drainage positions used in infants and children.[13] Other versions incorporating minor variations have also been published.[2,19,20] Postural drainage can be performed with or without percussion or vibration. When accompanied by percussion or vibration, each position is maintained for 1 to 5 minutes, depending on the severity of the patient's condition. When percussion or vibration is omitted, longer periods of simple postural drainage can be performed.

Percussion

Percussion is believed to loosen secretions from the bronchial walls. While the patient is in the various postural drainage positions, the clinician percusses the chest wall, using a cupped hand (see Figure 12-5). The areas to be percussed are illustrated in Figures 12-3 and 12-4. Clinicians should not percuss over bony prominences; over the spine, sternum, abdomen, last few ribs, sutured areas, drainage tubes, kidneys, or liver; or below the rib cage. The ideal frequency of percussion is unknown; however, some reports recommend a frequency of 5 to 6 Hz (300-360 blows per minute), whereas others recommend slow, rhythmic clapping.[19,21] Several devices can be used for percussion, including soft face masks as well as those commercially designed, such as "palm cups" and mechanical percussors (Figure 12-6). Infants and children may have percussion performed in the lap of the clinician. However, if the patient is mechanically ventilated or has multiple tubes and intravenous lines in place, it may be preferable to perform therapy with the patient in the bed. Catheters, tubes, and indwelling lines are easily dislodged in infants and young children, and appropriate care must be taken.

Postural Drainage and Percussion

Many investigations have been conducted to determine the relative importance of percussion, vibration, and postural drainage. In a study designed to determine the

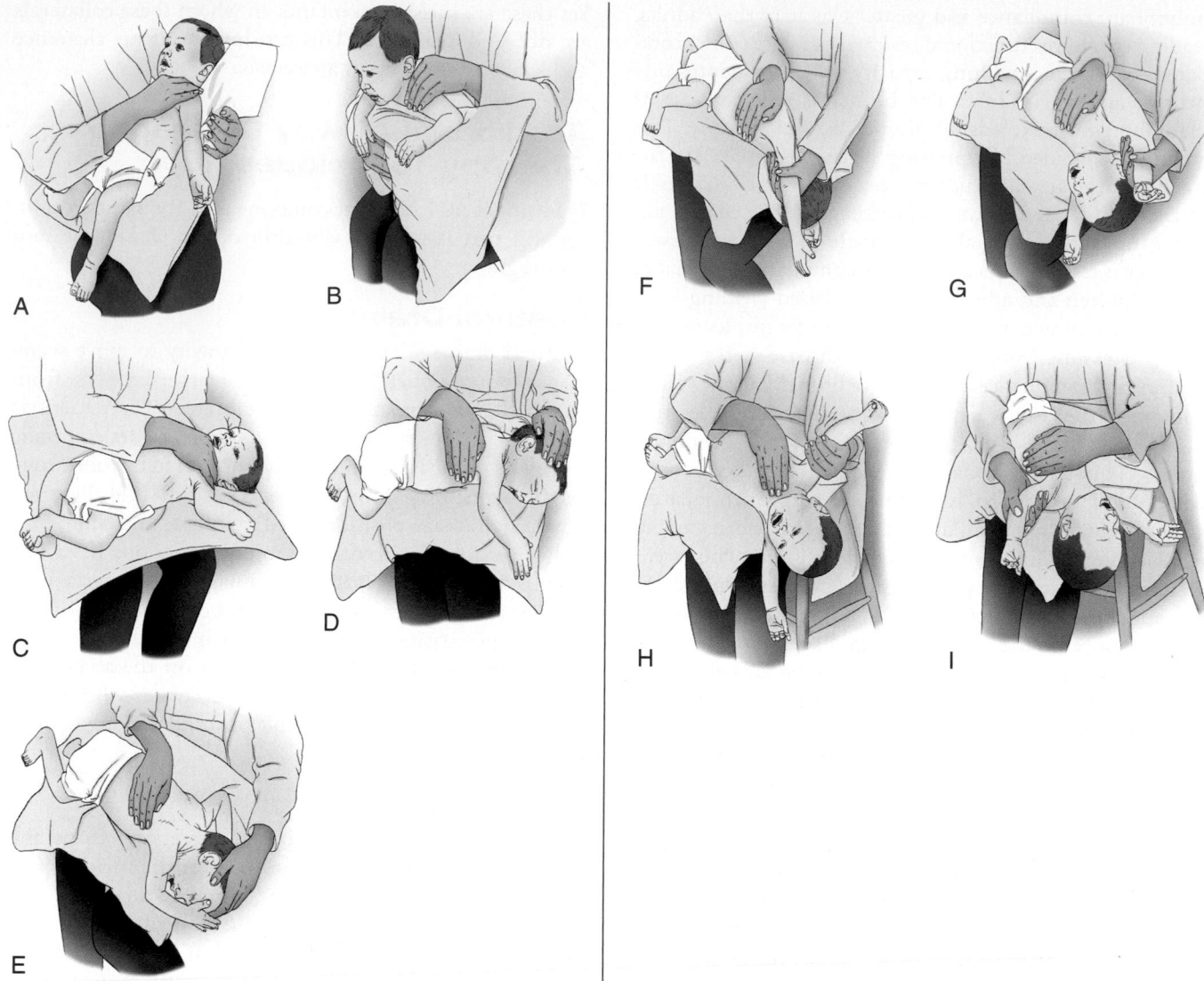

FIGURE 12-3 Postural drainage positions for infants and younger children. **A,** Apical segment of the right upper lobe and apical subsegment of the apical–posterior segment of the left upper lobe. **B,** Posterior segment of the right upper lobe and posterior subsegment of the apical–posterior segment of the left upper lobe. **C,** Anterior segments of right and left upper lobes. **D,** Superior segments of both lower lobes. **E,** Posterior basal segments of both lower lobes. Postural drainage positions for infants. **F,** Lateral basal segment of the right lower lobe. Lateral basal segment of the left lower lobe is drained in a similar fashion but with the right side down. **G,** Anterior basal segment of the right lower lobe. The segments on the left side are drained in a similar fashion but with the right side down. **H,** Right middle lobe. **I,** Left lingular segment of lower lobe.

contribution of these maneuvers to clearance of mucus, there was no demonstration of improvement in clearance of mucus from the lung when percussion, vibration, or breathing exercises were added to postural drainage.[22] These investigators also showed that FET was superior to simple coughing and when combined with postural drainage was the most effective form of treatment.[23] Other studies[24-26] have reported the following:

1. Percussion without postural drainage or cough produced minimal change in the clearance of mucus.

2. When compared with simple postural drainage, chest percussion actually reduced the amount of sputum mobilized.

3. Manual self-percussion did not increase the amount of sputum expectorated compared with simple postural drainage in a group of patients with cystic fibrosis (CF).

Vibration of the Chest Wall

Vibrations represent an additional method of transmitting energy through the chest wall to loosen or move bronchial

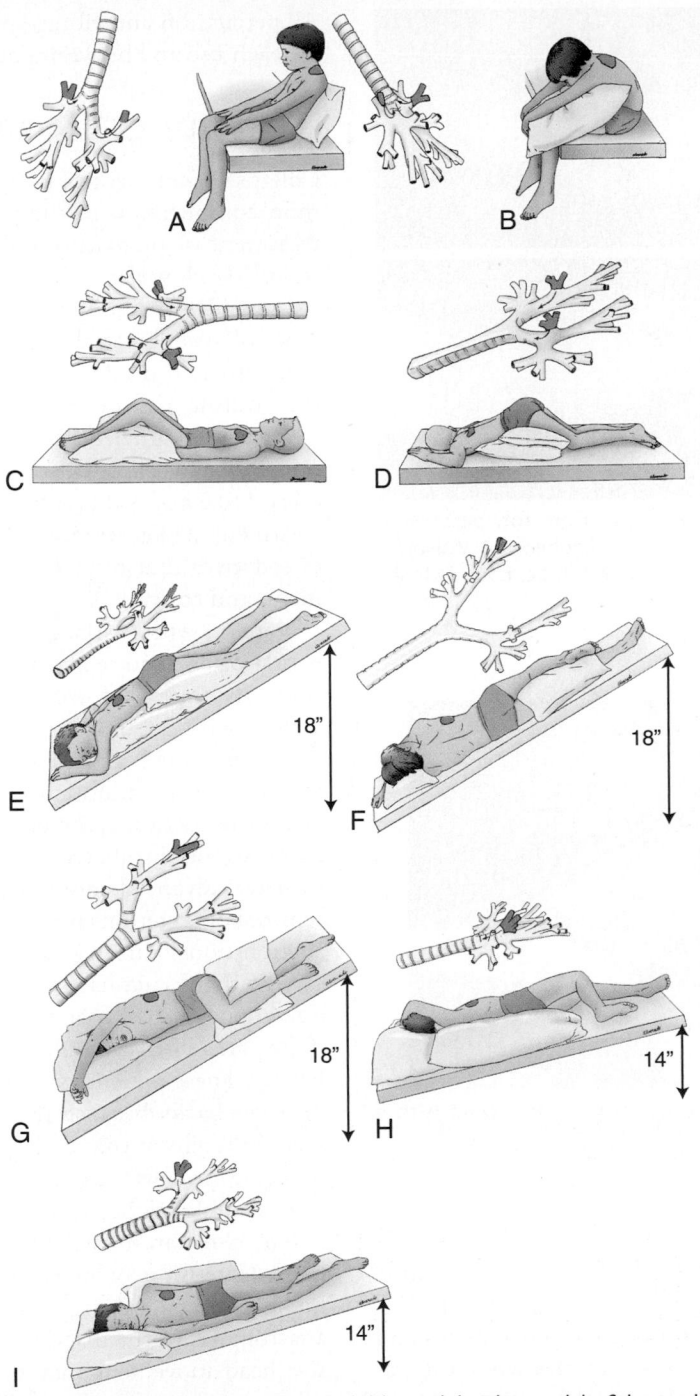

FIGURE 12-4 Postural drainage positions for the child or adult. The model of the tracheobronchial tree next to or above the child illustrates the segmental bronchi being drained. The shaded area on the child's chest illustrates the area to be percussed or vibrated. **A,** Apical segment of right upper lobe and apical subsegment of apical–posterior segment of left upper lobe (area between the clavicle and top of the scapula). **B,** Posterior segment of right upper lobe and posterior subsegment of apical–posterior segment of left upper lobe (area over the upper back). Postural drainage positions for the child or adult. The model of the tracheobronchial tree next to or above the child illustrates the segmental bronchi being drained. The stippled area on the child's chest illustrates the area to be percussed or vibrated. **C,** Anterior segments of right and left upper lobes (area between clavicle and nipple). **D,** Superior segments of both lower lobes (area over middle of back at tip of scapula, beside spine). **E,** Posterior basal segments of both lower lobes (area over lower rib cage, beside spine). **F,** Lateral basal segment of right lower lobe. Segment on left is drained in a similar fashion but with the right side down (area over middle portion of rib cage). **G,** Anterior basal segment of left lower lobe. Segment on right is drained in a similar fashion but with the left side down (area over lower ribs, below the armpit). **H,** Right middle lobe (area over right nipple; below breast in developing females). **I,** Left lingular segment of lower lobe (area over left nipple; below breast in developing females).

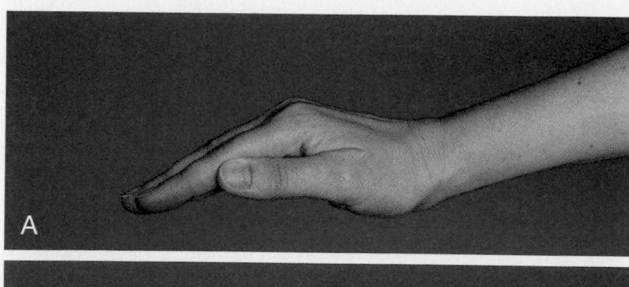
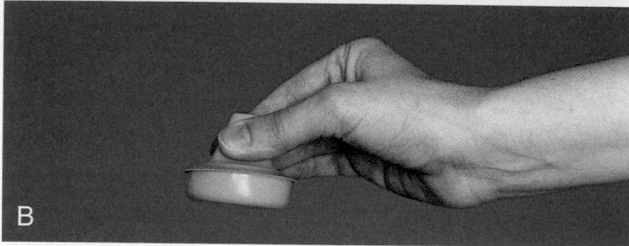

FIGURE 12-5 A, Cupped hand position for percussion. **B,** Device for infant percussion. From Hockenberry M, Wilson D: *Wong's nursing care of infants and children,* ed 9, St. Louis: Mosby, 2011.

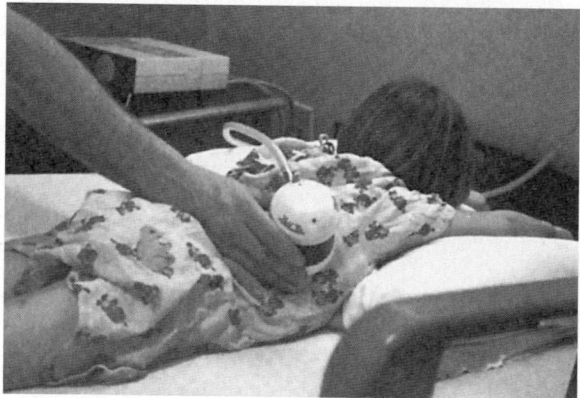

FIGURE 12-6 Percussion being performed on a child with a pneumatic percussor.

secretions. Unlike in percussion, the clinician's hand does not lose contact with the chest wall during the procedure. Vibrations are performed by placing both hands (one over the other) over the area to be vibrated and tensing and contracting the shoulder and arm muscles while the patient exhales. To prolong exhalation, the patient may be asked to breathe through pursed lips or make a "hissing" sound. As with percussion, the ideal frequency is unknown, although some recommend 10 to 15 Hz.[27] It is unclear how well clinicians are able to perform vibrations at this frequency. Several mechanical vibrators are commercially available. Some models of mechanical percussors or vibrators are appropriate only for the newborn or premature infant, whereas other models are appropriate for the larger child. When evaluating such devices, the clinician should consider whether the appearance and sound of the device will be frightening and whether the amount of force is appropriate for the size of the patient.

All percussion and vibration devices should be cleaned after each use and between patients.

AIRWAY CLEARANCE THERAPY

Collapse of the right upper lobe after extubation is a common complication in the premature infant, and routine treatment of premature infants after extubation is common.[28,29] However, most treatments are not required because little respiratory compromise is seen with a single-lobe collapse. Treatment may be given to the right upper lobe only and need not be prolonged, nor does it require the routine use of percussion. A treatment length of 5 minutes is sufficient, and vibration is applied to the right upper lobe in one of the three standard drainage positions every 4 to 6 hours for 24 to 48 hours.[29] The most beneficial treatment is likely frequent position changes and weaning of sedatives that return the patient's natural sigh, movement, and cough.

Patients with esophageal atresia and tracheoesophageal fistula often require assistance in mobilizing thick secretions. Aspiration of oropharyngeal secretions, leading to atelectasis or pneumonia, is common. If surgical repair has been performed, deep endotracheal suctioning (beyond the tip of the endotracheal tube) is contraindicated because the suction catheter may reopen the closed fistula. Likewise, nonintubated patients should rarely have the catheter advanced more than 7 cm because this makes removal of secretions more difficult. On occasion, tracheal suction under direct vision with a laryngoscope is necessary. If the fistula has been closed, Trendelenburg (head-down) positioning may be used. This is especially helpful if the patient has difficulty clearing oral secretions by swallowing. These patients should not be routinely placed flat on their backs because this promotes aspiration of oral secretions. Given that a thoracotomy has been performed to repair the defect, use of a small mechanical vibrator may be preferable to chest percussion.

The clinician must be careful to avoid excessive movement (extension or extreme turning) while treating the infant. Esophageal atresia is repaired by performing an anastomosis of the distal and proximal esophagus. Excessive head movement may result in its disruption. Many other patients often require ACT in the neonatal intensive care unit. Usually, such patients have been intubated for some time and have responded to prolonged intubation with excessive production of secretions.

Behavioral Issues

When missing the key component of cooperation, airway clearance becomes much more difficult. The potential for harm during airway clearance modalities increases as transpulmonary pressure swings increase.[13] When forceful crying occurs during airway clearance, these swings create an environment suitable for lung damage. All efforts to decrease crying, such as facilitated tucking or modified

ACT, should be incorporated. In modalities that administer pressure to aid airway clearance, less pressure should be administered to a noncooperative child. For older patients, a multidisciplinary approach can increase airway clearance quantity and quality by 50%.[30] This approach, utilized by Ernst et al., involves allowing for patient selection of airway clearance protocol, creating a reward system for the patient, and scheduling priority given to airway clearance.[30] When performing ACT on young children, the clinician must make a special effort to secure the patient's confidence and cooperation. Spending a few moments to gain the child's confidence is well worth the effort. Assigning the same clinician to treat the child as often as is practical may be useful in establishing a rapport. Likewise, allowing the child as much control over the situation as possible, such as deciding which lobes will be treated first, may increase the child's sense of control and reduce hospitalization-related anxiety. Having a parent available during therapy, especially when the child is unfamiliar with ACT, is useful as well.

ACT may be extremely uncomfortable for the postoperative patient, and routine use of ACT in these patients may actually promote atelectasis. Some patients, however, suffer from excessive secretions or mucous plugging and atelectasis. Performing ACT in these patients can be difficult. Adequate analgesia is essential, and attempts should be made to schedule ACT shortly after pain medication is administered. Coughing is also a considerable source of discomfort in pediatric patients postoperatively. Cough efficacy can be improved if the patient is taught to splint the wounds when coughing. Holding a pillow over the incision may also be useful in minimizing movement of the incision when coughing.

ADVERSE CONSEQUENCES

Several conditions common to the full-term or preterm newborn suggest that these infants may be at risk for increased complications from ACT; therefore, modification of routine ACT procedures is advisable. Because the newborn has high chest wall compliance, the loss of lung volume caused by chest wall compression (e.g., from percussion) may be greater in the infant than in the adult.[31] For this reason, some institutions routinely omit chest wall percussion in neonatal ACT treatments, opting instead for the use of small vibrators. Because an infant's chest wall is not as thick as an adult's and the infant's ribs are more cartilaginous, a gentler touch is required during therapy.[32] Hypoxemia has been reported after ACT in the newborn.[33-36] Handling infants, for whatever reason, often results in hypoxemia. It is therefore essential that oxygenation be monitored during ACT in infants.

Routine application of ACT in the preterm infant has been associated with an increased risk of intraventricular hemorrhage (IVH).[37] The preterm infant is unable to adequately regulate cerebral blood flow, and changes in blood pressure often lead to increased intracranial pressure and volume, with rupture of immature blood vessels. Trendelenburg positioning and chest wall percussion would seem likely to increase cerebral blood flow and to reduce venous return, further increasing the risk of IVH. Therefore these procedures should be used sparingly, if at all, in infants at risk. If possible, ACT should be withheld from infants at high risk for IVH (i.e., very premature infants in the first few days of life).

Critically ill newborns are unable to adequately maintain body temperature and are therefore routinely placed in incubators or under radiant warmers. Caregiver interventions of any kind, including ACT, interfere with maintaining temperature stability, especially for infants in closed incubators. Treatment time with these patients should be kept to a minimum, usually between 5 and 10 minutes. If a patient is in a temperature-regulated environment, special attention must be given to preventing heat loss during therapy.

The trachea and bronchi of the newborn appear especially vulnerable to damaging effects from endotracheal tubes and suction catheters. Consequences of deep endotracheal suctioning include the development of bronchial stenosis and granulomas. Avoiding deep endotracheal suctioning minimizes risks.[38] Therefore, when suctioning intubated infants after ACT, the suction catheter should not be routinely advanced beyond the end of the endotracheal tube. If there is evidence of persistent secretion retention despite adequate suction of the endotracheal tube, the suction catheter can be carefully and slowly advanced 1 or 2 cm beyond the tip of the endotracheal tube.

Many infants in the neonatal intensive care unit are sensitive to handling. This is especially true of the preterm infant as well as the full-term infant with pulmonary hypertension, who may develop hypoxemia or bradycardia in response to excessive stimulation. Many clinicians believe that clustering as many caregiver interventions as possible can minimize the adverse consequences of handling, thereby leaving the infant undisturbed for longer periods. Minimizing excessive light and sound associated with therapy is also desirable.

Cough

All ACT sessions should end with a period of deep breathing and coughing. Patients with minimal lung disease should be able to clear the lungs after one or two attempts. Those with severe lung disease or neuromuscular weakness may need more prolonged coughing periods or coughing assistance (e.g., tussive squeezes, insufflator-exsufflator, abdominal compression). Prolonged periods of unproductive coughing should be avoided because they may tire the patient. The clinician should emphasize effective, productive coughing. Infants may require nasopharyngeal suction to stimulate a cough, whereas patients with artificial airways may require endotracheal suctioning.

The following procedures are sometimes incorporated into ACT treatments, or used independently, with the aim of promoting bronchial drainage: (1) FET, (2) PEP therapy with Cough Assist, (3) AD, and (4) automatic high frequency chest wall compression (HFCWC)/high-frequency chest wall oscillation (HFCWO).

Forced Expiration Technique

FET is also known as "huff" coughing. This maneuver requires the patient to forcibly exhale, from middle to low lung volumes, with an open glottis. This is repeated several times, after which the patient coughs to remove any loosened mucus.[39] It requires extreme cooperation and cannot be performed on infants or young children. FET can be used alone or in conjunction with other forms of therapy. It is designed to prevent dynamic airway collapse by preventing the explosive pressure changes associated with coughing.[8,39] Studies have documented that patients with long-standing lung disorders characterized by destruction or weakening of the bronchial wall, such as CF and bronchiectasis, have ineffective coughing secondary to dynamic airway compression while coughing.[40] The developers of this technique now use the term *active cycle of breathing* to refer to FET. They emphasize the importance of interspersing "huff" coughs with periods of deep, relaxed breathing. This helps prevent bronchospasm and ensures sufficient lung volume to promote an effective cough.

Coughing and Forced Expiration Technique

Over the years, a number of investigators have demonstrated that the single most important component of ACT is vigorous coughing.[41-45] Simple postural drainage has been reported to improve secretion clearance, whereas the addition of percussion did not.[42] Several other studies in patients with CF and other chronic lung diseases likewise support the notion that vigorous coughing, especially when used in conjunction with FET, may be as effective as postural drainage and percussion.[43,44,46]

Many clinicians, however, are reluctant to abandon postural drainage, percussion, or vibration in favor of simple FET, especially in patients needing lifelong assistance with secretion removal, such as those with CF. A 3-year prospective study in children with CF demonstrated that conventional ACT, performed twice a day, was more effective than FET used at the same frequency.[47] Patients performing FET in this study had an average age of slightly younger than 12 years. In contrast, patients in studies that showed FET to be successful were older.[44,46] This suggests that forms of self-care may be more effective in adolescents than in younger children, who perhaps require more supervision. Likewise, comparison of studies on the efficacy of exercise as pulmonary therapy in CF suggests that self-therapy is more effective in older patients.[48,49]

Positive Expiratory Pressure Therapy

PEP therapy uses an expiratory resistor, coupled with the patient's active expiration, to generate positive airway pressure throughout expiration. This prevents dynamic airway collapse and improves clearance of mucus.[50] It is widely used in Europe, and increasingly in the United States, as an adjunct or substitute for conventional ACT in the treatment of CF or bronchiectasis, and to a lesser extent in postoperative patients. Various devices are available to serve as expiratory resistors: anything from simple high-resistance 2.5 endotracheal tube (ETT) adapters attached to a mask or mouthpiece, to a Flutter (Axcan Pharma, Mont-Saint-Hilaire, PQ, Canada), acapella (blue; Smiths Medical, Weston, MA), or Quake device (Thayer Medical, Tucson, AZ) that requires hand motion and breathing coordination. PEP therapy is essentially the same as the "blow bottles" that have been used to prevent postoperative atelectasis.[51] Both PEP therapy and FET are advocated as forms of simple self-treatment for patients with CF. PEP therapy is better tolerated by children than conventional IPPB.

Cough Assist

The insufflator–exsufflator, or Cough Assist, has shown to be beneficial in patients with neuromuscular weakness by simply supporting their cough effort. This blower-driven device provides positive airflow and pressure to increase their FRC and allow air distal to the mucus. The increase in FRC allows their weak muscles the best advantage possible to create a cough. Then it creates a negative flow and pressure to help simulate a cough.[52] Streigl et al. demonstrated in an infant lung model with a tracheostomy tube that insufflation time of 1 second or more is required for the insufflattor–exsufflator to achieve equilibration of alveolar pressure to insufflation pressure. They also discovered that longer exsufflation time does not significantly alter maximum expiratory flowrate.[52] Vienello et al.[53] showed that the insufflator–exsufflator in conjunction with traditional chest physiotherapy therapy (CPT) may improve the management of airway secretions.

Manual Rib Cage Compression. Manual rib cage compression (MRCC), or tussive squeezes as some may call them, can be used to increase the expiratory flow rate and facilitate the expectoration of mucus. Although most studies have not shown a benefit,[54-57] a recent publication has brought to light that the procedure may be to blame.[58] In order for MRCC to be effect, the expiratory flow rates generated must be higher than inspiratory flow rates. Daniel Marti and colleagues[58] were able to demonstrate in animals that hard and brief MRCC synchronized with early expiratory phase was superior to soft and gradual rib cage compression applied late in the expiratory phase. If the goal is to mimic a cough for those who cannot cough for themselves, it must be similar. Coughs are violent bursts of flow that exceed inspiratory flow rates and are

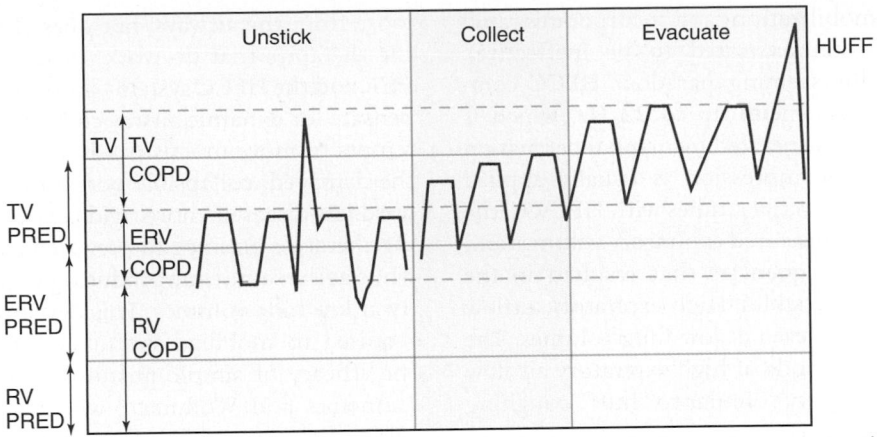

FIGURE 12-7   Graphic illustration of the depth of successive breaths by lung volumes, using the autogenic drainage technique. *ERV,* Expiratory reserve volume; *HUFF,* huff maneuver; *PRED,* predicted; *RV,* residual volume; *TV,* tidal volume.

extremely effective in the strong patient. The MRCC must be similar in order to be effective.

Autogenic Drainage

AD is a series of breathing exercises designed to mobilize secretions in patients with bronchiectasis or CF.[59-61] To loosen secretions from the smallest airways, the patient begins breathing in a slow, controlled manner, first at the expiratory reserve volume level. The volume of ventilation is then increased, with the patient breathing in the normal tidal volume range but exhaling approximately halfway into the expiratory reserve volume. This moves secretions from the peripheral to the middle airways. Finally, the depth of inspiration is increased, with the patient inhaling maximally to total lung capacity and exhaling as before about halfway into the expiratory reserve volume. Figure 12-7 graphically illustrates the autogenic drainage technique. Advocates of AD claim that its simplicity (no devices or clinicians are needed) and efficacy make it an ideal form of self-treatment for patients with CF.

Positive Expiratory Pressure Therapy and Autogenic Drainage

PEP therapy and AD have been shown to be highly effective. PEP therapy, especially, has been shown by a number of researchers to be beneficial in mobilizing secretions and preserving pulmonary function in patients with CF, and with FET it was marginally superior to simple FET and postural drainage.[62-69] Less information is available on AD, although a few reports indicate it is highly effective and that compliance is improved.[59-61,70]

High-Frequency Chest Wall Compression

Commercially available devices have been developed that compresses the entire chest wall at high frequencies by means of a snug-fitting inflatable vest connected to a high-performance air compressor (Figure 12-8). Intermittent

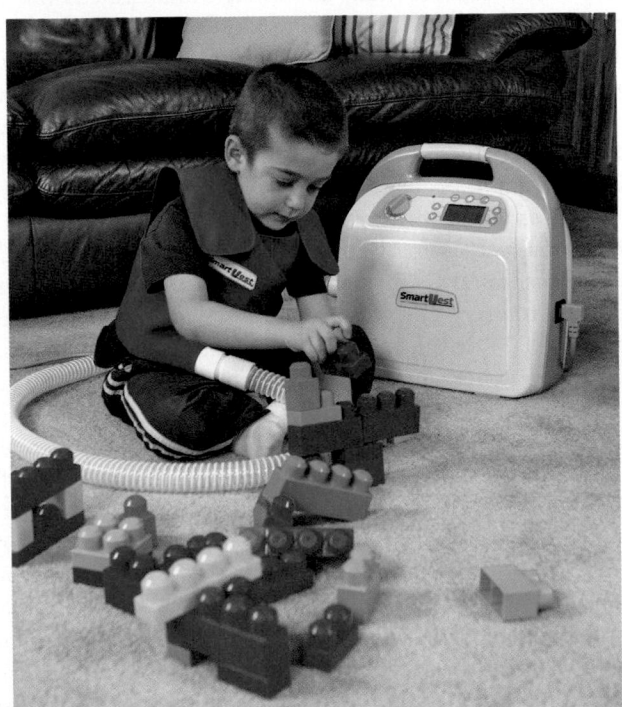

FIGURE 12-8   Patient wearing an inflatable vest during high-frequency chest compression therapy in the hospital. (Used with permission of Electromed, Inc.)

chest wall compression produces brief periods of high expiratory airflow, which loosens and mobilizes mucus from bronchial walls.[71] The device is widely used in patients with CF.

HFCWC has also been evaluated in a long-term study. After a 22-month period of using HFCC as the sole form of ACT, patients experienced a small but significant improvement in pulmonary function. In contrast, after a similar period on conventional manual ACT, pulmonary function declined somewhat.[71] HFCWC does not require the patient to perform postural drainage (known to be effective for sputum mobilization) and incorporates rapid percussion (generally demonstrated to be ineffective). What accounts for this seeming paradox? HFCC compresses the chest at frequencies up to 22 Hz, which is much higher than can be generated by manual percussion (5-8 Hz). Furthermore, compression is usually applied only on exhalation. In the initial studies with HFCWC, the developers of this device measured expiratory volumes and flows and selected the frequencies that resulted in the highest values for these variables. High expiratory airflow is maintained with HFCC, even at low lung volumes. The result is multiple, brief periods of high expiratory air flow (or more precisely air velocity), similar to "huff" coughing or FET.[72]

High expiratory air velocity at low lung volumes produces the greatest air–mucus interaction and hence mucus mobilization. HFCWC does not directly dislodge mucus from the bronchial wall, as conventional percussion is thought to do, but instead simulates multiple coughs or FETs by generating high expiratory air velocities. Because the compressive phase of HFCC is brief (as short as 0.02 second at a frequency of 22 Hz) and the glottis remains open during therapy, it is unlikely that dynamic airway collapse occurs, as happens with natural coughing in patients with bronchiectasis or CF.

Manual percussion bears little resemblance to HFCWC. In contrast to HFCWC, manual percussion is rarely, if ever, adjusted to produce optimal expiratory airflow to simulate cough or FET. In addition, it is given during inspiration as well as expiration, which may limit the deep breathing that is essential for producing high expiratory air velocities. Finally, manual percussion is applied only to a small portion of the chest wall at one time, which may be insufficient to generate adequate expiratory flows.

High-Frequency Chest Wall Oscillation

High-frequency chest wall oscillation (HFCWO) is similar to HFCC with the exception that the device provides positive (compression/push) as well as negative pressure (pulls) oscillations to the chest wall. It that has not been well studied nor compared to HFCC, but likely has similar results to HFCC.[53,73] Plioplys et al.[73] showed a reduction in pneumonias and respiratory-related hospitalizations in a study of seven quadriplegic cerebral palsy patients. This negative extrathoracic pressure swing may prove to be more beneficial in infants and toddlers, who are more prone to airway collapse.

Effectiveness of Techniques

Proponents of conventional ACT techniques often describe the problem that ACT aims to treat as abnormal (excessive, thick, tenacious) secretions. Although this is partially correct, therapies that would seem to attack this problem directly have proved disappointing. Manual, low-frequency chest percussion does not seem to jar mucus

loose from the airways, nor does chest wall vibration. Of the therapies that do work—postural drainage, PEP, AD, FET, and the HFCC system—all attempt to prevent or compensate for dynamic airway collapse. Postural drainage attempts to move mucus passively, by force of gravity, past the damaged, collapsible portions of the airways and toward less diseased, more rigid central airways. The remaining therapies attempt to prevent dynamic airway collapse while at the same time producing high expiratory air velocity at low lung volumes. This develops the shearing forces required to mobilize sputum.[4] A novel explanation for the efficacy of simple postural drainage is suggested by Lannefors and Wollmer,[74] who demonstrated improved mucous clearance in the dependent lung of patients undergoing postural drainage. For most patients, lung volumes and airway diameter are reduced in the dependent lung but ventilation is increased. These factors result in increased air movement at high velocity, which increases turbulence and shearing in small airways and results in greater mobilization of mucus.

Deep breathing associated with vigorous exercise has also been shown to be an effective technique for mobilization of secretions in patients with CF.[75,76] To accommodate the increased ventilatory demands of exercise, rate and depth of breathing are increased and active exhalation may occur. Hence, vigorous exercise produces a ventilatory pattern that, like AD or FET, increases air velocity at low lung volumes and promotes sputum mobilization.

"Take a deep breath and you'll feel better." This is a sound piece of advice that was given long before the advent of incentive spirometry or IPPB. Taking a deep breath to total lung capacity, either by sighing or yawning, is a normal, unconscious maneuver performed periodically to keep the lungs inflated and to avoid ventilation–perfusion mismatch.[77] When the breathing pattern becomes one of tidal ventilation without periodic maximal inflation, atelectasis ensues within a few hours.[78] Variations in the normal pattern of breathing may result in respiratory complications and an increase in postoperative morbidity and mortality. Changes in the breathing patterns of pediatric patients are most often caused by increased sedation, narcotics, pain, fluid overload, parenchymal lung damage, fear and anxiety, and abdominal or thoracic surgery. It has been estimated that 10% to 40% and even as many as 70% of patients undergoing abdominal or thoracic surgery experience postoperative pulmonary complications,[79,80] consisting of atelectasis, pneumonia, pulmonary embolism, and hypoxemia. These conditions are believed to be caused by reduced diaphragmatic movement (especially after upper abdominal surgery), changes in chest wall muscle tone, and secretion retention, all of which result in decreased lung volumes.[81]

The modalities and methods used to increase a child's lung volume can be classified as (1) voluntary, using the patient's own effort and initiative to sustain a deep breath (incentive spirometry); and (2) applied, providing the patient with a positive-pressure–generated breath to achieve an increase in lung volume (IPPB). In this chapter these methods of lung volume expansion therapy are discussed as they relate to the pediatric patient.

COMPLICATIONS OF AIRWAY CLEARANCE THERAPY

Numerous studies have demonstrated that ACT can be detrimental, especially when applied in patients with little or no sputum production. Reported complications of ACT range from rare reports of complete airway obstruction and respiratory arrest to bronchospasm and hypoxemia.

Hypoxemia

The most commonly cited adverse effect of ACT is hypoxemia. Several studies have reported hypoxemia in infants receiving ACT.[33-36] Hypoxemia has also been documented in studies of adolescent and adult patients receiving ACT and was reported to occur more often in patients with preexisting cardiovascular complications, with minimal sputum production, and when mucoid rather than mucopurulent secretions were present. It occurred in patients with good pulmonary function and also when supplemental oxygen was being used.[82-87] Tachypnea and tachycardia may occur in patients who experience hypoxemia during ACT.

There may be a variety of reasons why ACT often causes hypoxemia. Among the proposed mechanisms are ventilation–perfusion abnormalities caused by postural changes, atelectasis, bronchospasm, alterations in cardiac output and oxygen consumption, and incomplete expectoration of mobilized secretions. In addition, each of the ACT techniques may contribute to hypoxemia to differing degrees.

Position

Most studies of the effects of posture on oxygenation in adults would suggest that putting the diseased portion of the lung uppermost, as in postural drainage therapy, improves oxygenation.[88-90] This is a consequence of improved perfusion of the healthy, dependent lung tissue at the expense of the diseased, elevated lung segments. Thus, at least for patients with localized, unilateral lung disease, abnormalities secondary to postural changes are an unlikely explanation for ACT-associated hypoxemia in patients outside of infancy. Infants, however, have better oxygenation when the affected side is dependent (i.e., the good lung is up).[91] This may in part be the result of higher baseline pulmonary artery pressures, which would mitigate the effects of gravity on pulmonary blood flow. Hence, alterations in relationships as a direct result of postural changes are a possible explanation for CPT-associated hypoxemia in infants. Patients with generalized lung disease may respond differently to postural changes, however, and careful monitoring of oxygenation with position

changes may be warranted. Positional changes during ACT may also result in hypotension or hypertension.

Percussion

Several studies report that chest percussion, rather than postural changes, is responsible for ACT-associated hypoxemia.[35,82-84] These studies suggest that chest percussion causes significant abnormalities, and unless counterbalanced by removal of a substantial quantity of mucus and improvement in ratios, the net change will be a deterioration in relationships and hypoxemia.

Atelectasis

Both human and animal studies have shown an increase in atelectasis when ACT was given.[81,92] Vigorous chest percussion has been noted to produce pressure swings in the chest of up to 30 cm H_2O. Such pressures generated by intermittent compression or percussion of the chest wall would seem sufficient to expel appreciable quantities of air from the lung, especially if chest wall compliance is high. Chest wall vibration, in contrast to percussion, has been associated with hypoxemia in some studies.[34-36,93,94] This reflects the fact that vibration may or may not be associated with chest wall compression, depending on the techniques or equipment used, whereas chest percussion invariably causes chest wall compression.

Bronchospasm

An additional explanation for the association of chest percussion with hypoxemia is the observation that chest percussion can cause bronchospasm in susceptible patients, especially when sputum production is minimal. Administering bronchodilators before therapy may be desirable, especially when ACT is applied in patients with reactive airway disease.

Increased Oxygen Consumption

Oxygen consumption is increased during ACT.[95,96] If significant shunting is present, or if an increase in cardiac output is not produced, increased oxygen consumption can be manifested by decreased PaO_2 (partial pressure of oxygen in the arterial blood).

Gastroesophageal Reflux

Gastroesophageal reflux (GER) is a common cause of respiratory problems in infants and children, and ACT is often ordered for patients who have GER. One study found that in patients with GER, ACT resulted in a fivefold increase in reflux episodes compared with periods when ACT was not given.[97] This increase in GER was seen even though treatments were withheld up to 3.5 hours after the infant's last feeding. The study did not link the increase in reflux episodes to any particular aspect of ACT, such as head-down positioning. GER may cause severe esophagitis, bronchospasm, or pneumonia and has been linked to apnea and sudden infant death syndrome.[98] Therefore ACT should be given only when the benefits of treatment clearly outweigh the risks of aggravated GER. Although withholding treatment as long as possible after an infant's feeding is advisable, it clearly will not eliminate the risks involved.

Airway Obstruction and Respiratory Arrest

Although ACT can be an effective means of removing bronchial foreign bodies in children, it may also result in acute upper airway obstruction and death.[99] This is especially true when the foreign body consists of organic material, such as seeds or nuts, that may increase in size (secondary to water absorption) after a period of time in the lung. Vomiting and aspiration may also occur during ACT, especially if therapy is given soon after the patient has eaten. Therefore at least 1 hour should be allowed after the last meal or feeding before beginning ACT. Patients receiving continuous feedings through gastric tubes should have the feedings turned off at least 30 minutes before therapy. More time may be needed in patients with a history of vomiting or reflux. For patients in whom feedings cannot be interrupted, Trendelenburg (head-down) positioning should not be used.

Intracranial Complications

Studies in preterm infants have reported that certain positions of the infant's head may increase intracranial pressure and that routine application of ACT, especially in the first few days of life, can significantly increase the risk of IVH.[37,100] ACT procedures in the child or adult with a recent head injury can also increase intracranial pressure.[101] Because of these concerns, many institutions do not place premature infants or patients with head injuries in the Trendelenburg position during ACT.

Rib Fractures and Bruising

Rib fractures have been reported as a complication of chest percussion in preterm infants with bronchopulmonary dysplasia.[102] The infants in this study suffered from rickets secondary to long-term parenteral nutrition. Improvement in nutritional therapy for preterm infants, however, should make rickets a rare finding in the infant with bronchopulmonary dysplasia. Infants with the rare condition osteogenesis imperfecta are also at high risk of rib fractures. Bruising may occur in some patients, especially in the very small premature infant and the child with vitamin K deficiency. Most patients are more comfortable if percussion or vibration is performed with the skin covered by a pajama top or T-shirt. If the patient is not wearing pajamas or clothing, a lightweight blanket or towel should be placed on the chest and back. Excessive padding, however, should be avoided.

Airway Trauma

In all patients, extreme care must be taken to maintain a proper airway. Infants and children with artificial airways

in place can be accidentally extubated during ACT, especially if they are being mechanically ventilated. The ventilator tubing or endotracheal tube, or both, are easily pulled during position changes, and extubation may result. When turning the patient, condensation in the ventilator tubing can be inadvertently drained into the patient's airway, which may result in bronchospasm and respiratory distress. Special attention should also be given to patients who receive ACT during the first 24 hours after a tracheostomy because hemorrhage may occur if therapy is given too vigorously.[32] Therefore, for patients in intensive care units or those with artificial airways in place, suction equipment as well as a manual resuscitator and mask should be readily available, preferably at the patient's bedside.

SELECTION OF PATIENTS FOR AIRWAY CLEARANCE THERAPY

ACT is ordered for a multiplicity of conditions, including acute respiratory infections, postoperative complications, CF, and asthma, to name a few. Evidence is increasing, however, that ACT is required in only a limited number of conditions, all of which are characterized by chronic excessive sputum production.

Conditions in Which Airway Clearance Therapy May Not Be Beneficial

Various studies in children and adults have demonstrated that ACT may not be beneficial in certain conditions.

Asthma

In studies of the effects of ACT in children hospitalized with severe exacerbation of asthma, no difference was found in the rate of improvement of pulmonary function, even in the most severe cases.[89] Other studies in adults with reactive airway disease have shown that chest percussion can cause bronchospasm and hypoxemia.[84,103,104] Selected patients with asthma may benefit from ACT, especially when copious secretions or obstructive atelectasis is present. However, bronchospasm and hypoxemia should be well controlled before treatment. ACT is no substitute for adequate treatment with bronchodilating agents. It is also essential that a patient with asthma be well hydrated before ACT is begun.

Bronchiolitis

Although bronchiolitis is characterized by increased secretions, studies have reported ACT to be of minimal value. CPT made no difference in the length of hospital stay or the severity or duration of symptoms in patients with bronchiolitis, even when associated pneumonia or atelectasis was present.[105] It also produced no beneficial changes in lung mechanics or work of breathing in patients with bronchiolitis.[106] The failure of CPT to produce an effect in bronchiolitis most likely results from the fact that the disease affects the smaller, peripheral airways, where ACT techniques are generally not effective.[8]

Pneumonia

Several studies have evaluated the role of CPT in pneumonia and have reported that CPT either had no effect or actually delayed resolution, especially in young adults.[105,107,109]

Postsurgical Patients

In a study of a group of closely matched pediatric cardiac surgery patients, Reines and colleagues[108] reported that those treated with ACT had twice the incidence of atelectasis as did the control group (68% vs. 32%), which received deep-breathing instruction, coughing, or suction as appropriate. Moreover, atelectasis was more severe and the duration of hospitalization was prolonged in the ACT group.

Percussion to the right upper lobe every 1 to 2 hours for 24 hours after extubation is a common practice in many neonatal intensive care units. This practice is based on a report by Finer and associates[109] that claimed a dramatic reduction in the risk of right upper lobe atelectasis after extubation when ACT was given. However, it is unclear from the study if suctioning alone or ACT was responsible for the results.

Conditions in Which Airway Clearance Therapy May Be Beneficial

In contrast to the reports criticizing its effectiveness, ACT has been shown to be beneficial in patients with acute and chronic conditions characterized by excessive secretion production or mucous plugging of large airways that does not clear with coughing or suction. "Excessive secretions" usually means 30 ml of sputum per day in adults. Obviously, lesser amounts would qualify as excessive secretions in children. ACT is also useful in the treatment of obstructive atelectasis. Figure 12-9 illustrates the process of evaluation of the pediatric patient for ACT.

Acute Lobar Atelectasis

The majority of patients with acute atelectasis secondary to mucous plugs respond with one ACT treatment.[28,112,113] If patients fail to respond to several ACT treatments, the atelectasis most likely is caused by conditions not amenable to ACT and therapy should be discontinued. The presence of an air bronchogram, suggesting no mucous obstruction of the airways, has been shown to predict a poor response to ACT.[28,113] Although a period of ACT after resolution of the atelectasis may be warranted, prolonged ACT should not be necessary. As discussed earlier, ACT is not useful in preventing the return of atelectasis, except in patients with large amounts of secretions.

Cystic Fibrosis

ACT has been widely employed as a mainstay of treatment for the pulmonary complications of CF. In fact, much of our knowledge of ACT comes from studies conducted in patients with CF.[47,111,113] Current issues in the application of ACT in these patients include the following questions:
1. Which techniques are most effective?
2. How can self-care be promoted?
3. How can compliance with therapy be improved?

Effective techniques are those that foster high expiratory air velocity at low lung volume, such as FET, PEP therapy, HFCC, vigorous exercise, and AD. Postural drainage is also a useful adjunct to PEP therapy or FET. Although little evidence is available to support the routine use of manual chest percussion in the treatment of CF, and although some CF centers (especially in Europe) have abandoned the routine use of manual chest percussion, most CF treatment centers in the United States still consider it an integral component of ACT. Many patients will expect percussion to be a part of their ACT treatments, especially when hospitalized. Therefore elimination of chest percussion from routine ACT treatments should not be carried out arbitrarily. Radical changes in ACT practice for patients facing a lifelong battle with excessive pulmonary secretions should be made only after careful deliberation and consultation with the pulmonary physicians responsible for their care.

The issue of promoting self-care is especially important when dealing with patients with CF and their families. Patients with CF differ from most patients receiving ACT in that they need to employ some technique or techniques for removal of bronchial secretions on a daily basis for the rest of their lives. Current practices, especially those that require the routine application of chest percussion by a second person, often give the message that ACT is a passive technique, that it is something that is done "to" rather than "by" the patient. This may promote passivity and dependence on parents or other caregivers. As a result, compliance is often poor and treatments become a frequent source of arguments in families of patients with CF, with difficulties increasing as the patients grow older.[46,114] Also, because ACT must be administered by a parent two or more times a day, it may interfere with normal adolescent developmental processes, such as increasing autonomy and separation from parents. Therefore increasing the patient's ability to perform self-care is essential. All patients with CF, especially as they approach adolescence, should be well instructed in one of the forms of self-care, such as PEP, AD, FET with or without postural drainage, or HFCC. Vigorous exercise, such as running or swimming, is also an effective form of self-therapy in well-motivated patients. The techniques selected will depend on patient preference and learning ability, the preferences of the attending physician, and, in the case of certain technologies, the ability to arrange financing. Patients and their families often report improved compliance with self-care over

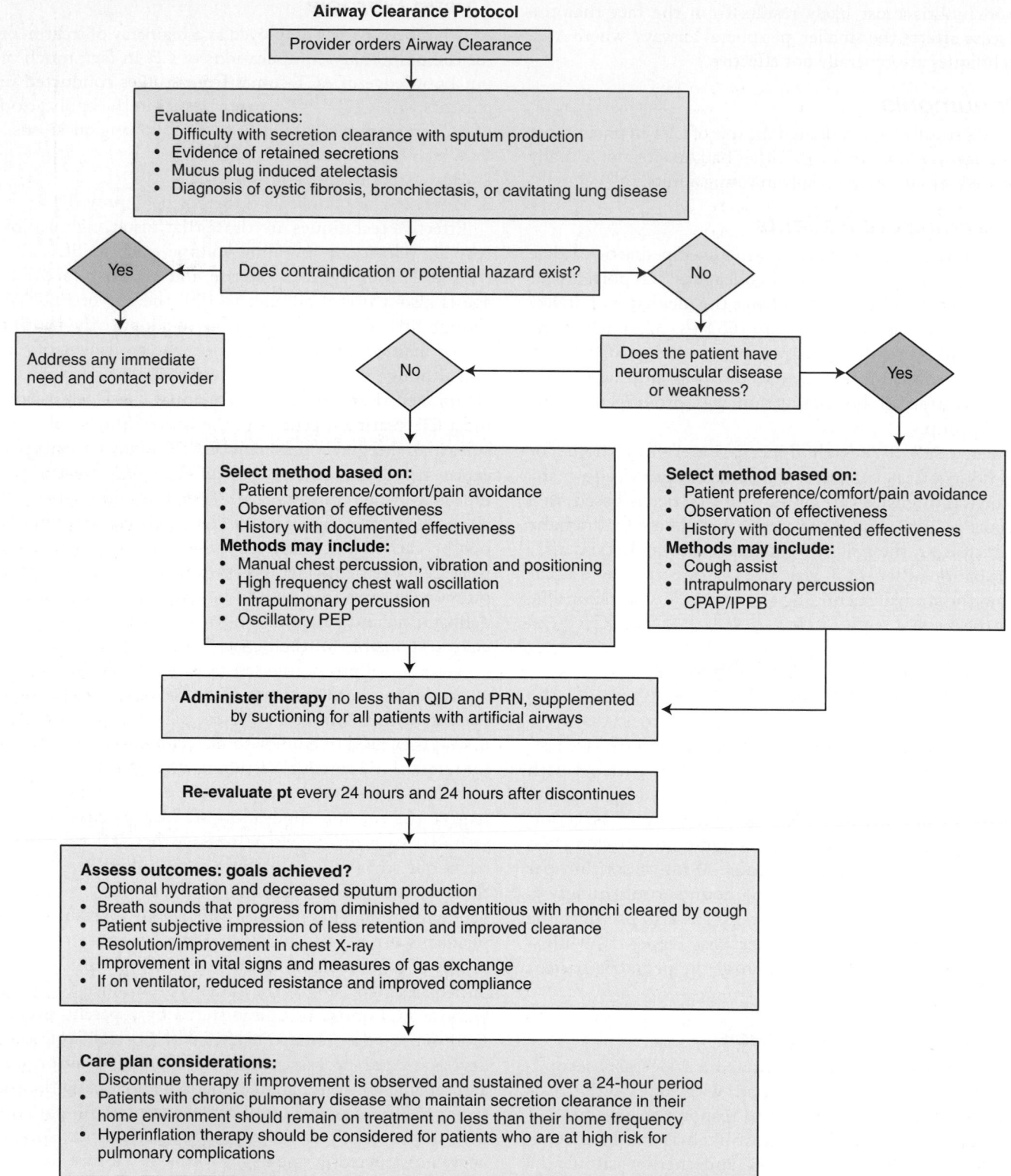

Airway Clearance Protocol

Provider orders Airway Clearance

Evaluate Indications:
• Difficulty with secretion clearance with sputum production
• Evidence of retained secretions
• Mucus plug induced atelectasis
• Diagnosis of cystic fibrosis, bronchiectasis, or cavitating lung disease

Does contraindication or potential hazard exist?

Yes → Address any immediate need and contact provider

No → Does the patient have neuromuscular disease or weakness?

No → **Select method based on:**
• Patient preference/comfort/pain avoidance
• Observation of effectiveness
• History with documented effectiveness
Methods may include:
• Manual chest percussion, vibration and positioning
• High frequency chest wall oscillation
• Intrapulmonary percussion
• Oscillatory PEP

Yes → **Select method based on:**
• Patient preference/comfort/pain avoidance
• Observation of effectiveness
• History with documented effectiveness
Methods may include:
• Cough assist
• Intrapulmonary percussion
• CPAP/IPPB

Administer therapy no less than QID and PRN, supplemented by suctioning for all patients with artificial airways

Re-evaluate pt every 24 hours and 24 hours after discontinues

Assess outcomes: goals achieved?
• Optional hydration and decreased sputum production
• Breath sounds that progress from diminished to adventitious with rhonchi cleared by cough
• Patient subjective impression of less retention and improved clearance
• Resolution/improvement in chest X-ray
• Improvement in vital signs and measures of gas exchange
• If on ventilator, reduced resistance and improved compliance

Care plan considerations:
• Discontinue therapy if improvement is observed and sustained over a 24-hour period
• Patients with chronic pulmonary disease who maintain secretion clearance in their home environment should remain on treatment no less than their home frequency
• Hyperinflation therapy should be considered for patients who are at high risk for pulmonary complications

FIGURE 12-9   Algorithm for evaluating and providing airway clearance.

parent-administered ACT, and treatment-related conflicts are minimized.[46]

Follow-up and consistency are essential when teaching bronchial drainage techniques. Reteaching may be necessary at intervals, and most patients with CF and their families are interested in learning new developments in ACT. Families often need assistance in adapting ACT practices to changing life circumstances, such as the patient entering school, traveling, entering college, and leaving home. Figure 12-8 demonstrates the use of HFCC while the child continues daily activities of life. Having a younger child play a game or continue some type of fun activity can be vitally important to ensure compliance.

Patients with advanced CF often have hemoptysis. ACT is usually withheld until the bleeding is controlled because vigorous coughing may aggravate the bleeding or dislodge clots. Likewise, ACT may need to be withheld in patients with pneumothorax, another common complication of advanced CF. Patients with end-stage disease may be especially reluctant to cooperate with ACT, especially the Trendelenburg positioning that is required. Supplemental oxygen may allow some patients with advanced disease to tolerate postural drainage. Withholding percussion may also improve the patient's ability to maintain the Trendelenburg position. Some investigators have reported that PEP therapy is better tolerated than postural drainage and percussion in patients with end-stage disease.[50]

Neuromuscular Disease or Injury

ACT is often used in many patients with neuromuscular injury or disease, and survival is often improved when ACT, coughing, turning, and deep breathing are incorporated into routine care (see Chapter 33, Neurological and Neuromuscular Disorders).[10,115-117] The goal is to return the patient with neuromuscular disease or injury to airway clearance that is as normal as possible. This may require hyperinflation type of therapies to return FRC levels to normal or assist with the patient's natural cough. Prolonged postural drainage is often especially helpful. However, patients with acute head injury should have well-controlled intracranial pressures before ACT is initiated.

Lung Abscess

Some patients with lung abscesses, especially older children, may be successfully treated with ACT.[118] Fearing that discharge of large amounts of infected material may spread the infection and lead to acute respiratory distress, some clinicians are reluctant to use ACT in the treatment of lung abscess.[27] Likewise, hemoptysis is a common complication in patients with lung abscess, and ACT may increase this risk. These concerns must be balanced against the knowledge that alternative treatments for lung abscess, such as lung resections, are also risky.

Though there is not enough evidence to definitively evaluate the role of ACT in many acute childhood diseases, it has become routine care for the CF patient. ACT appears likely to be of benefit in the maintenance or prevention of respiratory-related neuromuscular disease complications and is probably of benefit in treating atelectasis in mechanically ventilated children. ACT appears to be of minimal to no benefit in the treatment of acute asthma, bronchiolitis, neonatal respiratory distress, or those requiring mechanical ventilation for acute respiratory failure, and it is not effective in preventing atelectasis in the immediate postoperative period. Caution should be used given that the conclusions are based on very limited data (Figure 12-10).

Proven	Possible
Cystic fibrosis - no one specific ACT superior	Reduction in reintubation rate post-extubation in neonates CPT
Probable	**Minimal to no benefit**
Neuromuscular disease - hyperinflation therapy (Cough Assist, IPV) Atelectasis during mechanical ventilation IPV	Asthma Bronchiolitis Neonatal RDS Acute resp. failure Post-op atelectasis

FIGURE 12-10 Effectiveness of airway clearance techniques.

CONTRAINDICATIONS

Frank hemoptysis, empyema, foreign body aspiration, and untreated pneumothorax are often considered contraindications to all components of ACT. Withholding ACT, especially percussion, is sometimes recommended when the platelet count is low (less than 50,000 cells/mm^3). ACT is also usually withheld in the immediate postoperative period after tracheostomy, tracheobronchial reconstruction, and selected other conditions in which postoperative movement is extremely dangerous. Chest percussion should not be performed directly over fractured ribs, areas of subcutaneous emphysema, or recently burned or grafted skin. Some conditions may require modification of therapy or omission of certain components of ACT.

LENGTH AND FREQUENCY OF THERAPY

Treatments for patients with CF or bronchiectasis should be performed for at least 30 minutes, with many patients benefiting from therapy lasting 45 minutes or longer. Patients with severe dyspnea may require rest periods, which will further prolong therapy. Most pediatric respiratory care departments limit routine ACT treatments to 15 to 20 minutes.[119] ACT is rarely needed more than every 4 hours, although selected patients may benefit from more frequent suctioning or coughing. ACT orders should be evaluated at least every 48 hours for patients in intensive care units, at least every 72 hours for acute care patients, or whenever there is a change in a patient's status.[120]

CLINICAL HIGHLIGHT

Regardless of your approach, standardization supported by clinical practice guidelines or protocols may be of assistance. Figure 12-9 is an example of a protocol used to guide therapy.

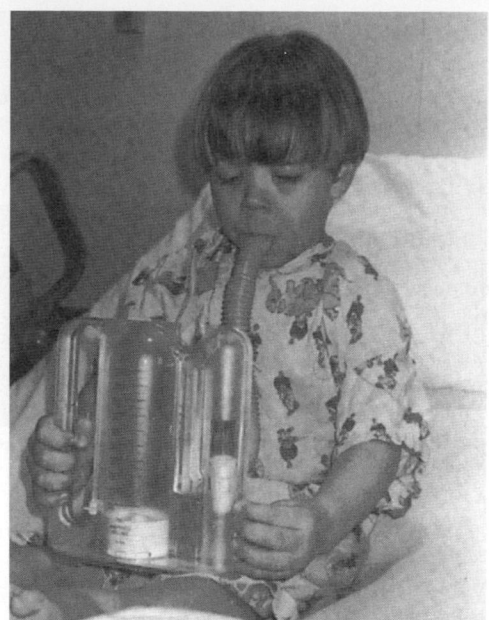

FIGURE 12-11   Child using incentive spirometry device.

THERAPY MODIFICATION

Many patients require modification of therapy because of medical or surgical procedures. Percussion may be extremely painful for patients postoperatively, and the use of manual vibration or mechanical vibrators is sometimes better tolerated. Also, clinicians should be careful to avoid percussion over implanted devices, such as ventricular–peritoneal shunts or implantable venous access devices (often used in patients with CF). Percussion is also omitted in patients with brittle bones—for example, in those with rickets or osteogenesis imperfecta.

Many patients may not tolerate Trendelenburg positioning. Included in this group are those with severe GER, recent intracranial trauma or surgery, increased intracranial pressure, abdominal distention or ascites, compromised diaphragm movement, uncontrolled hypertension, and severe cardiopulmonary failure.[120] With careful monitoring, simple side-to-side positioning may be attempted in these patients. The patient with a gastrostomy tube or chest tube, or both, may also require modifications in drainage positions.

Patients receiving ACT often have a disorder affecting only one lobe. These patients do not need ACT in all 11 positions but rather an abbreviated ACT treatment that uses postural drainage positions for the affected lobe only.

Infants and small children are unable to perform maneuvers such as FET or AD. Some clinicians have attempted to mimic these techniques with gentle chest wall compression during the expiratory phase, allowing the child to exhale to less than functional residual capacity. Like AD or FET performed in cooperative older patients, this technique results in increased expiratory air velocity at low lung volumes, improving mucus mobilization.

MONITORING DURING THERAPY

Patients in an intensive care unit who require ACT should have continuous monitoring of arterial oxygen saturation (Sao_2), heart rate, and respiratory rate. Breathing pattern, skin color, and breath sounds should also be noted.[120] Patients not in an intensive care unit who require high oxygen concentrations or who have a condition presenting a high risk of respiratory or cardiac failure should also have these variables monitored. Other patients with mild respiratory distress should have pulse and respiratory rate as well as breathing pattern, skin color, and breath sounds measured before and after therapy. This is especially true for younger patients who cannot verbalize complaints of distress. Routine monitoring of heart rate and respiratory rate for patients with chronic respiratory disorders, such as CF, is probably not warranted and may inadvertently give the message that ACT is harmful. When performing percussion or vibration on patients who are connected to cardiopulmonary monitors, the alarm on the monitor may become activated because of interference from the percussion or vibration. It is best to refrain from turning the monitor alarms completely off.

EVALUATION OF THERAPY

Because the goal of ACT is to promote the removal of excessive bronchial secretions, the single most important variable in evaluating the effectiveness of ACT is the amount of secretions expectorated with therapy; however, this cannot be done in a vacuum and the basics should not be forgotten. The hydration status of the patient, and whether or not the patient's lungs are acidic, can play a huge role in the success of airway clearance.[121,122] Mucus changes from sol to gel if the lungs are acidic. Changes in sputum production, breath sounds, vital signs, chest radiographic findings, blood gas values, and lung mechanics may indicate a positive response to the therapy.[120] The removal of excessive bronchial secretions is not always associated with an immediate change in blood gases, breath sounds, or lung mechanics. Patients with advanced CF, for example, almost always have audible rales before and after therapy, whereas pulmonary function and blood gas determinations change little.

Patients undergoing mechanical ventilation may have measurements of lung mechanics as well as noninvasive blood gas monitoring data readily available. If so, the clinician should note any changes associated with therapy. Deterioration in these variables, especially if unaccompanied by removal of secretions, suggests that therapy should be modified or discontinued.

DOCUMENTATION OF THERAPY

When charting ACT treatments, the clinician should describe the techniques used (e.g., postural drainage, percussion, and AD), which lobes were treated, and what positions the patient was placed in. If certain segments or positions are omitted, this should be documented, as well as the reason why this was done. The clinician should also note if suctioning was performed. To document the response to therapy, pretreatment and posttreatment breath sounds, vital signs, and the amount and quality of sputum expectorated should be noted.

HYPERINFLATION THERAPY

Incentive Spirometry

Incentive spirometry, also referred to as *sustained maximal inspiration,* was introduced in the early 1970s in an effort to prevent postoperative pulmonary complications.[92,123] It was designed to encourage patients to improve their inspiratory volumes while visualizing their inspiratory effort. Forced expiratory maneuvers using devices such as blow bottles, blow gloves, and balloons have been prescribed in the past to prevent postoperative complications; however, they have been associated with the development of atelectasis and do not result in the same physiological effects as incentive spirometry.[124-126] Although it is still debated which methods are most effective for the prevention and management of postoperative pulmonary complications, it is estimated that incentive spirometry is prescribed in 95% of all U.S. hospitals for prophylaxis and treatment of postoperative atelectasis.[127-131] The objectives of incentive spirometry are to prevent or reverse atelectasis, improve lung volumes, and improve inspiratory muscle performance (including use of the diaphragm).[124]

Indications, Contraindications, and Complications

Clinical conditions that may benefit from incentive spirometry are listed in Box 12-1.[124] Clinical symptoms often include fever, increased work of breathing, tachypnea, hypoxia, and evidence of atelectasis on the chest radiograph. For incentive spirometry to be effective in the pediatric patient, he or she must be able to cooperate

and understand the procedure and to be able to breathe volumes exceeding his or her normal tidal volume.

Incentive spirometry is contraindicated in patients who cannot cooperate or follow instructions concerning the proper use of the device. The child may be uncooperative, physically disabled, or simply too young to effectively perform the maneuvers. Alternative methods such as walking, getting up in a chair, frequent changes in position, and singing, to name a few, may help to improve lung volumes and should then be considered.[132,133]

The majority of problems that patients experience with incentive spirometry are the result of inadequate supervision or instruction, or both. These two factors account for a large number of ineffective treatments.[134] Hyperventilation may occur in the patient who performs the maneuvers too rapidly, and he or she may complain of lightheadedness or tingling in the fingers. The patient may also complain of fatigue during the procedure. These complaints can be alleviated by coaching the patient to slow down and rest between each maneuver. Pain from surgical incisions is often encountered postoperatively and can be decreased by splinting the surgical area with a pillow during deep breathing and coughing. Airway closure and bronchospasm may occur if the patient exhales forcefully to less than functional residual capacity before taking a deep inspiration. Again, this can be avoided with proper coaching by the clinician. Hypoxia may develop if the patient's oxygen therapy is interrupted, especially when a mask is used. This can be prevented by using a nasal cannula during therapy.

Devices

The original Bartlett-Edwards incentive spirometer operated on a piston–bellows principle and was designed to fall open by gravity at a preset volume. A battery-operated light was activated when the patient inhaled from the spirometer and the preset volume was reached. To keep the light on, the patient had to continue to inhale. The light went off when the patient's glottis closed or total lung capacity was reached.[135] There are many different types and brands of incentive spirometers, including disposable and nondisposable devices. They are classified according to how inhalation is activated: (1) volume oriented or (2) flow oriented.

Most of the current volume-oriented incentive spirometers are based on the original Bartlett-Edwards spirometer. A volume is preset as a goal, and the patient is instructed to inhale until the preset goal is reached. The spirometer volume is measured according to the amount of volume displaced during the inhalation. Flow-oriented spirometers operate by using a floating ball or bar that is raised by the negative flow generated with inspiration. The more rapid and forceful the inspiratory flow, the higher the ball rises. Although differences in the inspiratory work of breathing among the various incentive spirometers have been reported, in terms of clinical outcome the differences

Box 12-1	Indications for Incentive Spirometry

- Abdominal surgery
- Thoracic surgery
- Surgery in patients with pulmonary disease
- Atelectasis
- Restrictive lung defects associated with quadriplegia
- Restrictive lung defects associated with a dysfunctional diaphragm

among the devices appear to be negligible.[136,137] The device used will vary from one institution to another and may even vary among patients within the institution. Regardless of the type, the operator's instructions should be read and universal precautions followed.[138]

The number of maneuvers to be performed per session should be either prescribed by the physician or set by departmental policy. Several sources have suggested 5 to 10 *effective* breaths per treatment as an adequate frequency.[124] The patient should cough during the session whenever it is felt necessary and then again when the maneuvers have been completed. The postoperative patient may need assistance with splinting of the incision during coughing as well as during deep breathing. A pillow or folded blanket can be placed over the incision area. The inspiratory volume goal may be increased when the patient reaches the preset goal repeatedly. Breath sounds should be assessed after coughing, and the incentive spirometer should be left within the patient's reach before the clinician leaves the room. The patient should be encouraged to perform the maneuvers independently between scheduled sessions. The frequency of sessions varies with the patient and may be prescribed as often and specifically as once per hour or as variably as three times per day.[21,22]

Assessment of Therapy

Documentation of the patient's response during therapy should include the following:

· Heart rate
· Respiratory rate
· Breath sounds
· Inspiratory volume or flow achieved
· Number of goals achieved
· Description of cough and sputum production
· Patient effort and tolerance
· How many maneuvers the family has tried/agreed to get the patient to do per hour
· Any patient complaints or adverse reactions, or both, and the corrective action taken

Therapy is considered effective if atelectasis is prevented or resolved and inspiratory muscle performance is improved.[124] Clinical signs of this would include a decreased respiratory rate, normal temperature, normal pulse rate, normal or improved breath sounds that were previously absent or diminished, a normal chest radiograph, improved oxygenation, and increased vital capacity and peak expiratory flows.[124]

Although there have been numerous studies evaluating the therapeutic value of incentive spirometry, it is difficult to compare them because of the variation in patients and study design.[139] However, a number of studies have indicated that incentive spirometry, along with other deep breathing maneuvers, is effective in reducing pulmonary complications when used correctly.[129,131,140-142] A study comparing the efficacy of postoperative incentive spirometry between children and adults concluded

that incentive spirometry is as effective in reducing the incidence of atelectasis in children who have undergone cardiac surgery.[143]

INTERMITTENT POSITIVE-PRESSURE BREATHING

IPPB is the intermittent, short-term delivery of positive pressure to a patient for the purpose of improving lung expansion, delivering aerosolized medications, and assisting ventilation.[144] Since its inception in 1947 and its introduction into the medical arena in 1948, IPPB has been one of the most controversial topics in respiratory care.[145] It was one of the most popular therapeutic modalities prescribed in the 1960s and 1970s and was regarded as the panacea to all pulmonary ailments. Not until the American College of Chest Physicians' conference on oxygen therapy in September 1983, when both its overuse and its doubtful efficacy were discussed, did IPPB decline as a treatment modality.[146] Today newly practiced modalities, such as bilevel positive airway pressure and incentive spirometry, have rendered the prescription of IPPB more selective than in the past.[147,148]

Indications, Contraindications, and Complications

Clinically, IPPB (Figure 12-12) is given to provide a significantly larger inhaled volume at a physiologically advantageous inspiratory to expiratory pattern than the patient can produce with spontaneous ventilation. If this goal is met, there should be improvement in the cough mechanism, distribution of ventilation, and delivery of medication.[149] In the pediatric population, however, the hazards and potential complications that can result from its use render it unpopular and ineffective among infants

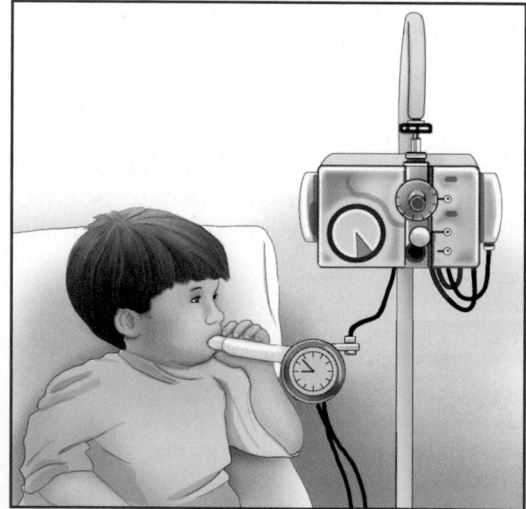

FIGURE 12-12   Intermittent positive-pressure breathing (IPPB) therapy being administered to a child, with a respirometer attached to the exhalation valve for exhaled volume monitoring.

and children.[150] It is indicated most often in the older patient who needs increased lung expansion but has failed to respond to other modes of treatment, such as incentive spirometry, chest physiotherapy, deep-breathing exercises, and bilevel positive airway pressure. This includes patients with neuromuscular disease or chest wall deformity that inhibits maximal inspiratory efforts. Medication can also be delivered via IPPB to these patients. However, studies have continued to report that the delivery of medications via IPPB depends on the technique and that the first mode of choice for aerosolized medication therapy should be a small-volume nebulizer or metered-dose inhaler.[151-153]

The absolute contraindication to IPPB is a tension pneumothorax; however, there are other factors that should be considered carefully before IPPB therapy is recommended. Because the effectiveness of applying IPPB therapy hinges on the cooperation of the patient, any infant or child who most likely would not cooperate and who has difficulty coordinating deep breathing should not be considered for this therapy. (Asynchronous breathing as well as breathing against the high positive pressure could result in increased work of breathing.) According to the American Association for Respiratory Care's clinical practice guideline for IPPB, other clinical contraindications include increased intracranial pressures (greater than 15 mm Hg); recent facial, oral, or skull surgery; tracheoesophageal fistula; recent esophageal surgery; active hemoptysis; active, untreated tuberculosis; radiographic evidence of blebs; hemodynamic instability; nausea; and swallowing of air.[144] Because IPPB is so rarely used in pediatrics, it is possible that the clinician may be inexperienced in administering the therapy and unable to provide optimal respiratory care. When this situation arises, the objective of providing a safe, effective treatment may be unattainable, and it is in the patient's best interest not to have the treatment administered.

Complications associated with IPPB therapy are listed in Box 12-2.[144,154,155] This list demonstrates the need for an experienced clinician to administer the therapy and to monitor the patient and the equipment closely. Should adverse reactions occur, the treatment should be discontinued and the physician notified of the situation.

Equipment

The equipment used during an IPPB treatment includes the IPPB device, the circuit, the patient application device, and the volume measuring device. Although the addition of a humidifier is not essential, it is recommended in patients with mucus retention. The most popular IPPB devices used in pediatric patients are the Bird series (Cardinal Health, Dublin, OH), the Puritan Bennett series (Puritan Bennett, Boulder, CO), and the Monaghan 515 (Monaghan Medical, Plattsburgh, NY). The devices vary in design and in flow, volume, and pressure capabilities.[156] The patient application devices are dependent on the patient's needs and include a mouthpiece, lip–mouth seal, mask, or endotracheal tube/tracheostomy adapter. A nose clip should be available for the patient who uses either a mouthpiece or lip seal. The volume measuring can be obtain by a spirometer. Suctioning equipment should be available, as should containers for collecting or disposing of sputum.[144]

Monitoring

The patient and equipment should be monitored closely during therapy. The heart rate and respiratory rate should be obtained before, during, and after each treatment. Breath sounds should be assessed before and after each treatment and any time the patient complains of respiratory difficulty or chest pains. With the goal of therapy being to generate a tidal volume during IPPB that is at least 15 ml/kg or to exceed one third of inspiratory capacity, it is essential that tidal volume be monitored.[157] To determine whether lung volume is being augmented, the patient's tidal volume should be monitored before (spontaneous breathing) and several times during therapy. The exhaled gas is measured during therapy at the exhalation valve with either a respirometer or spirometer. If the tidal volume delivered during IPPB therapy is not greater than that during spontaneous breathing, the therapy is of little, if any, value to the patient. The patient's peak flow should also be monitored before and after treatment.

Assessment of Therapy

Document the following with each IPPB treatment:
· Heart rate
· Respiratory rate
· Breath sounds
· Pressure used (beginning and end of therapy)
· Tidal volume obtained (before and during therapy)
· Machine controls used (i.e., sensitivity, flow)
· Fraction of inspired oxygen (FiO_2) values
· Medication aerosolized
· Peak flow

Box 12-2	**Complications Associated with Intermittent Positive-Pressure Breathing**

- Bronchospasm
- Gastric distention and ileus
- Nosocomial infection
- Decreased venous return
- Hyperventilation
- Hypoventilation
- Impaction of secretions
- Fatigue
- Air trapping
- Volutrauma, pneumothorax
- Hemoptysis

- Description of cough and sputum production
- Patient cooperation and tolerance
- Duration of therapy
- Any patient complaints or adverse reactions and the corrective action taken

IPPB therapy is believed to be effective if the therapeutic goals are met, including the following:

- An augmented tidal volume during IPPB (15 ml/kg or more than one third of the inspiratory capacity)
- An increase in peak flow or forced expiratory volume in 1 second (FEV$_1$)
- A more effective cough
- Secretion clearance
- Improved breath sounds
- An improved chest radiograph[144]

When compared with other aerosol delivery devices, IPPB in the pediatric patient is both equipment and labor intensive.[104] With this in mind, perhaps thought should be given *not* to whether IPPB is effective in delivering aerosols but rather to whether IPPB is the most effective method of delivery.[119] However, although there are other less expensive and less invasive lung expansion maneuvers, there remain patients who fail to respond to these maneuvers but who do benefit from IPPB. If there are no observable benefits from the therapy, however, its use cannot be justified.

INTRAPULMONARY PERCUSSIVE VENTILATION

Intrapulmonary percussive ventilation (IPV) is a technique that utilizes **hyperinflation therapy** and airway clearance therapy in one. The IPV device uses high-frequency oscillatory ventilation to produce percussion. The percussions are high-flow jets of gas that are delivered to the airways by a flow interrupter called a Phasitron. Activation of the Venturi system within the Phasitron creates bursts of gas at frequencies of 100 to 300 bursts per minute within a tightly controlled ratio of gas delivery and passive exhalation. The relationship between the gas bursts and exhalation determines the intrapulmonary "wedge" pressure. It is this wedge pressure that may provide mobilization and clearance of pulmonary secretions.

Indications, Contraindications, and Complications

IPV is designed to both treat active pulmonary disease and to prevent the development of disease caused by secretion retention. Specific goals of therapy include promoting the mobilization of bronchial secretions, improving the efficiency and distribution of ventilation, providing an alternative delivery system for bronchodilator therapy, providing intrathoracic percussion and vibration, and providing an alternative system for the delivery of positive pressure to the lungs. The Phasitron may be manually triggered during IPV therapy in nonintubated, spontaneously breathing patients or may be set to continuous percussion for use in intubated patients. IPV may be applied via mouthpiece, mask, artificial airway, or through a ventilator.

If you take a least aggressive to most aggressive approach, the primary indication for a combination therapy like IPV is a patient refractory to traditional bronchial hygiene methods. Other indications are similar to other airway clearance procedures, such as patients with atelectasis, bronchitis, bronchiectasis, and bronchopneumonia. Patients who have aggressive secretion-producing disease coupled with muscle weakness are likely the best candidates.

Contraindications are not that different than positive pressure and airway clearance and include untreated pneumothorax, hemoptysis, active tuberculosis, and fractured ribs or unstable chest

Monitoring

The patient and equipment should be monitored closely during therapy. The heart rate and respiratory rate should be obtained before, during, and after each treatment. Breath sounds should be assessed before and after each treatment and any time the patient complains of respiratory difficulty or chest pains, with the goal of therapy being to clear secretions and improve the efficiency of breathing.

Assessment of Therapy

Document the following with each IPV treatment:

- Heart rate
- Respiratory rate
- Breath sounds
- Pressure used (beginning and end of therapy)
- Machine controls used
- Medication aerosolized
- Peak flow (if applicable)
- Description of sputum production
- Patient cooperation and tolerance
- Duration of therapy
- Any patient complaints or adverse reactions and the corrective action taken

IPV therapy is believed to be effective if the therapeutic goals are met, including the following:

- Secretion clearance
- Improved breath sounds
- Improved gas exchange
- Medication delivery
- An improved chest radiograph[158]

CLINICAL HIGHLIGHT

Hyperinflation therapy maybe the only airway clearance a patient needs.

FUTURE OF AIRWAY CLEARANCE THERAPY

The future of airway clearance will center on normalization of physiological airway clearance mechanisms. This will be accomplished by new and novel drug and device therapies such as hypertonic saline or such simple devices as the Cough Assist (Emerson), which helps neuromuscular patients mimic a stronger cough. Because of the understood benefits of deep breathing and coughing, paralytics in acute lung injury are no longer common practice. Gene therapy for CF is just around the corner. Advances in technology will continue to give us tools that allow us to accomplish the basics while reducing the overall physical size and power consumption. Many of these new devices will provide a user-friendly interface that can be utilized by non–health care providers in the home care setting. This will allow us to customize our therapy for the best outcome depending on the social, economic, and educational needs of the patient and family.

CASE STUDY

You are assigned to treat a 10-year-old with CF who is struggling with secretion management. You are requested by the physician to assess and treat the patient with what you feel is the most appropriate ACT. After further assessment, you determine that the patient is hypoxic, requiring a dry high-flow oxygen device; has inspissated secretions and adventitious breath sounds; and is fatiguing. What should be your first actions?

1. Provide humidity as soon as possible.
2. Determine the patient's home regimen and what has worked in the past.
3. Consider an ACT with hyperinflation therapy to support fatiguing muscles.
4. Call physician to report fatigue.
   A. 4, 2, 1, 3
   B. 4 only and wait for direction
   C. 1, 2, 3, 4
   D. 2, 3

See Evolve Resources for answers.

KEY POINTS

- The primary use of ACT should be limited to those who cannot clear their airway secretions.
- The most effective ACT is that which mimics or supports normal physiology.
- ACT should target symptoms. See the table here for a list of ACTs to best target various symptoms.

Symptom	Possible cause	Initial ACT
Weak or poor cough	• Neuromuscular disease	Combination ACT and hyperinflation therapy. Clinician choice as to which therapy creates the highest expiratory flow rate. This requires increasing the FRC.
	• Oversedation	Wean sedation if possible and support with hyperinflation therapy.
	• Pain	Support pain management and encourage deep breathing and coughing with mobilization if possible.
Inspissated secretions	• Poor humidification	Hydration and chest physical therapy.
Airway collapse that leads to retained secretions	• External forces or defects within the airway	Solve external force issues if possible. PEP for obstructions that lead to atelectasis. CPT for those obstructed secretions that lead to distal hyperinflation.
Expectorating a large volume of secretions	• Infection	Treat infection or possible cause of sputum production and support with chest physical therapy.

- All ACT should have an objective outcome to determine effectiveness and be reevaluated frequently.

ASSESSMENT QUESTIONS

See Evolve Resources for answers.

1. Many institutions found that the routine use of IPPB was replaced with routine use of ACT in what two decades?
   A. 1900s and 1910s
   B. 1920s and 1930s
   C. 1960s and 1970s
   D. 1980s and 1990s

2. Postural drainage was used as early as:
   A. 1901
   B. 1911
   C. 1940
   D. 1953

3. When doing percussion therapy, what is the recommended frequency?
   A. 1 to 2 Hz
   B. 3 to 4 Hz
   C. 5 to 6 Hz
   D. 7 to 8 Hz

4. When providing vibration chest physiotherapy, what is the recommended frequency?
   A. 6 to 7 Hz
   B. 8 to 9 Hz
   C. 10 to 15 Hz
   D. >20 Hz
5. The four components of *traditional*[159] ACT are:
   A. Postural drainage, percussion, vibration, and coughing
   B. FET, IS, IPPB, and HFFC
   C. PEP, position, AD, and resistance
   D. Hydration, percussion, deep breathing, and FET
6. Premature infants may be at risk for increased complications from ACT. Why?
   A. The high chest wall compliance of premature infants can cause loss of lung volume.
   B. ACT is associated with IVH.
   C. Prolonged handling can interfere with the temperature-regulated environment of these patients.
   D. A, B, and C are correct.
7. What hyperinflation therapy was introduced in the 1970s to prevent postoperative pulmonary complications?
   A. Deep breath and cough
   B. Incentive spirometry
   C. CPT
   D. PEP
8. ACT is required in only a limited number of conditions, all of which are characterized by which of the following?
   A. Chronic, excessive sputum production
   B. Disease state
   C. Patient age and disease state
   D. None of the above
9. Treatments for patients with CF or bronchiectasis should be performed for at least _____ and reevaluated every _____ for acute care.
   A. 10 minutes, 24 hours
   B. 15 minutes, 48 hours
   C. 20 minutes, 96 hours
   D. 30 minutes, 72 hours
10. What are the contraindications for ACT?
    A. Frank hemoptysis
    B. Empyema
    C. Foreign body aspiration
    D. All of the above

References

1. Ewart W: The treatment of bronchiectasis and of chronic bronchial infections by posture and respiratory exercises, *Lancet* 2:70, 1901.
2. Gaskell DV, Webber BA: *The Brompton Hospital guide to chest physiotherapy*, Oxford, 1973, Blackwell Scientific Publications.
3. Murray JF: The ketchup-bottle method, *N Engl J Med* 300:1155, 1979.
4. Sutton PP, et al: Chest physiotherapy: a review, *Eur J Respir Dis* 63:188, 1982.
5. Kirilloff LH, et al: Does chest physical therapy work? *Chest* 88:436, 1985.
6. Sutton P: Chest physiotherapy: time for a reappraisal, *Br J Dis Chest* 82:127, 1988.
7. Selsby Jones JG, Chest physiotherapy may be harmful in some patients, *BMJ* 298:541, 1989.
8. Selsby, Jones JG: Chest physiotherapy: physiological and clinical aspects, *Br J Anaesth* 64:621, 1990.
9. Pavia D: The role of chest physiotherapy in mucus hypersecretion, *Lung* 168(suppl):614, 1990.
10. Stiller KR: Chest physiotherapy for the medical patient: are current practices effective? *Aust N Z J Med* 20:183, 1990.
11. Eid N, et al: Chest physiotherapy in review, *Respir Care* 36:270, 1991.
12. Lewis RM: Chest physical therapy: time for a redefinition and a renaming, *Respir Care* 37:419, 1992.
13. Oberwaldner B: Physiotherapy for airway clearance in paediatrics, *Eur Respir J* 15(1):196–204, 2000.
14. Papastamelos C, Panitch HB, England SE, Allen JL: Developmental changes in chest wall compliance in infancy and early childhood, *J Appl Physiol* 78(1):179–184, 1995.
15. Lai-Fook SJ, Hyatt RE: Effects of age on elastic moduli of human lungs, *J Appl Physiol* 89(1):163–168, 2000.
16. Penn RB, Wolfson MR, Shaffer TH: Developmental differences in tracheal cartilage mechanics, *Pediatr Res* 26(5):429–433, 1989.
17. Hall GL, Hantos Z, Wildhaber JH, Sly PD: Contribution of nasal pathways to low frequency respiratory impedance in infants, *Thorax* 57(5):396–399, 2002.
18. Hough: *Physiotherapy in respiratory care: a problem solving approach*, London, 1991, Chapman & Hall.
19. Cystic Fibrosis Foundation: *Consumer fact sheet: an introduction to chest physical therapy*, Bethesda, MD, 1992, Cystic Fibrosis Foundation.
20. Mellins RB: Pulmonary physiotherapy in the pediatric age group, *Am Rev Respir Dis* 110(2 suppl):137, 1974.
21. Sutton PP, et al: Assessment of percussion, vibratory shaking, and breathing exercises in chest physiotherapy, *Eur J Respir Dis* 66:147, 1985.
22. Sutton PP, Parker RA, Webber BA: Assessment of the forced expiration technique, postural drainage and directed coughing in chest physiotherapy, *Eur J Respir Dis* 64:62, 1983.
23. van der Schans CP, Piers DA, Postma DS: Effect of manual percussion on tracheobronchial clearance in patients with chronic airflow obstruction and excessive tracheobronchial secretion, *Thorax* 41:448, 1986.
24. Murphy MB, Concannon D, FitzGerald M: Chest percussion: help or hindrance to postural drainage, *Ir Med J* 76:189, 1983.
25. Webber, et al: Evaluation of self-percussion during postural drainage using the forced expiration technique, *Physiother Pract* 1:42, 1985.
26. Faling LJ: Chest physical therapy. In Burton GG, Gee GN, Hodgkin JE, editors: *Respiratory care: a guide to clinical practice*, ed 3, Philadelphia, 1991, JB Lippincott, pp 625–654.
27. Marini JJ, Pierson DJ, Hudson LD: Acute lobar atelectasis: a prospective comparison of fiberoptic bronchoscopy and respiratory therapy, *Am Rev Respir Dis* 19:971, 1979.
28. Finer NN, Boyd J: Chest physiotherapy in the neonate: a controlled study, *Pediatrics* 61:282, 1978.
29. Ernst MM, Wooldridge JL, Conway E, et al: Using quality improvement science to implement a multidisciplinary behavioral intervention targeting pediatric inpatient airway clearance, *J Pediatr Psychol* 35(1):14-24. doi: jsp013 [pii] 10.1093/jpepsy/jsp013.
30. O'Bradovich HM, Chernick V: The functional basis of respiratory pathology. In Chernick V, editor: *Kendig's disorders of the*

respiratory tract in children, ed 5, Philadelphia, 1990, WB Saunders pp 3–47.

31. Walters P: Chest physiotherapy. In Levin DL, Morris FC, Moore GC, editors: *A practical guide to pediatric intensive care*, St. Louis, 1979, Mosby, pp 395–403.

32. Holloway R, et al: Effect of chest physiotherapy on blood gases of neonates treated by intermittent positive pressure respiration, *Thorax* 24:421, 1969.

33. Fox WW, Schwartz JG, Schaffer TH: Pulmonary physiotherapy in neonates: physiologic changes and respiratory management, *J Pediatr* 92:977, 1978.

34. Curran CL, Kachoyeanos MK: The effects on neonates of two methods of chest physical therapy, *MCN Am J Matern Child Nurs* 4:309, 1979.

35. Walsh CM, et al: Controlled supplemental oxygenation during tracheobronchial hygiene, *Nurs Res* 36:211, 1987.

36. Raval D, et al: Chest physiotherapy in preterm infants with RDS in the first 24 hours of life, *J Perinatol* 7:301, 1987.

37. Green CG: Assessment of the pediatric airway by flexible bronchoscopy, *Respir Care* 36:555, 1991.

38. Pryor JA: The forced expiration technique. In Pryor JA, editor: *International perspectives in physical therapy*, vol 7, Edinburgh, 1991, Churchill Livingstone, pp 79–100.

39. Zapletal A, et al: Chest physiotherapy and airway obstruction in patients with cystic fibrosis: a negative report, *Eur J Respir Dis* 64:426, 1983.

40. Oldenburg FA, et al: Effects of postural drainage, exercise, and cough on mucus clearance in chronic bronchitis, *Am Rev Respir Dis* 120:739, 1979.

41. Rossman CM, et al: Effect of chest physiotherapy on the removal of mucus in patients with cystic fibrosis, *Am Rev Respir Dis* 126:131, 1982.

42. DeBoeck C, Zinman R: Cough versus chest physiotherapy, *Am Rev Respir Dis* 129:132, 1984.

43. Bain J, Bishop J, Olinsky A: Evaluation of directed coughing in cystic fibrosis, *Br J Dis Chest* 82:138, 1988.

44. van Hengstum M, et al: Conventional physiotherapy and forced expiratory manoeuvres have similar effects on tracheobronchial clearance, *Eur Respir J* 1:758, 1988.

45. Klig S, et al: A biopsychosocial examination of two methods of pulmonary therapy [abstract], *Pediatr Pulmonol* 4(suppl):145, 1989.

46. Reisman J, et al: Role of conventional physiotherapy in cystic fibrosis, *J Pediatr* 113:632, 1988.

47. Holzer FJ, Schnall R, Landau LI: The effect of a home exercise programme in children with cystic fibrosis, *Aust Paediatr J* 20:297, 1984.

48. Blomquist M, et al: Physical activity and self treatment in cystic fibrosis, *Arch Dis Child* 61:362, 1986.

49. Mahlmeister MJ, et al: Positive-expiratory-pressure mask therapy: theoretical and practical considerations and a review of the literature, *Respir Care* 36:1218, 1991.

50. Iverson LIG, et al: Comparative study of IPPB, the incentive spirometer and blow bottles: the prevention of atelectasis following cardiac surgery, *Ann Thorac Surg* 25:197, 1978.

51. Striegl AM, Redding GJ, Diblasi R, et al: Use of a lung model to assess mechanical in-exsufflator therapy in infants with tracheostomy, *Pediatr Pulmonol* 2010. doi: 10.1002/ppul.21353.

52. Vianello A, Ragazzi R, Mirri L, Arcaro G, Cutrone C, Fitta C: Tracheoinnominate fistula in a Duchenne muscular dystrophy patient: successful management with an endovascular stent, *Neuromuscul Disord* 15(8):569–571, 2005. doi: 10.1016/j.nmd.2005.04.010.

53. Avena Kde M, Duarte AC, Cravo SL, Sologuren MJ, Gastaldi AC: [Effects of manually assisted coughing on respiratory mechanics in patients requiring full ventilatory support], *J Bras Pneumol* 34(6):380–386, 2008.

54. Unoki T, Kawasaki Y, Mizutani T, et al: Effects of expiratory rib-cage compression on oxygenation, ventilation, and airway-secretion removal in patients receiving mechanical ventilation, *Respir Care* 50(11):1430–1437, 2005.

55. Unoki T, Mizutani T, Toyooka H: Effects of expiratory rib cage compression and/or prone position on oxygenation and ventilation in mechanically ventilated rabbits with induced atelectasis, *Respir Care* 48(8):754–762, 2003.

56. Unoki T, Mizutani T, Toyooka H: Effects of expiratory rib cage compression combined with endotracheal suctioning on gas exchange in mechanically ventilated rabbits with induced atelectasis, *Respir Care* 49(8):896–901, 2004.

57. Marti JD, Li Bassi G, Rigol M, et al: Effects of manual rib cage compressions on expiratory flow and mucus clearance during mechanical ventilation, *Crit Care Med* 41(3):850–856, 2013. doi: 10.1097/CCM.0b013e3182711b52.

58. Schoni MH: Autogenic drainage: a modern approach to physiotherapy in cystic fibrosis, *J R Soc Med* 82(16 suppl):32, 1989.

59. David: Autogenic drainage—the German approach. In Pryor JA, editor: *International perspectives in physical therapy*, vol 7, Edinburgh, 1991, Churchill Livingstone, pp 65–78.

60. Davidson AGF, et al: Long-term comparison of conventional percussion and drainage physiotherapy versus autogenic drainage in cystic fibrosis [abstract], *Pediatr Pulmonol* 8(suppl):298, 1992.

61. Falk M, et al: Improving the ketchup bottle method with positive expiratory pressure, PEP, in cystic fibrosis, *Eur J Respir Dis* 65:423, 1984.

62. Tonnesen P, Stovring S: Positive expiratory pressure (PEP) as lung physiotherapy in cystic fibrosis: a pilot study, *Eur J Respir Dis* 65:419, 1984.

63. Tyrell JC, Hiller EJ, Martin J: Face mask physiotherapy in cystic fibrosis, *Arch Dis Child* 61:598, 1986.

64. Oberwaldner B, Evans JC, Zach MS: Forced expirations against a variable resistance: a new chest physiotherapy method in cystic fibrosis, *Pediatr Pulmonol* 2:358, 1986.

65. Van Asperen PP, et al: Comparison of a positive expiratory pressure (PEP) mask with postural drainage in patients with cystic fibrosis, *Aust Paediatr J* 23:283, 1987.

66. Falk M, Andersen JB: Positive expiratory pressure (PEP) mask. In Pryor JA, editor: *International perspectives in physical therapy*, vol 7, Edinburgh, 1991, Churchill Livingstone, pp 51–63.

67. Oberwaldner B, et al: Chest physiotherapy in hospitalized patients with cystic fibrosis: a study of lung function effects and sputum production, *Eur Respir J* 4:152, 1991.

68. Mortensen J, et al: The effects of postural drainage and positive expiratory pressure physiotherapy on tracheobronchial clearance in cystic fibrosis, *Chest* 100:1350, 1991.

69. Lindemann H, et al: Autogenic drainage: efficacy of a simplified method, *Acta Univ Carol* 36:210, 1990.

70. Warwick WJ, Hansen LG: The long-term efficacy of high-frequency chest compression on pulmonary complications of cystic fibrosis, *Pediatr Pulmonol* 11:265, 1991.

71. Warwick WJ: High frequency chest compression moves mucus by means of sustained staccato coughs [abstract], *Pediatr Pulmonol* 6(suppl):283, 1991.

72. Plioplys AV: Correspondence on "safety, tolerability, and efficacy of high-frequency chest wall oscillation in pediatric patients with cerebral palsy and neuromuscular diseases: an exploratory randomized controlled trial." *J Child Neurol* 25(12):1598, 1991, author reply 1598. doi: 10.1177/0883073810384614.

73. Lannefors L, Wollmer P: Mucus clearance with three chest physiotherapy regimes in cystic fibrosis: a comparison between postural drainage, PEP, and physical exercise, *Eur Respir J* 5:748, 1992.

74. Zach M, et al: Cystic fibrosis: physical exercise versus chest physiotherapy, *Arch Dis Child* 57:587, 1982.

75. Andreasson B, et al: Long-term effects of physical exercise on working capacity and pulmonary function in cystic fibrosis, *Acta Paediatr Scand* 76:70, 1987.

76. Bartlett RH, et al: Physiology of yawning and its application to postoperative care, *Surg Forum* 21:223, 1970.

77. Bartlett RH: Incentive spirometry. In Kacmarek R, Stoller J, editors: *Current respiratory care: techniques and therapy,* St. Louis, 1988, Mosby.

78. Bartlett RH: Post-traumatic pulmonary insufficiency. In Cooper P, Nyhus L, editors: *Surgery annual,* New York, 1971, Appleton-Century-Crofts.

79. Ali J, et al: Consequences of postoperative alterations in respiratory mechanics, *Am J Surg* 128:376, 1974.

80. Meyers JR, et al: Changes in residual capacity of the lung after operation, *Arch Surg* 110:567, 1975.

81. McDonnell T, McNicholas WT, Fitzgerald MX: Hypoxaemia during chest physiotherapy in patients with cystic fibrosis, *Ir J Med Sci* 155:345, 1986.

82. Gormezano J, Branthwaite MA: Pulmonary physiotherapy with assisted ventilation, *Anaesthesia* 27:249, 1972.

83. Gormezano J, Branthwaite MA: Effects of physiotherapy during intermittent positive pressure ventilation, *Anaesthesia* 27:258, 1972.

84. Huseby J, et al: Oxygenation during chest physiotherapy [abstract], *Chest* 70:430, 1976.

85. Tyler ML, et al: Prediction of oxygenation during chest physiotherapy in critically ill patients [abstract], *Am Rev Respir Dis* 121:218, 1980.

86. Dhainaut JF, Bons J, Bricard C: Improved oxygenation in patients with extensive unilateral pneumonia using the lateral decubitus position, *Thorax* 35:792, 1980.

87. Emolina C, et al: Positional hypoxemia in unilateral lung disease, *N Engl J Med* 304:523, 1981.

88. Rivara: Positional hypoxemia during artificial ventilation, *Crit Care Med* 12:436, 1984.

89. Heaf DP, et al: Postural effects on gas exchange in infants, *N Engl J Med* 308:1505, 1983.

90. Holody B, Goldberg HS: The effect of mechanical vibration physiotherapy on arterial oxygenation in acutely ill patients with atelectasis or pneumonia, *Am Rev Respir Dis* 124:372, 1981.

91. Mohsenifar Z, et al: Mechanical vibration and conventional chest physiotherapy in outpatients with stable chronic obstructive lung disease, *Chest* 87:463, 1985.

92. Weissman C, et al: Effect of routine intensive care interactions on metabolic rate, *Chest* 86:815, 1984.

93. Weissman C, Kemper M: The oxygen uptake–oxygen delivery relationship during ICU interventions, *Chest* 99:430, 1991.

94. Vandenplas Y, et al: Esophageal pH monitoring data during chest physiotherapy, *J Pediatr Gastroenterol Nutr* 13:23, 1991.

95. Orenstein SR, Orenstein DM: Gastroesophageal reflux and respiratory disease in children, *J Pediatr* 112:847, 1988.

96. Kosloske: Tracheobronchial foreign bodies in children: back to the bronchoscope and a balloon, *Pediatrics* 66:321, 1980.

97. Emery JR, Peabody JL: Head position affects intracranial pressure in newborn infants, *J Pediatr* 103:950, 1983.

98. Ersson U, et al: Observations on intracranial dynamics during respiratory physiotherapy in unconscious neurosurgical patients, *Acta Anaesth Scand* 343:99, 1990.

99. Purohit DM, Caldwell C, Levkoff AH: Multiple rib fractures due to physiotherapy in a neonate with hyaline membrane disease, *Am J Dis Child* 129:1103, 1975.

100. Asher MI, et al: Effects of chest physical therapy on lung function in children recovering from acute severe asthma, *Pediatr Pulmonol* 9:146, 1990.

101. Campbell AH, O'Connell JM, Wilson F: The effects of chest physiotherapy upon the FEV_1 in chronic bronchitis, *Med J Aust* 1:33, 1975.

102. Wollmer P, et al: Inefficiency of chest percussion in the physical therapy of chronic bronchitis, *Eur J Respir Dis* 66:233, 1985.

103. Webb MSC, et al: Chest physiotherapy in acute bronchiolitis, *Arch Dis Child* 60:1078, 1985.

104. Quittell LM, et al: The effectiveness of chest physical therapy (CPT) in infants with bronchiolitis [abstract], *Am Rev Respir Dis* 137:406, 1988.

105. Graham WGB, Bradley DA: Efficacy of chest physiotherapy and intermittent positive-pressure breathing in the resolution of pneumonia, *N Engl J Med* 299:624, 1978.

106. Britton S, Bejstedt M, Vedin L: Chest physiotherapy in primary pneumonia, *BMJ* 290:1703, 1985.

107. Reines HD, et al: Chest physiotherapy fails to prevent postoperative atelectasis in children after cardiac surgery, *Ann Surg* 195:451, 1982.

108. Finer NN, et al: Postextubation atelectasis: a retrospective review and a prospective controlled study, *J Pediatr* 94:110, 1979.

109. Stiller K, et al: Acute lobar atelectasis: a comparison of two chest physiotherapy regimens, *Chest* 98:1336, 1990.

110. Currie DC, et al: Practice, problems and compliance with postural drainage: a survey of chronic sputum producers, *Br J Dis Chest* 80:249, 1986.

111. Hammon W, Martin RJ: Chest physiotherapy for acute atelectasis, *Phys Ther* 61:217, 1981.

112. MacKenzie CF, Shing B, McAslun TC: Chest physiotherapy: the effect on arterial oxygenation, *Anesth Analg* 57:28, 1978.

113. Connors AF, et al: Chest physical therapy: the immediate effect on oxygenation in acutely ill patients, *Chest* 79:559, 1980.

114. McMichan JC, Michel L, Westbrook PR: Pulmonary dysfunction following traumatic quadriplegia, *JAMA* 243:528, 1980.

115. Kosloske, et al: Drainage of pediatric lung abscess by cough, catheter, or complete resection, *J Pediatr Surg* 21:596, 1986.

116. Lewis R: Chest physical therapy in pediatrics: a national survey [abstract], *Respir Care* 36:1307, 1991.

117. American Association for Respiratory Care: Clinical practice guideline: postural drainage therapy, *Respir Care* 36:1418, 1991.

118. Holma B, Hegg PO: pH- and protein-dependent buffer capacity and viscosity of respiratory mucus: their interrelationships and influence on health, *Sci Total Environ* 84:71, 1989.

119. Zelenina M, et al: Nickel and extracellular acidification inhibit the water permeability of human aquaporin-3 in lung epithelial cells, *J Biol Chem* 278:30037, 2003.

120. Bartlett RH, Gazzaniga AB, Geraghty TR: Respiratory maneuvers to prevent postoperative pulmonary complications: a critical review, *JAMA* 224:1017, 1973.

121. Bakow ED: Sustained maximal inspiration: a rationale for its use, *Respir Care* 22:379, 1977.

122. American Association for Respiratory Care: Clinical practice guideline: incentive spirometry, *Respir Care* 36:1402, 1991.

123. Harken DE: A review of the activities of the thoracic center for the III and IV hospital groups, 160th general hospital European theater of operations, June 10, 1944. to Jan 1, 1945, *J Thoracic Cardiovasc Surg* 15:31, 1946.

124. Iverson LIG, et al: A comparative study of IPPB, the incentive spirometer and blow bottles: the prevention of atelectasis following cardiac surgery, *Ann Thoracic Surg* 35:197, 1978.

125. O'Donohue WJ: National survey of the usage of lung expansion modalities for the prevention and treatment of postoperative atelectasis following abdominal and thoracic surgery, *Chest* 87:76, 1985.

126. Oikkonen M, et al: Comparison of incentive spirometry and intermittent positive pressure breathing after coronary artery bypass graft, *Chest* 99:60, 1991.

127. Stock MC, et al: Prevention of postoperative pulmonary complications with CPAP, incentive spirometry, and conservative therapy, *Chest* 87:151, 1985.

128. Stock MC, et al: Comparison of continuous positive airway pressure, incentive spirometry, and conservative therapy after cardiac operations, *Crit Care Med* 12:969, 1984.

129. Celli BR, Rodriguez KS, Snider GL: A controlled trial of intermittent positive pressure breathing, incentive spirometry, and deep breathing exercises in preventing pulmonary complications after abdominal surgery, *Am Rev Respir Dis* 130:12, 1984.

130. Craven JL, et al: The evaluation of incentive spirometry in the management of postoperative pulmonary complications, *Br J Surg* 61:793, 1974.

131. Bartlett RH: Respiratory therapy to prevent pulmonary complications of surgery, *Respir Care* 29:667, 1984.

132. Scuderi J, Olsen GN: Respiratory therapy in the management of postoperative complications, *Respir Care* 34:281, 1989.

133. Bartlett RH, et al: Studies on the pathogenesis and prevention of postoperative pulmonary complications, *Surg Gynecol Obstet* 137:925, 1973.

134. Mang H, Obermayer A: Imposed work of breathing during sustained maximal inspiration: comparison of six incentive spirometers, *Respir Care* 34:1122, 1989.

135. Lederer DH, Van de Water JM, Indech RB: Which deep breathing device should the postoperative patient use? *Chest* 77:610, 1980.

136. Centers for Disease Control and Prevention: Update: universal precautions for prevention of transmission of human immunodeficiency virus, hepatitis B virus, and other bloodborne pathogens in health care settings, *MMWR Morb Mortal Wkly Rep* 37:377, 1988.

137. Schwieger, et al: Absence of benefit of incentive spirometry in low-risk patients undergoing elective cholecystectomy, *Chest* 89:652, 1986.

138. Davies BL, Macleod JP, Ogilvie HM: The efficacy of incentive spirometers in postoperative protocols for low-risk patients, *Can J Nurs Res* 22:19, 1990.

139. Gale GD, Sanders DE: Incentive spirometry: its value after cardiac surgery, *Can Anaesth Soc J* 27:475, 1980.

140. Jung R, et al: Comparison of three methods of respiratory care following upper abdominal surgery, *Chest* 78:31, 1980.

141. Gooding JM, et al: Is incentive spirometry valuable as an addition to traditional respiratory maneuvers? [abstract], *Respir Care* 22:414, 1977.

142. Krastins, et al: An evaluation of incentive spirometry in the management of pulmonary complications after cardiac surgery in the pediatric population, *Crit Care Med* 10:525, 1982.

143. American Association for Respiratory Care: Clinical practice guideline: intermittent positive pressure breathing, *Respir Care* 48:540, 2003.

144. Motley HL, et al: Use of intermittent positive pressure breathing combined with nebulization in pulmonary disease, *Am J Med* 5:853, 1948.

145. Eubank DH, Bone RC: Intermittent positive pressure breathing. In Eubank DH, Bone RC, editors: *Comprehensive respiratory care: a learning system module,* St. Louis, 1985, Mosby, pp 430–450.

146. Chang N, Levison H: The effect of nebulized bronchodilator administration with or without IPPB on ventilatory function in children with cystic fibrosis and asthma, *Am Rev Respir Dis* 106:867, 1972.

147. Baker JP: Magnitude of usage of intermittent positive pressure breathing, *Am Rev Respir Dis* 110:S170, 1974.

148. Handelsman H: Agency for Health Care Policy and Research. *Health technology reports: intermittent positive pressure breathing (IPPB) therapy,* AHCPR Pub. No. 92-0013. Rockville, Md, 1991, Office of Health Technology, U.S. Department of Health and Human Services, Public Health Service.

149. Burgess WR, Chernick V: Humidity and aerosol therapy. In Burger WR, Chernick V, editors: *Respiratory therapy in newborn infants and children,* New York, 1982, Thieme-Stratton, pp 74–84.

150. Jasper AC, et al: Cost–benefit comparison of aerosol bronchodilator delivery methods in hospitalized patients, *Chest* 91:614, 1987.

151. Summer W, et al: Aerosol bronchodilator delivery methods: relative impact on pulmonary function and cost of respiratory care, *Arch Intern Med* 149:618, 1989.

152. American Association for Respiratory Care Clinical practice guideline: selection of a device for delivery of aerosol to the lung parenchyma, *Respir Care* 41:647, 1996.

153. Bierman CW: Pneumomediastinum and pneumothorax complicating asthma in children, *Am J Dis Child* 114:43, 1967.

154. Moore RB, Cotton EK, Dinnery MA: The effect of IPPB on airway resistance in normal and asthmatic children, *J Allergy Clin Immunol* 49:137, 1972.

155. McPherson SP: *Respiratory therapy equipment,* ed 7, St. Louis, 2004, Mosby.

156. Chatburn RL: High-frequency assisted airway clearance, *Respir Care* 52(9):1224–1235; discussion 1235–1237, 2007.

157. American Association for Respiratory Care: AARC clinical practice guideline. Postural drainage therapy, *Respir Care* 36(12):1418–1426, 1991.

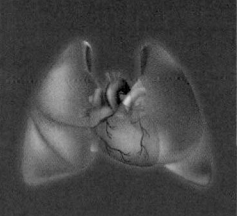

Chapter 13

Airway Management

AMY BRENSKI, PAUL SHEERAN

OUTLINE

LEARNING OBJECTIVES

After reading this chapter the reader will be able to:
1. Identify four general indications for intubation
2. Explain how to perform orotracheal intubation
3. Explain how to perform nasotracheal intubation
4. Select the correctly sized endotracheal tube for patients of different ages
5. Describe the complications of intubation
6. Explain the criteria for extubation
7. Appraise the reasons for failed extubation and treatment strategies
8. List the indications for tracheotomy
9. Describe the major complications of tracheotomy
10. List the criteria for decannulation
11. Describe the setup and list the equipment needed for tracheostomy tube changes

KEY TERMS

Tracheotomy   Suctioning

Recognizing the child who is in respiratory distress or failure is an integral step in caring for the critically ill child. Ensuring adequate oxygenation, ventilation, and airway protection is a major goal in managing any ill child. Bag-mask ventilation ensures adequate oxygenation and ventilation. Endotracheal intubation ensures airway protection and the prevention of aspiration of either gastric contents or oral secretions. Establishment of a secure airway is one of the unique and challenging procedures associated with neonatal and pediatric critical care that has a profound impact on life and death.

INTUBATION

Rapid and unencumbered intubation of the trachea depends on knowledge of upper airway anatomy, the indications for intubation, the appropriate use of airway equipment, and the medications available to facilitate intubation. Before attempting to intubate any patient, the patient's history and physical appearance must be assessed with respect to the patient having a difficult airway. The parent should be asked if the patient was difficult to intubate in the past. Any old anesthesia records should be reviewed. A history of burn injury or radiation to the head or neck makes airway manipulation difficult. The presence of a small jaw, limited mouth opening, decreased neck extension, or a space-occupying lesion of the mouth makes intubation more difficult. If airway manipulation is expected to be difficult, airway techniques other than direct laryngoscopy may be needed (see Approaches to the Difficult Airway later in this chapter).

Indications

The specific indications for endotracheal intubation are numerous; however, all can be placed in one of four broad categories, which can be defined by the four "Ps":

1. Pulmonary function
2. Provide an airway
3. Protect the airway
4. Pulmonary hygiene

The need for intubation because of a lack of pulmonary function results from deficits in oxygenation, ventilation, or both, taken in concert with the patient's clinical condition. Acute ventilatory dysfunction can be defined as an arterial partial pressure of carbon dioxide ($PaCO_2$) greater than 50 to 60 mm Hg with a pH less than 7.3. Pulmonary dysfunction as a result of hypoxemia is defined as an arterial partial pressure of oxygen (PaO_2) less than 60 mm Hg with a fraction of inspired oxygen (FiO_2) greater than or equal to 0.60. These definitions assume that there is no intracardiac right to left shunt resulting from a congenital cardiac defect.

It is difficult to reliably administer an FiO_2 greater than 0.8 using traditional devices for the administration of supplemental oxygen. Therefore, a patient with decreasing oxygen saturation who is unresponsive to increases in oxygen concentration is a candidate for an escalation of care that may include both noninvasive and invasive methods of providing support, such as noninvasive positive pressure or intubation and mechanical ventilation.

Respiratory failure in children is most commonly caused by pneumonia or bronchiolitis. Upper airway obstruction may also cause respiratory failure. Examples that are included in this category are diseases such as laryngotracheobronchitis (i.e., croup), epiglottitis, laryngeal papillomatosis, and severe subglottic stenosis. Intubation is necessary in patients who have loss of airway reflexes and in patients with weakness. Loss of airway reflexes occurs in patients with head injury and drug overdose. Weakness occurs in patients with such diseases as botulism and Guillain-Barré syndrome. Patients who have penetrating or crush injury to the midface, tongue, both mandibles, or the neck may need to be intubated for airway protection. Paralysis of these patients must be avoided because of the presence of acquired anatomical abnormalities. Intubation of these patients is most safely performed in the operating room by a surgeon and anesthesiologist in attendance. And finally, patients who have infection of the anterior neck (Ludwig's angina) or hematoma of the neck (as may occur in patients with bleeding disorders) have airway deviation and should be intubated in the operating room.

Equipment

Anticipating and preparing for intubation by collecting the proper equipment are essential components of a successful endotracheal intubation. The equipment necessary for intubation is listed in Table 13-1. Using the mnemonic *MSMAID* facilitates preintubation preparation so that essential equipment is not inadvertently omitted.

Endotracheal Tubes

Once a decision has been made to undertake intubation, the appropriate size and type of endotracheal tube (ETT) must be identified. The ETTs most commonly used are sterile, disposable, and made of clear nontoxic plastic or polyvinyl chloride. The tubes have markings placed longitudinally 1 cm apart and can be used as reference points for proper placement once endotracheal intubation is accomplished (Figure 13-1). The distal end of the ETT may contain a side hole, a Murphy eye, to prevent complete

TABLE 13-1	
Essential Equipment for Intubation	
Mnemonic	**Equipment**
Monitors	ECG, pulse oximeter, BP, end-tidal CO_2 detector, stethoscope
Suction	Yankauer suction catheter, ETT suction catheters
Machine	Oxygen source, functioning bag and mask
Airway	Masks, oral airways, nasal trumpets, endotracheal tubes, appropriate stylet, laryngoscopes (handles, curved and straight blades, bulbs, batteries), McGill forceps, tape, benzoin
Intravenous	One patent intravenous line
Drugs	Anesthetic and resuscitative agents

BP, Blood pressure; *ECG,* electrocardiogram.

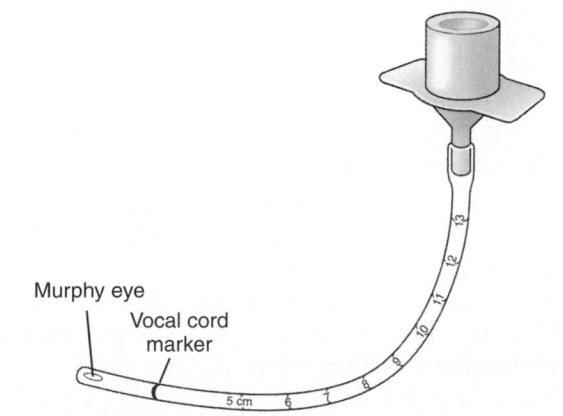

Murphy eye
Vocal cord marker
5 cm

FIGURE 13-1 Endotracheal tube with distance markings.

obstruction of the ETT if mucoid secretions occlude the distal end of the endotracheal tube. The Microcuff endotracheal tubes are cuffed endotracheal tubes that have a small, very thin cuff that sits well below the vocal cords when it is positioned properly. The Microcuff endotracheal tubes do not have a Murphy eye. The appropriate ETT size is determined by the patient's age and size. The appropriate ETT for any child 1 year of age or older may be determined by the following formula.[1]

$$\text{Internal diameter (mm)} = (\text{age [yr]} \div 4) + 4$$

Using this formula, a 4-year-old would need a 5.0-mm ETT, an 8-year-old child would need a 6.0-mm ETT, and so on.

Accurate selection of an ETT takes into consideration the child's weight (Table 13-2), size, and length.[2-4] Comparing the size of the pinky of the patient with the size of the ETT is a method that can be used to approximate the appropriate size ETT for a child. ETT one-half size smaller and one-half size larger than the estimated or calculated size should always be available. The appropriate adult endotracheal tube size for an adult female is 7 mm and for an adult male is 8 mm.

Cuffed and Uncuffed Tubes

Because the cricoid cartilage is the narrowest portion of the pediatric airway until about 8 years of age, use of an uncuffed ETT was traditionally recommended until that time. In 2005 the American Heart Association's Pediatric Advance Life Support program (PALS) stopped recommending uncuffed tubes because there was no evidence to support one over the other. Today it is left up to the clinician to determine whether a cuff is needed for patients less

than 8 years of age. As a child grows, the airway becomes more adultlike and tubular, with the vocal cords, not the subglottic space, becoming the smallest cross-sectional area of the airway.[5] A cuffed ETT helps create a seal to occlude unwanted air leaks during positive-pressure ventilation. The cuff also reduces the likelihood of pulmonary aspiration, although this not guaranteed simply by placing a cuffed ETT. However, with the advent of low-profile cuffs in smaller endotracheal tubes (as low as 3.0 mm), more anesthesiologists at children's hospitals are using low-profile cuffs in the operating room in small children and infants. The deflated cuff on the distal end of the ETT increases the outer diameter of the tube by approximately 0.5 mm when compared with uncuffed tubes. To compensate for the increased diameter of the cuff on the ETT, a smaller tube, 0.5 to 1 mm, is inserted when the cuff is present.

Laryngoscope Blades and Handles

The laryngoscope is the instrument used to expose the glottic opening during intubation. It consists of two parts: a handle and a blade. The handle is available in two sizes: large and small. The handle also contains batteries that power a light source incorporated into the blade. The large handle is recommended for an adult, but it may also be suitable for an infant, child, or adolescent depending on operator preference and patient characteristics. Because of its size and ease of manipulation, the small handle should be used for a premature infant or newborn. Before commencing the process of intubation, the blade and handle should be tested to ensure that they fit together properly and lock in place. The lightbulb should be functional and screwed in place securely.

Many types of laryngoscope blades are available. The Miller blade is a straight blade that is available in multiple sizes. The Philips blade comes in sizes 1 and 2 and is a straight blade that has the advantages of being wider than the Miller blade and having a small curve at its tip. The Philips blade is especially useful in children who have laryngomalacia because the floppy epiglottis can be lifted out of the way. The Macintosh blades are curved and wide. The Macintosh 2 blade can be used in children approximately 17 kg. The Macintosh 3 blade can be used in patients who weigh more than 25 kg. Each blade requires a different technique for exposing the glottis. When a straight blade is used, the epiglottis may be lifted with the tip of the blade and pressed against the base of the tongue (Figure 13-2). In contrast, the tip of the curved blade is placed in the vallecula, the space between the epiglottis and the base of the tongue. As the laryngoscope is pulled forward, it elevates the epiglottis and exposes the glottis (Figure 13-3).[6] Multiple blade types and sizes should be immediately available during any intubation procedure.

Laryngeal Mask Airway

The laryngeal mask airway (LMA; Figure 13-4)[7] is a useful alternative to a bag-mask apparatus. If endotracheal tube

TABLE 13-2	
Neonatal Resuscitation Program Guidelines for Pediatric Endotracheal Tube Size	
Child's Age	Internal Diameter (mm)
Premature	
Less than1000 g	2.5
1000-2000 g	3.0
2000-3000 g	3.5
Normal newborns	
3000-4000 g	3.5-4.0
Infants and children younger than 12 years	
6-12 mo	4.0-4.5
1-2 years	4.5
4 years	5.0
6 years	5.5
8 years	6.0
10 years	6.5
Children 12 years of age and older	
Female	7.0-8.5
Male	8.0-10.0

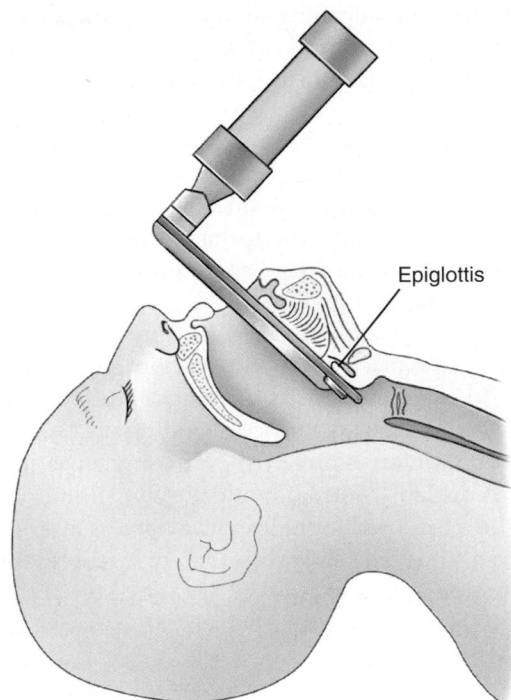

FIGURE 13-2 Direct laryngoscopy using a straight (Miller) blade.

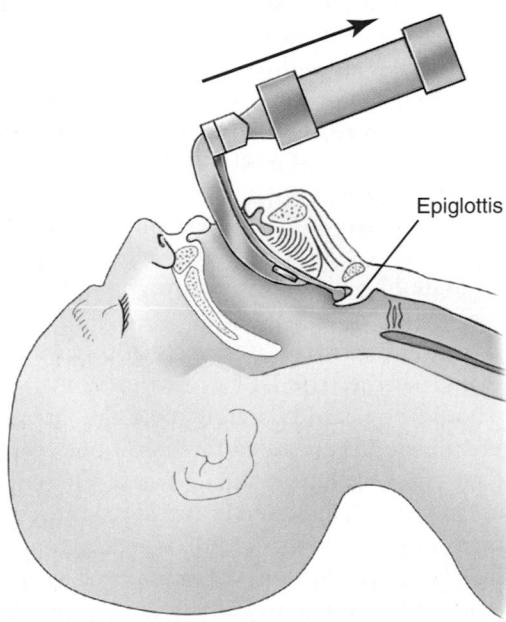

FIGURE 13-3 Direct laryngoscopy using a curved (MacIntosh) blade and demonstrating proper lifting technique. Note the upward and forward lift while the wrist is held straight.

placement is unsuccessful, placement of an LMA can be used as a temporizing measure. It is essential to realize that the LMA does not provide a secure airway and that it may permit aspiration of gastric or oral secretions.

The lubricated LMA is placed by itself into the pharynx above the epiglottis and can be used for gentle (<20 cm H_2O)

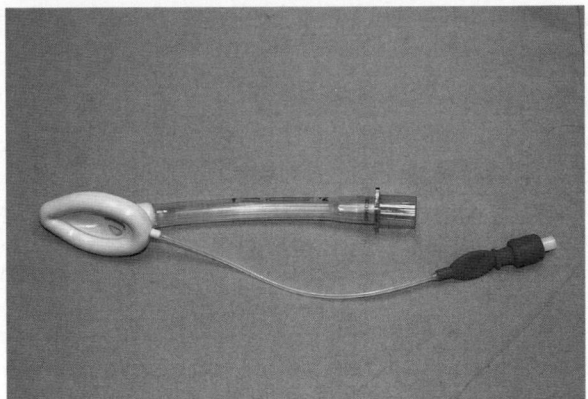

FIGURE 13-4 A laryngeal mask airway (LMA).

TABLE 13-3	
Suggested Laryngeal Mask Airway Size Based on Weight	
Size	Weight (kg)
0.5	Infants up to 2.5
1	2.5-5
1.5	5-10
2	10-20
2.5	20-30
3	30-50
4	>50

positive-pressure ventilation. The deflated mask is manually inserted into the patient's mouth and guided blindly along the hard palate. It is advanced until resistance is encountered. (The distal tip of the LMA rests against the upper esophageal sphincter at this point.) The balloon is inflated to form a seal in the pharynx (the volume air to inflate in the balloon is stated on the outside of the LMA package). The LMAs come in different sizes, including 1, 1.5, 2, 2.5, 3, and 4. Every emergency airway cart should have all sizes of LMAs available (Table 13-3).

Suction Equipment

Suctioning of the mouth and posterior pharynx before direct laryngoscopy facilitates viewing of the vocal cords if secretions are present. Suctioning of the endotracheal tube once placed clears the lower airway of secretions. Suction equipment should include a tonsil-tip suction catheter (e.g., Yankauer) and several standard sterile suction catheters.

INTUBATION PROCEDURE

The indication for endotracheal intubation will determine the most appropriate technique to use during the process of providing an airway for the patient. The options available to the clinician are orotracheal intubation, nasal intubation, or awake intubation. Universal precautions (i.e., the use of gloves, a mask, and eye protection) should be observed with all intubation procedures to reduce the risk of transmitting infectious diseases.

Orotracheal Intubation

The height of the patient's bed should be such that the patient's head is level with the laryngoscopist's xiphoid process. This will allow direct visualization of the airway without putting undue physical stress or strain on the clinician. The occiput of babies and infants is larger than that of older children. A small roll placed under the shoulders of these younger patients facilitates viewing of the vocal cords during laryngoscopy. Direct laryngoscopy may be facilitated by placing a roll under the shoulders of any patient lying on a soft mattress.

If the patient is breathing spontaneously, the application of 100% oxygen for 5 minutes with a bag and mask with 5 cm H_2O of PEEP is sufficient to fully oxygenate the lungs in the absence of lung disease. An amnestic agent, an analgesic agent, and a neuromuscular blocker are then administered to facilitate intubation. The use of external cricoid pressure by an assistant is controversial.[8] Properly held pressure over the cricoid pressure may or may not occlude the esophagus[9] and may or may not prevent the aspiration of gastric contents. Improperly held cricoid pressure may lead to distortion of the larynx and so make visualization of the larynx more difficult.

If the patient has been adequately preoxygenated, then bag-mask ventilations should be avoided for the 45 to 60 seconds that are needed for the neuromuscular blocker to provide muscle relaxation. Positive-pressure ventilation at this point may lead to insufflations of the stomach, which in turn lead to regurgitation and aspiration. Cricoid pressure is not needed if the patient does not receive bag-mask ventilations while he or she is paralyzed. The mouth and oropharynx are suctioned as needed. Laryngoscopy is then performed.

Figure 13-5 illustrates the glottic structures as viewed through the laryngoscope. After visualizing the glottic opening, the appropriate-sized ETT is held in the right hand and is introduced into the right side of the patient's mouth to avoid obstructing the view of the glottic opening while placing the ETT. The tip of the ETT is advanced

through the glottic opening so that the single black ring is just distal to the opening of the glottis. If the ETT is marked with three rings, the ETT should be inserted until the double black ring is distal to the glottic opening. When inserting a cuffed ETT, the tube is advanced until the cuff is distal to the vocal cords. Any single attempt at intubation should not exceed 30 seconds. In the event that intubation cannot be readily performed, the patient's airway should be reestablished by bag-and-mask ventilation to ensure adequate oxygenation.

The presence of vapor in the ETT is not an accurate test for proper ETT placement. Proper endotracheal, and not esophageal, placement of the endotracheal tube is confirmed with sustained presence of end-tidal CO_2. Capnography via a monitor is preferred over a single-use end-tidal device (Pedi-Cap; Nellcor, Boulder, CO). End-tidal CO_2 should be monitored for at least five breaths after intubation. Even endotracheal tubes placed in the esophagus may have transient detection of CO_2 as a result of the presence of CO_2 in the stomach (which can occur because of bag-mask ventilations).

The proper ETT position is in the midtrachea—that is, below the clavicle and 1 to 2 cm above the carina. The proper depth of the endotracheal tube can be estimated based on the size of the endotracheal tube used. Multiply the internal diameter of the endotracheal tube by 3 and tape the ETT at that centimeter mark at the lip (e.g., a 4.0-mm ETT should be taped at 12 cm at the lip). The proper length of the endotracheal tube can be estimated in premature infants according to their weight: add 6 to their weight in kg (e.g., in a 1- kg baby the ETT should be taped at 7). This formula cannot be used in children greater than 3 kg. Confirmation of the proper position of the endotracheal tube should be confirmed with X-ray. Endotracheal tube depth formulas may not be accurate in patients with micrognathia or midface hypoplasia.

The chest is auscultated after intubation as a method for assessing whether the ETT is in the trachea. Breath sounds should be heard bilaterally over the lateral chest wall. If breath sounds are auscultated over both the stomach and the chest wall, then the ETT is in the esophagus and should be pulled. It should be noted that auscultation is not the most accurate method of assessing proper ETT placement. The most accurate assessment of whether the ETT has passed into the trachea is direct visualization. Because direct visualization is not always reliable as a result of the presence of secretions or airway swelling, obtaining carbon dioxide via the use of a disposable end-tidal carbon dioxide (ETCO_2) detector or by capnography is essential.

The ETT is secured by preparing the skin with benzoin. Two strips of tape are cut long enough to reach from the lateral aspect of the right eye to the lateral aspect of the left eye. Each piece is split into a Y shape with the arms of the Y two thirds the length of the tape. The tape should have a width that will easily fit on the upper

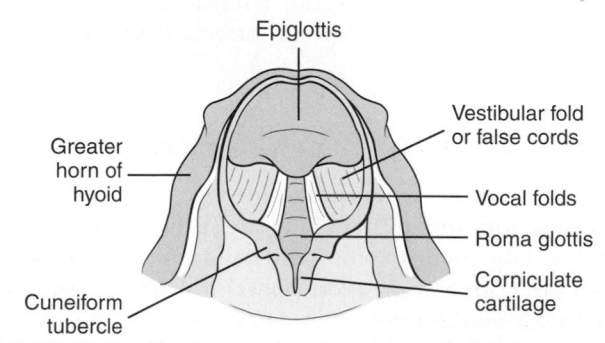

FIGURE 13-5 Glottic structures viewed through the laryngoscope.

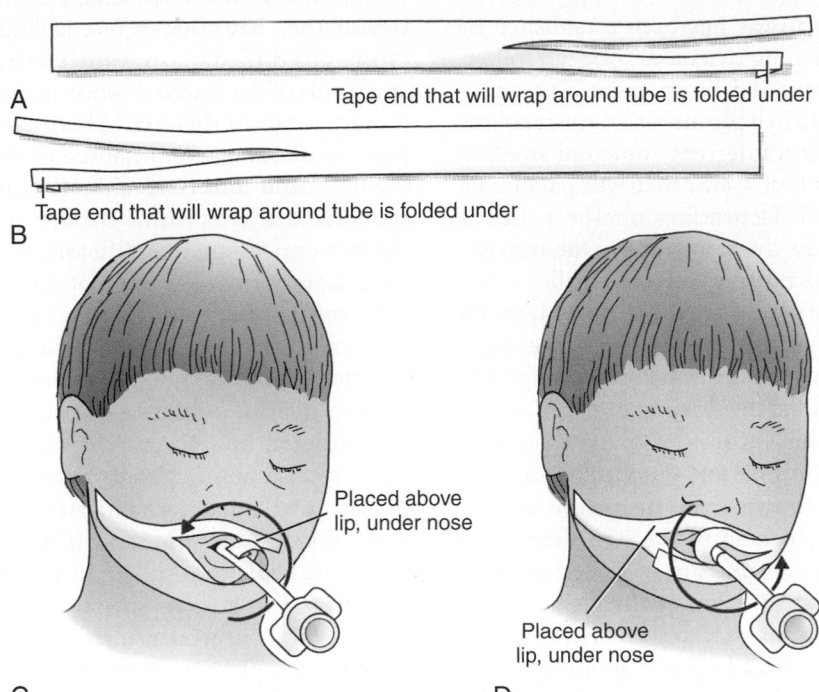

A Tape end that will wrap around tube is folded under

B Tape end that will wrap around tube is folded under

Placed above
lip, under nose

Placed above
lip, under nose

C   D

FIGURE 13-6   Steps used to secure an endotracheal tube (ETT) with tape. **Steps A and B,** Slit two pieces of tape, making a Y on one end of each piece (as shown). Turn under the end of the tape that will be wrapped around the ETT. This will make tape removal easier. **Step C,** Apply benzoin to the area below the nose and across the cheeks (where tape will be placed). Attach one piece of tape to the cheek and below the nose, wrapping the bottom of the Y around the ETT. The tape should be placed under the tube (chin side) first, and then wrapped around the top of the tube. **Step D,** Repeat step C on the other side of the face.

Box 13-1	Equipment for Endotracheal Tube Stabilization

- Alcohol
- Tincture of benzoin
- Scissors
- Adhesive tape
- Two precut Y-shaped pieces

lip and around the ETT. One end of the tape is secured to the cheek and wrapped around the tube in "barber pole" fashion (Figure 13-6). The necessary equipment (Box 13-1) for securing the ETT is assembled before attempting intubation. Other taping methods may be used to secure the ETT, as long as the method can be performed by all personnel involved in airway care and is fast and secure. The centimeter mark at which the ETT is secured must be recorded to allow assessment of proper position at a later time if needed.

Various devices are available to secure the ETT as an alternative to using tape. Figure 13-7 illustrates an example of one of these devices. When selecting a device to secure the tube, it is important that it does not occlude access to the mouth, provides minimal tube movement when the head moves, and secures without creating ulcers at pressure points. In addition, the same rules apply as with taping

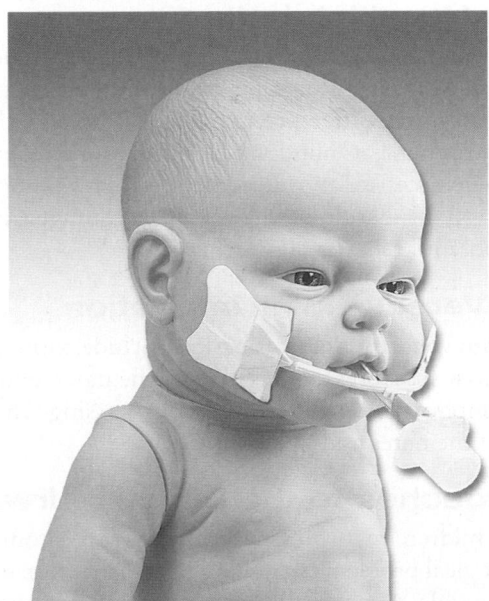

FIGURE 13-7   The NeoBar. A commercial adaptation of the Logan bow for stabilizing an infant endotracheal tube.

methods: fast, easy, and can be applied by all personnel. Evidence that these devices help reduce the incidence of accidental extubations is inconclusive. However, it does suggest that the devices may be more effective on a small infant than on a larger infant or child.[10,11]

Nasotracheal Intubation

Once a patent and stable airway has been established by the orotracheal route, switching to a nasal tube can follow. The patient's nares are prepared by spraying a vasoconstrictive agent, such as phenylephrine or oxymetazoline, into the opening. These drugs decrease mucosal swelling and inflammation. An ETT of a size that will pass easily through the nares is used. Depending on the patient's anatomy, this may either be the same size as the tube selected for orotracheal intubation or 0.5 mm smaller.

The tube is lubricated with either petroleum jelly or 2% lidocaine jelly. The tube is then inserted into the nares until approximately one half of it has passed through the nose. While an assistant holds the existing oral ETT in the left corner of the mouth, the glottis is exposed in the same manner as for orotracheal intubation. Once the nasal tube is visualized in the hypopharynx, the tip of the tube is grabbed with McGill forceps held in the right hand and the nasal tube is lifted up and in front of the opening to the larynx. When direct visualization of the glottic opening is ensured, the assistant is asked to remove the orotracheal tube while the nasotracheal tube is simultaneously advanced into the trachea. The centimeter mark at the nares is noted and the ETT is taped securely in place. The major contraindications to nasotracheal intubation are a bleeding diathesis, such as thrombocytopenia, abnormal clotting times, facial trauma, suspected basilar skull fracture, and abnormal anatomy such as choanal atresia.

Blind Nasal Intubation

The larynx of an infant or small child is anterior and cephalad, making intubation more difficult in general. This anatomical difference between adults and children makes attempts at blind nasal intubation almost uniformly unsuccessful. Wisdom dictates that attempts at a blind nasal intubation be vigorously discouraged, because of the potential for damaging the airway.

Oral Versus Nasal Intubation

Disadvantages to nasal intubation include a predisposition to sinusitis, pressure necrosis of the nares, and bleeding complications associated with passing the ETT through the nares and upper airway.

Approaches to the Difficult Airway

Some children may present challenging anatomical or physiological problems that may make intubation difficult or impossible. Congenital causes of a difficult airway include the presence of micrognathia, retrognathia, midface hypoplasia, limited mouth opening, space-occupying lesion of the mouth, and limited cervical spine mobility (e.g., as a result of Klippel-Feil syndrome). Patients with a mucopolysaccharidosis (Hunter's syndrome or Hurler's syndrome) may have several sites of airway obstruction and be extremely difficult to intubate. Children with craniofacial syndromes (e.g., Treacher Collins syndrome or Pierre Robin syndrome) are assumed to have a difficult airway, even if they have undergone jaw advancement. Acquired causes of a difficult airway include limited mouth opening as a result of decreased temporomandibular joint mobility (as may occur in rheumatoid arthritis or muscular dystrophy), orofacial trauma, trauma to the neck, hematoma of the neck, and infections either of the anterior neck or the epiglottis. Patients with a history of burns or radiation to the face or neck are very difficult to intubate. The clinician should always have additional options available to secure the airway in the event that orotracheal intubation is not successful. An LMA should be readily available during intubation attempts. A fiberoptic laryngoscope greatly facilitates intubation of patients with a difficult airway.[12] It is best to learn how to use the fiberoptic laryngoscope on patients with a normal airway before using this device on patients with an abnormal airway. This is true for any difficult airway adjunct device. If it is known that a patient will be difficult to intubate, it is best not to paralyze the patient and to have an anesthesiologist or ear, nose, and throat (ENT) surgeon available to assist intubation if intubation attempts are unsuccessful. It is essential that no more than three attempts be made at direct laryngoscopy of any patient. A "cannot intubate" scenario can devolve into a "cannot ventilate" (i.e., cannot bag-mask ventilate) scenario if the airway is traumatized by multiple intubation attempts. Flexible fiberoptic intubation, retrograde intubation, and cricothyroidotomy require the advanced airway skills of either an anesthesiologist or ENT surgeon.

Emergency Tracheotomy

In the infant and small child it is preferred to perform a tracheotomy after the airway has been secured. Circumstances in which endotracheal intubation may be difficult or impossible include severe trauma or hemorrhage, craniofacial problems, and the newborn with complete laryngeal obstruction. Alternative approaches to securing the airway are dictated by the urgency of the clinical situation and the age of the patient. These include tracheotomy under local anesthesia, mask ventilation, or cricothyroidotomy.

Epiglottitis

Since the *Haemophilus influenzae* type B (Hib) vaccine was introduced in the United States in 1988, the frequency of epiglottitis has decreased dramatically. Between the years 1987 and 1995, the incidence of Hib disease in children younger than 5 years decreased by 96%.[13] Today epiglottitis is a rare disorder, and experience with its emergency management is declining.

Epiglottitis is a true pediatric emergency. The child with clinical manifestations of epiglottitis (drooling, stridor, and respiratory distress) should not undergo a visual examination in the emergency department. The child should not be stimulated and should be kept as calm as possible. If the patient is stable, a soft-tissue lateral neck

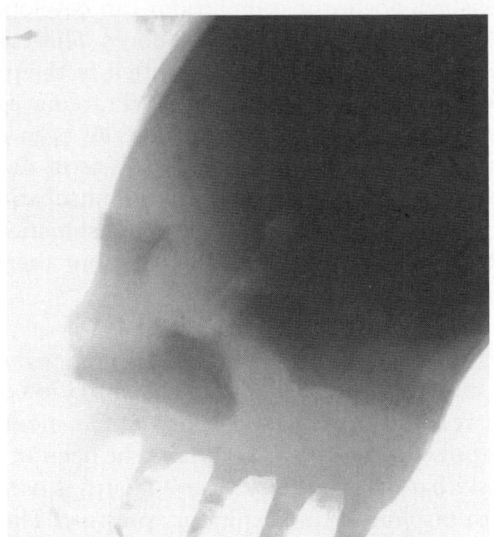

FIGURE 13-8 Lateral soft-tissue neck radiograph revealing epiglottitis.

radiograph (Figure 13-8) can be performed. Radiological findings include thickening of the epiglottis and aryepiglottic folds and the classic "thumbprint" sign. If the patient is not stable or if the diagnosis of epiglottitis has been made, then the patient should be immediately transported to the operating room to be managed by an ENT surgeon and an anesthesiologist.

Laryngotracheal Stenosis

Children with laryngotracheal stenosis who do not have a tracheotomy may require intubation. The severity of the stenosis may dictate the approach used to access the airway. Plain magnified soft-tissue radiographs may show subglottic narrowing or long-segment tracheal stenosis. In cases of mild subglottic stenosis the patient may be intubated orally, but it is essential to start with an endotracheal tube size at least one smaller than the age-appropriate tube and air leakage must be checked. A leak between 10 and 20 cm H_2O during the time of intubation is necessary so that further damage is not incurred. If the air leak is greater than 20 cm H_2O, a smaller tube should be placed. In cases of severe laryngotracheal stenosis, an LMA may be used; occasionally, as an alternative, an emergency tracheotomy may be performed.

Artificial Airway Cuff Management

If a cuffed ETT or tracheostomy is used, the cuff is inflated once proper placement of the artificial airway is ensured. If the patient has a large leak with the cuff deflated, then the cuff is inflated to minimal leak (see the next paragraph). To inflate the cuff, a 5- or 10-ml syringe is attached to the pilot balloon and gradually air is added to the cuff. Positive pressure applied through the ETT should produce an audible escape of air, or leak, at less than or equal to 20 cm H_2O. The larynx should be auscultated to confirm the leak. Intracuff pressures are maintained at less than 20 to 25 cm H_2O because higher pressures are associated with ischemia and necrosis of the tracheal mucosa and can lead to tracheal stenosis. Cuff inflation may cause vocal cord necrosis if the cuff is positioned at the level of the vocal cords as may occur with cuffed endotracheal tubes that are not Microcuff tubes.

Cuff pressures should be checked approximately every 8 hours to guarantee that the pressure does not exceed the recommended levels. If a cuff pressure–measuring device is not available, the minimal leak test can be performed. To inflate the cuff to minimal leak, the cuff is inflated until no air leak is noted during the application of positive pressure. Then a small amount of air is withdrawn from the cuff until a slight leak is auscultated.

If large amounts of air are required in the cuff and a leak persists, one of two possibilities exists: (1) The cuff is damaged or (2) it has not been completely advanced through the cords. The latter problem can be identified by direct laryngoscopy. In patients younger than 8 years, the cricoid cartilage, the narrowest portion of the airway, serves as a functional cuff. Once again, the clinical situation may direct the clinician to use a cuffed or uncuffed ETT, depending on need.

Patient Monitoring

Continuously evaluating the patient undergoing intubation is essential to ensure a safe and effective outcome. Before the airway is manipulated, the heart rate, blood pressure, and oxygen saturation should be monitored and recorded. The patient's heart rate, blood pressure, and oxygen saturation should be monitored continuously. A continuous electrocardiogram monitors the heart for arrhythmias. A single individual should be made responsible for the task of monitoring the patient continuously during the procedure. If, at any time, acceptable values or rhythms are breached, the clinician should be warned and attempts at intubation stopped. The airway should be reestablished using a bag and mask.

Complications

Serious complications from endotracheal intubation may occur at any time during or after the intubation procedure. Immediate complications include hypoxia caused by prolonged intubation attempts, loss of the airway, esophageal intubation, and mainstem intubation in a patient with lung disease. Airway trauma may occur during multiple attempts at intubation. Any patient with suspected perforation or laceration of the pharynx or larynx should be evaluated by an ENT surgeon. Bradycardia may occur during intubation attempts and usually is due to hypoxia. Stimulation of the carina by the endotracheal tube causes reflex bradycardia. Bronchospasm may occur during attempts at intubation. Laryngospasm is rare outside the operating room. Hypotension responds to the administration of crystalloid.

EXTUBATION

The most important question to consider when evaluating a patient for extubation is whether there has been improvement in or reversal of the disease process that initially mandated the intubation. Before extubation, the patient must be hemodynamically stable, must be able to breathe spontaneously with an adequate tidal volume and respiratory pattern, and must have adequate neurological integrity to protect the airway.

Hemodynamic stability is manifested by normal capillary refill, urine output, and blood pressure. The patient should be alert and awake with evidence of adequate muscle strength. In addition, adequate airway protective reflexes include being able to gag, swallow, and cough.

Accidental Extubation

Risk factors associated with accidental extubation include failure to secure the ETT properly, lack of adequate sedation, failure to provide adequate restraint, and the performance of a procedure, such as chest radiography, on a patient.

Equipment

As with the intubation procedure, anticipation and preparation are essential in accomplishing a smooth extubation. The equipment necessary for extubation includes a bag-and-mask setup, suction equipment, adhesive remover, and all the equipment previously listed for intubation (see Table 13-1). This ensures a proactive approach to patient care in the event that the patient does not tolerate extubation and requires reintubation.

Procedure

Pulmonary function is optimized by administering aerosolized β-agonists as needed and suctioning the oropharynx and trachea before extubation. If the patient has been receiving enteral feedings, the feedings are discontinued for at least 6 hours before the planned extubation.

If a cuffed tube is in place, the cuff should be deflated. While the ETT is held in place, the tape is removed from the face and tube with an adhesive remover. One large breath is administered, and the ETT is withdrawn from the trachea near peak inflation. The majority of patients will then cough and begin to breathe spontaneously. It is not unusual, especially in small children, for a short interval of breath holding to occur. Oxygen is administered by the most appropriate delivery device, such as a nasal cannula, face tent, face mask, or oxyhood. The oxygen concentration is titrated to maintain an oxygen saturation level that is clinically indicated.

Complications

Sore throat and hoarseness are common complaints after extubation. The presence of an ETT may cause edema of the laryngeal structures. Once extubation is successfully accomplished, postextubation stridor can develop within minutes and usually peaks within 8 hours. This condition has been well described and occurs often in the pediatric population. Corticosteroids, aerosolized racemic epinephrine, and helium-oxygen mixtures have all been used to treat this complication.[14,15] A meta-analysis of the use of corticosteroids in the prevention of reintubation and postextubation stridor did not show any statistically significant difference in reintubation rates, but there was a significant decrease in stridor.[14]

Nasal Mask Ventilation, Heliox

To ease the transition to spontaneous ventilation or when there is residual upper airway obstruction, noninvasive positive-pressure mask ventilation may be helpful. A nasal face mask that fits over the nose and mouth is used to deliver both inspiratory and expiratory pressure. The BiPAP (bilevel positive airway pressure) system may be a useful method to transition the patient to spontaneous respiration after extubation. In the event that a fixed narrow opening such as in subglottic stenosis is the cause of difficulty, then a helium–oxygen mixture (heliox) may be beneficial. Its lower density may reduce the viscosity of airflow and decrease airway resistance. Mixtures of helium to oxygen are available as 80% helium–20% oxygen and 70% helium–30% oxygen. Additional oxygen can be titrated into these mixtures; however, as the concentration of oxygen increases, the density of the gas decreases, and so does the agent's efficacy. When the upper airway obstruction has resolved, one can then gradually wean the heliox.

Extubation Failure

The best predictor of successful extubation is a successful spontaneous breathing trial.[16] Successful extubation appears to be inversely related to the duration of the intubation period.[16,17] A child who cannot successfully extubate may need to be evaluated for cause of failure and airway obstruction. Checking an air leak before extubation is often done to assess for airway edema but may not predict successful extubation.[18] Use of dexamethasone is often recommended, particularly when no air leak is audible at a pressure of 25 cm of H_2O before extubation, and may have some benefit in children, but the studies are inconclusive.[19,20] Consultation with a pediatric otolaryngologist may be indicated.

Evaluation of stridor may include examination of the airway in the operating room with direct laryngosocopy and bronchoscopy. The most common cause of extubation failure is soft tissue swelling of the larynx and subglottis or more chronic inflammation such as vocal cord granulatomata. Often these can be managed with conservative medical therapy and reintubation with a smaller tube followed by a repeat bronchoscopy. Persistent lesions can be managed with excision or balloon dilation in cases of isolated soft-tissue edema.[21] In some cases, it may be beneficial to perform an awake examination at the bedside before reintubation. This will allow for diagnosis of dynamic airway lesions such as laryngomalacia or vocal cord mobility problems. When injuries or inflammation progresses to a more mature stage, stenosis ensues. In the diagnosis of a lower airway lesion such as subglottic narrowing caused by edema, subglottic cysts, or subglottic stenosis, bronchoscopy is necessary.

The degree of subglottic stenosis is determined by using endotracheal tubes to estimate the size of the larynx. This is performed under general anesthesia at laryngoscopy or can be estimated if the patient is intubated with an uncuffed endotracheal tube. The appropriate size tube for a child of that age will leak at less than 25 cm of H_2O pressure. The Cotton-Myer grading chart estimates percent of airway obstruction. These are subdivided into grades I to IV, where four represents no detectable lumen. The degree of obstruction helps direct therapy and can predict success or failure of different treatment regimens. It also provides a framework to allow clinicians to compare data and outcomes.[22] In the specific case of neonates with isolated subglottic stenosis, anterior cricoids split can be effective at achieving extubation.[23] In cases of airway obstruction caused by subglottic stenosis and other critical airway obstructions, tracheostomy or laryngotracheal reconstruction may be indicated.

TRACHEOTOMY

The child who is not a candidate for extubation or airway reconstruction may require a tracheostomy. The term *tracheotomy* generally describes the actual incision into the trachea. A mature opening in the neck is usually described as a *tracheostomy*. Many names exist for the tube that is placed in the opening, but by general consensus a panel of experts agree on the term *tracheostomy tube*.[24] The decision to perform a tracheostomy is based on the future airway prognosis, as well as on the family's ability to care for an artificial airway at home. Before proceeding with a tracheotomy the risks as well as the significant burden for the family must be considered. Communication with the family and patient when appropriate is important early on in the decision making process. It is essential to provide families and patients with information about tracheostomy tubes, their care, complications as well as any alternatives that may exist to allow for the best decision making. Whenever possible, it is important to assess the family's ability to communicate and comprehend the implications of this life-changing event.[25] They should be given the opportunity to participate in the process whenever time and the patient's health status permits. Because these patients disproportionately have multiple medical problems, using a family-centered approach may have benefits for these patients. [26-28]

Tracheotomy Indications

The main indications for tracheotomy in infants and children are airway obstruction, long-term ventilation, and pulmonary hygiene or other neurological conditions necessitating pulmonary hygiene.[29,30] Children with congenital or acquired upper airway obstruction may require a tracheotomy at an early age if extubation cannot be accomplished. Congenital laryngeal stenosis, which varies in severity, may require a tracheotomy at an early age or even in the delivery room. Because many of these patients require intubation, many cases of presumed acquired subglottic stenosis may in fact be congenital in nature.[31] Nonetheless, laryngeal and subglottic stenosis are more often acquired after intubation and remain a common cause of subglottic stenosis, the most common site of airway obstruction leading to failure to extubate. This number has increased since the 1970s as a result of the increasing incidence of prolonged intubation of neonates.[32] Smaller airways in the very young are far more likely to be symptomatic with even mild areas of narrowing. In fact, the majority of tracheostomies are performed in the first year of life.[33-35]

True vocal cord paralysis is a common cause of stridor, airway obstruction, and failure to extubate in children. Bilateral vocal cord paralysis, is less common than unilateral and is usually idiopathic.[36] These children regularly experience severe airway obstruction and require tracheostomy. Spontaneous recovery does occur,[37] but often not within the first year.[38] However, the most common identifiable causes are usually secondary to central nervous system problems, such as Arnold-Chiari malformation This type of true vocal cord paralysis may resolve after correction of the Chiari malformation. Bilateral true vocal cord paralysis can be a manifestation of a neuromuscular disorder. The prognosis in these cases depends on the nature of the underlying cause.[39]

More often, vocal cord paralysis is unilateral and acquired after a surgical procedure somewhere along the route of the recurrent laryngeal nerve, from skull base to the upper chest.[36] The most common of these procedures are performed for congenital heart disease, usually involving repair of the aortic arch.[40] Rarely do these children require tracheostomy. The patients ultimately requiring tracheostomy were far more likely to require tracheostomy for other reasons, such as failure to wean from the ventilator, and had high rate of comorbidities.[41] Tracheostomy has a high mortality rate in patients undergoing surgeries for congenital heart disease, and this greatly impacts decision making in these complex patients.[41] In many cases the vocal cord paralysis resolves within months, but sometimes it takes as long as several years. Around one third will resolve spontaneously. Nearly half will experience aspiration but often with a good-quality voice.[42]

Premature children with bronchopulmonary dysplasia may require a tracheotomy for long-term ventilation. This is a common indication for tracheostomy in children younger than 1 year and has been increasing in the past few years as a result of increased survival of preterm infants.[43] Children with severe dysphagia and neuromuscular disease who have trouble managing secretions may be prone to chronic aspiration and recurrent pneumonia. These children may benefit from tracheostomy for pulmonary toilet and improved quality of life. Less commonly, tracheostomy is required in patients with severe airway obstruction leading to obstructive sleep apnea that cannot be relieved surgically or cannot be managed with noninvasive ventilation such as bilevel positive airway pressure (BiPAP) or continuous positive airway pressure (CPAP). In rare cases, critically ill children or children requiring multiple surgical procedures who are difficult to intubate because of complex airway anatomy may require tracheostomy. This is most common in children with complex craniofacial anomalies[44] or severe craniofacial trauma.[45]

The decision to perform tracheostomy is often complex and should involve multidisciplinary input from involved physicians and providers. These should include but are not limited to pediatric specialists in intensive care medicine, otolaryngology, pulmonology, sleep medicine, anesthesia, craniofacial surgery, and pediatric and cardiothoracic surgery. A multidisciplinary approach to the management of children requiring tracheostomy may lead to better patient outcomes. It has been shown that use of a tracheostomy care protocol developed with multidisciplinary input leads to decreased morbidity and mortality and reduced time to decannulation.[46,47] Use of the consultative services of a tracheostomy specialist in the decision-making process for the team, staff, and family is appropriate whenever available at your institution.

Tracheostomy Tubes

Tracheostomy tubes come in various dimensions and materials, and selecting an appropriately sized tracheostomy tube is an important issue before placement. The age, size, and medical condition of the patient, as well as the indication for the tracheostomy, determine the type of tracheostomy tube selected. Tracheostomy tubes come in various sizes, which are usually chosen on the basis of age. Tracheostomy tubes have three dimensions: inner diameter, outer diameter, and length. The size of the tracheostomy tube reflects the inner diameter of the tube similar to endotracheal tubes. The depth of the tube from the flange to its tip is the measurement of the length of the tube. Standard-sized tracheostomy tubes for children come in two groups based on different lengths. Neonatal tracheostomy tubes are shorter, ranging from 30 to 34 mm. Tubes intended for older children are longer, starting at 38 mm in length. When a longer or shorter length of tracheostomy tube is needed, a specialized or custom tracheostomy tube can be ordered. Other modifications are available in special-order tubes, such as various options for the shape of the flanges and different angles of the shaft of the tube.[48] Use of these custom tubes may warrant consultation with a tracheostomy specialist, a specialty nurse or nurse practitioner, or possibly a pediatric otolaryngologist or pulmonologist. The dimensions of three common brands of tracheostomy tubes are compared in Table 13-4.

When selecting a tube, in addition to the size, the shape and composition must be considered. Plastic tubes are generally used in pediatric patients.[25] Plastic tubes are made of polyvinyl chloride, which is rigid. Some studies suggest there may be slow leakage of phthalates from these types of substances, which may be toxic to a patient over time. [49,50] Another brand of tracheostomy tube is routinely made of silicone, which may be softer and is a relatively inert substance. However, some of these tubes require wire reinforcement, which may limit their utility during imaging, but they may be more flexible. Some clinicians will replace one material with another to try to combat problems such as pressure ulcers or granulation tissue. In a tortuous airway, a more flexible tube may reduce pressure in areas of contact; changing the arc of the tube may reduce pressure, specifically on the posterior wall, for example. In patients prone to forming granulation tissue, changing to a potentially less inflammatory material may reduce this complication.

A cuffed tracheostomy tube may be needed for a child requiring higher ventilatory pressures for chronic lung

TABLE 13-4

Dimensions of Three Commonly Used Brands of Tracheostomy Tube

Cannula	Inner Diameter (mm)	Outer Diameter (mm)	Length of Cannula (mm)
Shiley			
3.0 Neonatal	3.0	4.5	30
3.5 Neonatal	3.5	5.2	32
4.0 Neonatal	4.0	5.9	34
3.0 Pediatric	3.0	4.5	39
3.5 Pediatric	3.5	5.2	40
4.0 Pediatric	4.0	5.9	41
4.5 Pediatric	4.5	6.0	42
5.0 Pediatric	5.0	7.1	44
5.5 Pediatric	5.5	7.7	46
Portex			
3.0	3.0	5.0	36
3.5	3.5	5.8	40
4.0	4.0	6.5	44
4.5	4.5	7.1	48
5.0	5.0	7.7	50
5.5	5.5	8.3	52
Bivona Neonatal Cuffless*			
2.5	2.5	4.0	30
3.0	3.0	4.7	32
3.5	3.5	5.3	34
4.0	4.0	6.0	36
Bivona Pediatric*			
2.5	2.5	4.0	38
3.0	3.0	4.7	39
3.5	3.5	5.3	40
4.0	4.0	6.0	41
4.5	4.5	6.7	42
5.0	5.0	7.3	44
5.5	5.5	8.0	46

*From Smiths Medical (St. Paul, MN).

disease or acute pulmonary inflammation.[51] There are three basic types of cuffs: high volume, low pressure; foam; and tight to shaft. The first two are inflated with air, whereas the last requires sterile water.[25] The type of cuff to be used is decided by the team and ordered specifically for each patient. It is important to avoid overinflation of the cuff. This may lead to any number of complications. Initially, it may misalign the tube in the airway or eventually cause the cuff to leak. Over time, an overinflated cuff may create contact points in the distal airway, leading to ulcerations, granulation tissue, or ultimately stenosis or scarring. It may be helpful to visualize the tracheotomy endoscopically with the cuff inflated with the usual amount of water or air to avoid such positioning problems. If the cuff appears tight, then less air or saline should be used. Some cuffs may not inflate in a symmetrical way, particularly when partly inflated, which may lead to asymmetrical positioning in the airway. Foam cuffs are usually reserved for special ventilation situations such as jet or oscillating ventilation, which requires much higher pressures to reduce the leak during inspiration. The cuff inflation can be varied with the ventilator to allow for air exit during expiration. This greatly reduces the amount of time the trachea is exposed to pressure.[48] Prolonged exposure to increased pressure can lead to tracheal dilation or "tracheomegaly."[52] Careful management of the tube size and cuff may prevent this complication. Cuff pressure should be checked regularly and adjusted as needed. Near consensus was reached regarding this concept in a recent tracheostomy clinical consensus statement by an expert panel.[25] Use of minimal leak technique to minimize cuff pressures, as outlined earlier in the use of endotracheal tubes, is a way to determine adequate cuff inflation.

Several types of tracheostomy ties may be used by caregivers. These include tracheotomy string or cotton twill tape, synthetic fleece like material with a Velcro fastener (Figure 13-9), and metal chain. The latter two facilitate cleaning and are easier to remove in an emergency However, they may also be easier for the patient to remove and lead to inadvertent decannulation. Each has its advantages and disadvantages and depends on the preference of the caregiver and needs of the individual patient.

Procedure and Technique

There are special concerns with respect to tracheostomy in the infant and small child. Although percutaneous tracheostomy

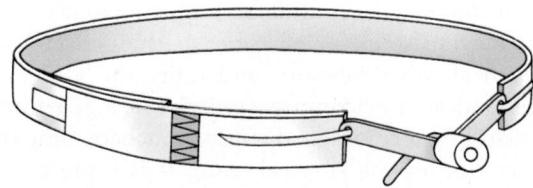

FIGURE 13-9 Diagram of a tracheostomy securing system with Velcro ties.

has been performed in few small series in pediatric patients, it has not been widely accepted because of the potential increase in complications.[53] First, the anatomical characteristics of this population make it more difficult to localize the trachea than in adults. The major landmarks, including the cricoid and thyroid cartilage, are not prominent and in very young infants are often completely covered by the hyoid bone. The trachea is smaller, is not as superficial, and is more mobile. In neonates, a large thymus may cover the anterior trachea, making surgical access more difficult. Rapid placement of a tracheostomy tube through the cricothyroid membrane or cricothyroidotomy is not advisable in an infant or small child because of the risk of vocal cord or laryngeal injury but may be performed in an emergency in an older child or adolescent.

Elective tracheostomy in infants and small children should be performed under controlled circumstances, usually with general anesthesia and ideally with an endotracheal tube in place. If the airway is not already established, or if the child has had prolonged intubation or has failed a trial of extubation, then the child may undergo bronchoscopy and intubation before tracheostomy. There may be instances, such as impeding airway compromise, when a tracheostomy is performed in older children or adolescents with the use of local anesthesia. A child may be maintaining his or her airway but may decompensate with induction of anesthesia or attempt at intubation. Cautious use of sedation and/or anxiolytics may be a useful adjunct in this situation. This should be avoided in small children. The airway can be managed by mask ventilation or by using a laryngeal mask airway in place of an endotracheal tube when intubation is not possible. This option may be particularly useful when performing a tracheostomy on a patient with a difficult airways, such as in patients with the Pierre Robin sequence. When flexible fiberoptic intubation is not possible because of a small jaw or reduced jaw opening, it can sometimes be successfully accomplished through a laryngeal mask airway in certain situations.[54] Challenging intubations such as these often require advanced airway management skills, and the most experienced people available should be notified.

Once the airway is established, the child is positioned for tracheotomy. A shoulder roll is used for hyperextension. The anesthesiologist is at the patient's head and has access to the airway at all times. An incision is made through the skin and subcutaneous tissue either in a transverse or vertical fashion. The strap muscles are separated to identify the midline, and careful midline dissection is performed to expose the trachea. The cricoid and then the upper tracheal cartilages are identified. Often the isthmus of the thyroid gland must be divided to expose the upper tracheal rings. The tracheostomy tube is usually placed between the second and fourth tracheal rings, depending on ease of exposure and size of the trachea and tube to be placed. Two stay sutures are placed on either side of the midline. These sutures are used to access the airway and readily locate the tracheostomy incision in the case of accidental decannulation and are usually removed at the time of the first tracheostomy tube change. A vertical midline incision is made through the middle of the tracheal rings between the sutures, which may expose the tip of the endotracheal tube. It is customary to have the anesthesiology team pull up the tube just above the tracheotomy site, maintaining intubation until the new airway is secure. This may not always be possible.

The tracheostomy tube is inserted and the obturator is removed. The anesthesia circuit is transferred from the endotracheal tube to the tracheosotomy tube. Bag ventilation may be used at this juncture. One should see a normal CO_2 tracing on the monitor as well as bilateral chest wall movement with ventilation. Anesthesia may auscultate in both axilla for bilateral breath sounds. Some surgeons prefer to immediately check the position of the tracheostomy tube above the carina using a flexible endoscope. This technique can also be used to estimate the distance of the tip of the tube from the carina. These examinations should be repeated after removing the shoulder roll and releasing the patient from neck extension because this may reposition the tracheostomy tube lower in the airway. Intraoperative flexible endoscopy examination through the tube may obviate the need for postoperative chest X-ray examination barring any signs of respiratory difficulty or complications.[55] The tracheostomy is usually secured with cotton twill ties in pediatric patients. Less commonly, some surgeons prefer to suture new tracheostomy tubes in place until the first tracheostomy change. The first tracheostomy tube change is usually done within the first week after the procedure.[25]

Postoperative Care

It is customary to obtain a chest radiograph immediately after surgery; however, this may not be necessary for all patients.[55] Immediate postoperative problems include bleeding, pneumothorax, subcutaneous emphysema with expansion of soft tissues, and, rarely, pulmonary edema. Any of these can lead to respiratory distress and ventilation problems. Chest radiographs should certainly be considered in the face of any respiratory problems or other serious immediate postoperative complication. If the patient required mechanical ventilation before the procedure, the ventilator settings may need to be adjusted to accommodate the changes in the patient's airway physiology after tracheosotomy tube placement.

It is during the immediate postoperative period, before healing of the surgical site and formation of the fistula tract from the skin to the trachea, that the child is at the highest risk for inadvertent decannulation. This is best avoided by admission to an intensive care unit with sedation as needed to avoided agitation and thrashing. Analgesia is also appropriate in the first few days after a potentially painful surgical procedure. Antibiotics are not routinely recommended unless there is evidence of an underlying infection or there is another indication for perioperative use. Postoperative care should include regular suctioning as needed. There are often more secretions and blood in the trachestomy tube in the postoperative period. If the patient is able to be weaned from the ventilator, humidified air can help reduce the risk of tracheostomy secretions drying in the lumen of the tube. Excellent pulmonary hygiene and secretion management is important to avoid mucous plugging that might necessitate an early urgent tracheostomy tube change.

Pressure sores or skin breakdown can occur at the superior border of the sternum, under the chin or circumferentially around the neck, which can lead to serious complications, especially in the critically ill child. The stoma site should be cleaned with care. Usually, normal saline is all that is needed. This practice varies widely from institution to institution. However, wound care is essential to successful healing in the postoperative period, with suctioning of the tracheostomy tube as well as around the trach site as needed to avoid skin breakdown. Padding or dressings placed under the flanges of the tracheostomy tube may need to be avoided to allow visualization of the surgical site and to prevent early decannulation. However, skin padding or dressings may become necessary to prevent progression of skin breakdown. Multiple devices are available that can be safely employed to minimize pressure on the skin at the tracheostomy site and, when used as part of a standardized practice, readily prevent skin breakdown.[56] At the discretion of the surgical service who placed the tracheostomy tube, the ties can be changed if they become excessively soiled or crusted or if swelling occurs and they become too tight.

The surgical team who performed the procedure are usually the ones who perform the first tracheostomy tube change about 1 week postoperatively. They can then determine that adequate healing and tract formation have occurred, allowing for staff to begin family education and performance of routine tracheostomy tube changes and tracheostomy care. Should respiratory distress, ventilation problems, inadvertent decannulation, or any respiratory emergency arise before this planned tracheostomy tube change, notification of the surgical team who placed the tracheostomy tube is appropriate. It is important that appropriate equipment is readily available at the bedside or immediately within reach to the providers in such an instance.[57] These include but are not limited to the obturator of the tracheostomy tube that is in place, spare inner cannulas if applicable, spare tracheostomy tubes of the same size and smaller if available, appropriately sized suction catheters useful for all tubes at the bedside, saline, endotracheal tubes, scissors, and lubricant. Other items may be requested or common practice at a given institution, including a complete operative tracheostomy tray at the discretion of the surgical team. It is important that these needs be communicated to the team caring for the patient.

Once the first tracheostomy change has occurred and it has been determined that the stoma is healed, bedside tracheostomy care and parental teaching usually can begin. Using a standardized protocol and checklists simplifies parental teaching. It is important that caregivers demonstrate competency before discharge home. It is also important that parents understand under what conditions they should urgently return to the hospital. Particularly in ventilated patients, this may be more important.[58] Ventilated patients with new tracheostomies are highly likely to be readmitted to the hospital within the first 6 months of their discharge, and it is helpful to clearly outline emergency notification parameters for the caregivers.[29]

Complications

In the 1970s the mortality rate from tracheotomy was reported to be as high as 24%.[53] More recent reports indicate mortality rates ranging from 0.5% to 3%.[33,54-59] This may be attributed to improvements in monitoring techniques such as pulse oximetry, as well as frequency of medical follow-up visits and heightened vigilance.[33] Avoidable deaths can be prevented by a thorough education program for all persons caring for a child in the hospital and the home.[28] Children who require long-term ventilation may experience more complications and seem to have a higher mortality rate overall. In fact, in patients requiring ventilation who have undergone tracheostomy, mortality increases precipitously after 30 days of continued hospital stay.[30] Overall, however, mortality for intensive care unit (ICU) patients who undergo tracheostomy tube placement compared with other ICU patients is comparable.[60]

The ability to replace the tracheostomy tube in case of accidental decannulation, proper airway assessment, good hygiene, and adequate systemic hydration and nutrition are important factors for a successful long-term outcome for an infant or child with a tracheostomy tube. Caregivers should demonstrate competency at both emergency and routine tracheostomy tube care before discharge.[58] Teaching the parents or caregivers to teach others caring for the child how to care for the tracheotomy site is a critical component of this training.[58]

The two most common reasons for death of a tracheostomy tube–dependent child are plugging of the tube with mucus and accidental decannulation. Plugging with mucus occurs when thick, viscous mucus obstructs the lumen of the tracheostomy tube. Factors that lead to this problem include dehydration, infection, and lack of humidity. Many children with bronchopulmonary dysplasia develop frequent exacerbations of mucous plugging with increased bronchorrhea. Viral or bacterial tracheitis may also lead to an increase in thick secretions. These problems can be avoided with appropriate hydration and pulmonary hygiene. Antibiotic therapy may be necessary in the case of infection. Sometimes the use of a humidifier or passive humidification device may help alleviate thick secretions. Acute mucous plugging requires emergency suctioning.

The tube is changed immediately if suctioning does not relieve the obstruction. Once the obstruction is relieved and the patient is out of danger, appropriate treatments are initiated to help prevent a recurrence of the problem.

If the obstruction is not relieved by tracheostomy tube change, steps should be taken to ensure that the tube is in the trachea and additional resources mobilized. If time and patient status permit, a chest X-ray examination may help visualize the location of the tracheostomy tube in the trachea. One can attempt to pass a suction catheter and bag ventilate the patient while assessing the chest wall mobility to assess the tube placement. One should take steps to ensure adequate delivery of oxygen in the case of hypoxia. If ventilation is not successful through the tracheostomy tube and the patient continues to deteriorate, one may attempt to place a different tube in the stoma or to perform oral mask ventilation or oral intubation. These may not be options in all patients and require staff to be aware of the status of the airway before the tracheostomy tube was placed and the original indications for it.

Another serious complication is accidental dislodgment of the tracheostomy tube. This accounts for most tracheotomy-related deaths.[33,59,60] Accidental dislodgment may occur during play activity, tracheotomy care, or when the child is alone. Immediate reinsertion is required.[25] This may be difficult during an emergency situation. If the same size tracheostomy tube cannot be inserted, then an attempt should be made to insert a tube that is one size smaller. If this is unsuccessful, the patient should be ventilated with a bag and mask if in distress until additional medical help arrives. Parents are usually sent home with a mask and bag for use in case of such an emergency. When the tube cannot be reinserted, similar steps to those outlined earlier should be taken if the child is in distress, including bag-mask ventilation, attempt at oral intubation, or even resuscitation through the stoma if necessary. It is important to remember to cover the stoma during any attempt at oral ventilation to prevent air escaping through the stoma. When there is a critical airway and there is no reserve airway around the tracheostomy tube, then insertion of an endotracheal tube into the tracheostomy site is an acceptable alternative in securing the airway. If this is not possible and the patient experiences full arrest, rescue breaths can be delivered into the stoma directly if mouth-to-mouth breaths do not achieve adequate ventilation.[61]

Other complications associated with tracheostomy use include bleeding, granulation tissue, tracheal erosion, tracheomalacia, and distal airway stenosis. External granulations may be managed conservatively if they do not interfere with tracheostomy tube changes or care. If granulation causes bleeding or difficulty with tube changes occurs, it can be cauterized or should be removed surgically. Suprastomal granulation is not routinely removed during endoscopy unless there is bleeding. Granulation tissue causing obstruction beyond the distal end of the tracheostomy tube often requires removal because it can mobilize into the airway with suctioning or tracheostomy tube changes, leading to complete airway obstruction. Suprastomal granulation may need to be removed just before decannulation because it can contribute to airway obstruction after tracheostomy tuberemoval.[62] Suprastomal tracheomalacia may also need to be repaired at the time of decannulation.

Bleeding from the tracheostomy tube is usually related to suction trauma or inflammation as a result of infection or tracheitis, but on occasion it may be caused by granulation or even erosion of the tracheal wall. Bleeding from suction trauma is usually self-limited and often occurs after a period of increased secretions or respiratory illness. Suctioning beyond the end of the tracheostomy tube should be avoided to prevent direct tracheal trauma and bleeding. Recurrent bleeding with increased secretions may indicate erosion of the posterior wall into the esophagus. This complication may also be associated with difficulties with tracheostomy tube changes or ventilation problems. Excessive bleeding or intermittent brisk bleeding may indicate that a major vessel has been eroded by the tracheostomy tube.[63] Most commonly this involves the innominate artery. Innominate arterial bleeding can be life threatening and may require intervention by a thoracic or pediatric surgeon. Both these complications are more commonly seen in adult patients.

Surveillance of the airway may help prevent such serious complications. Routine care of a tracheostomy includes regular interval bronchoscopies to ensure there are no major problems developing with the tracheotomy site. However, there is no consensus on the frequency with which these should occur and practice varies widely. Certainly if a patient is exhibiting any of the symptoms outlined earlier, it is generally agreed upon that bronchoscopy is indicated. In fact, patients with long-standing tracheostomies who were having symptoms at the time of their bronchoscopy were far more likely to have abnormal findings at bronchoscopy compared with those who were asymptomatic.[64]

Distal tracheal narrowing as a result of scarring is a serious complication and is best avoided. Appropriate management of granulations and mechanical tracheostomy tube problems such as contact ulcerations before scarring sets in may prevent this problem. As a distal obstruction develops, one may bypass it using a longer tube.[48] However, it is prudent to address the cause of the scar tissue formation because it can recur in the more distal trachea. Once the carina is involved with scarring or stenosis, bypassing may no longer be an option and surgical intervention may become necessary.[63] Regular surveillance bronchoscopy and treatment of distal airway problems as they arise may prevent these severe long-term complications of tracheostomy tubes.[65] Consultation with a tracheostomy specialist, pediatric otolaryngologist, or pediatric pulmonologist is appropriate before increasing the length or size of a tracheostomy tube in many instances, depending on the complexity of these problems.

Other problems encountered with a chronic tracheotomy include speech delay and difficulty with phonation. The tracheostomy is designed to bypass the larynx and therefore often interferes with speech production. Some children can phonate around the tracheostomy by occluding the opening, allowing air to pass around the tracheostomy tube through the vocal cords. This does require that the airway is patent above the tracheostomy tube. Use of a cuff usually precludes this option.[66] For children who require their tracheostomy only during sleep, such as children with central sleep apnea using a nighttime ventilator, they may be able to cap their tracheostomy tube completely during the day. They will need to breathe around the tracheostomy on both inspiration and expiration when the tube is capped. The child with a tracheostomy may be fitted for a Passey-Muir speech valve. This one-way valve allows flow of air into the tracheostomy tube but occludes it during expiration, redirecting air up around the tracheostomy tube and through the glottis to allow phonation. These can be used in certain patients in conjunction with a ventilator as well. Consultation with a tracheostomy specialist or speech therapist is appropriate in these situations.[67]

Children with tracheostomy all have significant reduction in laryngeal elevation during swallowing. The tracheostomy tube fixes the larynx in a more stationary position in the neck because of scarring of the tract. This can contribute to swallowing difficulties. The underlying medical condition necessitating the tracheostomy tube placement may also contribute to the swallowing dysfunction. Neuromuscular problems or degenerative diseases can lead to motor weakness, reduced reflexes, and diminished coordination of the complex functions involved in swallowing. Children who have prolonged intubations at a young age often experience oral aversion, which may require intensive oromotor therapy to overcome. Finally, the sense of smell and therefore taste may be altered in a child when the nasal airway is bypassed. Close work with a speech and swallowing therapist can be very important for the young child or infant with a tracheostomy.[57,67]

Routine Tracheostomy Tube Changes

The first tracheostomy tube change is customarily done only by the surgeon who performed the surgery or another physician from the surgical service. Generally, after the first change, the stoma has healed adequately to allow for routine tracheostomy care and changes and teaching of family members to perform them as well. Safe tracheostomy tube changes are an important part of routine tracheostomy care. It is essential that the child's parents or caregivers learn proper tracheostomy tube care before the child is discharged.[25] Tracheostomy tube changes can be routine, perhaps once weekly in a child, although the frequency varies according to the patient's needs. Children generally require more frequent changes of their tracheostomy than adults because pediatric tubes do not usually have an inner cannula.

| Box 13-2 | Equipment Needed for Tracheostomy Tube Changes |

- Correct size tracheostomy tube and obturator
- Smaller size tracheostomy tube
- Blanket roll
- Lubricant
- Tracheotomy ties
- Scissors
- Clean wet and dry gauze
- Resuscitation bag with mask
- Oxygen source

A change will be made urgently when there is suspected obstruction or respiratory distress. Preparation is the key to safety. It is always imperative to have proper equipment around for the tracheostomy tube change. (Recommended equipment is listed in Box 13-2.) It is also important to perform routine tracheostomy tube changes during daytime hours when everyone is alert and a "partner" is available. It is best to perform a routine tube change with two people. Proper lighting and position are essential. One must always communicate with the helper, be prepared for the worst, and remain calm, especially during an emergency.[68,69] Perform proper hand hygiene before any manipulation of the tracheostomy tube when possible (i.e., unless the situation is an emergency).

Ideally, at least 2 hours should have passed after the last feeding before the tracheostomy tube is changed to minimize the risk of vomiting or aspiration during the change. All supplies and emergency equipment are prepared. The role of the partner is determined and then the child is placed in the supine position on a shoulder roll with the neck hyperextended to make tube insertion easier. It is important to be prepared for any emergency such as a difficult insertion, inability to reaccess the airway, significant respiratory distress, bradycardia, or desaturation.

If at all possible, try to calm the child if he or she is agitated. Tracheostomy tube changes can be much more difficult if the child is agitated or fighting. Provide supplemental oxygen or bag ventilation if needed. Suction the tracheostomy tube if needed. Deflate the cuff fully if one is present on both the tracheostomy tube in place and the new one to be replaced. Release the tracheostomy ties and remove them. One person will hold the tracheostomy tube in place. The other person will perform routine tracheostomy site care, including cleaning the peristomal area or the neck skin. When both caregivers are ready, the lead caregiver counts to three. One caregiver removes the old tracheostomy tube and the other immediately replaces the new tube with obturator in place. Remove the obturator and assess for breathing by watching for respiratory efforts and chest wall motion. Auscultation with a stethoscope may also be performed when necessary. Secure the ties. Repeat suctioning if indicated or if there is any concern that the tracheostomy tube is not in place or may be occluded. The ties are threaded and secured and then checked for correct tension: The ties should be tight enough to hold the tube in place without movement yet not bind or pinch the neck.[69]

Tracheotomy Home Care

Many of the complications of tracheotomy take place in the home. Therefore an optimal home-care environment is essential. Parents and caregivers should be able to smoothly and quickly perform tracheostomy tube changes even in an urgent situation both with a partner and alone if necessary. These skills should be demonstrated to appropriate staff before discharge home from hospital or extended care facility.[70] It may be advisable that caregivers of patients with tracheostomy tubes be trained in cardiopulmonary resuscitation; however, this recommendation did not reach consensus in a recent consensus panel.[25] They must be able to perform routine functions such as suctioning and cleaning. Adequate tracheostomy equipment should always be available. This includes such items as the obturator of the tube in place, a spare tracheostomy tube, a smaller size tracheostomy tube, tracheostomy ties, dressing, suction catheters, suction machine, humidity devices, and monitors, if indicated.[68,70] Home nursing care may also be required based on the patient's need. This should be determined by discharge planning before discharge from the hospital. Each patient and family has unique needs, resources, and capabilities and these should be assessed before the child's discharge from the hospital

Decannulation

A patient may be considered for decannulation or removal of the tracheostomy when the following conditions have been met.

1. The original indication for the tracheostomy tube has resolved or been corrected.
2. The patient is tolerating either a cap during most or all waking hours or tolerating a Passy-Muir valve most of the day. The patient should not require removal of either for suctioning or respiratory complaints.

If these conditions have not been met, the patient should at a minimum tolerate downsizing of the tracheostomy tube. The child should have adequate level of consciousness and pharyngeal function to protect the airway from aspiration of food or secretions. The child should have an effective cough to clear secretions. The child should have had some evaluation of the airway with endoscopy before the tracheostomy removal. If the child has a difficult airway or is difficult to intubate, consideration should be made for the need for future surgeries.[25] Some physicians recommend a capped sleep study to ensure resolution of upper airway obstruction manifesting as obstructive sleep apnea or to ensure resolution of any central apnea that may have been present.[71]

Downsizing, use of a speaking valve, and ultimately capping can allow for a gradual transition to breathing through the nose and upper airway after a long period of breathing through a tracheostomy. An abrupt change in the airway such as tracheostomy removal can lead to anxiety and even respiratory distress, resulting in failed decannulation.[72] Once the tube is removed, an occlusive dressing should be applied until the stoma has closed spontaneously. Many physicians prefer to observe the patient overnight on monitors after tracheostomy removal. In certain circumstances, an in-office removal with a short period of observation may be appropriate depending on the patient's age and original indication for tracheostomy placement. A small number of children may have a persistent tracheocutaneous fistula that may require surgical closure. It may be important to determine that the upper airway obstruction has completely resolved in a patient whose tracheostomy site does not close if it is considered like any other fistula in the body. This can be accomplished with bronchoscopy, upper airway endoscopy, and possible sleep study if suspicion is high or symptoms suggest a problem. These symptoms include snoring, stridor, recurrent respiratory infections, failure to thrive, and sleep disturbances.[73,74]

Laryngotracheal Reconstruction

The child with critical subglottic stenosis and adequate pulmonary function may be a good candidate for laryngotracheal reconstruction (LTR). There are many surgical approaches to LTR, again depending on the situation.[75,76] In general, LTR involves expansion of the airway with cartilage grafts or resection of the stenotic portion of the airway. Use of autologous, auricular, and costal cartilage grafts have been described.[32] However, for circumferential stenosis with good cartilaginous support, an anterior costal (rib) cartilage graft without stenting may be adequate (Figure 13-10). When there is posterior glottic stenosis,

then a posterior split and cartilage graft may be performed with a short stenting period.[77] If the posterior stenosis is associated with a significant loss of cartilage, a period of stenting may be required (Figure 13-11). Laryngotracheal reconstruction may be accomplished with a single-staged or double-staged procedure. In a single-staged procedure, the child is kept intubated for several days to weeks with the endotracheal tube acting as the stent in the newly reconstructed airway. Repeat endoscopy is usually performed to confirm successful healing of the repair before extubation. However, extubation in the intensive care unit may be recommended without an examination at the discretion of the surgeon.

In the single-stage technique, sedation and paralysis may be necessary to prevent premature extubation. Postoperative fevers are common in this period and children undergoing single-stage procedures are at higher risk, with the likelihood increasing with the duration of postoperative intubation. The usual cause of postoperative fevers in LTR patients is atelectasis, which may not be significant.[78] Chest physical therapy has been shown to increase atelectasis and have serious complications in some patient populations.[79] It is not generally recommended. After extubation, supportive respiratory care is provided, including supplemental oxygen, oral suctioning, and humidification. If the child develops stridor, inhaled epinephrine can be used to acutely relieve airway obstruction. Heliox may be helpful immediately after extubation in cases of persistent stridor or signs of obstruction. Evaluation with bronchoscopy may be indicated in instances in which a patient requires reintubation. Often a patient will require removal of granulation tissue to relieve obstruction and successfully extubate.[80] Less commonly, a secondary airway lesion is unmasked by relief of the previous critical airway stenosis and must be addressed to achieve extubation. This is

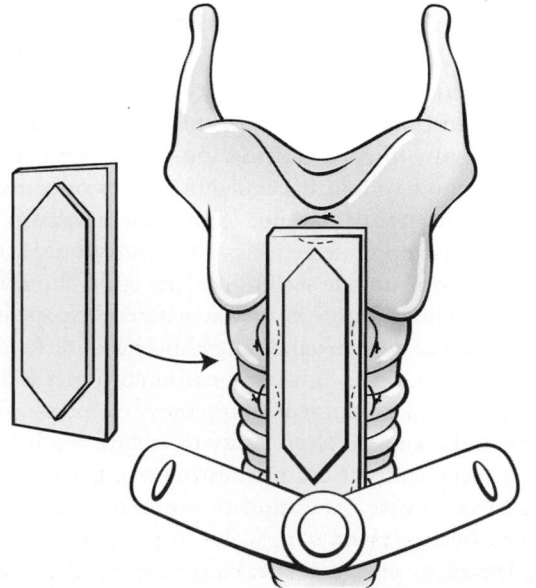

FIGURE 13-10 Laryngotracheoplasty using an anteriorly placed costal cartilage graft.

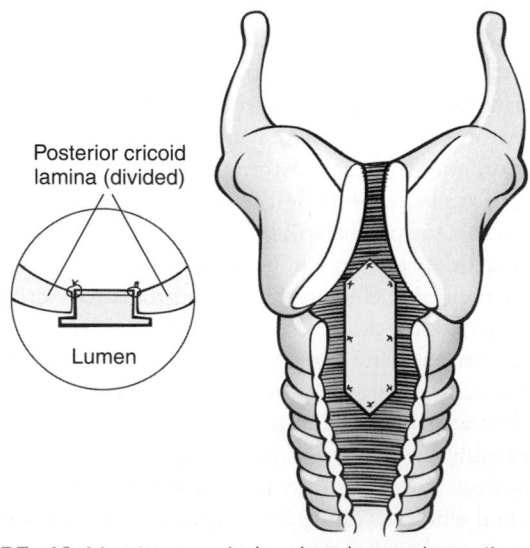

Posterior cricoid lamina (divided)

Lumen

FIGURE 13-11 A posteriorly placed costal cartilage graft maintains excellent expansion of the cricoid and glottis.

most often a dynamic lesion, such as laryngomalacia, that was disguised by the previously more dominant site of obstruction.[81]

In some instances a tracheostomy is already in place, or the reconstruction is more extensive and may require a longer period of stenting. This can be performed in a staged fashion.[80] Stenting and postoperative care depend on the situation. If the patient requires a short period of stenting, the procedure may be accomplished in a single-stage manner and the tracheostomy tube removed at the time of surgery. For longer periods of stenting, staged LTR may be performed with a synthetic stent secured into the airway for various periods of time. These devices contain both an airway stent that passes through the reconstructed area of the airway and larynx and an external port to the tracheostomy site. The patient must often breathe and be suctioned through the tracheostomy site. This type of device is known as a T tube, and its major disadvantage for most of these devices is that the tracheostomy component of the airway often cannot be removed in cases of plugging.[82] Exquisite postoperative care and hygiene is needed to prevent this complication.[82] In older children with a larger airway, a tracheostomy tube with an inner cannula can be incorporated into the stent, allowing for changing of the inner cannula in the case of plugging. For severe or total stenosis of the high trachea or subglottis, a partial cricotracheal resection (PCTR) rather than a traditional LTR may be indicated.[83] Some patients undergoing cricotracheal resection can undergo a single-stage procedure and will be left intubated nasally after the resection.[84] The success of the procedure varies proportionately with the severity of the stenosis present.[80]

Providing a safe and adequate airway while preserving normal laryngeal functions, such as voice and protection during swallowing, is the ultimate goal of LTR or PCTR.[85] It seems that many efforts aimed at expansion of the airway can negatively impact these functions of the larynx. Patients with complete airway obstruction or the most severe cases of obstruction may be more likely to require multiple procedures or require an indwelling stent.[84] An indwelling stent passing through the larynx greatly reduces laryngeal elevation during swallowing. These stents are sometimes open at the top to the hypopharynx, increasing likelihood of aspiration through the stent. The duration and severity of dysphagia are worse in patients undergoing more complex reconstructions in conjunction with indwelling T tubes, as well as those undergoing multiple procedures.[85] Therapy with a speech pathologist to develop compensatory strategies for better swallowing as well as diet modifications can improve swallowing.[86] Children with severe underlying disorders or oral aversion before undergoing reconstruction, regardless of procedure type, are more likely to continue with similar problems postoperatively.[85] A large number of patients have voice abnormalities after

one of these procedures, and further research is needed to evaluate long-term outcomes of voice in this patient population.[85,87]

SUCTIONING

Suctioning secretions from the airway or ETT maintains patency, prevents aspiration, assists an ineffective cough, and can be used to obtain specimens for diagnostic purposes. Because suctioning is not a benign procedure, recognizing when it is or is not indicated is important. Some specific indications include auscultating decreased breath sounds; implicating a possible mucous plug; difficulty during mechanical ventilation, possibly resulting from ETT occlusion or airway secretions; decreasing oxygen saturation; and the visible presence of secretions.[88] Although there are no absolute contraindications to suctioning, relative contraindications include patients with thrombocytopenia, epiglottitis, an unsecured airway, and labile cardiovascular or respiratory conditions. It is best to suction only when required and to avoid potential complications by repeatedly suctioning without indication.

Procedure

The necessary equipment for suctioning is gathered before initiating the procedure. This includes oxygen, a resuscitation bag and mask, suction catheters, sterile gloves, lavage fluid, a stethoscope, and a suction regulator to set the appropriate vacuum pressure. The vacuum pressure is set at 60 to 80 mm Hg for a neonate and at 80 to 100 mm Hg for a pediatric patient. The appropriate catheter length is determined by measuring the length of the ETT or tracheostomy tube against the suction catheter. The proper length should pass the end of the tube but not touch the carina.[89] Optimally, the catheter should be less than one half the size of the internal diameter of the ETT to avoid total obstruction of the tube, but this is often impossible in smaller inner diameter tubes.

The patient's breath sounds, heart rate and pattern, respiratory rate and pattern, arterial oxygen saturation, and excessive ventilator pressures are monitored continuously. As with all procedures, an adequate explanation of the process must be provided to the patient and family before the procedure. The patient is ventilated with an FiO₂ of at least 0.1 to 0.2 greater than the oxygen being delivered at the time of the intervention, or an FiO₂ of 1.0 when necessary. The same peak inspiratory pressures and positive end-expiratory pressure as set on the ventilator are used.

To suction, the catheter is moistened with saline (often the humidity alone is enough to lubricate) and, without applying suction, inserted into the airway to the predetermined length, or until resistance is met. It is pulled back 0.5 to 1.5 cm, and intermittent suction is applied, using the thumb port, while withdrawing and rotating the catheter.

Hypoxemia and atelectasis are avoided by keeping the duration of suctioning to less than 10 seconds per pass, and less than 5 seconds when applying the vacuum. The patient is oxygenated and ventilated between passes while observing the patient's vital signs on the monitors. Breath sounds are checked to evaluate the need for repeating the procedure. The need for further suctioning is reevaluated on the basis of the patient's clinical status. Potentially, rotating the head to the right facilitates entry into the left mainstem bronchus, whereas turning the head to the left facilitates entering the right mainstem bronchus, if required for aggressive suctioning.

Although not always required and somewhat controversial,[88,89] instilling a lavage solution may be necessary to remove mucous plugs or thick, tenacious secretions. Lavage or irrigating solutions include wetting agents such as normal saline, detergents such as sodium bicarbonate, and mucolytics such as *N*-acetylcysteine. For the neonatal patient, small incremental amounts are instilled to a volume of 0.5 to 1 ml. In the older child, 2 to 5 ml is instilled. Lavage is followed by manual ventilation and subsequent suctioning. Bagging the instilled solution into the ETT allows it to disperse throughout the lung fields to help liquefy and loosen secretions. If saline is to be used with suctioning, the clinician must remember there are potentially significant differences in the neonatal and adult airway chemistry. In particular, the antimicrobial component of airway mucus in the neonate is significantly different compared with an adult. A recent study in the neonatal population compared routine use of a low-sodium solution versus the use of normal saline. The low-sodium solution significantly reduced VAP and chronic lung disease.[91] In neonates the low-sodium solution may preserve the antimicrobial component of the airway mucus while still enhancing cough and secretion removal. The possible advantages of normal saline for adults and low-sodium saline solutions in neonates prompts careful consideration of routine saline use for suctioning in the pediatric population. Certain types of wetting agents, such as sterile water or hypertonic saline solution, cause mucosal irritation, bronchospasm, and overhydration.

Saline instillation after suctioning remains a controversial topic in pediatrics, particularly with neonates. Catheter insertion alone may dislodge thousands of bacteria located within the lumen of the ETT; a saline flush serves as a vehicle and potentially contributes to the distribution of bacteria distally into the lung—fostering the concern that routine saline instillation may increase the incidence of VAP. In contrast, new evidence suggests that the reservoir of bacteria within the lumen of the ETT may be eliminated or reduced with routine saline administration. In addition, sedated patients may benefit from a saline-stimulated cough. The patient's cough will always be our strongest ally in airway maintenance. Clearly, suctioning without a

cough will only clear the ETT. In 2009, Caruso studied 262 adult patients on the use of routine saline installation. Results demonstrated a 54% reduction in the risk of VAP with routine saline instillation.[92] A limitation of this study was that heat moisture exchangers (HMEs) were used to provide humidification, possibly necessitating saline instillation for secretion thinning.

Therefore the following suctioning algorithm (Figure 13-12) is recommended for use.

Nasotracheal Suction

Blind nasotracheal suctioning requires that all the previously mentioned equipment used for ETT suctioning be readily available.[90] The procedure for blind nasotracheal suctioning differs in that an ETT is not present. An infant is placed in the sniffing position, and the head and neck of an older child are slightly hyperextended. The suction catheter is lubricated with water or soluble jelly and placed in the nares. With the clinician facing the patient, the catheter is inserted slightly medial to the septum. The natural curve of the catheter is used as a guide to advance it over the top of the palate. When the catheter reaches the oropharynx, it is advanced into the tracheobronchial tree during inspiration. The catheter is pulled back 0.5 to 1.0 cm once resistance is felt, and suction is intermittently applied as previously described. Extreme caution must be taken when facial trauma is present.

Hypoxemia, bradycardia with resultant hypotension, bronchospasm, laryngospasm, airway trauma, hemorrhage, infection, and aspiration are all potential complications of blind nasotracheal suctioning. The most common complication in the neonatal patient is hypoxemia and subsequent bradycardia. The incidence of this complication can be reduced by frequent bagging between suctioning, limiting suction time, and increasing the FiO_2. Before the procedure is begun in the premature infant and unstable neonate, careful monitoring of the blood pressure is performed because hypertension associated with the procedure predisposes the patient to intracranial hemorrhage.

Bulb Suction

The bulb syringe is a manually operated device for use in the home or hospital and is extremely helpful to obligate nose breathers such as neonates or infants suffering from bronchiolitis. It is important to be gentle when using it because vigorous suctioning can lead to bleeding and airway swelling and damage. The bulb syringe is squeezed gently and held down. It is inserted in the area of mucus, and the pressure on the bulb is released to suction the mucus. Once the syringe is removed from the nasal passage, secretions are removed with a combination of squeezes and the syringe is cleansed with water and wiped with gauze pads. The bulb syringe should be

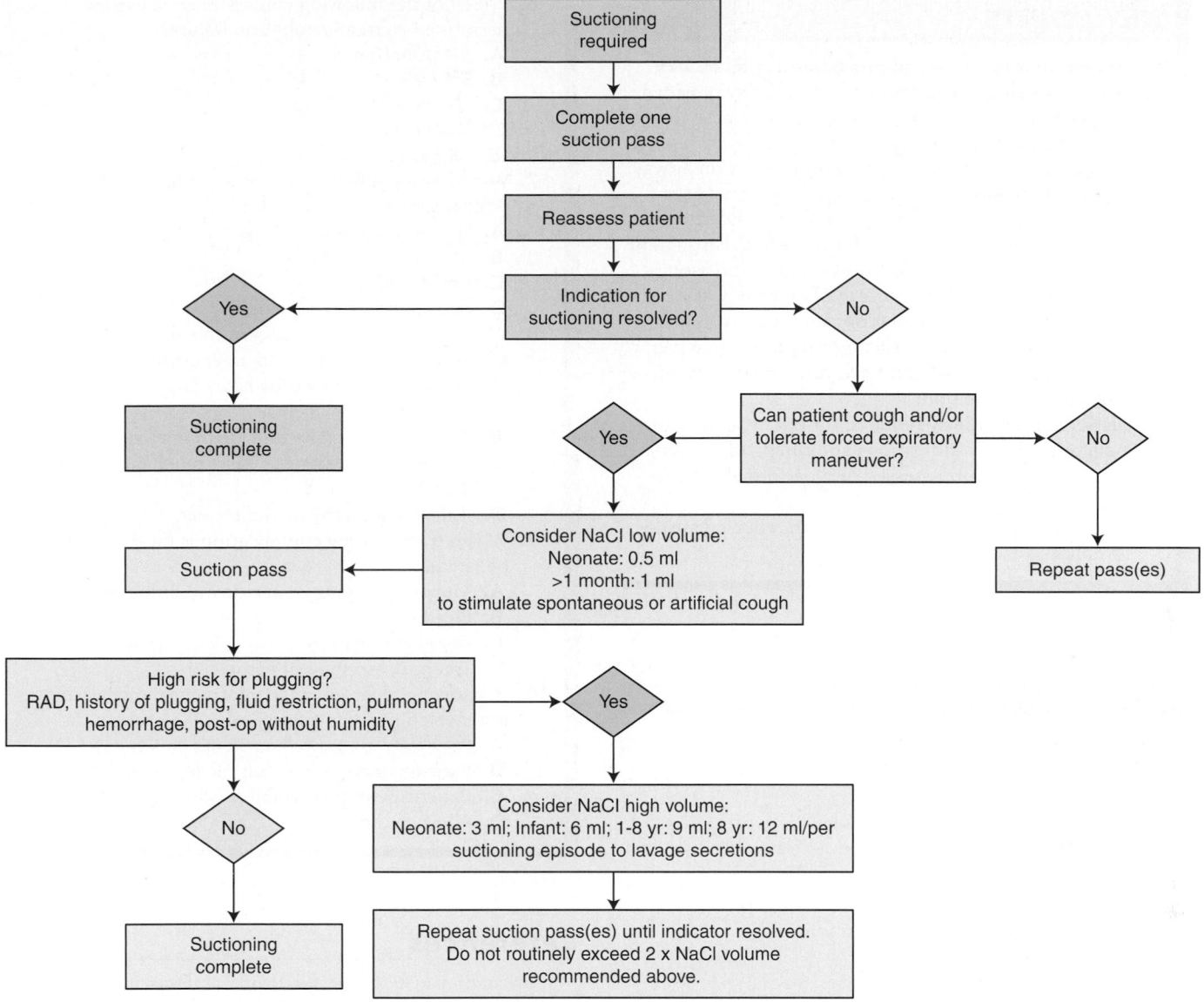

FIGURE 13-12   Suggested suctioning and saline use algorithm.

cleansed thoroughly after each use and allowed to air dry.

Closed Tracheal Suction Systems

As the frequency of suctioning increases, the need for a closed tracheal suction system or special suctioning adapter becomes imperative. These systems are necessary to prevent alveolar collapse associated with the loss of distention from positive end-expiratory pressure during suctioning and to reduce suction-related pulmonary complications. Closed tracheal suction systems are designed to allow minimal disruption with mechanical ventilation, to prevent the loss of positive end-expiratory pressure, and to avoid hypoxia. This system is added to an adapter, as well as an irrigation port, protective sleeve, closed lock, and

control valve, and markings on the suction catheter help determine the approximate depth of suctioning. Additional advantages include less contamination of the sheathed catheter, a decrease in airborne particles being introduced into the ETT, and a faster return to the preoxygenation baseline.

There are some disadvantages with these systems. Bacterial growth can occur if the catheter is not changed in a timely manner, but this is no different than with the ETT itself. Failure to pull the catheter back fully into the correct position can cause damage to or occlude the airway. Other disadvantages may be the possibility of leaving the continuous suction in the "on" position, causing hypoxemia and increased dead space if an inappropriate adapter size is used.

KEY POINTS

- Intubation is not a benign procedure; however, with proper care and preparation it can be safely provided.
- When complications of intubation occur, simple adjunct devices or techniques can provide life-sustaining results.
- Tracheostomies provide a stable and long-term airway. Proper education of staff and care providers can reduce adverse events when experts are not available.
- Tracheostomies are provided for a specific reason, and every care provider should be aware of that reason. This ensures proper care in case of an emergency.
- Proper timing of decannulation can reduce complications and the need for specialty equipment; however, it has its associated risks. Not everyone will be a candidate for decannulation.
- Suctioning is routinely required for tracheal tubes to maintain patency. Indications and timing of suctioning must be individually assessed and performed only when necessary.
- Proper humidification can assist with reducing airway complications.

ASSESSMENT QUESTIONS

See Evolve Resources for answers.

1. Which is not a reason for intubation?
   - **A.** Pulmonary function
   - **B.** Central apnea
   - **C.** Upper airway obstruction
   - **D.** Pulmonary hygiene
2. What is the age-appropriate ETT for a 1-year-old? A 2-year-old? A 4-year-old? A 6-year-old?
   - **A.** 4.0, 4.5, 5, 5.5
   - **B.** 3.5, 5, 5.5, 6
   - **C.** 4.0, 5, 6, 7
   - **D.** 4.5, 5.5, 6.5, 7
3. When would one consider an LMA instead of intubation?
   - **A.** Awake, short-term ventilation
   - **B.** To protect against aspiration
   - **C.** To protect the vocal cords
   - **D.** Unconscious, backup to intubation
4. What are the disadvantages of nasotracheal intubation?
   - **A.** Sinusitis
   - **B.** Pressure necrosis, bleeding
   - **C.** Postextubation atelectasis
   - **D.** All of the above
5. What intubation approach would one use in a larynx that is difficult or impossible to expose with a standard rigid laryngoscope?
   - **A.** LMA
   - **B.** Cricothyroidotomy
   - **C.** Flexible fiberoptic intubation
   - **D.** Tracheostomy
6. Which of the following choices may be used/performed to treat extubation failure?
   - **A.** Reintubation
   - **B.** Steroids
   - **C.** Heliox
   - **D.** Tracheostomy
   - **E.** All of the above
7. Which of the following is not an indication for a tracheotomy?
   - **A.** Severe subglottic stenosis
   - **B.** Mild laryngomalacia
   - **C.** Chronic ventilation
   - **D.** Poor pulmonary hygiene
8. What is the difference between the outside diameter of a tracheostomy tube and an endotracheal tube?
   - **A.** The tracheostomy tube has a larger outside diameter.
   - **B.** They have the same outside diameter.
   - **C.** The endotracheal tube has a much larger outside diameter.
   - **D.** It depends on the manufacturer.
9. Which tracheotomy complication is most likely to be lethal?
   - **A.** Mucous plugging or accidental dislodgement
   - **B.** Bleeding
   - **C.** Distal granulation
   - **D.** Tracheal–esophageal fistula
10. In patients undergoing laryngotracheal reconstruction, which patients have swallowing problems?
    - **A.** Patients with indwelling stents or T tubes
    - **B.** Patients undergoing multiple procedures
    - **C.** Patients with preexisting swallowing problems
    - **D.** All of the above

References

1. International Guidelines for Neonatal Resuscitation: An excerpt from the Guidelines 2005 for Cardiopulmonary Resuscitation and Emergency Cardiovascular Care International Consensus on Science, *Pediatrics*, 2005.
2. Keep PJ, Manford ML: Endotracheal tube sizes for children, *Anaesthesia* 29:181, 1974.
3. Hinkle AJ: A rapid and reliable method of selecting endotracheal tube size in children [abstract], *Anesth Analg* 67:S592, 1988.
4. Luten RC, et al: Length-based endotracheal tube and emergency equipment selection in pediatrics, *Ann Emerg Med* 21:900, 1992.
5. Berry FA, Yemen TA: Pediatric airway in health and disease, *Pediatr Clin North Am* 41:153, 1994.
6. Behar PM, Todd NW: Resuscitation of the newborn with airway compromise, *Clin Perinatol* 26:717, 1999.
7. Brain AIJ: The laryngeal mask: a new concept in airway management, *Br J Anaesth* 55:801, 1983.
8. Ovassapian A, Ramez Salem M: Sellick's maneuver: To do or not do, *Anesth Analg* 109:1360, 2009.
9. Boet S, et al: Cricoid pressure provides incomplete esophageal occlusion associated with lateral deviation: a magnetic resonance imaging study, *J Emerg Med* 42:606, 2012.
10. Brown MS: Prevention of accidental extubation in newborns, *Am J Dis Child* 142:1240, 1988.

11. Volsko TA, Chatburn RL: Comparison of two methods for securing the endotracheal tube in neonates, *Respir Care* 42:288, 1997.

12. Holm-Knudsen R: The difficult pediatric airway—a review of new devices for indirect laryngoscopy in children younger than two years of age, *Paediatr Anaesth* Feb 21: 98, 2011.

13. Lee AK, Crutcher JM: Oklahoma notes decline in *Haemophilus influenzae:* invasive *Haemophilus influenzae* disease among children aged < 5 years in Oklahoma, 1990-1997, *J Oklahoma State Med Assoc* 92:276, 1999.

14. Markovitz BP, Randolph AG: Corticosteriods for the prevention of reintubation and postextubation stridor in pediatric patients: a meta analysis, *Pediatr Crit Care* 3:223, 2002.

15. Duncan PG: Efficacy of helium–oxygen mixtures in the management of severe viral and postintubation croup, *Can Anaesth Soc J* 26:206, 1979.

16. Chavez A, dela Cruz R, Zaritsky A: Spontaneous breathing trial predicts successful extubation in infants and children, *Pediatr Crit Care Med* 7(4):324, 2006.

17. Kurachek SC, Newth CJ, Quasney MW, et al: Extubation failure in pediatric intensive care: a multiple-center study of risk factors and outcomes, *Crit Care Med* 31(11):2657, 2003.

18. Suominen PK, Touminen NA, Salminen JT, et al: The air-leak test is not a good predictor of postextubation adverse events in children undergoing cardiac surgery, *J Cardiothorac Vasc Anesth* 21(2):197–202, 2007.

19. Malhotra D, Gurcoo S, Qazi S, Gupta S: Randomized comparative efficacy of dexamethasone to prevent postextubation upper airway complications in children and adults in ICU, *Indian J Anaesth* 53(4):442, 2009.

20. Khemani RG, Randolph A, Markovitz B: Steroids for post extubation stridor: pediatric evidence is still inconclusive, *Intensive Care Med* 36(7):1276, 2010.

21. Whigham AS, Howell R, Choi S, Penña M, Zalzal G, Preciado D: Outcomes of balloon dilation in pediatric subglottic stenosis, *Ann Otol Rhinol Laryngol* 121(7):442, 2012.

22. Myer CM, O'Conner DM, Cotton RT: A proposed laryngotracheal stenosis grading system based on endotracheal tube size, *Ann Otol Rhinol Laryngol* 103;319, 2012.

23. Eze NN, Wyatt ME, Hartley BE: The role of the anterior cricoids split in facilitation extubation in infants, *Int J Pediatr Otorhinolaryngol* 69(6):843, 2005.

24. Rudnick EF, Mitchell RB: Tracheostomy in children. In Pereira KD, Mitchell RB, editors: *Pediatric otolaryngology for the clinician,* Totowa, NJ, 2009, Humana Press, pp 159–163.

25. Mitchell RB, Hussey HM, Setzen G, et al: Clinical consensus statement: tracheostomy care, *Otolaryngol Head Neck Surg* 148(1):6–20, 2013.

26. Srivastava R, Stone BL, Murphy NA: Hospitalist care of the medically complex child, *Pediatr Clin North Am* 52(4):1165, 2005.

27. Shields L, Zhou H, Pratt J, Taylor M, Hunter J, Pascoe E: Family-centred care for hospitalized children aged 0-12 years, *Cochrane Database Syst Rev* 10:CD004811, 2012.

28. Corbett HJ, Mann KS, Mitra I, Jesudason EC, Losty PD, Clarke RW: Tracheostomy—a 10-year experience from a UK pediatric surgical center, *J Pediatr Surg* 42(7):1251, 2007.

29. Graf JM, Montagnino BA, Hueckel R, McPherson ML: Pediatric tracheostomies: a recent experience from one academic center, *Pediatr Crit Care Med* 9(1):96–100, 2008.

30. Spentzas T, Auth M, Hess P, Minarik M, Storgion S, Stidham G: Natural course following pediatric tracheostomy, *J Intensive Care Med* 25(1):39–45, 2010.

31. Schroeder JW Jr, Holinger LD: Congenital laryngeal stenosis, *Otolaryngol Clin North Am* 41(5):865, 2008.

32. Santos D, Mitchell R: The history of pediatric airway reconstruction, *Laryngoscope* 120(4):815, 2010.

33. Wetmore RF, Marsh RR, Thompson ME, Tom LW: Pediatric tracheostomy: a changing procedure? *Ann Otol Rhinol Laryngol* 108(7 Pt 1):695, 1999.

34. Palmer PM, Dutton JM, McCulloch TM, et al: Trends in the use of tracheotomy in the pediatric patient: The Iowa experience, *Head Neck* 17:328–333, 1995.

35. Potsic WP, Cotton RT, Handler SD: *Surgical pediatric otolaryngology: head and neck surgery,* New York, 1997, Thieme Medical Publishers.

36. Daya H, Hosni A, Bejar-Solar I, Evans JN, Bailey CM: Pediatric vocal fold paralysis: a long-term retrospective study, *Arch Otolaryngol Head Neck Surg* 126(1):21, 2000.

37. Miyamoto RC, Parikh SR, Gellad W, Licameli GR: Bilateral congential vocal cord paralysis: a 16-year institutional review, *Otolaryngol Head Neck Surg* 133(2):241, 2005.

38. Berkowitz: Natural history of tracheostomy-dependent idiopathic congenital bilateral vocal fold paralysis, *Otolaryngol Head Neck Surg* 136(4):649, 2007.

39. Lapeña JF Jr, Berkowitz RG: Neuromuscular disorders presenting as congenital bilateral vocal cord paralysis, *Ann Otol Rhinol Laryngol* 110(10):952, 2001.

40. Khariwala SS, Lee WT, Koltai PJ: Laryngotracheal consequences of pediatric cardiac surgery, Arch *Otolaryngol Head Neck Surg* 131(4):336, 2005.

41. Cotts T, Hirsch J, Thorne M, Gajarski R: Tracheostomy after pediatric cardiac surgery: frequency, indications, and outcomes, *J Thorac Cardiovasc Surg* 141(2):413, 2011.

42. Truong MT, Messner AH, Kerschner JE, Scholes M, Wong-Dominguez J, Milczuk HA, Yoon PJ: Pediatric vocal fold paralysis after cardiac surgery: rate of recovery and sequelae, *Otolaryngol Head Neck Surg* 137(5):780, 2007.

43. Pereira KD, MacGregor AR, Mitchell RB: Complications of neonatal tracheostomy: a 5-year review, *Otolaryngol Head Neck Surg* 131:810, 2004.

44. Hasan RA, Nikolis A, Dutta S, Jackson IT: Clinical outcome of perioperative airway and ventilatory management in children undergoing craniofacial surgery, *J Craniofac Surg* 15(4):655, 2004.

45. Castilla DM, Dinh CT, Younis R: Pediatric airway management in craniofacial trauma, *J Craniofac Surg* 22(4):1175, 2011.

46. Garrubba M, Turner T, Grieveson C: Multidisciplinary care for tracheostomy patients: a systematic review, *Crit Care* 13:R177, 2009.

47. Cetto R, Arora A, Hettige R, et al: Improving tracheostomy care: a prospective study of the multidisciplinary approach, *Clin Otolaryngol* 36:482–488, 2011.

48. Arjmand, EM, Brenski AC: Advances in tracheostomy in the pediatric age group, *Adv Otolaryngol Head Neck Surg* 15:41–69, 2001.

49. Chiellini F, Ferri M, Latini G: Physical-chemical assessment of di-(2-ethylhexyl)-phthalate leakage from poly(vinyl chloride) endotracheal tubes after application in high risk newborns, *Int J Pharm* 409(1-2):57–61, 2011.

50. Mankidy R, Wiseman S, Ma H, Giesy JP: Biological impact of phthalates, *Toxicol Lett* pii:S0378-4274(12)01405, 2012.

51. Schroeder JW Jr, Schneider JS, Walner DL: The influence of peak airway pressure and oxygen requirement on infant tracheostomy, *Int J Pediatr Otorhinolaryngol* 76(6):869, 2012.

52. Keszler M, Nassabeh-Montazami S, Abubakar K: Evolution of tidal volume requirement during the first 3 weeks of life in infants <800 g ventilated with volume guarantee, *Arch Dis Child Fetal Neonatal Ed* 94(4):F279–82, 2009.

53. Sajjadian A, Isaacson G: Pediatric precutaneous revision tracheotomy, *Laryngoscope* 107:1550, 1997.

54. Hernandez MR, Klock PA Jr, Ovassapian A: Evolution of the extraglottic airway: a review of its history, applications, and practical tips for success, *Anesth Analg* 114(2):349, 2012.

55. Genther DJ, Thorne MC: Utility of routine postoperative chest radiography in pediatric tracheostomy, *Int J Pediatr Otorhinolaryngol* 74(12):1397, 2010.

56. Boesch RP, Myers C, Garrett T, et al: Prevention of tracheostomy-related pressure ulcers in children, *Pediatrics* 129(3):e792, 2012.

57. Gluth MB, Maska S, Nelson J, et al: Postoperative management of pediatric tracheostomy: results of a nationwide survey, *Otolaryngol Head Neck Surg* 35:11–17, 1996.

58. Kun SS, Davidson-Ward SL, Hulse LM, Keens TG: How much do primary care givers know about tracheostomy and home ventilator emergency care? *Pediatr Pulmonol* 45(3):270, 2010.

59. Tantinikorn W, Alper CM, Bluestone CD, Casselbrant ML: Outcome in pediatric tracheotomy, *Am J Otolaryngol* 24(3):131, 2003.

60. Wood D, McShane P, Davis P: Tracheostomy in children admitted to paediatric intensive care, *Arch Dis Child* 97(10):866, 2012.

61. American Heart Association: *Pediatric Advanced Life Support provider manual*, 2011.

62. Chen C, Bent JP, Parikh SR: Powered debridement of suprastomal granulation tissue to facilitate pediatric tracheotomy decannulation, *Int J Pediatr Otorhinolaryngol* 75(12):1558, 2011.

63. Das P, Zhu H, Shah RK, Roberson DW, Berry J, Skinner ML: Tracheotomy-related catastrophic events: results of a national survey, *Laryngoscopy* 122:30–37, 2012.

64. Kharasch VS, Dumas HM, Haley SM, et al: Bronchoscopy findings in children and young adults with tracheostomy due to congenital anomalies and neurological impairment, *J Pediatr Rehabil Med* 1(2):137, 2008.

65. Zuh H, Das P, Brereton J, Roberson D, Shah RK: Surveillance and management practices in tracheotomy patients, *Laryngoscope* 122:46–50, 2012.

66. Gereau SA, Navarro GC, Cluteria B, et al: Selection of pediatric patients for use of the Passy-Muir valve for speech production, *Int J Pediatric Otolaryngol* 35:11–17, 1996.

67. Baumgatener CA, Bewyer E, Bruner D: Management of communication and swallowing in intensive care: the role of the speech pathologist, *AACN Adv Crit Care* 19(4):433, 2008.

68. Cincinnati Children's Hospital Medical Center: *Tracheotomy care handbook.* Cincinnati, OH, 2010, Cincinnati Chileren's Hospital Medical Center, KN-00209.

69. Dallas Children's Medical Center: *Home instructions for the caregivers of a child with a tracheostomy: a guide for caring for your child*, Dallas, 2011, Dallas Children's Medical Center.

70. Joseph RA: Tracheostomy in infants: parent education for home care, *Neonatal Netw* 30(4):231, 2011.

71. Roland PS, Rosenfeld RM, Brooks LJ, et al: Clinical practice guideline: polysomnography for sleep-disordered breathing prior to tonsillectomy in children, *Otolaryngol Head Neck Surg* 145(suppl 1):S1–S15, 2011.

72. Black RJ, Baldwin DL, Johns AN: Tracheostomy "decannulation panic" in children: fact or fiction? *J Laryngol Otol* 98(3):297–304, 1984.

73. Tunkel DE, et al: Polysomnography in the evaluation of readiness for decannulation in children, *Arch Otolaryngol Head Neck Surg* 122:721, 1996.

74. Gallagher TQ, Hartnick CJ: Tracheocutaneous fistula closure, *Adv Otorhinolaryngol* 73:76, 2012.

75. Cotton RT, Gray SD, Miller RP: Update of the Cincinnati experience in pediatric laryngotracheal reconstruction, *Laryngoscope* 99:1111, 1989.

76. Holinger LD: Treatment of severe subglottic stenosis without tracheotomy, *Ann Otol Laryngol Rhinol* 91:407, 1982.

77. Rutter MJ, Cotton RT: The use of posterior cricoids grafting in managing isolated posterior glottis stenosis in children, *Arch Otolaryngol Head Neck Surg* 130(6):737, 2004.

78. Schraff SA, Brumbaugh C, Meinzen-Derr J, Willging PJ: The significance of post-operative fever following airway reconstruction, *Int J Ped Otorhinolaryngol* 74(5):520, 2010.

79. Reines HD, Sade RM, Bradford BF, Marshall J: Chest physiotherapy fails to prevent postoperative atelectasis in children after cardiac surgery, *Ann Surg* 195:451, 1982.

80. Hartnick CJ, Hartley BE, Lacy PD, et al: Surgery for pediatric subglottic stenosis: disease-specific outcomes, *Ann Otol Rhinol Laryngol* 110(12):1109, 2001.

81. Rutter MJ, Link DT, Liu JH, Cotton RT: Laryngotracheal reconstruction and the hidden airway lesion, *Laryngoscope* 110(11):1871–1874, 2000.

82. Stern Y, Willging JP, Cotton RT: Use of Montgomery T-tube in laryngotracheal reconstruction in children: is it safe? *Ann Otol Rhinol Laryngol* 107(12):1006, 1998.

83. Monnier P, Lang F, Savary M: Partial cricotracheal resection for severe pediatric subglottic stenosis: update of the Lausanne experience, *Ann Otol Laryngol Rhinol* 107:961, 1998.

84. Johnson RF, Rutter M, Cotton R, Vijayasekeran S, White D: Cricotracheal resection in children 2 years of age and younger, *Ann Otol Rhinol Larynhol* 117(2):110, 2008.

85. Miller CK, Linck J, Willging JP: Duration and extent of dysphagia following pediatric airway reconstruction, *Int J Pediatr Otorhinolaryngol* 73(4):573, 2009.

86. Smith LP, Otto SE, Wagner KA, Chewaproug L, Lacobs IN, Zur KB: Management of oral feeding in children undergoing airway reconstruction, *Laryngoscope* 119(5):967, 2009.

87. Baker S, Kelchner L, Weinrich B, et al: Pediatric laryngotracheal stenosis and airway reconstruction: a review of voice outcomes, assessment, and treatment issues, *J Voice* 20(4):631, 2006.

88. Hagler DA, Traver GA: Endotracheal saline and suction catheters: sources of lower airway contamination, *Am J Crit Care* 3:444, 1994.

89. Raymond SJ: Normal saline instillation before suctioning: helpful or harmful? A review of the literature, *Am J Crit Care* 4:267, 1995.

90. Gray RF, Todd NW, Jacobs IN: Tracheostomy decannulation in children: approaches and techniques, *Laryngoscope* 108:8, 1998.

91. Christensen RD, Henry E, Baer VL, et al: A low-sodium solution for airway care: results of a multicenter trial, *Respir Care* 55(12):1680–1685.

92. Caruso P, Denari S, Ruiz SA, Demarzo SE, Deheinzelin D: Saline instillation before tracheal suctioning decreases the incidence of ventilator-associated pneumonia, *Crit Care Med* 37(1):32–38, 2009.

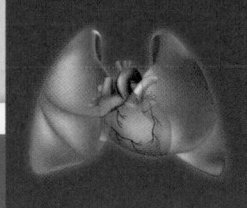

Chapter 14

Surfactant Replacement Therapy

SANTINA A. ZANELLI, DAVID KAUFMAN

LEARNING OBJECTIVES

After reading this chapter the reader will be able to:

1. Explain how surfactant affects surface tension and improves lung function
2. Identify disease processes associated with surfactant deficiency, dysfunction, or inactivation
3. Discuss the delivery, benefits, and adverse effects of surfactant replacement
4. Identify patients and disease processes that may benefit from surfactant replacement therapy

KEY TERMS

Compliance
Pulmonary surfactant

Respiratory distress syndrome
Surfactant proteins

Surfactant replacement therapy
Surface tension

The successful introduction of surfactant therapy into clinical care is one of the best examples of how discoveries in the laboratory can be directly translated into improved patient care. Basic scientific research linked relative or total lack of surfactant secondary to decreased production or inactivation to **respiratory distress syndrome** (RDS) in preterm infants. The phenomenal success of **surfactant replacement therapy** in RDS has prompted investigation into the possible role of surfactant therapy in other types of acute lung injuries, including acute RDS (ARDS).[1,2] It is clear that qualitative and quantitative surfactant abnormalities are present in many non-RDS types of acute lung injuries and that the expanding role of surfactant replacement must be explored.

THE DISCOVERY OF SURFACTANT

The seeds were sown in the early nineteenth century with the observations of Pierre Simon Laplace and Thomas Young.[3] In their theory of capillary action they described the relationship of transsurface pressure and surface tension at a gas–fluid interface in a sphere as P = 2 × ST/R (where P is the transsurface or distending pressure, ST is surface tension, and R is the radius of the sphere). More than a century later, in 1929, the Swedish physiologist Kurt von Neergaard,[4] while studying respiratory mechanics, discovered that the retractile force of the lung was dependent on the surface tension in the alveoli (Figure 14-1). Twenty years later, Macklin[5] postulated the existence of a "mucoprotein" lining in the lung that had the surface tension–lowering properties observed by von Neergaard. In the 1950s, Mead and co-workers[6,7] at the Harvard School of Public Health discovered that surface forces at the lung's air–liquid interface contributed to elastic recoil, especially at large lung volumes. Simultaneously, Clements[8] discovered the role of the alveolar lining layer in mediating surface tension changes with area, thereby stabilizing air-filled spaces at low lung volumes and augmenting elastic recoil at large lung volumes. He named the material "pulmonary surfactant" and established its role as an antiatelectasis factor. In 1955, Pattle[9] discovered that bubbles expressed from the lungs of fetal guinea pigs did not have the stability of those found in term mammalian lungs, stating that the immature lung of the premature baby may have increased surface forces. In 1959, Avery and Mead[10] noted from autopsies that the lungs of infants who died of hyaline membrane disease never had foam in their airways. They lacked foam because they lacked surfactant and therefore the capacity to reduce surface tension when surface area is reduced during exhalation. These findings identified surfactant deficiency as the cause of RDS. Finally, in 1980, Fujiwara and colleagues reported success in producing and using surfactant replacement for preterm infants with RDS.[11] The release of surfactant for clinical use in the United States by the U.S. Food and Drug Administration in 1990 resulted in a measurable reduction in perinatal mortality and morbidity. The use of exogenous surfactants for treatment of lung injury beyond the neonatal period is only now being studied and may offer similar promise.[12-14]

SURFACTANT PHYSIOLOGY
Function

A surfactant is any molecule that localizes on aqueous surfaces. In the lung, alveolar surfaces are lined by a layer of fluid, called surfactant. **Pulmonary surfactant** creates an air–liquid interface that reduces surface tension proportionally to alveolar size. **Surface tension** is created by the attraction of water molecules to one another. This is best illustrated by observing that water placed on a flat surface coalesces to form a droplet. During respiration, carbon dioxide and water are exhaled at the surface of the alveoli, creating a liquid interface with inhaled air. As indicated by the Laplace law, this attraction would lead to the collapse of alveoli as each alveolus becomes smaller. However, in the presence of surfactant, water molecules are pushed apart in the alveolus, preventing alveolar collapse during exhalation. Surface tension is reduced in proportion to the number of surfactant molecules per surface area. Surfactant displaces water from the air–liquid surface and lowers the surface tension from 75 to 25 dyn/cm (during inflation).[15]

The lung can be thought of as a large number of interconnected bubbles that form the interface between the gaseous environment and the wet alveolar surface. If this interface were without surfactant, two consequences would ensue: (1) Every breath would take a considerable amount of pressure to expand the lung, comparable to the 80 to 90 cm H_2O of pressure required for a newborn's first breath, and (2) the lung would rapidly collapse during exhalation.

Pulmonary surfactant lowers surface tension at all lung volumes, a critical function as alveolar surface decreases during expiration (Figure 14-2). If surface tension did not decrease with decreasing lung volume, alveoli of different sizes would require different distending pressures. Small alveoli would empty into large ones and there would be an overall tendency for the lung to coalesce into a smaller number of large alveoli as lung volume diminished. This would significantly decrease the surface area for gas exchange as well. Surfactant not only decreases surface tension but also reduces it to a greater degree at low lung volume, counteracting the effects of decreasing alveolar size.

Functionally, surfactant increases lung **compliance,** promotes homogeneous gas distribution during inhalation, and allows a residual volume of gas to be evenly distributed throughout the lung during exhalation; that is, it maintains functional residual capacity. In the absence of surfactant, distribution of ventilation becomes uneven, the lungs become stiff, and atelectasis ensues during exhalation. The result is increased work of breathing, hypoxia, and respiratory failure, the clinical picture exemplified

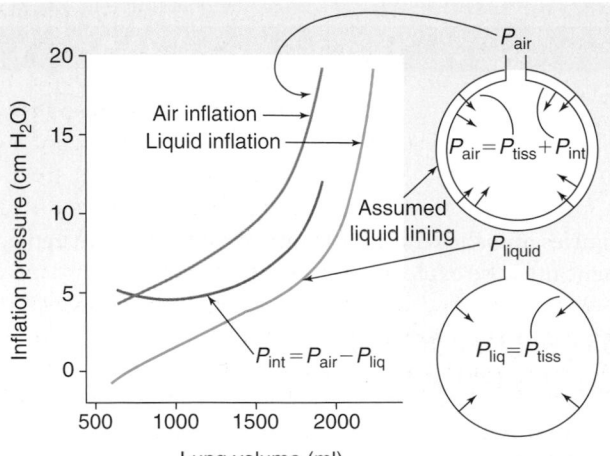

FIGURE 14-1   A, Pressure–volume relationship of air-filled versus liquid-filled lung from von Neergaard's original data (1929). **B,** The difference in recoil attributed to a liquid–air interface (i.e., "bubble lining") that is eliminated by a liquid-only interface. *P,* Pressure; *tiss,* tissue; *int,* air–liquid interface; *liq,* liquid.

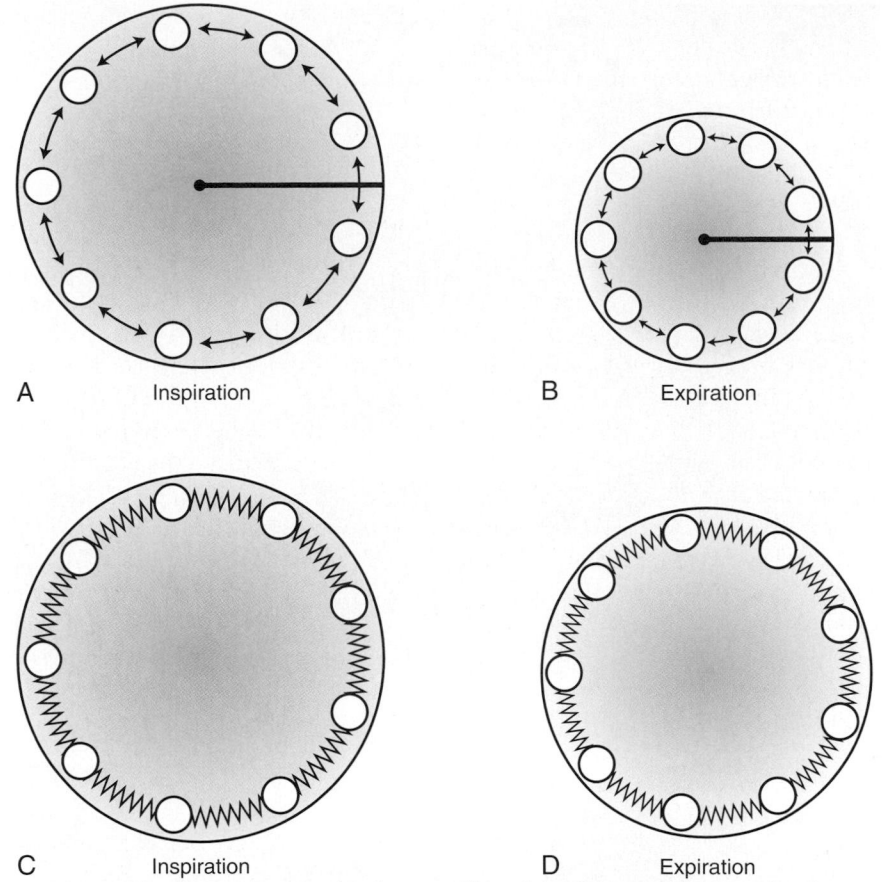

FIGURE 14-2 A, Alveolar surface tension is a manifestation of the strong attraction between molecules that are aligned on the surface of the alveoli. **B,** During expiration, when the alveolar radius is smaller, attraction between the molecules is stronger and there is a greater tendency to collapse. **C,** When surfactant is present, it spreads over the alveolus and dilutes the molecules. **D,** During expiration, the surfactant is compressed and the alveolar surface tension is lowered. This stabilizes the alveoli and prevents collapse of those alveoli with smaller radii.

Box 14-1	**Surfactant Function**

- Prevents collapse of lung during deflation (expiration)
- Lessens work of breathing (oxygen consumption)
- Optimizes surface area for gas exchange and ventilation–perfusion matching
- Optimizes lung compliance (high at low lung volumes and low at high lung volumes)
- Protects the lung epithelium and facilitates clearance of foreign material
- Prevents capillary leakage of fluid into alveoli
- Defends against microorganisms (infection)

by preterm infants with RDS. Surfactant functions are summarized in Box 14-1.

Surfactant Metabolism and Composition

Surfactant is produced by type II alveolar epithelial cells (pneumatocytes) in the lung (Figure 14-3). After synthesis, the surfactant components are packaged in the form of lamellar bodies and secreted into the fluid layer lining the alveoli in response to a variety of stimuli, including mechanical stretch (Figure 14-4). After secretion into the alveolar space, surfactant is transformed into tubular myelin, a highly organized, lipid-rich monolayer responsible for reducing surface tension. The half-time for turnover of human surfactant is not known, but in animals such as rats and rabbits it is 5 to 10 hours.[16] Secretion and clearance are balanced, with 90% of the surfactant being recycled by the type II pneumatocytes. Studies using labeled surfactant introduced into the airways have shown the majority being taken up directly by the pneumatocytes and being repackaged in lamellar bodies and eventually resecreted.[17] The remaining 10% are cleared by alveolar macrophages.

Surfactant composition is fairly constant among mammalian species. Surfactant is composed of approximately 90% lipids (of which 80% to 85% is phospholipids) and approximately 10% proteins (Table 14-1).[18] Phosphatidylcholine (PC) is the most abundant phospholipid (75% to 80%)

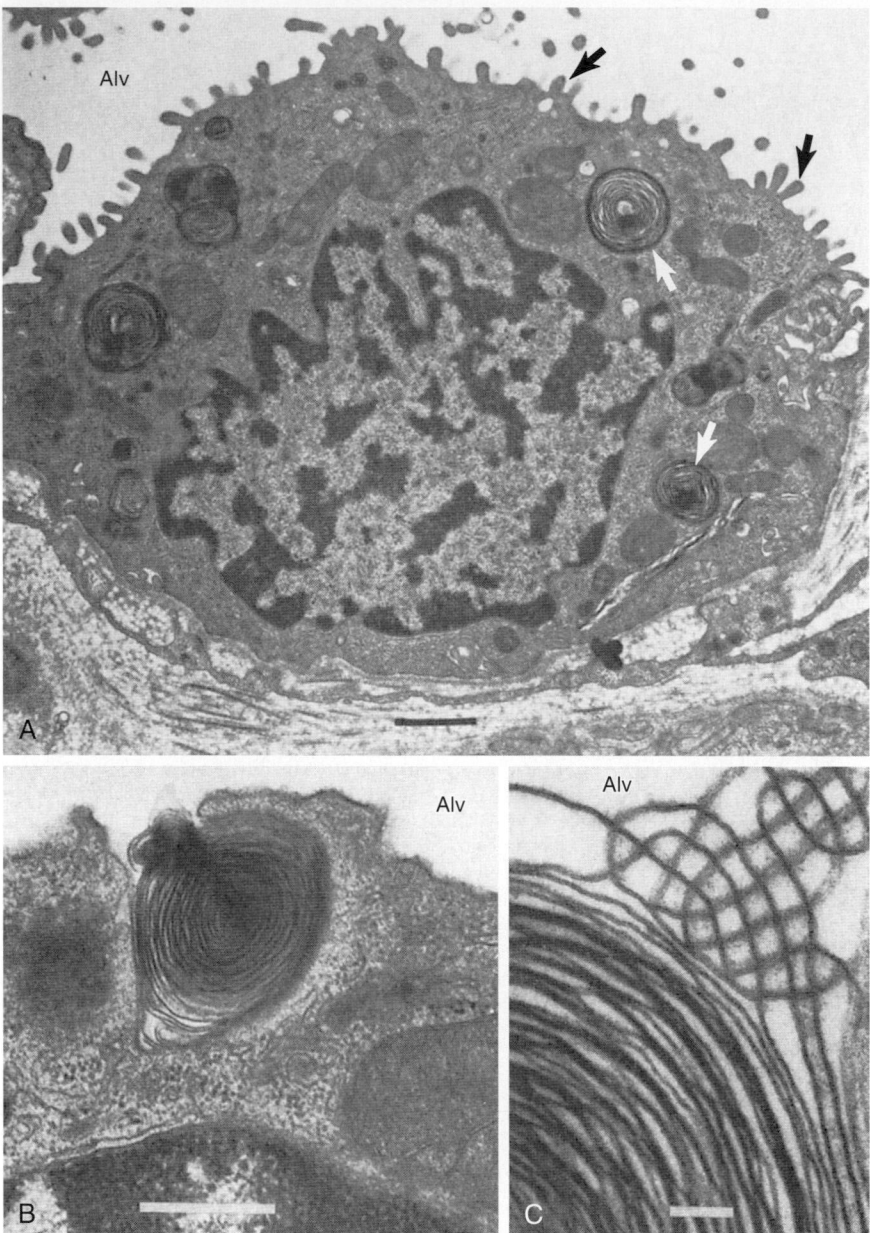

FIGURE 14-3 **A,** Type II cell from a human lung, showing characteristic lamellar inclusion bodies (*open arrows*) within the cell, which are the storage sites of intracellular surfactant. Microvilli (*solid arrows*) are projecting into the alveolus (*Alv*). **B,** Beginning exocytosis of a lamellar body into the alveolar space of a human lung. **C,** Secreted lamellar body and newly formed tubular myelin (appearing as a lattice) in the alveolar liquid in a fetal rat lung. Membrane continuities between outer lamellar bodies and adjacent tubular myelin provide evidence of intra-alveolar tubular myelin formation.

and is mostly saturated (40% to 55%) in the form of dipalmitoylphosphatidylcholine (DPPC). DPPC is the most important surfactant component in reducing surface tension and consists of two molecules of palmitic acid and one molecule of phosphatidylcholine attached to a glycerol backbone. DPPC has a hydrophobic end (fatty acids) and a hydrophilic end (nitrogenous base) and aligns itself in the air–liquid interface with the hydrophobic end toward the gas phase and the hydrophilic end toward the liquid phase (Figure 14-5). This configuration aligns

negative charges in the gas phase and positive charges in the liquid phase, allowing like charges to repel each other, displacing water and creating the pressure required to keep alveoli expanded during expiration. This alignment of DPPC is critical to the ability of surfactant to lower surface tension, and **surfactant proteins** B and C appear vital for this process. If proper alignment does not occur, positive and negative ends of DPPC attract and cause surfactant to clump together, rendering it ineffective and actually resulting in atelectasis.

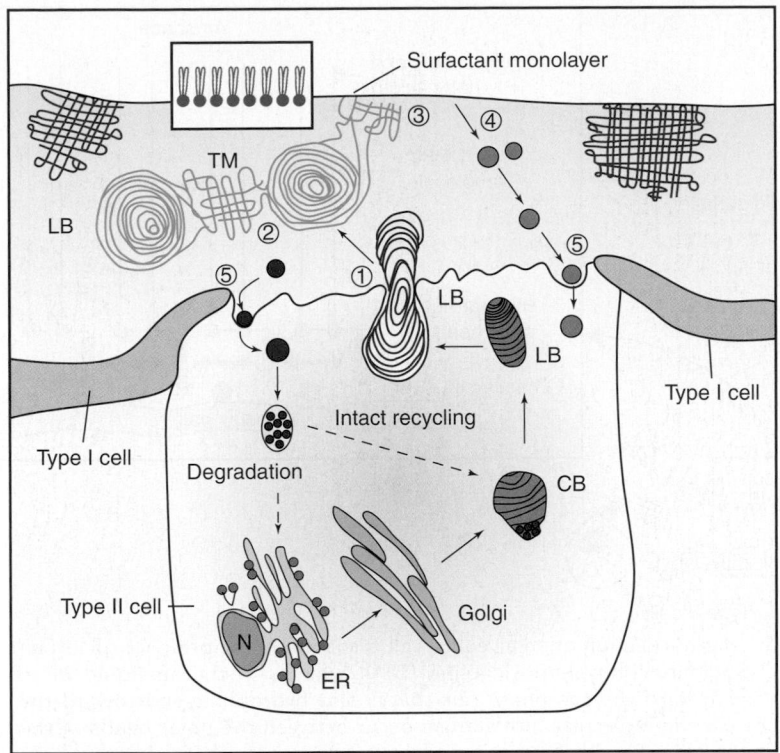

FIGURE 14-4   Schematic diagram of surfactant metabolism. *1,* secretion of LB; *2,* conversion of LB into TM; *3,* generation of monolayer from TM material; *4,* formation of small aggregate material from mono-layer; *5,* reuptake of surfactant material. In general, *solid arrows* indicate accepted pathways. Probable pathways are indicated by *dashed arrows*. *N,* nucleus; *ER,* endoplasmic reticulum; *CB,* composite body; *LB,* lamellar body; *TM,* tubular myelin.

TABLE 14-1

Components of Pulmonary Surfactant

Component	Amount	Function
Lipids	**90%-95%**	
1- Phospholipids	80%-85%	
1-1 Phosphatidylcholine (PC)	70%-75% of phospholipids	
Dipalmitoylphosphatidylcholine (DPCC, saturated)	50% of PC	Major surface-active species
1-palmitoyl-2-oleoyl-phosphatidylcholine (POPC, unsaturated)	50% of PC	Contributes to fluidify and improve dynamic behavior of surfactant
1-2 Anionic phospholipids: phosphatidylglycerol, phosphatidylinositol, phosphatidylserine	8%-15% of phospholipids	
1-2 Other phospholipids: phosphatidylethanolamine, sphingomyelin	5% of phospholipids	
2- Neutral lipids (mostly cholesterol [90%], diglycerides, triglycerides)	5%-10%	Antioxidant Membrane structure
3- Other lipids	2%	
Proteins	**5%-10%**	
1- Loosely associated (mainly serum)	0%-5%	
2- Surfactant apoproteins		
Hydrophilic proteins, SP-A, SP-D*	2%-4%	Participate in the innate host defense immune system
Hydrophobic proteins, SP-B, SP-C*	1%-2%	Enhances stability and spreading of lipids Critical for lamellar bodies formation (SP-B)

SP-A, Surfactant protein A; *SP-B,* surfactant protein B; *SP-C,* surfactant protein C; *SP-D,* surfactant protein D.

*Data from Rooney SA. The surfactant system and lung phospholipid biochemistry. *Am Rev Respir Dis* 1985;131:439; Young SL, et al. Pulmonary surfactant lipid production in oxygen-exposed rat lungs. *Lab Invest* 1982;46:570; Veldhuizen R, et al. The role of lipids in pulmonary surfactant. *Biochim Biophys Acta* 1998;1408(2-3):90–108; and Glasser, JR et al. Surfactant and its role in the pathobiology of pulmonary infection. *Microbes Infect* 2012;14(1):17–25.

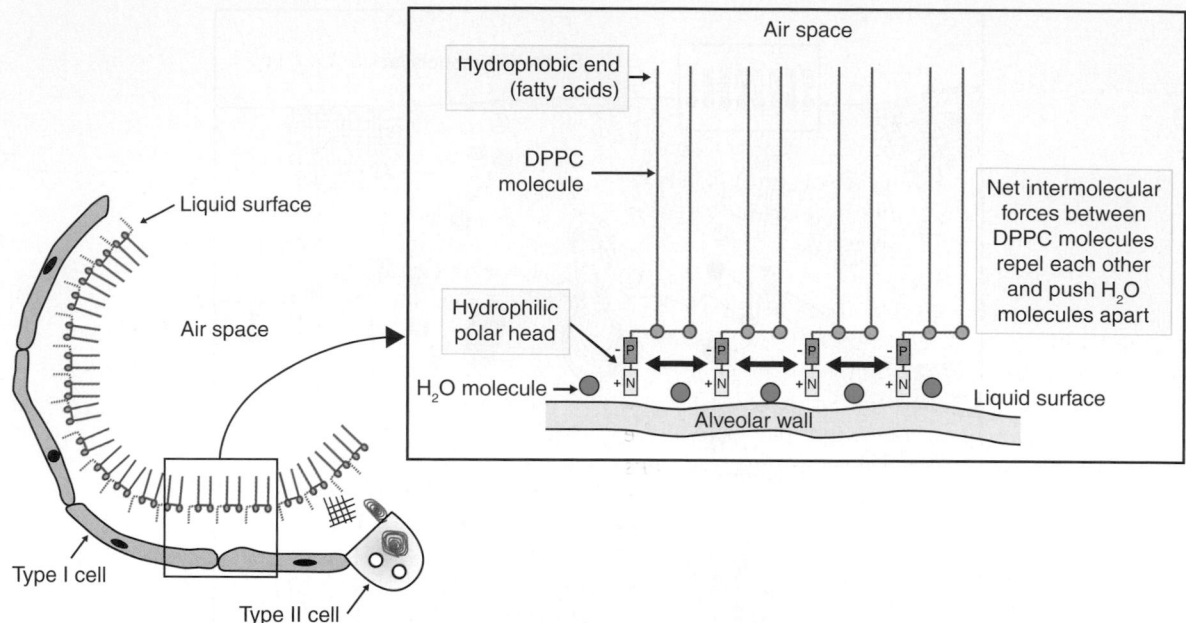

FIGURE 14-5 A cross-section of an alveolus wall is shown. In the presence of surfactant protein B (not shown), dipalmitoylphosphatidylcholine (DPPC) aligns in the air–liquid interface with the hydrophobic end toward the gas phase (air space) and hydrophilic end toward the liquid phase (liquid surface). Strong molecular interactions occur between the polar heads of the hydrophobic end. Note that the polar head has a positive charge associated with its nitrogenous base (*N*) and a negative charge associated with its phosphate group (*P*). This alignment creates electrostatic forces of repulsion, pushing water molecules apart, preventing atelectasis, and holding the airway open during exhalation.

Surfactant protein (SP)-A, SP-B, SP-C, and SP-D are the known proteins associated with surfactant.[13-22] SP-A and SP-D are hydrophilic (water soluble) and SP-B and SP-C are hydrophobic (lipid soluble and positively charged).

SP-A is a calcium-dependent collectin (collagen-like lectin). Collectins bind to the surface of microorganisms via polysaccharides, phospholipids, and glycolipids-dependent interactions and lead to aggregation, opsonization, and clearance of the organisms by alveolar macrophages in the lung. SP-A is the most abundant of the surfactant-associated proteins. It is thought to be important in the regulation of surfactant metabolism, as well as in tubular myelin formation.[23] The most important role of SP-A, however, is in innate host defense of the lung.[24] SP-A functions as an opsonin for bacteria, fungi, and viruses. In SP-A–deficient mice, tubular myelin is absent, but surfactant processing and function are intact. Despite relatively normal lung function, SP-A–deficient mice are highly susceptible to infections.

SP-D is also a collectin and enhances the binding, phagocytosis, and killing of microbes by alveolar macrophages.[24] In addition, SP-D has a role in the suppression of proinflammatory responses. Lack of SP-D in transgenic mice leads to emphysema, macrophage activation, accumulation of oxygen-reactive species, and increased surfactant alveolar pools. So SP-D also plays a key role in

surfactant homeostasis. Polymorphisms of the human genes for SP-A and SP-D have been documented and result in increased susceptibility to infections with respiratory syncytial virus and *Mycobacterium* tuberculosis.

SP-B is a membrane-associated protein that binds to the surface of lipid bilayers. SP-B, as discussed previously, is critical for alignment of surfactant at the air–liquid interface and for the formation of surfactant storage lamellar bodies in type II cells. SP-B is the only surfactant protein that humans cannot live without. SP-B protein deficiency is fatal in infancy without lung transplantation.

SP-C is necessary for the stability of the surfactant phospholipid film and for stability during dynamic compression in the respiratory cycle.[25] SP-C–deficient mice develop interstitial lung disease with emphysema, epithelial cell dysplasia, and inflammation. Infants with SP-C deficiency have RDS and pulmonary fibrosis. SP-C is not required for the formation of lamellar bodies or tubular myelin.

Other nonpulmonary surfactant-associated alveolar proteins are important in host defense: fibronectin, lysozyme, antiproteases, immunoglobulins (IgA), defensins, mucins, and Clara cell proteins. Excluding nonsurfactant proteins from the alveolus is critical to surfactant function and processing because surfactant homeostasis may be disrupted by blood proteins, albumin, fibrin, and edema, as well as other substances.

Hormonal Effects on Surfactant Production

Antenatal steroids have been extensively studied and have been shown to decrease RDS in infants between 24 and 34 weeks of gestation. There is no increased infection risk with rupture of membranes, including prolonged rupture of membranes or chorioamnionitis. A single course of corticosteroids is currently recommended by the American College of Obstetricians and Gynecologists (ACOG) for pregnant women between 24 weeks and 34 weeks of gestation who are at risk of preterm delivery within 7 days.[26] This course may consist of betamehasone (2 doses, 24 hours apart) or dexamethasone (4 doses, 12 hours apart). A single rescue course may be considered if the first course was given more than 2 weeks prior in women less than 32 6/7 weeks of gestation who are likely to deliver within the next week. Additional repeat courses have not demonstrated any benefit, may be associated with poorer outcomes, and are not recommended.[27,28] There is an increase in RNA within 2 hours of the first dose and an increase in protein secretion within 12 hours.[29] The full effect on surfactant production is present by 48 hours after the first dose. Antenatal steroid use in infants with less than 24 weeks of gestation has not been studied prospectively, but its use may be beneficial if resuscitation is planned.

Thyroid hormones, in addition to other hormones, are also important for lung development. Because thyroid hormones do not cross the placenta, several investigators examined antenatal thyrotropin-releasing hormone for the prevention of RDS in preterm infants. Unfortunately, no benefit was demonstrated in multicenter clinical trials.[30,31]

Fetal Lung Maturity Testing

Measurement of phospholipids in the amniotic fluid can be used to determine fetal lung maturity, because phosphatidylglycerol (PG) and phosphatidylcholine (lecithin) increase while sphingomyelin decreases during gestation. Available tests include quantification of phospholipids present in the amniotic fluid and measurement of surfactant characteristics as well as function and number of lamellar bodies (Table 14-2).[32] The first test used for this purpose was based on the lecithin-to-sphingomyelin ratio. PG measurement in the amniotic fluid is a more accurate test than lecithin-to-sphingomyelin ratios. PG is produced by type II pneumatocytes and is nearly undetectable until 35 weeks of gestation. Interestingly, PG is not required for surfactant function but correlates with pulmonary maturity. PG is now the basis of a rapid and inexpensive slide agglutination test (Amniostat-FLM-PG; Irvine Scientific, Santa Ana, Calif.) with 90% sensitivity. PG can be used for both amniotic fluid and vaginal pool samples in infants with premature rupture of membranes. False positives can occur if the samples are contaminated by bacteria containing PG in their cell wall. The TDx-FLMII (Abbott Diagnostics, Abbott Park, Ill.) a widely method to assess fetal lung

TABLE 14-2			
Fetal Lung Maturity Testing*			
Quantification of Surfactant Components	**Mature**	**Transitional**	**Immature**
Phospholipid measurement			
Lecithin-to-sphingomyelin ratio	>2.0	1.5-2.0	<1.5
Phosphatidylglycerol	Present	Trace	Absent
Desaturated phosphatidylcholine	>70	50-70	<50
Fluorescence detection	>50,000	15,000-70,000	<15,000
Microviscometer assay			
Lamellar bodies			
Lamellar body count	>32,000		
Surfactant characteristics			
Surfactant function			
Foam stability index	>48%	47%	<47%
Shake test			
Tap test			
Amniotic fluid turbidity			
Optical density			
Visual inspection			

*Includes testing values for the five most common tests.
From Geary CA, Whitsett JA. *Amniotic fluid markers of fetal lung maturity*. In: Spitzer AR, editor: Intensive care of the fetus and neonate, ed 2. St. Louis: Elsevier Mosby, 2005:122–132.

maturity is no longer available. The lamellar body count has now increased in popularity because it requires less than 1 ml of amniotic fluid, can be performed in 15 minutes, and retains a good specificity, with a count greater than 32,000 predicting a mature lecithin-to-sphingomyelin ratio in 99% of cases. Specific clinical settings need to be considered, because gestational diabetes delays maturation and PG is the preferred test. Fetal lung maturity may be accelerated in some but not all pregnancies with pregnancy-induced hypertension, intrauterine growth restriction, and in utero exposure to maternal smoking and cocaine.

SURFACTANT DYSFUNCTION IN ACUTE LUNG INJURY

Abnormalities in surfactant (quantity or pool size, function, composition, and metabolism), destruction or inactivation of surfactant, and direct type II cell damage have been described in ARDS and other types of acute lung injuries (Table 14-3).[34]

Altered Surfactant Quantity

The evidence related to altered surfactant pool size in acute lung injury is variable. Decreases, increases, and no changes in pool size have all been reported.[35-38] This confusion reflects the difficulty in quantifying surfactant material

TABLE 14-3

Diseases That Affect Surfactant

Surfactant Deficiency	Surfactant Inactivation/Inhibition	Surfactant Dysfunction
Respiratory distress syndrome	Aspiration syndromes Meconium	SP-C deficiency
SP-B deficiency	Blood Amniotic fluid	ABCA3 deficiency
	Pulmonary hemorrhage	Congenital diaphragmatic hernia
	Infections Pneumonia	Smoking and COPD
	Respiratory syncytial virus	Lung transplantation
	Sepsis	
	ARDS caused by: Near drowning Smoke inhalation Transfusions Trauma Sepsis	
	Pulmonary diseases Asthma Cystic fibrosis	

ARDS, Adult respiratory distress syndrome; *ABCA3,* member A3 of the ATP binding cassette family of proteins; *COPD,* chronic obstructive pulmonary disease; *SP-B,* surfactant protein B; *SP-C,* surfactant protein C.

obtained from bronchoalveolar lavage. Different clinical factors or types of lung injuries may affect the lung and surfactant function differently. For example, prolonged exposure to 85% oxygen results in type II alveolar cell hyperplasia and increased surfactant secretion, whereas 100% exposure decreases alveolar cell numbers and surfactant secretion.[20,39] Direct type II cell injury or necrosis will result in a decreased surfactant pool. At present, no firm conclusions can be drawn regarding the effects of acute lung injury on the quantity of surfactant.

Altered Surfactant Composition

A consistent finding in studies of acute lung injury is that alterations in the composition of surfactant occur. These findings include a decrease in surfactant-associated proteins in patients with ARDS and decreases in the quantities of phosphatidylcholine and phosphatidylglycerol along with an increase in sphingomyelin and other phospholipids.[37,40] Furthermore, these abnormalities appear to reverse with recovery from acute lung injury.[41,42] The relationship of these abnormalities in surfactant composition to lung dysfunction is unknown, but surfactant isolated from animal models of lung injury has abnormal surface activity in vitro.[42,43]

Altered Surfactant Metabolism

Studies indicate that surfactant metabolism may be altered in acute lung injury. Animals injured by hyperoxia

have decreased incorporation of surfactant precursors into lung tissue that reverses with recovery.[44] Other animal models show more rapid conversion of large to small surfactant forms that have poor surface tension–lowering properties. Bronchoalveolar lavage specimens from patients with ARDS also support evidence of altered surfactant metabolism, showing increased levels of proteases and alterations in the density profiles of surfactant.[45]

Surfactant Inactivation

Inactivation by proteins is the most common surfactant abnormality seen in acute lung injury. These proteins competitively displace surfactant phospholipid from the alveolar monolayer and are less surface-active molecules than surfactant; this results in a decreased capacity to reduce surface tension.

Many etiologies are associated with increased capillary permeability leading to pulmonary edema and resulting in surfactant inactivation. Albumin, hemoglobin, fibrin, complement, blood, meconium, and other proteins may gain access to the alveolar space secondary to alveolar–capillary membrane damage and have been shown in vitro to diminish the surface tension–reducing properties of surfactant.[45-47] Proteins compete with surfactant for the air-fluid interface and interfere with monolayer formation.[48] Several blood components are strong inactivators of surfactant including hemoglobin, fibrin, fibrinogen, red blood cell membrane lipids, immunoglobulins, and plasma proteins. Similarly, several substances in meconium inactivate or alter surfactant function, including proteolytic enzymes, free fatty acids, phospholipases, bile salts, lanugo, squamous cells, bilirubin, steroid compounds, cholesterol, and triglycerides.[12] Regardless of the etiology, surfactant inactivation leads to diminished lung compliance, increased intrapulmonary shunting, and atelectasis characteristic of ARDS (Figure 14-6).[49]

CLINICAL APPLICATIONS AND REPLACEMENT

The typical clinical presentation of surfactant deficiency is summarized in Table 14-4. At present, exogenous surfactant administration is most commonly used for prophylaxis or treatment of preterm infants with RDS. It is also increasingly used in neonates as well as pediatric and adult patients in diseases associated with or leading to surfactant inactivation.

Respiratory Distress Syndrome
Incidence

Typically, RDS affects premature infants born at less than 35 weeks of gestation. Its incidence increases with lower gestational ages. RDS affects 86% of infants weighing 501 to 750 g at birth, 79% of infants weighing 751 to 1000 g, 48% of infants at 1000 to 1250 g, and 27% between 1251 and 1500 g.[50] Representative chest radiographs of a premature

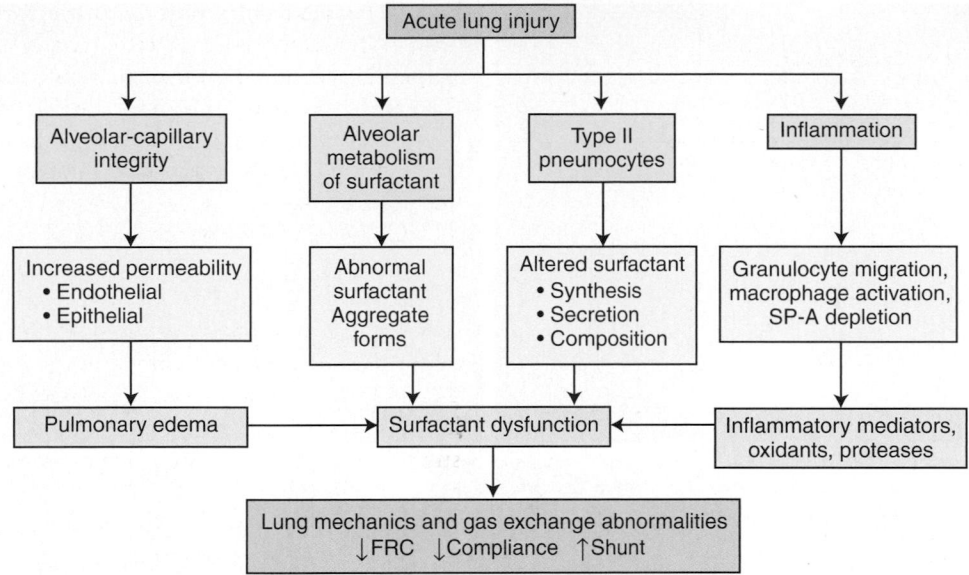

FIGURE 14-6 Four pathways that contribute to surfactant dysfunction during acute lung injury. *FRC*, Functional residual capacity; *SP-A*, surfactant protein A.

TABLE 14-4

Clinical Presentation of Surfactant Deficiency RDS and ARDS

Pathophysiology	Laboratory Changes	Physical Examination	Radiographic Changes
Atelectasis	↓ PO_2	Lung	Diffuse reticular granular pattern
↓FRC	↑ Carbon dioxide	Tachypnea	Air bronchograms
Ventilation–perfusion mismatch	Metabolic acidosis	Apnea	Atelectasis
		Increased work of breathing (nasal flaring, retractions, grunting)	
		↓ Breath sounds	
		Poor air entry	
		Cardiovascular	
		Cyanosis (oxygen requirement)	
		Pallor	
		Poor perfusion	

ARDS, Acute respiratory distress syndrome; *FRC*, functional residual capacity; *PO_2*, oxygen pressure; *RDS*, respiratory distress syndrome.

infant with RDS before and after surfactant administration as well as typical pathology findings in RDS are presented in Figure 14-7.

Treatment

Early experimental animal studies with administration of phospholipid mixtures showed some effect, but more dramatic and sustained improvements in oxygenation could be demonstrated only with natural surfactant complexes, harvested from the lavage of adult rabbit lungs, and later obtained from cows, pigs, and human amniotic fluid. Bioactivity of the synthetic preparations was improved with the addition of alcohols such as hexadecanol as well as tyloxapol (a formaldehyde polymer) to enhance dispersion and spread in the aqueous phase.

The first human trial in 1980 by Fujiwara and colleagues showed that natural animal-derived surfactant was effective in treating 10 premature infants with RDS.[11] The investigators instilled 3 to 5 ml of surfactant (from minced bovine extract and containing DPPC) directly to the trachea and enhanced distribution by changing the position of the infant. They demonstrated a prompt increase in oxygenation after one dose that was sustained for 2 to 3 days in some infants. This represented a marked improvement when compared with results obtained with synthetic DPPC.

Large controlled trials have since established that surfactant preparations greatly reduce mortality in preterm infants. Surfactant replacement for prophylaxis or treatment of RDS has reduced the risk of pneumothorax by 30% to 65% and death by about 40%.[51] Early analysis

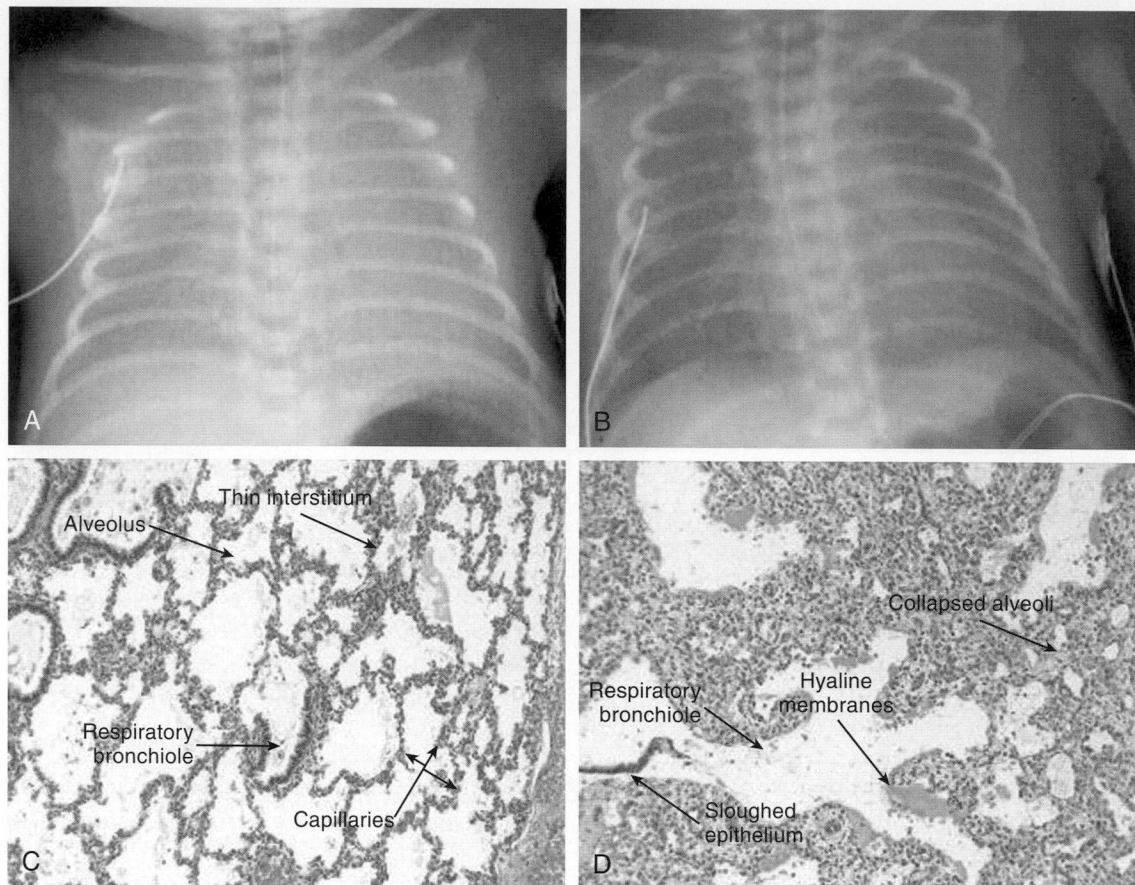

FIGURE 14-7   A, Chest radiograph of a premature infant with respiratory distress syndrome (RDS) demonstrating diffuse reticulogranular pattern (ground-glass appearance), air bronchograms, and low lung volume. **B,** Chest radiograph of the same premature infant after surfactant administration, demonstrating improved lung volumes. **C,** Photomicrograph of normal alveoli, demonstrating normal microscopic structure of the lung of a newborn infant. Clear areas are the air-containing expanded alveoli. The colored structures that form a honeycomb lattice are the walls that line the alveolar space. **D,** Microscopic structure of the lung from a premature infant who died of RDS. The normal honeycomb lattice is collapsed (atelectasis), the alveolar walls are adherent to each other, and the lung is almost airless. Those air-containing spaces (clear areas) that do remain are lined by a pink-staining layer of inflammatory protein termed the hyaline membrane. (Photos courtesy Drs. David Kaufman and Robin LeGallo.)

showed a possible decrease in bronchopulmonary dysplasia, but it is now accepted by experts in the field that surfactants do not reduce the overall incidence of chronic lung disease or bronchopulmonary dysplasia.[2] Surfactant administration is also not associated with significant changes in intraventricular hemorrhage (IVH), patent ductus arteriosus (PDA), or retinopathy of prematurity. However, in one study, infants weighing more than 1250 g had a lower incidence of IVH and PDA.[52]

Two clinical strategies are currently used: (1) prophylaxis within 15 to 30 minutes of birth in small premature infants and (2) rescue treatment in infants with clinical evidence of RDS.

Prophylactic Surfactant

Prophylactic surfactant administration grew out of animal data demonstrating decreased epithelial damage and

pulmonary edema when surfactant is given in the first 15 minutes of life.[53]

Prophylactic surfactant is administered after initial stabilization in the first 15 minutes after birth, compared with 1.5 to 7.4 hours in rescue strategies. Initial studies comparing prophylactic to rescue surfactant favored the former with noted decrease in mortality, pneumothorax, and pulmonary interstitial emphysema.[2] The majority of studies included larger premature infants (up to 30 weeks of gestation) and were conducted before the era of systematic antenatal steroid administration and routine postdelivery stabilization on continuous positive airway pressure (CPAP). All these factors are likely to have affected the rates of RDS, air leak, IVH, and mortality. Therefore, there is some debate as to whether a lower threshold for prophylaxis (e.g., less than 750 g, less than 1000 g, or less than 27 to 28 weeks of gestation) would define a higher risk group and avoid unnecessary prophylaxis of more mature infants.

Two large randomized controlled trials (the COIN and SUPPORT trials)[54,55] have examined the use of early stabilization with nasal CPAP (NCPAP) versus early intubation and surfactant administration in extremely low birth weight infants. In the COIN trial,[55] 610 extremely preterm infants (25 to 28 weeks of gestation), who were not intubated at 5 minutes of life, were randomized to either NCPAP or intubation with ventilation.[56] A distending pressure of 8 cm H_2O was used in the NCPAP group, notably higher than CPAP levels used in other centers. The authors' rationale to start with 8 cm was that distending pressure is important for maintaining functional residual capacity and for improving lung compliance and oxygenation, and 8 cm H_2O had been shown to be more effective than a lower pressure.[57] Forty-six percent of infants in the NCPAP group eventually required intubation (55% for infants born at 25 or 26 weeks of gestation and 40% for those born at 27 or 28 weeks of gestation). The total days requiring intubation and ventilation were less in the NCPAP group ($P < 0.001$). The need for surfactant use was 50% less in the NCPAP group (38% vs. 77%; $P < 0.001$). Pneumothorax was more common in the NCPAP group (9.1% vs. 3%; $P < 0.001$), with 98% of those infants needing intubation, but there was no increase in intracranial hemorrhage. There was no difference in oxygen requirement at 36 weeks postmenstrual age, mortality, or length of hospitalization. In the SUPPORT trial,[54] 1316 extremely

preterm infants (24 to 27 weeks of gestation) were randomly assigned to nasal CPAP in the delivery room or intubation and surfactant treatment (less than 1 hour after birth). Infants in the CPAP group less frequently required intubation or postnatal corticosteroids for bronchopulmonary dysplasia ($P < 0.001$), required fewer days of mechanical ventilation ($P = 0.03$), and were more likely to be alive and free from the need for mechanical ventilation by day 7 ($P = 0.01$). There was no difference in the rate of bronchopulmonary disease (BPD; 47.8 vs. 51%).

These studies suggest that for infants older than 24 weeks and demonstrating adequate respiratory effort, the use of early CPAP is a reasonable alternative to early intubation for prophylactic surfactant. However, clear guidelines for surfactant administration need to be in place if such strategies are to be applied successfully. It is also important to remember that in ventilated preterm infants, early surfactant administration results in decreased mortality (RR 0.84; 95% confidence interval [CI] 0.74 to 0.95) and chronic lung disease (RR 0.69; 95% CI 0.55 to 0.86).[58]

Strategies for surfactant administration are summarized in Table 14-5.

Rescue Surfactant and Repeat Doses

In patients to whom prophylactic surfactant is not given, clinical signs and symptoms of RDS can be used to determine the need for surfactant administration (see Table 14-4). However, specific criteria for surfactant administration for infants on CPAP are still an area of debate. A reasonable approach

TABLE 14-5

Surfactant Delivery

	Comments	Studies
Timing		
Prophylaxis	Surfactant given <15 minutes after birth, before symptoms appear	↓ PTX and mortality in infants <31 wk[72]
Rescue	At time of clinical signs and symptoms	↓ PTX and mortality[2]
Subsequent dosing	Required if inactivation or insufficient delivery of surfactant	Surfactant may be redosed in the first 48-96 h after presentation
		Usually one or two doses are sufficient. Third and fourth doses did not improve outcomes[73]
Administration		
Adapter	ETT with side adapter or Y-adapter attached to ETT	Minimizes desaturation caused by disconnection from positive pressure ventilation or the ventilator for administration
Delivery	Bolus intratracheal administration	Bolus administration ↓ homogeneous distribution
		Slow infusion ↓ nonhomogeneous distribution pattern in animals
		Aerosolization ↓ only small amounts of aerosolized surfactant are delivered to the lung[74]
		Efficacy currently being reevaluated as noninvasive ventilation becomes more common[64,75]
Dose	75-100 mg/kg	75-100 mg/kg to overcome destruction by macrophages and inhibition by plasma proteins
		100 and 120 mg/kg produced better results than 50 and 60 mg/kg[76,77]
		Equal efficacy of 100 and 200 mg/kg of porcine surfactant[78,79]

Continued

TABLE 14-5		
Surfactant Delivery—cont'd		
	Comments	Studies
Surfactant products and dose (phospholipid/dose)	Intratracheal administration	Calfactant: 3 ml/kg (105 mg) q6h up to four doses Poractant: 2.5 ml/kg (200 mg), then 1.25 ml/kg (100 mg) q12h Beractant 4 ml/kg (100) q6h up to four doses
Aliquots	To enhance delivery distribution in the lung	No difference if dose is divided into two or four aliquots[80]
Positioning	Position infant with either the right or left side dependent for administration in two aliquots Deliver as fast as possible for improved distribution Maintain the position for about 10 seconds NOTE: a four-position, four-aliquot technique is equivalent[80]	Although recommended, it is not necessary to move infant into different positions during instillation because exogenous surfactant has remarkable spreading properties
Monitoring		
	Oxygenation	Side effects include cyanosis, bradycardia, reflux of surfactant into the ETT, and airway obstruction Surfactant delivery should be paused until vital signs recover and ETT clears of visible surfactant Infant may need to be repositioned prone and positive pressure ventilation increased for lung inflation
	Heart rate Presence of surfactant in the ETT	

ETT, Endotracheal tube; *PTX,* pneumothorax.

would be to provide early rescue surfactant for those infants with evidence of moderate to severe RDS on chest radiograph and fraction of inspired oxygen (FiO_2) above 30% to 50% (depending on gestational age and whether or not antenatal steroids were used).[59] There is evidence that early rescue surfactant results in decreased need for mechanical ventilation, decreased BPD, and decreased pneumothoraces, particularly when given at a lower threshold ($FiO_2 < 0.45$).[60,61] Surfactant can be provided using the intubation-surfactant-extubation (INSURE) procedure. Risk factors for INSURE failure include weight less than 750 g, Po_2/FiO_2 less than 218, and arterial/alveolar oxygen tension ratio (a/Apo_2) less than 0.44.[62] The use of a laryngeal mask airway, obviating the need for intubation and possibly mechanical ventilation, has been shown to be effective in larger infants.[63] Additionally, other minimally invasive methods of surfactant administration, including aerolized surfactant[64] or via insertion of a thin catheter into the trachea,[65] are currently being investigated to facilitate the administration of surfactant in spontaneously breathing infants with RDS.

Redosing of surfactant in infants with RDS has been shown to result in improved oxygenation, decreased ventilatory requirement, and fewer pneumothoraces.[66] The criteria for surfactant redosing remains an area of controversy. A few studies have demonstrated some short-term but no long-term benefits with retreatment at a low threshold (still intubated, mean airway pressure greater

than 6 cm H_2O, with FiO_2 more than 0.030), versus high threshold (still intubated, mean airway pressure greater than 7 cm H_2O and FiO_2 more than 0.040) or an increase in FiO_2 up to 0.10.[51] Early rescue compared with late rescue strategies have demonstrated decreased mortality and decreased incidence of pneumothorax.[67]

Natural versus Synthetic Preparations

At present there are several different types of exogenous commercial surfactants[51,68] (Table 14-6): minced bovine lung lipid extracts enriched with synthetic lipids (beractant [Survanta, Abbott Nutrition, Columbus, OH, and surfactant TA [Surfacten, Mitsubishi Tokyo Tanabe Pharma, Tokyo, Japan]), bovine lung lavage lipid extracts (calfactant [Infasurf, ONY Inc., Amherst, NY] and bovactant SF-RI [Alveofact, Boehringer Ingelheim, Ingelheim, Germany]), minced porcine lung enriched by chromatography (poractant alpha [Curosurf; Chiesi Farmaceutici, Parma, Italy], and a mixture of synthetic lipids. The bovine surfactants contain SP-B and SP-C, but not SP-A. Calfactant contains much more SP-B and SP-C than does beractant. The synthetic surfactants contain no proteins. Compared with older synthetic surfactants, natural surfactants have a more rapid onset of action, allow the fraction of inspired oxygen to be reduced faster, and decrease the incidence of pneumothorax as well as mortality. Clinical trials comparing different natural surfactants have not clearly demonstrated

The use of dilute surfactant lavage has also been studied in severe MAS. The principle is that both surfactant delivery and meconium removal can be achieved by lavage, because surfactant facilitates the removal of foreign debris. A pilot trial using large volumes (48 ml/kg of lucinactant) reported not statistically significant trends toward more rapid extubation and decreased FiO$_2$ requirements for lucinactant-lavaged infants.[92] However, one third of the patients had bloody effluents, and more infants in the lavage group (one third) met failure criteria. In addition, surfactant–saline lavage was associated with significant oxygen desaturation during administration, resulting in interruption of the procedure in 20% of the subjects because of hypoxemia or hypotension. The effects of surfactant lavage with lower volume (15 ml/kg of lucinactant) were evaluated in a small randomized controlled trial (66 infants with MAS).[93] There was no change in duration of respiratory support, but the combined outcome of mortality or need for ECMO was reduced in the lung lavage group (10% vs. 31%, OR 0.24; 95% CI, 0.060 to 0.97). Tolerance was improved with this lower volume of lung lavage, with only transient desaturations and no associated changes in heart rate or blood pressure noted during administration.

Randomized trials are needed to compare surfactant lavage strategies versus standard surfactant administration, because they may have the same efficacy. In addition, saline may not be an ideal fluid for lung lavage and perfluorocarbons (used in liquid ventilation trials) may offer an attractive alternative because they have gas exchange properties.

In summary, for MAS, surfactant given early in patients meeting similar respiratory criteria as those with surfactant deficiency (intubated on more than 30% to 40% oxygen) and redosing using similar criteria is important to translating this evidence into clinical practice.

Pneumonia and Sepsis

Infection and inflammation are associated with inflammatory mediators (transforming growth factor β, tumor necrosis factor α, interleukin [IL]-1, IL-5, IL-6, and IL-8) that lead to surfactant alteration, some degree of capillary leak, and pulmonary edema.[94] The combination of edema and leak of plasma proteins into the alveolus leads to surfactant dysfunction. Microorganisms may also directly injure type II cells. Specific microbes may produce substances that downregulate SP-B and SP-C production, catalyze phospholipid hydrolysis (breakdown), and alter fatty acid composition. In animal studies of group B *Streptococcus* pneumonia, surfactant decreased bacterial proliferation and improved compliance compared with controls.[95,96]

A retrospective study of 118 infants with group B *Streptococcus* infection demonstrated improvement in oxygenation and mean airway pressure.[97] The authors compared the infected surfactant-treated group with infants with RDS and noted that the infected patients had a slower response and were more likely to need repeated doses. In the multicenter placebo-controlled trial in neonates by Lotze and co-workers discussed earlier, 30% of the enrolled infants in both groups had sepsis.[89] Surfactant decreased the need for ECMO, and the effect was greatest in the infants with an oxygen index between 15 and 22, suggesting that earlier treatment may improve outcomes. Randomized controlled trials are required to evaluate this issue further.[98]

Congenital Diaphragmatic Hernia

Infants with congenital diaphragmatic hernia (CDH) have immature lung development. In addition, relative surfactant deficiency has been demonstrated in animal models as well as in infants with CDH.[99,100] Exogenous surfactant replacement first demonstrated some efficacy in infants with CDH in a series of small case reports.[101-103] Several large series have reported improved outcomes (survival and no need for ECMO) in infants with CDH. In these studies patients received surfactant as part of a gentle ventilation strategy aimed at limiting barotraumas and volutrauma (with either conventional or high-frequency ventilation), with some patients also receiving nitric oxide.[104-108] The use of surfactant in infants with CDH has been incorporated into the treatment protocols of patients with CDH at many centers. Analysis of data from the CDH registry regarding surfactant use in infants with CDH did not demonstrate any benefit.[109-112] However, the subjects were not randomized, only a subset of the registry was analyzed, and there were no specific guidelines for surfactant use or criteria for ECMO. Therefore, it is possible that the more severely affected infants with CDH received surfactant, skewing the results. Randomized controlled trials in this area are still needed to clarify the potential benefits of surfactant replacement therapy in infants with CDH.

Extracorporeal Membrane Oxygenation

ECMO and cardiopulmonary bypass are associated with the development of an inflammatory-mediated capillary leak syndrome. This leads to fluid and neutrophil accumulation in the lungs and interstitial tissues, resulting in pulmonary edema and in turn prolonging time receiving ECMO. Inflammatory mediators attract and activate white blood cells, possibly contributing to lung injury and edema. Some infants receiving ECMO are unable to wean and may benefit from surfactant administration if surfactant inhibition is contributory to their respiratory failure. A blinded, randomized, controlled study of multiple-dose surfactant therapy demonstrated decreased ECMO duration as well as reduced disease complications.[113] Four doses of modified bovine lung surfactant extract (beractant) were administered to the surfactant group (n = 28), and an equal volume of air was administered to the control group (n = 28). The ECMO treatment period was significantly shorter in the surfactant group (P = 0.023). The overall incidence of complications after ECMO was also decreased in the surfactant group (18% vs. 46%; $P = 0.025$).

Infants with CDH requiring ECMO are a challenging patient group to manage. After surgery, failure to wean off of ECMO may be due to:

· Severe pulmonary hypoplasia (as indicated by ECMO requirement for their management)
· Severe pulmonary hypertension
· Pulmonary edema
· Surfactant inactivation
· Complications of surgery

One study examined whether surfactant administration could improve outcomes and decrease the duration of ECMO for infants with CDH.[114] These infants received either four doses of surfactant (beractant, n = 9) or an equal volume of air (control group, n = 8). Tracheal aspirate SP-A concentrations were initially low, and then increased over time in both CDH groups. Lung compliance, time to extubation, time on oxygen, and total number of hospital days were not different between the two groups.

Acute Respiratory Distress Syndrome

Significant impairments of surfactant production and composition have been demonstrated in the lungs of patients with ARDS. Surfactant alterations include reduced phospholipid content and, in particular, reduced DPPC levels, as well as decreased levels of surfactant-associated proteins.[37,115,116] These changes lead to decreased surface activity, resulting in the atelectasis and decreased lung compliance characteristic of ARDS.

Three large trials failed to demonstrate a benefit of surfactant therapy in adult patients with ARDS.[117-119] In children with ARDS, the efficacy of surfactant therapy has been assessed in several pilot studies. Calfactant administration to children with hypoxemic respiratory failure resulted in immediate improvement in oxygenation, as well as a 32% reduction in time requiring mechanical ventilation and a 30% reduction in stay in the pediatric intensive care unit.[120]

In a separate study, 20 children with an acute pulmonary disease and severe hypoxemia (13 with systemic or pulmonary disease and 7 with cardiac disease) received poractant alpha. There was a moderate improvement in oxygenation among patients with systemic or pulmonary disease but not in children with hypoxemic pulmonary pathology in the postoperative period of cardiovascular surgery. The improvement in oxygenation of the patients who survived was greater than that of those who died.[121]

A multicenter, randomized control trial was published comparing 153 children with respiratory failure from acute lung injury and assigned to 2 doses of calfactant 12 hours apart versus placebo.[122] Calfactant acutely improved oxygenation, with a decrease in the oxygen index from 20 to 13.9. In addition, there was a significant decrease in mortality in the calfactant group, with an odds ratio of 2.32 (95% CI, 1.15 to 4.85). In this study, no difference in duration of mechanical ventilation, intensive care unit stay, or hospital stay was noted. Adverse effects of the therapy were minimal, and in those patients who did not benefit it did not cause harm. The authors of this study have discussed that although this treatment is still under investigation, patients with direct lung injury such as near drowning, pneumonia, or trauma with severe pulmonary compromise, may benefit, whereas patients with diseases involving ongoing capillary leak (e.g., sepsis) do not respond.

Although promising, the results of these studies are confounded by variability in dosing, time of administration, and type of surfactant. In addition, attention to patient population, immune status, and mechanism of lung injury should be integrated into the design of future surfactant trials for ARDS.

Viral Bronchiolitis

Impairment in surfactant function has been reported in patients with viral bronchiolitis,[123] including reduced levels of SP-A, SP-B, and SP-D as well as decreased DPPC.[124,125] In a small randomized controlled trial of poractant alpha in 20 infants with severe RSV bronchiolitis surfactant therapy appeared to improve gas exchange, reduce peak inspiratory pressure, and shorten time on conventional ventilation and duration of intensive care unit stay.[126] In a second randomized trial 19 ventilated infants with RSV bronchiolitis received beractant or placebo. Again, patients in the surfactant group had improved oxygenation, improved lung compliance, and shortened time on ventilation.[127] A recent Cochrane review concluded that larger trials are required to evaluate the efficacy of surfactant replacement in bronchiolitis.[128]

Asthma

Decreased SP-A levels have been reported in sputum from patients with acute asthma.[129] In addition, antigen challenge of patients with asthma results in altered phospholipid properties and increased surface tension.[130] A pilot placebo-controlled trial of surfactant replacement therapy (Surfactant TA) was conducted in 11 adult patients with acute asthma. Respiratory functions were significantly improved in all patients in the surfactant group, including forced vital capacity, forced expiratory volume in 1 second, and arterial partial pressure of oxygen. No difference was detected in arterial partial pressure of carbon dioxide.[131] However, in 12 children with asthma, there was no significant improvement in airflow obstruction and bronchial responsiveness to histamine after surfactant nebulization (Bovactant SF-RI).[132] Additional studies, particularly focusing on synthetic surfactant to avoid a potential immune response to natural surfactant, are necessary to clarify the benefits of surfactant replacement in asthma.[133]

Cystic Fibrosis

Multiple studies have looked at surfactant in patients with CF, with contrasting results that may be explained in part by the age of the patients. In young patients, no difference in SP-A levels are noted; however, with the development of inflammation, increased levels are observed.[134] In patients with more chronic CF, SP-A levels decrease.[135,136] Griese and co-workers also demonstrated deficient surface tension ability of phospholipids in patients with CF when compared with healthy control subjects.[137] In contrast, Postle and co-workers found no difference in phospholipids.[136] In 2005 the surfactant function of 20 patients with CF was studied longitudinally. The study demonstrated a progressive loss of surfactant function, which correlated with increased inflammation and decreased lung function. In this study, the concentrations of SP-A, SP-C, and SP-D did not change, whereas that of SP-B increased.[138]

No therapeutic trials in children have been published. A pilot study of Bovactant SF-RI versus placebo in adults with severe CF showed no improvement in lung function or oxygenation.[137]

FUTURE DIRECTIONS

Today, thanks to surfactant replacement therapy, RDS is an uncommon cause of death in the preterm infant. Annual deaths from RDS in the United States have decreased from 10,000 to 15,000 per year in the 1950s to less than 1000 in 2002. If surfactant replacement is unequivocally effective in treating surfactant-deficient preterm infants, current evidence suggests that it may prove useful as an adjunctive therapy when surfactant dysfunction is a contributing factor in acute respiratory failure. Thus surfactant replacement offers promise to improve disturbed lung physiology and allow moderation of ventilator support in children with acute respiratory failure.

However, challenges remain in the area of surfactant uses and delivery. Technical aspects, including timing of delivery, number of doses, and mode of delivery, need to be studied in relation to specific disease type. The development of less invasive modes of surfactant delivery is currently being evaluated and will likely change clinical practice in the near future. Other future developments are likely to focus on increased use of synthetic surfactants containing genetically engineered surfactant-associated proteins. These synthetic surfactants are potentially more effective because of their constant and known composition, but they also offer less risk to the patient.

Finally, increased understanding of individual genetic polymorphisms regarding surfactant-associated proteins[130,140] may lead to the identification of patients who will or will not benefit from surfactant administration.

KEY POINTS

- Pulmonary surfactant is a complex mixture of lipids and protein that lowers surface tension proportionally to alveolar size and prevents alveolar collapse during expiration.
- Surfactant proteins A and D are important components of innate immunity for inhaled pathogens.
- Surfactant deficiency, dysfunction, or inactivation underlies the pathophysiology of many respiratory disorders including, RDS, ARDS, and MAS.
- Exogenous surfactant replacement therapy was first used successfully to treat neonatal RDS.
- Surfactant replacement therapy is an active area of research, with studies investigating its efficacy in other patient populations, including those with ARDS, asthma, and cystic fibrosis.

CASE STUDY 1

An 800-g baby boy is born by spontaneous vaginal delivery at 26 weeks of gestation as a result of cervical incompetence. The infant is active, with Apgar scores of 5 and 6, and needs positive pressure ventilation to establish regular respirations. Grunting occurs immediately, and a nasal continuous positive airway pressure (NCPAP) of 5 cm H_2O is applied after positive pressure ventilation at 5 minutes. The chest radiograph demonstrates a homogeneous ground-glass pattern. The infant's first arterial blood gas determination at 30 minutes of life on 70% oxygen produces the following results: pH 7.10; PCO_2, 78 mm Hg; PO_2, 52 mm Hg.

What would you do at this point? (NOTE: More than one answer may be acceptable.)

A. Continue NCPAP.
B. Perform endotracheal intubation.
C. Perform endotracheal intubation and administer surfactant.
D. Increase the FIO_2.

See Evolve Resources for answers.

CASE STUDY 2

A full-term infant is delivered by STAT cesarian section for fetal heart rate decelerations. Thick meconium is noted when membranes are ruptured during the C section. The obstetrician suctions the infant and then the pediatrician performs endotracheal intubation and suctions the airway. On physical examination, the infant has significant grunting and intercostal retractions. The trachea is reintubated and the infant is placed on high-frequency oscillatory ventilation. He requires an FIO_2 of 1.0 and has preductal saturations of 90% and postductal saturations of 85%. The chest radiograph demonstrates bilateral streaky densities throughout the lung fields.

What is this infant at risk for? (NOTE: More than one answer may be acceptable.)
- **A.** Pneumothorax
- **B.** Persistent pulmonary hypertension of the newborn
- **C.** Respiratory distress syndrome
- **D.** Aspiration pneumonia

See Evolve Resources for answers.

ASSESSMENT QUESTIONS

See Evolve Resources for answers.

1. What is/are the most abundant components of surfactant?
   - **A.** Dipalmitoylphosphatidylcholine (DPPC)
   - **B.** Surfactant protein B
   - **C.** SP-C
   - **D.** Phosphatidylglycerol
2. Surfactant inactivation and dysfunction have not been described in which of the following diseases?
   - **A.** Meconium aspiration syndrome
   - **B.** Asthma
   - **C.** Cystic fibrosis
   - **D.** Congenital heart disease
   - **E.** Sepsis
3. Natural surfactant preparations come from which of the following mammals (select all that apply)?
   - **A.** Pigs
   - **B.** Cows
   - **C.** Calves
   - **D.** Horses
   - **E.** Whales
4. Which air sac in the following diagram requires higher pressure to inflate (assuming similar surface tension)?

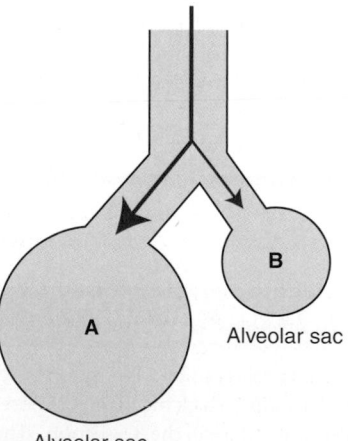

Alveolar sac

Alveolar sac

   - **A.** Air sac A
   - **B.** Air sac B
5. Which surfactant-associated protein deficiency is fatal in infancy without lung transplantation?
   - **A.** SP-A deficiency
   - **B.** SP-B deficiency
   - **C.** SP-C deficiency
   - **D.** SP-D deficiency

6. Which surfactant protein(s) is/are important in defense against infection (pick all that apply)?
   - **A.** SP-A
   - **B.** SP-B
   - **C.** SP-C
   - **D.** SP-D
7. What is the most common complication of surfactant administration in the preterm neonate?
   - **A.** Hypoxemia
   - **B.** Airway obstruction
   - **C.** Pulmonary hemorrhage
   - **D.** Infection
   - **E.** Hypotension
8. What are the benefits of surfactant replacement therapy in infants with RDS (pick all that apply)?
   - **A.** Reduction in the severity of RDS
   - **B.** Reduction in the incidence of air leaks (pneumothorax and pulmonary interstitial emphysema)
   - **C.** Reduction in mortality from RDS by 40% to 60%
   - **D.** Reduction in the incidence of bronchopulmonary dysplasia
   - **E.** Reduction in the incidence of intraventricular hemorrhage
9. What component(s) of natural surfactant increase(s) efficacy compared with synthetic surfactants (pick all that apply)?
   - **A.** SP-B
   - **B.** Percentage of DPPC
   - **C.** SP-C
   - **D.** Cholesterol
10. What radiographic findings are typical of a child with RDS (pick all that apply)?
    - **A.** Large lung volume
    - **B.** Atelectasis
    - **C.** Air bronchograms
    - **D.** Pulmonary interstitial emphysema
    - **E.** Ground-glass pattern

References

1. Pfister RH, Soll RF: New synthetic surfactants: the next generation? *Biol Neonate* 87:338–344, 2005.
2. Suresh GK, Soll RF: Overview of surfactant replacement trials, *J Perinatol* 25(Suppl 2):S40–S44, 2005.
3. Obladen M: History of surfactant up to 1980, *Biol Neonate* 87:308–316, 2005.
4. Von Neergaard K: Neue Auffassugen uber einen Grundbegriff der Atemmechanik: Die Retraktionskraft der Lunge, abhangig von der Oberflachenspannung in den Alveolen, *Z Gesamte Exp Med* 66:373, 1929.
5. Macklin CC: The pulmonary alveolar mucoid film and the pneumonocytes, *Lancet* 266:1099–1104, 1954.
6. Mead J, Lindgren I, Gaensler EA: The mechanical properties of the lungs in emphysema, *J Clin Invest* 34:1005–1016, 1955.
7. Avery ME: Surfactant deficiency in hyaline membrane disease: the story of discovery, *Am J Respir Crit Care Med* 161:1074–1075, 2000.
8. Clements JA: Surface tension of lung extracts, *Proc Soc Exp Biol Med* 95:170–172, 1957.
9. Pattle RE: Properties, function and origin of the alveolar lining layer, *Nature* 175:1125–1126, 1955.

10. Avery ME, Mead J: Surface properties in relation to atelectasis and hyaline membrane disease, *AMA J Dis Child* 97: 517–523, 1959.
11. Fujiwara T, Maeta H, Chida S, et al: Artificial surfactant therapy in hyaline-membrane disease, *Lancet* 1:55–59, 1980.
12. Wiswell TE: Expanded uses of surfactant therapy, *Clin Perinatol* 28:695–711, 2001.
13. Poynter SE, LeVine AM: Surfactant biology and clinical application, *Crit Care Clin* 19:459–472, 2003.
14. Finer NN: Surfactant use for neonatal lung injury: beyond respiratory distress syndrome, *Paediatr Respir Rev* 5(Suppl A): S289–S297, 2004.
15. Jobe AH, Ikegami M: Biology of surfactant, *Clin Perinatol* 28:655–viii, 2001.
16. Fujiwara T, Konishi M, Chida S, et al: Surfactant replacement therapy with a single postventilatory dose of a reconstituted bovine surfactant in preterm neonates with respiratory distress syndrome: final analysis of a multicenter, double-blind, randomized trial and comparison with similar trials. The Surfactant-TA Study Group, *Pediatrics* 86:753–764, 1990.
17. Williams MC: Uptake of lectins by pulmonary alveolar type II cells: subsequent deposition into lamellar bodies, *Proc Natl Acad Sci U S A* 81:6383–6387, 1984.
18. Glasser JR, Mallampalli RK: Surfactant and its role in the pathobiology of pulmonary infection, *Microbes Infect* 14: 17–25, 2012.
19. Rooney SA: The surfactant system and lung phospholipid biochemistry, *Am Rev Respir Dis* 131:439–460, 1985.
20. Young SL, Crapo JD, Kremers SA, et al: Pulmonary surfactant lipid production in oxygen-exposed rat lungs, *Lab Invest* 46:570–576, 1982.
21. Veldhuizen R, Nag K, Orgeig S, et al: The role of lipids in pulmonary surfactant, *Biochim Biophys Acta* 1408. 90–108, 1998.
22. Creuwels LA, van Golde LM, Haagsman HP: The pulmonary surfactant system: biochemical and clinical aspects, *Lung* 175:1–39, 1997.
23. Chung J, Yu SH, Whitsett JA, et al: Effect of surfactant-associated protein-A (SP-A) on the activity of lipid extract surfactant, *Biochim Biophys Acta* 1002:348–358, 1989.
24. Bersani I, Speer CP, Kunzmann S: Surfactant proteins A and D in pulmonary diseases of preterm infants, *Expert Rev Anti Infect Ther* 10:573–584, 2012.
25. Curstedt T: Surfactant protein C: basics to bedside, *J Perinatol* 25(Suppl 2):S36–S38, 2005.
26. ACOG Committee Opinion No. 475: Antenatal corticosteroid therapy for fetal maturation, *Obstet Gynecol* 117: 422–424, 2011.
27. Lee MJ, Davies J, Guinn D, et al: Single versus weekly courses of antenatal corticosteroids in preterm premature rupture of membranes, *Obstet Gynecol* 103:274–281, 2004.
28. Banks BA, Macones G, Cnaan A, et al: Multiple courses of antenatal corticosteroids are associated with early severe lung disease in preterm neonates, *J Perinatol* 22:101–107, 2002.
29. Zimmermann LJ, Janssen DJ, Tibboel D, et al: Surfactant metabolism in the neonate, *Biol Neonate* 87:296–307, 2005.
30. Ballard RA, Ballard PL, Cnaan A, et al: Antenatal thyrotropin-releasing hormone to prevent lung disease in preterm infants. North American Thyrotropin-Releasing Hormone Study Group, *N Engl J Med* 338:493–498, 1998.
31. Australian collaborative trial of antenatal thyrotropin-releasing hormone (ACTOBAT) for prevention of neonatal respiratory disease, *Lancet* 345:877–882, 1995.
32. Geary CA, Whitsett JA: Amniotic fluid markers of fetal lung maturity. In Spitzer AR, editor: *Intensive care of the fetus and neonate*, 2nd ed Philadelphia, 2005, Elsevier Mosby, pp 122–132.
33. O'Neill E, Thorp J: Antepartum evaluation of the fetus and fetal well being, *Clin Obstet Gynecol* 55:722–730, 2012.
34. Jobe AH, Ikegami M: Surfactant and acute lung injury, *Proc Assoc Am Physicians* 110:489–495, 1998.
35. Pison U, Seeger W, Buchhorn R, et al: Surfactant abnormalities in patients with respiratory failure after multiple trauma, *Am Rev Respir Dis* 140:1033–1039, 1989.
36. Pison U, Obertacke U, Brand M, et al: Altered pulmonary surfactant in uncomplicated and septicemia-complicated courses of acute respiratory failure, *J Trauma* 30:19–26, 1990.
37. Gregory TJ, Longmore WJ, Moxley MA, et al: Surfactant chemical composition and biophysical activity in acute respiratory distress syndrome, *J Clin Invest* 88:1976–1981, 1991.
38. Low RB, Adler KB, Woodcock-Mitchell J, et al: Bronchoalveolar lavage lipids during development of bleomycin-induced fibrosis in rats. Relationship to altered epithelial cell morphology, *Am Rev Respir Dis* 138:709–713, 1988.
39. Holm BA, Notter RH, Siegle J, et al: Pulmonary physiological and surfactant changes during injury and recovery from hyperoxia, *J Appl Physiol* 59:1402–1409, 1985.
40. Pison U, Gono E, Joka T, et al: Phospholipid lung profile in adult respiratory distress syndrome—evidence for surfactant abnormality, *Prog Clin Biol Res* 236A:517–523, 1987.
41. Lewis JF, Jobe AH: Surfactant and the adult respiratory distress syndrome, *Am Rev Respir Dis* 147:218–233, 1993.
42. Veldhuizen RA, McCaig LA, Akino T, et al: Pulmonary surfactant subfractions in patients with the acute respiratory distress syndrome, *Am J Respir Crit Care Med* 152:1867–1871, 1995.
43. Ueda T, Ikegami M, Jobe A: Surfactant subtypes. In vitro conversion, in vivo function, and effects of serum proteins, *Am J Respir Crit Care Med* 149:1254–1259, 1994.
44. Holm BA, Matalon S, Finkelstein JN, et al: Type II pneumocyte changes during hyperoxic lung injury and recovery, *J Appl Physiol* 65:2672–2678, 1988.
45. Seeger W, Gunther A, Walmrath HD, et al: Alveolar surfactant and adult respiratory distress syndrome. Pathogenetic role and therapeutic prospects, *Clin Investig* 71:177–190, 1993.
46. Kobayashi T, Nitta K, Ganzuka M, et al: Inactivation of exogenous surfactant by pulmonary edema fluid, *Pediatr Res* 29:353–356, 1991.
47. Bruni R, Fan BR, vid-Cu R, et al: Inactivation of surfactant in rat lungs, *Pediatr Res* 39:236–240, 1996.
48. Holm BA, Enhorning G, Notter RH: A biophysical mechanism by which plasma proteins inhibit lung surfactant activity, *Chem Phys Lipids* 49:49–55, 1988.
49. Holm BA, Matalon S: Role of pulmonary surfactant in the development and treatment of adult respiratory distress syndrome, *Anesth Analg* 69:805–818, 1989.
50. Hack M, Wright LL, Shankaran S, et al: Very-low-birth-weight outcomes of the National Institute of Child Health and Human Development Neonatal Network, November 1989 to October 1990, *Am J Obstet Gynecol* 172:457–464, 1995.
51. Suresh GK, Soll RF: Current surfactant use in premature infants, *Clin Perinatol* 28:671–694, 2001.
52. Long W, Corbet A, Cotton R, et al: A controlled trial of synthetic surfactant in infants weighing 1250 g or more with respiratory distress syndrome. The American Exosurf Neonatal Study Group I, and the Canadian Exosurf Neonatal Study Group, *N Engl J Med* 325:1696–1703, 1991.
53. Jobe AH, Mitchell BR, Gunkel JH: Beneficial effects of the combined use of prenatal corticosteroids and postnatal surfactant on preterm infants, *Am J Obstet Gynecol* 168:508–513, 1993.
54. Finer NN, Carlo WA, Walsh MC, et al: Early CPAP versus surfactant in extremely preterm infants, *N Engl J Med* 362:1970–1979, 2010.

55. Morley CJ, Davis PG, Doyle LW, et al: Nasal CPAP or intubation at birth for very preterm infants, *N Engl J Med* 358: 700–708, 2008.

56. Morley CJ, Davis PG: Continuous positive airway pressure: scientific and clinical rationale, *Curr Opin Pediatr* 20:119–124, 2008.

57. Elgellab A, Riou Y, Abbazine A, et al: Effects of nasal continuous positive airway pressure (NCPAP) on breathing pattern in spontaneously breathing premature newborn infants, *Intensive Care Med* 27:1782–1787, 2001.

58. Bahadue FL, Soll R: Early versus delayed selective surfactant treatment for neonatal respiratory distress syndrome, *Cochrane Database Syst Rev* 11:CD001456, 2012.

59. Halliday HL: Surfactants: past, present and future, *J Perinatol* 28(Suppl 1):S47–S56, 2008.

60. Stevens TP, Harrington EW, Blennow M, et al: Early surfactant administration with brief ventilation vs. selective surfactant and continued mechanical ventilation for preterm infants with or at risk for respiratory distress syndrome, *Cochrane Database Syst Rev* 4:CD003063, 2007.

61. Dani C, Bertini G, Pezzati M, et al: Early extubation and nasal continuous positive airway pressure after surfactant treatment for respiratory distress syndrome among preterm infants <30 weeks' gestation, *Pediatrics* 113:e560–e563, 2004.

62. Dani C, Corsini I, Poggi C: Risk factors for intubation-surfactant-extubation (INSURE) failure and multiple INSURE strategy in preterm infants, *Early Hum Dev* 88(Suppl 1): S3–S4, 2012.

63. Trevisanuto D, Grazzina N, Ferrarese P, et al: Laryngeal mask airway used as a delivery conduit for the administration of surfactant to preterm infants with respiratory distress syndrome, *Biol Neonate* 87:217–220, 2005.

64. Mazela J, Merritt TA, Finer NN: Aerosolized surfactants, *Curr Opin Pediatr* 19:155–162, 2007.

65. Gopel W, Kribs A, Ziegler A, et al: Avoidance of mechanical ventilation by surfactant treatment of spontaneously breathing preterm infants (AMV): an open-label, randomised, controlled trial, *Lancet* 378:1627–1634, 2011.

66. Soll R, Ozek E: Multiple versus single doses of exogenous surfactant for the prevention or treatment of neonatal respiratory distress syndrome, *Cochrane Database Syst Rev* 1:CD000141, 2009.

67. Yost CC, Soll RF: Early versus delayed selective surfactant treatment for neonatal respiratory distress syndrome, *Cochrane Database Syst Rev* 2:CD001456, 2000.

68. Lacaze-Masmonteil T: Exogenous surfactant therapy: newer developments, *Semin Neonatol* 8:433–440, 2003.

69. Curstedt T, Johansson J: New synthetic surfactants—basic science, *Biol Neonate* 87: 332–337, 2005.

70. Moya FR, Gadzinowski J, Bancalari E, et al: A multicenter, randomized, masked, comparison trial of lucinactant, colfosceril palmitate, and beractant for the prevention of respiratory distress syndrome among very preterm infants, *Pediatrics* 115:1018–1029, 2005.

71. Sinha SK, Lacaze-Masmonteil T, Soler A, et al: A multicenter, randomized, controlled trial of lucinactant versus poractant alfa among very premature infants at high risk for respiratory distress syndrome, *Pediatrics* 115:1030–1038, 2005.

72. Soll RF, Morley CJ: Prophylactic versus selective use of surfactant in preventing morbidity and mortality in preterm infants, *Cochrane Database Syst Rev* 2:CD000510, 2001.

73. Early versus delayed neonatal administration of a synthetic surfactant—the judgment of OSIRIS. The OSIRIS Collaborative Group (open study of infants at high risk of or with respiratory insufficiency—the role of surfactant), *Lancet* 340: 1363–1369, 1992.

74. Berggren E, Liljedahl M, Winbladh B, et al: Pilot study of nebulized surfactant therapy for neonatal respiratory distress syndrome, *Acta Paediatr* 89:460–464, 2000.

75. Donn SM, Sinha SK: Aerosolized lucinactant: a potential alternative to intratracheal surfactant replacement therapy, *Expert Opin Pharmacother* 9:475–478, 2008.

76. Gortner L, Pohlandt F, Bartmann P, et al: High-dose versus low-dose bovine surfactant treatment in very premature infants, *Acta Paediatr* 83:135–141, 1994.

77. Konishi M, Fujiwara T, Naito T, et al: Surfactant replacement therapy in neonatal respiratory distress syndrome. A multicentre, randomized clinical trial: comparison of high- versus low-dose of surfactant TA, *Eur J Pediatr* 147:20–25, 1988.

78. Halliday HL, Tarnow-Mordi WO, Corcoran JD, et al: Multicentre randomised trial comparing high and low dose surfactant regimens for the treatment of respiratory distress syndrome (the Curosurf 4 trial), *Arch Dis Child* 69:276–280, 1993.

79. Herting E, Tubman R, Halliday HL, et al: [Effect of 2 different dosages of a porcine surfactant on pulmonary gas exchange of premature infants with severe respiratory distress syndrome], *Monatsschr Kinderheilkd* 141:721–727, 1993.

80. Zola EM, Gunkel JH, Chan RK, et al: Comparison of three dosing procedures for administration of bovine surfactant to neonates with respiratory distress syndrome, *J Pediatr* 122:453–459, 1993.

81. Lin TW, Su BH, Lin HC, et al: Risk factors of pulmonary hemorrhage in very-low-birth-weight infants: a two-year retrospective study, *Acta Paediatr Taiwan* 41:255–258, 2000.

82. Pandit PB, Dunn MS, Colucci EA: Surfactant therapy in neonates with respiratory deterioration due to pulmonary hemorrhage, *Pediatrics* 95:32–36, 1995.

83. Aziz A, Ohlsson A: Surfactant for pulmonary haemorrhage in neonates, *Cochrane Database Syst Rev* 7:CD005254, 2012.

84. Moses D, Holm BA, Spitale P, et al: Inhibition of pulmonary surfactant function by meconium, *Am J Obstet Gynecol* 164:477–481, 1991.

85. Sun B, Curstedt T, Song GW, et al: Surfactant improves lung function and morphology in newborn rabbits with meconium aspiration, *Biol Neonate* 63:96–104, 1993.

86. Halliday HL, Speer CP, Robertson B: Treatment of severe meconium aspiration syndrome with porcine surfactant. Collaborative Surfactant Study Group, *Eur J Pediatr* 155:1047–1051, 1996.

87. Khammash H, Perlman M, Wojtulewicz J, et al: Surfactant therapy in full-term neonates with severe respiratory failure, *Pediatrics* 92:135–139, 1993.

88. Findlay RD, Taeusch HW, Walther FJ: Surfactant replacement therapy for meconium aspiration syndrome, *Pediatrics* 97:48–52, 1996.

89. Lotze A, Mitchell BR, Bulas DI, et al: Multicenter study of surfactant (beractant) use in the treatment of term infants with severe respiratory failure. Survanta in Term Infants Study Group, *J Pediatr* 132:40–47, 1998.

90. Chinese Collaborative Study Group for Neonatal Respiratory Diseases: Treatment of severe meconium aspiration syndrome with porcine surfactant: a multicentre, randomized, controlled trial, *Acta Paediatr* 94:896–902, 2005.

91. El Shahed AI, Dargaville P, Ohlsson A, et al: Surfactant for meconium aspiration syndrome in full term/near term infants, *Cochrane Database Syst Rev* CD002054, 2007.

92. Wiswell TE, Knight GR, Finer NN, et al: A multicenter, randomized, controlled trial comparing Surfaxin (Lucinactant) lavage with standard care for treatment of meconium aspiration syndrome, *Pediatrics* 109:1081–1087, 2002.

93. Dargaville PA, Copnell B, Mills JF, et al: Randomized controlled trial of lung lavage with dilute surfactant for meconium aspiration syndrome, *J Pediatr* 158:383–389, 2011.

94. Merrill JD, Ballard RA: Pulmonary surfactant for neonatal respiratory disorders, *Curr Opin Pediatr* 15:149–154, 2003.

95. Herting E, Sun B, Jarstrand C, et al: Surfactant improves lung function and mitigates bacterial growth in immature ventilated rabbits with experimentally induced neonatal group B streptococcal pneumonia, *Arch Dis Child Fetal Neonatal Ed* 76:F3–F8, 1997.

96. Herting E, Gan X, Rauprich P, et al: Combined treatment with surfactant and specific immunoglobulin reduces bacterial proliferation in experimental neonatal group B streptococcal pneumonia, *Am J Respir Crit Care Med* 159: 1862–1867, 1999.

97. Herting E, Gefeller O, Land M, et al: Surfactant treatment of neonates with respiratory failure and group B streptococcal infection. Members of the Collaborative European Multicenter Study Group, *Pediatrics* 106:957–964, 2000.

98. Tan K, Lai NM, Sharma A: Surfactant for bacterial pneumonia in late preterm and term infants, *Cochrane Database Syst Rev* 2:CD008155, 2012.

99. Wilcox DT, Glick PL, Karamanoukian HL, et al: Contributions by individual lungs to the surfactant status in congenital diaphragmatic hernia, *Pediatr Res* 41:686–691, 1997.

100. Moya FR, Thomas VL, Romaguera J, et al: Fetal lung maturation in congenital diaphragmatic hernia, *Am J Obstet Gynecol* 173:1401–1405, 1995.

101. Glick PL, Leach CL, Besner GE, et al: Pathophysiology of congenital diaphragmatic hernia. III: Exogenous surfactant therapy for the high-risk neonate with CDH, *J Pediatr Surg* 27:866–869, 1992.

102. Bos AP, Tibboel D, Hazebroek FW, et al: Surfactant replacement therapy in high-risk congenital diaphragmatic hernia, *Lancet* 338:1279, 1991.

103. Bae CW, Jang CK, Chung SJ, et al: Exogenous pulmonary surfactant replacement therapy in a neonate with pulmonary hypoplasia accompanying congenital diaphragmatic hernia—a case report, *J Korean Med Sci* 11: 265–270, 1996.

104. Dubois A, Storme L, Jaillard S, et al: [Congenital hernia of the diaphragm. A retrospective study of 123 cases recorded in the Neonatal Medicine Department, URHC in Lille between 1985 and 1996], *Arch Pediatr* 7:132–142, 2000.

105. Somaschini M, Locatelli G, Salvoni L, et al: Impact of new treatments for respiratory failure on outcome of infants with congenital diaphragmatic hernia, *Eur J Pediatr* 158:780–784, 1999.

106. Kays DW, Langham MR Jr, Ledbetter DJ, et al: Detrimental effects of standard medical therapy in congenital diaphragmatic hernia, *Ann Surg* 230:340–348, 1999.

107. Langham MR Jr, Kays DW, Beierle EA, et al: Twenty years of progress in congenital diaphragmatic hernia at the University of Florida, *Am Surg* 69:45–52, 2003.

108. Boloker J, Bateman DA, Wung JT, et al: Congenital diaphragmatic hernia in 120 infants treated consecutively with permissive hypercapnea/spontaneous respiration/elective repair, *J Pediatr Surg* 37:357–366, 2002.

109. Colby CE, Lally KP, Hintz SR, et al: Surfactant replacement therapy on ECMO does not improve outcome in neonates with congenital diaphragmatic hernia, *J Pediatr Surg* 39:1632–1637, 2004.

110. Doyle NM, Lally KP: The CDH Study Group and advances in the clinical care of the patient with congenital diaphragmatic hernia, *Semin Perinatol* 28:174–184, 2004.

111. Lally KP, Lally PA, Langham MR, et al: Surfactant does not improve survival rate in preterm infants with congenital diaphragmatic hernia, *J Pediatr Surg* 39: 829–833, 2004.

112. Van MK: Is surfactant therapy beneficial in the treatment of the term newborn infant with congenital diaphragmatic hernia? *J Pediatr* 145:312–316, 2004.

113. Lotze A, Knight GR, Martin GR, et al: Improved pulmonary outcome after exogenous surfactant therapy for respiratory failure in term infants requiring extracorporeal membrane oxygenation, *J Pediatr* 122:261–268, 1993.

114. Lotze A, Knight GR, Anderson KD, et al: Surfactant (beractant) therapy for infants with congenital diaphragmatic hernia on ECMO: evidence of persistent surfactant deficiency, *J Pediatr Surg* 29:407–412, 1994.

115. Greene KE, Wright JR, Steinberg KP, et al: Serial changes in surfactant-associated proteins in lung and serum before and after onset of ARDS, *Am J Respir Crit Care Med* 160: 1843–1850, 1999.

116. Baker CS, Evans TW, Randle BJ, et al: Damage to surfactant-specific protein in acute respiratory distress syndrome, *Lancet* 353:1232–1237, 1999.

117. Anzueto A, Baughman RP, Guntupalli KK, et al: Aerosolized surfactant in adults with sepsis-induced acute respiratory distress syndrome. Exosurf Acute Respiratory Distress Syndrome Sepsis Study Group, *N Engl J Med* 334:1417–1421, 1996.

118. Gregory TJ, Steinberg KP, Spragg R, et al: Bovine surfactant therapy for patients with acute respiratory distress syndrome, *Am J Respir Crit Care Med* 155:1309–1315, 1997.

119. Spragg RG, Lewis JF, Walmrath HD, et al: Effect of recombinant surfactant protein C-based surfactant on the acute respiratory distress syndrome, *N Engl J Med* 351:884–892, 2004.

120. Willson DF, Zaritsky A, Bauman LA, et al: Instillation of calf lung surfactant extract (calfactant) is beneficial in pediatric acute hypoxemic respiratory failure. Members of the Mid-Atlantic Pediatric Critical Care Network, *Crit Care Med* 27:188–195, 1999.

121. Lopez-Herce J, de LN, Carrillo A, et al: Surfactant treatment for acute respiratory distress syndrome, *Arch Dis Child* 80:248–252, 1999.

122. Willson DF, Thomas NJ, Markovitz BP, et al: Effect of exogenous surfactant (calfactant) in pediatric acute lung injury: a randomized controlled trial, *JAMA* 293: 470–476, 2005.

123. Dargaville PA, South M, McDougall PN: Surfactant abnormalities in infants with severe viral bronchiolitis, *Arch Dis Child* 75:133–136, 1996.

124. Skelton R, Holland P, Darowski M, et al: Abnormal surfactant composition and activity in severe bronchiolitis, *Acta Paediatr* 88:942–946, 1999.

125. Kerr MH, Paton JY: Surfactant protein levels in severe respiratory syncytial virus infection, *Am J Respir Crit Care Med* 159:1115–1118, 1999.

126. Luchetti M, Casiraghi G, Valsecchi R, et al: Porcine-derived surfactant treatment of severe bronchiolitis, *Acta Anaesthesiol Scand* 42:805–810, 1998.

127. Tibby SM, Hatherill M, Wright SM, et al: Exogenous surfactant supplementation in infants with respiratory syncytial virus bronchiolitis, *Am J Respir Crit Care Med* 162:1251–1256, 2000.

128. Jat KR, Chawla D: Surfactant therapy for bronchiolitis in critically ill infants, *Cochrane Database Syst Rev* 9:CD009194, 2012.

129. Kurashima K, Fujimura M, Matsuda T, et al: Surface activity of sputum from acute asthmatic patients, *Am J Respir Crit Care Med* 155:1254–1259, 1997.

130. Hite RD, Seeds MC, Bowton DL, et al: Surfactant phospholipid changes after antigen challenge: a role for phosphatidylglycerol in dysfunction, *Am J Physiol Lung Cell Mol Physiol* 288:L610–L617, 2005.

131. Kurashima K, Ogawa H, Ohka T, et al: A pilot study of surfactant inhalation in the treatment of asthmatic attack, *Arerugi* 40:160–163, 1991.

132. Oetomo SB, Dorrepaal C, Bos H, et al: Surfactant nebulization does not alter airflow obstruction and bronchial responsiveness to histamine in asthmatic children, *Am J Respir Crit Care Med* 153:1148–1152, 1996.

133. Erpenbeck VJ, Krug N, Hohlfeld JM: Therapeutic use of surfactant components in allergic asthma, *Naunyn Schmiedebergs Arch Pharmacol* 379:217–224, 2009.

134. Hull J, South M, Phelan P, et al: Surfactant composition in infants and young children with cystic fibrosis, *Am J Respir Crit Care Med* 156:161–165, 1997.

135. Griese M, Birrer P, Demirsoy A: Pulmonary surfactant in cystic fibrosis, *Eur Respir J* 10:1983–1988, 1997.

136. Postle AD, Mander A, Reid KB, et al: Deficient hydrophilic lung surfactant proteins A and D with normal surfactant phospholipid molecular species in cystic fibrosis, *Am J Respir Cell Mol Biol* 20:90–98, 1999.

137. Griese M, Bufler P, Teller J, et al: Nebulization of a bovine surfactant in cystic fibrosis: a pilot study, *Eur Respir J* 10:1989–1994, 1997.

138. Griese M, Essl R, Schmidt R, et al: Sequential analysis of surfactant, lung function and inflammation in cystic fibrosis patients, *Respir Res* 6:133, 2005.

139. Hallman M, Haataja R: Genetic basis of respiratory distress syndrome, *Front Biosci* 12:2670–2682, 2007.

140. Silveyra P, Floros J: Genetic variant associations of human SP-A and SP-D with acute and chronic lung injury, *Front Biosci* 17:407–429, 2012.

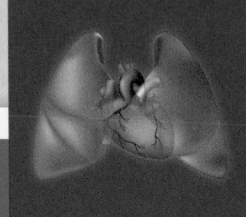

Chapter 15

Continuous Positive Airway Pressure (CPAP)

ASHOK K. DEORARI, ANU THUKRAL

LEARNING OBJECTIVES

After reading this chapter the reader will be able to:

1. Provide a brief history of the various methods used to generate CPAP in infants
2. Describe the various physiological effects of CPAP
3. Describe the indications/contraindications for CPAP
4. Identify commonly used delivery systems and nasal interfaces for delivering CPAP
5. Discuss potential differences in the operation and patient response between gas delivery systems and CPAP interfaces
6. Determine various strategies used to manage patients receiving CPAP and how these may impact outcomes
7. Describe monitoring strategies for determining positive and negative responses to CPAP
8. Identify common complications and how they can be avoided when using CPAP
9. Review bedside care procedures, performed by clinicians, that contribute to the successful use of CPAP in infants
10. Describe various weaning strategies that have been used for withdrawing CPAP in infants

KEY TERMS

Chronic lung disease
Continuous positive airway pressure (CPAP)
Functional residual capacity (FRC)

High-flow nasal cannulas (HFNC)
Mechanical ventilation
Partial pressure of carbon dioxide in arterial blood ($PaCO_2$)

Partial pressure of oxygen in arterial blood (PaO_2)
Work of breathing

Continuous positive airway pressure (CPAP), also called continuous distending pressure (CDP), refers to application of continuous pressure during both inspiration and expiration in a spontaneously breathing neonate. By providing constant airway pressure, the alveoli are kept open, which increases the **functional residual capacity (FRC)** of the lung, thus resulting in better gas exchange.[1] CPAP has been a standard of care for managing critically ill infants for nearly four decades now and has had a significant impact on improving patient outcomes, particularly when considering the morbidity and mortality of low-birth-weight, premature infants.

CPAP use in neonates was first described by Gregory and colleagues[2] in 1971 during an era when efforts to mechanically ventilate infants with respiratory distress often resulted in pulmonary air leaks and death. Their rationale

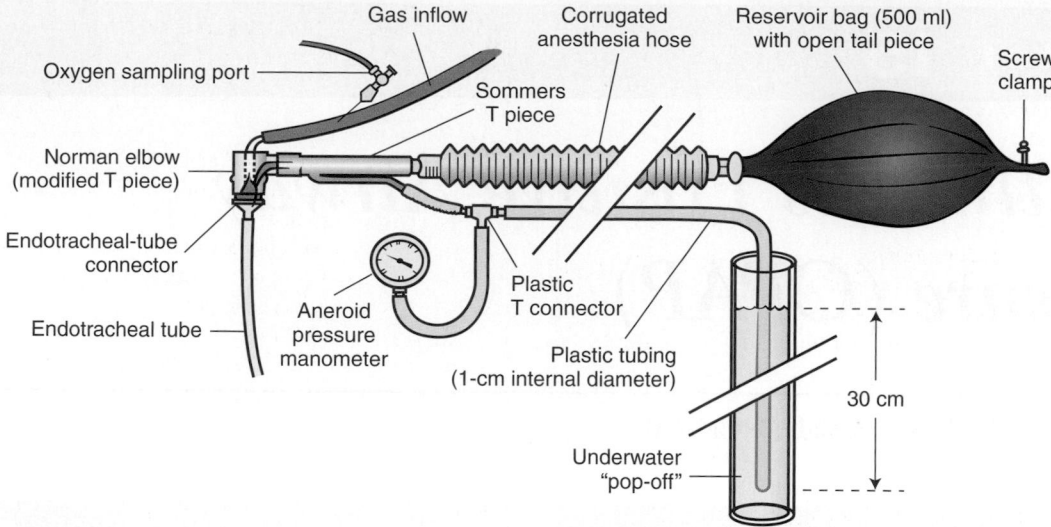

FIGURE 15-1 Early system used for applying continuous positive airway pressure (CPAP) to infants through an endotracheal tube.

for applying CPAP was to reproduce the physiological effects of expiratory grunting, exhibited by infants in respiratory distress, to maintain their FRC. They accomplished this by allowing intubated subjects to breathe spontaneously through a modified T-piece system using a blended, humidified gas source and a flow-inflating resuscitation bag with a screw-clamp at the tail of the bag, which maintained pressure by restricting flow to the atmosphere (Figure 15-1). In another method, nonintubated subjects were placed into a sealed head chamber that was pressurized with fresh gas to produce effects similar to endotracheal tube CPAP but without the potential risks associated with the use of an endotracheal tube.[2]

Early attempts were made to provide a noninvasive form of CPAP to the lung; for example, infants were placed in a box with their head out through a loose-fitting cuff around the neck and negative pressure was applied continuously to the infant's chest wall.[3-5] Further efforts to avoid intubation were accomplished with the application of nasal prong CPAP, which was first described by Kattwinkel and colleagues in 1973.[6] Today, nasal prong CPAP is the most common method by which CPAP is delivered to spontaneously breathing infants with respiratory disease.

This discussion focuses primarily on nasal CPAP delivery systems and interfaces that are most commonly used in clinical practice for newborn infants. These systems include ventilator-derived CPAP (V-CPAP), bubble CPAP (B-CPAP), and Infant Flow CPAP (IF-CPAP). Box 15-1 lists terms that are often used to describe these modes and methods described in this chapter.

Chapter 17 (Invasive Mechanical Ventilation of the Neonatal and Pediatric Patient) discusses CPAP delivery through the mechanical ventilator when using an endotracheal or tracheostomy tube. Chapter 16 (Noninvasive Mechanical Ventilation of the Infant and Child) discusses

Box 15-1	**Terms Used to Describe Noninvasive Pressure**

CPAP: Continuous positive airway pressure
V-CPAP: Ventilator-derived continuous positive airway pressure
B-CPAP: Bubble continuous positive airway pressure
IF-CPAP: Infant Flow continuous positive airway pressure
IF-SiPAP: Infant Flow "sigh" positive airway pressure

noninvasive forms of support, including CPAP, that are commonly used in larger infants and pediatric patients.

PHYSIOLOGICAL EFFECTS

CPAP increases functional residual capacity in patients with respiratory distress syndrome. It improves **partial pressure of oxygen in arterial blood (Pao$_2$)**,[7] improves lung mechanics,[8,9] reduces thoracoabdominal asynchrony,[10,11] stabilizes the chest wall,[12] improves the ventilation-to-perfusion ratio,[13] and improves the distribution of ventilation.[7] CPAP in spontaneously breathing infants with respiratory failure improves the breathing strategy as reflected by improved **work of breathing,** increased tidal volume, and a reduction in "labor breathing index."[11] CPAP decreases the respiratory rate and increases the expiratory time and the time constant of the respiratory system.[14] The characteristic protective expiratory braking observed in premature newborn infants is abolished by CPAP.[14] A decreased respiratory rate is not due to altered ventilatory response to carbon dioxide.[15] The decrease in minute volume is likely due to reductions in alveolar dead space.[2] Box 15-2 shows physiological effects that are commonly associated with CPAP.

Box 15-2	Physiological Effects of Continuous Positive Airway Pressure

- Increases functional residual capacity and tidal volume
- Decreases intrapulmonary shunt
- Increases pulmonary compliance
- Decreases airway resistance
- Stabilizes the chest wall and the upper airways, thus preventing obstructive apnea
- Improves the distribution of ventilation, ventilation-to-perfusion ratio, and gas exchange
- Decreases work of breathing and reduces alveolar dead space
- Protects the developing lung
- Better type 2 pneumocyte function and even recycling of surfactant, thus contributing to early recovery from **hyaline membrane disease (HMD)**
- Decreases cellular indicators of lung injury
- Reduces the need for intubation and mechanical ventilation
- Stimulates the J receptors in the pleura and provides positive feedback to the respiratory center by Hering-Breuer reflex

Box 15-3	Indications and Contraindications of Continuous Positive Airway Pressure

INDICATIONS
1. Premature infants
   - Delivery room CPAP and prophylactic CPAP[21,44-51,53]
   - Respiratory distress syndrome[21,42]
   - Apnea of prematurity
   - After extubation from mechanical ventilation[43]
   - Early surfactant administration followed by NCPAP[52]
2. Obstructive airway diseases
   - Obstructive apnea
   - Laryngeal or tracheal malacia
   - Bronchopulmonary dysplasia
   - Viral bronchiolitis
3. Pneumonia
   - Viral or bacterial
   - Aspiration
4. Transient tachypnea of the newborn[55]
5. Meconium aspiration syndrome[67]
6. Other possible indications
   a. Used in conjunction with:
      - Surfactant administration
      - Nitric oxide administration
      - Extracorporeal membrane oxygenation
   b. Paralysis of a hemidiaphragm
   c. Congestive heart failure, pulmonary edema, pulmonary hemorrhage

CONTRAINDICATIONS
1. Criteria for CPAP failure requiring mechanical ventilation
   - $Pa_{CO_2} > 60$ mm Hg consistently
   - pH < 7.25
2. Upper airway abnormalities
   - Choanal atresia
   - Cleft palate
   - Tracheoesophageal fistula
3. Untreated congenital diaphragmatic hernia
4. Neuromuscular disorders
5. Central nervous system depressant medications
6. Central or frequent apnea

An increasing body of evidence demonstrates that by using CPAP, mechanical ventilation can be avoided, resulting in a lower incidence of lung injury and hence chronic lung disease.[16,17] By applying CPAP, the airways can be protected from mechanical injury and colonization related to the endotracheal tube.[18] Infants treated with CPAP have been found to have a lower incidence of complications related to mechanical ventilation, including respiratory-related nosocomial infections, apnea, intraventricular hemorrhage, retinopathy of prematurity, and chronic lung disease, when compared with infants who were intubated and treated with mechanical ventilation. Although a thorough discussion describing the effects of ventilator-induced lung injury in infants is beyond the scope of this chapter, it is important to realize that a major goal of CPAP is to eliminate or reduce the need for prolonged ventilator support.

Postnatal lung development in low-birth-weight infants—specifically, primary and secondary septation-forming saccules and alveoli and angiogenesis[18-23]—may be arrested or altered by mechanical ventilation, placing the infant at risk for developing **chronic lung disease.**[19] CPAP decreases indicators of lung injury.[20] Early application of CPAP reduces the need for intubation and counters the arrest of postnatal lung development in infants, and hence may decrease the incidence of chronic lung disease.

INDICATIONS

CPAP is clinically indicated in infants with both obstructive and restrictive lung diseases. Box 15-3 lists the indications and contraindications regarding CPAP use. The use of CPAP can clinically impact lung disease predominantly to improve oxygenation, counter atelectasis,[7,21-25] and stabilize the chest wall.[12] CPAP is also used to stent open airways and hence lower airway resistance to gas flow in patients with obstructive lung disease and apnea.[26-31] CPAP is often used to maintain airway patency in infants with obstructive apnea[29,10,32-34] and obstructive airway diseases.[28,35-38] Figure 15-2 shows the effect of CPAP on the anatomical structures of the upper airways.

According to American Association for Respiratory Care (AARC) clinical practice guidelines,[39] neonates presenting with respiratory rate greater than 30% of normal and paradoxical chest wall movement[40] with suprasternal and substernal retractions, grunting, nasal flaring, and cyanotic skin color[41] should be considered for CPAP administration as long as they are able to demonstrate adequate ventilation, as defined by a **partial pressure of carbon**

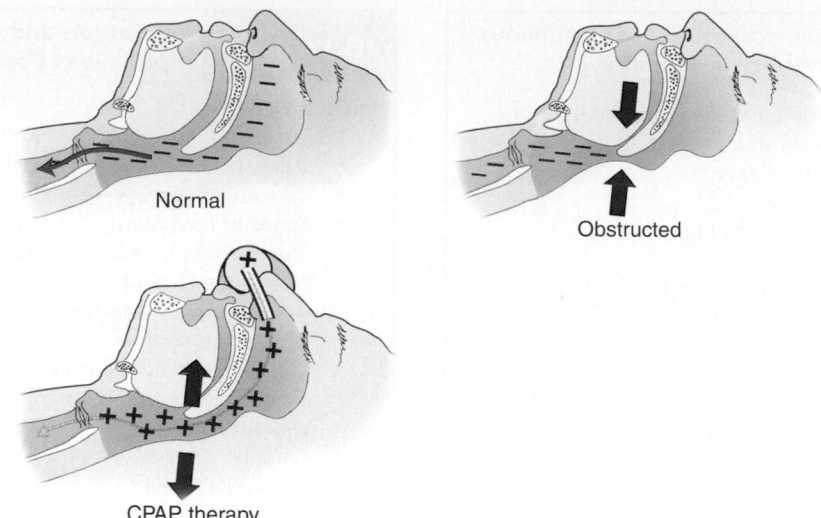

FIGURE 15-2   *Top left,* Normal patent upper airway. *Top right,* Tongue obstructing upper airway. *Bottom,* CPAP distending structures of oropharynx, preventing obstruction by the tongue and soft palate.

dioxide in arterial blood (Paco₂) less than 60 mm Hg and a pH greater than 7.25.[39]

Nasal CPAP has been used as the primary modality in respiratory distress syndrome.[21,42] In addition, CPAP is an effective option for prevention of extubation failure.[43] It is also used as a primary modality in the delivery room[21,44-51] and following early surfactant delivery.[52] Recent trials on CPAP utility in the delivery room have focused on smaller and more immature neonates. The Surfactant Positive Pressure and Pulse Oximetry Randomized Trial (SUPPORT) compared[48] delivery room CPAP with limited ventilation strategy with ventilation and surfactant administration within 60 minutes of birth and demonstrated CPAP as an effective initial ventilatory strategy. The COIN (CPAP or Intubation) trial reported a trend toward a lower rate of death or bronchopulmonary disease (BPD) at 36 weeks in infants who received CPAP.[51] Similar findings were also reported, in addition to a reduction in the need of mechanical ventilation after early CPAP, in the recent trial published by the South American Neocosur Network.[53] Overall, CPAP started soon after birth appears to reduce BPD and death and is an acceptable alternative to endotracheal intubation in the delivery room. CPAP has also been successful in the treatment of pneumonias,[54] transient tachypnea of the newborn,[55] meconium aspiration syndrome,[56-58] and paralysis of the hemidiaphragm. It has been employed for infants with pulmonary edema and patent ductus arteriosus.[59]

CPAP has been shown to improve lung function in patients with postoperative congenital heart disease[60,61] and after surgical repair of abdominal wall defects; however, increased abdominal pressure may adversely affect pulmonary function.[62] CPAP use in infants with diaphragmatic hernia is indicated only after surgical repair. CPAP is used in conjunction with the administration of surfactant[16,52,63-65] and

nitric oxide[66] and as a source of high airway pressure in infants receiving extracorporeal membrane oxygenation.[67]

CPAP is an effective option for preventing extubation failure.[43] In addition, it is used as a primary modality in respiratory distress syndrome,[21-42] as a modality in the delivery room[21,44-51] and immediately following early surfactant delivery.[52]

CONTRAINDICATIONS

Infants with persistent apneic episodes who are unable to maintain Paco₂ less than 60 mm Hg and pH greater than 7.25 should not be given CPAP; if they are already receiving CPAP, then mechanical ventilation is indicated.[39] Infants with congenital anomalies such as choanal atresia, cleft palate, tracheoesophageal fistula, or preoperative diaphragmatic hernia should not receive CPAP. CPAP is contraindicated in infants with neural muscular disorders, infants receiving central nervous system (CNS) depressants, and infants with central apnea or frequent apneic episodes resulting in desaturation or bradycardia.[39] In addition, severe cardiorespiratory instability and poor respiratory drive are also contraindications to the initiation of CPAP.

HAZARDS AND COMPLICATIONS

Noninvasive application of CPAP is considered a "gentler" method of support when compared with mechanical ventilation; however, CPAP is still associated with some of the same hazards and complications that are often associated with mechanical ventilation. Pneumothorax is a complication that is occasionally reported in infants receiving CPAP.[69] This is a result of inadvertent positive end-expiratory pressure related to gas trapping when infants are tachypneic and do not have a sufficient expiratory time. This may also occur after surfactant replacement therapy, when pulmonary compliance improves and the infant has not been weaned appropriately and thus is exposed to excessive airway and hence alveolar pressure. Other forms of air leak caused by inappropriately high CPAP levels may include pulmonary interstitial emphysema, pneumomediastinum, and pneumatocele.[70-76] Although extremely rare, vascular air embolism has been described in infants receiving CPAP.[75] This occurs when a laceration in the lung parenchyma introduces air into the cardiovascular system. Increased intracranial pressures related to lung overdistention may also occur as a result of CPAP.[76] CPAP has been reported as having an adverse impact on renal effects, including decreased urine output and glomerular filtration rate.[77] Decreased gastrointestinal blood flow has been cited as a potential complication of endotracheal CPAP and may well manifest similarly in nasal CPAP.[78] Bowel distention is often noted with CPAP.[79] Infants may swallow gas, which can result in bulging flanks, increased abdominal girth, and visibly dilated intestinal loops on radiographs.

A study comparing spontaneously breathing unassisted premature infants with infants receiving CPAP showed that there were no detectable differences in hemodynamic values, including stroke volume and cardiac output as measured by echocardiogram.[80] This implies that there is no need to withhold CPAP support to prevent circulatory complications; however, hemodynamic compromise should always be considered as a factor when using any positive pressure device. Complications that have been described regarding problems with equipment include desaturation as a result of loss of airway pressure caused by inappropriate fit of nasal prongs or leak around a face mask. Face masks may also result in leaks around the eyes and damage to facial tissue from improper fixation. An open mouth can lead to a loss in airway pressure as a result of leaks.[81] Obstruction of nasal prongs from mucous plugging or tips pressed against the nasal mucosa can lead to losses in airway pressure unmeasured by low-pressure alarm systems and can increase work of breathing.[81] Leaks or obstruction can also lead to a loss in the inspired fraction of oxygen (FiO_2). Fluctuations in baseline pressure and increase in work of breathing can be caused by insufficient gas flow.[82]

Local irritation and trauma[83] to the nasal septum may occur because of misalignment or improper fixation of nasal prongs.[84] Nasal snubbing and circumferential distortion (widening) of the nares can be caused by nasal prongs, especially if CPAP is being used for more than just a few days.[85] Breakdown and erosion low on the septum at the base of the philtrum can occur when using nasal masks.[85,86] Columella necrosis has been reported after only a few days of CPAP use (Figure 15-3). Inadequate humidification can lead to nasal mucosal damage.[87,88] Skin irritation of the head and neck from improperly secured bonnets or CPAP head harnesses can also occur.[39] Equipment failure and dysfunction should always be considered as potential

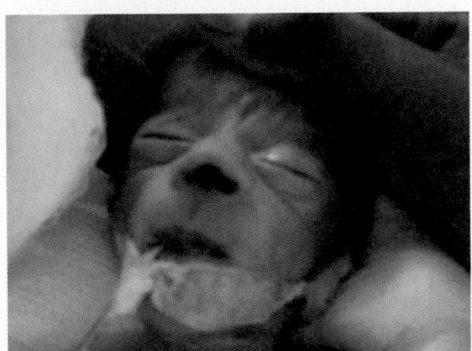

FIGURE 15-3 Columella necrosis resulting from short-term nasal CPAP.

sources of complication for an infant's condition when providing CPAP.

DELIVERY SYSTEMS AND PATIENT INTERFACES

The term *delivery system* describes the mechanism by which fresh gas flow is generated and positive pressure is maintained at the patient's airway. A number of devices are commonly used to deliver CPAP to infants. They are characterized by their ability to provide either a constant or variable flow source. The system also includes a humidifier, circuit, and oxygen analyzer. Gas temperature and humidity are important aspects when maintaining the neutral thermal environment of a newborn infant and thus should be adjusted to provide a temperature between 37° C and 39° C and 100% humidity to the patient. The humidifier servoregulates temperature on the basis of measurements acquired at the humidifier probe and thus should not be placed within an incubator or directly beneath a radiant warmer. The circuit should be constructed of flexible and lightweight material to prevent traction and torque on the nasal interface. This helps minimize patient discomfort and nasal injury.[88] The delivery system should include a "pop-off device" placed close to the airway to protect the patient from overpressurization, thereby limiting excessive volume delivery to the respiratory system.

The term *patient interface device* describes the mechanism by which gas flow from the delivery system is delivered to the airway of the infant. Historically, various interface devices have been applied to administer CPAP to infants. These include enclosure of the head in a plastic pressure chamber, a pressurized plastic bag fitted over the infant's head, face chambers, face masks, tight-fitting face masks, devices requiring a neck seal, endotracheal tubes, nasopharyngeal tubes, and long and short binasal pharyngeal prongs.[89]

Today, CPAP is most often administered through short binasal prongs, and this method is considered the most effective interface option for delivering CPAP to infants.[89,90] This is attributed primarily to infants being regarded as obligate nose breathers, resulting in CPAP delivering relatively constant airway pressures. Nasal prongs also facilitate mobilization and oral feeding.[90] Because the other methods are used infrequently in the clinical setting, this chapter focuses primarily on short binasal prongs and nasal masks for interfacing with these systems. The short binasal prongs include argyle nasal prongs, Hudson prongs, Fisher and Paykel prongs, Infant Flow driver or Aladdin (Arabella) generators, INCA prongs, and Medijet prongs.

Clinicians have often speculated that differences in the level of imposed resistance and hence imposed work of breathing (WOB) between the systems are clinically relevant to infants and may contribute to CPAP failure. Nasal prongs have been reported to have lower resistance to gas flow when compared with other commonly used nasal interfaces. These differences are related to the length and internal diameters of the interfaces but are also associated with the delivery system and how CPAP is maintained by this system. Table 15-1 shows the pressure drop at various flow rates in the devices that have traditionally been used to interface with CPAP delivery systems. The WOB is related to the resistance to gas flow when breathing through the various elements imposed by the CPAP system and interface. The WOB is superimposed on the physiological WOB; which in turn increases the total amount of WOB done by the patient.[91] Imposed expiratory resistance can also impact the inspiratory WOB in spontaneously breathing infants.[92] Exhalation is considered active in infants with lung disease and therefore expiratory resistance is an important consideration.[93] This also becomes important because most infants, especially premature infants, do not have adequate energy stores and high caloric requirements often resulting in rapid deterioration of the respiratory status.

Early systems that used flow resistors (screw clamp; see Figure 15-1) for exhalation were associated with higher resistance, and hence a higher amount of energy was expended to breathe; currently available systems, on the other hand, use low-resistance threshold-type resistors. In theory, a threshold resistor produces no resistance to exhalation and maintains CPAP by applying an opposing force that is equal to the amount of the desired system pressure. Infant mechanical ventilators have been shown to have higher imposed expiratory resistance compared with an endotracheal tube. However, imposed resistance and hence WOB are likely to be lower when breathing through a ventilator with nasal prongs than with an endotracheal tube.[94] The water seal in B-CPAP functions as a pure threshold-type resistor and has been shown to have low imposed expiratory resistance. The IF-CPAP device has been shown in a lung model to have one quarter of the imposed WOB compared with other forms of CPAP.[95] IF-CPAP has also been shown to significantly reduce inspiratory WOB in preterm infants and to improve compliance better compared with mechanical ventilator CPAP.[96-98] In another study comparing differences in the WOB for infants randomized to B-CPAP or IF-CPAP, resistive WOB was lower for infants treated with IF-CPAP; however, these results did not reflect any clinically significant differences in the total inspiratory WOB done by the patient.[99]

TABLE 15-1

Dimensions of Nasal Continuous Positive Airway Pressure Devices and Pressure Drop at Various Flows[93]

Device	Size	Prong Length*	Int. Diameter*[†]	Ext. Diameter*[†]	PRESSURE DROP AT DIFFERENT FLOWS				
					4 L/min	5 L/min	6 L/min	7 L/min	8 L/min
Duotube	2.5	40	1.4	2.5	9.7	15	21	29	38
	3.0	40	1.8	3.0	3.0	4.5	6.2	8.3	10.5
	3.5	40	2.5	3.5	1.1	1.7	2.3	3.1	3.9
Single prong[‡]	2.5	50	2.5	3.8	2.2	3.3	4.4	5.9	7.3
	3.0	50	3.0	4.3	1.1	1.5	2.1	2.7	3.3
	3.5	50	3.5	4.9	0.6	0.9	1.2	1.6	1.9
Argyle prong	Extra small	6	1.8	3.1	1.7	2.6	3.6	4.8	6.2
	Small	8	2.3	4.0	0.9	1.4	1.9	2.5	3.2
	Large	10	2.3	4.8	0.7	1.1	1.5	2.1	2.6
Hudson prong	0	11	2.3	3.7	1.4	2.2	3.1	4.2	5.4
	1	11	2.6	3.9	0.8	1.3	1.8	2.5	3.3
	2	11	3.0	4.6	0.3	0.5	0.6	0.9	1.1
	3	12	3.5	4.9	0.2	0.3	0.4	0.5	0.6
	4	15	4.0	5.4	0.1	0.2	0.3	0.5	0.6
Infant Flow driver	Small	6	3.0	3.9	0.2	0.2	0.3	0.4	0.5
	Medium	7	3.5	4.3	−0.1	−0.2	−0.3	−0.4	−0.5
	Large	7	4.0	4.6	−0.2	−0.3	−0.5	−0.7	−0.9

*Outer diameter, inner diameter, length in mm, does not include the length proximal to the bridge between the prongs.
[†] Internal and outer diameters were measured at the prong tip.
[‡]Refers to Mallinckrodt endotracheal tube cut down to 5 cm in length and attached to a standard endotracheal tube adapter with pressure side port.

Mechanical Ventilator CPAP

Time-cycled, pressure-limited, constant-flow infant ventilators were introduced in the mid-1970s and are still a simple and efficient method for nasal CPAP delivery to infants. Ventilator CPAP (V-CPAP), often described as "conventional CPAP," has been accomplished by placing ventilators in the CPAP mode and setting a constant flow rate while interfacing with the system using binasal prongs, a single nasopharyngeal tube, or an endotracheal tube inserted into the nasopharynx. Time-cycled, pressure-limited ventilators use exhalation valves to maintain CPAP. The convenience of a blended gas source, alarm options, and low cost made this a popular choice among clinicians. The advantage of such a system is that if intubated patients failed V-CPAP, or if the patient was extubated from conventional ventilation, then the ventilator was available at the bedside without having to set up a separate delivery system.

Today, a number of commercially available microprocessor-controlled infant ventilators allow noninvasive application of V-CPAP. In these systems CPAP is maintained with a variable demand–flow system. Flow rate and airway pressure are regulated by servo controlling the aperture size of the exhalation valve. These ventilators also include the following:

· Highly responsive demand–flow systems
· Leak compensation
· Airway graphics monitoring
· Apnea backup breaths

The interface that is most commonly used with this delivery system is the Fisher and Paykel nasal prongs (Fisher & Paykel Healthcare, Auckland, NZ) (Figure 15-4A) and the Hudson nasal prongs (Hudson RCI/Teleflex, Research Triangle Park, NC, Figure 15-4B). The prongs are adjusted so that there is never contact between the prongs and the nasal septum.[84] The prong size is established on the basis of weight, using a sizing chart provided by the manufacturer (Table 15-2, Hudson nasal prongs) or the head circumference, nasal orifice and nasal septum size in Fisher and Paykel nasal prongs. The prongs stay in place by attaching the circuitry to a premade hat, using safety pins and rubber bands. A proximal pressure line or "pop-off" can be attached at a Luer adapter at the nasal interface, or this can also be plugged.

Bubble Nasal CPAP

B-CPAP (also known as the "water seal" or "bubbly bottle" method) is a simple, safe, inexpensive constant flow delivery system that has been used for nearly four decades to deliver CPAP.[100-103] This method was implemented by Jen-Tien Wung in the 1970s at Columbia University Medical Center (New York, NY). It is constructed with readily available equipment and materials that can usually be found in most respiratory care equipment storage areas. A commercially available version of this system (Fisher & Paykel Healthcare, Auckland, New Zealand) is currently being

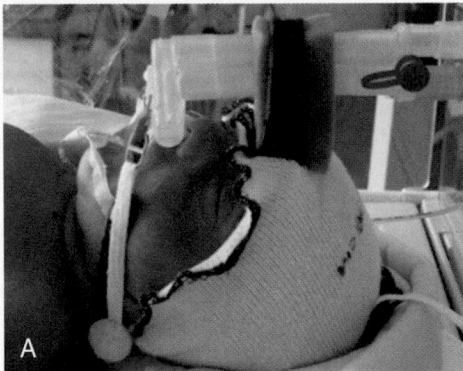
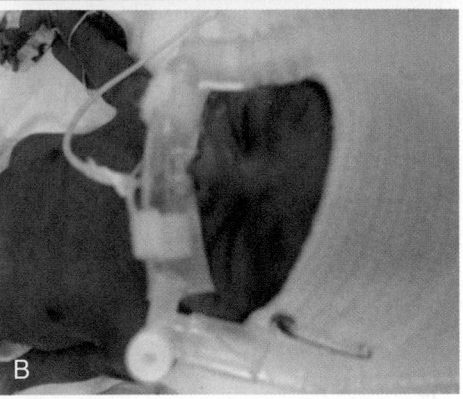

FIGURE 15-4 Hudson RCI infant nasal prong interface with bonnet fixation.

TABLE 15-2

Sizing Chart for Hudson RCI Infant Nasal Prong CPAP

Weight Range (g)	Suggested Cannula Size
Less than 700	0
700 to 1250	1
1250 to 2000	2
2000 to 3000	3
More than 3000	4
1 to 2 years of age	5

used in Europe and Australia. Materials include the following (Figure 15-5)[78,87]:

· An infant dual-limb heated wire ventilator circuit
· A humidifier and blended gas source
· A pressure transducer
· A water column filled to 10 cm with either sterile water or a 25% acetic acid solution

A measuring tape is attached to the outside of the water column. The CPAP level is maintained by submerging the distal end of expiratory circuit straight down into the fluid from the surface of the water line to a measured depth in centimeters, thus creating the amount of CPAP in centimeters of water. If a higher level of CPAP is needed, the tube can be advanced farther down into the fluid column. The flow rate of humidified gas (6 to 10 L/min) is set to meet the inspiratory flow rate requirements of the patient, maintain the CPAP level, and rinse the system of exhaled

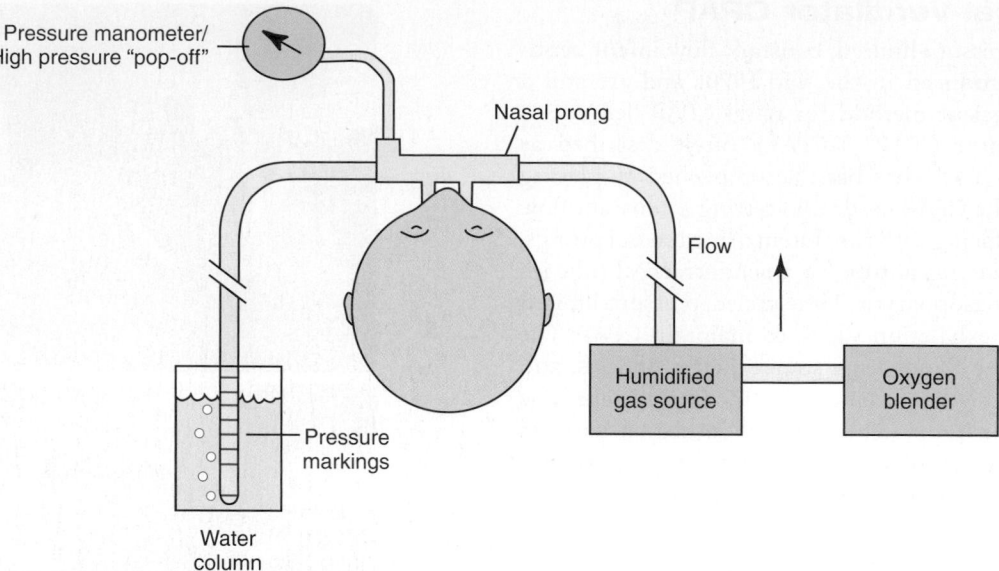

FIGURE 15-5   A simple system for delivering bubble nasal CPAP.

carbon dioxide.[87] The pressure measured at the nasal prong could be slightly higher than the submersion depth of the expiratory tubing below the water surface when higher flow rates are used; therefore, airway pressure should always be monitored at the nasal prong to ensure proper CPAP levels. A high-pressure pop-off can be placed as close to the patient as possible should the expiratory limb become occluded. This system has few alarms or monitoring options and therefore it is extremely important to evaluate patients frequently, because vital signs may be the only effective alarm for alerting clinicians to airway disconnects, prong occlusion, and mechanical system failure.

The use of B-CPAP in infants has been shown to significantly reduce minute volume and respiratory rate with no changes in transcutaneous carbon dioxide or oxygen saturation compared with mechanical ventilator CPAP. Small pressure fluctuations created by the back pressure of bubbles in the underwater seal are transmitted to the airway, thereby producing a noisy component that may enhance lung recruitment and gas mixing in a fashion similar to mechanisms that are present during high-frequency oscillatory ventilation.[104-106]

Subjective accounts of a visible "thoracic wiggle" from these bubble effects are often reported by clinicians caring for infants supported with B-CPAP. The use of higher flow rates can result in more vigorous bubbling and hence higher pressure fluctuations in the delivery system; however, this does not appear to improve gas exchange.[107] In premature animals, the use of B-CPAP has resulted in improvements in gas exchange, lung mechanics, and lung volume, which suggest enhanced alveolar recruitment when compared with V-CPAP.[105] B-CPAP may be associated with reduced extubation failure.[108]

Infant Flow Nasal CPAP

Infant Flow CPAP (IF-CPAP) (Cardinal Health, Dublin, OH) is a commercially available variable flow device that is specifically designed to deliver CPAP in newborns. The "flow driver" provides the source gas (Figure 15-6) and consists of an internalized flow metering system, a blender with an FiO_2 control knob, a digitalized pressure LED, an alarm system, and a pressure relief system.[109] An external auxiliary gas flow meter is used to provide gas source identical to the set FiO_2 for nebulizers and manual resuscitators. Blended gas is humidified and delivered to the nasal interface "flow generator" (Figure 15-7), using a proprietary patient circuit. Despite setting a constant flow on the flow driver, the unique geometric design of the flow generator incorporates unique physical properties that allow control of gas delivery to and from the patient and is thus

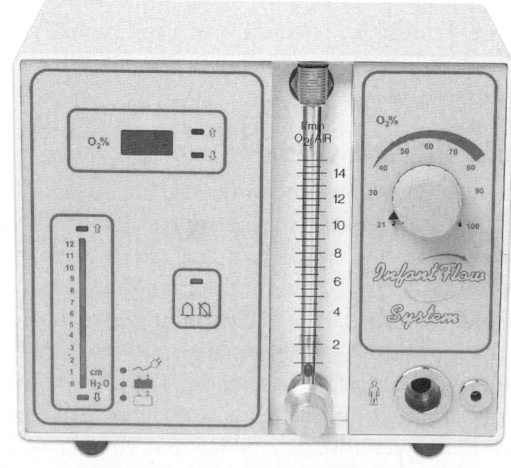

FIGURE 15-6   Infant Flow driver.

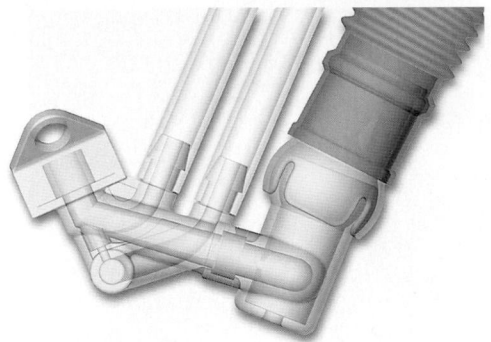

FIGURE 15-7 Infant Flow generator nasal interface device.

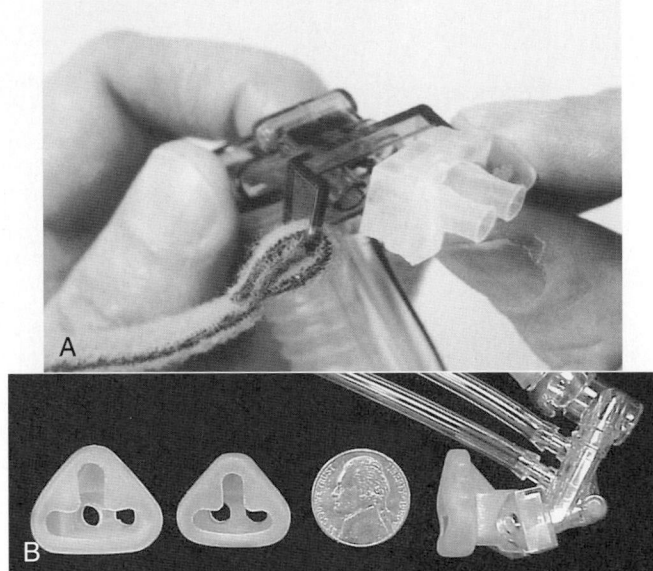

FIGURE 15-8 Silicone nasal prongs (**A**) and masks (**B**) attached to an Infant Flow driver.

considered variable. The set flow rate is based on the fluctuation of the baseline pressure measurement, which is made at the flow generator, as indicated by the light-emitting diode bars on the front panel of the flow driver. If the nasal prongs or mask are sized and fitted properly, a flow rate of 8 L/min should maintain a CPAP level of approximately 5 cm H_2O.

The design of the flow generator uses a fluidic flip valve, which is designed with nonmoving parts and provides fresh gas to the infant during inhalation and directs flow away from the infant during exhalation. Gas delivery is accomplished on the basis of the Bernoulli effect, whereby gas flow is provided to each nostril through the fresh gas inlet and passes through twin nasal jet injector nozzles at high velocity, which in turn converts the flow into a constant pressure.[109] If the patient requires any additional inspiratory flow, a Venturi-type effect created by the jet injector nozzles entrains more gas to be delivered. When the infant makes a spontaneous expiratory effort, exhaled gas passes freely and unimpeded by the flow of incoming air. This is accomplished by the Coanda and abreve; effect, which triggers the "fluidic flip" and redirects incoming flow and exhaled gases through the expiratory channel simultaneously. Once the expiratory effort stops and expiratory flow ceases, the flow immediately switches back to the inspiratory position[109] (Figure 15-8).

The IF-CPAP system has been shown to deliver more consistent pressure, lowering the WOB, being less sensitive to leaks, and being more effective at alveolar recruitment compared with other forms of CPAP.[96,110] IF-CPAP use has also been shown to reduce the need for supplemental oxygenation in extremely low birth weight infants after extubation compared with infants randomized to receive V-CPAP with nasal prongs.[111] The ability of the Infant Flow driver to provide consistent pressure at the airway lowers WOB by applying greater stability to the infant respiratory system mechanics for a given change in intrapleural pressure.[95] The decreased variability of the airway pressure and fast response times of the IF-CPAP may also be due to the fact that the flow regulation mechanism is located at the nasal interface device, whereas other CPAP devices (i.e., V-CPAP) regulate flow downstream from the patient (exhalation valve).

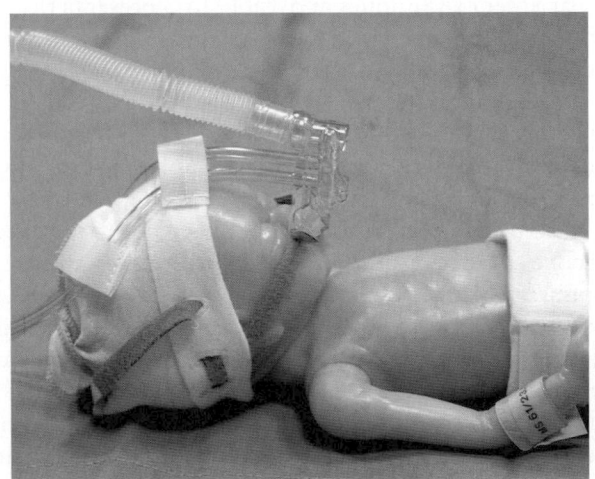

FIGURE 15-9 Proper fixation for the Infant Flow CPAP system.

IF-CPAP is delivered to infants by using either a proprietary nasal mask or nasal prongs (Figure 15-9). The nasal prongs and masks are made from a soft silicone-based elastomer and are attached directly to the Infant Flow generator, which is then held in place once the interface is fastened by attachment to a soft cap or bonnet (see Figure 15-9). The thin, soft material that constructs these nasal devices may provide important mechanical effects when using nasal prongs by flaring out during gas inflow, thus increasing the effective internal diameter and decreasing the leak around the prongs. A mask does not rely on a prong entering the nares and may be more beneficial when trying to secure the nasal device onto an infant with craniofacial abnormalities. Nasal prongs have been shown to result in nasal and septal wall skin breakdown, whereas nasal masks have been associated with breakdown low on the septum or at the base of the

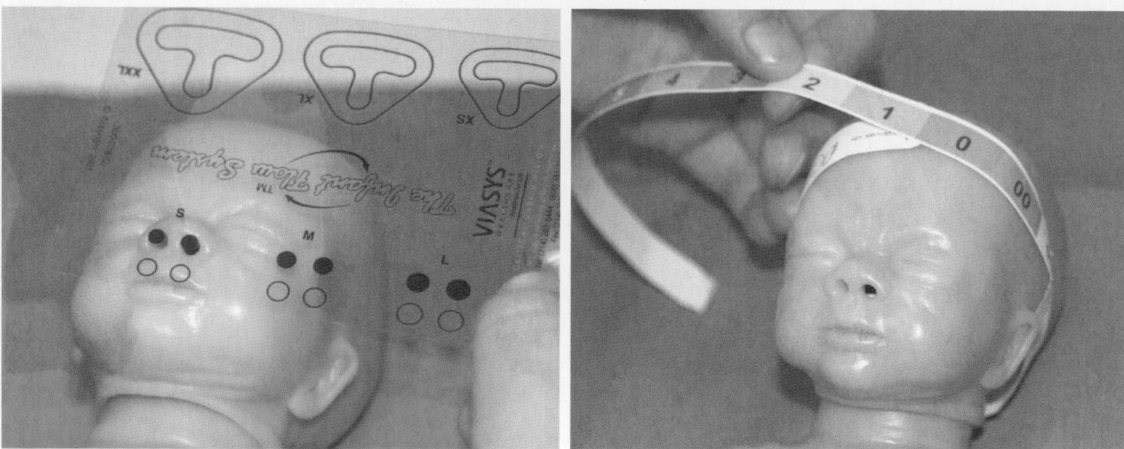

FIGURE 15-10   Nasal prong (*left*) and head circumference (*right*) measurements for the Infant Flow CPAP system.

philtrum.[85] Some clinicians prefer switching back and forth when using nasal masks and prongs to eliminate these soft tissue injuries. Figure 15-10 shows the proper measurement techniques and Table 15-3 presents the sizing chart used to select the properly sized bonnet and nasal interface for use with the IF-CPAP device.

High-Flow Nasal Cannulas

Nasal cannulas with an outer diameter of 3 mm and flows up to 2 L/min have been reported to deliver CPAP.[112] Studies of CPAP via nasal cannulas have found it to be as effective as conventional CPAP prongs in the treatment of respiratory distress and apnea of prematurity.[113,114]

The pressures delivered with this technique when measured are highly variable and depend on the flow rate, the size of leak around the cannulas and the degree of mouth opening.[112,115] A recent Cochrane review could not find an adequate number of trials and concluded that there was insufficient evidence to establish the safety or effectiveness of high-flow nasal cannulas as a form of respiratory support in preterm infants.[116] Safe and effective use of **high-flow nasal cannulas (HFNC)** requires careful selection of an appropriate nasal prong-to-nares ratio even with an integrated pressure relief valve.[117]

MANAGEMENT STRATEGIES

Initiation

CPAP is often used in newborn intensive care to avoid endotracheal intubation and mechanical ventilation. **Mechanical ventilation** in preterm infants is associated with increased risk of sepsis, lung injury, arrested lung development, and chronic lung disease.[118,119] There is no consensus regarding the most effective management strategy or delivery system to administer CPAP in newborn infants.[94] Management is based more on clinical experience than research trials. In one institution, where elective B-CPAP has been the initial form of support for newborn infants for nearly four decades, this practice has resulted in less frequent use of mechanical ventilation and surfactant replacement therapy.[102] This practice has been associated with significant reductions in chronic lung disease compared with other centers that use mechanical ventilation as an initial strategy for managing infants. Some institutions support early elective surfactant therapy, brief ventilation, and extubation to nasal CPAP. This practice is also associated with significant reductions in the need for mechanical ventilation, fewer air leak syndromes, and lower incidence of chronic lung disease compared with a strategy of selective surfactant administration and continued ventilator support.[120]

The steps of initiation include:
1. Preparing the circuit, the bubble chamber (in B-CPAP), and the machine
2. Fixing the cap
3. Securing nasal prongs
4. Connecting the circuit
5. Insertion of orogastric tube
6. Setting of pressure, FiO₂, and flow

TABLE 15-3		
Cardinal Health Infant Flow Nasal CPAP Bonnet Sizing		
Bonnet Size	**Bonnet Color**	**Tape Measurement (cm)***
000	White	18-20
00	Gray	20-22
0	Pink	22-24
1	Light brown	24-26
2	Yellow	26-28
3	Light blue	28-30
4	Gold	30-32
5	Light green	32-34
6	Light burgundy	34-36
7	Orange	36-38
8	Dark green	38-40
9	Navy	40-42

*Tape measurement indicates the measured head circumference.
Courtesy Cardinal Health (Dublin, OH).

Application

CPAP is effective at reducing the incidence and duration of severe apneic episodes.[121] However, before CPAP can be applied, it is important to emphasize that infants experiencing frequent and sustained apneas or severe respiratory failure should not be considered for this form of support. It is essential that infants have a sufficient stimulus to breathe because CPAP is intended only for spontaneously breathing infants. Infants who do not respond to CPAP and continue to have frequent unresponsive apnea have failed this form of support.

The primary clinical objectives for managing infants with CPAP are to *recruit* collapsed lung units, *stabilize* the lung volume, *maintain* adequate lung expansion, *avoid* hyperinflation and apnea, *improve* gas exchange, and *eliminate* the need for mechanical ventilation. This practice requires a team of clinicians who are properly trained in the technical aspects of the CPAP equipment as well as understand the pathophysiology of the infant pulmonary system. This team usually consists of the respiratory therapist and the nurse caring for the patient. Patients receiving CPAP are often more time consuming than patients requiring mechanical ventilation.

CPAP of 4 to 6 cm H_2O is a common starting point for initiating CPAP.[34,122,123] Infants with obstructive lung disease may initially require higher CPAP levels in order to stent the airways open while allowing adequate ventilation.[37,38] Once CPAP is applied, it may take some time for patients to adjust to breathing through this system. Often, they resist the initial placement of the equipment but then relax once they have become used to it. If the infant continues to appear anxious, agitated, and inconsolable, it is very important to rule out hypoxia and airway obstruction. It is important to adopt "minimal handling" awareness and whenever possible cluster the patient care duties to limit infant stress.

The flow should be minimal to produce bubbling in the bubble chamber. It varies depending upon the pressure set, the lung disease, the weight of the baby, and the leaks in the circuit or from the patient's mouth. In the absence of a blender, first set the total flow and then set the air and the oxygen flow to get the desired FiO_2.

At first the FiO_2 should be set at the same level the patient was receiving before CPAP administration. Higher levels may be used to maintain adequate oxygen saturations or PaO_2.

During the *recruitment* stage, it is not uncommon for the patient to remain at a higher FiO_2 until the lung volumes are stabilized. Often an increase in FiO_2 may have no effect on oxygenation because of intrapulmonary shunting, and thus additional pressure is required. A 40% increase in FiO_2 during the first 24 hours of nasal CPAP may represent a useful clinical marker to identify infants at high risk for developing a pneumothorax.[68] Physiological changes associated with pneumothorax include decreased arterial blood pressure, increased heart rate, and increased respiratory rate; narrowed pulse pressure; and decreased PaO_2.[69]

Once recruitment occurs, FiO_2 should be weaned promptly in order to avoid complications caused by hyperoxemia.[124] The CPAP level is generally increased in increments of 1 or 2 cm H_2O; very rarely pressures up to 12 cm H_2O may be required when applying CPAP. The pressure and FiO_2 are increased to attain the desired PaO_2. However, it is best to change only one parameter at a time.

The patient is thought to be approaching *stabilization* once an adequate level of CPAP is attained. Oxygenation, ventilation, and chest radiograph appearance begin to improve. Reductions in the work of breathing, respiratory rate, and incidence of apnea are also important findings that indicate that the patient is improving.[125] Box 15-4 lists the signs indicating clinical *stabilization* of patients supported with CPAP. More tolerant guidelines for pH and $PaCO_2$ or "permissive hypercapnia" have become widely accepted clinical practices when treating critically ill infants.[126] This alone has likely reduced the number of intubations in infants receiving CPAP. However, it is also important to evaluate ventilation frequently by means of capillary blood gas readings or with a calibrated transcutaneous monitor, because extreme hypercapnia increases the risk for developing intraventricular hemorrhage in small infants.[127]

If the patient is not responding to CPAP, it is usually because the lungs are not opening with the amount of support the clinician has chosen. If the CPAP level is set below the opening pressure of the terminal respiratory units, then *recruitment* is unlikely to occur.[109] Breathing at low functional residual capacity can also lead to atelectrauma.[128] Proper assessment of tissue perfusion is vital. Increased intrathoracic pressure may result in worsening hemodynamic status. This is common when patients have low intravascular blood volumes or poor cardiac output. Intravenous fluid bolus can help eliminate this problem. If the patient develops apnea that does not require intubation, a loading dose of caffeine citrate (20 mg/kg) followed by a daily maintenance dose of 5 mg/kg (up to 10 mg/kg) can reduce the incidence of apnea.[129]

A rise in $PaCO_2$, or fall in PaO_2, after increasing the CPAP pressure may indicate that the optimal CPAP level has

---

Box 15-4	Indicators of Stabilization with Continuous Positive Airway Pressure Support

- Comfortable infant
- Reduced respiratory rate
- Minimal or no chest retractions
- SpO_2 between 88% to 95%
- Improvement in chest radiograph appearance
- Reduction in severity and frequency of apneic episodes
- Blood gas suggests PaO_2 50 to 80 mm, $PaCO_2$ 40 to 60 mm, pH 7.35 to 7.45 (with bubbling in the bubbling chamber and bubbling heard in the chest*)

*If on B-CPAP.

been exceeded.[13,130] An increase in mean airway pressure can result in increased alveolar dead space as a result of mechanical compression of the pulmonary microvasculature. If gas exchange worsens in a patient who appeared to be improving, the pressure can first be reduced; otherwise intubation is indicated.

Criteria used to recognize when a patient has failed CPAP and requires intubation and mechanical ventilation should be established by the medical team before placing a patient on CPAP. There are no definitive recommendations at this time and most institutions rely on anecdotal experience when identifying respiratory failure in infants receiving CPAP support. Box 15-5 lists some clinical signs indicating that CPAP has failed and that intubation and mechanical ventilation are indicated. Extremely low birth weight (less than 1000 g) infants, born at less than 26 weeks of gestation, are among the patients who most commonly fail nasal CPAP.[45] Other risk parameters include moderate or severe respiratory distress syndrome, septicemia, pneumothorax,[131] need of positive pressure ventilation, alveolar–arterial oxygen gradient ($AaDo_2$) greater than 180 in the first arterial blood gas,[129] lack or partial exposure to antenatal steroids,[132] need for oxygen in resuscitation and maintained in first hours of life, male gender, higher CPAP pressures (more than 5 cm of H_2O), and respiratory distress syndrome with criteria for surfactant adminisatration.[133] CPAP is only about 50% effective at eliminating the need for ventilation in infants born at less than 26 weeks of gestation.[134] Recognizing CPAP failure, and the need for intubation and mechanical ventilation, is paramount for the neonatal patient because failure can ensue rapidly as the result of respiratory muscle failure, worsening gas exchange, and apnea.

Monitoring

Monitoring is an essential component in managing patients receiving CPAP. The patient and CPAP system should be assessed frequently and at regular intervals to evaluate the effectiveness of the level of support and plan for subsequent care.

The physical assessment can be helpful when identifying early warning signs of respiratory impairment. Frequent assessment and measurements of vital signs and gas exchange can aid in the early diagnosis of air leak (e.g., pneumothorax) and other complications associated with the use of CPAP. Physical assessment should include documentation of breath sounds, heart rate, blood pressure, skin color, work of breathing, chest rise, level of activity, condition of the nares and nasal septum, secretions, oxygen saturation, transcutaneous carbon dioxide, and periodic arterial blood gas analyses. Brief disconnection from a bubble CPAP device may be indicated in order to properly assess breath sounds. Blood gases should be obtained if there is an acute deterioration in status but only after the patient becomes stabilized. If the $PaCO_2$ correlates closely or trends with the transcutaneous carbon dioxide, then blood gas monitoring should be minimized because of the low circulating blood volume in infants and the possibility for contamination with pathogens. Oxygen can be weaned on the basis of measurements obtained with a pulse oximeter.

Equipment monitoring should be incorporated into this assessment in order to verify proper function and eliminate equipment failure as a variable, should the patient's condition deteriorate.

Equipment monitoring includes assessment of pressure at the patient airway and verification of the presence of an attached low-pressure or disconnect alarm. However, besides loss of pressure to the patient, back pressure from the resistance across the prongs may prevent the low-pressure or disconnect alarm from sounding. A high-pressure "pop-off" (at least 15 cm H_2O) should be placed in line with the system and assessed for proper function. Other monitors with alarms, such as a pulse oximeter, transcutaneous monitor, or bradycardia alarm, should also be used with a low-pressure, or disconnect, alarm.

When using a B-CPAP device, the frequency of "bubbling" should be evaluated. A continuous bubbling usually indicates adequate gas delivery to the patient. If bubbling ceases during the breath cycle, this may indicate gas loss or a large leak at the patient interface or the patient circuit. Small fluctuations in pressure are common because of the frequency and amplitude of the bubbles; however, if large fluctuations are noted and coincide with the infant's

---

Box 15-5	**Recognizing Failure of Continuous Positive Airway Pressure Support**

Before considering CPAP failure, check the following conditions:
- Baby is not fighting CPAP interface
- Nasal prongs are of correct size
- Adequate humidification without any condensation in the circuit
- Adequate pressure and FiO_2 were delivered (check neck position, clear nostrils and airway)
- Surfactant has been administered in case of respiratory distress syndrome (RDS)

Markers of CPAP failure include the following:
- Increased WOB, nasal flaring, and retractions
- Decreasing pH (<7.25)
- $PaCO_2$ greater than 60 mm Hg*
- FiO_2 requirement exceeding 0.6 to 0.7 with PaO_2 less than 50 to 60 mm Hg†
- Nasal CPAP exceeding 8 to 10 cm H_2O
- Frequent apnea with cyanosis and bradycardia (not responding to caffeine therapy)

CPAP, Continuous positive airway pressure; *FiO_2*, fraction of inspired oxygen; *PaCO_2*, arterial partial pressure of carbon dioxide; *PaO_2*, arterial partial pressure of oxygen; *WOB*, work of breathing.
*Higher ranges may apply in infants with chronic carbon dioxide retention.
†Range should be consistent with clinical state and the presence of congenital heart disease or persistent pulmonary hypertension of the newborn.

inspiratory phase, then additional flow should be added to the system. Frequent monitoring of the water level height should be done to prevent changes in system pressure caused by condensation and evaporation. Water should be added or suctioned out to accommodate the desired CPAP level.

In the IF-CPAP and mechanical ventilator CPAP systems, low-pressure alarms usually indicate a leak caused by nasal prongs that are too small or an excessive oropharyngeal leak. The oropharynx acts as a safety valve preventing excessive accumulation of pressure in the airway. Oropharyngeal leaks are more common when using CPAP levels exceeding 8 to 10 cm H_2O. A chin strap, or pacifier, can be helpful at gently sealing the leak and reestablishing the CPAP level.[87] The set flow rate delivered by the CPAP device should not be increased until large leaks have been identified and resolved. The flow rate should then be adjusted to minimize large fluctuations in the system pressure as measured by a pressure manometer placed at the airway.

A functional manual resuscitator with the proper positive end-expiratory pressure setting as well as intubation equipment should be at the bedside in the event that the patient requires manual ventilation or intubation. Transcutaneous carbon dioxide monitors should be calibrated on the basis of manufacturer specifications. Humidification devices should also be documented as being on and set at the proper temperature and humidity levels. Water levels should also be frequently evaluated and maintained when using B-CPAP.

Chest radiographs are a valuable clinical tool for estimating lung expansion during the recruitment phase and for visualizing potential air leaks in the lung parenchyma.[135] Chest radiographs can also be helpful in determining whether the patient has any gastric distention from air entering the abdomen, which is more common when using CPAP levels exceeding 10 to 12 cm H_2O. This can decrease respiratory compliance, limit contraction of the diaphragm, and add significantly to respiratory distress. Gastric distention can be alleviated or prevented by inserting an oral gastric tube or by applying suction via a properly sized suction catheter.

Bedside Care and Airway Management

The proper bedside care of an infant receiving CPAP is perhaps the single most important aspect regarding outcomes and successful use of CPAP therapy.[84] It has also been recognized that these improved outcomes correlate well with the level of skill, familiarity, and experience of the clinicians after implementation of a new CPAP strategy in infants.[123] This includes caregivers who are adequately trained and are proficient at troubleshooting and selecting the proper-sized hat and nasal prongs or mask. The prongs should fill the entire nares without blanching the external nares.[84] Selecting prongs that are too small can result in

increased resistance and WOB, prong displacement, and excessive leaks.[103]

The fixation technique is also an important aspect of airway care in infants receiving CPAP support. The hat should be tight fitting, covering the ears and extending to the base of the neck.[84] Lateral attachment of straps should provide equal and gentle tension to avoid pressure points on the skin while securing the nasal interface to the infant.[87] The lack of stabilization and, hence, excessive movement of the prongs could result in worsening nasal injury, airway displacement, and loss of system pressure.

Another important consideration regarding bedside care that relates to airway management includes proper positioning of the infant. Infants can be positioned prone, supine, or on their side and should be turned every 2 to 4 hours.[87] The use of a small folded towel roll beneath the shoulders or chest can help support the infant and help maintain a patent airway.[87]

On occasion, the nasal prongs should be removed from the infant, and delicate suctioning through the mouth and nasopharynx should be done with a 5-Fr suction catheter. Nasal resistance is elevated in the neonate compared with the adult and is therefore rapidly elevated by a partial airway obstruction caused by mucous accumulation or swelling.[95] Therefore, infants who are suctioned usually have noticeable changes in WOB afterward. After suctioning, the nose should be evaluated for any signs of skin breakdown or nasal trauma and the prongs should be checked for the presence of kinking or mucus. Table 15-4 shows a nasal breakdown scoring system used for premature infants requiring CPAP.

The safe and effective delivery of aerosolized medications has been accomplished in-line using various delivery methods.[136] These drugs include bronchodilators, corticosteroids, surfactant, and ribavirin. Often, clinicians remove patients from the CPAP system to deliver bronchodilators. This should be done only if the patient tolerates being without CPAP; otherwise the risks of giving the medications outweigh their intended benefit. In addition to the appropriate airway management, some important key principles like optimal positioning, swaddling and containment of the infant, promoting day–night cycling of lights, minimizing sound levels in the intensive care unit, and involving parents in nursing care are some factors that may play an important role in improving brain function and subsequent development.[137]

Weaning

Attempts at weaning patients from CPAP should be considered when the patient is stable, has no incidents of apnea, and exhibits acceptable vital signs, blood gas values, and chest radiographic findings. Ideally, the Fio_2 should be weaned aggressively. If infants require oxygen chronically (because of pulmonary hypertension), then it is helpful to wean to an oxygen level that can be maintained reasonably with a separate oxygen delivery device. Some institutions

TABLE 15-4

Nasal Breakdown Scoring System for Premature Infants on Continuous Positive Airway Pressure*

	SCORE				
	0 = Normal	1 = Pale or Pink/Red	2 = Bleeding, Ulcer, Eschar	3 = Skin Tear	Nasal Compression (+ if Present)
Internal nares					
External nares					
Philtrum					
Bridge					
Septum					

Courtesy Walsh BK, Kaufman D, Zanelli S, Hicks T, University of Virginia Medical Center (Charlottesville, VA).

wean FiO_2 to 0.21 and then pressure is weaned in increments of 1 to 2 cm H_2O to a level between 3 and 5 cm H_2O. Birth weight may be a significant factor related to the time to successful NCPAP weaning.[138] Several weaning strategies have been described. The most common methods for weaning and withdrawal include (1) decreasing CPAP to a predefined level of airway pressure and then stopping CPAP completely; (2) removing CPAP for a predetermined number of hours each day (also known as "CPAP holidays"[139]) and gradually increasing the amount of time off CPAP each day until it can be stopped completely; and (3) stopping CPAP and starting high-flow heated humidified air (and oxygen if required) via nasal cannula. A trial is under way comparing the efficacy of bilevel nasal CPAP and conventional CPAP in extubation of infants less than 30 weeks of gestation.[140] A recent randomized controlled trial compared three methods for weaning CPAP in preterm infants. In method 1 (M1), the infant was taken off CPAP with the view to stay off. In method 2 (M2) the infant was cycled on and off CPAP with incremental time off. In method 3 (M3) the infant was cycled on and off CPAP but during off periods was supported by a 2-mm nasal cannula at a flow of 0.5 L/min. It was inferred that the first method significantly shortened CPAP weaning time, CPAP duration, and oxygen duration; reduced the incidence of bronchopulmonary dysplasia; and shortened admission time. However, further trials are required to confirm these results.[141]

ADVANCING CONCEPTS

Infant Flow SiPAP

Infant Flow "sigh" positive airway pressure (IF-SiPAP) (Cardinal Health) is a new device that uses the Infant Flow driver design and a new flow generator (Figure 15-11) to allow the infant to breathe spontaneously at two separate CPAP levels. This is accomplished by setting the baseline CPAP level, followed by a slow, unsynchronized secondary pressure (sigh breath) set at approximately 2 to 3 cm H_2O higher than the baseline pressure. The inspiratory time is set at about 1 to 3 seconds. The respiratory rate controls

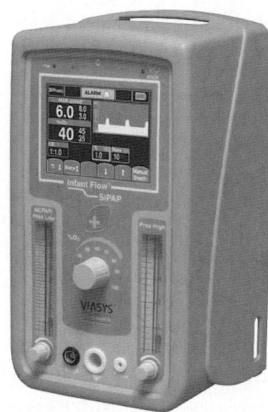

FIGURE 15-11   IF SiPAP flow generator.

the frequency of the intermittent "sigh" breaths. The infant is thus allowed to breathe spontaneously throughout the complete cycle of the sigh breath. Figure 15-12 shows the sequence of spontaneous breathing of a low-birth-weight infant during the pressure sigh created by the IF-SiPAP.

This concept is not intended to serve as a noninvasive pressure support mode but rather to aid in the recruitment and stabilization of unstable alveoli and thus preserve functional residual capacity. Unlike pressure support, the small delta pressure is held in the lung longer and the patient is not allowed to terminate the breath on the basis of certain criteria; rather, the patient breathes spontaneously throughout the entire respiratory cycle. In theory, these "sigh" breaths should also improve gas exchange and work of breathing and serve as a stimulant for apneic infants. The application of spontaneous breathing, as compared with the absence of spontaneous breathing, during a sustained pressure-hold has been shown to promote reopening of atelectatic lung regions and improve end-expiratory lung volume.[142] To date, there is only one published report that shows that the use of bilevel nasal CPAP results in significant improvements in gas exchange compared with standard nasal CPAP (Figure 15-13) in preterm infants.[143]

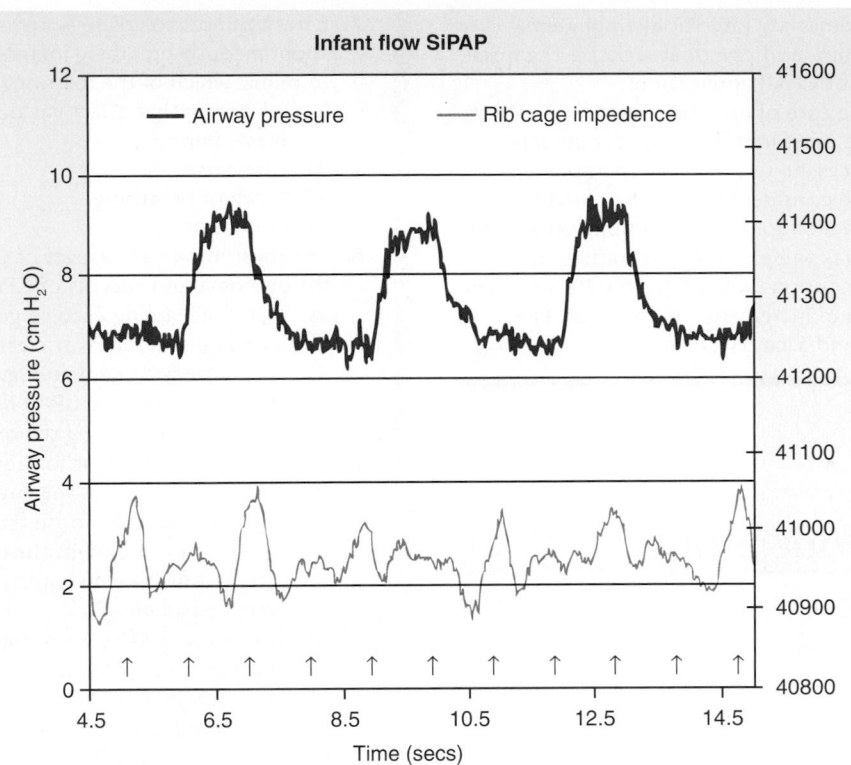

FIGURE 15-12   IF SiPAP: spontaneous breathing measurements made in a low-birth-weight infant. Airway pressure was obtained at the nasal interface, and the rib cage impedence (relative volume change) measurements were obtained with respiratory impedance plethysmography bands. The *arrows* indicate spontaneous breathing efforts made by the patient.

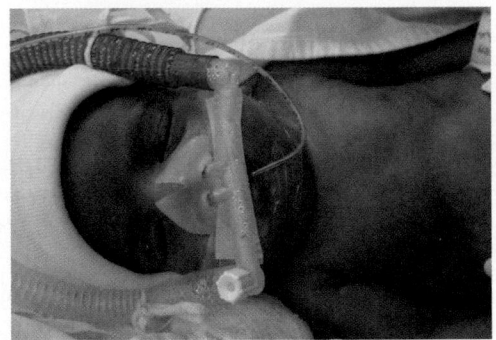

FIGURE 15-13   Infant comfortably positioned on CPAP.

KEY POINTS

- Early attempts at CPAP included placing infants in boxes with their head out through a loose-fitting cuff around the neck while negative pressure was applied continuously to the infant's chest wall. Later it changed to the application of nasal prong CPAP, which is still the most common method of CPAP delivery today.
- CPAP opens alveoli, thus increasing the functional residual capacity (FRC) of the lung, resulting in better gas exchange.

- CPAP can be given for both obstructive and nonobstructive diseases. The primary indications in preterm infants are respiratory distress syndrome, apnea of prematurity, delivery room prophylactic CPAP, after extubation from mechanical ventilation, and surfactant administration followed by NCPAP. The contraindications of CPAP include choanal atresia, cleft palate, tracheoesophageal fistula, and preoperative diaphragmatic hernia.
- The delivery system for CPAP can be a ventilator, bubble CPAP device, Infant Flow driver, or high-flow nasal cannula. Endotracheal tubes, nasopharyngeal prongs, and long and short binasal prongs are the common interfaces used for CPAP delivery.
- Among the delivery systems available, current evidence does not support a single device for CPAP delivery. A short binasal prong, however, is the most effective interface option for delivering CPAP to infants.
- There is no consensus regarding the most effective management strategy to administer CPAP in newborn infants. Management is based more on clinical experience than research trials.
- Monitoring and bedside care with supportive management are the key parameters that decide success with CPAP. Stabilization is judged as a comfortable infant with reduced respiratory rate and minimal or no chest retractions, in addition to other important key features.

- Pneumothorax, pulmonary interstitial emphysema, pneumomediastinum, and pneumatocele are the possible complications of CPAP application.
- The proper bedside care of an infant receiving CPAP is, perhaps, the single most important aspect influencing outcomes and successful use of CPAP therapy.
- Weaning should be considered when the patient is stable, has no incidents of apnea, and exhibits acceptable vital signs, blood gas values, and chest radiographic findings. Some institutions wean FiO_2 to 0.21 and then pressure is weaned in increments of 1 to 2 cm H_2O to a level between 3 and 5 cm H_2O.

ASSESSMENT QUESTIONS

See Evolve Resources for answers.

1. The most common interface used to deliver CPAP to spontaneously breathing infants is:
   A. Infant hood
   B. Nasal prongs
   C. Nasopharyngeal endotracheal tube
2. Physiological effects of CPAP include all of the following *except*:
   A. Improved respiratory system compliance and resistance
   B. Stabilization of the chest wall
   C. Increased mucus production
   D. Less lung injury than with mechanical ventilators
3. CPAP is contraindicated in infants with which of the following congenital anomalies?
   A. Preoperative congenital diaphragmatic hernia
   B. Postoperative heart surgery
   C. Postoperative congenital diaphragmatic hernia
4. CPAP levels greater than 8 cm H_2O are commonly associated with which of the following conditions?
   A. Gastric distention
   B. Oropharyngeal leaks
   C. Acute pulmonary edema
   D. Both A and B
5. Which of the following clinical indicators best describes methods for detecting early pneumothorax while monitoring infants receiving nasal CPAP?
   A. Persistent coughing and nasal flaring
   B. Widened pulse pressure
   C. An increased FiO_2 over the first day of CPAP support
   D. A significant increase in respiratory distress
   E. Diminished bilateral breath sounds
6. The following factors are essential when constructing a B-CPAP system *except*:
   A. A positive end-expiratory pressure/exhalation valve
   B. Hudson nasal prongs
   C. A blended gas source

7. Early attempts to create systems to provide CPAP to spontaneously breathing infants were aimed at trying to mimic which of the following important physiological factors that affect gas delivery to the lung?
   A. Nasal flaring
   B. Chest rise
   C. Work of breathing
   D. Grunting
8. The most important aspect of CPAP that can impact the outcome and success of CPAP is:
   A. The device being used to generate CPAP
   B. Suctioning and airway clearance techniques
   C. Proper bedside care and level of experience of clinicians using the CPAP device
   D. The physician writing the orders
9. The proper arrangement for any nasal CPAP system includes all of the following *except*:
   A. The hat should be loose fitting, covering the nose and extending to the base of the neck.
   B. Lateral attachment should provide gentle tension on the nasal interface.
   C. The prongs should be properly sized to eliminate migration from the nares.
   D. The hat should be tight fitting, covering the ears and extending to the base of the neck.
10. All of the following devices are considered acceptable for measuring and delivering nasal CPAP safely to infants *except*:
    A. V-CPAP
    B. B-CPAP
    C. IF-SiPAP
    D. High-flow nasal cannula

References

1. Courtney SE, Barrington KJ: Continuous positive airway pressure and noninvasive ventilation, *Clin Perinatol* 34(1):73–92, vi, 2007.
2. Gregory GA, Kitterman JA, Phibbs RH, Tooley WH, Hamilton WK: Treatment of the idiopathic respiratory-distress syndrome with continuous positive airway pressure, *N Engl J Med* 284(24):1333, 1971.
3. Bancalari E, Gerhardt T, Monkus E: Simple device for producing continuous negative pressure in infants with IRDS, *Pediatrics* 52(1):128, 1973.
4. Chernick V, Vidyasagar D: Continuous negative chest wall pressure in hyaline membrane disease: one year experience, *Pediatrics* 49(5):753, 1972.
5. Bancalari E, Garcia OL, Jesse MJ: Effects of continuous negative pressure on lung mechanics in idiopathic respiratory distress syndrome, *Pediatrics* 51(3):485, 1973.
6. Kattwinkel J, Fleming D, Cha CC, Fanaroff AA, Klaus MH: A device for administration of continuous positive airway pressure by the nasal route, *Pediatrics* 52(1):131, 1973.
7. Richardson CP, Jung AL: Effects of continuous positive airway pressure on pulmonary function and blood gases of infants with respiratory distress syndrome, *Pediatr Res* 12(7):771, 1978.
8. Saunders RA, Milner AD, Hopkin IE: The effects of continuous positive airway pressure on lung mechanics and lung volumes in the neonate, *Biol Neonate* 29(3–4):178, 1976.
9. Greenspan JS, Abbasi S, Bhutani VK: Sequential changes in pulmonary mechanics in the very low birth weight (less than or equal to 1000 grams) infant, *J Pediatr* 113(4):732, 1988.

10. Locke R, Greenspan JS, Shaffer TH, Rubenstein SD, Wolfson MR: Effect of nasal CPAP on thoracoabdominal motion in neonates with respiratory insufficiency, *Pediatr Pulmonol* 11(3):259, 1991.

11. Elgellab A, Riou Y, Abbazine A, et al: Effects of nasal continuous positive airway pressure (NCPAP) on breathing pattern in spontaneously breathing premature newborn infants, *Intensive Care Med* 27(11):1782, 2001.

12. Heldt GP: Development of stability of the respiratory system in preterm infants, *J Appl Physiol* 65(1):441, 1988.

13. Landers S, Hansen TN, Corbet AJ, Stevener MJ, Rudolph AJ: Optimal constant positive airway pressure assessed by arterial alveolar difference for CO_2 in hyaline membrane disease, *Pediatr Res* 20(9):884, 1986.

14. Magnenant E, Rakza T, Riou Y, et al: Dynamic behavior of respiratory system during nasal continuous positive airway pressure in spontaneously breathing premature newborn infants, *Pediatr Pulmonol* 37(6):485, 2004.

15. Durand M, McCann E, Brady JP: Effect of continuous positive airway pressure on the ventilatory response to CO_2 in preterm infants, *Pediatrics* 71(4):634, 1983.

16. Kamper J, Wulff K, Larsen C, Lindequist S: Early treatment with nasal continuous positive airway pressure in very low-birth-weight infants, *Acta Paediatr* 82(2):193, 1993.

17. De Klerk AM, De Klerk RK: Nasal continuous positive airway pressure and outcomes of preterm infants, *J Paediatr Child Health* 37(2):161, 2001.

18. Narendran V, Donovan EF, Hoath SB, Akinbi HT, Steichen JJ, Jobe AH: Early bubble CPAP and outcomes in ELBW preterm infants, *J Perinatol* 23(3):195, 2003.

19. Jobe AH, Bancalari E: Bronchopulmonary dysplasia, *Am J Respir Crit Care Med* 163(7):1723, 2001.

20. Jobe AH, Kramer BW, Moss TJ, Newnham JP, Ikegami M: Decreased indicators of lung injury with continuous positive expiratory pressure in preterm lambs, *Pediatr Res* 52(3):387, 2002.

21. Ho JJ, Subramaniam P, Henderson-Smart DJ, Davis PG: Continuous distending pressure for respiratory distress syndrome in preterm infants, *Cochrane Database Syst Rev* (2): CD002271, 2002.

22. Krouskop RW, Brown EG, Sweet AY: The early use of continuous positive airway pressure in the treatment of idiopathic respiratory distress syndrome, *J Pediatr* 87(2):263, 1975.

23. Harris H, Wilson S, Brans Y, Wirtschafter D, Cassady G: Nasal continuous positive airway pressure. Improvement in arterial oxygenation in hyaline membrane disease. *Biol Neonate* 29 (3–4):231, 1976.

24. Yu VY, Rolfe P: Effect of continuous positive airway pressure breathing on cardiorespiratory function in infants with respiratory distress syndrome, *Acta Paediatr Scand* 66(1):59, 1977.

25. Polin RA, Sahni R: Newer experience with CPAP, *Semin Neonatol* 7(5):379, 2002.

26. Miller MJ, DiFiore JM, Strohl KP, Martin RJ: Effects of nasal CPAP on supraglottic and total pulmonary resistance in preterm infants, *J Appl Physiol* 68(1):141, 1990.

27. Gaon P, Lee S, Hannan S, Ingram D, Milner AD: Assessment of effect of nasal continuous positive pressure on laryngeal opening using fibre optic laryngoscopy, *Arch Dis Child Fetal Neonatal Ed* 80(3):F230, 1999.

28. Miller RW, Pollack MM, Murphy TM, Fink RJ: Effectiveness of continuous positive airway pressure in the treatment of bronchomalacia in infants: a bronchoscopic documentation, *Crit Care Med* 14(2):125, 1986.

29. Miller MJ, Carlo WA, Martin RJ: Continuous positive airway pressure selectively reduces obstructive apnea in preterm infants, *J Pediatr* 106(1):91, 1985.

30. Jones RA: Apnoea of immaturity. 1. A controlled trial of theophylline and face mask continuous positive airways pressure, *Arch Dis Child* 57(10):761, 1982.

31. Henderson-Smart DJ, Subramaniam P, Davis PG: Continuous positive airway pressure versus theophylline for apnea in preterm infants, *Cochrane Database Syst Rev* (4):CD001072, 2001.

32. Robertson NJ, Hamilton PA: Randomised trial of elective continuous positive airway pressure (CPAP) compared with rescue CPAP after extubation, *Arch Dis Child Fetal Neonatal Ed* 79(1):F58, 1998.

33. Kattwinkel J: Neonatal apnea: pathogenesis and therapy, *J Pediatr* 90(3):342, 1977.

34. Kurz H: Influence of nasopharyngeal CPAP on breathing pattern and incidence of apnoeas in preterm infants, *Biol Neonate* 76(3):129, 1999.

35. Speidel BD, Dunn PM: Effect of continuous positive airway pressure on breathing pattern of infants with respiratory-distress syndrome, *Lancet* 1(7902):302, 1975.

36. Davis S, Jones M, Kisling J, Angelicchio C, Tepper RS: Effect of continuous positive airway pressure on forced expiratory flows in infants with tracheomalacia, *Am J Respir Crit Care Med* 158(1):148, 1998.

37. Panitch HB, Allen JL, Alpert BE, Schidlow DV: Effects of CPAP on lung mechanics in infants with acquired tracheobronchomalacia, *Am J Respir Crit Care Med* 150(5 Pt 1):1341, 1994.

38. Weigle CG: Treatment of an infant with tracheobronchomalacia at home with a lightweight, high-humidity, continuous positive airway pressure system, *Crit Care Med* 18(8):892, 1990.

39. American Association for Respiratory Care (AARC): Application of continuous positive airway pressure to neonates via nasal prongs or nasopharyngeal tube, *Respir Care* 39(8):817, 1994.

40. Kiciman NM, Andréasson B, Bernstein G, et al: Thoracoabdominal motion in newborns during ventilation delivered by endotracheal tube or nasal prongs, *Pediatr Pulmonol* 25(3): 175, 1998.

41. Jonson B, Ahlström H, Lindroth M, Svenningsen NW: Continuous positive airway pressure: modes of action in relation to clinical applications, *Pediatr Clin North Am* 27(3):687, 1980.

42. Buckmaster AG, Arnolda GR, Wright IM, Henderson-Smart DJ: CPAP use in babies with respiratory distress in Australian special care nurseries, *J Paediatr Child Health* 43(5):376, 2007.

43. Davis PG, Henderson-Smart DJ: Nasal continuous positive airways pressure immediately after extubation for preventing morbidity in preterm infants, *Cochrane Database Syst Rev* (2):CD000143, 2003.

44. Sandri F, Plavka R, Ancora G, et al: Prophylactic or early selective surfactant combined with nCPAP in very preterm infants, *Pediatrics* 125(6):e1402, 2010.

45. Finer NN, Carlo WA, Duara S, et al: Delivery room continuous positive airway pressure/positive end-expiratory pressure in extremely low birth weight infants: a feasibility trial, *Pediatrics* 114(3):651, 2004.

46. Sandri F, Ancora G, Lanzoni A, et al: Prophylactic nasal continuous positive airways pressure in newborns of 28-31 weeks gestation: multicentre randomised controlled clinical trial, *Arch Dis Child Fetal Neonatal Ed* 89(5):F394, 2004.

47. Han VK, Beverley DW, Clarson C, et al: Randomized controlled trial of very early continuous distending pressure in the management of preterm infants, *Early Hum Dev* 15(1): 21–32, 1987.

48. Finer NN, Carlo WA, Walsh MC, et al: Early CPAP versus surfactant in extremely preterm infants, *N Engl J Med* 362(21):1970, 2010.

49. Subramaniam P, Henderson-Smart DJ, Davis PG: Prophylactic nasal continuous positive airways pressure for preventing morbidity and mortality in very preterm infants, *Cochrane Database Syst Rev* (3):CD001243, 2005.

50. Rojas MA, Lozano JM, Rojas MX, et al: Very early surfactant without mandatory ventilation in premature infants treated with early continuous positive airway pressure: a randomized, controlled trial, *Pediatrics* 123(1):137, 2009.

51. Morley CJ, Davis PG, Doyle LW, Brion LP, Hascoet J-M, Carlin JB: Nasal CPAP or intubation at birth for very preterm infants, *N Engl J Med* 358(7):700, 2008.

52. Stevens TP, Blennow M, Soll RF: Early surfactant administration with brief ventilation vs selective surfactant and continued mechanical ventilation for preterm infants with or at risk for RDS, *Cochrane Database Syst Rev* (2):CD003063, 2002.

53. Tapia JL, Urzua S, Bancalari A, et al: Randomized trial of early bubble continuous positive airway pressure for very low birth weight infants, *J Pediatr* 161(1):75-80.e1, 2012.

54. Jeena P, Pillay P, Adhikari M: Nasal CPAP in newborns with acute respiratory failure, *Ann Trop Paediatr* 22(3):201, 2002.

55. Yurdakok M, Ozek E: Transient tachypnea of the newborn: the treatment strategies, *Curr Pharm Des* 18(21):3046, 2012.

56. Lin H-C, Su B-H, Lin T-W, Tsai C-H, Yeh T-F: System-based strategy for the management of meconium aspiration syndrome: 198 consecutive cases observations, *Acta Paediatr Taiwan* 46(2):67, 2005.

57. Fox WW, Berman LS, Downes JJ Jr, Peckham GJ: The therapeutic application of end-expiratory pressure in the meconium aspiration syndrome, *Pediatrics* 56(2):214, 1975.

58. Goldsmith JP: Continuous positive airway pressure and conventional mechanical ventilation in the treatment of meconium aspiration syndrome, *J Perinatol* 28(Suppl 3):S49, 2008.

59. Robertson NR: Prolonged continuous positive airways pressure for pulmonary oedema due to persistent ductus arteriosus in the newborn, *Arch Dis Child* 49(7):585, 1974.

60. Gregory GA, Edmunds LH Jr, Kitterman JA, Phibbs RH, Tooley WH: Continuous positive airway pressure and pulmonary and circulatory function after cardiac surgery in infants less than three months of age, *Anesthesiology* 43(4):426, 1975.

61. Cogswell JJ, Hatch DJ, Kerr AA, Taylor B: Effects of continuous positive airway pressure on lung mechanics of babies after operation for congenital heart disease, *Arch Dis Child* 50(10):799, 1975.

62. Buyukpamukcu N, Hicsonmez A: The effect of C.P.A.P. upon pulmonary reserve and cardiac output under increased abdominal pressure, *J Pediatr Surg* 12(1):49, 1977.

63. Verder H, Albertsen P, Ebbesen F, et al: Nasal continuous positive airway pressure and early surfactant therapy for respiratory distress syndrome in newborns of less than 30 weeks' gestation, *Pediatrics* 103(2):E24, 1999.

64. Verder H, Robertson B, Greisen G, et al: Surfactant therapy and nasal continuous positive airway pressure for newborns with respiratory distress syndrome. Danish-Swedish Multicenter Study Group, *N Engl J Med* 331(16):1051, 1994.

65. Kribs A, Vierzig A, Hünseler C, et al: Early surfactant in spontaneously breathing with nCPAP in ELBW infants—a single centre four year experience, *Acta Paediatr* 97(3):293, 2008.

66. Horbar JD, Badger GJ, Carpenter JH, et al: Trends in mortality and morbidity for very low birth weight infants, 1991-1999, *Pediatrics* 110(1 Pt 1):143, 2002.

67. Keszler M, Ryckman FC, McDonald JV Jr, et al: A prospective, multicenter, randomized study of high versus low positive end-expiratory pressure during extracorporeal membrane oxygenation, *J Pediatr* 120(1):107, 1992.

68. Goldsmith JP: Continuous positive airway pressure and conventional mechanical ventilation in the treatment of meconium aspiration syndrome, *J Perinatol* 28(Suppl 3):S49, 2008.

69. Migliori C, Campana A, Cattarelli D, Pontiggia F, Chirico G: [Pneumothorax during nasal-CPAP: a predictable complication?], *Pediatr Med Chir* 25(5):345, 2003.

70. Ogata ES, Gregory GA, Kitterman JA, Phibbs RH, Tooley WH: Pneumothorax in the respiratory distress syndrome: incidence and effect on vital signs, blood gases, and pH, *Pediatrics* 58(2):177, 1976.

71. Hall RT, Rhodes PG: Pneumothorax and pneumomediastinum in infants with idiopathic respiratory distress syndrome receiving continuous positive airway pressure, *Pediatrics* 55(4):493, 1975.

72. Gessler P, Toenz M, Gugger M, Pfenninger J: Lobar pulmonary interstitial emphysema in a premature infant on continuous positive airway pressure using nasal prongs, *Eur J Pediatr* 160(4):263, 2001.

73. Gürakan B, Tarcan A, Arda IS, Coşkun M: Persistent pulmonary interstitial emphysema in an unventilated neonate, *Pediatr Pulmonol* 34(5):409, 2002.

74. De Bie HMA, Van Toledo-Eppinga L, Verbeke JIML, Van Elburg RM: Neonatal pneumatocele as a complication of nasal continuous positive airway pressure, *Arch Dis Child Fetal Neonatal Ed* 86(3):F202, 2002.

75. Wong W, Fok TF, Ng PC, Chui KM, To KF: Vascular air embolism: a rare complication of nasal CPAP, *J Paediatr Child Health* 33(5):444, 1997.

76. Palmer KS, Spencer SA, Wickramasinghe YA, Wright T, Southall DP, Rolfe P: Effects of positive and negative pressure ventilation on cerebral blood volume of newborn infants, *Acta Paediatr* 84(2):132, 1995.

77. Tulassay T, Machay T, Kiszel J, Varga J: Effects of continuous positive airway pressure on renal function in prematures, *Biol Neonate* 43(3–4):152, 1983.

78. Furzan JA, Gabriele G, Wheeler JM, Fixler DE, Rosenfeld CR: Regional blood flows in newborn lambs during endotracheal continuous airway pressure and continuous negative pressure breathing, *Pediatr Res* 15(5):874, 1981.

79. Jaile JC, Levin T, Wung JT, Abramson SJ, Ruzal-Shapiro C, Berdon WE: Benign gaseous distension of the bowel in premature infants treated with nasal continuous airway pressure: a study of contributing factors, *AJR Am J Roentgenol* 158(1):125, 1992.

80. Moritz B, Fritz M, Mann C, Simma B: Nasal continuous positive airway pressure (n-CPAP) does not change cardiac output in preterm infants, *Am J Perinatol* 25(2):105, 2008.

81. De Paoli AG, Morley C, Davis PG: Nasal CPAP for neonates: what do we know in 2003? *Arch Dis Child Fetal Neonatal Ed* 88(3):F168, 2003.

82. Bonta BW, Uauy R, Warshaw JB, Motoyama EK: Determination of optimal continuous positive airway pressure for the treatment of IRDS by measurement of esophageal pressure, *J Pediatr* 91(3):449, 1977.

83. Peck DJ, Tulloh RM, Madden N, Petros AJ: A wandering nasal prong—a thing of risks and problems, *Paediatr Anaesth* 9(1):77, 1999.

84. Loftus BC, Ahn J, Haddad J Jr: Neonatal nasal deformities secondary to nasal continuous positive airway pressure, *Laryngoscope* 104(8 Pt 1):1019, 1994.

85. McCoskey L: Nursing Care Guidelines for prevention of nasal breakdown in neonates receiving nasal CPAP, *Adv Neonatal Care* 8(2):116, 2008.

86. Yong S-C, Chen S-J, Boo N-Y: Incidence of nasal trauma associated with nasal prong versus nasal mask during continuous positive airway pressure treatment in very low birth-weight infants: a randomised control study, *Arch Dis Child Fetal Neonatal Ed* 90(6):F480, 2005.

87. Lee S-Y, Lopez V: Physiological effects of two temperature settings in preterm infants on nasal continuous airway pressure ventilation, *J Clin Nurs* 11(6):845, 2002.

88. Bonner KM, Mainous RO: The nursing care of the infant receiving bubble CPAP therapy, *Adv Neonatal Care* 8(2): 78–95; quiz 96–97, 2008.

89. De Paoli AG, Davis PG, Faber B, Morley CJ: Devices and pressure sources for administration of nasal continuous positive airway pressure (NCPAP) in preterm neonates, *Cochrane Database Syst Rev* (1):CD002977, 2008.

90. Davis P, Davies M, Faber B: A randomised controlled trial of two methods of delivering nasal continuous positive airway pressure after extubation to infants weighing less than 1000 g: binasal (Hudson) versus single nasal prongs, *Arch Dis Child Fetal Neonatal Ed* 85(2):F82, 2001.

91. Banner MJ, Kirby RR, Blanch PB: Differentiating total work of breathing into its component parts. Essential for appropriate interpretation, *Chest* 109(5):1141, 1996.

92. Moomjian AS, Schwartz JG, Wagaman MJ, Shutack JG, Shaffer TH, Fox WW: The effect of external expiratory resistance on lung volume and pulmonary function in the neonate, *J Pediatr* 96(5):908, 1980.

93. Emeriaud G, Beck J, Tucci M, Lacroix J, Sinderby C: Diaphragm electrical activity during expiration in mechanically ventilated infants, *Pediatr Res* 59(5):705, 2006.

94. De Paoli AG, Morley CJ, Davis PG, Lau R, Hingeley E: In vitro comparison of nasal continuous positive airway pressure devices for neonates, *Arch Dis Child Fetal Neonatal Ed* 87(1):F42, 2002.

95. Pandit PB, Courtney SE, Pyon KH, Saslow JG, Habib RH: Work of breathing during constant- and variable-flow nasal continuous positive airway pressure in preterm neonates, *Pediatrics* 108(3):682, 2001.

96. Courtney SE, Pyon KH, Saslow JG, Arnold GK, Pandit PB, Habib RH: Lung recruitment and breathing pattern during variable versus continuous flow nasal continuous positive airway pressure in premature infants: an evaluation of three devices, *Pediatrics* 107(2):304, 2001.

97. Lee KS, Dunn MS, Fenwick M, Shennan AT: A comparison of underwater bubble continuous positive airway pressure with ventilator-derived continuous positive airway pressure in premature neonates ready for extubation, *Biol Neonate* 73(2):69, 1998.

98. Liptsen E, Aghai ZH, Pyon KH, et al: Work of breathing during nasal continuous positive airway pressure in preterm infants: a comparison of bubble vs variable-flow devices, *J Perinatol* 25(7):453, 2005.

99. Chernick V: Continuous distending pressure in hyaline membrane disease: of devices, disadvantages, and a daring study, *Pediatrics* 52(1):114, 1973.

100. Kaur C, Sema A, Beri RS, Puliyel JM: A simple circuit to deliver bubbling CPAP, *Indian Pediatr* 45(4):312, 2008.

101. Avery ME, Tooley WH, Keller JB, et al: Is chronic lung disease in low birth weight infants preventable? A survey of eight centers, *Pediatrics* 79(1):26, 1987.

102. Kahn DJ, Courtney SE, Steele AM, Habib RH: Unpredictability of delivered bubble nasal continuous positive airway pressure: role of bias flow magnitude and nares-prong air leaks, *Pediatr Res* 62(3):343, 2007.

103. Pillow JJ, Travadi JN: Bubble CPAP: is the noise important? An in vitro study, *Pediatr Res* 57(6):826, 2005.

104. Pillow JJ, Hillman N, Moss TJM, et al: Bubble continuous positive airway pressure enhances lung volume and gas exchange in preterm lambs, *Am J Respir Crit Care Med* 176(1):63, 2007.

105. Suki B, Alencar AM, Sujeer MK, et al: Life-support system benefits from noise, *Nature* 393(6681):127, 1998.

106. Morley CJ, Lau R, De Paoli A, Davis PG: Nasal continuous positive airway pressure: does bubbling improve gas exchange? *Arch Dis Child Fetal Neonatal Ed* 90(4):F343, 2005.

107. Moa G, Nilsson K, Zetterström H, Jonsson LO: A new device for administration of nasal continuous positive airway pressure in the newborn: an experimental study, *Crit Care Med* 16(12):1238, 1988.

108. Yadav S, Thukral A, Sankar MJ, et al: Bubble vs conventional continuous positive airway pressure for prevention of extubation failure in preterm very low birth weight infants: a pilot study, *Indian J Pediatr* 79(9):1163, 2012.

109. Wiswell TE, Srinivasan P: Continuous positive airway pressure [Internet]. ed 4. In Goldsmith JP, Karotkin EH, editors: *Assisted ventilation of the neonate*, ed 4, Philadelphia, 2003, WB Saunders, 127 [cited 2012. Sep 15].

110. Stoll BJ, Gordon T, Korones SB, et al: Late-onset sepsis in very low birth weight neonates: a report from the National Institute of Child Health and Human Development Neonatal Research Network, *J Pediatr* 129(1):63, 1996.

111. Thomson MA, Yoder BA, Winter VT, Giavedoni L, Chang LY, Coalson JJ: Delayed extubation to nasal continuous positive airway pressure in the immature baboon model of bronchopulmonary dysplasia: lung clinical and pathological findings, *Pediatrics* 118(5):2038, 2006.

112. Locke RG, Wolfson MR, Shaffer TH, Rubenstein SD, Greenspan JS: Inadvertent administration of positive end-distending pressure during nasal cannula flow, *Pediatrics* 91(1):135, 1993.

113. Sreenan C, Lemke RP, Hudson-Mason A, Osiovich H: High-flow nasal cannulae in the management of apnea of prematurity: a comparison with conventional nasal continuous positive airway pressure, *Pediatrics* 107(5):1081, 2001.

114. Saslow JG, Aghai ZH, Nakhla TA, et al: Work of breathing using high-flow nasal cannula in preterm infants, *J Perinatol* 26(8):476, 2006.

115. Kubicka ZJ, Limauro J, Darnall RA: Heated, humidified high-flow nasal cannula therapy: yet another way to deliver continuous positive airway pressure? *Pediatrics* 121(1):82, 2008.

116. Wilkinson D, Andersen C, O'Donnell CP, De Paoli AG: High flow nasal cannula for respiratory support in preterm infants, *Cochrane Database Syst Rev* (5):CD006405, 2011.

117. Sivieri EM, Gerdes JS, Abbasi S: Effect of HFNC flow rate, cannula size, and nares diameter on generated airway pressures: an in vitro study, *Pediatr Pulmonol* 48(5):506–14, May 2013

118. Hillman NH, Moss TJM, Kallapur SG, et al: Brief, large tidal volume ventilation initiates lung injury and a systemic response in fetal sheep, *Am J Respir Crit Care Med* 176(6):575, 2007.

119. Martin RJ, Nearman HS, Katona PG, Klaus MH: The effect of a low continuous positive airway pressure on the reflex control of respiration in the preterm infant, *J Pediatr* 90(6): 976, 1977.

120. Stevens TP, Harrington EW, Blennow M, Soll RF: Early surfactant administration with brief ventilation vs. selective surfactant and continued mechanical ventilation for preterm infants with or at risk for respiratory distress syndrome, *Cochrane Database Syst Rev* (4):CD003063, 2007.

121. Lindner W, Vossbeck S, Hummler H, Pohlandt F: Delivery room management of extremely low birth weight infants: spontaneous breathing or intubation? *Pediatrics* 103(5 Pt 1): 961, 1999.

122. Thia LP, McKenzie SA, Blyth TP, Minasian CC, Kozlowska WJ, Carr SB: Randomised controlled trial of nasal continuous positive airways pressure (CPAP) in bronchiolitis, *Arch Dis Child* 93(1):45, 2008.

123. Flynn JT, Bancalari E, Snyder ES, et al: A cohort study of transcutaneous oxygen tension and the incidence and severity of retinopathy of prematurity, *N Engl J Med* 326(16):1050, 1992.

124. Miller JD, Carlo WA: Safety and effectiveness of permissive hypercapnia in the preterm infant, *Curr Opin Pediatr* 19(2):142, 2007.

125. Fabres J, Carlo WA, Phillips V, Howard G, Ambalavanan N: Both extremes of arterial carbon dioxide pressure and the magnitude of fluctuations in arterial carbon dioxide pressure are associated with severe intraventricular hemorrhage in preterm infants, *Pediatrics* 119(2):299, 2007.

126. Clark RH, Gerstmann DR, Jobe AH, Moffitt ST, Slutsky AS, Yoder BA: Lung injury in neonates: causes, strategies for prevention, and long-term consequences, *J Pediatr* 139(4):478, 2001.

127. Schmidt B, Roberts RS, Davis P, et al: Long-term effects of caffeine therapy for apnea of prematurity, *N Engl J Med* 357(19):1893, 2007.

128. Andréasson B, Lindroth M, Svenningsen NW, et al: Measurement of ventilation and respiratory mechanics during continuous positive airway pressure (CPAP) treatment in infants, *Acta Paediatr Scand* 78(2):194, 1989.

129. Ammari A, Suri M, Milisavljevic V, et al: Variables associated with the early failure of nasal CPAP in very low birth weight infants, *J Pediatr* 147(3):341, 2005.

130. AARC clinical practice guideline: Patient-ventilator system checks. American Association for Respiratory Care, *Respir Care* 37(8):882, 1992.

131. Boo NY, Zuraidah AL, Lim NL, Zulfiqar MA: Predictors of failure of nasal continuous positive airway pressure in treatment of preterm infants with respiratory distress syndrome, *J Trop Pediatr* 46(3):172, 2000.

132. Koti J, Murki S, Gaddam P, Reddy A, Reddy MDR: Bubble CPAP for respiratory distress syndrome in preterm infants, *Indian Pediatr* 47(2):139, 2010.

133. Rocha G, Flôr-de-Lima F, Proença E, et al: Failure of early nasal continuous positive airway pressure in preterm infants of 26 to 30 weeks gestation, *J Perinatol* [Internet] 2012. Aug 30 [cited 2012. Sep 17]. Available from: http://www.ncbi.nlm.nih.gov/pubmed/22935774.

134. Giedion A, Haefliger H, Dangel P: Acute pulmonary X-ray changes in hyaline membrane disease treated with artificial ventilation and positive end-expiratory pressure (PEP), *Pediatr Radiol* 1(3):145, 1973.

135. Greenough A, Premkumar M, Patel D: Ventilatory strategies for the extremely premature infant, *Paediatr Anaesth* 18(5):371, 2008.

136. Jardine LA, Inglis GD, Davies MW: Strategies for the withdrawal of nasal continuous positive airway pressure (NCPAP) in preterm infants, *Cochrane Database Syst Rev* (2):CD006979, 2011.

137. Als H, Duffy FH, McAnulty G, et al: NIDCAP improves brain function and structure in preterm infants with severe intrauterine growth restriction, *J Perinatol* 32(10):797, 2012.

138. Rastogi S, Rajasekhar H, Gupta A, Bhutada A, Rastogi D, Wung J-T: Factors affecting the weaning from nasal CPAP in preterm neonates, *Int J Pediatr* 2012. 416073, 2012.

139. Shoemaker MT, Pierce MR, Yoder BA, DiGeronimo RJ: High flow nasal cannula versus nasal CPAP for neonatal respiratory disease: a retrospective study, *J Perinatol* 27(2):85, 2007.

140. Victor S: EXTUBATE: a randomised controlled trial of nasal biphasic positive airway pressure vs. nasal continuous positive airway pressure following extubation in infants less than 30 weeks' gestation: study protocol for a randomised controlled trial, *Trials* 12:257, 2011.

141. Todd DA, Wright A, Broom M, et al: Methods of weaning preterm babies <30 weeks gestation off CPAP: a multicentre randomised controlled trial, *Arch Dis Child Fetal Neonatal Ed* 97(4):F236, 2012.

142. User experience network. Supply gas failure alarm on Cardinal Health Infant Flow SiPAP units may not activate, *Health Devices* 38(7):232, 2009.

143. Migliori C, Motta M, Angeli A, Chirico G: Nasal bilevel vs. continuous positive airway pressure in preterm infants, *Pediatr Pulmonol* 40(5):426, 2005.

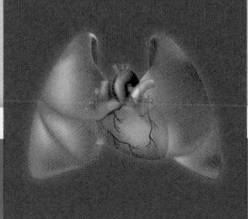

Chapter 16

Noninvasive Mechanical Ventilation of the Infant and Child

W. GERALD TEAGUE, DENISE THOMPSON-BATT

OUTLINE

Definitions and Introduction
  Factors for the Respiratory Care Professional to
    Consider Before Starting NPPV in a Child
Objectives of NPPV and CPAP
Objectives of High-Flow Nasal Cannula
**Experience with NPPV Treatment in Pediatric Respiratory
  Disorders**
  Acute Respiratory Distress
  Chronic Respiratory Failure
  Obstructive Sleep Apnea Syndrome and Morbid Obesity
Noninvasive Ventilation with Positive-Pressure Devices
  Bilevel Pressure-Targeted Ventilators
  Adaptive Servoventilation (ASV) and Proportional Assist
    Ventilation (PAV)
  Volume-Regulated Ventilators

Noninvasive Ventilation with Negative-Pressure Devices
NPPV Adjustment: Modes and Pressure Titration
  Modes
  Pressure Titration
Interface Selection and Fit
Monitoring the Patient and Ventilator Circuit
Complications and Contraindications to NPPV
  Complications
  Contraindications
Future of Noninvasive Ventilation in Pediatrics

LEARNING OBJECTIVES

After reading this chapter the reader will be able to:
  1. Describe the effects of NPPV on respiratory function
  2. Differentiate the effects of NPPV from CPAP on
     respiratory function
  3. Identify pediatric respiratory disorders amenable to a
     trial of NPPV
  4. Identify clinical scenarios in children less amenable to a
     trial of NPPV

  5. Explain the inspiratory pressure support feature of
     commercial bilevel pressure ventilators
  6. Discuss how adjustments in inspiratory and expiratory
     positive airway pressures affect respiratory function
  7. Recall the principles of interface selection so as to
     optimize the effectiveness and comfort of NPPV
  8. Discuss common complications and contraindications
     to NPPV

KEY TERMS

Noninvasive positive airway pressure
  (NPPV)
Negative pressure–assisted ventila-
  tion (NPAV)

Continuous positive airway pressure
  (CPAP)
High-flow nasal cannula (HFNC)

Inspiratory positive airway pressure
  (IPAP)
Expiratory positive airway pressure
  (EPAP)

DEFINITIONS AND INTRODUCTION

Methods of respiratory assistance that do not require an indwelling artificial airway are collectively termed *noninvasive* (Box 16-1). This chapter addresses noninvasive ventilation in children in general, but the focus is primarily on **noninvasive positive airway pressure (NPPV).** Interest in NPPV treatment in infants and children over the past three decades has grown, in part because of the pervasive belief that NPPV is a safe alternate to invasive assisted ventilation via endotracheal tube. Although the cumulative experience with NPPV treatment of children in the acute settings is promising, the evidence that NPPV is superior to standard treatment in preventing intubation is inconclusive. A trial of NPPV treatment may delay intubation and actually worsen clinical outcomes as suggested by its use in adults with simple community-acquired pneumonia.[1] Improved survival of children with severe lung injury who are left with long-term respiratory dysfunction has fostered the use of NPPV in the pediatric intensive care unit. NPPV is used in this setting to facilitate early extubation and transition to ambulatory care. The evidence in support of NPPV as a means of early extubation in children with severe lung disease is not conclusive.[2] NPPV is also commonly used in the emergency department and general care areas of the hospital to treat children with acute respiratory distress.[3] The safety and effectiveness of NPPV therapy in children outside the intensive care unit (ICU) for acute respiratory disorders have not been well studied or validated despite this common practice.

NPPV treatment of infants and children with chronic respiratory disorders in the outpatient setting has also steadily grown. Caregivers of children with chronic respiratory

failure managed at home by tracheostomy and positive pressure ventilation often seek NPPV as a means to tracheal decannulation so as to ameliorate the social disadvantages associated with a tracheostomy.[4] There are no clear guidelines for monitoring of children treated with NPPV in either the hospital or ambulatory setting. These and other issues pertaining to the use of NPPV in the pediatric patient are addressed in this chapter.

Factors for the Respiratory Care Professional to Consider Before Starting NPPV in a Child

Foremost, the clinician should assess the age and pattern of respiratory dysfunction in the child and the clinical setting to decide whether a trial of NPPV is even warranted. Are sedation and electronic monitoring going to be necessary? A second consideration is whether or not the available equipment for NPPV has the necessary performance features to meet the ventilatory demand of the child. Commercially available bilevel pressure ventilators with inspiratory pressure support are designed to respond to the mechanical properties and respiratory time constants of adults,[5] and the tidal volume by NPPV is dependent on the level of respiratory impedance.[6] Furthermore, small children and infants with respiratory distress often cannot attain the predefined levels of inspiratory flow or pressure required to trigger the inspiratory support feature. After initiation of NPPV, the child must be assessed immediately to be certain that the work of breathing has decreased and that there is sufficient improvement in respiratory gas exchange.

OBJECTIVES OF NPPV AND CPAP

The broad objectives of assisted ventilation are addressed elsewhere (see Chapter 17, Invasive Mechanical Ventilation of the Neonate and Pediatric Patient). The primary objectives of NPPV in children with acute respiratory distress are to decrease the work of breathing and improve respiratory gas exchange (Box 16-2). To determine the effectiveness of NPPV in achieving these objectives, the respiratory therapy professional must complete a thorough examination of the child. Children with acute respiratory distress typically breathe rapidly and shallowly, use the accessory muscles of respiration, and present with thoracic/abdominal retractions. Therefore the therapist's primary objective is to evaluate the work of breathing before and after initiation of NPPV and document in the medical record that the goals of treatment have been achieved.

Children with respiratory failure from neuromuscular weakness or central alveolar hypoventilation may not demonstrate the signs and symptoms of respiratory distress despite severe derangement in respiratory gas exchange. In such patients and in young infants, an arterial blood gas is necessary to assess the degree of respiratory dysfunction

---

Box 16-1	**Noninvasive Ventilation: Broad Purpose and Definitions**

The broad purpose of noninvasive ventilation is to treat respiratory dysfunction and restore respiratory gas exchange in a range of clinical settings.

Noninvasive positive pressure ventilation (NPPV): A method of respiratory assistance that involves an external interface and cyclical positive pressure device.

Negative pressure–assisted ventilation (NPAV): A method of respiratory assistance based on intermittent application of subatmospheric pressure external to the chest wall through a tank or mold.

Continuous positive airway pressure (CPAP): A method of respiratory assistance based on application of a distending flow via an external interface to attain a defined constant positive pressure.

High-flow nasal cannula (HFNC): A means of respiratory assistance that utilizes a soft nasal cannula interface and high humidified flow source to raise the intraluminal pharyngeal pressure.

The primary objectives of NPPV are to decrease the work of breathing and improve respiratory gas exchange.
- Decreased work of breathing manifested by
  - Decreased respiratory rate
  - Decreased retractions
  - Decreased use of accessory muscles of breathing
- Improved respiratory gas exchange manifested by
  - Decreased arterial Pa_{CO_2}
  - Increased arterial Pa_{O_2}
  - Increased arterial pH
- Increased functional residual capacity (FRC)
- Increased patency of the oral-pharyngeal airway and decreased intrinsic auto-PEEP

and to determine the effectiveness of NPPV. A venous blood gas is often used to assess the acid/base status of a child in the acute setting but is not a reliable estimate of respiratory gas exchange. Thus arterial or capillary blood samples are the preferred method of collection. The attending physician of record should be notified when, in the opinion of the therapist, a child has failed a trial of noninvasive ventilation.

The clinical objectives of **continuous positive airway pressure (CPAP)** therapy are similar to those of NPPV but through different mechanisms. An appropriate level of CPAP must increase end-expiratory lung volume (functional residual capacity) and thereby improve oxygenation. CPAP therapy may or may not improve tidal volume and alveolar ventilation. In children and neonates with restrictive respiratory dysfunction and decreased lung compliance, CPAP therapy can raise tidal volume. However, in children with lung overexpansion from air trapping and increased compliance, CPAP therapy may actually decrease tidal volume. Two clinical trials have compared intermittent nasal NPPV to CPAP in neonates with respiratory distress syndrome.[7,8] A significant decrease in treatment failure, defined as the need for rescue invasive ventilation, was found in NPPV-treated infants, but NPPV did not decrease in the prevalence of chronic lung disease. In daily practice, CPAP is likely as good a choice as NPPV in situations in which the predominant respiratory derangement is hypoxemia from ventilation–perfusion inequality but the child has adequate alveolar ventilation. NPPV is preferred when hypoventilation is present and the child has sufficient inspiratory effort to trigger the inspiratory pressure support function of the NPPV device.

NPPV can be applied to children with both acute and chronic respiratory disorders to achieve other benefits on lung function (see Box 16-2). Children with restrictive lung disorders, including atelectasis, pneumonia, neuromuscular weakness, and morbid obesity, typically present with hypoxemia and a reduction in functional residual capacity.

Both NPPV and CPAP are effective in this setting to restore end-expiratory lung volume. NPPV is offered to patients with chronic hypoventilation disorders as a clinical benefit used at night to reduce the severity of daytime symptoms associated with chronic hypercarbia—headache and fatigue.[9] The daytime Pa_{CO_2} (arterial partial pressure of carbon dioxide) should decrease 1 to 2 weeks after initiation of nocturnal NPPV treatment. This is likely explained by decreased blood pH through nocturnal carbon dioxide elimination, diminution of renal bicarbonate reabsorption, and restoration of the central ventilatory responsiveness to changes in pH. We have found that intermittent NPPV treatment in pediatric patients with chronic hypoventilation disorders effectively improves daytime carbon dioxide elimination for at least a period of 1 year and that this improvement is associated with a decrease in total serum levels of bicarbonate.[10,11]

Likewise, in children with intermittent or chronic upper airway obstruction NPPV or CPAP can raise the intraluminal pharyngeal and hypopharyngeal pressures to impede collapse and maintain the patency of the laryngeal inlet. Assessment of the effectiveness of NPPV or CPAP in both these functions is important and involves a detailed respiratory examination and appropriate monitoring of gas exchange. The sleep laboratory is an ideal location to assess the effectiveness of NPPV and CPAP in the treatment of upper airway dysfunction and sleep-disordered breathing. There is an important role for the respiratory therapist in optimal interface selection, adjustment, and monitoring of NPPV in the polysomnography laboratory.

OBJECTIVES OF HIGH-FLOW NASAL CANNULA

High-flow nasal cannula (HFNC) systems are commonly used in the neonatal (NICU) and pediatric intensive care units (PICU) to treat acute respiratory distress. HFNC treatment is often selected as an alternative to NPPV and CPAP to avoid the relative discomfort of a mask interface. The goal is to administer a threshold level of nasal gas flow to raise the intraluminal nasopharyngeal pressure sufficient to increase functional residual capacity and maintain upper airway patency. The effectiveness of HFNC in meeting these objectives is not well studied in children.[12] In premature infants the minimal level of HFNC treatment to improve respiratory status was found in one systematic review to be greater than 2 lpm.[13] In a study of infants with bronchiolitis, nasopharyngeal pressures increased linearly (0.45 cm H_2O for each 1 L/min increase) with HFNC rates up to 6 lpm.[14] In an uncontrolled study of children in the ICU, treatment with HFNC was associated with acute improvement in respiratory distress and aeration on chest film.[15] Children presenting to the emergency department with acute respiratory distress treated with HFNC per an institutional protocol had a significant reduction in intubation rates compared with children not treated in this way during an earlier period, but this observation was retrospective and not controlled.[16] For more details on suggested flow settings, please refer to Chapter 10.

EXPERIENCE WITH NPPV TREATMENT IN PEDIATRIC RESPIRATORY DISORDERS

Acute Respiratory Distress

NPPV is widely used in the ICU setting to treat infants and children with acute respiratory distress associated with a broad spectrum of disorders (Box 16-3). Whereas the cumulative evidence is highly supportive of an early trial of NPPV in adults with acute cardiogenic pulmonary edema[17] and acute exacerbations of COPD,[18] evidence in support of NPPV treatment in adults with acute asthma is not conclusive.[19] Furthermore, there is no comparable level of evidence to support or refute NPPV use in acute respiratory disorders of children. This topic was last reviewed in 2003,[20] and the fundamental question from that review is the same today: Does NPPV treatment prevent or just delay intubation in children with acute respiratory distress at risk for respiratory failure? The physiological benefits of NPPV in children with acute respiratory failure associated with hypercarbia were recently described.[21] Application of NPPV led to a 33% increase in tidal volume, and a 56% decrease in the diaphragmatic pressure–time product. These changes indicate a significant decrease in work of breathing as well as improved respiratory gas exchange. Unfortunately, short-term physiological improvements after NPPV application in children with acute respiratory distress have not been linked to improved clinical outcomes confirmed by controlled trials. The studies to date are observational and include children with diverse causes of respiratory distress.

In a recent observational study of 151 small children in acute respiratory distress who were treated with NPPV, there were clear improvements in gas exchange and work of breathing, but the study was uncontrolled and the intubation failure rate was nearly 25%.[22] Risk factors for NPPV failure (i.e., need for intubation) were premature birth and pneumonia. Improvements in oxygenation occurred in both the NPPV success and NPPV failure groups in the first 4 hours of treatment, but indices in the work of breathing improved only in the NPPV success group. A 5-year review of NPPV use in children in the ICU setting again supported its effectiveness (77% success rate in preventing intubation), but these observations are both uncontrolled and retrospective.[23] These reports do highlight disorders wherein NPPV treatment in children was not effective, including acute respiratory distress syndrome (ARDS).[23,24] In case series NPPV has been applied with mixed results to children with respiratory distress from status asthmaticus,[20] acute chest syndrome,[25] and congenital heart disease.[26] With acute asthma, NPPV may be an effective adjunct therapy to improve lung function when applied in combination with nebulized bronchodilators.[27] An important note to the interpretation of these reports for the respiratory care professional is the need for sedation to comfortably apply NPPV in the acute setting, especially for children with status asthmaticus.[20]

Guide for the Practicing Respiratory Care Professional: Acute Respiratory Distress

The practicing respiratory professional should consider several factors before initiating a trial of NPPV in an infant or child with acute respiratory distress (Box 16-4). Foremost the therapist must evaluate the setting and available resources to monitor and treat the child. Monitoring requirements and availability of skilled ancillary personnel are as important with NPPV as they are in a child who requires intubation and mechanical ventilation. Case reports do not support a trial of NPPV in patients with cardiovascular instability and fulminant respiratory failure—for example, children with rapidly evolving hypoxemia from ARDS.[23] Pediatric disorders that lead to a low likelihood of successful response to NPPV include ARDS, status asthmaticus, pulmonary hemorrhage with hemoptysis, and sepsis with cardiovascular instability. NPPV should not be initiated based on the assumption that it will necessarily decrease the likelihood of endotracheal intubation and thus should be restricted to a practice environment also conducive to immediate airway management and critical care support of the child. Consideration should also be given to whether or not the child will need sedation to tolerate NPPV. Agitation with placement of the mask interface is an important cause of treatment failure in children with status asthmaticus treated with NPPV.[20]

Chronic Respiratory Failure

NPPV is often used to treat children with chronic respiratory disorders in two settings—as rescue therapy, based on

---

Box 16-3	Acute Respiratory Disorders of Infancy and Childhood Amenable to Treatment with NPPV

- Early phase of ARDS
- Acute chest syndrome
- Congenital heart disease
- Complicated community-acquired pneumonia
- Pulmonary edema
- Fat or bone marrow embolism
- Status asthmaticus
- Postextubation respiratory distress
- Acute pulmonary hemorrhage
- Near drowning lung injury
- Acute lung aspiration syndromes
- Bronchiolitis
- Acute respiratory distress post bone marrow transplantation

Box 16-4	Factors Informing the Success or Failure of NPPV in the Treatment of Acute Respiratory Distress in Children

- Assignment of skilled personnel to monitor and manage a critically ill child
- Availability of appropriate NPPV equipment and monitoring devices
- Level of postnatal development and status of airway protective reflexes
- Exclusion of children with rapidly evolving hypoxemia: cardiovascular instability, ARDS, severe asthma

the belief that it can prevent endotracheal intubation in acute exacerbations, and as a long-term clinical benefit. In a recent European review, outpatient NPPV use in children was concentrated among a few centers specializing in pediatric respiratory care.[28] Long-term use of NPPV can provide substantial clinical benefit in children with a range of respiratory disorders complicated by chronic respiratory failure (Box 16-5).[29-32] The physiological benefits of NPPV treatment in the ambulatory setting have been reviewed earlier in this chapter. Perhaps the most successful experience with NPPV as a rescue therapy is its use in acute exacerbations of hypercarbic respiratory failure in children with chronic neuromuscular disorders.[33] Children with myelomeningocele are at risk for a number of life-threatening respiratory complications for which NPPV has been used effectively in combination with other respiratory therapies.[34] In children with advanced cystic fibrosis (CF) lung disease, long-term NPPV has been successful as a bridge therapy to lung transplantation.[35] In a single uncontrolled case series, long-term NPPV use was associated with stabilization of lung function in advanced CF lung disease,[36] but the short-term use of NPPV was no more beneficial than standard therapies in clearing airway secretions.[37] Nonetheless, in a systematic review of available trials of NPPV, the current recommendation is to consider its use as an adjunct therapy for airway secretion clearance in patients with cystic fibrosis lung disease.[38]

Box 16-5	Pediatric Chronic Respiratory Disorders Amenable to Long-Term NPPV Treatment

- Chronic respiratory failure associated with neuromuscular weakness or chest wall dysfunction
- Cerebral palsy and other severe neurobehavioral abnormalities
- Respiratory complications of myelomeningocele
- Advanced cystic fibrosis lung disease (as a bridge to transplantation)
- Alternate to tracheostomy in congenital central alveolar hypoventilation syndrome

Standard treatment for congenital central alveolar hypoventilation syndrome (CCHS) is long-term assisted ventilation via tracheostomy, with and without supplemental diaphragmatic pacing. CCHS is an especially high-risk disorder when considering treatment with NPPV because of the failure of autonomic ventilatory drive during quiet sleep. These children are at high risk of central hypoventilation. Nonetheless, because of the social and medical disadvantages of a tracheostomy, caregivers of children with CCHS increasingly seek noninvasive modes of ventilation as a means to facilitate tracheal decannulation.[11,30] NPPV has been used to treat children with CCHS with standard mask interfaces and as a bridge to long-term treatment with negative-pressure assisted ventilation.[39] In regard to effective settings, a recent modification of the pressure-support mode to facilitate assured volume delivery was used to treat a teenager with CCHS.[40]

Guide for the Practicing Respiratory Care Professional: Chronic Disorders

Respiratory care professionals involved in the treatment with NPPV of children with chronic respiratory disorders should make sure that appropriate monitoring is in place. In the home setting NPPV should be viewed as a treatment with a probable clinical benefit, and not for the purposes of life support. Hence monitoring requirements may be less stringent in the home setting than in the hospital but, most importantly, is determined by the acuity of the child's condition. The selection of a comfortable mask interface that fits appropriately is especially important for long-term NPPV use in children. In about one fifth of children an interface change is necessary, primarily because of patient discomfort.[41] CCHS is a special disorder in which careful monitoring is necessary whenever the child is asleep. The device used to apply NPPV must be set to deliver effective and consistent minute ventilation, and a backup ventilatory rate is mandatory. The sleep laboratory is an ideal setting to assess the adequacy of meeting these goals in children, and such studies should be done on a regular basis. A best practice advisory is available from the American Academy of Sleep Medicine to adjust NPPV settings via polysomnography in adults and children with stable alveolar hypoventilation syndromes.[42] Although there are certainly neonates with CCHS who have been treated with NPPV alone since birth, the safety of this practice as an alternative to standard treatment with regard to long-term developmental and cardiopulmonary outcomes has not been rigorously studied.

Obstructive Sleep Apnea Syndrome and Morbid Obesity

NPPV is often selected as an alternate to nasal CPAP in children with complicated obstructive sleep apnea syndrome (OSAS) and in children with obesity hypoventilation syndrome. The advantage of NPPV in these disorders is the pressure support function, which will assist the respiratory muscles during inspiration to overcome resistance imposed by a collapsed upper airway and stiff chest wall. Although there are no clear guidelines, selection of NPPV over CPAP in children with OSAS is typically made in OSAS complicated by alveolar hypoventilation and hypercarbia. OSAS often complicates a restrictive pattern of respiratory dysfunction in a number of so-called overlap syndromes, including cerebral palsy, myelomeningocele, Down syndrome, and morbid obesity. In these disorders NPPV confers a distinct advantage over CPAP to decrease the work of the respiratory muscles, increase tidal volume, and thereby reverse alveolar hypoventilation. A distinct pattern of periodic central apnea during sleep is an important complication of sleep-disordered breathing in congestive heart failure patients. Application of a sufficient level of CPAP to reduce the apnea-hypopnea index in heart failure patients below 15 events per hours was associated with improved cardiac function.[43] NPPV is widely touted as a means to improve nocturnal ventilation and sleep quality in patients with obesity hypoventilation syndrome. However, in a recent controlled trial, although NPPV did improve daytime CO_2 elimination, it did not alter a panel of inflammatory and metabolic disturbances in obesity hypoventilation syndrome.[44]

NONINVASIVE VENTILATION WITH POSITIVE-PRESSURE DEVICES

Bilevel Pressure-Targeted Ventilators

NPPV is accomplished in children using either pressure-support or volume-regulated devices.[28] Bilevel devices deliver pressure-supported assisted ventilation, a mode in which a step threshold change in inspiratory flow or pressure triggers the unit to deliver a preset level of positive pressure during the inspiratory effort. The result is an increase in tidal volume that is dependent on the compliance and resistance of the respiratory system and the gradient between the inspiratory and expiratory pressure adjustments.[6,45] Most bilevel ventilators available for commercial use are adept at delivering sufficient flow to reach the targeted level of inspiratory pressure.[5] These devices also have a flow compensation feature so that small leaks around the interface or through the mouth do not seriously impair performance. However, the capacity of NPPV devices to compensate for severe leaks is limited and the result is greater patient/ventilation asynchrony, cited as a common reason for NPPV failure in the acute setting.[29]

Other features that are standard on bilevel pressure-targeted ventilators include an **expiratory positive airway pressure (EPAP)** adjustment, backup ventilatory rate, and mode selection. Some devices introduced recently feature an integrated blender to titrate supplemental oxygen delivery (such as the BiPAP Vision ventilator support system; Philips Respironics, Murrysville, PA). Other more recent adaptations of bilevel ventilators include integrated alarm systems, graphic display, memory chip for recording events, and internal battery packs.

Regulatory Issues with Bilevel Ventilators

Despite widespread publications citing their effectiveness and safety, the U.S. Food and Drug Administration (FDA) does not approve bilevel devices as an invasive mode of mechanical ventilation in children. Instead these devices are in the FDA category of noncontinuous ventilator and as such are primarily intended to augment patient ventilation. The position of most managed care agencies and home respiratory vendors is that bilevel positive airway pressure with backup rate is not appropriate for use with a tracheostomy or as a substitute for an FDA-approved portable home ventilator. Although this has not been an issue for inpatient application, it is a major impediment for outpatient use. Most home care companies require that physicians sign an indemnification agreement releasing them from liability should the device fail.

Adaptive Servoventilation (ASV) and Proportional Assist Ventilation (PAV)

The adaptive servoventilator (AutoSet CS; ResMed, Sydney, Australia) is a modified bilevel pressure ventilator suitable for NPPV. The device provides a baseline level of ventilatory support (end-inspiratory pressure of 9 cm H_2O) superimposed on 5 cm H_2O CPAP. The subject's ventilation is servocontrolled with a high-gain integral controller (0.3 cm H_2O per L/min per second, clipped to 4 to 10 cm H_2O) to equal a moving target ventilation of 90% of the long-term average ventilation (time constant 3 min).[46] If the subject suddenly ceases all central respiratory effort, the device will increase the inspiratory pressure amplitude from a minimum of 4 cm H_2O up to whatever is required to maintain ventilation at 90% of the long-term average. In comparison to nocturnal CPAP, ASV decreased central apnea and Cheyne-Stokes breathing and improved sleep quality in adults with congestive heart failure. Although use of ASV in children is limited, its design features are amenable to long-term disorders complicated by central alveolar hypoventilation, including Chiari malformation, myelomeningocele, and even CCHS.

Proportional assist ventilation (PAV, BiPAP Vision Ventilator, Respironics Inc, Pittsburgh, PA) is a modification of pressure-support ventilation (PSV) to match ventilator responsiveness to patient breathing effort. Unlike PSV that uses a preset inspiratory pressure, PAV provides inspiratory flow and pressure in proportion to the patient's spontaneous breathing effort as determined by instantaneous feedback from an in-line pneumotachometer.[47] Cycles from inspiration to expiration are not dependent on a predetermined reduction in inspiratory flow, as is the case with PSV. PAV, when properly adjusted, terminates delivery of inspiratory assistance with cessation of inspiratory effort. In this way, PAV has the potential of enhancing patient–ventilator synchrony. PAV performed better in regards to patient preference and some physiological variables than standard PSV by nasal mask in a comparison trial of adults with acute respiratory failure.[48]

Volume-Regulated Ventilators

NPPV can be accomplished through portable ventilators designed to cycle in the volume mode. The features of these ventilators are reviewed in Chapter 35 (Home Care). The potential advantages of volume-regulated devices for NPPV include superior performance when used in the synchronized intermittent mandatory ventilation mode for patients who, with significant neuromuscular weakness or central hypoventilation, may not trigger bilevel ventilators. However, this limitation of standard bilevel ventilators may be overcome with modern devices with the technical features to provide ASV and PAV.

Major drawbacks of portable volume-regulated ventilators for NPPV in pediatric patients include their relative size, limited portability, and, most importantly, limited attainment of high levels of inspiratory flow to support spontaneous respiratory efforts. Newer generations of portable ventilators are smaller and provide flow rates that support spontaneous breathing, including pressure support.

To appropriately adjust a volume-regulated ventilator for NPPV, the delivered tidal volume should be approximately twice that of the child's physiological tidal volume to accommodate the dead space of the nasopharynx and conducting airways. Setting the tidal volume above the physiologic range and adjusting the peak inspiratory pressure until the required tidal volume is achieved can accomplish this. This method, originally referred to as *pressure plateau ventilation*, is commonly used for invasive long-term mechanical ventilation in pediatric patients.[49] Probably because of enhanced patient comfort and lower costs with pressure-device NPPV, there is a modern trend away from volume-regulated and toward pressure-supported devices to accomplish NPPV in the ambulatory setting.[50]

NONINVASIVE VENTILATION WITH NEGATIVE-PRESSURE DEVICES

Negative pressure–assisted ventilation (NPAV) is a form of respiratory assistance in which subatmospheric pressure is applied intermittently through a cuirass or tank (iron lung) device external to the chest wall. Expiration occurs as the pressure around the chest wall is allowed to return to atmospheric levels. This method of assisted ventilation has a long tradition of being effective in pediatric patients with hypoventilation associated with acquired neurological injury from trauma or infection and chronic restrictive lung disorders.[51,52] However, large tank ventilators are difficult to transport and have gradually fallen out of use. Instead modern cuirass devices

(United Hayek RTC, London United Kingdom) are FDA approved and being utilized on a limited bases. The advantage of these devices is a beneficial effect on cardiac filling pressures and volumes, a benefit found even in healthy individuals.[53] In a highly novel application, negative pressure applied to the abdomen in combination with nasal CPAP has been studied as an effective means to recruit atelectatic lung, although this approach has not been used in humans.[54] An important drawback of negative-pressure ventilation is significant disruption of sleep in patients with neuromuscular disorders and poor control of the muscle group supporting the upper airway. In these patients, treatment with negative-pressure ventilation can be complicated by recurrent episodes of obstructive apnea/hypopnea culminating in transient hypoxemia.

NPPV ADJUSTMENT: MODES AND PRESSURE TITRATION

Modes

Most bilevel pressure-targeted ventilators suitable for NPPV feature CPAP, spontaneous, timed, and spontaneous/timed operating modes (Box 16-6). In the CPAP mode, these devices provide constant flow to maintain a target level of continuous positive airway pressure. Inspiratory pressure support is not provided. In the spontaneous mode, the ventilator responds to a threshold level of inspiratory flow or to a change in volume that is initiated by the patient's spontaneous respiratory effort. At the inspiratory flow threshold, the ventilator delivers additional gas flow to reach the preset **inspiratory positive airway pressure (IPAP).** Exhalation occurs after the inspiratory flow peaks and then decreases to a threshold level. In the timed mode, the ventilator does not flow trigger but delivers intermittent pulses of positive airway pressure at a set rate. In the spontaneous/timed mode, the flow-trigger feature is activated. The ventilator cycles in the timed mode only in the event of prolonged apnea.

Guide for the Practicing Respiratory Care Professional: NPPV Adjustment

Pediatric patients are typically managed with NPPV in the spontaneous/timed mode. The chief advantage of this mode is patient comfort. This results when the child's

---

Box 16-6   NPPV Modes

CPAP: Continuous flow with no inspiratory pressure assist or rate

Spontaneous: Patient-triggered inspiratory pressure assist with no backup rate

Timed: Device-initiated pulse of preset positive pressure at a set rate

Spontaneous/Timed: Patient-triggered inspiratory pressure assist and timed mode cycling in the event of prolonged apnea

inspiratory efforts are assisted with the inspiratory pressure support feature. Significant barriers to effective NPPV in pediatric patients treated with NPPV are ineffective triggering[55-56] and patient/ventilator asynchrony.[29] The best way for the practicing therapist to promote effective triggering and prevent asynchrony with NPPV is to minimize leaks around the mask interface. In the presence of a significant leak, the inspiratory pressure target is never reached, resulting in a long inflation time as the unit delivers massive amounts of inspiratory flow in an attempt to attain the preset inspiratory pressure. This may require application of an oral-nasal mask in a child with significant mouth leak. Some modern bilevel ventilators (VPAP III ST, ResMed, Poway, CA; BiPAP Vision, Philips Respironics) designed for NPPV feature an adjustable inflation time that can be set to prevent this problem. There is little published experience with pediatric patients treated with NPPV exclusively in the timed mode. Recent guidelines recommend consideration of the timed mode or use of a backup rate in children with evidence of central alveolar hypoventilation.[42] In this mode the ventilator essentially functions as a time-cycled, pressure-limited device. It is important for therapists to be aware that many ventilators available for NPPV in children have significant performance limitations; hence the need for appropriate bedside assessment and monitoring.[57]

Pressure Titration

With modern bilevel pressure ventilators, the IPAP adjustment determines the target distending airway pressure attained during flow-triggered or timed ventilator inflations (Box 16-7). The IPAP should be set above the EPAP to raise the child's tidal volume, "unload" the respiratory muscles, and decrease respiratory distress. The differential between the IPAP and EPAP adjustment determines the tidal volume. Detailed guidelines for the adjustment of NPPV settings in the polysomnography laboratory are provided by the American Academy of Sleep Medicine.[42] Although modern bilevel devices are capable of achieving IPAP levels of 30 cm H_2O, children younger than 12 years typically do not tolerate pressures higher than 20 cm H_2O without some type of sedation.[20] There may be a delay of several hours before a step increase in IPAP achieves a reduction in $PaCO_2$. In this event, other factors can be used to determine the effectiveness in NPPV (Table 16-1). In day-to-day clinical practice, an IPAP setting of between 8 and 12 cm H_2O is typically sufficient to achieve the goals of NPPV in pediatric patients.

Box 16-7	NPPV Pressure Adjustments

Inspiratory positive airway pressure (IPAP): Determines the tidal volume
Expiratory positive airway pressure (EPAP): Raises end-expiratory lung volume and impedes upper airway collapse

TABLE 16-1	
Methods to Determine the Clinical Effectiveness of Noninvasive Ventilation	
Outcome Expected	**Method and Limitations**
Decrease in work of breathing	*Physical examination:* Acute decrease in respiratory rate, retractions, and use of accessory muscles. Not reliable in young infants and children with neuromuscular and central disorders.
Improvement in respiratory gas exchange	*Pulse oximetry:* Acute improvement in SaO_2. Not a reliable metric in the assessment of hypoventilation. Interpretation obscured by concurrent O_2 treatment. *Blood gas sampling:* Increase in pH, decrease in $PaCO_2$, increase in PaO_2; invasive—$PaCO_2$ may not decrease for hours if at all in some disorders. *End-tidal CO_2 monitoring:* Acute reduction in end-tidal CO_2. High background flow in NPPV circuit can wash out expired CO_2. *Transcutaneous CO_2 monitoring:* Subacute reduction in transcutaneous CO_2 monitoring; accuracy dependent on careful electrode placement; changes lag minutes behind change in actual $PaCO_2$.
Increase in FRC	*Routine chest radiography:* Increased lung expansion, decreased atelectasis; difficult to accomplish during therapy; changes can lag days behind.
Maintenance of upper airway patency	*Sleep polysomnography:* Subacute reductions in the number of airway-occlusive episodes decrease with the degree of thoracoabdominal asynchrony. Not amenable to acute clinical setting.

FRC, Functional residual capacity; *NPPV*, noninvasive positive pressure ventilation; *$PaCO_2$*, arterial partial pressure of carbon dioxide; *PaO_2*, arterial partial pressure of oxygen; *SaO_2*, arterial oxygen saturation.

The EPAP adjustment with NPPV primarily determines the end-expiratory lung volume and maintains the stability of the upper airway. In a typical pediatric application of NPPV, EPAP levels of 6 to 8 cm H_2O are effective in improving oxygenation and preventing obstructive apnea. Most children, regardless of the setting or indication, poorly tolerate EPAP levels above 10 cm H_2O.

Overtitration of airway pressures is a common mistake when NPPV is attempted in pediatric patients. In children with normal lung compliance, typically those with neuromuscular lung diseases, optimal results are seen at relatively low distending pressures. Raising the pressure to compensate for leaks around the nasal mask or through the mouth often is poorly tolerated in children and can lead to central hypoventilation. The mechanism behind this is uncertain, but it is also seen in adult patients with obesity hypoventilation syndrome treated with nasal CPAP.[58]

In negative pressure–assisted ventilation, the applied subatmospheric pressure is decreased incrementally to raise the tidal volume. A significant hazard in exposing patients with neuromuscular disorders to intermittent external subatmospheric pressures while leaving the head and neck exposed to ambient atmospheric pressure is episodic obstructive apnea and hypopnea. In clinical practice this can be minimized by concomitant nasal CPAP therapy with negative pressure–assisted ventilation.

INTERFACE SELECTION AND FIT

Interface devices appropriate for NPPV include nasal masks, nasal–oral masks, and nasal plugs or pillows.[41] Recent advances in interface design have led to assisted ventilation with a helmet device. Administration of CPAP via a helmet was compared with conventional mask interface in children with acute respiratory distress and was well tolerated, with some physiological advantages.[59] One study in adults compared different interfaces and showed that although nasal masks are more acceptable to patients, facial masks and nasal plugs delivered higher minute ventilation with better carbon dioxide elimination than nasal masks.[60]

In most clinical scenarios the nasal mask is the preferred interface in pediatric patients (Box 16-8). Newer-generation nasal masks have a soft gel cushion (e.g., the Phantom nasal mask, SleepNet, Manchester, NH) that conforms to the contours of the face and forehead and are thus more comfortable. These models also minimize air leaks and facial trauma. However, in critically ill patients even small oral air leaks are undesirable. Nasal–oral masks should be considered when absolute avoidance of an oral air leak is necessary. However, nasal–oral masks may pose a significant risk of aspiration of gastric contents in the event of emesis and also may increase anxiety in young children. Under these conditions, sedation is often necessary, and the child should not be fed.

Nasal masks are commercially available in a wide range of sizes and shapes to fit children and adolescents. However, soft nasal masks are not widely available for small infants and in one case series children younger than 2 years treated with NPPV required custom-made masks. Custom masks may also be indicated in children with midfacial syndromes associated with maxillary hypoplasia. The nasal mask should fit snugly around the nasal margins. When the mask is too large, significant tension on the head straps is necessary to prevent mask leaks, thereby promoting dermal ulceration at the nasal bridge. Long-term intermittent NPPV by means of a nasal mask may impair maxillary bone growth.[61] This concern, although not clearly supported by available evidence, is considered significant by caregivers of children treated with NPPV.

Nasal plugs or pillows can be substituted for nasal masks in children who complain of discomfort with the nasal mask. Nasal plugs or pillows are not used as often because most children eventually adapt to the nasal mask very well. They may have some role treating teenagers because they place no pressure on the face and do not interfere with vision.

MONITORING THE PATIENT AND VENTILATOR CIRCUIT

Selection of patient and ventilator monitors with NPPV is based primarily on the clinical setting and the acuity of the patient. In critically ill children, NPPV serves a life support function. The optimal location for patients receiving NPPV depends on the capacity for adequate monitoring, staff skill, experience with and knowledge of the equipment used, and awareness of potential complications. The patient should thus be monitored with arterial oxygen saturation (SaO_2), arterial blood gases, work of breathing, development of hemodynamic instability or altered mental status, and failure to tolerate the device. Each monitor device should have alarm limits set by an experienced respiratory therapist.

Often, NPPV is used for stable patients with respiratory dysfunction as a clinical benefit. A hospital ward, sleep laboratory, or step-down unit is an appropriate setting for NPPV in this capacity. A pulse oximeter alone may be sufficient monitoring provided the child is clinically stable and not likely to decompensate in the event of equipment failure or removal of the interface. Novel monitoring of compliance, leak, and selected physiological variables is available through software integrated into modern bilevel devices. In one observational study, this type of monitoring provided helpful information for the clinician in regard to respiratory events but was prone to artifacts; hence the need for independent validation.[62]

Intermittent NPPV can be accomplished safely at home without any patient or ventilator monitors. However, children with stable long-term disorders treated with NPPV in the home setting have frequent episodes of hypercarbia in the absence of hypoxemia.[63] In children with these hypercarbic episodes, daytime capillary arterialized carbon dioxide levels were normal in nearly all of them. Thus routine continuous carbon dioxide monitoring is advised for children at risk for hypoventilation and treated with NPPV. This is often a challenge with NPPV because of dilution of exhaled carbon dioxide by the continuous flow present between the nasal opening and mask interface. An alternate

Box 16-8	Guide to Interface Selection in Pediatric Patients Treated with NPPV

- Consider the setting: acute respiratory distress versus long-term use for a chronic disorder.
- Consider the acuity: A complete seal is important if gas exchange is compromised by leak.
- Soft nasal masks are more comfortable, better tolerated, and have a relative safety advantage.
- Nasal oral masks are indicated when a complete seal is necessary and the child is in acute distress.
- The most common error in pediatrics is to select an overly large mask in the interest of comfort. These pose greater risks of leak and skin irritation.

to nasal sampling devices is the recent introduction of ear CO_2 monitoring systems, but these have not been adequately studied in children in the ambulatory setting.

COMPLICATIONS AND CONTRAINDICATIONS TO NPPV

Complications

Pediatric patients are at relatively higher risk for complications to NPPV as a result of unique physiological differences from adults (Table 16-2). Because NPPV is often used in the long-term treatment of young children, it may well affect the postnatal growth of the mid-face and jawbone. Long-term NPPV use is associated with a facial flattening in a majority of children and retraction of the mandible in some.[64] An important confounding issue is whether or not children at risk for mid-facial hypoplasia are more likely to be treated with NPPV and whether the disorders themselves promote abnormal facial growth versus the effects of the mask interface per se. Whatever the mechanism, this is an important cosmetic consideration and should be shared with the caregivers of children in advance of a course of long-term NPPV. A fatal complication of NPPV has been reported in an adult patient who died from hypoventilation and failure of the battery pack device.[65]

Approximately half of children experience one or more minor complications of NPPV. The most common minor complication reported is skin irritation as a result of the nasal mask (48%), leading to skin necrosis in up to 8%.[64] Other minor but important side effects of NPPV in children include nasal dryness or discomfort, epistaxis, and eye irritation. One study found that prolonged use of maintenance steroids was an additional risk factor for development of skin ulcers during NPPV.[66] Epistaxis can be prevented by humidification, whereas conjunctival irritation may be prevented by selection of appropriate-sized nasal mask.

Contraindications

The only absolute contraindication to a trial of NPPV in pediatric patients with acute respiratory distress is cardiovascular instability. Relative contraindications include nasopharyngeal obstruction, massive hemoptysis, poor clearance of or profuse oral secretions, and extreme agitation or anxiety.

FUTURE OF NONINVASIVE VENTILATION IN PEDIATRICS

A major impediment to the future of NPPV in infants and children is the reluctance of companies that manufacture bilevel ventilators to seek FDA approval of their devices for pediatric patients. This is primarily because of the cost of FDA approval and the relatively low volume of units expected to be sold in the pediatric market. The result is that clinicians who care for children with chronic hypoventilation disorders and who are attracted to NPPV as an alternative to invasive tracheostomy with positive pressure ventilation become involved in funding disputes and legal conflicts with companies that dispense durable medical equipment.

Despite these constraints, the future for NPPV in pediatric patients is promising. Smaller interfaces and flow-triggered, pressure-targeted units suitable for small children are appearing for home use. Modern bilevel units already can achieve target inspiratory pressures of 30 cm H_2O and are equipped with independent oxygen adjustment settings. These units also come with a maximal inspiratory time setting so as to prevent prolonged inflations in the presence of uncompensated leaks. Proportion assist ventilation, a method of assisted ventilation that is responsive to the resistive and elastic properties of the respiratory system, can be administered by means of a nasal mask. This method of assisted ventilation is well beyond preliminary trials in adults and may have significant advantages over NPPV with current bilevel devices. At present, NPPV treatment should be restricted to carefully selected children and only in centers equipped with the appropriate equipment and experienced personnel. Randomized trials comparing early NPPV versus standard treatment in well-characterized patient populations are needed to clearly define the role of NPPV in children.

TABLE 16-2

Factors Unique to Pediatric Patients That Promote Complications of NPPV

Complication	Factor Unique to Children
Aspiration	Immaturity of airway protective reflexes
Reflux	Impaired gastroesophageal sphincter function during infancy
Upper airway obstruction	Anatomical factors, difficulty clearing secretions
Large oral leak	Tendency to mouth breathe
Agitation	Anxiety, incomplete understanding, developmental disorders

---

CLINICAL HIGHLIGHT

CS is an 11-year-old girl with advanced cystic fibrosis lung disease and CF-associated diabetes. She was hospitalized four times in the past year for treatment of pulmonary exacerbations with systemic broad-spectrum antibiotics, chest physiotherapy, inhaled hypertonic saline, and inhaled Colistin. CS's sputum is infected with pan-resistant *Burkholderia cepacia*, and despite the hospitalizations her FEV_1 has decreased over time to 20% of predicted. Her SaO_2 in room air is 85% but increases to 95% with 2 lpm nasal cannula oxygen. A recent echocardiogram showed moderate pulmonary artery hypertension with enlargement of the right ventricle. CS was referred to a regional center for evaluation for lung transplant. However, she was not listed for transplant and asked to return for reevaluation in 6 months. In the interim, CS developed morning headaches. A capillary blood gas in room air showed a pH of 7.41, $PaCO_2$ of 53 torr, and PaO_2 of 74 torr. Because of the headaches, pulmonary hypertension, and hybercarbia, CS was offered nocturnal NPPV as a bridge therapy during the transplant evaluation period. She preferred a face mask interface and was treated with a pressure-targeted bilevel device adjusted to the spontaneous/timed mode, a backup rate of 12 breaths per minute, IPAP of 14 cm, EPAP of 8 cm, and FiO_2 of 0.21. After a few months of NPPV the patient's morning headaches cleared, her pulmonary artery pressure as estimated by echocardiogram stabilized, and her body mass index reached a plateau. The plan is to continue nocturnal NPPV pending evaluation for lung transplantation.

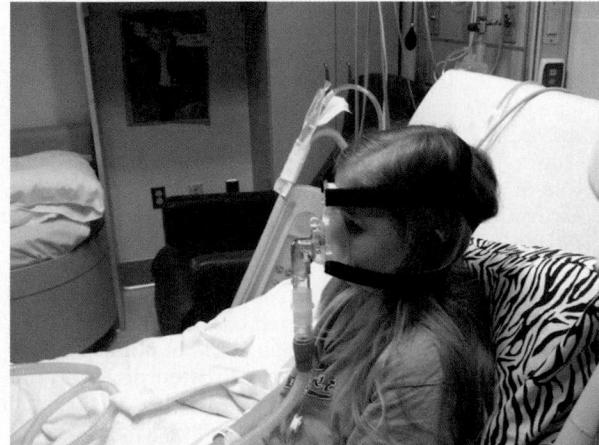

Adolescent with advanced cystic fibrosis lung disease treated with face mask NPPV.

KEY POINTS

- NPPV is a noninvasive mode of respiratory assistance administered by an external interface device for the purposes of improving alveolar ventilation and oxygenation, decreasing the spontaneous work of breathing, and relieving respiratory distress.
- In contrast to CPAP, NPPV in most applications will raise the child's tidal volume and hence increase CO_2 elimination.
- Various respiratory disorders of childhood may be treated with NPPV, but the available evidence best supports NPPV use in some forms of acute respiratory distress and long-term for treatment of chronic restrictive disorders.
- NPPV is less effective in children with cardiopulmonary instability and severe lung injury such as evolving ARDS. Its use in children with acute asthma, while promising, is not supported by clinical studies.
- In bilevel pressure devices suitable for use with NPPV, the inspiratory pressure support feature is triggered when the child makes a spontaneous respiratory effort and can therefore decrease the work of breathing.

- The tidal volume attained during NPPV is positively correlated with the pressure gradient between the IPAP and EPAP settings.
- The optimal interface for NPPV in most children is a soft nasal mask that fits snugly over the child's nose and does not require undue tension on the attachment straps to remain in place.
- The most common complication of NPPV in children is skin irritation at the interface margins, but serious life-threatening complications have also been reported.

ASSESSMENT QUESTIONS

See Evolve Resources for answers.

1. An absolute contraindication to a trial of NPPV in a child with respiratory distress is:
   A. Status asthmaticus
   B. Absence of a nasogastric tube to ventilate the stomach
   C. Cardiovascular instability
   D. Tracheoesophageal fistula
2. True or false:
   The required level of monitoring for a child with long-term respiratory failure treated with nocturnal NPPV in the ambulatory setting as a probable clinical benefit should include a cardiorespiratory monitor and pulse oximeter.
3. The following pediatric respiratory disorders may be treated with a trial of NPPV in the acute setting *except:*
   A. ARDS with sepsis
   B. Bronchiolitis
   C. Acute exacerbation of cystic fibrosis lung disease
   D. Pneumonia in a child with muscular dystrophy
4. True or false:
   Current evidence supports a trial of NPPV to prevent endotracheal intubation and invasive mechanical ventilation in children with acute respiratory distress.
5. You are called by the floor nurse to evaluate a child with cerebral palsy and pneumonia treated with NPPV who is agitated. The child's heart rate is elevated and he is moving around the bed. The best response in this situation is to:
   A. Reassure the nurse and the child's parents that NPPV takes some time to get used to and simply observe the child over time.
   B. Notify the attending physician that the child is not tolerating NPPV and needs to be sedated so that the NPPV can be effective.
   C. Do a complete respiratory examination paying attention to the child's work of breathing and vital signs before and after application of NPPV
   D. Replace the nasal mask interface with a full face mask interface that covers the mouth and nose so as to prevent oral leak.

References

1. Ferrar M, Cosentini R, Nava S: The use of non-invasive ventilation during acute respiratory failure due to pneumonia, *Eur J Intern Med* 23:420, 2012.

2. Keenan SP, Powers C, McCormack DG, Block G: Noninvasive positive-pressure ventilation for postextubation respiratory distress: a randomized controlled trial, *JAMA* 287:3238, 2002.

3. Thys F, Roeseler J, Delaere S, et al: Two-level non-invasive positive pressure ventilation in the initial treatment of acute respiratory failure in an emergency department, *Eur J Emerg Med* 6(3):207, 1999.

4. Make BJ, Hill NS, Goldberg AI, et al: Management of pediatric patients requiring long-term ventilation, *Chest* 113:289S, 1998.

5. Kacmarek RM: Characteristics of pressure-targeted ventilators used for noninvasive positive pressure ventilation, *Respir Care* 42:380, 1997.

6. Adams AB, Bliss PL, Hotchkiss J: Effects of respiratory impedance on the performance of bilevel pressure ventilators, *Respir Care* 45:390, 2000.

7. Meneses J, Bhandari V, Alves JG: Nasal intermittent positive pressure ventilation versus nasal continuous positive airway pressure for preterm infants with respiratory distress syndrome: a systematic review and meta-analysis, *Arch Pediatr Adolesc Med* 166:372, 2012.

8. Gizzi C, Papoff P, Campelli M, Cerasaro C, Agostino R, Moretti C: Surfactant and noninvasive ventilation for preterm infants, *Acta Biomed* 83(Suppl 1):24, 2012.

9. Hill NS, et al: Efficacy of nocturnal nasal ventilation in patients with restrictive thoracic disease, *Am Rev Respir Dis* 145:365, 1992.

10. Teague WG: Long term mechanical ventilation in infants and children. In Hill NS, editor: *Long-term mechanical ventilation*, New York, 2001, Marcel Dekker, pp 177.

11. Teague WG, Harsch A, Lesnick B: Non-invasive positive pressure ventilation as a long-term treatment for pediatric patients with chronic hypoventilation disorders, *Am J Respir Crit Care Med* 159:297[abstract], 1999.

12. Lee JH, Rehder KJ, Williford L, Cheifetz IM, Turner DA: Use of high flow nasal cannula in critically ill infants, children, and adults: a critical review of the literature, *Intensive Care Med* 39(2):247-57, 2012 Nov 10. [Epub ahead of print]

13. Manley BJ, Dold SK, Davis PG, Roehr CC: High-flow nasal cannulae for respiratory support of pre-term infants: a review of the evidence, *Neonatology* 102:300–308, 2012.

14. Arora B, Mahajan P, Zidan MA, Sethuraman U: Nasopharyngeal airway pressures in bronchiolitis patients treated with high-flow nasal cannula oxygen therapy, *Pediatr Emerg Care* 28:1179–1184, 2012.

15. Spentzas T, Minarik M, Patters AB, Vinson B, Stidham G: Children with respiratory distress treated with high flow nasal cannula, *J Intensive Care Med* 24:323–328, 2009.

16. Wing R, James C, Maranda LS, Armsby CC: Use of high-flow nasal cannula support in the emergency department reduces the need for intubation in pediatric acute respiratory insufficiency, *Pediatr Emerg Care* 28:1117–1123, 2012.

17. Vital FM, Saconato H, Ladeira MT, et al: Non-invasive positive pressure ventilation (CPAP or bilevel NPPV) for cardiogenic pulmonary edema, *Cochrane Database System Rev* (3):CD005351, 2008.

18. Ram FS, Picot J, Lightowler J, Wedzicha JA: Non-invasive positive pressure ventilation for treatment of respiratory failure due to acute exacerbations of chronic obstructive pulmonary disease, *Cochrane Database System Rev* (3):CD004104, 2004.

19. Ram FS, Wellington S, Rowe BH, Wedzicha JA: Non-invasive positive pressure ventilation for treatment of respiratory failure due to acute exacerbations of asthma, *Cochrane Database System Rev* (1):CD004360, 2005.

20. Teague WG: Noninvasive ventilation in the pediatric intensive care unit for children with acute respiratory failure, *Pediatr Pulmonol* 35:418, 2003.

21. Essouri S, Durand P, Chevret L, et al: Physiological effects of noninvasive positive ventilation during acute moderate hypercapnic respiratory insufficiency in children, *Intensive Care Med* 34:2248, 2008.

22. Abadesso C, Nunes P, Silvestre C, Matias E, Loureiro H, Almeida H: Non-invasive ventilation in acute respiratory failure in children, *Pediatri Rep* 4(2):Epub.e16, 2012. doi: 10.4081/pr.2012.e16.

23. Essouri S, Chevret L, Durand P, Haas V, Fauroux B, Devictor D: Noninvasive positive pressure ventilation: five years of experience in a pediatric intensive care unit, *Pediatr Crit Care Med* 7:329, 2006.

24. Mayordomo-Colunga, Medina A, Rey C, Diaz JJ, Concha A, Los Arcos M, Menendez S: Predictive factors of non-invasive ventilation failure in critically ill children: a prospective epidemiological study, *Intensive Care Med* 35:527, 2009.

25. Padman R, Henry M: The use of bilevel positive airway pressure for the treatment of acute chest syndrome of sickle cell disease, *Del Med J* 76:199, 2004.

26. Gupta P, Kuperstock JE, Hashmi S, et al: Efficacy and predictors of success of noninvasive ventilation for prevention of extubation failure in critically ill children with heart disease, *Pediatr Cardiol* 34(4):964-77, 2012. (Epub ahead of print).

27. Galindo-Filho VC, Domelas-de-Andrade A, Brandao DC, et al: Noninvasive ventilation coupled with nebulization during asthma crises: a randomized controlled trial, *Respir Care* 58(2):241-9, 2012 July 10. (Epub ahead of print).

28. Fauroux B, Boffa C, Desquerre I, Estournet B, Trang H: Long-term noninvasive mechanical ventilation for children at home: a national survey, *Pediatr Pulmonol* 35:119, 2003.

29. Hess DR: The growing role of noninvasive ventilation in patients requiring prolonged mechanical ventilation, *Respir Care* 57:900, 2012.

30. Teague WG: Non-invasive positive pressure ventilation: current status in paediatric patients, *Paediatr Respir Rev* 6:52, 2005.

31. Faroux B, Lofaso F: Domiciliary non-invasive ventilation in children, *Rev Mal Respir* 22:289, 2005.

32. Matsui S, Nakagawa G, Takei S, et al: The effect of noninvasive positive pressure ventilation in children with severe motor and intellectual disability with respiratory insufficiency, *No To Hattatsu* 44:284, 2012.

33. Piastra M, Antonelli M, Caresta E, Chiaretti A, Polidori G, Conti G: Noninvasive ventilation in childhood acute neuromuscular respiratory failure: a pilot study, *Respiration* 73:791, 2006.

34. Kirk VG, Morielli A, Gozal D, et al: Treatment of sleep-disordered breathing in children with myelomeningocele, *Pediatr Pulmonol* 30:445, 2000.

35. Padman R, et al: Noninvasive positive pressure ventilation in end-stage cystic fibrosis: a report of seven cases, *Respir Care* 39:736, 1994.

36. Faroux B, Le Roux E, Ravilly S, Bellis G, Clement A: Long-term noninvasive ventilation in patients with cystic fibrosis, *Respiration* 76:168, 2008.

37. Placidi G, Cornacchia M, Polese G, Zanolla L, Assael BM, Braggion C: Chest physiotherapy with positive airway pressure: a pilot study of short-term effects on sputum clearance in patients with cystic fibrosis and severe airway obstruction, *Respir Care* 51:1145, 2006.

38. Moran F: Bradley JM, Piper AJ: Non-invasive ventilation for cystic fibrosis, *Cochrane Database Syst Rev* 21:CD002769, 2009.

39. Tibballs J, Henning RD: Noninvasive ventilatory strategies in the management of a newborn infant and three children with congenital central hypoventilation syndrome, *Pediatr Pulmonol* 36:544, 2003.

40. Vagiakis E, Koutsourelakis I, Perraki E, et al: Average volume-assured pressure support in a 16-year-old girl with congenital central hypoventilation syndrome, *J Clin Sleep Med* 6:609, 2010.

41. Ramirez A, Delord V, Khirani S, et al: Interfaces for long-term noninvasive positive pressure ventilation in children, *Intensive Care Med* 38:655, 2012.

42. Berry RB, Chediak A, Brown LK, et al: Best clinical practices for the sleep center adjustment of non-invasive positive pressure ventilation (NPPV) in stable chronic alveolar hypoventilation syndromes, *J Clin Sleep Med* 6:491, 2010.

43. Arzt M, Floras JS, Logan AG, et al: Suppression of central sleep apnea by continuous positive airway pressure and transplant-free survival in heart failure: a post hoc analysis of the Canadian Continuous Positive Airway Pressure for Patients with Central Sleep Apnea and Heart Failure Trial (CANPAP), *Circulation* 115:3173, 2007.

44. Borel JC, Tamisier R, Gonzalez-Bermejo J, et al: Noninvasive ventilation in mild obesity hypoventilation syndrome: a randomized controlled trial, *Chest* 141:692, 2012.

45. Strumpf DA, et al: An evaluation of the Respironics BiPAP bilevel CPAP device for delivery of assisted ventilation, *Respir Care* 35:415, 1990.

46. Teschler H, Dohring J, Wang YM, Berthon-Jones M: Adaptive pressure support servo-ventilation: a novel treatment for Cheyne-Stokes respiration in heart failure, *Am J Respir Crit Care Med* 164:614, 2001.

47. Younes M, Puddy A, Roberts D, et al: Proportional assist ventilation: results of an initial clinical trial, *Am Rev Respir Dis* 145:121, 1992.

48. Gay PC, Hess DR, Hill NS: Noninvasive proportional assist ventilation for acute respiratory insufficiency: Comparison with pressure support ventilation, *Am J Respir Crit Care Med* 164:1606, 2001.

49. Keens TG, Jansen MT, DeWitt PK: Home care for children with chronic respiratory failure, *Semin Respir Med* 11:269, 1990.

50. Janssens JP, Derivaz S, Breitenstein E, et al: Changing patterns in long-term noninvasive ventilation: a 7-year prospective study in the Geneva Lake area, *Chest* 123:67, 2003.

51. Hartmann H, et al: Negative extra thoracic pressure ventilation in central hypoventilation syndrome, *Arch Dis Child* 70:418, 1994.

52. Linton DM: Cuirass ventilation: a review and update, *Crit Care Resusc* 7(1):22, 2005.

53. McBride WT, Ranaldi G, Dougherty MJ, et al: The hemodynamic and respiratory effects of cuirass ventilation in healthy volunteers: Part 1, *J Cardiothorac Vasc Anesth* 26:868, 2012.

54. Chierichetti M, Engelberts D, El-Khuffash A, Babyn P, Post M, Kavanagh BP: Continuous negative abdominal distension augments recruitment of atelectatic lung, *Crit Care Med* 40:1864, 2012.

55. Nava S, Ceriana P: Patient-ventilator interaction during noninvasive positive pressure ventilation, *Respir Care Clin N Am* 11:281, 2005.

56. Cuvelier A, Achour L, Rabarimanantsoa H, Letellier C, Muir JF, Fauroux Bl: A noninvasive method to identify ineffective triggering in patients with noninvasive pressure support ventilation, *Respiration* 80:198, 2010.

57. Fauroux B, Leroux K, Desmarais G, et al: Performance of ventilators for noninvasive positive pressure ventilation in children, *Eur Respir J* 31:1300, 2008.

58. Piper AJ, Sullivan CE: Effects of short-term NIPPV in the treatment of patients with severe obstructive sleep apnea and hypercapnia, *Chest* 105:434, 1994.

59. Chidini G, Calderini E, Cesana BM, Gandini C, Prandi E, Pelosi P: Noninvasive continuous positive airway pressure in acute respiratory failure: helmet versus facial mask, *Pediatrics* 126(2):e330, 2010.

60. Navales P, et al: Physiologic evaluation of noninvasive mechanical ventilation delivered with three types of mask in patients with chronic hypercapnic respiratory failure, *Crit Care Med* 28:1785, 2000.

61. Villa MP, Pagani J, Ambrosio R, Ronchetti R, Bernkopf E: Mid-face hypoplasia after long-term nasal ventilation, *Am J Respir Crit Care Med* 166:1142, 2002.

62. Pasquina P, Adler D, Farr P, Bourqui P, Bridevaux PO, Janssens JP: What does built-in software of home ventilators tell us? An observational study of 150 patients on home ventilation, *Respiration* 83:293, 2012.

63. Paiva R, Krivec U, Aubertin G, Cohen E, Clement A, Fauroux B: Carbon dioxide monitoring during long-term noninvasive respiratory support in children, *Intensive Care Med* 35:1068, 2009.

64. Fauroux B, Lavis JF, Nicot F, et al: Facial side effects during noninvasive positive pressure ventilation in children, *Intensive Care Med* 31:965, 2005.

65. Lechtzin N, Weiner CM, Clawson L: A fatal complication of noninvasive ventilation, *N Engl J Med* 344:533, 2001.

66. Meecham Jones DJ, Braid GM, Wedzicha JA: Nasal masks for domiciliary positive pressure ventilation: patient usage and complications, *Thorax* 49:811, 1994.

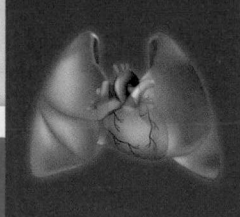

Chapter 17

Invasive Mechanical Ventilation of the Neonate and Pediatric Patient

BRIAN K. WALSH, KEVIN L. CREZEE

OUTLINE

LEARNING OBJECTIVES

After reading this chapter the reader will be able to:

1. Explain when mechanical ventilation is indicated in neonates and pediatrics
2. Describe the basic fundamentals for managing patients undergoing mechanical ventilation
3. Identify complications associated with mechanical ventilation
4. Explain various approaches for minimizing complications with ventilators

5. Compare differences in operation between pressure, volume, and adaptive control breathe types
6. Provide reasons why one mode of ventilation would be chosen over another for certain conditions
7. Determine initial ventilator settings for various patient sizes
8. Recognize factors that could improve interaction between the patient and the mechanical ventilator
9. Define and discuss various weaning strategies
10. Define *high-frequency ventilation*
11. Describe how gas is delivered and exhaled during high-frequency jet ventilation
12. Describe how gas is delivered and exhaled during high-frequency oscillatory ventilation
13. Describe the relative role frequency and tidal volume play during high-frequency ventilation
14. Explain the relationship between lung volume and oxygenation during high-frequency ventilation
15. Identify lung volume strategies for a given pathophysiology

KEY TERMS

Adaptive control ventilation
Adaptive pressure ventilation
Assist/control ventilation
Atelectrauma
Barotrauma
Control ventilation

High-frequency jet ventilation
High-frequency oscillatory ventilation
High-frequency percussive ventilation
High-frequency ventilation

Low-frequency ventilation
Pressure control ventilation
Pressure support ventilation
Trigger
Volume ventilation
Volutrauma

INTRODUCTION

Neonatal and pediatric mechanical ventilation presents some of the most clinically challenging situations in respiratory care. The neonatal and pediatric population encompasses a broad range of weights, ages, sizes, and diseases; therefore, ventilator practices can vary widely. In this chapter a *neonate* is defined as any newborn infant younger than 44 weeks of gestation and a *pediatric patient* represents any child older than 1 month of age. We also identify **low-frequency ventilation** (LFV) as ventilation modes that provide breaths per minute of 150 or less and **high-frequency ventilation** (HFV) as modes of ventilation that provide breaths per minute of more than 150. Some use the term *conventional ventilation* to generally describe all modes of ventilation that do not provide rates above 150, leaving clinicians to believe that HFV modes are nonconventional or nontraditional. The authors do not support this concept and believe that all invasive modes provided in this chapter are routinely used in the neonatal and pediatric respiratory care environment.

Children are not small adults, and infants are not small children.[1] Most of the concepts presented in this chapter are the same for both pediatric and neonatal applications; however, there are other situations that are quite unique to the neonatal or pediatric patient. Like the similarities and differences in neonatal and pediatric populations, low- and high-frequency ventilation share some of the same. Where there are differences, for simplicity we will label them as low- or high-frequency ventilation. Please pay careful attention to the section headings as you read.

At present, there is no consensus regarding optimal ventilator strategies for this patient population. A tremendous amount of research still needs to be done to determine best practices for managing neonatal and pediatric patients receiving mechanical ventilation. To manage neonatal and pediatric mechanical ventilation effectively, the clinician must combine the principles described in this chapter with the knowledge of how airway anatomy and pulmonary pathophysiology are impacted by various diseases. It is beyond the scope of this chapter to provide an in-depth review of ventilator equipment or guidelines for disease-specific ventilator management. These aspects are more than adequately covered elsewhere in this book or by your ventilator manufacturer's website resources for clinicians.

We have witnessed the development and implementation of several exciting modalities for the respiratory care of newborns and pediatric patients. These new tools range from enhancements in the pharmacological management of distinct cardiopulmonary disorders to tremendous strides in mechanical ventilation (MV). Critical to the successful application of these new treatments is the development of disease-specific strategies, which also include ways in which some therapies may positively interact with others. Low- and high-frequency ventilation continues to play an important role in this growth.[2-5]

The link between mechanical ventilation, oxygen, and subsequent acute and chronic lung disease was made in both pediatric and adult patients shortly after the introduction of LFV into clinical practice.[6,7] More recent trials indicate that ventilating patients with acute respiratory distress syndrome with higher tidal volumes contributes to further lung damage.[8,9] The various techniques of HFV emerged later from efforts to develop methods of managing respiratory failure that would minimize the negative pulmonary consequences of ventilatory support. At that time, our understanding of the mechanisms of these injuries was limited to the observed interactions between oxygen, pressure, and time.[10] This gap in the fundamental understanding of concepts of ventilator-induced lung injury explains both the early controversies regarding HFV strategies and the conflicting clinical reports.[11,12] The finding, at least in animal models, that a lung-protective ventilator strategy is possible helped spawn a growing body of data describing lung injury mechanisms, and, therefore, prevention techniques.[13] These remain the focus of ongoing research and commentary.[14,15]

This chapter reviews (1) basic concepts of LFV and HFV, (2) current understanding of mechanisms of gas exchange for LFV and HFV, (3) basic approaches of each mode of ventilation, (4) basic disease-specific strategies, and (5) special patient care considerations. This chapter also introduces the emerging understanding of the interaction between modes of ventilation, monitoring, and strategies.

INDICATIONS FOR MECHANICAL VENTILATION

General and Physiological

The physiological objectives for mechanical ventilation in a neonatal or pediatric patient are as follows:

- To manipulate alveolar ventilation
- To improve oxygenation
- To optimize lung volume
- To reduce the work of breathing
- To minimize risks associated with ventilator-induced lung injury

In general, mechanical ventilation is initiated to increase oxygenation, correct respiratory acidosis, reduce respiratory distress, prevent or reverse atelectasis, reduce respiratory muscle fatigue, manage intracranial pressure, lower oxygen consumption, and stabilize the chest wall for adequate lung expansion. Box 17-1 lists clinical situations in which mechanical ventilation is indicated.[1,16]

High-Frequency Ventilation
Neonatal Patients

The bulk of clinical data regarding appropriate application of HFV devices has been acquired from neonatal humans and animals. From these studies, two clear indications for HFV use during either routine or rescue circumstances have evolved. They include diffuse, homogeneous lung disease (or the atelectasis-prone lung), in which LFV management is failing or may lead to increased risk of pulmonary

---

Box 17-1	**Clinical Indications for (but Not Limited to) Mechanical Ventilation**

PULMONARY DISORDERS
Restrictive Process
- Respiratory distress syndrome
- Acute respiratory distress syndrome
- Pulmonary hemorrhage
- Pulmonary hypoplasia/agenesis
- Congenital pneumonia
- Pneumothorax/air leaks
- Pleural effusion/chylothorax
- Aspiration syndromes (blood, amniotic fluid)
- Flail chest
- Bronchopleural fistula
- Abdominal distention
- Diaphragmatic hernia
- Congenital lung cysts, tumors
- Rib cage anomalies
- Extrinsic masses

Obstructive Process
- Meconium aspiration
- Congenital lobar emphysema
- Asthma
- Bronchiolitis
- Cystic fibrosis
- Bronchopulmonary dysplasia

Airway
- Laryngomalacia
- Tracheomalacia
- Choanal atresia
- Pierre Robin syndrome
- Micrognathia
- Nasopharyngeal tumor
- Subglottic stenosis

EXTRAPULMONARY DISORDERS
Neurological/Muscular
- Myasthenia gravis
- Muscular dystrophy
- Guillain-Barré syndrome
- Cerebral edema
- Cerebral hemorrhage
- Spinal cord injury/disease
- Phrenic nerve damage

Hypoventilation
- Sleep apnea
- Overdose/poisoning
- Postoperative recovery

Increased Intracranial Pressure
- Infection
- Head trauma
- Near-drowning
- Reye's syndrome

Cardiovascular Dysfunction
- Cardiac shunting
- Cyanotic heart disease
- Circulatory collapse
- Hypovolemia
- Anemia
- Polycythemia
- Congestive heart failure
- Postoperative cardiac surgery
- Persistent pulmonary hypertension

Metabolic
- Acidosis
- Hypoglycemia
- Hypothermia
- Hyperthermia

morbidity, and existing pulmonary air leak syndromes (e.g., pneumothorax and pulmonary interstitial emphysema (PIE). Diffuse homogeneous lung disease includes natural surfactant deficiency (respiratory distress syndrome), shock lung in the newborn, and diffuse pneumonia. Other diagnoses, including congenital pulmonary hypoplasia (both the congenital diffuse variety and that associated with congenital diaphragmatic hernia), may be additional indications. The efficacy of HFV for pulmonary hypoplasia is promising but not yet clearly established.[17]

Each of the lung diseases just mentioned has been successfully managed with extracorporeal membrane oxygenation (ECMO).[18] The role of pre-ECMO HFV has been the subject of wide debate, with at least one published report describing a 50% reduction in the need for ECMO among infants referred to an ECMO center and who met ECMO criteria and began high-frequency oscillatory ventilation (HFOV) on admission.[19] However, there are also data that imply an increased risk of pulmonary morbidity among infants avoiding ECMO with HFV. The timing of HFV intervention, the parameters determining HFV failure, and the decision to discontinue HFV and initiate ECMO are currently empirical.[20]

HFV continues to be indicated for infants in whom air leak syndromes develop, but, gratefully, the incidence of intractable air leak has decreased. This is probably the result of surfactant use, improved ventilatory techniques and devices, and better patient monitoring. Other conditions common to the neonate but not clearly benefited by HFV include particulate meconium aspiration, congenital lobar emphysema, bronchopulmonary dysplasia, and viral pneumonia. Further data from controlled trials with defined patient populations and treatment strategies are needed to offer clearer recommendations about HFV use in these conditions.

Pediatric Patients

Controlled trials in pediatric patients have been fairly limited.[21] However, as would be anticipated, proper strategic HFV use has had positive results in children with acute respiratory distress syndrome (ARDS) and pulmonary air leak. In general, HFOV is applied as a rescue therapy in those failing LFV. An additional interesting HFV application is high-frequency jet ventilation (HFJV) use during and

after cardiac surgery, especially for children undergoing right ventricular outflow tract diversion or repair. At least two groups of investigators have reported improved hemodynamic measurements in children managed with the HFJV in both intraoperative and postoperative environments.[22,23] The ability to provide adequate ventilation with low mean and peak pressures in children with otherwise normal lungs offers a substantial advantage of HFJV over HFOV and LFV. Furthermore, this feature makes HFJV a more efficacious method of treating traumatic or acquired bronchopleural fistulas than other forms of respiratory support.

TYPES OF MECHANICAL VENTILATION

Mechanical ventilator breath types have traditionally been classified by the type of mechanical ventilator being used but can now be employed in a variety of ways, which are defined mainly by the control variable.[24] The two most common breath types are pressure and volume. Figure 17-1 compares the differences between the flow and pressure waveforms of volume and pressure ventilation. Modern microprocessor ventilators incorporate gas delivery systems that can produce a wide variety of flow and pressure waveforms and are capable of delivering volume and pressure ventilation as well as hybrid modes that combine various aspects of volume and pressure.

Another determinate is the breath frequency of the mechanical ventilator. Traditionally the type of ventilator must change to provide HFV. However, currently all high-frequency ventilators provide pressure-type breath, so we will discuss this further in the pressure mode of ventilation section of this chapter.

Pressure Ventilation

Pressure ventilation uses a pressure setting as the main feature to define inflation. Pressure ventilators are classified as positive pressure or negative pressure.[24] Positive-pressure ventilators use a high external pressure gradient to drive a gas mixture into the lungs and produce inflation.

Negative-pressure ventilation permits gas flow into the lungs by using a vacuum to externally expand the thorax.

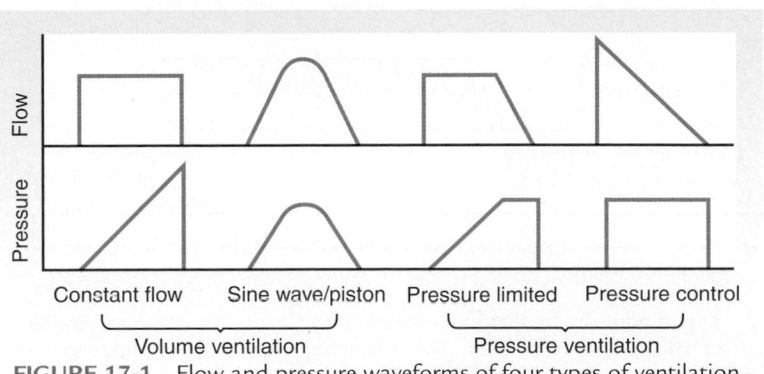

FIGURE 17-1   Flow and pressure waveforms of four types of ventilation.

The chest wall pressure drops, thereby creating a decrease in pleural pressure that is less than the airway opening pressure, and air flows into the lungs. The main advantage of a negative-pressure ventilator is that it may avoid endotracheal intubation or tracheotomy. Because negative-pressure ventilation is provided without an artificial airway, it is sometimes referred to as *noninvasive ventilation*; however, it should be understood that all forms of mechanical ventilation provide ventilation in an "unnatural" form. In addition, both positive- and negative-pressure ventilation produce positive transpulmonary pressures and may have similar complications as a result.

Microprocessor ventilators are also capable of delivering preset pressure breaths and are useful for neonate and pediatric ventilation. This form of pressure ventilation is called pressure-controlled ventilation (PCV). Usually a preset pressure level, inspiratory time, and frequency are chosen by the operator. Flow, however, is variable and is a function of driving pressure and peaks almost instantly to attain the defined pressure level. Constant pressure is maintained throughout the inspiratory time, and flow decelerates rapidly.[25,26] However, the total flow delivered to the respiratory system is regulated by the ventilator to ensure that pressure is maintained throughout the entire inspiratory time. The majority of the tidal volume is delivered early in the inflation stage, while pressure is held constant. Compared with other types of ventilation, the resulting distribution of alveolar pressures sustained by tidal volume may lead to a lower dead space–to–tidal volume (V_D/V_T) ratio, improved ventilation, and improved oxygenation.[27,28] PCV can offer lower work of breathing and improved comfort for patients with increased and variable respiratory demand.[29] Although the peak pressure level is constant or nearly constant, PCV results in a higher mean airway pressure ($\overline{Paw}$) than do other types of ventilation. The disadvantages or advantages of a higher $\overline{Paw}$ should be considered when instituting PCV. Another disadvantage when using any type of pressure ventilation is that tidal volume will vary with changes in lung compliance and constant alveolar minute ventilation may be difficult to obtain.

High-Frequency Ventilation

High-frequency ventilation is a general term used to describe mechanical ventilation using tidal volumes less than or equal to the dead space volume and delivered at supraphysiological rates. Tidal volume, dead space volume, and breathing rate magnitude vary with patient age and size (tidal and dead space volumes vary inversely with increasing age, whereas breathing rate varies directly). The U.S. Food and Drug Administration (FDA) has chosen to define HFV devices as those that provide breathing rates exceeding 150 breaths per minute. These ventilators operate at breathing rates of 4 to 15 Hz (1 Hz = 60 breaths per minute or 1 cycle per second) and deliver the requisite small tidal volumes. HFV discussion is limited to those devices currently cleared by the FDA for use in neonates and/or pediatric patients. Several types of HFV devices have been tested and reported in the literature. They differ functionally by the way each breath is generated, their relationship to conventional ventilator settings (if any), the range of breathing rates, and the nature of the expiratory portion of the respiratory cycle. Figure 17-2 compares

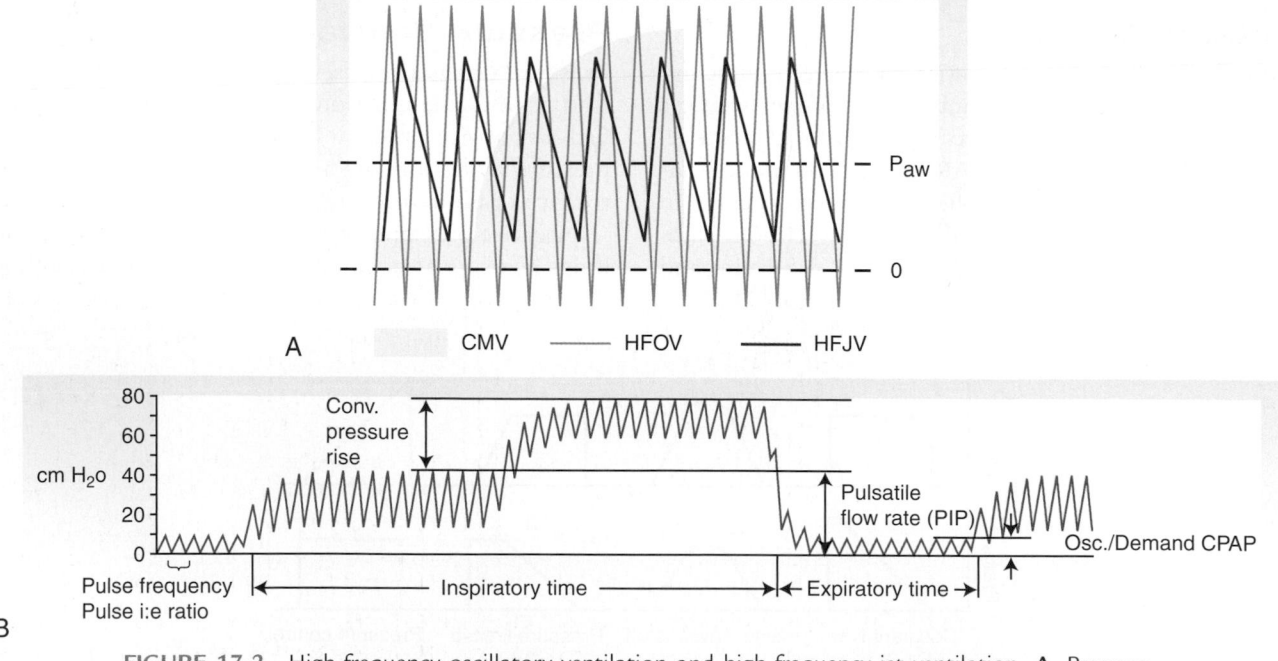

FIGURE 17-2   High-frequency oscillatory ventilation and high-frequency jet ventilation. **A,** Pressure time waveform of HFOV and HFJV with LFV in the background for comparison. **B,** Pressure time waveform of HFPV. Settings on HFPV are clearly labeled.

pressure waveforms of each of the high-frequency ventilation modes.

Mid-Frequency Positive Pressure Ventilation. Mid-frequency positive pressure ventilation (MFPV) is a modification of time-cycled, pressure-limited infant ventilators that provides breathing rates up to 150 breaths per minute (2.5 Hz).[30] Typically rates are between 60 and 150. The limitations of this approach include larger delivered tidal volumes than with HFV and the potential for intrapulmonary gas trapping. High-frequency positive-pressure ventilation (HFPPV) was first described in the anesthesia literature as a tool for managing patients during bronchoscopic or laryngeal surgery.[31] HFPPV subsequently received brief exposure as a management tool for more chronic conditions in adults and underwent brief trials in a small series of infants with respiratory distress.[32,33] These definitions are included here for completeness only because the use of FDA-approved HFV devices has generally replaced the routine use of these techniques in infants.

High-Frequency Percussive Ventilation. High-frequency percussive ventilation (HFPV) delivers short bursts of gas to a sliding Venturi valve. The burst may entrain air to deliver high-frequency distending pressure at peak inspiratory pressure (PIP) and positive end-expiratory pressure (PEEP). High-frequency breaths are active at both levels of pressure. Decreased compliance equals increased resistance and decreased movement of the valve. The most common models require a minimum number of low-frequency, time-cycled, pressure-limited breaths to operate. HFPV generates a $\overline{Paw}$ by stacking high speed bursts in combination with flow and expiratory system resistance instead of a common exhalation valve on most ventilators. The $\overline{Paw}$ builds filling the lung while maintaining HFV. The lack of an exhalation valve makes the actively created to maintain pressurization. Percussive ventilators are pneumatically powered and controlled; batteries or electricity are used for monitoring systems. Pneumatic cartridges time-cycle pressure-limited breaths that build in pressure over time, filling the lung as pressurization occurs in conjunction with high-frequency breaths.

High-Frequency Jet Ventilation. High-frequency jet ventilation devices deliver short-pulsed jets distal to the proximal end of the endotracheal tube (ETT). Functional tidal volumes are a combination of the jet breath and entrainment volumes that are "dragged" along with each jet. Original techniques using a modified triple-lumen ETT and those employing catheters placed in a standard ETT have been described.[34,35] Modern adaptations use a special connector (Figure 17-3) that replaces the ETT adapter to allow the combination of the HFJV and LFV. These devices combine LFV breaths with jet breaths and rely on passive chest recoil for gas egress. Baseline pressures are provided by continuous flow from the LFV. Tandem use with an LFV is usually required dependent of the ventilation strategies applied. The short time for pulse delivery generally results in longer I:E times with HFJV.

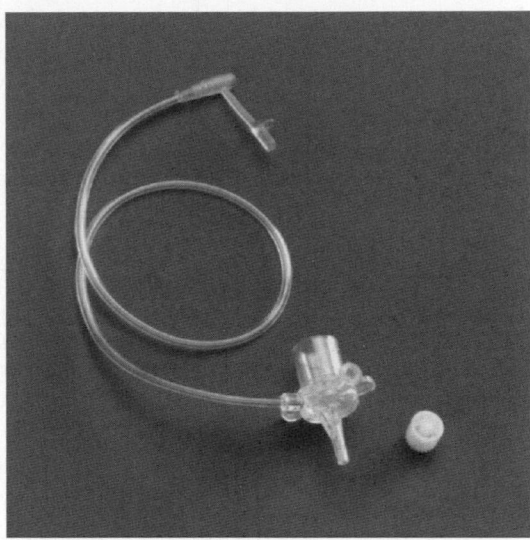

FIGURE 17-3 LifePort ETT adapter. Jet pulses are delivered through the side lumen of the ETT, and servocontrol over jet pressures is maintained by feedback from pressures sampled at the distal ETT lumen. Connection to a conventional ventilator is provided at the proximal ETT opening. This ETT adapter is made specifically for use with this device. (Courtesy Bunnell Inc., Salt Lake City, Utah.)

High-Frequency Oscillatory Ventilation. Of all HFV techniques, **high-frequency oscillatory ventilation** devices may be the most variable. Initial techniques included loudspeakers whose output was attached to the ETT and a host of piston pump devices with various performance characteristics.[36-39] Common to all of these devices is the provision of extremely small tidal volumes and very high rates of 8 to 30 Hz, as well as the presence of a continuous distending pressure (CDP) or mean airway pressure $\overline{Paw}$. The outward flow of expiratory gases is enhanced by the active exhalation phase of the piston cycle. This last feature distinguishes HFOV from all other HFV methods. All current devices use a standard ETT, allow precise control over $\overline{Paw}$ and pressure amplitude, and in general are not used in tandem with conventional ventilators. The ability to accurately adjust continuous (or mean) and phasic pressures and the inspiratory-to-expiratory (I/E) ratio varies among devices. Ventilator output is delivered to the proximal ETT (at the ETT circuit connection). Because the ETT behaves as a low-pass filter at these rapid breathing rates, pulmonary structures experience markedly dampened phasic pressures.

Volume Ventilation

Volume control ventilation (VCV) is most often used in adult patients and is chosen when ventilating a pediatric patient. Adult volume-cycled ventilators were used initially in newborn intensive care in the early 1970s and fell from favor with the invention of pressure-controlled ventilators that were designed specifically for use in neonates. Because of improved sensor and ventilator technology, it is now possible to use volume ventilation in all patients.[40] A constant tidal volume and flow rate characterize **volume ventilation,** and the resulting peak inspiratory pressure varies with changes in respiratory system compliance and resistance. When a flow-controlling valve is used, tidal volume is calculated by measuring the flow delivered over a preset inflation time.[41]

VCV with a constant flow has the advantage of a lower $\overline{Paw}$ compared with pressure ventilation. This is often a critical factor after cardiac surgery in infants and children. Many currently available ventilators offer the option of delivering this constant flow with either a traditional square-wave flow pattern or a 50% decelerating flow pattern in VCV. In theory, tidal volume does not vary with changing lung compliance or airway resistance during volume ventilation. As lung impedance increases, however, tidal volume may decrease if the ventilator cannot correct for volume losses resulting from gas compression in the patient circuit. Delivered tidal volume may also be affected by leaks from cuffless endotracheal tubes, which are commonly used during neonatal mechanical ventilation. When ventilating a larger patient, the volume loss may be negligible; however, in a small child or infant it may be a significant portion of the delivered tidal volume. Failure to consider this volume loss may result in hypoventilation and hypercapnia of the patient. The compressed volume can also affect the calculations of respiratory compliance, oxygen consumption, carbon dioxide production, and dead space volume.[42] To account for this loss, an effective tidal volume should be calculated (Box 17-2).[43] Newer generation ventilators that utilize internal transducers calculate tubing compliance during pre-use checks. A piston-driven volume ventilator also delivers a constant volume with a variable peak pressure. Because of the piston action, flow peaks in the middle of the inflation when stroke speed is the greatest. Although piston ventilators are seldom used in the pediatric critical care setting, they become an inexpensive and practical choice for the nonacute care or home setting.

Many home ventilators also allow the use of pressure limitation by setting a desired maximal pressure level. Using this feature decreases tidal volume from the volume set on the ventilator, but exactly how it affects volume depends on the specific ventilator and inflation time settings. A piston-generated pressure preset mode is not appropriate for the pediatric or infant home setting. Using a microprocessor-based turbine-driven portable ventilator is a better home care choice in such a situation.

CASE STUDY 1

You are called to assist with a full-term neonate who was transferred to your facility for further evaluation. The patient is an infant of a diabetic mother who tested positive for group B streptococcus infection. He is 5 kg, has received one dose of surfactant, and has extremely low lung volumes on AP chest radiograph. The transport team has the infant on LFV, pressure control, rate of 60, PIP of 38, PEEP of 8, and FiO_2 of 1.0. These ventilator settings are producing an SpO_2 of 85%, with an admission blood gas of 7.2/65/66/23. What mode of ventilation would you suggest for this patient and why?

See Evolve Resources for answers.

Adaptive Ventilation

Advances in ventilator sensors, response times, and microprocessor technologies have introduced new features into mechanical ventilators. **Adaptive control** or *volume-targeted* refers to a ventilation mode that allows the clinician to set a volume target while the ventilator delivers pressure-controlled breaths.[44] Although it is impossible to control two variables simultaneously (volume and pressure), this form of ventilation can be thought of simply as a pressure controller that servocontrols the pressure levels automatically in response to measurements of volume or compliance. These modes are commonly used in the neonatal and pediatric populations. These "hybrid modes" allow the comfort of pressure control with the maintenance of a tidal volume target by servocontrolling pressure on the basis of feedback obtained at the ventilator pneumotachometer. As lung compliance and airway resistance improve or worsen, the microprocessor will measure these changes and increase or decrease the pressure level on the basis of a breath-to-breath analysis, a multiple-breath average, or within-breath measurement. Some of these modes use more than one flow control signal at the flow valve and may switch from PCV to VCV within a single breath to establish a minimal tidal volume goal. These modes can provide the

---

Box 17-2	Calculation of Effective Tidal Volume

$$V_{Teff} = V_{Tset} - [(Pstatic^* - PEEP) \times Circuit]$$

DETERMINATION OF COMPLIANCE FACTOR OF CIRCUIT

1. With the circuit assembled and connected to the ventilator, the patient connection to the circuit is occluded.
2. A known volume of gas is delivered into the circuit through the ventilator, and the resulting peak inspiratory pressure is noted.
3. The resulting pressure is divided by the delivered volume to obtain the compliance factor of the circuit. This is generally 1 ml/cm H_2O for infant circuits and 2 to 3 ml/cm H_2O for larger circuits.

V_{Teff}, Effective tidal volume; V_{Tset}, tidal volume set on ventilator; *Pstatic*, static (plateau) pressure measured during inflation; *PEEP*, positive end-expiratory pressure set on ventilator; *circuit*, compliance or compression factor of circuit.

*If static or plateau pressure measurement cannot be obtained because of airway leaks, the peak inspiratory pressure may be used as an approximation.

patient with some of the best features of PCV and VCV. Adaptive-control modes can be effective at maintaining a more consistent tidal volume and hence alveolar minute ventilation in patients who are prone to abrupt changes in pulmonary compliance.

Limited data exist concerning whether these modes are superior to traditional approaches to mechanical ventilation of humans. On the basis of these limited data, the future of these modes looks promising. A meta-analysis of trials comparing PCV with various volume-targeted modes in premature infants resulted in trends favoring volume targeting for reduction in duration of ventilation, rates of pneumothorax, severe intraventricular hemorrhage, and (to a lesser degree) incidence of bronchopulmonary dysplasia.[45] These modes have also been shown to be effective in avoiding hypocapneic/hypercapneic episodes in premature infants, in whom cerebral blood flow is impacted by small changes in carbon dioxide.[46] Future randomized controlled clinical trials are necessary to determine clinical significance in improving survival without complications in premature infants when using adaptive-control modes over other modes of ventilation.

MODES OF MECHANICAL VENTILATION

The mode of ventilation is defined by how a ventilator is going to interface with the patient's breathing efforts. These modes can use pressure, flow, or other signals to trigger. The main control variables may be volume, pressure, or flow and may use either positive or negative pressure as the driving force. Most ventilators are capable of providing multiple modes, and some even combine modes to enhance the patient–ventilator interface. Figure 17-4 illustrates various modes of ventilation and how they interface with spontaneous breathing.

Low-Frequency Ventilation
Control Mode
The control mode is used when the clinician needs to maintain complete control over a patient's ventilation variables. To attain complete control, the patient-triggering mechanism is made inactive and all breaths are delivered at a preset volume or pressure, frequency, and inspiratory flow rate.[47] The patient should be sedated to apnea and/or paralyzed to avoid asynchrony between ventilator inflations and patient breathing efforts. **Control ventilation** may be desirable when extreme ventilation variables are required, and asynchrony may result in complications such as pneumothorax but this is rare.

Assist/Control Mode
Like the control mode, the **assist/control ventilation** (A/C) mode allows the clinician control over most of the patient's ventilation variables except for frequency. The

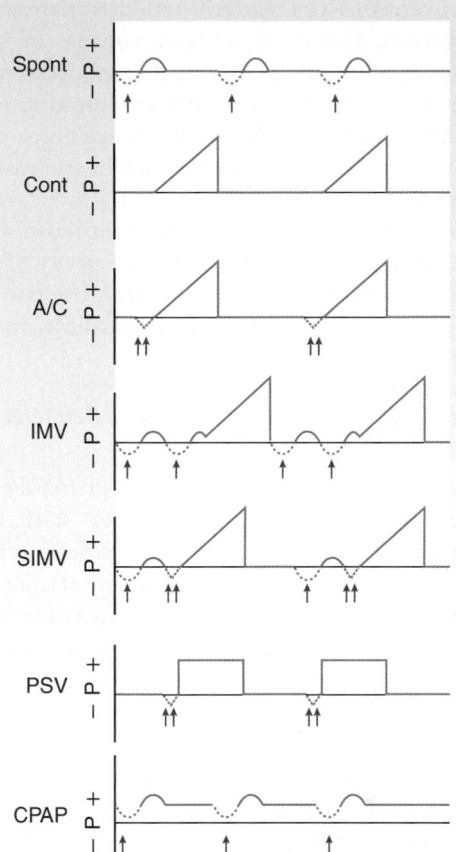

FIGURE 17-4   Pressure waveforms of seven modes of ventilation. *Single arrows* denote spontaneous inspiratory efforts. *Double arrows* denote ventilator breaths triggered by inspiratory efforts. *Spont,* Spontaneous breathing; *Cont,* controlled ventilation; *A/C,* assist/control ventilation; *IMV,* intermittent mandatory ventilation; *SIMV,* synchronized intermittent mandatory ventilation; *PSV,* pressure support ventilation; *CPAP,* continuous positive airway pressure.

volume or pressure, frequency, and inspiratory flow rate are preset, and the ventilator supports every breath. However, the patient is allowed to use his or her own ventilatory drive to trigger the ventilator and receive a breath at the preset volume or pressure. If the patient fails to take a breath during a specific period, the ventilator delivers the defined breath at a preset rate. Control and A/C are then defined as machine-triggered and patient-triggered continuous mandatory ventilation.[48] Some ventilators have control and A/C as the same mode, with the sensitivity setting being the only difference. The sensitivity of the triggering mechanism is set sufficiently low to be activated by any attempted breath. The sensitivity must also be set sufficiently high to prevent activation (autocycling) by artifacts such as cardiac activity, airway leaks, or patient care procedures. The A/C mode may be useful for older children or adolescents. It is being used more often in neonates and small children who are more susceptible to lung injury, especially when using volume and adaptive-control modes. The advantage of the A/C mode is that every breath delivered to the patient, whether patient or machine triggered, has a guaranteed volume or pressure. There are several disadvantages to this mode. In neonates, infants, or small children with high respiratory rates, hyperventilation, hyperinflation, and respiratory alkalosis may occur. The work of breathing may be increased, especially for patients who are not breathing in synchrony with the machine or who are "fighting the ventilator." Sedating the patient may alleviate this. If the sensitivity of the triggering mechanism is not set adequately, the patient's inspiratory effort may be increased and result in an increase in oxygen consumption.[2]

Synchronized Intermittent Mandatory Ventilation

Early models of mechanical ventilators primarily used intermittent mandatory ventilation (IMV). With IMV the ventilator was incapable of sensing patient effort and would deliver mandatory breaths on top of spontaneous breaths. To avoid patient–ventilator asynchrony, a sensing mechanism is built into most modern ventilators. The ventilator presets a rate for the delivery of mandatory breaths (of preset volume or pressure and flow rate) and attempts to synchronize the breaths with the patient's spontaneous effort. If no patient effort is sensed within a specific window of time, a mandatory breath is given. Airway pressure or flow is the usual triggering mechanism for synchronized intermittent mandatory ventilation (SIMV). Small volumes and rapid rates characterize an infant's spontaneous breathing effort, which makes synchronizing ventilator inflation difficult. With the latest advances in sensor technology, SIMV is now a feasible option in neonates and infants.[49-51] Advantages of this mode are that it allows the patient to perform part of the ventilatory work while maintaining a backup of mandatory ventilation and that it is useful in weaning the patient from mechanical ventilation (Box 17-3). Hyperventilation and respiratory alkalosis are risks just as with the A/C mode, but they are less likely to occur. Another risk associated with SIMV is increased work of breathing during spontaneous ventilation. This may be the result of inadequate inspiratory flow, ventilator response to the patient's inspiratory effort, ventilator circuitry, or endotracheal tube resistance.[2] Today, most all mechanical ventilators will allow you to add a form of pressure support to augment the patient's spontaneous breaths.

Adaptive Control

Pressure-Regulated Volume Control. Pressure-regulated volume control (PRVC) attempts to maintain a minimal target tidal volume with a constant pressure by manipulating the flow waveform. The ventilator initially performs a test breath sequence, which measures dynamic or static system compliance. Subsequent adjustments in pressure or tidal volume are made on the basis of the previous breath or a historical average of breaths. Some ventilators initiate a "test breath" sequence during PRVC by implementing a brief inspiratory pause during a volume-controlled breath. The static pressure measured during the pause will be the pressure control level for the next breath. The following breaths will increase or decrease the pressure control level to try to achieve the set tidal volume with the lowest possible pressure. Within a few sequential breaths, the tidal volume goal may be reached. Certain conditions can restart the test breath sequence for optimal accuracy, including high-pressure limitation. Other modes that implement similar volume strategies as PRVC are volume support ventilation (VSV), Vsynch, VC plus, and auto-flow. Most new microprocessor ventilators can provide these modes within assist/control and synchronized intermittent mandatory ventilation.

Machine Volume. Another form of adaptive-controlled ventilation in neonatal and pediatric mechanical ventilation is machine volume (MV), which uses an intrabreath pressure adjustment to target volume. This mode is further classified as auto-set-point control. Auto-set-point control is a more advanced version of an adaptive-control mode. The breath can start out as pressure controlled and automatically switch to volume controlled within the same breath.[52] The ventilator flow control valve measures compliance every 2 milliseconds within the breath and can increase or decrease the pressure adjustment within this time by manipulating the flow rate if the delivered volume is not being met or if the patient requires more flow. The ventilator calculates a target flow rate on the basis of the minimal volume set at the ventilator and the inspiratory time. The breath begins as a PCV breath with a variable-decelerating flow signal and once the minimal tidal volume has been met; the breath is terminated at the preset inspiratory time and ends as a PCV breath. If the minimal tidal volume goal has not been delivered, then the ventilator transitions from a decelerating flow to a continuous flow signal to reach the tidal volume goal within the preset inspiratory time. The high-pressure limit must be set appropriately to protect against high pressure. The operator can set a volume limit feature, which will terminate the

---

Box 17-3	Benefits of Synchronized Intermittent Mandatory Ventilation

- Better distribution of ventilation by coordinating air flow with respiratory muscle effort
- Improved oxygenation by reducing ventilation–perfusion mismatch
- Better tidal volume at the same positive inspiratory pressure
- Improved minute ventilation through the minimization of ineffective breaths
- Reduced incidence of pneumothorax
- Reduced incidence of intraventricular hemorrhage because of less variation in cerebral blood flow
- Decreased use of sedation and paralysis
- Reduced length of ventilation

breath once this preset volume is exceeded either at the proximal flow sensor or at the ventilator flow control valve. This mode is similar to VAPS and pressure augmentation but different in that the inspiratory time will not be increased in order to deliver the set tidal volume. The clinician must set an uncorrected minimal tidal volume when using this mode in neonates. This includes the volume of gas delivered to the patient as well as the volume of gas delivered to the ventilator circuit.

Volume Guarantee. Volume guarantee (VG) is another form of adaptive-control ventilation that is used in one type of neonatal ventilator. The operator sets a tidal volume, inspiratory time, and flow rate. This mode can also be applied to pressure support ventilation. The ventilator incorporates a proximal flow sensor at the patient airway. The microprocessor assesses an eight-breath historical average of expired tidal volume and will increase pressure on the basis of these measurements up to the pressure limit to deliver the target volume. If compliance or resistance improves dramatically, then the ventilator will terminate breath delivery if the delivered tidal volume exceeds 130% of the set tidal volume. Pressure will also wean as the result of improving compliance, based on the breath average. Because the ventilator makes manipulations on the basis of expiratory tidal volume, this mode can correct for compressible volume loss of inspired gases and small endotracheal tube leaks and is useful in the neonatal population. The practitioner should be careful when using this mode with excessive endotracheal tube leaks. "In the presence of a substantial leak around the endotracheal tube, there are concerns that this system will falsely underestimate the actual tidal volume delivered to the lung and overcompensate the subsequent breaths with excessive tidal volumes."[53]

Pressure Support Ventilation

Continuous Positive Airway Pressure. While traditionally not consider a mode of ventilation, continuous positive airway pressure (CPAP), also termed *constant or continuous airway pressure,* can facilitate ventilation by maintaining lung volumes and preventing airway collapse often seen in our younger patients. CPAP is a constant, above-ambient pressure applied to the airways and maintained through the entire respiratory cycle.[54] Respiratory efforts are spontaneous and not supported by mandatory ventilator inflations.[47] However, many ventilators provide a "backup" mode of ventilation that provides full support in the event that the patient becomes apneic. In the pediatric setting, CPAP is applied to improve oxygenation by increasing the functional residual capacity, as in aspiration pneumonitis, or to stent floppy anatomical structures, as in tracheomalacia or disorders associated with sleep apnea.[55,56] CPAP should be considered as a primary mode to improve lung compliance and oxygenation in spontaneously breathing patients when the potential adverse effects of high peak airway pressures and **volutrauma** must be

avoided.[55,57-59] It is commonly used in intubated and tracheostomy patients when weaning from mechanical ventilation. High levels of CPAP may overdistend the lungs, increase the work of breathing, and reduce compliance. See Chapter 15 for a discussion on the most population use of CPAP.

Pressure Support Ventilation. Pressure support ventilation (PSV) is a spontaneous ventilation mode in which each breath must be triggered by the patient. It incorporates a constant pressure inflation that is triggered by the patient and terminated when inspiratory flow decays to a certain threshold (usually a percentage of peak flow). PSV improves the efficiency of inspiratory work of breathing, decreases the respiratory rate, reduces the oxygen cost of breathing, and is associated with faster weaning times.[60,61] It may be associated with an improved sense of breathing comfort by the patient.[62,63] PSV is popularly used to augment breaths in conjunction with SIMV or as a mode for weaning patients from mechanical ventilation.[64] Combining PSV with SIMV may help reduce some of the work associated with demand valves and small endotracheal tubes, but it may also increase $\overline{Paw}$. Caution should be used in clinical situations in which increased $\overline{Paw}$ may be harmful. PSV is useful as a standalone mode or for weaning patients receiving short- and long-term mechanical ventilation. If the patient develops an endotracheal tube leak, the flow termination criteria may not be met, thereby creating a "breath hold." Ventilators have been introduced that allow adjustment of the flow termination criteria, which may help alleviate this problem. Current ventilators have incorporated a preset or adjustable backup time termination setting that will cycle the breath into exhalation should a leak occur and the flow-cycling criteria are not met.

Effective PSV can result in adequate tidal volume and minute ventilation at a lower respiratory rate.[65] Other modes that adapt PSV to meet tidal volume or minute volume criteria are also available. Such modes provide true pressure support inflation but then alter an inflation to meet a minimal tidal volume if not met during the PSV inflation.[47]

Adaptive Pressure Support Ventilation.

Volume-Assured Pressure Support. Volume-assured pressure support (VAPS) uses pressure support ventilation while maintaining a minimal tidal volume with each breath. If the patient does not receive the minimal tidal volume during a breath, the flow rate is held constant and the pressure is increased until the volume is received.[47] This mode is useful in patients who have good respiratory effort but may rely on the ventilator to ensure a steady volume goal when pulmonary compliance and resistance are variable.

Volume Support. Volume support (VS) is a spontaneous drive pressure support mode of ventilation (see pressure support section for more details); however, like volume guarantee or PRVC, it targets a tidal volume. By adjusting the PS level to achieve the tidal volume it can be used in patients with changing compliance and effort. It incorporates a constant pressure inflation that is triggered by the patient and terminated when inspiratory flow decays to a certain threshold (usually a percentage of peak flow). Depending on the device, the mode of ventilation will look at the previous tidal volume or average of tidal volumes and adjust the pressure up or down in a predetermined algorithm in an effort to maintain the targeted tidal volume.

Many clinicians maintain that constant pressure ventilation is superior to other types of ventilation in neonates or pediatric patients who have leaks around a cuffless endotracheal tube. However, a leak around an endotracheal tube reduces ventilation during constant pressure ventilation just as it does with other types of ventilation.[66]

Neurally Adjusted Ventilatory Assist. Neurally adjusted ventilatory assist allows the patient full neurological control of the triggering, magnitude, and timing of the mechanical support provided, regardless of changes in respiratory drive, mechanics, and muscle function.[67] Neurally adjusted ventilatory assist uses a nasogastric tube with specialized sensors that obtain signals from the electrical activity of the diaphragm to control the timing and pressure of the ventilation delivered.[68] In theory, this form of triggering and support is particularly useful for patients with gas trapping and auto-PEEP who have high work of breathing because of triggering or asynchrony.

Adaptive Support Ventilation. Adaptive support ventilation uses a combination of pressure and flow to maintain targeted minute ventilation established by a preset weight and percent of minute ventilation.[69] Adaptive support allows the patient to determine optimal comfort level and enhances the patient-preferred respiratory rate or volume to achieve volume targets for tidal volume and minute ventilation along a precalculated support curve.[70,71] The patient's lung mechanics, expiratory time constants, and lung compliance are used to determine optimal targets for tidal volume and rate along the curve. The algorithm adjusts breath to breath to meet the patient's variable demands or lack of demands by providing safety backup ventilation.[72]

Airway Pressure Release Ventilation

Airway pressure release ventilation (APRV) is another form of CPAP, in which a CPAP level and a pressure release level are set along with the frequency and time of the pressure release. This mode of ventilation is usually indicated when a patient has intrapulmonary shunting from respiratory distress syndrome (RDS) or acute respiratory distress syndrome (ARDS) that is not responding to traditional approaches with a conventional mechanical ventilator. A high level of CPAP is held in the lung for up to 2 seconds for infants and 4 seconds for pediatrics, and the patient is able to breathe spontaneously during this pressure hold. The ventilator will continue to provide inspiratory flow to the patient during spontaneous breathing in order to maintain the high CPAP level. This is accomplished

because the expiratory valve is active throughout inhalation and exhalation and the patient is allowed to exhale during inspiration as long as the inflation pressure is still being held in the ventilator system. Spontaneous breathing at a higher pressure not only aids in alveolar recruitment but through the application of pleural pressure change, improvements in the distribution of lung volume to diseased lung units may improve functional residual capacity (FRC) and pulmonary compliance.[73] The short intermittent decreases in the CPAP level allow alveolar emptying of gases. Unlike conventional CPAP, however, the intermittent release of pressure augments ventilation and allows elimination of carbon dioxide.[74,75] APRV has been used in neonatal, pediatric, and adult forms of respiratory failure.[73] APRV has been referred to as *bilevel positive airway pressure* (BiPAP) but is inherently different in that it is usually implemented in an intubated patient who is failing conventional mechanical ventilation because of refractory hypoxemia. Noninvasive BiPAP does not require that a patient be tracheally intubated. In this mode the pressure level changes between inspiration and expiration. Although its use in preventing sleep apnea is similar to that of conventional CPAP, it may be helpful in overcoming ventilation difficulties and avoiding tracheotomy in individuals afflicted with neuromuscular diseases, such as spinal muscular atrophy.[76]

MECHANISMS OF GAS EXCHANGE

The mechanical ventilation (MV) techniques previously described represent different locations on the ventilation spectrum. On this spectrum, LFV occupies one extreme with relatively large tidal volumes and low breathing rates and HFOV resides at the other extreme with very small tidal volumes and high breathing rates. The techniques of LFV breath rates up to 150, HFPV, and HFJV lie in between. As one traverses this ventilatory spectrum, the classic roles of convection to deliver bulk gas to small airways and diffusion to distribute the gas among the gas-exchanging surfaces become blurred. Most of the research attempting to refine our understanding of gas transport and exchange during LFV and HFV has been accomplished in adult or animal models with normal or injured lungs. At best, the injured states mimic secondary (not natural) surfactant deficiency, and adult pulmonary time constants and airway rigidity differ significantly from those of the neonatal lung.

Enhanced diffusion is found in large and medium airways in which alterations in gas flow velocity profiles occur. This is thought to be responsible for delivery of gas farther into the lung than can be explained by pure convection.[77] There is significant interdependence between adjacent alveolar units because the walls of any alveolar unit are shared with juxtaposed alveoli, each providing stability to the other. Once inflated, these units, which may have different time constants, can equilibrate gases by swinging ventilation between them. This phenomenon, called *pendelluft,* tends to equilibrate gas concentrations in conducting airways and serves to improve gas exchange from distal pulmonary units. In addition, the impact of enhanced diffusion, the product of tidal volume and rate, and the relationship between pulmonary units may all vary depending on the HFV technique used, the settings chosen, the patient's lung size, and pathological conditions.[78] Obviously, our understanding of this complex set of gas exchange dynamics remains incomplete.

FLOW AND PRESSURE WAVEFORM PATTERNS IN LOW-FREQUENCY VENTILATION

To fully understand mechanical ventilation, the clinician should relate each change in a ventilator setting with the effect it will have on respiratory variables. Using this approach helps the clinician to understand the relationship of each ventilator setting to the respiratory system, rather than memorizing a long list of cause-and-effect relationships.[25] The concepts of flow and pressure as they relate to time are helpful in relating ventilator settings to the goals of mechanical ventilation. The pressure and flow waveforms are altered each time a ventilator setting is changed. These waveforms can be viewed as two-dimensional pictures of the changes that occur in the lungs as the ventilator settings are adjusted. Tidal volume and $\overline{Paw}$ as they relate to flow and pressure waveforms are shown in Figure 17-5. Assuming constant lung conditions and inflation time, an increase in the inspired volume per unit time results in an increase in peak pressure and an increase in

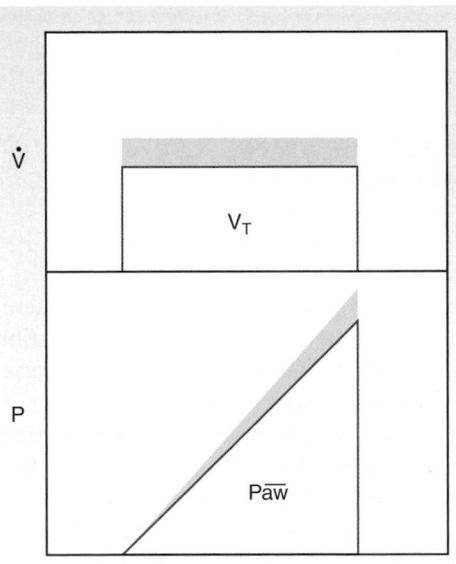

FIGURE 17-5 Flow $(\dot{V})$ and pressure (P) waveforms during constant flow–volume ventilation. The *unshaded area* below each waveform represents tidal volume (V_T) and mean airway pressure $(\overline{Paw})$. The *shaded area* represents the increase in V_T $\overline{Paw}$ and when flow is increased.

both tidal volume and $\overline{Paw}$. Similarly, if the tidal volume control on a ventilator increases, flow, peak pressure, and $\overline{Paw}$ also increase. Note that once a change occurs in one variable it results in changes in other variables. Two-dimensional images such as this help to illustrate concepts as they relate to ventilator management or other ventilator functions. The clinician would embrace flow and pressure waveform pattern and measurements of tidal volumes in HFV if practical ways of measuring existed.

TIME CONSTANTS

The concept of a time constant in the lung represents how fast pressure equilibrates between the circuit and the alveoli. Conversely, it represents the maximal rate at which exhalation occurs. The time constant is a mathematic and physiological concept that is not consistently applied clinically. Previously, accurately obtaining the values necessary for calculating a time constant was technically difficult. Advances in pulmonary function measurement techniques have made these data more available.

A time constant is the product of multiplying compliance and resistance. The time constant relates to both inspiratory filling and expiratory emptying of the lungs. Mouth pressure or proximal airway pressure equilibrates with alveolar pressure in three to five time constants.[79] In a healthy newborn this is 0.33 second. In severely premature infants with respiratory distress syndrome with decreased lung compliance, one time constant can be as short as 0.05 second.[80] This means that pressure equilibration will occur in 0.15 to 0.25 second, which is the minimal inspiratory time required to ensure complete delivery of the tidal volume. When airway resistance is high, such as in meconium aspiration syndrome, the time constant is longer. This would indicate using longer inspiratory times, lower inspiratory flows, and longer exhalation times to ventilate these infants.

Monitoring respiratory system mechanics to derive time constants assists in properly adjusting adequate inspiratory time and expiratory time during ventilation. The time component is important when using rapid rates to allow adequate exhalation without developing breath stacking and automatic positive end-expiratory pressure (auto-PEEP) and to minimize iatrogenic lung damage. Using serial measurements of resistance and compliance directs the setting of ventilator parameters to match the changing pathophysiology of the patient.[81]

TRIGGERING AND SYNCHRONIZATION IN LOW-FREQUENCY VENTILATION

Patient triggering is one of the most important links to the LFV ventilator. Proper triggering can reduce work of breathing, allows a patient to be more comfortable, reduces oxygen consumption, and can result in a shorter duration of ventilation.[82] There are three types of sensing: flow, pressure, and electrical activity of the diaphragm (Table 17-1). Many ventilators can do one if not two of the types of sensing. When types of triggering are considered, the placement of the triggering device and its effects on the patient are evaluated. Flow triggering is the most commonly used in the neonatal patient population.

Flow Sensing

Many ventilators now offer flow triggering as the primary mechanism by which a breath is initiated by a patient from the ventilator. A pneumotachometer between the circuit and the patient senses effort by measuring inspiratory flow. Two types of pneumotachometers can be used to sense flow: the heated-wire anemometer and the variable-orifice pneumotachometer. These units have fast response times, usually in the 30- to 70-millisecond range, and provide reliable synchronization at all rates.[83,84] However, flow sensors add dead space to the airway, and the potential increase in tidal volume associated with SIMV may be negated by an increase in carbon dioxide retention. Flow sensors may also be affected by secretions and require frequent cleaning. Flow sensing and triggering can also be done with the internal ventilator pneumotachometer and can be sensitive enough for most patients. With these improvements in making the ventilator more receptive to patient effort, problems associated with secretions, condensation, system/patient leaks, and active cardiac pulsation could lead to erroneous triggering of the ventilator (auto-cycling).

Pressure Sensing

Some ventilators use a drop in the pressure signal sensed at the airway to trigger the ventilator with the patient's breath. For the pressure in the circuit to drop to less than the trigger level, or sensitivity setting, approximately 2 ml of volume must be displaced. This often accounts for a large portion of the neonatal tidal volume and thus is not well tolerated. A low-birth-weight infant may not consistently produce the level of effort necessary to trigger the ventilator. During pressure sensing, the response time tends to be slow because of delay from the progression of the pressure drop through the ventilator tubing. Because of this, synchronization is difficult to achieve at ventilator rates greater than 35 to 40 breaths per minute.

Electrical Activity of the Diaphragm

Neurally adjusted ventilatory assist (NAVA) uses a nasogastric tube with specialized sensors that obtain signals from the electrical activity of the diaphragm (EAdi) to control the timing and pressure of the ventilation delivered.[67] In theory, this form of triggering and support is particularly useful for patients with gas trapping and auto-PEEP who have high work of breathing as a result of triggering. This form of triggering is not affected by leaks and secretions; therefore, auto-cycling and hypocapnia in newborns can be eliminated. However, this modality is invasive and placement of the nasogastric tube could be initially uncomfortable to the patient, yet it may lead to increased synchrony and earlier liberation.

CASE STUDY 2

You are called by your nursing colleague to assess a patient who does not appear to be comfortable and doesn't appear to be triggering the ventilator. What steps would you take to solve this problem?

See Evolve Resources for answers.

MANAGING VENTILATOR SETTINGS

Low-Frequency Ventilation
Initial Setup

Clinical protocols guiding decisions to implement MV techniques should be in place in each institution before these devices are used. Personnel involved in patient management must demonstrate proficiency in the use of the device and clinical expertise to ensure patient safety. Active training programs within each institution should be mandatory and include a demonstration by personnel that they understand ventilator controls and circuit design, basic troubleshooting, and management strategies. Before the initiation of MV, each device and circuit should be inspected to ensure proper calibration and function. Specific care should be taken to ensure that (1) proper gas temperature and humidity are present, (2) ventilator and circuit position is such that a smooth transition can

---

TABLE 17-1

Synchronizing Systems for Mechanical Ventilators

Type	Source	Advantages/Disadvantages
Flow sensor	Pneumotachometer (heated wire, variable orifice, differential pressure)	Fast response; provides volume measurement; adds dead space; affected by secretions
Pressure sensor	Proximal airway, ventilator demand valve	No dead space; requires good patient effort; low transit time
Electrical activity of the diaphragm (EAdi)	Nasogastric tube with electrodes that determine the electrical activity of the diaphragm	No dead space; unaffected by secretions, auto-PEEP, and leaks; requires catheter (invasive); no volume measurement

TABLE 17-2

Initial Mechanical Ventilator Settings

	Premature Infant	Infant	Toddler	Small Child	Child	Adolescent
Respiratory rate (breaths/min)	40-60	25-40	20-35	20-30	18-25	12-20
V_T (ml/kg)	4-6	5-8	5-8	6-9	7-10	7-10
Inspiratory time (s)	0.25-0.4	0.3-0.5	0.6-0.7	0.7-0.8	0.8-1	1-1.2
PEEP (cm H_2O)	5	5	5	5	5	5
FIO_2	*	*	*	*	*	*

FIO_2, Fraction of inspired oxygen; *PEEP*, peak end-expiratory pressure; V_T, tidal volume.
*Start 10% higher than preintubation FIO_2 or 100% unless contraindicated.

occur, and (3) initial settings are lower than anticipated requirements to allow a slow increase toward desired levels and prevention of inadvertent injury. Finally, other appropriate primary therapies (e.g., surfactant replacement for surfactant deficiency and vasopressor support for impaired myocardial function), good pulmonary toilet are not replaced by MV and should be optimized along with ventilatory management.

Proper management of ventilator settings requires monitoring of noninvasive monitors, arterial blood gases, chest radiographs, and ventilator waveforms and physical assessment of the patient. Table 17-2 shows commonly used initial ventilator settings suggested for different patient sizes; however, certain conditions or severity of disease may require a different initial approach.

High-Frequency Ventilation

Until more recently, HFV use was limited to patients in whom LFV was failing. The literature and experience with neonates through adults are changing this impression, so that HFV is increasingly being used before rescue situations develop. These developments are changing current protocols for moving patients from LFV to HFV. Because of this, it is necessary to focus on the concepts that need to be considered when applying HFV to patients, rather than describing specific ventilator settings. The evolving literature and device-specific manufacturer's recommendations should be consulted for more details. Successful application of any HFV device requires accurate comprehension of individual patient pulmonary pathophysiology and selection of an appropriate ventilatory strategy. At present, there are two fundamentally differing strategies that are designed to approach contrasting pulmonary pathophysiological processes.

Each HFV device was initially developed for specific lung disease states. Because of ethical, scientific, and legal constraints, use in human infants was at first confined to rescue patients in whom conventional methods were failing. With increasing anecdotal success noted by several groups, it became apparent that strategies applied to these infants were unique to each device. Subsequently, refinements in patient management led to tailoring device design, with a resultant narrowing of the spectrum of lung diseases to which they could be applied. For example,

HFJV was directed toward air leak syndromes and HFOV toward diffuse alveolar disease. Studies have now shown that $\overline{Paw}$ recruitment of the atelectasis-prone lung can be accomplished with different HFV types with similar successes in gas exchange, histological evidence of uniform gas distribution, and decreased hyaline membrane formation.[85,86] Conversely, Clark and associates[87] reported successful HFOV treatment of a series of infants with PIE and supported the value of HFOV use in patients with air leaks. In another study of infants with PIE, Keszler and coworkers[88] reported a clear superiority of HFJV over low frequency ventilation in a carefully controlled multicenter trial. Keszler and coworkers[89] have subsequently had success in managing infants with RDS with HFJV. These findings imply that successful management of infants with significant pulmonary disorders is best accomplished by device-specific strategies directed toward specific lung pathophysiological processes rather than by specific HFV types.

Management Strategies

High-Volume Strategy. For the patient with an atelectasis-prone lung (e.g., natural or acquired surfactant deficiency), the primary therapeutic goal is to optimize lung inflation so that ventilation–perfusion mismatching is minimized while reducing inflation–deflation breathing patterns that initiate a cascade of events leading to lung tissue injury.[11,89] This has been termed the *high-volume strategy*. Two separate means of achieving this goal have evolved.

One method is to increase the distending pressures ($\overline{Paw}$ or CDP) in small increments (1 to 2 cm H_2O) while watching for improvement in oxygenation (arterial blood gas determinations, transcutaneous carbon dioxide, or pulse oximetry saturations) and mean lung volumes (MLV) determined by chest radiograph. Mean airway pressure is increased until oxygenation improves significantly or until MLV reaches desired levels, or both, which may be determined by the presence of a well-inflated lung on a radiograph (Figure 17-6). While using this method, care must be taken to anticipate silent lung recruitment and to reduce $\overline{Paw}$ as appropriate to avoid serious impairment to venous return and reduction in cardiac output. Silent lung recruitment is gradual lung inflation taking place with static $\overline{Paw}$ settings (Figure 17-7). Clinical clues heralding this include

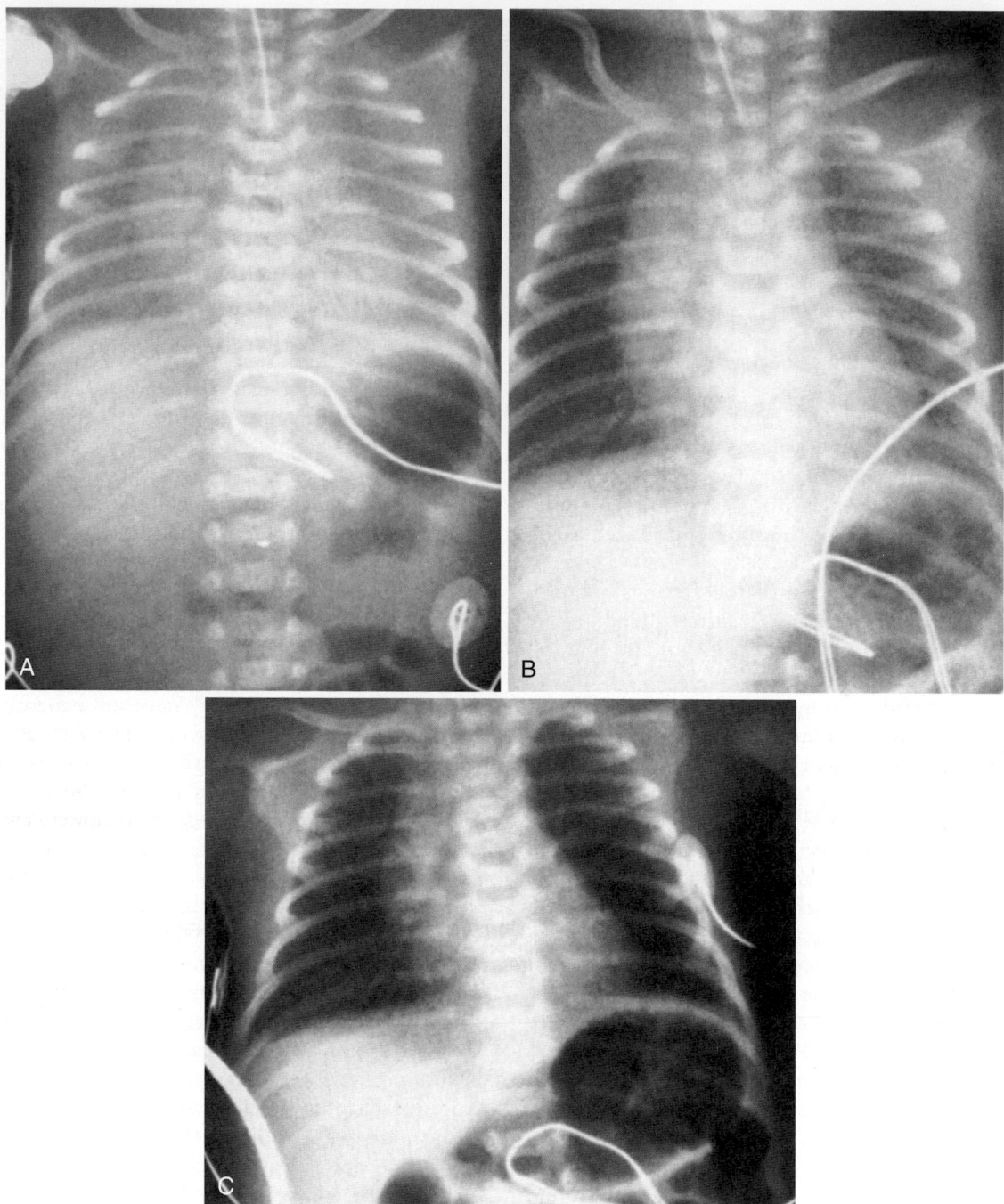

FIGURE 17-6 Radiographs during the first day of life for a 30-week premature infant with respiratory distress syndrome (RDS) managed with HFOV to achieve optimal mean lung volume (MLV). **A,** Initial $\overline{Paw}$ equal to 10 cm H_2O, fraction of inspired oxygen (FiO_2) equal to 1. **B,** At 12 hours of age, with $\overline{Paw}$ equal to 15 cm H_2O and FiO_2 equal to 0.45. **C,** At 24 hours of age with $\overline{Paw}$ equal to 12 cm H_2O and FiO_2 equal to 0.28.

rapid improvements with subsequent unexplained decrements in oxygenation, decreasing $PaCO_2$ without changes in oscillatory amplitude (improving compliance), and, finally, clinical changes in perfusion. These problems often can be avoided with diligence and anticipation. Silent recruitment, although more common during initial HFV management, can occur any time attempts are made to optimize MLV. Data confirm the pulmonary, central nervous system, and cardiovascular safety and efficacy of this technique.[13,90-93]

The other approach to recruiting the collapsed lung is the use of sustained inflations (SIs), that is, applying plateau pressures at levels in excess of expected alveolar opening pressures for periods of 5 to 30 seconds. This technique should result in incremental improvement in oxygenation if pressure levels are adequate. Furthermore, because of lung hysteresis, the inter-SI $\overline{Paw}$ can often be reduced to levels slightly less than can be achieved with the other lung inflation method. SIs are usually repeated until no change in

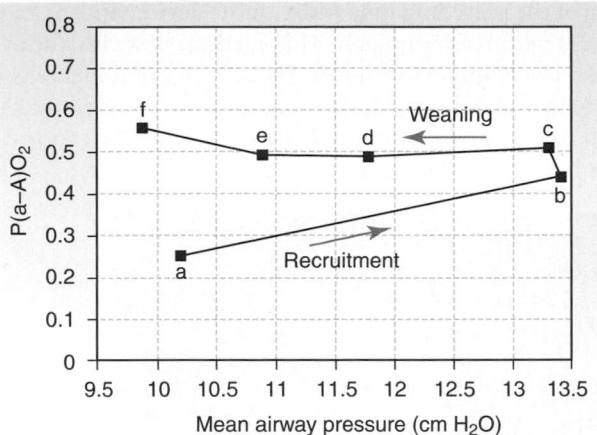

FIGURE 17-7   Mean arterial-to-alveolar oxygen tension ratio [P(a–A)O$_2$] and $\overline{\text{Paw}}$ of 21 premature infants managed with HFOV immediately after surfactant replacement. Note that increasing $\overline{\text{Paw}}$ initially results in increased P(a–A)O$_2$ (alveolar recruitment); subsequent $\overline{\text{Paw}}$ weaning does not reduce oxygenation but is associated with gradual improvement in P(a–A)O$_2$. The line between points *b* and *c* represents silent lung recruitment as assessed by improving P(a–A)O$_2$ with essentially stable $\overline{\text{Paw}}$. (*a*) Surfactant replacement; (*b*) 12 hours later; (*c*) 12 to 24 hours later; (*d*) 24 to 48 hours later; (*e*) 48 to 72 hours later; and (*f*) 72 to 96 hours later.

oxygenation is noted or until oxygenation decreases. Both imply that the lung is at the upper limits of lung capacity. The need for repeat SI maneuvers is determined by the level of inter-SI $\overline{\text{Paw}}$ used and the amount of subsequent alveolar derecruitment. The SI method may achieve optimal MLV more rapidly and, because of the lower inter-SI $\overline{\text{Paw}}$, avoid silent recruitment. However, potential disadvantages include the risk of using too little pressure (minimal recruitment) or too much pressure (airway injury, air leak, and reductions in cardiac output). Data from excised baboon lungs suggest that lung recruitment responses to SI maneuvers are

dependent on lung pathophysiology. Thus there is a difference in the response of surfactant-sufficient collapsed lungs and uninjured surfactant-deficient lungs.[4] This method has been used successfully in infants with minimal complications.[3,92] Definite superiority of one technique over the other has not been demonstrated.

Note the contrast between LFV and HFV. With LFV, lung recruitment is achieved by increasing inspiratory time, end-expiratory pressure, and the resultant mean airway pressure, whereas HFV uses $\overline{\text{Paw}}$ alone to achieve lung recruitment. Supplying adequate oscillatory amplitude around the baseline $\overline{\text{Paw}}$ provides ventilation during HFPV and HFOV. With HFJV, ventilation is determined by changes in jet-pulse tidal volume delivery and by the amount of background CV used. It is critical to avoid the temptation to use HFV phasic pressure to recruit underinflated lung units. Table 17-3 suggests an algorithm for implementation of the high-volume strategy.

Low-Volume Strategy.   In contrast to the lung inflation strategies described, management of infants with PIE, pneumothorax, or air trapping requires the employment of alternative strategies because attempts to achieve optimal mean lung volume (MLV) in these patients will exaggerate existing lung overinflation or serve to further damage the injured lung. Here the primary objective should be to offer a ventilatory strategy that allows the lung to slowly deflate, or one that minimizes ongoing air leakage while providing tolerable ventilation and accepting higher FIO$_2$. This is accomplished with all HFV systems by using a lower $\overline{\text{Paw}}$ than that creating the problem. (These patients are usually undergoing CV before being switched to HFV.) This allows the lung to derecruit and isolates damaged areas from inflation pressures. The consequence of this, however, is the frequent requirement for a higher FIO$_2$. In addition, tidal volume delivery must be decreased to further reduce tidal volume exposure while using I/E ratios and ventilatory frequencies

TABLE 17-3

Generic Oxygenation and Ventilation Strategies for Use During High-frequency Ventilation in Patients with Diffuse Lung Disease

Oxygenation Strategies

PaO$_2$	Increased	Normal	Decreased
Lung inflation	Normal	Normal	Normal
Primary response	Decrease FIO$_2$	None	Increase FIO$_2$
Secondary response	None	None	None
PaO$_2$	Increased	Normal	Decreased
Lung inflation	Decreased	Decreased	Decreased
Primary response	Increase $\overline{\text{Paw}}$	Increase $\overline{\text{Paw}}$	Increase $\overline{\text{Paw}}$
Secondary response	Decrease FIO$_2$	None	Increase FIO$_2$
PaO$_2$	Increased	Normal	Decreased
Lung inflation	Increased	Increased	Increased
Primary response	Decrease $\overline{\text{Paw}}$	Decrease $\overline{\text{Paw}}$	Decrease $\overline{\text{Paw}}$
Secondary response	Decrease FIO$_2$	None	Increase FIO$_2$

Ventilation Strategies

PaCO$_2$	Increased	Normal	Decreased
Primary response	Increase OA	None	Decrease OA
Secondary response frequency	Decrease frequency	None	Increase

OA, oscillatory amplitude.

that maximize gas egress. A $PaCO_2$ between 50 and 60 mm Hg is often tolerated in these patients as long as the arterial pH exceeds 7.25 (these parameter limits will likely vary among institutions). Once there is radiographic evidence that the lung has adequately deflated and air leaks have resolved (for at least 12 to 24 hours), the lung is reinflated by one of the preceding lung inflation strategies. Air leak rarely recurs with this approach. This method is successful in at least 66% of infants with PIE. Those with PIE under tension and myocardial compromise are more difficult to manage and have poorer outcomes (Figure 17-8).[12,94] This approach has been dubbed the *low-volume strategy*.

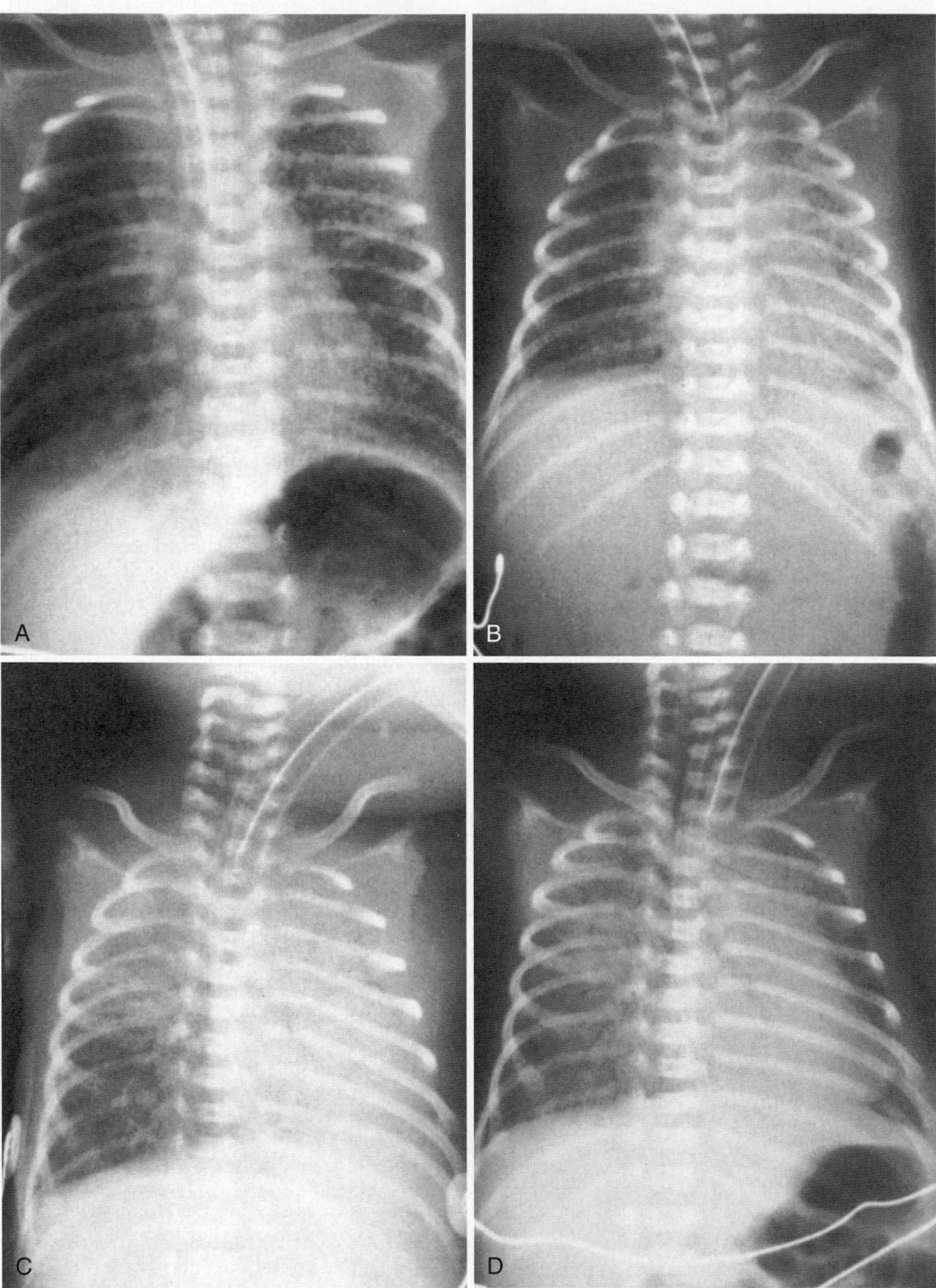

FIGURE 17-8 Radiographs of a 2-day-old preterm infant with pulmonary interstitial emphysema (PIE). **A,** Paw equal to 16 cm H_2O and FiO_2 equal to 0.65. **B,** Six hours later, Paw equal to 8 cm H_2O and FiO_2 equal to 1. **C,** Twelve hours later, settings were unchanged, PIE was resolved, and lung was nearly totally deflated. **D,** Thirty-six hours later, reinflation was beginning, Paw was equal to 12 cm H_2O, and FiO_2 was equal to 0.45.

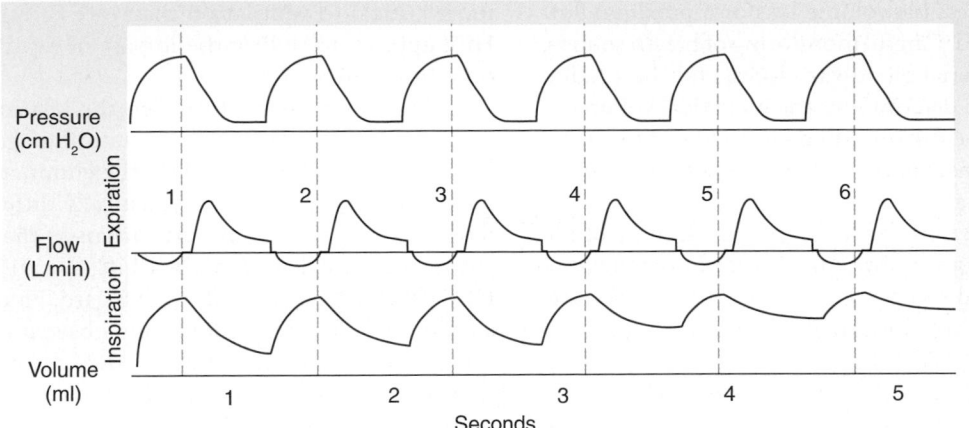

FIGURE 17-9 Air trapping illustrated in a flow (L/min) over time scalar. Expiratory flow never returns to baseline before the ventilator cycles again.

MANIPULATING VENTILATION

Low-Frequency Ventilation

One of the main goals of mechanical ventilation is to manipulate the arterial carbon dioxide tension ($PaCO_2$), which is affected by changing the minute ventilation. The minute ventilation is directly related to ventilation frequency and tidal volume and is inversely related to the $PaCO_2$.

Frequency

Frequency or rate is generally the first method used to increase minute ventilation. At low rates and conventional I/E ratios or during weaning, adjusting frequency is the most desirable option. Two disadvantages exist when manipulating frequency at higher rates or inverse I/E ratios. The first is that as frequency increases, air trapping is likely to occur.[95,96] Figure 17-9 illustrates this in a flow/time scalar graphic. Notice that flow does not come back to baseline. The second is that when the I/E ratio is kept constant, minute ventilation does not change.

Tidal Volume

An alternative to adjusting frequency is to change any variable that affects tidal volume and hence affects minute ventilation and $PaCO_2$. The goal is to select a variable that will increase the area under the flow waveform. This is accomplished by increasing flow or inspiratory time. The tidal volume control on a microprocessor ventilator adjusts flow or times to derive an increase in tidal volume. Another variable that is available on some ventilators is the I:E ratio. Adjusting it to provide a longer inspiratory time may also improve elimination of carbon dioxide. Altering tidal volume variables is useful in situations such as severe asthma, in which the goal is to minimize the rate and air trapping while maximizing exhalation time and ventilation. Figure 17-10 illustrates the three ways in which the flow waveform can change to increase tidal volume and minute ventilation.

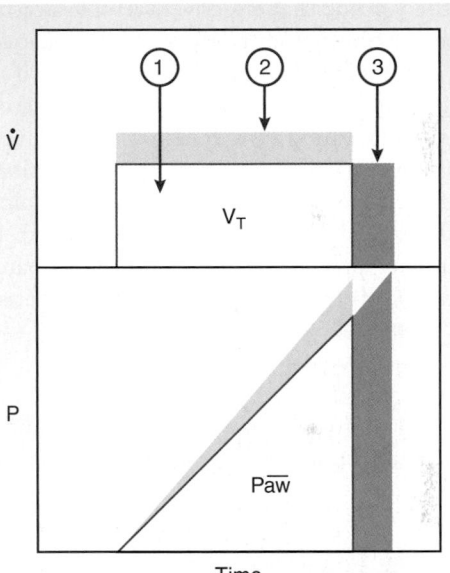

FIGURE 17-10 Control variables that affect minute ventilation by increasing the area under the flow ($\dot{V}$) waveform to increase tidal volume (V_T). *1,* Increase V_T or rate; *2,* increase inspiratory flow; *3,* increase inspiratory time. Also shown is the associated change in mean airway pressure ($\overline{Paw}$). *P,* Pressure.

Research has shown that the largest contribution to ventilator-induced lung injury results from lung overdistention caused by excessive tidal volume (volutrauma), followed by the repetitive opening and closing of the terminal lung units (**atelectrauma**).[97] Therefore, more emphasis is being placed on setting lower tidal volumes, improvements in tidal volume monitoring, and setting adequate PEEP levels. The tidal volume setting in neonates varies from 4 to 6 ml/kg in low-birth-weight premature infants, to 5 to 8 ml/kg in term infants, and to 7 to 10 ml/kg in pediatric and adolescent patients.[53,97] Lower volumes have been shown to be effective for patients with restrictive lung disease such as RDS and ARDS.[98,99] Tidal volume should be corrected for compressible volume loss or a proximal flow sensor should be used. Careful monitoring of breath sounds, chest expansion, arterial blood gas values, and chest radiographs is essential in determining adequate tidal volume.

During pressure ventilation, increasing the pressure limit may also increase tidal volume. When the pressure limit is reached, flow decelerates. The increase in tidal volume is the result of the delay in flow deceleration and widening of the area under the flow waveform. An increase in the pressure limit during PCV and PSV causes the initial flow to increase. The result is a larger decelerating flow waveform and larger tidal volume. Figure 17-11 illustrates the way a change in the pressure limit affects both forms of pressure ventilation.

High-Frequency Ventilation

Classic physiology teaches that elimination of carbon dioxide is directly related to the product of breathing rate and tidal volume (minute ventilation, where $\dot{V}CO_2 = f \times V_T$); however, the volume that effectively removes carbon dioxide is alveolar volume that is, the difference between tidal and dead space volumes. On the basis of this, if tidal volume is less than dead space, this difference, zero, and its product with breathing rate does not yield a meaningful number. Because all of the HFV methods described are effective means of ventilation, even with tidal volumes less than dead space, a new explanation is needed. Fredberg and coworkers[37] provided insight into this apparent paradox by describing elimination of carbon dioxide as follows:

$$(\dot{V}_{CO_2}) = (f)^x \times (V_T)^y$$

where x is 0.5 to 1 and y is 1.5 to 2.2 (depending on the device). From this relationship we see that tidal volume is

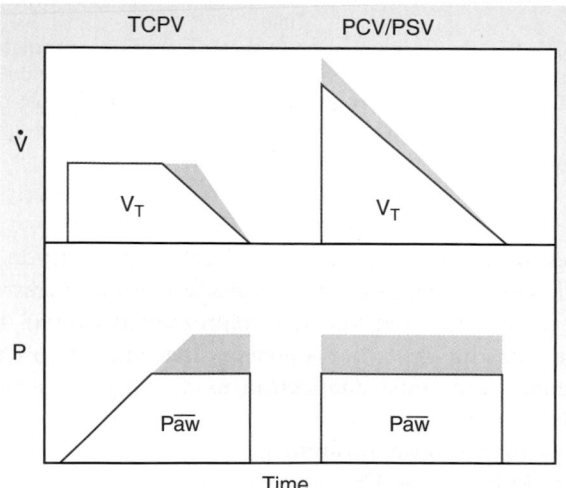

FIGURE 17-11 Waveforms comparing the mechanism of increasing tidal volume (V_T) by adjusting pressure limit during time-cycled pressure-limited ventilation (TCPV) to pressure-control or pressure-support ventilation (PCV/PSV). Flow changes during PCV/PSV, but only the length of time changes before flow decelerates during TCPV. *Paw,* Mean airway pressure; $\dot{V}$, flow.

more critical to ventilation than rate is during HFV, and HFV appears to reduce the impact of dead space volume on ventilation.

Unlike oxygenation, in which the relationship of $\overline{Paw}$ to MLV and subsequent optimization of gas exchange is similar between LFV and HFV, the elimination of carbon dioxide by LFV and HFV is drastically different. This difference lies not only in the alterations to the minute ventilation equation just described but also in the nature of HFV devices themselves. In this regard, Fredberg and colleagues[37] made several interesting observations during an evaluation of multiple neonatal HFV devices. They noted that not only is carbon dioxide elimination during HFV more sensitive to changes in tidal volume than in rate but also the tidal volume output of HFV devices is sensitive to changes in ETT diameter and lung compliance. As ETT dimensions and compliance decreased, so did tidal volume output from the HFV tested. This occurred in the presence of stable ventilator settings. Therefore any clinical change causing a decrease in ETT diameter, such as reintubation with a different-sized ETT or partial ETT obstruction with tracheal secretions, alters the delivered tidal volume. Furthermore, improvements in lung compliance (e.g., volume recruitment) and decrements in lung compliance (e.g., patent ductus arteriosus or alveolar derecruitment) have a direct effect on tidal volume.

In addition, the relationship between ventilator frequency and carbon dioxide elimination is nonintuitive. Changes in ventilator rate at a given pressure amplitude cause an inverse change in tidal volume. Thus when ventilation must be improved, a reduction in breathing frequency improves ventilation because the increased volume output per stroke has a greater impact on ventilation than does the decrease in stroke frequency. The converse is also true. When less ventilation is needed and pressure amplitude is already minimized, increasing breathing frequency will further decrease tidal volume and allow weaning from ventilation. Figure 17-12 depicts data collected during volume measurement experiments with a CareFusion 3100A high-frequency oscillator (Cardinal Health, Dublin, Ohio). Observe that although varying $\overline{Paw}$ (10 and 20 cm H_2O) had no impact on tidal volume output at any given oscillatory amplitude, there was a substantial difference in tidal volume with differing frequencies. Volumes at 10 Hz are much higher than those at 15 Hz for each oscillatory amplitude tested.

Frequency

Breathing frequency ranges between 2 and 28 Hz, depending on the device. Rates lower than 4 Hz and greater than 15 Hz are rarely used. The impact of the breathing rate on ventilation during HFV is less than the impact of tidal volume. Frequency is therefore not usually changed, and management of ventilation occurs with changes in delivered volume. Changes in frequency are made when operating at machine limits of tidal volume (both low and high

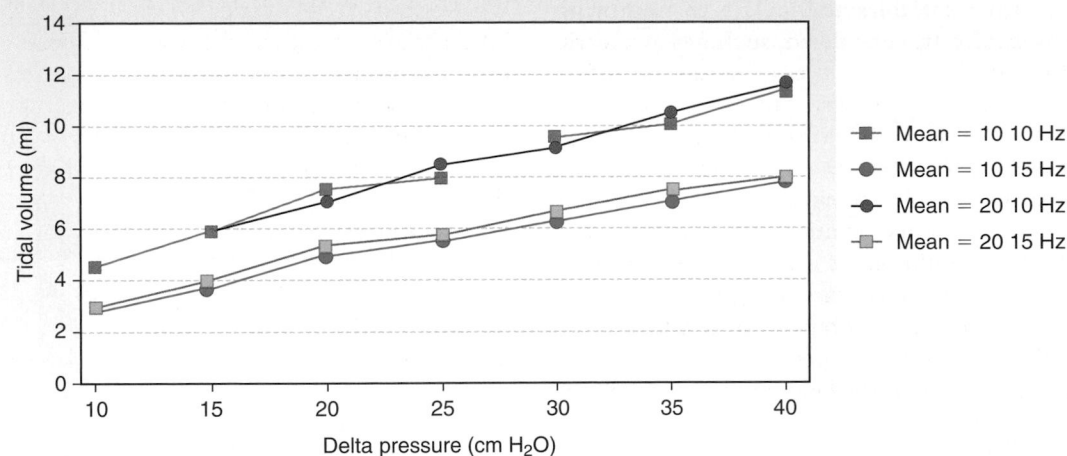

FIGURE 17-12 Tidal volume output measured during high-frequency oscillatory ventilation (HFOV) with a CareFusion 3100A at a mean airway pressure ($\overline{Paw}$) equal to 10 and 20 cm H_2O and a frequency equal to 10 and 15 Hz. There is a nearly linear relationship between oscillatory amplitude and tidal volume. At each oscillatory amplitude tested, tidal volume at 10 Hz is higher than at 15 Hz. $\overline{Paw}$ has no effect.

limits). Choices of breathing frequency depend on understanding optimal functional characteristics of each device and the nature of the patient and the disease treated. For example, with a similar disease, such as acute RDS, neonatal and pediatric patients are managed with different frequencies during HFOV. The smaller child requires a lower tidal volume and therefore a higher frequency. Preliminary data in mature animals suggest that, at an equivalent arterial partial pressure of carbon dioxide ($PaCO_2$), higher frequencies during HFOV are less damaging to airways than lower frequencies.[100]

Oscillatory Amplitude or Peak Pressure

Each of the ventilators available in the United States is pressure limited. Changes in delivered pressure amplitude have a direct influence on tidal volume delivery. The purpose of measuring peak inspiratory pressure is to offer both patient safety and ease of adjustment of delivered tidal volume. Although HFJV provides separate control and displays an estimate of distal ETT peak pressure, the HFOV does not. The oscillatory amplitude (the peak-to-trough pressure difference). Measurement of pressures (whether peak or peak-to-trough) distal to the insertion point of HFV breaths in the patient circuit is important to avoid underestimation of pressures seen by pulmonary structures. Transducers, amplifiers, and measuring circuit fidelity must be adequate and unfiltered to properly measure peak-to-peak pressures at these breathing frequencies.

During HFOV, peak and trough pressures are measured, although they are not usually displayed. Because of the impact of the ETT on transmitted pressure, these values have only relative significance. Of more importance is the difference between peak and trough pressures, known as *oscillatory amplitude* or simply the *delta P*. Delivered volume

is directly proportional to this peak–trough difference, and adjustments result in changes in tidal volume (see Figure 17-12). During HFOV, the relationship between oscillatory amplitude and tidal volume actually delivered to the lung is subject to the same constraints as peak-to-end-expiratory pressure differences during pressure-limited LFV. Changes in downstream compliance and impingement on the ETT lumen cause tidal volumes to vary without changes in displayed pressure amplitudes. Control over tidal volume during HFJV occurs by modifications in distally measured peak pressures. Although this measurement is less vulnerable to variations in the ETT lumen, total volume delivery during HFJV is a combination of jet pulse and gas entrained with each breath from the proximal ETT connection. This entrainment volume is vulnerable to reductions in the ETT lumen.

MANIPULATING OXYGENATION

Fraction of Inspired Oxygen

The most obvious way to improve oxygen delivery is to increase the alveolar oxygen tension by increasing the fraction of inspired oxygen (FIO_2). A simple method to determine the FIO_2 needed for a desired arterial oxygen tension (PaO_2) is derived from the arterial-to-alveolar oxygen tension ratio. Assuming constant barometric pressure, $PaCO_2$, and stable lung conditions, the equation simplifies to:

$$FIO_2 \text{ desired} = PaO_2 \text{ desired} \times FIO_2 \text{ known}/PaO_2 \text{ known}$$

Because prolonged exposure to high levels of oxygen may be toxic, the lowest acceptable FIO_2 should be used.[101] However, high levels of oxygen may be necessary to correct hypoxemia when treating severe lung disease or persistent pulmonary hypertension of the newborn. To avoid these complications, other variables that relate to improving oxygenation must also be considered, such as $\overline{Paw}$, nitric oxide, and PEEP.

Low-Frequency Ventilation
Mean Airway Pressure

Improvement in PaO_2 is directly related to an increase in $\overline{Paw}$. (It may have an inverse relationship in right-to-left cardiac shunts or in pulmonary volutrauma.[102,103]) This improvement is believed to be caused by recruitment of collapsed alveoli or the redistribution of lung fluid, or both.[42] $\overline{Paw}$ is the area under the pressure waveform from the beginning of inflation to the beginning of the next inflation divided by the total cycle time. A simple equation for estimating $\overline{Paw}$ is as follows:

$$\overline{Paw} = 1/2 \times \text{peak pressure} \times$$
$$(\text{inspiratory/time/inspiratory} + \text{expiratory times})$$

Several control variables affect $\overline{Paw}$, including inspiratory time, peak pressure, frequency, flow, and PEEP. The denominator of the equation for $\overline{Paw}$ is cycle time or frequency. As frequency increases, cycle time decreases so that the result is an increase in the value of $\overline{Paw}$. Figure 17-13 demonstrates how the pressure waveform can be altered by these variables to increase $\overline{Paw}$. The desired $\overline{Paw}$ is one in which both oxygenation and ventilation are optimized and the risks of pulmonary volutrauma, impaired hemodynamics, and fluid retention are minimized.

Flow Rate

The flow rate will directly affect $\overline{Paw}$. Ideally, inspiratory flow should be set to match the patient's peak inspiratory demands and depends largely on the following:
· The patient's spontaneous effort
· The work of breathing
· Patient–ventilator synchrony

Too much or not enough flow can increase the work of breathing or cause dyssynchrony.[104,105] Figure 17-14 presents a flow–volume loop illustrating when there is inadequate flow. Flow and pressure waveforms vary among ventilators. The flow required for spontaneous breathing is provided by means of continuous flow or a demand valve that is triggered by the patient's inspiratory effort.[16]

Inspiratory Time and I:E Ratio

The inspiratory time and I/E ratio also directly affect $\overline{Paw}$. Although there are few specific data regarding guidelines for inspiratory time and I:E ratio, it is suggested that the appropriate inspiratory time and I:E ratio depend on the patient's ventilation and oxygenation status as well as on the level of spontaneous breathing. Ventilators are often set at an inspiratory time of 0.25 to 0.5 second for neonates, 0.6 to 0.9 second for toddlers and children, and 1 to 1.2 seconds for adolescents, with an I/E ratio of 1:2 to 1:3.

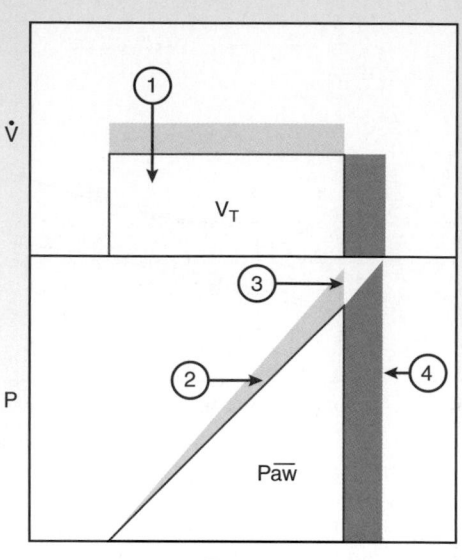

FIGURE 17-13 Control variables that alter mean airway pressure ($\overline{Paw}$) by increasing the area under the pressure waveform. *1,* Increase tidal volume (V_T) or rate; *2,* increase inspiratory flow; *3,* increase peak pressure; *4,* increase inspiratory time. Also shown is the associated change in V_T. *P*, Pressure; $\dot{V}$, flow.

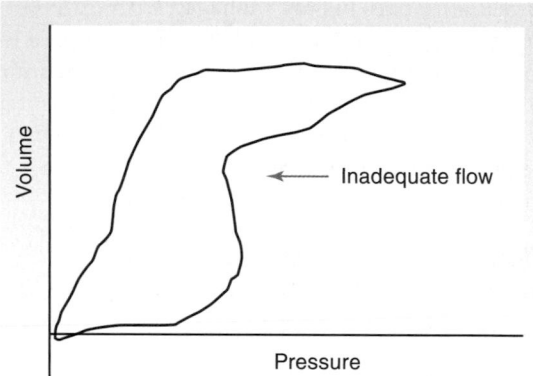

FIGURE 17-14 Inadequate flow support on flow–volume loop. A normal loop should look like a football at a 45-degree angle. The inspiratory phase of this loop is concave, owing to inadequate flow.

Increasing the inspiratory time or I/E ratio is performed in an effort to increase $\overline{Paw}$ and improve oxygenation. When this is carried out, however, the impact on patient comfort, the need for sedation, and the development of auto-PEEP, hemodynamic compromise, and breath stacking must be considered.[106] Figure 17-15 presents what is seen on the ventilator graphics if the inspiratory time is excessive.

Positive End-Expiratory Pressure

The most significant variable affecting $\overline{Paw}$ is PEEP. Figure 17-16 shows the relationship of PEEP to the pressure waveform and $\overline{Paw}$. PEEP affects pressure

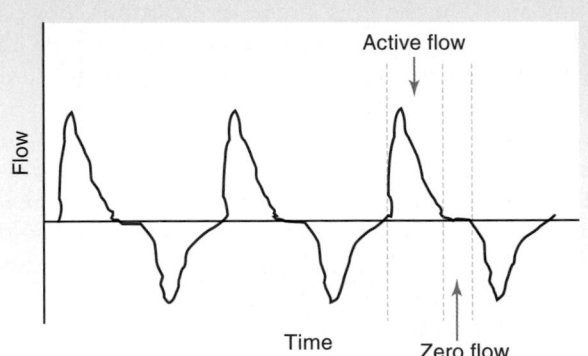

FIGURE 17-15 Excessive inspiratory time on flow/time scalar. Flow returns to baseline before the ventilator cycles into expiration.

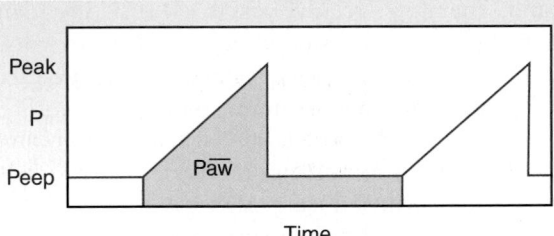

FIGURE 17-16 The relationship of positive end-expiratory pressure (PEEP) to the pressure waveform. Note that mean airway pressure (Paw) is the area under the waveform during the entire respiratory cycle. *P*, Pressure.

throughout the entire respiratory cycle and alters the simple formula given previously for $\overline{Paw}$ to

$$\overline{Paw} = 1/2 \times (\text{Peak pressure} - \text{PEEP}) \times$$
$$(\text{Inspiratory time/Inspiratory time} + \text{Expiratory time})$$
$$+ \text{PEEP}$$

PEEP improves gas exchange by improving PaO_2, maintenance of recruited alveoli, increasing functional lung volume, decreasing intrapulmonary shunting, and improving lung compliance.[107-109] Simply stated the goal of PEEP therapy is to improve oxygenation by increasing FRC through maintenance of airway patency and alveolar recruitment.

An adequate PEEP level is the amount of PEEP necessary to attain an acceptable PaO_2 at the lowest FiO_2, although avoidance of high PEEP levels is desirable.[110] It is determined by many physiologic factors, which may or may not be monitored in any given clinical situation. A conservative but acceptable PaO_2 is 45 to 65 mm Hg for neonates younger than 33 weeks of gestation and 60 to 80 mm Hg for pediatric patients at an FiO_2 of 0.4 to 0.5. PEEP usually begins at 3 to 5 cm H_2O, with increases made in increments of 2 cm H_2O.[111,112] A method of judging adequate PEEP levels is to monitor static lung compliance or to calculate it by dividing the effective tidal volume

formula by the end-inspiratory pause pressure minus PEEP. When the functional residual capacity is low, static compliance increases as PEEP increases because of shifting of the ventilating volume to the optimal point on the compliance curve. When optimal distention is reached, lung compliance is maximal. If PEEP is increased further, overdistention, reduced compliance, and decreased oxygen transport may result.[107] A static compliance measurement can be difficult to obtain in patients with cuffless endotracheal tubes that have a leak.

Monitoring the $PaCO_2$ to end-tidal carbon dioxide gradient may also be useful in judging PEEP levels (see Chapter 8, Invasive Blood Gas Analysis and Cardiovascular Monitoring). Overdistention and reduced cardiac output resulting from excessive PEEP cause the gradient to widen. Caution must be exercised with this method because other abnormalities causing a low cardiac output may also increase this gradient.[28,113] Because excessive levels of PEEP can affect cardiac function, monitoring mean blood pressure, central venous pressure, mean pulmonary artery pressure, and other hemodynamic variables is also important while monitoring PEEP levels. When pulmonary artery catheters are used, cardiac output and the pulmonary shunt fraction are useful measures. A reduction of the shunt fraction, normally to less than 15%, is the goal when applying PEEP in patients with ARDS.[108] When using this variable to adjust PEEP and the shunt fraction is reduced to less than 15%, levels of PEEP in excess of 25 cm H_2O are usually required.[109] This aspect of using PEEP in the pediatric population is generally prohibited in patients with a cuffless endotracheal tube because of the leakage around the tube.

Not only can PEEP be applied as a ventilating variable, but it also can be present in the form of auto-PEEP (intrinsic, occult, or inadvertent PEEP).[114,115] Auto-PEEP is the difference between alveolar pressure and external airway pressure at end expiration.[26] Causes include impedance to exhalation related to airway resistance, expiratory muscle activity, imposed resistance caused by endotracheal tubes and exhalation valves, water obstructing the exhalation circuit, rapid breathing frequency, and inverse I/E ratio.[16] Auto-PEEP has the same clinical effects as therapeutically applied PEEP. The two possible goals to managing auto-PEEP are either (1) to minimize it or (2) to use it as a ventilation variable in manipulating $\overline{Paw}$. In either case, recognizing and monitoring auto-PEEP are clinically important. The use of PEEP in obstructive lung disease, such as asthma, is controversial, with some investigators reporting improved gas exchange and decreased airway resistance, whereas others found increased air trapping and hemodynamic compromise.[116,117] More recent research has shown that higher set PEEP levels can be helpful in decreasing the work of breathing in mechanically ventilated, spontaneously breathing pediatric patients with obstructive airway disease.[118] In theory, external PEEP holds the airways open and allows better exhalation, thus reducing the auto-PEEP and making it easier for patients to trigger ventilator breaths. Multiple variables affect ventilation and oxygenation. It must be understood that manipulating a ventilator setting with the objective of improving one condition may result in undesirable effects on another.[16] Balancing these variables allows the clinician to meet the goals of mechanical ventilation, as well as to optimize oxygen delivery, recruit lung volume, improve gas distribution, and alter minute ventilation.

High-Frequency Ventilation

Although from a mechanistic perspective gas exchange remains complex, the clinical management of oxygenation is more straightforward than LFV. Excluding adjustments of FiO_2, oxygenation is improved during LFV and HFV by recruiting or maintaining lung volume. In fact, there is a direct and linear relationship between lung volume and oxygenation (Figure 17-17). The exception to this occurs when the lung is either under- or overinflated. In each circumstance the relationship between ventilation and perfusion is disturbed and oxygenation is impaired. Achieving an optimal MLV, then, optimizes ventilation–perfusion matching while avoiding impaired cardiac output. As discussed earlier, adjusting several LFV settings, such as tidal volume, peak pressure, inspiratory time, and end-expiratory pressure, accomplishes this. The resulting $\overline{Paw}$ is an indirect expression of the pressure effort required to achieve and sustain the desired MLV. Phasic pressures delivered with LFV during attempts to recruit lung volumes can damage the fragile, yet noncompliant, infant airways and lung parenchyma. Sometime this is referred to as tidal recruitment. Thus conventional tidal volume breathing applied to lungs with nonuniform compliances, as in the premature surfactant-deficient lung, results in nonhomogeneous gas distribution, with overinflation of compliant areas and underinflation of oncompliant regions. During spontaneous or conventional mechanical breathing, the lung swings past the MLV and mean $\overline{Paw}$ during the cycles of inspiration and expiration, residing at the MLV (and $\overline{Paw}$) for only brief periods. With normal lung mechanics, a stable FRC is maintained and oxygenation is

not impaired. In the lung prone to atelectasis, however, residual lung volumes are dynamic. Although volume may seem adequate at peak inflation, stable lung volumes may not exist and oxygenation will be significantly impaired (even in the presence of positive end-expiratory pressures).[119,120]

The methods used to create and maintain $\overline{Paw}$ (or CDP during HFOV) therefore have a profound effect on the consequences of reaching the MLV. Conventional methods require the use of relatively high peak pressures to recruit collapsed noncompliant pulmonary units. The potential negative impact has already been described. The approach taken during HFV strategies, in contrast, is the application of a CDP without the use of high phasic pressures. In fact, direct control over CDP ($\overline{Paw}$) is possible, with ventilation occurring around a relatively fixed intrapulmonary pressure and, therefore, relatively stable MLV. The danger of this technique, as mentioned earlier, is lung overdistention and resultant decreases in venous return and cardiac output. This can occur without changes in ventilation pressures during LFV and HFOV when lung volume is silently recruited as compliance improves.

The optimal MLV, during high-volume strategies, is reached when distending pressure exceeds alveolar opening pressures, and, as a result, the arterial-to-alveolar oxygen tension ratio [$P(a–A)O_2$] is maximized. This measure of oxygenation is useful because it normalizes measured arterial partial pressure of oxygen (PaO_2) for delivered FiO_2.[121] Perfect oxygenation, unobtainable in nature, yields a ratio of 1:1. The safe application of pressures adequate to achieve a stable MLV during management of the uninjured, atelectasis-prone lung is the goal of mechanical ventilation. Data from both animal and human infant studies suggest that improved oxygenation, with acceptable ventilation, does occur safely with HFV techniques while using distending pressures that are initially higher than in LFV controls.[12,90,91] Attempts to achieve improved oxygenation using mean pressures lower than those used in LFV, although attractive in theory, have not proved fruitful except in short-term studies and in patients with pulmonary interstitial emphysema in whom low-volume strategies are desired and intentional. Experiments performed by McCulloch and coworkers,[122] using the surfactant-deficient rabbit model, elegantly demonstrated the relationship between lung inflation strategy and resultant lung volume and gas exchange. In this work, animals with similar pressure–volume relationships after lavage were managed for a 7-hour study period with conventional mechanical ventilation, HFOV with a low lung volume strategy, or HFOV with a high lung volume strategy. Figure 17-18 graphically demonstrates the impact of these approaches on lung volumes. Note the significantly higher volumes obtained in the animals receiving HFOV and a high lung volume at an equivalent $\overline{Paw}$. As anticipated, this group also had a fivefold higher PaO_2 and less evidence of significant bronchiolar epithelial injury.[122]

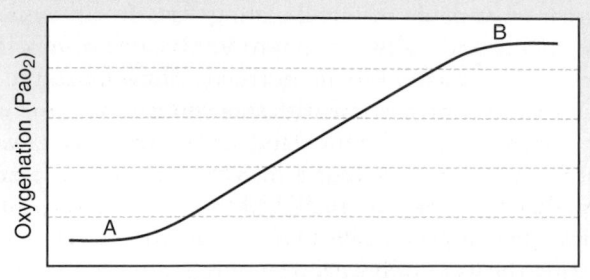

FIGURE 17-17 Relationship between mean lung volume and oxygenation (by inference, between $\overline{Paw}$ or CDP and MLV). **A,** Unopened lung. **B,** Overinflated lung.

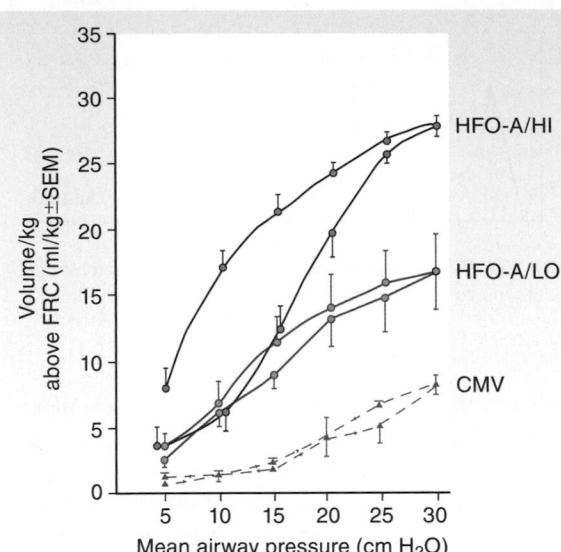

FIGURE 17-18 Respiratory system pressure–volume curves obtained after 7 hours of ventilation in surfactant-depleted rabbits. Note the intergroup differences in total respiratory system compliance and lung volumes. The differences in hysteresis (inflation–deflation limb separation) are also significant between groups. *CMV,* Conventional mechanical ventilation; *FRC,* functional residual capacity; *HFO-A,* high-frequency oscillatory ventilation with an active expiratory phase; *HFO-A/HI,* HFO-A at a high lung volume; *HFO-A/LO,* HFO-A at a low lung volume.

Figure 17-18 also illustrates that an equivalent $\overline{\text{Paw}}$ does not imply equivalent lung volumes. As patient compliance changes, so does the $\overline{\text{Paw}}$ required to maintain optimal MLV. Obviously, a direct measure of MLV or compliance during HFV would be extremely useful; however, neither is currently available for routine bedside use. Clinical measures to properly wean patients and avoid inadvertent overdistention are discussed later in this chapter.

Positive End-Expiratory Pressure

Like peak pressure, the attempt to apply a conventional setting to an HFV technique can lead to confusion. One can easily measure trough pressures during HFV, but the meaning and value are unclear. With LFV, we relate oxygenation to levels of end-expiratory pressure because this setting contributes so significantly to $\overline{\text{Paw}}$. With HFJV this remains true because end-expiratory pressure is set by adding it from the LFV. During HFOV, however, it is set directly, and true end-expiratory pressure (or trough pressure) is meaningless. In fact, to avoid confusion some authors suggest that CDP (rather than $\overline{\text{Paw}}$) be used to describe the constant pressure delivered during HFOV.

Mean Airway Pressure or Continual Distending Pressure

Mean airway pressure or CDP controls MLV. During LFV, this setting is the consequence of a combination of ventilator settings, and although it is a true mathematical average of pulmonary pressures, the lung maintains this

pressure (and hence volume) for only brief periods. During HFV, especially HFOV, this pressure is directly controlled by the combination of bias flow and expiratory valve aperture. In this circumstance, the HFV static pressure (or CDP) truly creates a static lung volume, the magnitude of which depends on lung compliance. All the devices described provide a display of $\overline{\text{Paw}}$. During HFJV and HFPV, control over this parameter is achieved by changing the settings of the tandem or built-in LFV. It cannot be overstated that as lung volume increases, so does compliance. In fact, at the very lung volume where oxygenation is optimized, compliance is as well. The importance of this concept is that ventilation is influenced if lung volume is too high, or too low, during HFV. Thus $\overline{\text{Paw}}$ facilitates oxygenation *and* permits optimal ventilation (see Figure 17-17). Therefore using $\overline{\text{Paw}}$ to maintain the correct lung volume is doubly critical.

Flow

The use of flow to control ventilator settings is variable among the devices described. During HFJV, jet pulses are delivered by means of a timing circuit with minimal control of flow. Pressures, and therefore volumes, are determined by variations of jet on-time and frequency. HFPV incorporates multiple solenoid technology to determine rate of pressure rise and end-expiratory pressures during LFV, which has little impact on HFV functions. HFOV CDP is determined by the combination of circuit bias flow and the back pressure created by the expiratory valve opening. Even though desired CDP may be achieved with complete valve closure, care should be taken to avoid this because rapid rebreathing followed by circuit (and patient) overpressurization will occur.

Inspiratory Time

Inspiratory time adjustments result in alterations in ventilator rate, I/E ratio, and tidal volume, all of which are significant to differing degrees for each type of HFV. Inspiratory time during HFJV is adjusted by changing jet on-time. Depending on ventilator frequency, this alters the I/E ratio and influences tidal volume output. Jet on-times of 20 to 34 msec are common. With HFOV, inspiratory time varies with ventilator rate but the I/E ratio is singularly meaningful. The recommendation is a 33% inspiratory time for the HFOV devices approved in the United States. The result is that for each completed respiratory cycle, one third is inspiratory and two thirds is expiratory. The importance of this lies in the enhancement of gas egress during exhalation because the 1:2 ratio favors the expiratory phase, thereby reducing inadvertent air trapping or breath stacking. This becomes a more significant factor as ventilator frequencies increase. Increases in inspiratory time at any given rate will increase tidal volume, but there is an obligatory reduction in I/E ratio that may offset any desirable effects. Changes in ventilator rate are made with changes in expiratory time, and the I/E ratio varies with frequency.

In comparison with the other ventilators, adjustments in tidal volume cannot be made by increasing inspiratory time, and I/E ratios will vary with frequency.

PATIENT-VENTILATOR INTERFACE

Understanding the ventilator circuit is an integral aspect of ventilator management. The *circuit* is the interface between the ventilator and the patient system.[123] There are five major factors to consider when assessing the impact of the circuit on ventilation:

· Compressible volume
· Air leak
· Dead space
· Resistance
· Humidification

Compressible Volume

The influence of compressible volume on effective tidal volume during volume ventilation was discussed earlier (see Adaptive Ventilation). Ventilator circuit compression influences tidal volume during pressure ventilation as well.[66] When the ventilator delivers a breath, pressure inside the circuit increases and compresses the gas volume delivered. This compressed volume never reaches the patient, and the inspired volume is less than the set volume. During expiration, however, the compressed volume passes through the exhalation valve and is measured as part of the patient's exhaled volume. This results in the patient's actual inflation volumes being less than that recorded as exhaled volume. If the actual volume delivered to the lungs of critically ill infants and young children is not accurately known, the patient may be at risk for atelectasis, hypoxia, and hypercapnia.[124] A circuit compliance or compression factor can be calculated, as illustrated in Box 17-2. Thus some clinicians describe this as volume "lost" in the tubing. The compressible volume of disposable tubing is generally greater than that of reusable tubing.[125] The humidifier also represents a source for gas compression and is included in calculating compressible volume. Using a constant-level self-feeding humidifier is necessary to minimize variations in compressible volume in all pediatric ventilation situations. When tidal volumes are measured with a proximal flow sensor placed at the endotracheal tube, ventilator circuit compliance and the confounding circuit variables are no longer pertinent factors.[124]

Air Leak

In the pediatric clinical setting, it is important not to confuse compressible volume losses with air leaks. Air leaks are most notable around a cuffless endotracheal or tracheostomy tube. Accurately monitoring tidal volume is difficult in the presence of an air leak. An excessive air leak compromises tidal volume delivery, reduces

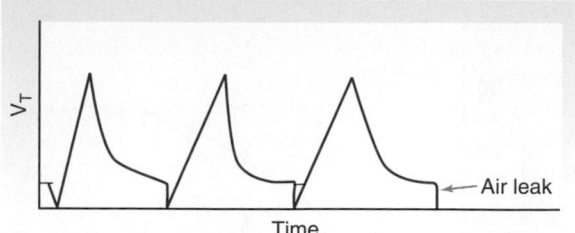

FIGURE 17-19   Air leak shown on a volume/time scalar. Volume never returns to baseline before ventilator cycles again. V_T, Tidal volume.

lung-distending pressures, and may adversely affect the ventilator triggering mechanism. In general, air leaks are monitored by the difference between the tidal volume delivered by the ventilator to the patient and the patient's exhaled tidal volume.[66] Another way to identify an air leak is via flow graphics. Figure 17-19 illustrates an air leak on a volume–time scale. In most clinical situations, an air leak greater than 15% of the delivered tidal volume makes volume ventilation difficult. Even though the leak still occurs during constant pressure ventilation, switching to a higher flow rate and pressure setting may deliver a satisfactory tidal volume. Usually reintubation is necessary to maintain consistent volume ventilation and adequate triggering of the ventilator.

Dead Space and Resistance

Dead space is the portion of the circuit distal to the main bias flow or circuit where gas can be rebreathed. This includes the volume of the circuit wye connector, elbow, any monitoring device attached to the endotracheal tube connector, the endotracheal tube, and the conducting airways. The conducting airways are known as *anatomical dead space* and are not influenced by the circuit. However, the dead space added to the circuit is *mechanical dead space*. With smaller pediatric volumes, mechanical dead space may result in undesired rebreathing of carbon dioxide. Specially designed pediatric or infant monitoring devices and circuits help minimize this. Overzealous application of low dead space monitoring devices may result in increased resistance at the airway if the proper size is not used. Another component to evaluate as a choke point for gas flow is the adaptor connecting the tubing to the elbow or the endotracheal tube. A rule of thumb is that the endotracheal tube should be the point of highest circuit resistance. If a circuit component is smaller in cross-sectional area than the endotracheal tube, another circuit or component should be used.[126]

HIGH-FREQUENCY CIRCUIT CONSIDERATIONS

To achieve adequate gas exchange for both oxygenation and ventilation, high-frequency ventilators have unique design requirements. With the exception of MFV, all HFV devices have special patient circuit considerations. Each of them must do the following:

· Use very low circuit compliance to reduce compressible volume and increase precision of control over the small volumes delivered
· Have intrinsic timing mechanisms to allow breathing frequencies between 4 and 28 Hz (varying by device)
· Provide control over inspiratory times and circuit design to allow sufficient time for gas egress during exhalation
· Adequately humidify gases
· Include alarms and fail-safe devices for patient safety

As a consequence of these considerations, circuit configurations cannot be altered without careful investigation because function and safety are extremely sensitive to small changes in engineering. Please see manufacturer's manual and clinical user website for more details specific to the HFV you may be using.

HUMIDIFICATION

The humidification system is an integral part of the patient-ventilator system. When the normal heating and humidification systems of the body are bypassed or are inadequate, it is necessary to artificially heat and humidify the inhaled gases. Optimal humidity and temperature are dependent on the clinical situation. Usually a temperature of 37° C and a water content of 44 mg/L are adequate.[127] Servocontrolled, heated humidifiers that possess a small compressible volume are used most often in neonatal and pediatric patients who require mechanical ventilation.

Complications associated with these humidifiers include overheating and nosocomial infection. Water condensation in the ventilator circuit may also lead to nosocomial infection as well as to the accidental drainage of water into the patient's lungs. With the use of a servocontrolled heated wire circuit, complications are not as common as they once were. However, awareness of the operational characteristics of the humidifier and its controlling mechanisms is important in the ventilator management.

CARE OF THE PATIENT

Positioning

As mentioned earlier, patient positioning is constrained with the use of invasive ventilation. The unique nature of the patient circuit challenges caregivers to ensure ETT stability. Positioning the patient appropriately by rotating among supine, prone, and left and right lateral decubitus positions remains as important during mechanical ventilation. Protocols describing approaches to positioning have been described.[128]

Patient positioning is believed to play a role in reducing ventilator-associated complications (VAC). For example, semi-recumbent body positioning in adult intensive care unit (ICU) patients was associated with a reduction of common risk factors for VAC, such as gastroesophageal reflux and subsequent aspiration.[129] In addition, semi-recumbent positioning (30 to 45 degrees) was associated with a decrease in VAC cases. However, the evidence on this topic is mixed. In 2006, van Nieuwenhoven et al. found no significant difference in the incidence of VAC related to elevation of the head (specifically 28 degrees vs. 10 degrees).[130] Further, lateral rotation therapy was tested and demonstrated a 12% reduction in the incidence of VAC.[131]

Although evidence on head of bed (HOB) elevation in pediatric patients is very limited, HOB elevation between 30 to 45 degrees for intubated infants and children is encouraged. In neonates, a similar effect may be achieved by positioning the incubator or radiant warmer mattresses in the reverse Trendelenburg position at an angle of 15 to 30 degrees (rather than 30 to 45 degrees) because the greater angle is difficult to maintain in very small patients.[132] To facilitate head-of-bed elevation in pediatric patients, beds and cribs with adequate positioning features should be used. Furthermore, the degree of elevation should be measured using validated instruments or bed markings and documented. Because patient positioning is thought to play an important role in VAC prevention and can be achieved with little to no negative implications, unless contraindications exist, elevating the HOB as outlined in Table 17-4 is recommended.

Endotracheal Tube

Nasal intubation is associated with an increase in sinusitis, a concern for adolescent and older patients who have fully developed sinuses. Sinusitis is associated with increased VAP rates.[133] Therefore the oral route is the preferred intubation site.[133] Aspiration of oropharyngeal or gastric secretions contaminated with potentially pathogenic organisms can occur around the ETT. Colonization of the ETT with bacteria encased in biofilm may result in embolization into the alveoli during suctioning. To minimize this risk, patients who are expected to have a lengthy duration of mechanical ventilation may benefit from placement of subglottic suction endotracheal tubes.[134] These specialty tubes, however, are not currently available in all sizes. The use of subglottic suctioning with available ETT sizes (currently 6.0 and higher) when the ventilator course is anticipated to be greater than 48 hours is recommended.

In adults, ETT cuff inflation pressure greater than 20 cm H_2O has been shown to protect the lower airway

TABLE 17-4	
Patient Positioning	
Age of Patient	Position of Bed
Neonate (<44 weeks GA)	15-30 degrees
Pediatric (≥44 weeks GA)	30-45 degrees

GA, gestational age.

from drainage of upper airway secretions. However, a European multicenter randomized trial comparing uncuffed ETTs to the Microcuff (cuffed ETT) demonstrated that the Microcuff ETT could safely seal the airway at an average cuff pressure of 10 cm H_2O and certainly 20 cm H_2O or less without a higher incidence of postextubation stridor.[135] Maintaining a cuff pressure of 5 to 15 cm H_2O will obtain a proper seal with Microcuff ETT and 15 to 25 cm H_2O with traditional cuffed ETT is recommended. On admission and before extubation, the cuff should be lowered to assess for the presence of a leak. If there is no leak, the provider should be notified. If pressures are greater than 15 cm H_2O for the Microcuff ETT or greater than 25 cm H_2O for the non-Microcuff ETT, the provider should be notified. The use of cuffed ETT in neonates less than 40 weeks gestation age is not recommended because smaller cuffed tubes are not currently available (currently 3.0 or higher). The smallest cuffed ETT would translate into a 3.5 uncuffed ETT with current sizing recommendation cuffed versus uncuffed ETT.

Suctioning

Suctioning techniques vary among institutions. One technique consists of quickly disconnecting the patient from the HFV circuit, performing suctioning, and reapplying HFV without bagging between disconnections. Because suctioning can reduce lung volume by the sudden drop in airway pressure at disconnection and by the negative pressures applied during the procedure, lung derecruitment can occur. For some patients, this requires a temporary increase in $\overline{Paw}$ to regain baseline oxygenation. Closed tracheal suction systems with connections appropriate for the ventilator circuit used may be used.

Ventilator Circuit

Changing of ventilator circuits need only occur when visibly soiled or malfunctioning.[136] Condensate should be removed routinely, taking care to drain away from the patient to avoid contaminating any inline nebulizers. When performing ventilator care, proper hand hygiene should be performed before and after each intervention and gloves should be worn.[136]

Airway Maintenance

The mere presence of an ETT impairs the cough reflex and may increase mucus production. The *suctioning smarter* philosophy consists of suctioning only when a clinical indication arises, not on a scheduled basis.[137] Standards for tracheal suctioning should address catheter size, length of time suction is applied, suction pressure, deep versus shallow techniques, open versus closed techniques, saline instillation, lung pathology, and ventilatory mode.

Suctioning

Suctioning should only be considered when secretions are present *or* clinical assessment is consistent with inspissations of secretions. In preparation for suctioning, selection of an appropriate catheter size is important. It is recommended that the hypopharynx is suctioned before ETT suctioning. Some patients may require limited preoxygenation. In the neonatal population, limiting preoxygenation to 10% to 20% above baseline F_{IO_2} is recommended.[137]

Suction Equipment
Open vs. Closed System Suctioning

Research supports the use of closed system suctioning. Use of closed system suctioning is associated with increased catheter size and suction pressure, which contribute to additional lung volume loss. In contrast, the use of open system suctioning resulted in volume loss independent of catheter size.[138] The potential benefits of using closed system suctioning include continued delivery of oxygen, supportive positive pressure, reduced risk of nosocomial infection, and reduced staff exposure.

Inline suction catheters have been shown to be just as effective without breaking the ventilator circuit while allowing quicker resumption of ventilation and F_{IO_2}. Currently, inline suction manufacturers recommend a 1- to 3-day change frequency. When compared with weekly suction catheter changes, there was no difference in the development of VAP using the 1- to 3-day change frequency. Further, the increased change frequency may increase the cost of care.[139] Therefore it is recommended that inline suction catheters are changed weekly and when malfunctioning or visibly soiled.

To prevent volume loss, health care providers should limit overall procedure time, not just actual suction time. A study of 200 neonates, weighing less than 1000 g, revealed twice the recovery time with the use of open suctioning versus closed suctioning.[140] In a smaller pediatric-based study, results were similar, supporting the benefit of using closed suctioning. In neonates receiving high-frequency oscillatory ventilation, open versus closed suctioning techniques produced essentially equal decreases in saturation and heart rate. Recovery time, however, from these decreases was significantly longer in the open suction group. Not surprisingly, open suctioning produced a greater lung volume loss.[138]

COMPLICATIONS OF MECHANICAL VENTILATION

Each of the physiological effects of mechanical ventilation has an associated risk. Box 17-4 lists the complications associated with mechanical ventilation.[16]

Volutrauma/Atelectrauma/Barotrauma

Alveolar overdistention is a primary cause of complications encountered during mechanical ventilation and is a result of high ventilating pressures (**barotrauma**), large tidal volumes (volutrauma), and repetitive opening and

Box 17-4	Complications of Mechanical Ventilation

- Barotrauma
- Volutrauma
- Atelectrauma
- Biotrauma
- Pulmonary interstitial emphysema
- Subcutaneous emphysema
- Pneumothorax
- Pneumomediastinum
- Pneumopericardium
- Pneumoperitoneum
- Bronchopulmonary dysplasia
- Nosocomial infection
  - Acute respiratory distress syndrome
  - Pneumonia
- Patient–ventilator asynchrony
  - Auto-PEEP
  - Hyperventilation
  - Respiratory alkalosis
  - Increased work of breathing
- Noncardiopulmonary complications
  - Psychological distress
  - Renal dysfunction
  - Fluid retention
- Gastrointestinal dysfunction
  - Vomiting
  - Ulceration and bleeding
  - Increased intracranial pressure
- Interventricular hemorrhage
- Periventricular leukomalacia
- Airway complications
  - Sinusitis
  - Vocal cord injury
  - Inadvertent extubation
  - Retention of secretions
  - Glottic injury
  - Glottic edema
  - Glottic stenosis
  - Glottic erosion
- Tracheal injury
- Tracheal erosion
- Tracheomalacia
- Tracheal dilation
- Tracheal-innominate artery fistula
- Airway obstruction
  - Mainstem intubation
  - Kinking of endotracheal tube
- Plugging of endotracheal tracheostomy tube
- Cardiovascular compromise
  - Decreased venous return
  - Decreased cardiac output
- Oxygen toxicity
- Retinopathy of prematurity
- Positive end-expiratory pressure (PEEP)

closing of the terminal lung units at low lung volumes (atelectrauma). Extrapulmonary air leaks, in the form of pneumothorax, pneumomediastinum, pneumoperitoneum, and subcutaneous emphysema, are the most notable complications and are the result of overdistention of alveolar and peribronchial tissues.[141] Treatment consists of detecting the leak, decreasing tidal volume, and decreasing the PEEP, relieving the leak with a chest tube if necessary. Permissive hypercapnia could also be a useful tool in the treatment of an air leak.[142] Rescue modes such as high-frequency jet ventilation, high-frequency oscillatory ventilation, and extracorporeal membrane oxygenation are implemented for excessive air leakage that is not responding during LFV.

Overdistention also causes a decrease in static compliance, an increase in the work of breathing, an increase in anatomical dead space, an increase in the air leak around the endotracheal tube, and possible difficulties in weaning. As compliance diminishes, the $PaCO_2$ may rise or fail to improve. To counter this, ventilation is increased, which may lead to further distention.

Because volumes are smaller in the neonatal and pediatric patient than in the adult, avoiding and detecting overdistention are critical aspects of ventilator management. Alarms that may help detect this are indirect and can be activated by other problems. These alarms may include

high $\overline{Paw}$; exhaled minute ventilation and tidal volumes, which is useful during SIMV and other spontaneous modes; high peak pressure; high PEEP; high respiratory frequency; and inverse I/E ratio. Measures such as using an end-expiratory pause to look for incomplete exhalation and an increase in PEEP or to detect auto-PEEP, measuring optimal static compliance, inspecting pressure–volume loops to determine overdistention or exhaled resistance, monitoring changes in $\overline{Paw}$, and obtaining a chest radiograph all help to detect overdistention.

The formation of a bronchopleural fistula presents an especially challenging clinical situation. Because the volume of gas delivered by the ventilator will follow the path of least resistance, a substantial part of the tidal volume will move into the pleural space during inspiration and escape through the chest tube. This volume is seen as the air bubbles through the water seal chamber of the chest tube drainage system, and the amount may be determined by noting the difference between the inspiratory and expiratory volumes. Although most bronchopleural fistulas are insignificant, if the leak is large enough it may result in inadequate ventilation and lead to ventilation–perfusion mismatch and further hypoxemia. Conventional treatment consisting of low pressures and volumes allowing permissive hypercapnia and allowing the patient to breathe spontaneously as much as possible may aid in decreasing flow through the fistula and facilitate its closure. When this is not possible in patients with severe ventilation problems, nonconventional modes of treatment may be needed. Independent lung ventilation or high-frequency ventilation may be considered, as may the use of valves to occlude the chest tube during inspiration.[143,144]

Cardiovascular Complications

Reduced cardiac output from cardiac septal deviation, increased pulmonary vascular resistance, reduced venous return, and reduced myocardial blood flow is a complication of mechanical ventilation. In most cases, it is a result of increased intrathoracic pressures. In the neonatal and pediatric patient it can usually be prevented by increasing the circulating fluid volume.[109,145] Vasopressor drugs may also be used to maintain cardiac output during ventilation regimens that include high distending volumes.[102] An increase in intrathoracic pressure may be applied in some clinical situations to reduce left-to-right shunting, raise pulmonary vascular resistance, and impede pulmonary blood flow. See Chapter 24 for more details.

Oxygen Toxicity

Oxygen toxicity is another concern during mechanical ventilation. High FIO_2 levels that have been applied for an extended period may result in tissue injury that alters lung function and gas distribution.[101] High FIO_2 levels have also been associated with an increase in chronic lung disease and retinopathy of prematurity among low-birth-weight infants.[146] Incorporating a high FIO_2 alarm and minimizing the FIO_2 to the level necessary to attain adequate tissue oxygenation, as well as using pulse oximetry and blood gas monitoring, are essential in attempting to prevent tissue damage. Most use an FIO_2 algorithm to help them determine the need to make mechanical ventilation interventions.

Hypoventilation/Hyperventilation

The primary cause of hypoventilation during mechanical ventilation is disconnection from the ventilator and accidental extubation.[147,148] Care must be used when moving the patient connected to a ventilator, especially during transport and patient care procedures such as chest physiotherapy. A low-pressure or disconnect alarm is essential to alert the clinician when this occurs. Hypoventilation may also result from high impedance to inflation, which can be due to high resistance (resulting from anatomical, pathological, or circuit design) or loss of pulmonary compliance.[149] A low-volume monitor will detect these changes. Underventilation can be avoided by calculating effective tidal volume or airway monitoring of ventilation variables, routinely monitoring or calculating compliance and resistance, monitoring pressure–volume and flow–volume loops, and using sufficient driving or working pressures to minimize attenuation of

the inflating flow waveform. An AP chest radiograph also may be helpful in detecting underaeration.

Hypoventilation may also be related to "operator error" in establishing ventilation. Hypoventilation caused by minute ventilation, frequency, volume, or flow rate that is insufficient to meet inspiratory demand results in increased work of breathing and muscle fatigue. These conditions may also be present when weaning from the ventilator and may cause weaning failure. The alert patient may communicate feelings of respiratory distress. Retractions, use of accessory muscles, head bobbing, and a 10% to 20% increase in heart rate and spontaneous respiratory frequency are clinical signs of insufficient ventilation. In a sedated, paralyzed, or critically ill patient, however, this problem may not be as evident. Using pressure–volume and flow–volume loops, monitoring carbon dioxide production and oxygen consumption, and obtaining other measurements such as a diaphragm electromyogram may help detect this problem. Ensuring that the initial inspiratory flow rate meets the patient's inspiratory demand is usually the best method of avoidance.[150,151] An example of a pressure–volume loop demonstrating insufficient flow caused by insufficient driving pressure during PSV is shown in Figure 17-20. Figure 17-21 shows the effect of a faulty flow transducer on a diaphragm electromyogram tracing during PSV, leading to increased work of breathing.

Hyperventilation can also be a problem if the patient's lung compliance improves (i.e., through surfactant administration or prone/supine positioning) in a pressure control or pressure support mode. Autocycling of the ventilator as a result of endotracheal tube leak, secretions in the circuit

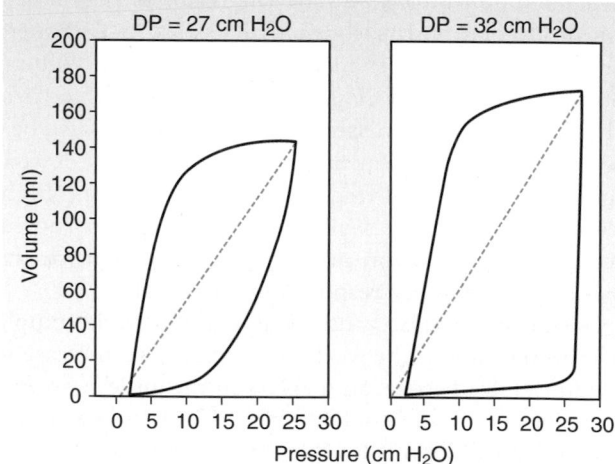

FIGURE 17-20 An example of a pressure–volume loop demonstrating insufficient flow caused by setting the driving pressure (DP) too low during pressure-support ventilation of a child. With DP set at 27 cm H_2O, the peak pressure (*top right-hand corner of the loop*) is reached at the end of inflation. With the DP set at 32 cm H_2O, the peak pressure is reached early during inflation (*lower right-hand corner of the loop*). Note the perpendicular right side of the loop.

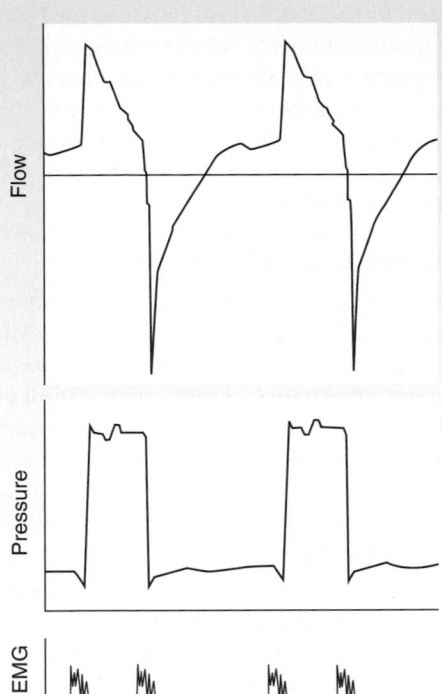

FIGURE 17-21 A recording of the electromyographic (EMG) signal shows muscle activity to initiate inflation during pressure-support ventilation. The flow transducer on this ventilator is defective, and the electromyogram shows abnormal muscle activity, not seen by clinical observation, at the end of inflation to stop the breath. Transdiaphragmatic pressure measurements would also help detect this situation.

or flow sensor, and inappropriate sensitivity setting can lead to hyperventilation. Hyperventilation and low carbon dioxide in low-birth-weight infants can result in cerebral vasoconstriction, which can cause a cystic brain lesion called periventricular leukomalacia.[152] Close monitoring of transcutaneous carbon dioxide levels, sensitivity, tidal volume, and minute ventilation with alarms has proved to be useful in reducing this problem.

MONITORING DURING LOW-FREQUENCY MECHANICAL VENTILATION

Monitoring effective ventilation is accomplished by using the techniques discussed previously. Box 17-5 lists monitoring applications as they apply to pediatric mechanical ventilation. Most ventilators monitor airway pressures, flow, ventilatory frequency, tidal volume, and minute volume. Essential aspects of monitoring include the following:

- Calculation of effective tidal volume or ensuring a properly calibrated ventilator
- Close observation of the patient for clinical signs of adequate ventilation as well as respiratory distress, such as chest expansion and retractions
- Noninvasive methods of determining oxygenation and ventilation status, such as pulse oximetry, transcutaneous monitoring, and end-tidal carbon dioxide monitoring
- Direct measurement of blood gas values

Figure 17-22 demonstrates possible problems detected with an end-tidal carbon dioxide monitor.[115,153]

Esophageal Pressure Monitoring

Some ventilators have the ability to monitor esophageal pressure. Esophageal pressure monitoring uses an air-filled, balloon-tipped catheter placed in the midsection of the esophagus, where pleural pressure measurements can be closely estimated. Esophageal pressure measurements can be extremely helpful in understanding the physiology of the respiratory system during mechanical ventilation.[154] It is essential that proper placement of the balloon catheter be confirmed in order to accurately measure esophageal pressure. These pressure measurements can be displayed

---

| **Box 17-5** | **Monitoring Applications in Neonatal and Pediatric Mechanical Ventilation** |

MEASURED VENTILATOR VARIABLES
- Effective tidal volume (calculated — LFV only)
- Minute ventilation (calculated – LFV only)
- Mean airway pressure ($\overline{Paw}$) (Directly measured — All)
- Low–high positive end-expiratory pressure (PEEP) (Directly Measured — LFV, HFPV, and HFJV only)
- High peak pressure (Directly measured — LFV, HFPV, and HFJV only)
- Fraction of inspired oxygen (FiO_2) (Directly measured — All)
- Pause pressure (Directly measured — LFV only)
- Inspiratory-to-expiratory ratio (Directly measured — all)
- Pressure waveform (Directly measured and displayed — LFV and HFPV only)
- Flow waveform (Directly measured and displayed — LFV only)
- Static compliance (Calculated — LFV only)
- Dynamic compliance (Calculated — LFV only)
- Airway resistance (Calculated — LFV only)
- Maximal inspiratory occlusion pressure (Measured — LFV only)

- Maximal expiratory occlusion pressure (Measured — LFV only)
- Maximal minute ventilation (Measured — LFV only)
- Vital capacity (Measured — LFV only)
- Oscillatory/amplitude/jet peak inspiratory pressure (Measured — HFV only)

SUPPLEMENTAL MONITORS
- Pulse oximetry
- End-tidal carbon dioxide with or without volumetric
- End-tidal carbon dioxide to $PaCO_2$ gradient
- Transcutaneous carbon dioxide
- Pressure–volume loop
- Esophageal pressure
- Transpulmonary pressure
- Dead space-to–tidal volume ratio
- Ineffective-to-effective tidal volume ratio
- Work of breathing
- Pressure–time product
- Pressure–time index

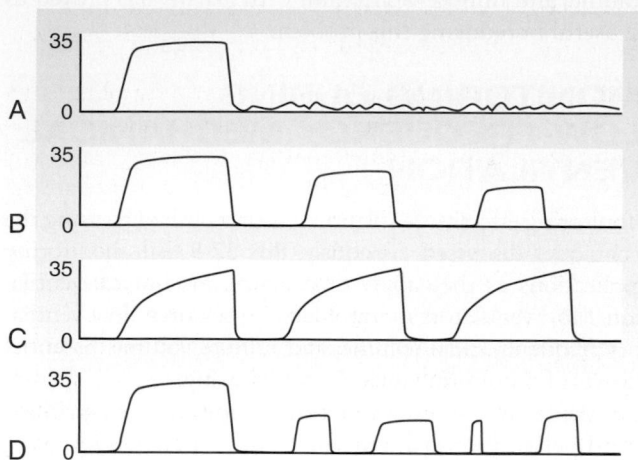

FIGURE 17-22 End-tidal carbon dioxide recordings. **A,** Abrupt disconnection from the ventilator. **B,** Falling partial pressure of end-tidal carbon dioxide (PETCO₂), possibly from an increase in tidal volume or, if PaCO₂ is unchanged, a reduction in pulmonary blood flow from overdistention or low cardiac output. **C,** Dampened waveform from severe air flow obstruction or side stream sampling tube obstruction. **D,** System leak or secretions in the sampling chamber.

graphically or incorporated into a number of pulmonary mechanics calculations. Calculations that require esophageal pressure include chest wall compliance, lung compliance, transpulmonary pressure, work of breathing, change in esophageal pressure, and auto-PEEP. In adults with ARDS, management of ventilation and PEEP by transpulmonary pressures has been shown to be superior to the ARDSNET protocol.[155]

Evaluation of the esophageal pressure waveform can be compared graphically with other ventilator graphics and provides important clinical information regarding interactions between the patient and the ventilator. Esophageal balloon technology can also guide the clinician during difficult weaning from mechanical ventilation without increased patient intolerance.[156]

Estimating Lung Volumes

At present, the ability to determine whether ventilator breaths are delivered at, below, or above their ideal functional residual capacity is deduced from surrogate measurements, including lung appearance on the chest radiograph, vital sign trends (particularly oxygenation), and dynamic pressure–volume (P-V) curves generated by modern ventilators.

Automated Slow Flow Rate Pressure–Volume Curves

Pressure–volume curves can provide important information about the compliance of the respiratory system when supporting mechanically ventilated patients with restrictive lung diseases. Ventilators have incorporated automated slow-flow or "quasi-static" P-V curves that use a slow inspiratory flow rate delivered during a single breath. This method reduces the pressure increase caused by the resistive elements (endotracheal tube, high flow rates) and more closely approximates the alveolar pressure.

The slope of the line is measured to determine compliance of the respiratory system (line C, Figure 17-23). These technologies also provide algorithms that measure the upper and lower inflection points of a nonlinear respiratory system compliance curve. These points represent areas on the P–V

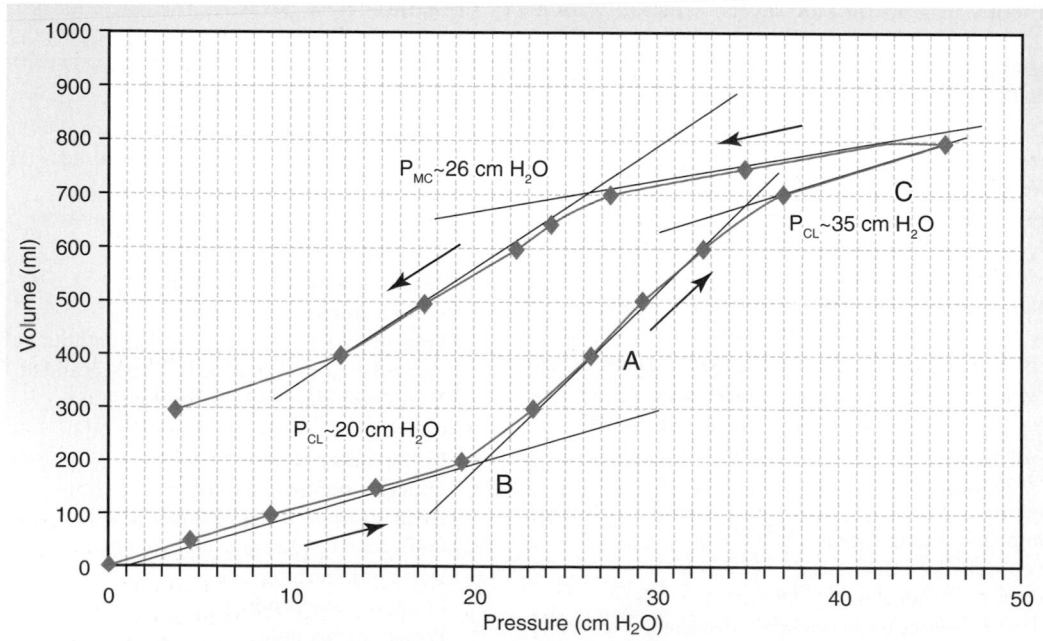

FIGURE 17-23 Pressure–volume curve as determined by the super-syringe method.

loop during lung inflation and deflation, where there is a substantial decrease in compliance. Figure 17-23 shows three lines that comprise the inflation limb (lower curve) of a static P–V curve. Line B represents an area of low compliance related to the opening of atelectatic lung units early during inflation of the lung. The point at which the slope of the line changes (where line A intersects line B) reflects an area where there is an acute improvement in compliance; this is known as the *lower inflection point*. Mechanical ventilator practices that adopt an "open lung approach" set PEEP to a pressure just above the lower inflection point. In theory, as long as the PEEP is set above the lower inflection point on the inflation or deflation limb, then oxygenation improves by resolving atelectasis and increasing the functional residual capacity. Lung injury can also be reduced because the patient is ventilated above the closing pressure of the lung and thus repetitive cycling of the lung at low volumes decreases atelectrauma. Figure 17-23 also distinguishes a second point where compliance decreases (where line A intersects line C); this is known as the *upper inflection point*. This point represents overdistension of the respiratory system. Ventilator pressures and/or tidal volume settings can be set below this point to avoid lung overdistension or volutrauma.

Nitrogen Multiple Breath Washout Technique

Nitrogen multiple breath washout technique has been used in a number of clinical studies and is considered to be the "gold standard" in the measurement of lung volume.[157-160] At present, the most accurate way to measure the volume of the lung is through dilution of a known amount of a gas with low solubility by rebreathing in a closed system. The changes in concentration with sequential breaths allow calculation of the volume of distribution of the gas. One gas that has been used for this purpose is nitrogen,[161] appealing because of its ubiquitous presence in the environment. Measurement of nitrogen gas concentrations, however, is available only by gas chromatography or mass spectrometry, neither of which is clinically practical. A technique has been validated by which the partial pressure of nitrogen is calculated as the residual of partial pressures of oxygen gas, carbon dioxide gas, and nitrogen gas, which together comprise the only three important gases in a ventilator circuit. The former two gases are readily measured in a ventilator circuit in real time but of course vary widely with the metabolic state of the patient. Olegård and coworkers have developed the nitrogen multiple breath washout technique to calculate FRC on the basis of changes in exhaled oxygen and carbon dioxide, manipulating inspired oxygen concentration to alter fraction of inspired nitrogen.[162] Measurement of FRC by this methodology in a lung model of known oxygen consumption and lung volumes[162] revealed excellent precision (mean FRC, 103% ± 5%) even when using incremental changes in FiO_2 from 0.9 to 1.0. Measurement in adult patients with respiratory insufficiency also revealed excellent precision.

MONITORING DURING HIGH-FREQUENCY VENTILATION

As during CV, the frequency of blood gas sampling is related to the patient's clinical status. Blood gas measurements should be obtained frequently during the early course of ventilatory management and in patients in extremis (e.g., every 1 to 4 hours). Intervals between samples should be increased as clinical conditions improve. For trending purposes, pulse oximetry and transcutaneous Po_2 and Pco_2 monitoring should be used. Because of rapid changes in $PaCO_2$ noted especially during initial HFV management, transcutaneous monitoring is strongly recommended. There is no alteration in performance of these noninvasive gas exchange methods for patients receiving HFV.[163]

WEANING FROM MECHANICAL VENTILATION

Low Frequency
Initiation

Weaning is the gradual process by which mechanical ventilation is discontinued and the patient resumes spontaneous breathing. The process may be rapid or slow, depending on the individual clinical situation. It is difficult to define at exactly what point during mechanical ventilation the weaning process should begin; however, most would agree that ideally it is after significant resolution or reversal of the pathological condition for which it was initiated. Before weaning begins, the patient's condition should be stable and the patient should be receiving adequate nourishment and be able to breathe spontaneously and maintain a clinically acceptable $PaCO_2$. The ventilator should be on acceptable settings: usually PEEP less than 8 cm H_2O; peak pressure less than 30 cm H_2O; ventilator rate less than 20 breaths per minute for a neonate, 15 breaths per minute for an infant/toddler, and 10 breaths per minute for a child or adolescent; and FiO_2 less than 0.4 to 0.5.[26,149,153,164,165]

Various methods exist for measuring respiratory muscle endurance and predicting successful weaning. Simple observations such as accessory or paradoxical muscle activity, respiratory rate, tidal volume, and minute ventilation are the first indicators of weaning readiness.[166,167] An increase in respiratory frequency of 15% to 20% or a reduction in tidal volume is associated with impending fatigue. Maintaining normal or clinically acceptable $PaCO_2$ with normal minute ventilation (0.5 to 1 L/min for an infant to 4 to 9 L/min for an adult) would indicate that the patient might tolerate weaning. Normal carbon dioxide production in an infant is 6 ml/kg/min, and it is 3 ml/kg/min in an adult.[168] Excessive carbon dioxide production indicates a hypermetabolic state and may be corrected by adjusting nutritional elements to lower the respiratory quotient. Another helpful determinant of the ability to wean is the V_D/V_T ratio. The normal value is 0.3; however, intubation and mechanical ventilation may alter this. A value of less than 0.6 to 0.7 may predict successful weaning. Another clinically measurable variable that roughly approximates the V_D/V_T ratio is the ineffective-to-effective tidal volume ratio. Abnormal values may indicate continued pulmonary or cardiac dysfunction. Measurement of the end-tidal carbon dioxide to $Paco_2$ gradient may also help detect continued pulmonary or cardiac dysfunction. In this case, cautious weaning may be indicated, although resolution of the clinical condition is most likely indicated.[164]

Other predicting factors may also be considered. A flow–volume loop may help discover impedance to inspiratory or expiratory flow that will precipitate fatigue. A pressure–volume loop may help determine work of breathing and evaluate various weaning modes. Measurements of dynamic and static compliance, resistance, transpulmonary pressure tracing, work of breathing, respiratory time fraction, the pressure time product (PTP), and the pressure time index (PTI) are useful variables in monitoring the course of weaning. The PTP reflects the metabolic work of the respiratory system and is an electronically integrated value derived from tidal volume, compliance, esophageal pressure, and duration of the breath.[169] The PTI combines the PTP and the respiratory time fraction and correlates directly with muscle fatigue and oxygen consumption.[170] Spontaneous maximal inspiratory and expiratory occlusion pressures may also be of value. These measurements are routine weaning values in many adult units, along with maximal spontaneous minute ventilation and vital capacity measurements. Unlike these measurements, however, occlusion pressure measurements do not require that a patient understand the breathing techniques necessary to effectively determine the values.

Concepts of Weaning

The basic weaning techniques used in neonates and pediatric patients include CPAP, SIMV, and PSV. Using CPAP during weaning is common among pediatric patients. The positive airway pressure is used to provide the physiological PEEP, which is bypassed when the patient is intubated.[171] Two techniques for using CPAP are practiced. The first is applied when there is sufficient respiratory drive and endurance but the physiological effects of PEEP are still required. In this case, the CPAP is gradually reduced during the weaning process. The second technique is a postoperative weaning technique. The usefulness of this technique in pediatrics may be limited, however, because of the high resistance of the small-diameter airways. It may occasionally be employed to build respiratory muscle endurance by using a bias flow during short-duration exercises alternating with long periods of complete rest. The exercise periods are slowly increased as the resting periods are decreased. The process continues until the patient can breathe without support for a specified time. This technique is typically used only when the goal is to wean the patient to intermittent periods off the ventilator,

such as with certain neuromuscular diseases or quadriplegia or in preparation for phrenic nerve pacing.

SIMV involves a gradual decrease in the ventilator frequency, usually in increments of 2 to 5 breaths per minute. As the ventilator rate is reduced, the patient is required to contribute more spontaneous efforts to the overall ventilation frequency. How quickly the SIMV rate is decreased depends on assessment of the patient's clinical status and blood gas values. The more slowly the process is performed, the more time the patient has to acclimate to less ventilator support. Factors such as ventilator system resistance, a sluggish demand valve, an inappropriately sized endotracheal tube, or insufficient inspiratory flow may affect the success of weaning with SIMV. Weaning with SIMV is generally uncomplicated and is usually successful in older patients with endotracheal tube sizes large enough to minimize excessive inspiratory resistance. When weaning patients with smaller tube sizes, the goal is to wean to a rate of 20 breaths per minute for an endotracheal tube less than 3.5 mm (internal diameter), 15 breaths per minute for endotracheal tube sizes of 4.0 to 5.0 mm, and 10 breaths per minute for anything greater than a 5.0-mm tube, and then extubate. When using continuous flow, a common practice is to set a standard flow rate on all ventilators in the neonatal patient population. Figure 17-24 shows the relationship of continuous flow to resistance. The smaller the diameter of the endotracheal tube, the more likely that changes in flow rate influence exhaled resistance. Using a rate less than those just stated is thought to contribute to fatigue and unsuccessful weaning because of endotracheal resistance.

Weaning with PSV provides sufficient positive pressure to minimize the metabolic requirements for ventilation during weaning.[26,61,164,167] In addition, PSV allows the patient to initiate the breath, preventing atrophy of the inspiratory muscles. Figure 17-25 illustrates a pressure–volume loop and other respiratory variables used to evaluate the

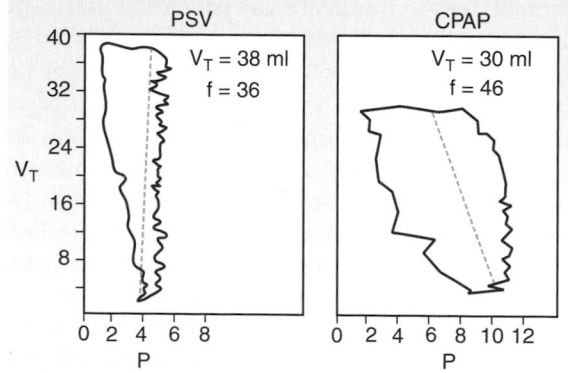

FIGURE 17-24 Pressure–volume loops of an infant during weaning, demonstrating the effectiveness of using 5 cm H_2O of PEEP and 1 cm H_2O of pressure-support ventilation instead of using 10 cm H_2O of continuous positive airway pressure (CPAP). *f,* Frequency (breaths/min); *P,* pressure; *PSV,* pressure-support ventilation; V_T, tidal volume.

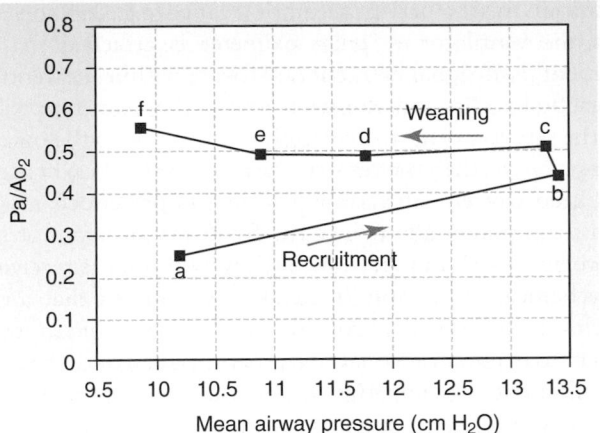

FIGURE 17-25 Mean arterial-to-alveolar oxygen tension ratio [P(a–a)O$_2$] and $\overline{\text{Paw}}$ of 21 premature infants managed with HFOV immediately after surfactant replacement. Note that increasing $\overline{\text{Paw}}$ initially results in increased P(a–a)O$_2$ (alveolar recruitment); subsequent $\overline{\text{Paw}}$ weaning does not reduce oxygenation but is associated with gradual improvement in P(a–a)O$_2$. The line between points b and c represents silent lung recruitment as assessed by improving P(a–a)O$_2$ $\overline{\text{Paw}}$ with essentially stable. (*a*) Surfactant replacement; (*b*) 12 hours later; (*c*) 12 to 24 hours later; (*d*) 24 to 48 hours later; (*e*) 48 to 72 hours later; and (*f*) 72 to 96 hours later.

effect of PSV and CPAP on an infant who is proving difficult to wean. Once weaning is indicated and PSV is selected, the pressure support level should be adjusted to deliver a tidal volume of 3 to 4 ml/kg. Frequency should be monitored and the driving pressure adjusted to attain an appropriate flow rate. Once satisfactory volume, flow, and frequency are set, the pressure support level can be reduced in increments of 2 to 5 cm H$_2$O. While at a higher pressure level, the patient contributes only the muscle work required to trigger the inflation. As the pressure is reduced, the patient progressively shares more of the work of breathing.[142] The pressure support should be weaned at a rate that is reasonable for each clinical situation. Endotracheal or tracheostomy tube leaks can hinder this progress. The patient who has been mechanically ventilated for only a short time, such as the stable postoperative patient, can be weaned at a rapid pace. The patient who has undergone long-term mechanical ventilation requires patience and persistence in reducing the support level by only 1 or 2 cm H$_2$O over a longer period, such as a day or even a week. In these patients, weaning can be slowed by clinical events such as a viral illness or fluid and electrolyte imbalance. Once these clinical conditions are resolved, usually weaning can be continued with a successful outcome.[26]

High Frequency

Initiation

At this stage of HFV development, weaning remains a challenge. Weaning ventilation is for the most part simple. Minute ventilation can be weaned by reducing oscillatory amplitude during HFOV and by decreasing peak pressure

and on-time with HFJV. Changes in ventilation rarely have an impact on oxygenation because lung volume is preserved. Conversely, weaning $\overline{\text{Paw}}$ with improving compliance and increasing lung inflation is less straightforward. Radiographic assessment of lung volume and F$_{IO_2}$ may provide empirical information guiding management sufficiency. The well-inflated lung requires a reduction in mean pressure to avoid the negative consequences of excessive lung volumes. However, too rapid a reduction in distending pressures can cause alveolar derecruitment in the unstable lung, and reinflation will be necessary. In general, $\overline{\text{Paw}}$ should be reduced slowly (1 to 2 cm H$_2$O) every 2 to 3 hours as long as there are no signs of overdistention (suggesting much more rapid decreases are necessary) or alveolar derecruitment (decrements in oxygenation). By taking advantage of lung hysteresis, gradual reductions in mean pressure generally do not cause significant changes in oxygenation or, by inference, lung volume (see Figure 17-25). Simple and reproducible bedside measures of lung volume are on the horizon. The application of these techniques to weaning may be useful in the future.

Radiographic assessment of lung volume takes considerable practice. The novice is cautioned that although, in general, lung volume can be assessed by counting the number of posterior ribs seen above the diaphragm, radiographs of neonates are usually anterior-to-posterior views and counting ribs requires the juxtaposition of an anterior structure (the diaphragm) against a posterior structure (the rib interfacing with the diaphragm). This method assesses a three-dimensional object (the lung) with a two-dimensional picture (the radiograph) and is vulnerable to technician-selected focus angles. It is possible, then, to underestimate or overestimate inflation.

The present inability to routinely measure lung volume or compliance at the bedside and the ease with which acceptable oxygenation is achieved with relatively high $\overline{\text{Paw}}$ can confuse the clinician about the speed with which weaning should occur. Experience seems to be the best teacher in this situation. The consequences of failing to wean the patient quickly enough are significant pulmonary overdistention and impairment of cardiac output. In neonates, this complication can increase the risk of intracranial hemorrhage because venous return from vessels draining the head is impeded and venous hypertension and vessel rupture can ensue. Conversely, rapid weaning of $\overline{\text{Paw}}$ can result in alveolar derecruitment requiring reinitiation of lung recruitment procedures.

TROUBLESHOOTING

The approach to troubleshooting does not differ from that of LFV or HFV. Either deterioration of the patient's vital signs or a ventilator alarm may alert the clinician. In either circumstance, it is necessary to ensure that the patient is in no further jeopardy before proceeding with a detailed troubleshooting procedure. High-frequency ventilators are dependent on patient airway caliber for adequate volume delivery. A change in airway diameter (e.g., by accumulation of secretions or by migration of the tip of the ETT against the tracheal wall) may significantly reduce delivered volumes. The first step should be a quick assessment of chest wall movement. If chest wall motion is substantially decreased, a brief use of manual ventilation while troubleshooting the airway and ventilator may dramatically improve the situation. Steps should be taken to correct any problems with the ETT lumen or position (i.e., suctioning, chest radiograph).

Like LFV, there are conditions in which HFV techniques are not uniformly successful. HFV seems especially vulnerable to the state of myocardial performance. In patients with poor cardiac output (e.g., decreased intravascular volume or reduced contractility), lung inflation with high $\overline{Paw}$ can result in abrupt and serious cardiac output impairment. Ensuring the adequacy of cardiac output before initiating HFV can mitigate this. Low-volume strategies will have less impact on cardiac output. For this reason, HFJV is successful during cardiac surgery and in circumstances in which lung compliance is normal and cardiac output is reduced.[22,23]

Because a relatively high MLV is necessary for HFOV, this technique is not optimal for use in normal lungs. Furthermore, in conditions in which airway resistance is increased, such as fresh particulate meconium aspiration, bronchopulmonary dysplasia, and reactive airway disease, HFOV may not be optimal. Because of the tremendous impedance to flow created by reductions in airway lumen with these disorders (thus increasing pulmonary time constants), decreases in delivered tidal volume or gas trapping, or both, cause derangement in gas exchange. In contrast, HFJV or HFPV using larger tidal volumes and lower breathing frequencies may be more efficacious in conditions in which airway time constants are pathologically prolonged. These impressions are based on theoretical considerations and anecdotal experiences. Extensive controlled data supporting these contentions are not currently available.

Each ventilator manufacturer has developed detailed approaches to troubleshooting the mechanical problems of its own device, and these recommendations should be followed, tempered by actual clinical experience. A regular preventive maintenance program will help reduce mechanical failures.

ADVANCING CONCEPTS

Low-Frequency Ventilation

Advances and improvements in technologies and practices such as high-frequency ventilation, nitric oxide, corticosteroids, prone positioning, permissive hypercapnia, extracorporeal membrane oxygenation, and surfactant replacement all influence future design and approaches to conventionally ventilating the neonate and pediatric patient.

Automated regulation of the inspired oxygen (closed-loop FIO_2) is a novel concept that is likely to be on the horizon for use in the near future. This feature requires the

clinician to set a patient saturation range (e.g., 85% to 92%) on the ventilator. A pulse oximeter is attached to the patient, and signal extraction software within the ventilator obtains these measurements from the oximeter probe. If the saturation measurement increases above or below the target range, then the ventilator will adjust the FIO_2 in order to keep oxygen saturations within the prescribed range. This can potentially reduce the frequency of hypo- or hyperoxic episodes in very low birth weight infants receiving mechanical ventilation. It has been speculated that long-term closed-loop FIO_2 control may reduce clinician time spent to maintain adequate oxygenation and reduce the risks of morbidity (retinopathy of prematurity and bronchopulmonary dysplasia) associated with supplemental oxygen and frequent episodes of hypoxemia and hyperoxemia.[170]

Ventilators are increasingly becoming "partial support" in that they must work dynamically with the patient. Proportional assist ventilation is an innovative new mode of ventilation that is currently being investigated for neonatal and pediatric mechanical ventilation. This mode uses an algorithm that varies pressure support or pressure control levels on the basis of patient effort and changes in patient elastic and resistive loads during inhalation and exhalation. Preliminary work suggests that this mode may result in improvements in patient synchrony, oxygenation index, and overall cardiovascular stability. New-generation ventilator companies are incorporating many modes, triggers, and graphics to help the clinician pick and choose what is best for an individual patient's needs. This fosters a dynamic relationship between the ventilator and patient. Negative-pressure ventilation is also finding its way back into the critical care setting. Cardiopulmonary interactions are being investigated in children after simple cardiac surgery.[172]

Electrical impedance tomography (EIT) capitalizes on changes in impedence in air-filled versus tissue-filled spaces to characterize and quantify regional distribution of lung volumes at the bedside. Significant work has been done to validate this technology in animals[173] and in humans.[174,175] This monitoring system uses a series of 16 electrodes placed across the patient's chest (Figure 17-26). Through complex algorithms, the impedance signal is

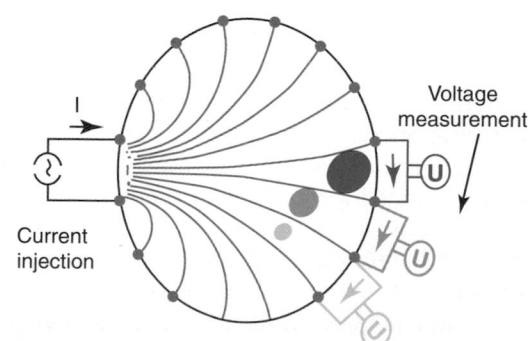

FIGURE 17-26 Electrical impedance tomographic images are created with a series of electrodes placed across the chest, each of which sends and receives electrical impulses from one another.

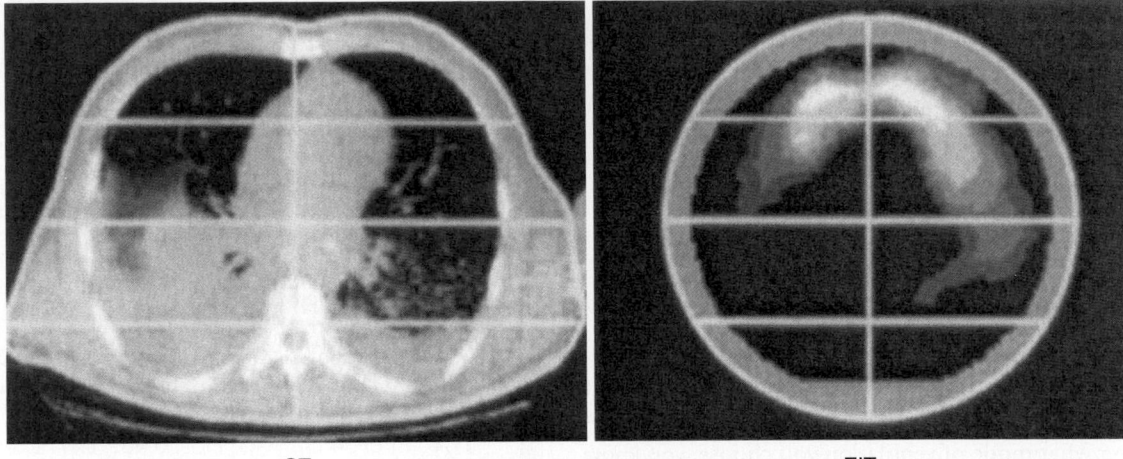

CT   EIT

FIGURE 17-27   Computed tomography (CT) and electrical impedance tomography (EIT) images in a patient with acute lung injury. Note that the EIT image provides functional and anatomical information regarding the presence of ventilated lung fields.

extracted and integrated to show a two-dimensional image (Figure 17-27). This has been shown to correlate with clinical and radiographic changes in patients.[174] In 10 mechanically ventilated adults with ARDS, end-expiratory lung volume as determined by nitrogen washout correlated well with end-expiratory lung impedance.[174] The ability to estimate lung volume noninvasively and in real time may aid in mechanical ventilator techniques designed to improve outcomes in patients with lung injury. Wolf and colleagues published the finding of their EIT-guided ventilation in an acute lung injury animal model.[176] This guided ventilation technique shows promise and will be studied further in humans.

There is a growing body of evidence regarding exhaled breath condensate changes in airway lining fluid (ALF) pH in acute and chronic respiratory diseases that are characterized, at least in part, by inflammation. It has been demonstrated that the pH of ALF is low (acidic) in multiple pulmonary inflammatory diseases, including asthma,[177] cystic fibrosis,[178] pneumonia, and ARDS.[179-181] This pH measurement can be detected continuously, safely, and noninvasively in exhaled breath condensate (EBC).[182] The pH of EBC may be a safe, noninvasive screening tool for progression of ARDS and of lung recruitment. It has been shown to predict respiratory failure and impending respiratory infection.[117] Figure 17-28, a histogram of a patient with severe asthma, demonstrates an acidic EBC pH that improves as the patient's exacerbation subsides. A continuous exhaled breath condensate pH collection and assay system (ALFA monitor; Respiratory Research, Austin, TX) consists of a condenser attached to the expiratory limb of the ventilator. Exhaled breath condensate is collected continuously from the expiratory port and condensed in a cooling chamber, and carbon dioxide is removed and collected in an inferior chamber where pH is continuously read. This yields a continuous, responsive measure from

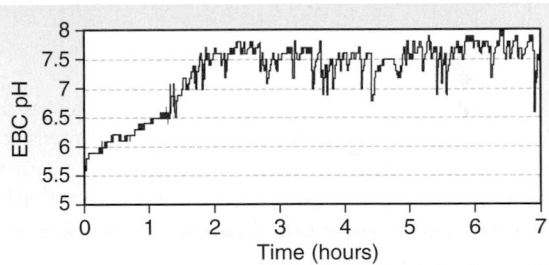

FIGURE 17-28   Sample tracing of exhaled breath condensate (EBC) pH over time in an intubated 14-year-old child with asthma. Note the responsiveness of EBC pH to the patient's improving condition.

ventilated patients, which (1) takes samples from an exhaust port on the outside of the ventilator circuit and (2) adds no measurable resistance to the ventilator circuit. The measurement of EBC in patients with lung injury may serve as an early marker of lung health.

High-Frequency Ventilation

The learning curve for these techniques continues to progress. Clinicians using HFV early in patients with respiratory distress syndrome believe that hospital courses are reduced and significant pulmonary morbidity is decreased.[12,90,183,184] The impact of HFJV on patients with PIE has been clearly demonstrated.[88] The precise role of HFV with respect to long-term outcome and cost of care continues to be defined. The availability of exogenous surfactant replacement, newer modes of CV for primary management, and ECMO and inhalational nitric oxide for patients with intractable respiratory failure continue to affect HFV use.[18,184-187] Ongoing investigations into the field of liquid ventilation, particularly partial liquid ventilation, are likely to stimulate new applications and enhance patient outcomes.

KEY POINTS

- The mechanical ventilator is a lifesaving piece of equipment and should be maintained as if your life depended on it. Remember that ventilators require calibration, preventative maintenance, and proper cleaning to ensure the best respiratory support.
- An ounce of prevention is worth a pound of a cure. Mechanical ventilation should only be provided for as long as it is needed. All steps should be taken by the respiratory care practitioner to minimize ventilator-associated lung injury or adverse events.
- No one mode of ventilation has been shown to be superior to another. It is vitally important that no matter what mode of ventilation you choose, you know all the management strategies associated with good outcomes.
- The HFV choice of strategy (high or low lung volumes) is lung disease specific. Although simplistic, it is reasonable to try to inflate an underinflated lung and deflate an overinflated or air-trapped one.
- Auto-PEEP is the difference between alveolar pressure and external airway pressure at end expiration.
- Simply stated, the goal of PEEP therapy is to improve oxygenation by increasing FRC through maintenance of airway patency and alveolar recruitment.
- Lowering the HFV frequency may improve ventilation.

ASSESSMENT QUESTIONS

See Evolve Resources for answers.

Low-Frequency Ventilation

1. Which of the following issues would most likely explain why a newborn infant's measured respiratory rate would rise from 40 to 100 breaths/minute on a ventilator after the patient was turned and an audible endotracheal tube leak was heard?
   A. Pneumothorax
   B. Auto-cycling
   C. Secretions
   D. Bradypnea

2. A 10-year-old child is intubated and receiving mechanical ventilation. The tidal volume is set at 280 ml, the peak airway pressure is 38 cm H_2O, the plateau pressure is 20 cm H_2O, and the PEEP is 5 cm H_2O. The tubing compliance factor is 1.5 ml/cm H_2O. What is the actual delivered V_T to this patient if the ventilator did not compensate for compressible volume loss?
   A. 255 ml
   B. 157 ml
   C. 230 ml
   D. 330 ml

3. A term infant is being invasively ventilated in pressure-targeted SIMV mode of ventilation, set rate is 16, PIP pressure is 18, PEEP 4, inspiratory time is 0.4, and FIO_2 is .30, and the physician would like to wean the infant from the ventilator. The clinician has tried turning the patient's set rate on SIMV down to 10 breaths/minute, but the infant immediately becomes tachypneic and desaturates to 85%. Which of the following should be done at this time?
   A. Increase the PEEP
   B. Initiate pressure support ventilation
   C. Increase the inspiratory time
   D. Extubate to nasal CPAP

4. A 600-g neonate is being mechanically ventilated in pressure control ventilation with the following ventilator settings: peak inspiratory pressure (PIP), 24 cm H_2O; PEEP, 4 cm H_2O; FIO_2, 0.45; respiratory rate, 40 breaths/minute. Which inspiratory time should the clinician recommend?
   A. 0.6 second
   B. 0.3 second
   C. 0.8 second
   D. 1.0 second

5. The physician would like to begin dual-control ventilation of a 500-g infant. What would be the initial corrected volume target?
   A. 5 ml/kg
   B. 7 ml/kg
   C. 8 ml/kg
   D. 10 ml/kg

6. While observing a ventilator flow graphic for a 12-year-old patient with asthma on a rate of 10 breaths per minute, the clinician notices that expiratory flow does not return to baseline and the patient's auto-PEEP level is 6 cm H_2O. Which ventilator manipulation might help this patient the most?
   A. Increase the respiratory rate by 8 breaths/minute
   B. Decrease the inspiratory time
   C. Decrease the peak inspiratory flow
   D. Increase the PEEP

7. A neonatal patient with respiratory syncytial virus (RSV) is receiving mechanical ventilation in the pressure control mode with the following current settings: PIP, 14 cm H_2O; PEEP, 5 cm H_2O; FIO_2, 0.50; respiratory rate, 28 breaths/minute. The patient has poor chest rise bilaterally, and breath sounds are underaerated with faint wheezes bilaterally. You notice that the measured tidal volume is 3 ml/kg and the respiratory rate is 80 breaths/minute. The patient has nasal flaring, retractions, and head bobbing. What should be suggested at this time?
   A. Placing the patient on a high-frequency oscillator
   B. Suctioning and then increasing the PIP
   C. Decreasing the respiratory rate
   D. Using a neuromuscular blocking agent

8. Which ventilator approach would be good for a 10-year-old boy with severe ARDS who is spontaneously breathing while undergoing ventilation?
   A. PCV
   B. APRV
   C. CPAP
   D. IRV

9. Which of the following factors does not affect mean airway pressure?
   A. PEEP
   B. I-time
   C. Time constant
   D. PIP

High-Frequency Ventilation

10. High-frequency ventilation is defined by the U.S. FDA as delivering more than:
    A. 150 breaths/minute
    B. 120 breaths/minute
    C. 100 breaths/minute
    D. 60 breaths/minute

11. High-frequency jet ventilation delivers gas by:
    A. Intermittently occluding a high flow of gas with a rotating vane
    B. Pulsing gas down the endotracheal tube at a high velocity
    C. Passing gas past the endotracheal tube and agitating it with a piston
    D. The same method as conventional ventilation, just at a higher frequency

12. High-frequency oscillatory ventilation delivers gas by:
    A. The same method as conventional ventilation, just at a higher frequency
    B. Pulsing gas down the endotracheal tube at a high velocity
    C. Alternating gas in and out via a rotating vane
    D. Passing gas past the endotracheal tube and agitating it with a piston.

13. The exhalation phase of HFOV differs from other forms of high-frequency ventilation because:
    A. Exhaled gas is actively pulled out via the patient as the piston moves back.
    B. Exhalation is passive, whereas on the HFJV gas is pulled out via a Venturi effect.
    C. Exhalation is active during HFOV due to a separate vacuum assist device.
    D. Exhaled gases passively exit the patient due to passive chest recoil.

14. Which of the following most accurately describe(s) the relationship of lung volume in a restrictive disease and $\overline{Paw}$:
    I. Increasing $\overline{Paw}$ increases lung volume and improves ventilation–perfusion matching.
    II. Increasing $\overline{Paw}$ increases the pressure gradient, allowing more oxygen to cross the alveolar capillary membrane.
    III. Increasing $\overline{Paw}$ improves the efficiency of the jet or piston.
    IV. At very high and very low lung volumes ventilation–perfusion matching is impaired.
    A. I
    B. II
    C. I, III, IV
    D. I and IV

15. The goal in treating atelectatic prone lung is:
    A. High lung volume to recruit alveolar lung units
    B. Low lung volumes to reduce the chance of barotrauma
    C. High tidal volumes during convention ventilation to assist in carbon dioxide removal
    D. High lung volume to recruit the lung and large tidal volumes to aid ventilation

16. The goal in treating infants with pulmonary interstitial emphysema or active air leak is:
    A. High lung volume to recruit alveolar lung units
    B. Low lung volume to reduce the chance of creating or worsening an air leak
    C. High lung volume to recruit the lung and large tidal volumes to aid ventilation
    D. Low tidal volumes combined with high lung volumes

17. A neonate is progressing satisfactorily on HFOV, with a mean airway pressure of 15 cm H_2O. The physician consults the respiratory clinician to determine in what increments the $\overline{Paw}$ should be weaned. What should the respiratory therapist recommend?
    A. 4–6 cm H_2O
    B. 3–4 cm H_2O
    C. 1–2 cm H_2O
    D. No increment; simply extubate

18. A clinician prepares to suction a patient undergoing HFV. What is the most likely consequence of suctioning?
    A. Hypoxia, requiring a temporary increase in $\overline{Paw}$ to resolve
    B. Pulmonary hemorrhage, requiring ETT epinephrine
    C. Negative-pressure pulmonary edema, requiring a temporary increase in $\overline{Paw}$ to resolve
    D. None of the above

19. An infant has just been placed on HFJV. What trending monitor(s) should be recommended?
    A. In-line blood gas analyzer
    B. Pulse oximetry
    C. Transcutaneous monitoring
    D. B and C

References

1. Mellins R, et al: *Respiratory care in infants and children*, New York, 1971, American Lung Association.
2. Bancalari E, Goldberg RN: High-frequency ventilation in the neonate, *Clin Perinatol* 14:581, 1987.
3. Froese AB, Bryan AC: High frequency ventilation, *Am Rev Respir Dis* 135:1363, 1987.
4. Gerstmann DR, deLemos RA: High-frequency ventilation: issues of strategy, *Clin Perinatol* 18:563, 1991.
5. Clark RH, Gerstmann DR: Controversies in high- frequency ventilation, *Clin Perinatol* 25:113, 1998.
6. Nash G, Blennerhassett JB, Pontoppidan H: Pulmonary lesions associated with oxygen therapy and artificial ventilation, *N Engl J Med* 276:368, 1967.

7. Northway WH, Rosan RC, Porter DY: Pulmonary disease following respirator therapy of hyaline membrane, *N Engl J Med* 276:357, 1967.

8. American Thoracic Society, European Society of Intensive Care Medicine, Societé de Réanimation de Langue Française: International Consensus Conferences in Intensive Care Medicine: ventilator-associated lung injury in ARDS, *Am J Respir Crit Care Med* 160:2118, 1999.

9. Acute Respiratory Distress Syndrome Network: Ventilation with lower tidal volumes as compared with traditional tidal volumes for acute lung injury and the acute respiratory distress syndrome, *N Engl J Med* 342:1301, 2000.

10. Taghizadeh, E.O.R. Reynolds: Pathogenesis of bronchopulmonary dysplasia following hyaline membrane disease, *Am J Pathol* 82:241, 1976.

11. HiFi Study Group: High-frequency oscillatory ventilation compared with conventional mechanical ventilation in the treatment of respiratory failure in preterm infants, *N Engl J Med* 320:88, 1989.

12. Clark RH, Null DM, Gerstmann DR, et al: Prospective randomized comparison of high-frequency oscillatory and conventional ventilation in respiratory distress syndrome, *Pediatrics* 89:5, 1992.

13. Meredith KS, Delemos RA, Coalson JJ, et al: Role of lung injury in the pathogenesis of hyaline membrane disease in premature baboons, *J Appl Physiol* 66:2150, 1989.

14. Jobe AH: Too many unvalidated new therapies to prevent chronic lung disease in preterm infants, *J Pediatr* 132:200, 1998.

15. Clark RH, Slutsky AS, Gertsmann DR: Lung protective strategies of ventilation in the neonate: what are they? *Pediatrics* 105:112, 2000.

16. American College of Chest Physicians: Consensus conference: mechanical ventilation, *Chest* 104:1835, 1993.

17. Gerstmann DR, et al: *Treatment of congenital diaphragmatic hernia with high-frequency oscillatory ventilation. Presented at the Eleventh Conference on High-Frequency Ventilation of Infants,* Snowbird, Utah, April 1994.

18. Bartlett RH, Roloff DW, Cornell RG, et al: Extracorporeal circulatory support in neonatal respiratory failure: a prospective randomized study, *Pediatrics* 76:479, 1985.

19. Carter JM, Gerstmann DR, Clark RH, et al: High-frequency oscillatory ventilation and extracorporeal membrane oxygenation for the treatment of acute neonatal respiratory failure, *Pediatrics* 85:159, 1990.

20. Paranka MS, Clark RH, Yoder BA, Nukk DM Jr: Predictors of failure of high-frequency ventilation in term infants with severe respiratory failure, *Pediatrics* 95:400, 1995.

21. Duval EL, Markhorst DG, Van Vught AJ, et al: High-frequency ventilation in pediatric patients, *Neth J Med* 56:177, 2000.

22. Dekeon MK, Markhorst DG, Van Vught AJ, et al: *High-frequency jet ventilation in post-operative Fontan patients. Presented at the Seventh Conference on High-frequency Ventilation of Infants,* Snowbird, Utah, April 1990.

23. Davis D, et al: *High-frequency jet ventilation: intraoperative application during neonatal cardiac surgery. Presented at the Ninth Conference of High-frequency Ventilation of Infants,* Snowbird, Utah, April 1992.

24. Chatburn R: A new system for understanding mechanical ventilators, *Respir Care* 36:1123, 1991.

25. Branson RD, et al: Altering flow rate during maximum pressure support ventilation: effects on cardiorespiratory function, *Respir Care* 35:1056, 1990.

26. Czervinske MP, et al: Effects of working pressure on respiratory pattern and airway pressure during pressure support ventilation in infants with chronic lung disease, *Respir Care* 33:930, 1988.

27. Bergman NA: Effect of varying respiratory waveforms on distribution of inspired gas during artificial ventilation, *Am Rev Respir Dis* 100:518, 1969.

28. Czervinske MP, Jiao JH, Teague WG: Improved effective to ineffective tidal volume ratio during pressure control ventilation of infant pigs, *Respir Care* 34:1067, 1989.

29. Campbell RS, Davis BR: Pressure-control versus volume-controlled ventilation: does it matter? *Respir Care* 47:416, 2002.

30. Bland RD, Kim MH, Light MJ, et al: High frequency mechanical ventilation in severe hyaline membrane disease, *Crit Care Med* 8:275, 1980.

31. Borg U, Eriksson I, Sjostrand U: High-frequency positive pressure ventilation (HFPPV): a review based upon its use during bronchoscopy and for laryngoscopic and microlaryngeal surgery under general anesthesia, *Anesth Analg* 59:594, 1980.

32. Sjostrand U: High-frequency positive pressure ventilation (HFPPV): a review, *Crit Care Med* 8:345, 1980.

33. Heijman L, Sjostrand U: Treatment of the respiratory distress syndrome: preliminary report, *Opusc Med* 19:235, 1974.

34. Boros SJ, Mammel MC, Coleman JM, et al: Neonatal high-frequency jet ventilation: four years' experience, *Pediatrics* 75:657, 1985.

35. Carlo WA, Chatburn RL, Martin RJ, et al: Decrease in airway pressure during high-frequency jet ventilation in infants with respiratory distress syndrome, *J Pediatr* 104:101, 1984.

36. Lunkenheimer PP, Frank I, Ising H, et al: Intrapulmonaler Gasweschsel unter simulierter Apnoe durch transtrachealen, periodischen intrathorakalen Druckwechsel, *Anaesthesist* 22:232, 1973.

37. Fredberg JJ, Glass GM, Boynton BF, et al: Factors influencing mechanical performance of neonatal high-frequency ventilators, *J Appl Physiol* 62:2485, 1987.

38. Jouvet P, Hubert P, Isabey D, et al: Assessment of high-frequency neonatal ventilator performances, *Intensive Care Med* 23:208, 1997.

39. Hatcher D, Wantanabe H, Ashbury T, et al: Mechanical performances of clinically available, neonatal, high-frequency, oscillatory-type ventilators, *Crit Care Med* 26:1081, 1998.

40. Singh J, Sinha SK, Clark P, et al: Mechanical ventilation of very low birth weight infants: is volume or pressure a better target variable? *J Pediatr* 149:308, 2006.

41. Hakanson DO: Positive pressure ventilation: volume-cycled ventilators. In Goldsmith JP, Karrotkin EH, editors: *Assisted ventilation of the neonate,* Philadelphia, 1981, WB Saunders, pp 161–179.

42. Tobin MJ: Monitoring of pressure, flow, and volume during mechanical ventilation, *Respir Care* 37:1081, 1992.

43. Demers RR, Pratter MR, Irwin RS: Use of the concept of ventilator compliance in the determination of static total compliance, *Respir Care* 26:644, 1981.

44. Branson RD, Johannigman JA: What is the evidence base for the newer ventilation modes? *Respir Care* 49:743, 2004.

45. McCallion N, Davis P, Morley CJ: Volume-targeted versus pressure-limited ventilation in the neonate, *Cochrane Database System Rev* 3:CD003666, 2005.

46. Dawson C, Davies MW: Volume-targeted ventilation and arterial carbon dioxide in neonates, *J Paediatr Child Health* 41:518, 2005.

47. Branson RD, Chatburn RL: Technical description and classification of modes of ventilator operation, *Respir Care* 37:1026, 1992.

48. Greenough A, Greenall F: Patient triggered ventilation in premature neonates, *Arch Dis Child* 63:77, 1988.

49. Greenough A, Dinitriou G, Prendergast M, et al: Synchronized mechanical ventilation for respiratory support in newborn infants, *Cochrane Database Syst Rev* 1:CD000456, 2008.

50. MacDonald K, et al: Effect of patient flow-triggered ventilation pulmonary mechanics in neonates, *Respir Care* 36:1315, 1991.

51. Sassoon CSH: Mechanical ventilator design and function: the trigger variable, *Respir Care* 37:1056, 1992.

52. Chatburn RL: Computer control of mechanical ventilation, *Respir Care* 49:507, 2004.

53. Sinah SK, Donn SM: Volume controlled ventilation. In Goldsmith JP, Karotkin EH, editor: *Assisted ventilation of the neonate*, Philadelphia, 2003, WB Saunders, pp 171–182.

54. American College of Chest Physicians–American Thoracic Society Joint Committee on Pulmonary Nomenclature: Pulmonary terms and symbols, *Chest* 67:583, 1975.

55. Abbey NC, Block AJ, Green D, et al: Measurement of pharyngeal volume by digitized magnetic resonance imaging: effect of nasal continuous positive airway pressure, *Am Rev Respir Dis* 140:717, 1989.

56. Waldhorn RE, Herrick TW, Nguyen MC, et al: Long-term compliance with nasal continuous positive airway pressure therapy of obstructive sleep apnea, *Chest* 97:33, 1990.

57. Katz JA, Marks JD: Inspiratory work with and without continuous positive airway pressure in patients with acute respiratory failure, *Anesthesiology* 63:598, 1985.

58. Chatburn RL: Similarities and differences in the management of acute lung injury in neonates (IRDS) and in adults (ARDS), *Respir Care* 33:539, 1988.

59. Smith RA, et al: Morphometric changes in a dog model of the adult respiratory distress syndrome after early therapy with continuous positive airway pressure, *Respir Care* 32:525, 1987.

60. Kacmarek RM: The role of pressure support ventilation in reducing work of breathing, *Respir Care* 33:99, 1988.

61. MacIntyre NR: Weaning from mechanical ventilatory support: volume-assisting intermittent breaths versus pressure-assisting every breath, *Respir Care* 33:121, 1988.

62. MacIntyre NR: Pressure support ventilation, *Respir Care* 31:189, 1986.

63. Brochard L, Harg A, Lorino H, et al: Inspiratory pressure support prevents diaphragmatic fatigue during weaning from mechanical ventilation, *Am Rev Respir Dis* 139:513, 1989.

64. Brochard L, Rua F, Lorino H, et al: Inspiratory pressure support compensates for the additional work of breathing caused by the endotracheal tube, *Anesthesiology* 75:739, 1991.

65. Forrette TL, et al: Changes in pediatric ventilatory dynamics during mechanical ventilation with PSV, *Respir Care* 35:1128, 1990.

66. Perez-Fontan JJ, Heldt GP, Gregory GG: The effect of a gas leak around the endotracheal tube on the mean tracheal pressure during mechanical ventilation, *Am Rev Respir Dis* 132:339, 1985.

67. Duyndam A, Bol BS, Kroon A, Tibboel D, Ista E: Neurally adjusted ventilatory assist: assessing the comfort and feasibility of use in neonates and children, *Nurs Crit Care* 18(2):86, 2013. doi: 10.1111/j.1478-5153.2012.00541.x

68. Sinderby C, Beck J, Sphija J, et al: Inspiratory muscle unloading by neurally adjusted ventilatory assist during maximal inspiratory efforts in healthy subjects, *Chest* 131:711, 2007.

69. Petter AH, Chiolero RL, Cassina T, Chassot PG, Muller XM, Revelly JP: Automatic "respirator/weaning" with adaptive support ventilation: the effect on duration of endotracheal intubation and patient management, *Anesth Analg* 97:1743, 2003.

70. Laubscher TP, Frutiger A, Fanconi S, Jutzi H, Brunner JX: Automatic selection of tidal volume, respiratory frequency and minute ventilation in intubated ICU patients as start up procedure for closed-loop controlled ventilation, *Int J Clin Monit Comput* 11:19, 1994.

71. Laubscher TP, Heinrichs W, Weiler N, Hartmann G, Brunner JX: An adaptive lung ventilation controller, *IEEE Trans Biomed Eng* 41:51, 1994.

72. Sulzer CF, Chiolero R, Chassot PG, Mueller XM, Revelly JP: Adaptive support ventilation for fast tracheal extubation after cardiac surgery: a randomized controlled study, *Anesthesiology* 95:1339, 2001.

73. NM Habashi NM: Other approaches to open lung ventilation: airway pressure release ventilation, *Crit Care Med* 3:229, 2005.

74. Stock MC, Downs JB: Airway pressure release ventilation: a new approach to ventilatory support during acute lung injury, *Respir Care* 32:517, 1987.

75. Stock MC, Downs JB, Frolicher DA: Airway pressure release ventilation, *Crit Care Med* 15:426, 1987.

76. Bach JR, Alba AS: Management of chronic alveolar hypoventilation by nasal ventilation, *Chest* 97:52, 1990.

77. Fredberg JJ: Augmented diffusion in the airways can support pulmonary gas exchange, *J Appl Physiol* 49:232, 1980.

78. Fredberg JJ, Keefe DH, Glass GM, et al: Alveolar pressure non-homogeneity during small amplitude high-frequency oscillation, *J Appl Physiol* 57:788, 1984.

79. Chatburn RL, McClellan LD: A heat and humidification system for high-frequency jet ventilation, *Respir Care* 27:1386, 1982.

80. Lunkenheimer PP, Frank I, Ising H, et al: Intrapulmonaler Gasweschsel unter simulierter Apnoe durch transtrachealen, periodischen intrathorakalen Druchkwechsel, *Anaesthesist* 22:232, 1973.

81. Reynolds EOR: Pressure waveform and ventilator settings for mechanical ventilation in severe hyaline membrane disease, *Int Anesthesiol Clin* 12:259, 1974.

82. Greenough A, Dinitriou G, Pendergast M, et al: Synchronized mechanical ventilation for respiratory support in newborn infants, *Cochrane Database Syst Rev* 1:CD000456, 2008.

83. Abbey NC, Block AJ, Green D, et al: Measurement of pharyngeal volume by digitized magnetic resonance imaging: effect of nasal continuous positive airway pressure, *Am Rev Respir Dis* 140:717, 1989.

84. Katz JA, Marks JD: Inspiratory work with and without continuous positive airway pressure in patients with acute respiratory failure, *Anesthesiology* 63:598, 1985.

85. Froese AB: *High-frequency ventilation: strategy and device differences. Presented at the Seventh Conference on High-frequency Ventilation of Infants*, Snowbird, Utah, April 1990.

86. Hamm CR, et al: High frequency jet ventilation preceded by lung volume recruitment decreases hyaline membrane formation in surfactant deficient lungs, *Pediatr Res* 27:305A, 1990.

87. Clark RH, Gerstmann DR, Null DM, et al: Pulmonary interstitial emphysema treated by high-frequency oscillatory ventilation, *Crit Care Med* 14:926, 1986.

88. Keszler M, Donn SM, Bucciarelli RL, et al: Multicenter controlled trial comparing high-frequency jet ventilation and conventional mechanical ventilation in newborns with pulmonary interstitial emphysema, *J Pediatr* 119:85, 1991.

89. Keszler M, Modnlou HD, Brudno DS, et al: Multicenter controlled trial of high-frequency jet ventilation in preterm infants with uncomplicated respiratory distress syndrome, *Pediatrics* 100:593, 1997.

90. HiFO Study Group: Randomized study of high-frequency oscillatory ventilation in infants with severe respiratory distress syndrome, *J Pediatr* 122:609, 1993.

91. Kinsella JP, et al: High-frequency ventilation versus intermittent mandatory ventilation: early hemodynamic effects in the premature baboon with hyaline membrane disease, *Pediatr Res* 29:160, 1991.

92. Ogawa Y, Miyasaka K, Kawano T, et al: A multicenter randomized trial of high-frequency oscillatory ventilation as compared with conventional ventilation in preterm infants with respiratory failure, *Early Hum Dev* 32:1, 1993.

93. Clark RH, Dykes FD, Bachman TE, et al: Intraventricular hemorrhage and high-frequency ventilation: a meta-analysis of prospective clinical trials, *Pediatrics* 98:1058, 1996.

94. Clark RH, Gerstmann DR, Null DM, et al: Pulmonary interstitial emphysema treated by high-frequency oscillatory ventilation, *Crit Care Med* 14:926, 1986.

95. Ramsden CA, Reynolds EOR: Ventilator settings for newborn infants, *Arch Dis Child* 62:529, 1987.

96. Boros SJ, Bing DR, Mammel MC, et al: Using conventional ventilators at unconventional rates, *Pediatrics* 74:487, 1984.

97. Kezler M: Volume-targeted ventilation, *Neoreviews* 7(5):250, 2006.

98. Clark RH, Slutsky AS, Gerstmann DR: Lung protective strategies of ventilation in the neonate: what are they? *Pediatrics* 105:112, 2000.

99. Eisner MD, Thompson T, Hudson LD, et al: Acute Respiratory Distress Syndrome Network: Efficacy of low tidal volume ventilation in patients with different clinical risk factors for acute lung injury and the acute respiratory distress syndrome, *Am J Respir Crit Care Med* 164:231, 2001.

100. Choong K: *Low frequency oscillation is potentially more injurious than high frequency oscillatory ventilation. Presented at the Seventeenth Conference on High-frequency Ventilation of Infants,* Snowbird, Utah, April 2000.

101. Jenkinson SG: Oxygen toxicity in acute respiratory failure, *Respir Care* 28:614, 1983.

102. Ciszek TA, Mondanlou HD, Owings D, et al: Mean airway pressure: significance during mechanical ventilation in neonates, *J Pediatr* 99:121, 1981.

103. Gallagher TJ, Banner MJ: Mean airway pressure as a determinant of oxygenation, *Crit Care Med* 8:244, 1980.

104. Kirby R: Improving ventilator patient interaction: reduction of flow dyssynchrony, *Crit Care Med* 25:10, 1997.

105. Amal J: Inspiratory flow rate: more may not be better, *Crit Care Med* 27:4, 1999.

106. Kacmarek RM: Essential gas delivery features of mechanical ventilators, *Respir Care* 37:1045, 1992.

107. Suter PM, Fairley HB, Isenberg MD: Optimum end-expiratory pressure in patients with acute pulmonary failure, *N Engl J Med* 292:284, 1975.

108. Kirby RR, Downs JB, Civetta JM, et al: High level positive end-expiratory pressure in acute respiratory insufficiency, *Chest* 71:18, 1977.

109. Kirby RR: Best PEEP: issues and choices in the selection and monitoring of PEEP levels, *Respir Care* 33:569, 1988.

110. Witte MK, Galli SA, Chatburn RL, et al: Optimal positive end-expiratory pressure therapy in infants and children with acute respiratory failure, *Pediatr Res* 24:217, 1988.

111. Carroll CG, Tuman KJ, Braverman B, et al: Minimal positive end-expiratory pressure (PEEP) may be "best PEEP." *Chest* 93:1020, 1988.

112. Nelson LD, Civetta JM, Hudson-Civetta J: Titrating positive end-expiratory pressure therapy in patients with early moderate arterial hypoxemia, *Crit Care Med* 15:14, 1987.

113. Bilen Z, Colhen IL: Auto-PEEP characterization and consequences, *Anesthesiol Rep* 3:255, 1990.

114. Benson MS, Pierson MD: Auto-PEEP during mechanical ventilation of adults, *Respir Care* 33:557, 1988.

115. Murray JP, Modell JH, Gallagher TJ, et al: Titration of PEEP by the arterial minus end tidal carbon dioxide gradient, *Chest* 85:100, 1984.

116. Marini JJ: Should PEEP be used in airflow obstruction? *Am Rev Respir Dis* 140:1, 1989.

117. Smith PG, El-Khatib MF, Carlo WA: PEEP does not improve pulmonary mechanics in infants with bronchiolitis, *Am Rev Respir Dis* 147:1295, 1993.

118. Graham AS, et al: Positive end-expiratory pressure and pressure support in peripheral airways obstruction: work of breathing in intubated children, *Intensive Care Med* 33:120, 2007.

119. Chang HK: Mechanisms of gas transport during ventilation by high-frequency oscillation, *J Appl Physiol* 56:553, 1984.

120. Robertson B: Pathology of neonatal surfactant deficiency, *Perspect Pediatr Pathol* 11:6, 1987.

121. Gilbert R, Keighley JF: The arterial/alveolar oxygen tension ratio: an index of gas exchange applicable to varying oxygen concentrations, *Am Rev Respir Dis* 109:142, 1974.

122. McCulloch PR, Forkert PG, Froese AB: Lung volume maintenance prevents lung injury during high-frequency oscillatory ventilation in surfactant deficient rabbits, *Am Rev Respir Dis* 137:1185, 1988.

123. Czervinske MP: Mechanical ventilator: a life support system [letter], *Crit Care Q* 7:1, 1984.

124. Hamel DS, Cheifetz IR: Measuring pediatric tidal volumes, *RT for Decision Makers in Respiratory Therapy,* 2002. June/July. Available from: http://www.rtmagazine.com/issues/articles/2002–06_05.asp. Retrieved October 2008.

125. Hess D, McCurdy S, Simmons M: Compression volume in adult ventilator circuits: a comparison of five disposable circuits and nondisposable circuits, *Respir Care* 36:1113, 1991.

126. Rasanen J, Leijala M: Breathing circuit respiratory work in infants recovering from respiratory failure, *Crit Care Med* 19:31, 1991.

127. Irlbeck D: Normal mechanisms of heat and moisture exchange in the respiratory tract, *Respir Care Clin North Am* 4:2, 1998.

128. Avila K, Mazza L, Morgan-Trujillo L, et al: High-frequency oscillatory ventilation: a nursing approach to bedside care, *Neonatal Network* 13:23, 1994.

129. Drakulovic MB, Torres A, Bauer TT, Nicolas JM, Nogue S, Ferrer M: Supine body position as a risk factor for nosocomial pneumonia in mechanically ventilated patients: a randomised trial, *Lancet* 354(9193):1851, 1999.

130. van Nieuwenhoven CA, Vandenbroucke-Grauls C, van Tiel FH, et al: Feasibility and effects of the semirecumbent position to prevent ventilator-associated pneumonia: a randomized study, *Crit Care Med* 34(2):396, 2006.

131. Staudinger T, Bojic A, Holzinger U, et al: Continuous lateral rotation therapy to prevent ventilator-associated pneumonia, *Crit Care Med* 38(2):486, 2010.

132. Curley MA, Schwalenstocker E, Deshpande JK, et al: Tailoring the Institute for Health Care Improvement 100,000 Lives Campaign to pediatric settings: the example of ventilator-associated pneumonia, *Pediatr Clin North Am* 53(6):1231, 2006.

133. Coffin SE, Klompas M, et al: Agency for Healthcare Research and Quality. *Strategies to prevent ventilator associated pneumonia in acute care hospitals.* http://www.guideline.gov/content.aspx?id=13396

134. Gentile MA, Siobal MS: Are specialized endotracheal tubes and heat-and-moisture exchangers cost-effective in preventing ventilator associated pneumonia? *Respiratory care* 55(2):184; discussion 196, 2010.

135. Weiss M, Dullenkopf A, Fischer JE, Keller C, Gerber AC: Prospective randomized controlled multi-centre trial of cuffed or uncuffed endotracheal tubes in small children, *Br J Anaesth* 103(6):867, 2009.

136. CDC and the Healthcare Infection Control Practices Advisory Committee: *Guidelines for preventing health-care-associated*

pneumonia 2003. http://www.cdc.gov/hicpac/pdf/guidelines/eic_in_hcf_03.pdf

137. Gardner DL, Shirland L: Evidence-based guideline for suctioning the intubated neonate and infant, *Neonatal Netw* 28(5):281, 2009.

138. Copnell B, Dargaville PA, Ryan EM, Kiraly NJ, Chin LO, Mills JF, et al: The effect of suction method, catheter size, and suction pressure on lung volume changes during endotracheal suction in piglets, *Pediatr Res* 66(4):405, 2009.

139. Stoller JK, Orens DK, Fatica C, et al: Weekly versus daily changes of in-line suction catheters: impact on rates of ventilator-associated pneumonia and associated costs, *Respir Care* 48(5):494, 2003.

140. Kalyn A, Blatz S, Sandra F, Paes B, Bautista C: Closed suctioning of intubated neonates maintains better physiologic stability: a randomized trial, *J Perinatol* 23(3):218, 2003.

141. Dreyfuss D, et al: High inflation pressure pulmonary edema: respective effects of high airway pressure, high tidal volume, and positive end expiratory pressure, *Am Rev Respir Dis* 137:1159, 1988.

142. MacIntyre NR: Pressure support ventilation: effects on ventilatory reflexes and ventilatory muscle workloads, *Respir Care* 32:447, 1987.

143. Gallagher TJ, Smith RA, Kirby RR, et al: Intermittent inspiratory chest tube occlusion to limit bronchopleural cutaneous airleaks, *Crit Care Med* 4:328, 1976.

144. Bevelaqua FA, Kay S: A modified technique for the management of bronchopleural fistula in ventilator-dependent patients: a report of two cases, *Respir Care* 31:904, 1986.

145. Walkinshaw M, Shoemaker WC: Use of volume loading to obtain preferred levels of PEEP, *Crit Care Med* 8:81, 1980.

146. STOP-ROP Multicenter Study Group: Supplemental Therapeutic Oxygen for Prethreshold Retinopathy Of Prematurity (STOP-ROP), a randomized, controlled trial. I. Primary outcomes, *Pediatrics* 105:295, 2000.

147. Dellinger PR: Complications of mechanical ventilation, *Pulmonol Crit Care Update* 5:2, 1989.

148. Strieter RM, Lynch JP: Complications in the ventilated patient, *Clin Chest Med* 9:127, 1988.

149. Mathewson HS, Linn RC, Gish GB: Pediatric mechanical ventilators, *J Kansas Med Soc* 84:255, 1983.

150. Marini JJ, Capps JS, Culver BH: The inspiratory work of breathing during assisted mechanical ventilation, *Chest* 87:612, 1985.

151. Shannon DC: Rational monitoring of respiratory function during mechanical ventilation of infants and children, *Intensive Care Med* 15:S13, 1989.

152. Fabres J, Carlo WA, Pillips, et al: Both extremes of arterial carbon dioxide pressure and the magnitude of fluctuations in arterial carbon dioxide pressure are associated with severe intraventricular hemorrhage in preterm infants, *Pediatrics* 119:299, 2007.

153. Harris K: Noninvasive monitoring of gas exchange, *Respir Care* 32:544, 1987.

154. Benditt JO: Esophageal and gastric pressure measurements, *Respir Care* 50:68, 2005.

155. NIH NHLBI ARDS Clinical Network: *Mechanical Ventilation Protocol Summary,* http://www.ardsnet.org/system/files/Ventilator%20Protocol%20Card.pdf. Accessed 9/8/13.

156. Gluck EH, Barkoviak JM: Medical effectiveness of esophageal balloon pressure manometry in weaning patients from mechanical ventilation, *Crit Care Med* 23:504, 1995.

157. Heinze H, et al: The accuracy of the oxygen washout technique for functional residual capacity assessment during spontaneous breathing, *Anesth Analg* 104:598, 2007.

158. Newth CJ, Enright P, Johnson RL: Multiple-breath nitrogen washout techniques: including measurements with patients on ventilators, *Eur Respir J* 10:2174, 1997.

159. Whiteley JP, Gavaghan DJ, Hahn CE: A mathematical evaluation of the multiple breath nitrogen washout (MBNW) technique and the multiple inert gas elimination technique (MIGET), *J Theor Biol* 194:517, 1998.

160. Zinserling J, Wrigge H, Varelmann D, et al: Measurement of functional residual capacity by nitrogen washout during partial ventilatory support, *Intensive Care Med* 29:720, 2003.

161. Wrigge H, et al: Determination of functional residual capacity (FRC) by multibreath nitrogen washout in a lung model and in mechanically ventilated patients: accuracy depends on continuous dynamic compensation for changes of gas sampling delay time, *Intensive Care Med* 24:487, 1998.

162. Olegård C, Söndergaard S, Houltz E, et al: Estimation of functional residual capacity at the bedside using standard monitoring equipment: a modified nitrogen washout/washin technique requiring a small change of the inspired oxygen fraction, *Anesth Analg* 101:206, 2005.

163. Meredith KS: *Clinical evaluation of non-invasive blood gas monitoring. Presented at the Eighth Conference on High-frequency Ventilation of Infants,* Snowbird, Utah, April 1991.

164. Pierson DJ: Weaning from mechanical ventilation in acute respiratory failure: concepts, indications, and techniques, *Respir Care* 28:646, 1983.

165. Venkataraman ST: Validation of predictors of extubation success and failure in mechanically ventilated infants and children, *Crit Care Med* 28:2991, 2000.

166. Manczur TI: Comparison of predictors of extubation from mechanical ventilated in children, *Pediatric Crit Care Med* 1:28, 2000.

167. Doershuk CF, Orenstein DM: Pulmonary function and exercise testing. In Lough MD, Doershuk CF, Stern RC, editors: *Pediatric respiratory therapy,* Chicago, 1979, Year Book Medical, pp 250.

168. Sassoon CS, Light RW, Lodia R, et al: Pressure–time product during continuous positive airway pressure, pressure support ventilation, and T-piece during weaning from mechanical ventilation, *Am Rev Respir Dis* 143:469, 1991.

169. Grassino A, Macklem P: Respiratory muscle fatigue and ventilator failure, *Annu Rev Med* 35:625, 1984.

170. Bancalari E, Gerhardt T, Everett R, et al: Closed-loop controlled inspired oxygen concentration for mechanically ventilated very low birth weight infants with frequent episodes of hypoxemia, *Pediatrics* 107:1120, 2001.

171. Berman LS, Foxx WW, Raphaely RC, et al: Optimum levels of CPAP for tracheal extubation of newborn infants, *J Pediatr* 89:109, 1976.

172. Shekerdemian LS: Cardiopulmonary interactions in healthy children and children after simple cardiac surgery: the effects of positive and negative pressure ventilation, *Heart* 78:587, 1997.

173. Frerichs I, Schmitz G, Pulletz S, et al: Reproducibility of regional lung ventilation distribution determined by electrical impedance tomography during mechanical ventilation, *Physiol Meas* 28:S261, 2007.

174. Hinz J, Hahn G, Neumann P, et al: End-expiratory lung impedance change enables bedside monitoring of end-expiratory lung volume change, *Intensive Care Med* 29:37, 2003.

175. Wolf GK, Grychtol B, van Genderingen, et al: Regional lung volume changes in children with acute respiratory distress syndrome during a derecruitment maneuver, *Crit Care Med* 35:1972, 2007.

176. Wolf GK, Gómez-Laberge C, Rettig JS, et al: Mechanical ventilation guided by electrical impedance tomography in experimental acute lung injury, *Crit Care Med* 2013. Mar 7. [Epub ahead of print.]

177. Hunt JF, Fang K, Malik R, et al: Endogenous airway acidification: implications for asthma pathophysiology, *Am J Respir Crit Care Med* 161:694, 2000.

178. Tate S, MacGregor G, Davis M, et al: Airways in cystic fibrosis are acidified: detection by exhaled breath condensate, *Thorax* 57:926, 2002.

179. Kostikas K, Papatheodorou G, Ganas K, et al: pH in expired breath condensate of patients with inflammatory airway diseases, *Am J Respir Crit Care Med* 165:1364, 2002.

180. Effros RM: Exhaled breath condensate acidification in acute lung injury, *Respir Med* 98:682; author reply 3, 2004.

181. Gessner C, Hammerschmidt S, Kuhn H, et al: Exhaled breath condensate acidification in acute lung injury, *Respir Med* 97:1188, 2003.

182. Walsh BK, Mackey DJ, Pajewski T, et al: Exhaled-breath condensate pH can be safely and continuously monitored in mechanically ventilated patients, *Respir Care* 51:1125, 2006.

183. Plavka R, et al: A prospective randomized comparison of conventional mechanical ventilation and very early high frequency ventilation in extremely premature newborns with respiratory distress syndrome, *Intensive Care Med* 25:68, 1999.

184. Courtney SE, Durand DJ, Asselin JM, et al: High-frequency oscillatory ventilation versus conventional mechanical ventilation for very-low-birth-weight infants, *N Engl J Med* 347:643, 2002.

185. Randel RC, Manning FL: One lung high-frequency ventilation in the management of an acquired neonatal pulmonary cyst, *J Perinatol* 9:66, 1989.

186. Bloom BT, et al: Respiratory distress syndrome and tracheoesophageal fistula: management with high-frequency ventilation, *Crit Care Med* 18:447, 1990.

187. Kinsella JP, Truog WE, Walsh WF, et al: Randomized, multicenter trial of inhaled nitric oxide and high-frequency oscillatory ventilation in severe, persistent pulmonary hypertension of the newborn, *J Pediatr* 131:55, 1997.

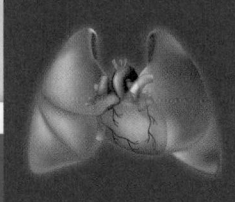

Chapter 18

Administration of Gas Mixtures

BRIAN K. WALSH

LEARNING OBJECTIVES

After reading this chapter the reader will be able to:

1. Identify the basic chemical properties of nitric oxide
2. Describe the process of smooth muscle contraction and relaxation
3. Differentiate between intravenous vasodilators (such as nitroprusside or prostaglandin E) and inhaled nitric oxide regarding ventilation-perfusion matching and shunt
4. Identify the potential side effects of inhaled nitric oxide
5. Describe the beneficial properties of helium when used medically
6. Describe how heliox affects nebulizers, flow meters, and mechanical ventilators
7. List the inhaled anesthetic agents that are commonly used to treat status asthmaticus
8. Identify which inhaled anesthetic agents are best tolerated by mask
9. List the physiological effects of inhaled anesthetic agents

KEY TERMS

Anesthetic mixtures
Enflurane
Halothane

Helium–oxygen mixture
Inhaled nitric oxide
Isoflurane

Pulmonary vasodilation
Sevoflurane
Therapeutic gas mixtures

One of the primary goals of critical care is to optimize oxygen delivery to the tissues. Often this entails the delivery of supplemental oxygen. However, other gases may be used to improve oxygen delivery, based on the patient's clinical diagnosis. The gases discussed in this chapter dilate the pulmonary vasculature, constrict the pulmonary vasculature, reduce airway resistance, and relax bronchial smooth muscle tone.

NITRIC OXIDE

Nitric oxide (NO) is a colorless, sweet-smelling, nonflammable toxic gas. Nitric oxide, not to be confused with *nitrous* oxide (N_2O, an anesthetic), is also an unstable, highly reactive, lipophilic, diatomic free radical. Because of its high reactivity, NO is often combined with nitrogen in various concentrations and stored in aluminum alloy cylinders. The most common concentration available commercially is 800 ppm, although higher and lower concentrations are available as well.

Physiological Basis of Action

Nitric oxide is a ubiquitous substance produced by nearly every cell and organ in the human body (Box 18-1). Directly or indirectly, NO performs numerous functions, including vasodilation, platelet inhibition, immune regulation, enzyme

Box 18-1	Organs and Cells Involved in the Endogenous Production of Nitric Oxide

- Brain
- Peripheral nerves
- Skeletal muscle
- Liver
- Myocytes

- Epithelium
- Platelets
- Adrenals
- Macrophages
- Lungs

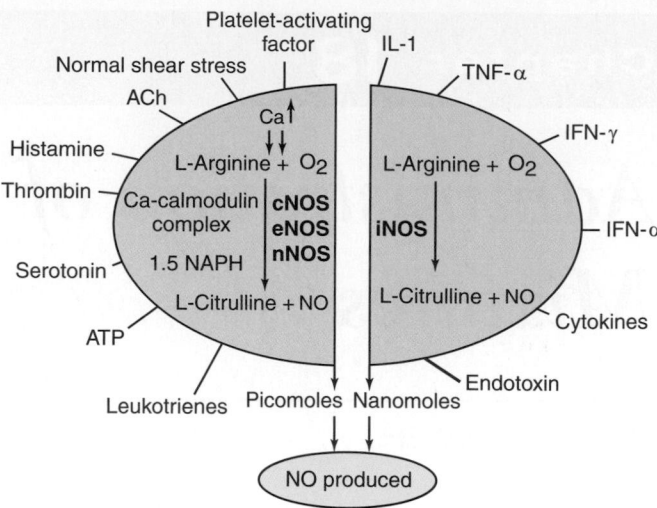

FIGURE 18-1   Endogenous nitric oxide (*NO*) production. Under normal conditions, picomoles of NO are produced. When inducible nitric acid synthase is activated in conditions of sepsis or inflammation, nanomoles of NO are produced. *ACh,* Acetylcholine; *ATP,* adenosine triphosphate; *cNOS,* constitutive nitric oxide synthase; *eNOS,* endogenous nitric oxide synthase; *IFN,* interferon; *IL,* interleukin; *iNOS,* induced nitric oxide synthase; *nNOS,* neuronal nitric oxide synthase; *TNF,* tumor necrosis factor.

regulation, and neurotransmission.[1] This chapter, however, focuses on smooth muscle relaxation of the pulmonary vascular bed.

Pulmonary Smooth Muscle Relaxation and Contraction

An understanding of the mechanism of smooth muscle relaxation in the pulmonary vascular bed is based on the regulation of smooth muscle tone. In general, smooth muscle tone is regulated by chemical, hormonal, nervous, and physical interactions.[2] Current understanding suggests that vascular smooth muscle is largely dependent on intracellular calcium ion (Ca^{2+}) concentration. Smooth muscle tissue comprises bundles of myofibrils, threadlike contractile fibers encased by the sarcoplasmic reticulum, a network of tubes or channels that store Ca^{2+}. Muscle contraction begins with the release of Ca^{2+} from the sarcoplasmic reticulum. Calcium ion binds with the protein calmodulin. The calcium–calmodulin complex activates the enzyme myosin light-chain kinase, enabling phosphorylation of the myosin, resulting in contraction of the cell. Contraction continues until Ca^{2+} is reabsorbed into the sarcoplasmic reticulum. Therefore, any process that inhibits the release of Ca^{2+} will interrupt smooth muscle contraction.

In the body, the process of smooth muscle relaxation uses cyclic guanosine monophosphate (cGMP) to reduce Ca^{2+} levels. In smooth muscle cells, cGMP activates cGMP-dependent kinase, preventing the release of Ca^{2+} from the sarcoplasmic reticulum, resulting in smooth muscle relaxation. In the early 1980s, researchers reported a potent smooth muscle–relaxing agent, endothelium-derived relaxing factor (EDRF),[3] now understood to be endogenous nitric oxide. Formation of EDRF results in increased levels of cGMP in smooth muscle cells. EDRF and cGMP are conceivably the two most important substances in regulating smooth muscle tone.[2,4]

Nitric Oxide Synthase and Endogenous Nitric Oxide Production

In the body, NO is produced by the combination of nitric oxide synthase (NOS) enzymes with the amino acid L-arginine and molecular oxygen. This combination results in the formation of the amino acid L-citrulline and NO (Figure 18-1). The two types of NOS enzymes are

constitutive and inducible. The *constitutive* NOS (cNOS) enzymes are normally expressed in tissues and consist of two isoforms: eNOS (endothelial in origin) and nNOS (neuronal in origin).[1] The one *inducible* NOS enzyme, iNOS, results from enzyme induction.[5] The cNOS enzymes, which are calmodulin dependent, produce relatively small amounts of NO (picomoles). The iNOS enzyme functions independently of calmodulin and produces relatively large amounts of NO (nanomoles). NO resulting from iNOS is most often produced in sepsis and is probably responsible for the pathological decrease in systemic vascular resistance observed in septic shock.

Once NO is formed and bound to hemoglobin, guanylyl cyclase is activated, which converts cyclic guanidine triphosphate to cGMP. This increased cGMP results in reduced Ca^{2+} and smooth muscle relaxation.

Inhaled Nitric Oxide

The underlying principle of inhaled nitric oxide (iNO) is its selectivity as a pulmonary vasodilator.[6] Inhaled NO will relax only pulmonary smooth muscle adjacent to functioning alveoli. Atelectatic or fluid-filled lung units will not participate in iNO uptake. Therefore, if the pulmonary vasculature is constricted in atelectatic regions of the lung, pulmonary blood flow will remain minimal in these regions, reducing intrapulmonary shunt (Figure 18-2). This is in contrast to intravenous vasodilators such as nitroprusside or prostacyclin. These drugs will relax pulmonary vasculature globally, reducing pulmonary vascular resistance but also increasing blood flow past nonfunctioning alveoli and intrapulmonary right-to-left shunt.

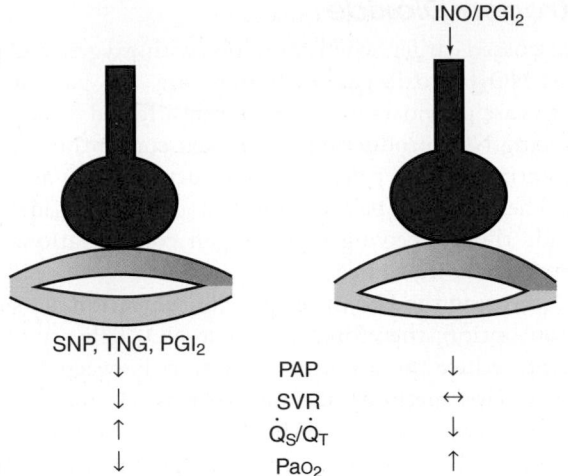

INO/PGI₂

SNP, TNG, PGI₂

↓	PAP	↓
↓	SVR	↔
↑	Q̇s/Q̇t	↓
↓	Pao₂	↑

FIGURE 18-2 Comparison of the vasodilator effects from systemic drugs and NO. Both reduce pulmonary artery pressure, but the systemic vasodilators also dilate the blood vessels not participating in gas exchange, thereby increasing the intrapulmonary shunt. *Pao₂*, Arterial partial pressure of oxygen; *PAP*, pulmonary artery pressure; *PGI₂*, prostacyclin; *S/T*, intrapulmonary shunt; *SNP*, sodium nitroprusside; *SVR*, systemic vascular resistance; *TNG*, nitroglycerin.

Newborn Hypoxic Respiratory Failure. The concept of treating pulmonary hypertension of term or near-term infants with iNO has been advocated in many early reports and randomized controlled trials. These studies confirmed that iNO improved oxygenation and reduced the need for extracorporeal membrane oxygenation. In 2000 the first U.S. Food and Drug Administration (FDA) approval of iNO as a noninvestigative drug was for the treatment of primary pulmonary hypertension of the term or near-term (>34 weeks gestational age) neonate with hypoxic respiratory failure associated with evidence of pulmonary hypertension. Hypoxic respiratory failure may be primary or a secondary effect of another disorder (meconium aspiration, congenital diaphragmatic hernia, pneumonia, etc.).

Dosing strategies should be focused on physiological end points.[7] This involves titrating the delivered NO in increments until a positive response is achieved. Several studies[8-13] have used an increase in oxygen saturation of 20% over baseline as an indication that the infant is responsive. These studies and others[14,15] have suggested that optimal dosing is usually in the 20- to 30-ppm range. Some infants will not respond positively. The Neonatal Inhaled Nitric Oxide Study (NINOS) trial[16] indicated that only 6% of nonresponders will demonstrate a positive response when given NO at 80 ppm. Typically, a response would be seen almost immediately; however, it is recommended[7] that determining an infant's response last no longer than 4 hours to limit the exposure to NO. Endogenous NO is downregulated when the patient receives iNO. This may result in a worsening of pulmonary hypertension and hypoxemia.[17,18]

Although there is strong evidence for the use of iNO in term or near-term infants, its efficacy in premature babies is less clear. Nitric oxide has been shown to improve oxygenation and outcomes in a few studies. However, larger randomized controlled trials[19-22] and a systematic review[23] have demonstrated similar improvements in oxygenation, but survival outcomes were unchanged. The preterm population is at increased risk for intraventricular hemorrhage and chronic lung disease. These larger, more recent trials did not show any increase in these comorbidities. Therefore, although its usefulness is still in question, NO does appear to be safe in the premature infant population. For detailed information on this subject, please refer to the American Association for Respiratory Care's *Evidence-Based Clinical Practice Guideline: Inhaled Nitric Oxide for Neonates With Acute Hypoxic Respiratory Failure*, located at http://www.rcjournal.com/contents/12.10/12.10.1717.pdf.

Acute Respiratory Distress Syndrome. Current research is investigating the use of NO in acute respiratory distress syndrome (ARDS) and acute lung injury. ARDS is a complex syndrome characterized by noncardiogenic pulmonary edema, diminished lung compliance, and pulmonary hypertension. Current therapy for ARDS is primarily supportive, allowing time for the lung to heal. Although no definitive studies show improved outcomes, iNO has been suggested to improve oxygenation and ventilation-perfusion (V/Q) matching, consequently lowering airway pressure and oxygen concentration. However, studies investigating the use of iNO for the treatment of ARDS or acute lung injury have failed to demonstrate improved outcomes. NO will reach more capillary endothelium by opening collapsed alveoli. In turn, a greater degree of vasorelaxation should occur. Studies have shown that responsiveness to iNO may be enhanced by the application of positive end-expiratory pressure, and perhaps turn nonresponders into responders (to iNO therapy).[24-26] In the pediatric population, Kinsella and colleagues[27] reported improved outcomes when using high-frequency oscillatory ventilation (HFOV) combined with iNO compared with HFOV or iNO alone. Mehta and colleagues[28] also studied the combined effects of iNO and HFOV, the rationale being that if lung volume were optimized they could further enhance the effects of iNO. They demonstrated that the use of HFOV did improve oxygenation response to iNO.[37] Further studies are warranted to determine whether this combination is clinically useful.

Application

Multiple methods have been advocated for the delivery of iNO.[29,30] Early systems were custom-built in-house and comprised two basic subsystems: delivery and monitoring. In these systems, NO is bled into the breathing circuit through a flow meter or blender. NO and NO₂ levels are monitored with an NO/NO₂ analyzer. These systems were cumbersome and were often difficult to assemble. Now that the use of iNO has increased, a few vendors have developed systems incorporating NO delivery with NO and NO_2 monitoring. These devices come in a variety of designs. Some are larger and designed for in-hospital use (Figure 18-3). Currently available systems can be battery operated, include a manual system, and may used for transport.

In general, NO is bled into the breathing circuit before the humidifier. To analyze *inspired* NO and NO_2 concentrations, gas is sampled before the patient–circuit interface. These devices provide alarms to monitor these values, as well as oxygen. The IKARA INOMAX DSIR (Clinton, NJ) and 12th Man Technologies (Garden Grove, CA) measure ventilator circuit gas flow. These flow measurements allow the device to modulate NO output to provide a stable concentration throughout the breath.

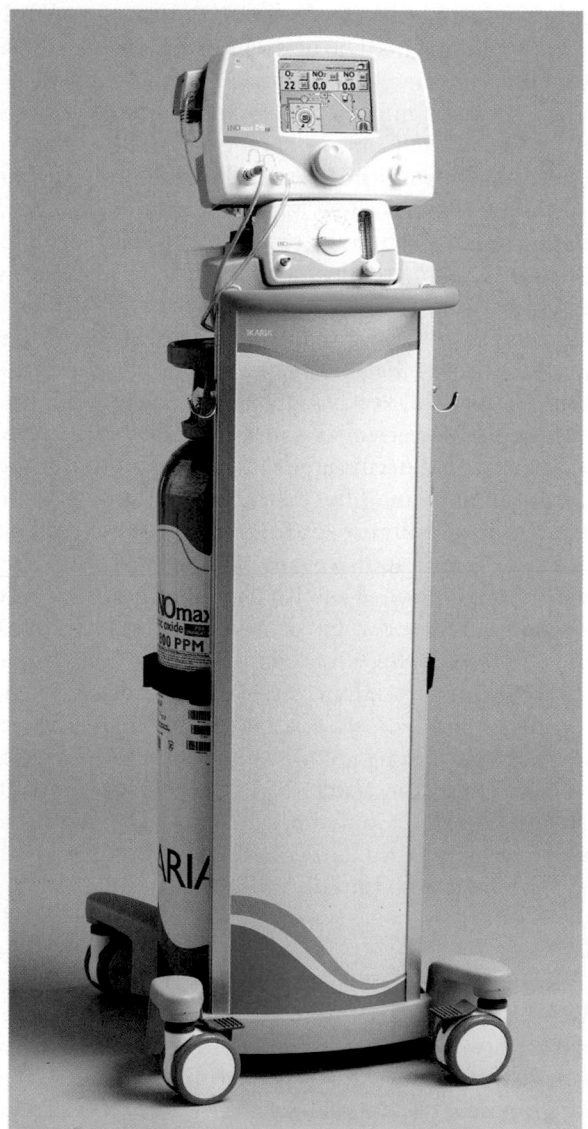

FIGURE 18-3 The INOMAX © DSIR drug-delivery system that is FDA-cleared for administration and monitoring of pharmaceutical-grade inhaled nitric oxide.

Nitrogen Dioxide

As discussed earlier, when combined with oxygen, NO produces NO_2, a toxic gas. Although rare, the patient and health care providers can be adversely affected. Factors influencing NO_2 production are oxygen concentration, NO concentration, and time of contact between NO and oxygen. Therefore the patients most at risk of NO_2 delivery include those receiving high oxygen concentrations and low ventilator flow rates.

Decreasing the NO or oxygen concentration is usually not an option; therefore, to reduce NO_2 delivery to the patient, reduce the duration of contact between NO and oxygen. Two methods accomplish this: (1) increase the inspiratory flow or (2) add the NO as close to the patient as possible. Each of these methods has practical limitations. Increasing the ventilator flow will reduce the time of contact between NO and oxygen before reaching the patient, but it may also affect inspiratory time, tidal volume, mean airway pressure, and so on. Adding NO into the inspiratory limb of the ventilator circuit close to the patient will reduce contact time, but it also creates monitoring difficulties. The practitioner must allow an adequate distance for proper mixing to ensure accurate NO measurement.

In addition, the local atmosphere could become contaminated with NO and NO_2. Although this is rare, early systems included means for the scavenging of expiratory and wasted gases. Usually this was accomplished by the collection of gases into a gas evacuation system similar in design to those used in anesthesia. Gas was collected in a large reservoir and removed continuously through the hospital's vacuum system. At first, scavenging was advocated to reduce the possible harmful inhalation of nitrogen dioxide by other personnel in the vicinity. Studies have shown this to be unnecessary because of the relatively small amounts of NO_2 present at the bedside. Modern hospitals have adequate room air exchange rates, and the chance of NO or NO_2 accumulation is remote. A possible caveat involves interfacility transport. Pressurized aircraft may not allow an adequate cabin air exchange rate to ensure safety. The aircraft crew must be made aware of this so that proper measures are taken to reduce this risk.

Methemoglobin

The half-life of iNO is extremely short, about 5 seconds. Once NO crosses the vascular endothelium, it is rapidly bound by hemoglobin, forming nitrosyl hemoglobin (methemoglobin). Methemoglobin production results from the oxidation of the iron in the hemoglobin.[31] The quantity of methemoglobin depends on iNO concentration and concurrent nitrate-based drug therapy (e.g., nitroprusside, nitroglycerin). If the methemoglobin level is excessive, a reduction in iNO or other nitro-based vasodilators is warranted. Ultimately, NO metabolites are excreted, primarily by the kidneys, as nitrates and nitrites.[32]

HELIUM–OXYGEN MIXTURES

Helium (He) was discovered in 1895 by Sir William Ramsay and independently by Langley and Cleve. Helium is one of the lightest elements, second only to hydrogen. It is a colorless, odorless, tasteless, and physiologically inert noble gas. Helium is present in dry air at a concentration of 0.0005%. At present, the majority of helium comes from natural gas mines in the United States. The supply is limited, and until the Helium Privatization Act of 1996, production was under the control of the U.S. government.

Helium is remarkable for its low density and high viscosity (Table 18-1). Pure helium gas has a density of 0.179 g/L, one seventh the density of air. A common misconception is that because of its low density, helium has low viscosity. Actually, helium is slightly more viscous than air. However, its kinematic viscosity (the ratio of absolute viscosity to density) is almost seven times greater than that of air. Therefore, from the standpoint of fluid dynamics, helium is much more viscous than air.[33]

Physiological Basis of Action

The use of helium–oxygen mixtures in treating airway obstruction was first described in 1934 by Barach.[34-37] Barach's studies reported a decrease in work of breathing in patients with both upper and lower airway obstruction. Helium is an inert gas, has no pharmacological properties of its own, and does not participate in or interfere with any biochemical activity in the body. Its sole purpose is to lower the total density of any gas mixture.

It is important to note that helium is not used to treat the underlying cause of increased airway resistance but rather to decrease the work of breathing until more definitive therapies are effective. When helium is combined with oxygen, the resulting gas mixture density is one third that of air. Poiseuille's law states that if the diameter of a tube is reduced by half, the pressure gradient to achieve the same flow increases 16 times. Graham's law states that the flow of gas through an orifice is inversely proportional to the square root of its density.[38] In other words, if the driving pressure remains constant, a gas with lower density will have higher flow than a gas with higher density. Alternatively, less pressure is required to maintain a given flow through a fixed orifice. This physical property of helium may be useful in overcoming airway resistance and obstruction.

In normal human anatomy, inspired gas is turbulent between the glottis and the tenth-generation airways, primarily

because of the high gas flow and larger radii of the airways. Physics dictates that greater pressure is required to move gas through a tube (or airway) under turbulent conditions compared with the same volume of gas during laminar flow. A quick review of Reynold's equation shows that decreasing density and increasing viscosity will reduce turbulent flow, decreasing the pressure and work required to move the gas (Box 18-2). Likewise, gas flow through a large, partially obstructed airway will create the same turbulent flow. Decreasing turbulent flow reduces the amount of pressure required to move the gas through the airways, decreasing the work required to breathe.

Application

Helium must be combined with oxygen when used clinically, thus the term *heliox*. Several concentrations of medical-grade helium are available commercially: 80% helium–20% oxygen heliox mixture (80:20), 70% helium–30% oxygen (70:30), and 100% helium–0% oxygen (100%). The 80:20 mixture has essentially the same concentration of oxygen as air; the nitrogen and trace gases are replaced with helium. The 70:30 mixture is useful for patients with airway obstruction who require increased oxygen concentration. The 100% helium concentration is rarely used, and it must be used with oxygen to be compatible with life. Clinicians who use 100% helium do so to reduce the number of tanks required to maintain a patient on heliox. Extreme caution and close monitoring must be employed when using this concentration as it is possible to deliver a hypoxic gas mixture to the patient, possibly resulting in asphyxiation and death.

For the purposes of this chapter, only the use of nonhypoxic gas mixtures is discussed. Heliox cylinders containing at least 20% oxygen are brown and white (or brown and green) and use a CGA-280 fitting.

Aerosol Delivery

Multiple studies have investigated the use of helium–oxygen mixtures and the deposition of aerosolized particles.[39-42] Anderson and colleagues[39] studied patients with stable asthma. Ten patients inhaled radiolabeled particles of Teflon suspended in air or a helium–oxygen mixture. The study concluded there was more aerosol deposition in the lung and less deposition in the upper airways when breathing helium–oxygen mixtures. In a similar study, 42 patients were randomly assigned to receive β-agonists with helium–oxygen mixtures or air.[43] Patients who used the helium–oxygen mixtures showed more improvement in expiratory peak flows

TABLE 18-1

Comparison of Inhaled Gas Densities and Viscosities

	Density (g/L)	Viscosity (μP)
Helium	0.179	188.7
Nitrogen	1.25	167.4
Air	1.29	170.8
Oxygen	1.42	192.6

than the group using air. These studies support the concept that aerosol has deeper and prolonged deposition in the lung when it is delivered with heliox as the carrier gas.

Heliox mixtures will cause pneumatic nebulizers to perform differently than if air or oxygen is used. When driving a pneumatic nebulizer with helium, the nebulizer will produce smaller particles, nebulize more slowly, and have reduced output compared with similar devices driven with air. When using a conventional pneumatic nebulizer driven with heliox, it is advisable to increase gas flow.[44] This will increase drug output by producing denser aerosol and larger particles. Newer generation of vibrating mesh nebulizers (Aerogen Micropump) may provide an alternative to gas driven nebulizers. If vibrating mesh nebulizers are used, heliox can be the carrier gas.

Oxygen Flow Meters

Helium is less dense and therefore more diffusible than oxygen. As a consequence, standard oxygen flow meters will indicate an incorrect flow when used with helium-containing mixtures. This error will cause the indicated flow to be erroneously low. An 80:20 heliox mixture is 1.8 times more diffusible than oxygen. To correct for the difference in gas density, the indicated flow on the flow meter is multiplied by 1.8. A 70:30 heliox mixture is 1.6 times more diffusible than oxygen. To obtain the accurate flow rate for this mixture, the indicated flow is multiplied by 1.6. This error will be present in most gas-measuring devices (see later discussion in this section).

Spontaneously Breathing Patients

Spontaneously breathing patients with upper or lower airway obstruction can be given heliox via mask. Because the goal of heliox therapy is to reduce the density of the inspired gas, it is important to deliver the greatest concentration of helium. Therefore the patient must be able to tolerate the lowest possible fractional concentration of inspired oxygen (Fio_2), and room air entrainment must be minimized, resulting in a higher fractional concentration of inspired helium (Fi_{He}). Nasal cannulas (with the exception of high-flow nasal cannulas) and simple masks allow far too much room air entrainment, thereby diluting the helium concentration. Therefore, a close-fitting nonrebreathing mask should be used. This limitation makes the treatment of young patients difficult. Children in distress may not tolerate the tightly fitting mask required to minimize air entrainment. Stillwell and colleagues[45] investigated the use of heliox mixtures delivered through an infant hood. Not surprisingly, they found a greater concentration of helium at the top of the hood (because of its lower gas density), away from the infant's nose and mouth. This resulted in a lower Fi_{He} and therefore a denser gas being delivered to the infant.

High-Flow Nasal Cannula

Heliox has been shown to reduce turbulence and improve aerosol delivery in a range of clinical settings. Ari and colleagues assessed the effects of heliox on medication delivery by comparing with 100% oxygen while testing the infant, pediatric cannulas running at flows of 3 and 6 lpm, and adult cannulas running at 10 and 30 lpm. At higher flows they found that heliox increased aerosol deposition compared with oxygen. At lower flows, there was less benefit from the use of heliox compared with oxygen in the pediatric and adult cannulas and no benefit for the infant. Aerosol delivery was significantly greater at lower flows with both heliox and oxygen in adults and pediatric ($p < 0.05$), the use of heliox at 6 lpm increased albuterol delivery by 40% compared with heliox at 3 L/min ($p = 0.049$) and oxygen at 6 L/min ($p = 0.043$) in infants. They surmised the use of heliox with high-flow nasal cannulas increased aerosol delivery more than oxygen at most flow rates.[46]

Mechanically Ventilated Patients

If the intent of heliox use is to prevent respiratory fatigue or failure, then it should be discontinued when mechanical ventilation is initiated. In this scenario the ventilator assumes the work of breathing. When mechanical ventilation is initiated, the patient will be in impending respiratory failure, hypoxic requiring high levels of oxygen, making heliox less effective. Once the patient is mechanically ventilated and continues to suffer from severe lower airway obstruction (as seen in status asthmaticus) and continues to have reduced expiratory flows and gas trapping. The use of heliox mixtures has been advocated to minimize air trapping, hemodynamic compromise, and to reduce peak inspiratory pressures.

The primary obstacle to heliox delivery via a mechanical ventilator is error in volume and flow measurement. Many mechanical ventilators rely on gas density to measure flows and volumes. Most errors result from underestimation of flow because of the low-density characteristics of helium. Volume is typically a mathematical integration of flow and time; therefore volumes will be equally affected. In one study the Servo 900C (Maquet, Bridgewater, NJ) demonstrated a statistically significant (approximately 10%) underestimation in volume measurement at a helium concentration of 50%, increasing to a 20% error at a helium concentration of 80%.[47] This error in flow and volume is also seen in external monitors as well. In the same study the VenTrak pulmonary monitor (Novametrix/Philips Respironics, Murrysville, PA) underestimated volume by 20% at a helium concentration of 20%, increasing to a 40% error at a helium concentration of 80%.

The safest method to deliver helium–oxygen mixtures via mechanical ventilation is to connect an 80:20 heliox mixture to the heliox-approved inlet of the mechanical ventilator. The practitioner then uses the ventilator's oxygen concentration control to adjust helium and oxygen to the desired mixture. This allows the practitioner to deliver a helium concentration up to the 80% helium. It is important to note that ventilators may not function properly with helium as a source gas. Please refer to the manufacturer's manual before attempting to add helium to the air inlet of any ventilator. It is never advisable to provide 100% helium through any ventilator.

This anomaly in volume calculations appears to be related to the heated-wire flow anemometer. The high thermal conductivity of helium rapidly cools the wires, simulating a high-flow condition. The microprocessor responds by closing the gas valves to such a degree that the ventilator will not function. As always, it is important to monitor oxygen concentration when using heliox. Three devices in the United States have been cleared by the U.S. FDA for use with helium mixtures: the AVEA (Cardinal Health, Dublin, OH), the Servo-*i* (Maquet, Bridgewater, NJ), and the Hamilton G5 (Hamilton Medical, Reno, NV).

Gas Mixtures in Extracorporeal Membrane Oxygenation

Some patients require extracorporeal membrane oxygenation to achieve adequate gas exchange (see Chapter 19, Extracorporeal Life Support). Gas from a blender passes through the oxygenator cartridge (artificial lung), gas exchange occurs. The oxygen in this gas oxygenates the blood. Carbon dioxide diffuses from the blood into the sweep gas. The membrane oxygenator in the extracorporeal membrane oxygenation circuit is efficient, and sometimes too efficient, in exchanging gases with the blood. When the sweep gas (blended gas flow through the membrane lung; usually CO_2 free) through the oxygenator removes too much CO_2 from the blood, carbogen may be substituted as the sweep gas to inhibit excessive CO_2 removal. Carbogen is a mixture of CO_2 and O_2, typically 95% oxygen and 5% carbon dioxide.

ANESTHETIC MIXTURES

Patients in status asthmaticus (SA) can be placed on helium–oxygen therapy as a temporizing measure to reduce the work of breathing until other therapy (β-agonists, methylxanthines, and corticosteroids) is effective. However, these patients often have bronchospasm that is refractory to conventional therapy. Certain volatile inhaled anesthetics are known for their bronchodilatory properties. Although no clinical trials have investigated the use of inhaled anesthetics (IAs) in the routine treatment of SA, several case reports exist.[48-55]

Of the several IAs used clinically for anesthesia, only a few (halothane, isoflurane, enflurane, and sevoflurane) have been widely reported as potential treatments for SA. *Halothane* is an alkane derivative and has been the volatile anesthetic of choice in reducing bronchospasm in asthmatic patients. Sevoflurane, a methyl ethyl ether, has been shown to be as effective as halothane in reducing lung resistance; however, safety studies for its use in children with asthma are needed.[49,56,57] Isoflurane and enflurane are also methyl ethyl ethers and are often used in the acute treatment of SA. Each has advantages and disadvantages in treating bronchospasm (Table 18-2).

TABLE 18-2

Comparison of Inhaled Anesthetic Agents

	Halothane	Isoflurane	Enflurane	Sevoflurane
Mean arterial pressure	↓	↓↓↓	↓↓	↓
Pulmonary vascular resistance	—	↓↓	↓	↓
Heart rate	↓	↑	↑↑	↑
Cardiac output	↓↓	—	↓↓↓	—
Airway irritant	—	↑↑;	↑↑	—
Respiratory depression	↑	↑	↑↑	↑
Myocardial sensitization to catecholamines	↑↑↑↑	—	—	—
Risk of explosion	—	—	—	—

Physiological Basis of Action

Volatile IAs reduce bronchospasm through a number of pathways: β-adrenergic receptor stimulation, direct smooth muscle relaxation, antagonism of acetylcholine and histamine, and inhibition of hypocapneic bronchoconstriction.[58] In essence, they reduce central afferent parasympathetic activity.[59] Therefore a patient receiving standard bronchodilators may see an additional response with the addition of an IA.[60]

Application

Qualified individuals must perform the setup and delivery of IAs. Respiratory care practitioners can be properly trained in the setup and operation of closed-loop (rebreathing circuit) anesthetic ventilators for the primary purpose of bronchodilation. In general, the anesthesiologist or specialty trained intensivist performs the initial setup and troubleshooting. Adjustments are usually done by protocol or RCP under the direct supervision of the intensive care physician or anesthesiologist. The bedside caregiver handles routine monitoring procedures. All caregivers must understand the pharmacology of the IA being delivered and its side effect profile.

The two ways to deliver IAs are by face mask for the spontaneously breathing patient and through a mechanical ventilator. In either system the setup is similar to that used in the operating room. Both methods require similar equipment: vaporizers for the volatile anesthetic, scavenging devices, anesthetic gas analyzers, and vital sign monitoring.

Inhaled Anesthetics via Face Mask

To avoid intubation and mechanical ventilation, treating the spontaneously breathing patient with an IA could be advantageous. The systems used for spontaneous breathing of IAs are complicated but are similar to full-face noninvasive continuous positive airway pressure circuits. The expiratory gases pass through a carbon dioxide absorber and then return to the inspiratory limb, creating a circle. A fresh gas supply (including the IA) is introduced after the carbon dioxide absorber. This design is called a *rebreathing circuit*.

The face mask must be tight fitting to prevent the leakage of the IA into the room and to ensure that the patient receives the IA. Because patients may be somewhat awake, they must be cooperative enough not to remove the mask. The IA must also be compatible with face mask administration. Enflurane and isoflurane are irritants to the upper airway and are unpleasant to breathe while conscious, especially for the pediatric patient. These vapors may produce laryngospasm and fighting. Isoflurane and enflurane are more suited for use with an intubated and mechanically ventilated patient. Conversely, halothane and sevoflurane are neutral-smelling vapors and may be accepted more readily via mask.

Typically, halothane is the IA of choice when delivering to a conscious, spontaneously breathing patient. The dose range for halothane is approximately 0.25% to 0.5%. The patient usually is sufficiently awake to communicate in short sentences. Bronchodilation is usually rapid (15 to 20 minutes). The patient benefits by the reduced resistance as well as the sedative effect.

Inhaled Anesthetics via Mechanical Ventilation

Almost universally, the Servo 900C has been used to deliver IAs to mechanically ventilated patients, but it is no longer supported. Most modern anesthesia ventilator or systems can be transported to the ICU and provide modern modes of ventilation such as pressure support ventilation.

Waste anesthetic agent may pose a risk for staff and visitors. Therefore, exhaled and waste gases need to be scavenged from the circuit. These waste gases are typically collected via waste anesthetic gas (WAG) outlets connected to the hospital vacuum system. Most ICUs are not outfitted with WAG suction outlets.

CASE STUDY

A 12-year-old boy with known persistent severe asthma has been admitted to the intensive care unit for further management of a severe exacerbation. He has received an appropriate dose of steroids and has been given continuous albuterol, 15 mg/hour for the last 4 hours, in the emergency department. There is a concern for respiratory fatigue. SPO_2 is 96% on 0.21 FiO_2.

What would you recommend at this point?

1. Heliox 80/20
2. Noninvasive ventilation
3. Intravenous β agonist
4. Volatile inhaled anesthetics

See Evolve Resources for answers.

KEY POINTS

- Nitric oxide can improve oxygenation and reduce the need for ECMO in the clinically indicated patient population.
- Inhaled endothelium relaxing factor (NO) can vasodilate the pulmonary capillary bed ventilated lung units and improve gas exchange.
- Inhaled nitric oxide is a selective vasodilator which improves it side effect profile.
- A helium-oxygen gas mixture can reduce the patient's work of breathing during severe obstructive airways disease such as status asthmaticus or croup. By reducing fatigue heliox enables medications such as steroids the time required to become effective without escalating to positive pressure ventilation.
- Heliox can be provided through most modern mechanical ventilators while accurately measuring tidal volumes.
- Inhaled anesthetics such as isoflurane and sevoflurane are potent bronchodilators.
- Modern anesthetic ventilators can adequately ventilate pediatric patients while safely providing, monitoring, and conserving volatile anesthetic agent.

ASSESSMENT QUESTIONS

See Evolve Resources for answers.

1. Which of the following is/are chemical properties of nitric oxide?
   A. Lipophilic
   B. Highly reactive
   C. Unstable free radical
   D. All of the above
2. Which chemical is most associated with smooth muscle contractility?
   A. Iron
   B. Calcium
   C. Citric acid
   D. L-Arginine
3. Inhaled nitric oxide reduces shunt by:
   A. Vasodilating only pulmonary capillaries adjacent to atelectatic lung units
   B. Decreasing pulmonary vascular resistance
   C. Increasing systemic oxygenation
   D. Vasodilating only pulmonary capillaries adjacent to functioning lung units
4. Which of the following are potential side effects of iNO administration?
   A. Nitrous oxide formation in the ventilator circuit
   B. Fetal hemoglobin formation
   C. Decrease in guanylyl cyclase in the sarcoplasmic reticulum
   D. Methemoglobin formation

5. Which of the following are useful properties of helium when used to treat patients in status asthmaticus?
   I. Lower density
   II. Lower viscosity
   III. Higher viscosity
   IV. Low thermal conductivity
   A. I and II
   B. I and III
   C. I, II, and IV
   D. I, III, and IV

6. All of the following are effects of heliox on mechanical ventilation *except:*
   A. Measured flow is falsely low when using a differential pneumotachometer.
   B. Nebulizer output is decreased.
   C. Actual flow from the flow meter is lower than indicated.
   D. Measured flow is falsely high when using a hot-wire anemometer.

7. Which of the following is *not* an inhaled anesthetic agent used to treat status asthmaticus?
   A. Halothane
   B. Sevoflurane
   C. Enflurane
   D. Nitrous oxide

8. Which of the following inhaled anesthetic agents are best tolerated by the patient when breathing spontaneously from a mask?
   A. Isoflurane and enflurane
   B. Halothane and sevoflurane
   C. Enflurane and sevoflurane
   D. Isoflurane, halothane, and sevoflurane

9. What IA should *not* be used in patients receiving catecholamines?
   A. Enflurane
   B. Isoflurane
   C. Sevoflurane
   D. Halothane

References

1. Hurford WE: The biological basis of inhaled nitric oxide, *Respir Care Clin North Am* 3:357, 1997.
2. Dagby RM, Corey-Kreyling MD: Structural aspects of the contractile machinery of smooth muscle: is the organization of contractile elements compatible with a sliding filament mechanism? In Stephens NL, editor: *Smooth muscle contraction*, New York, 1984, Marcel Dekker, pp 47–74.
3. Furchgott RF, Zawadzki JV: The obligatory role of endothelial cells in the relaxation of arterial smooth muscle by acetylcholine, *Nature* 288:373, 1980.
4. Miller CC, Miller J: Pulmonary vascular smooth muscle regulation: the role of inhaled nitric oxide gas, *Respir Care* 37:1175, 1992.
5. Aranda A, Pearl RG: The biology of nitric oxide, *Respir Care* 44:156, 1999.
6. Bigatello LM, Hurford WE, Hess D: Use of inhaled nitric oxide for ARDS, *Respir Care Clin North Am* 3:437, 1997.
7. Macrae DJ, et al: Inhaled nitric oxide therapy in neonates and children: reaching a European consensus, *Intensive Care Med* 30:372, 2004.
8. Barefield ES, et al: Inhaled nitric oxide in term infants with hypoxemic respiratory failure, *J Pediatr* 129:279, 1996.
9. Clark RH, et al: Clinical Inhaled Nitric Oxide Research Group: Low-dose nitric oxide therapy for persistent pulmonary hypertension of the newborn, *N Engl J Med* 342:469, 2000.
10. Davidson D, et al: Inhaled nitric oxide for the early treatment of persistent pulmonary hypertension of the newborn: a randomized, doublemasked, placebo-controlled, dose-response, multicenter study, *Pediatrics* 101:325, 1998.
11. Day RW, et al: Acute response to inhaled nitric oxide in newborns with respiratory failure and pulmonary hypertension, *Pediatrics* 98:698, 1996.
12. Neonatal Inhaled Nitric Oxide Study Group (NINOS): Inhaled nitric oxide in full-term and nearly full-term infants with hypoxic respiratory failure, *N Engl J Med* 336:597, 1997.
13. Roberts JD Jr, et al: Inhaled Nitric Oxide Study Group: Inhaled nitric oxide and persistent pulmonary hypertension of the newborn, *N Engl J Med* 336:605, 1997.
14. Finer NN, et al: Inhaled nitric oxide in infants referred for extracorporeal membrane oxygenation: dose response, *J Pediatr* 124:302, 1994.
15. Demirakça S, et al: Inhaled nitric oxide in neonatal and pediatric acute respiratory distress syndrome: dose response, prolonged inhalation and weaning, *Crit Care Med* 24:1913, 1996.
16. Neonatal Inhaled Nitric Oxide Study Group (NINOS): Inhaled nitric oxide in full-term and nearly full-term infants with hypoxic respiratory failure, *N Engl J Med* 336:597, 1997.
17. Dötsch J, et al: Recovery from withdrawal of inhaled nitric oxide and kinetics of nitric oxide–induced inhibition of nitric oxide synthase activity in vitro, *Intensive Care Med* 26:330, 2000.
18. Black SM, et al: Inhaled nitric oxide inhibits NOS activity in lambs: potential mechanism for rebound pulmonary hypertension, *Am J Physiol* 277:H1849, 1999.
19. Kinsella JP, et al: Inhaled nitric oxide in premature neonates with severe hypoxemic respiratory failure: a randomised controlled trial, *Lancet* 354:1061, 1999.
20. Franco-Belgium Collaborative NO Trial Group: Early compared with delayed inhaled nitric oxide in moderately hypoxemic neonates with respiratory failure: a randomised controlled trial, *Lancet* 354:1066, 1999.
21. KP Van Meurs, et al: Preemie Inhaled Nitric Oxide Study: Inhaled nitric oxide for premature infants with severe respiratory failure, *N Engl J Med* 353:13, 2005.
22. D Field, et al: INNOVO Trial Collaborating Group: Neonatal ventilation with inhaled nitric oxide versus ventilatory support without inhaled nitric oxide for preterm infants with severe respiratory failure: the INNOVO Multicentre Randomised Controlled Trial (ISRCTN 1782. 339), *Pediatrics* 115:926, 2005.
23. Barrington KJ, Finer NN: Inhaled nitric oxide for respiratory failure in preterm infants, *Cochrane Database Syst Rev* 1:CD000509, 2006.
24. Puybasset L, et al: Factors influencing cardiopulmonary effects of inhaled nitric oxide in acute respiratory failure, *Am J Respir Crit Care Med* 152:318, 1995.
25. Okamoto K, et al: Combined effects of inhaled nitric oxide and positive end-expiratory pressure during mechanical ventilation in acute respiratory distress syndrome, *Artif Organs* 24:390, 2000.
26. Johannigman JA, et al: Positive end-expiratory pressure and response to inhaled nitric oxide: changing nonresponders to responders, *Surgery* 127:390, 2000.
27. Kinsella JP, et al: Randomized, multicenter trial of inhaled nitric oxide and high-frequency oscillatory ventilation in severe, persistent pulmonary hypertension of the newborn, *J Pediatr* 131:55, 1997.

28. Mehta S, et al: Acute oxygenation response to inhaled nitric oxide when combined with high-frequency oscillatory ventilation in adults with acute respiratory distress syndrome, *Crit Care Med* 31:383, 2003.

29. Hess D, Ritz R, Branson RD: Delivery systems for inhaled nitric oxide, *Respir Care Clin North Am* 3:371, 1997.

30. Branson RD, et al: Inhaled nitric oxide systems and monitoring, *Respir Care* 44:281, 1999.

31. Curry S: Methemoglobinemia, *Ann Emerg Med* 11:214, 1982.

32. Jacob TD, et al: Hemodynamic effects and metabolic fate of inhaled nitric oxide in hypoxic piglets, *J Appl Physiol* 76:1794, 1994.

33. Papamoschou D: Theoretical validation of the respiratory benefits of helium–oxygen mixtures, *Respir Physiol* 99:183, 1995.

34. Barach AL: Use of helium as a new therapeutic gas, *Proc Soc Exp Biol Med* 32:462, 1934.

35. Barach AL: The therapeutic use of helium, *JAMA* 107:1273, 1936.

36. Barach AL: The use of helium in the treatment of asthma and obstructive lesions of the larynx and trachea, *Ann Intern Med* 9:739, 1935.

37. Barach AL: The use of helium as a new therapeutic gas, *Anesth Analg* 14:210, 1935.

38. Nunn JF: Diffusion and alveolar/capillary permeability. In *Applied respiratory physiology*, London, 1987, Butterworth, pp 184–206.

39. Anderson M, et al: Deposition in asthmatics of particles inhaled in air or helium–oxygen, *Am Rev Respir Dis* 147:524, 1993.

40. Svartengren M, et al: Human lung deposition of particles suspended in air or in helium/oxygen mixture, *Exp Lung Res* 15:575, 1989.

41. Bandi V, et al: Deposition pattern of heliox-driven bronchodilator aerosol in the airways of stable asthmatics, *J Asthma* 42:583, 2005.

42. Corcoran TE, et al: Aerosol drug delivery using heliox and nebulizer reservoirs: results from an MRI-based pediatric model, *J Aerosol Med* 16:263, 2003.

43. Melmed A, et al: The use of heliox as a vehicle for β-agonist nebulization in patients with severe asthma [abstract], *Am J Respir Crit Care Med* 151:A269, 1995.

44. Hess DR, et al: The effect of heliox on nebulizer function using a β-agonist bronchodilator, *Chest* 115:184, 1999.

45. PC Stillwell, et al: Effectiveness of open-circuit Oxyhood delivery of helium–oxygen, *Chest* 95:1222, 1989.

46. Ari A, Harwood R, Sheard M, Dailey P, Fink JB: In vitro comparison of heliox and oxygen in aerosol delivery using pediatric high flow nasal cannula, *Pediatr Pulmonol* 46(8):795, 2011. doi: 10.1002/ppul.21421.

47. Rogers MS, et al: Volume accuracy of the Siemens Servo 900C and Novametrix Ventrak when delivering helium oxygen mixtures [abstract], *Respir Care* 40:1206, 1995.

48. Wheeler DS, et al: Isoflurane therapy for status asthmaticus in children: a case series and protocol, *Pediatr Crit Care Med* 1:55, 2000.

49. Restrepo RD, Pettignano R, DeMeuse P: Halothane, an effective infrequently used drug, in the treatment of pediatric status asthmaticus: a case report, *J Asthma* 42:649, 2005.

50. Bishop MJ, Rooke GA: Sevoflurane for patients with asthma [letter], *Anesth Analg* 91:245, 2000.

51. Habre W, et al: Respiratory mechanics during sevoflurane anesthesia in children with and without asthma, *Anesth Analg* 89:1177, 1999.

52. Padkin AJ, Baigel G, Morgan GA: Halothane treatment of severe asthma to avoid mechanical ventilation, *Anesthesia* 52:994, 1997.

53. Miyagi T, et al: Prolonged isoflurane anesthesia in a case of catastrophic asthma, *Acta Paediatr Jpn* 39:375, 1997.

54. Carroll, CL, Smith SR, Collins MS, Bhandari A, Schramm CM, Zucker AR: Endotracheal intubation and pediatric status asthmaticus: site of original care affects treatment, *Pediatr Crit Care Med* 8(2):91, 2007. doi: 10.1097/01.PCC.0000257115.02573.FC.

55. Shankar V, Churchwell KB, Deshpande JK: Isoflurane therapy for severe refractory status asthmaticus in children, *Intensive Care Med* 32(6):927, 2006. doi: 10.1007/s00134-006-0163-0.

56. Rooke GA, Choi JH, Bishop MJ: The effect of isoflurane, halothane, sevoflurane, and thiopental/nitrous oxide on respiratory system resistance after trachea intubation, *Anesthesiology* 86:1294, 1997.

57. Habre W, Wildhaber JH, Sly PD: Prevention of methacholine induced changes in respiratory mechanics in piglets with sevoflurane and halothane, *Anesthesiology* 87:585, 1997.

58. Hirschman CA, et al: Mechanism of action of inhalational anesthesia on airways, *Anesthesiology* 56:107, 1982.

59. Stoelting R: *Pharmacology and physiology in anesthetic practice*, Philadelphia, 1987, JB Lippincott, p 45.

60. Johnson RG, et al: Isoflurane therapy for status asthmaticus in children and adults, *Chest* 97:698, 1990.

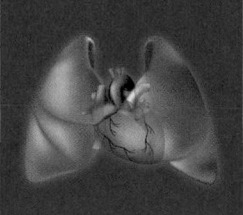

Chapter 19

Extracorporeal Membrane Oxygenation

PETER BETIT

LEARNING OBJECTIVES

After reading this chapter the reader will be able to:

1. Describe the extracorporeal membrane oxygenation systems
2. Explain the rationale for the use of extracorporeal membrane oxygenation in the management of respiratory and cardiac failure in newborns, infants, and children
3. Compare and contrast the various modes of support for extracorporeal membrane oxygenation
4. Describe the elements of monitoring the extracorporeal membrane oxygenation functions and patient response.
5. Identify complications associated with extracorporeal membrane oxygenation

KEY TERMS

Centrifugal pump
Extracorporeal membrane
  oxygenation

Hemofiltration
Oxygenation index
Roller pump

Sweep gas
Venoarterial
Venovenous

Extracorporeal membrane oxygenation (ECMO) is an invasive technique in which blood is drained from the venous system, mechanically pumped through an artificial lung, and reinfused to the patient through either the pulmonary or systemic systems. Components of an ECMO system are essentially modifications of cardiopulmonary bypass machines and are designed for longer duration of support, typically applied in an intensive care setting. The primary aim of ECMO is to support organ function in patients with respiratory or cardiorespiratory failure in order to provide time for the disease process to reverse or to further evaluate the underlying condition and determine if medical or surgical treatment options are available.[1]

BACKGROUND

The earliest forms of artificial gas exchange and mechanical circulatory support have been attributed to Gibbon, when in 1937 he reported the use of cardiopulmonary bypass during pulmonary artery occlusion in animals and in 1953 he successfully performed extracorporeal circulation in a human.[2,3] Gibbon's invention was a roller pump used as a substitute for the heart, and to achieve gas exchange, blood was distributed in a film along stainless steel screens vertically suspended in a plastic chamber.

The concept of artificial perfusion was further advanced by Lillehei and associates in 1955 when they reported a series of eight pediatric patients in whom cardiac surgery was performed, using the parent as the oxygenator.[4] Subsequently a bubble oxygenator was designed and successfully used in seven patients; however, the use of bubble oxygenators limited the duration of bypass to a few hours because the direct blood–gas interface resulted in hemolysis, denatured plasma proteins, and thrombus formation.[5]

There was further interest in developing a membrane oxygenator when the observation was made that blue venous blood entering a hemodialysis membrane turned red when the blood exited the membrane.[6] In 1956, Clowes reported the first clinical use of a membrane for gas exchange.[7] The membrane oxygenator was constructed of polyethylene and Teflon and for the first time eliminated the direct blood–gas interface; however, gas exchange was limited and the size of the membrane hindered its clinical application.

Subsequently silicone rubber was found to have gas transfer characteristics far superior to polyethylene, and in 1963 a silicone membrane was developed.[8] With this device the first extended bypass procedure was performed in animals, which demonstrated minimal hematological effect for up to 1 week.[9] This development paved the way for further interest in the application of long-term extracorporeal support.

The first successful use of ECMO was reported in 1972 when a 24-year-old man with multiple trauma and respiratory failure was maintained on extracorporeal support for 75 hours, during which time his lung injury resolved.[10] This prompted a multicenter, randomized prospective study of ECMO in adults with acute respiratory failure, and a collaborative study was published in 1979.[11] The results were discouraging, with only eight survivors: four in the conventional mechanical ventilation group and four in the ECMO group. The authors were forced to conclude that although ECMO could support gas exchange, it could not improve survival of patients with acute respiratory distress syndrome (ARDS). A number of factors may have led to the poor results of this trial. Some of the centers had limited or no experience with ECMO and a significant proportion of the patients had irreversible lung injury. Additionally this study took place in an era when lung protective ventilation was not fully appreciated.

Despite the disappointing results of the adult trial, the search continued to identify a population with reversible lung disease that could potentially benefit from ECMO. In 1976 Bartlett and Harken successfully used ECMO to support a neonate with meconium aspiration syndrome and essentially pioneered neonatal ECMO.[12] Their success continued, and in 1982 they reported a 55% survival rate in a series of 45 neonates treated with ECMO.[13]

By the mid-1980s, two prospective randomized trials comparing ECMO to conventional mechanical ventilation (CMV) were published. The study by Bartlett and colleagues reported 100% survival of the 11 patients receiving ECMO and 0% survival in the control group, albeit only one patient constituted the control group.[14] O'Rourke and colleagues subsequently reported 100% survival for nine ECMO patients, compared with 33% for six newborns treated conventionally.[15]

In early 1990s, ECMO emerged as a standard mode of support for newborns with acute respiratory failure unresponsive to maximal medical treatment. This acceptance occurred despite the limited number of randomized controlled trials. In 1996 the UK Collaborative ECMO Trial Group reported the results of a trial that assessed whether a policy of ECMO referral was beneficial on survival to 1 year without severe disability when compared with conventional management.[16] Recruitment to the trial was stopped early because an interim analysis of the data suggested a clear advantage with ECMO. The results of this study left little doubt that ECMO was and remains an effective lifesaving treatment for neonates with severe respiratory failure.

Throughout the eighties and nineties, a number of neonatal ECMO programs were established and in 1989 the Extracorporeal Life Support Organization (ELSO, Ann Arbor, MI), was formed.[17] The mission of this organization is to coordinate clinical research in extracorporeal techniques, to develop guidelines, and to maintain an ECMO registry. Although ELSO is based in the United States, a number of centers from around the world have joined this collaborative organization, which has a membership of more than 150 active ECMO centers. The ELSO Registry collects and compiles data, including demographic, complication, and outcome statistics for neonatal, pediatric and adult applications and has entries for more than 50,000 ECMO cases.[17]

USES OF EXTRACORPOREAL MEMBRANE OXYGENATION

ECMO continues to be a vital component of newborn and pediatric critical care medicine. It is used to support newborns, infants, and children with near fatal respiratory and cardiac failure and continues to serve as the ultimate safety net as advance therapies, medications, and surgical options are explored.[1] Table 19-1 summarizes the use of ECMO in neonates and pediatrics.

TABLE 19-1

Overall Summary of ECMO Use in Neonates and Pediatrics: Extracorporeal Life Support Organization, ECLS Registry Report[17]

Neonates	Total Cases	Survival (%)
Respiratory support	25,746	19,232 (75%)
Cardiac support	4797	1912 (40%)
Pediatrics		
Respiratory Support	5475	3061 (56%)
Cardiac Support	5976	2913 (49%)
Total	41,994	27,118 (65%)

Neonatal Hypoxemic Respiratory Failure

More than 26,000 newborns with respiratory failure have been reported in the ELSO Registry, which represents the bulk of the neonatal ECMO experience.[17] This includes patients with the diagnosis of persistent pulmonary hypertension of the newborn (PPHN), meconium aspiration syndrome (MAS), respiratory distress syndrome (RDS), sepsis, and air leak syndromes, all reversible conditions, which is a key element for positive outcomes when providing ECMO.

The classic trajectory of neonatal hypoxemic respiratory failure typically begins with evidence of respiratory distress shortly after birth, which progresses to a point where tracheal intubation, assisted ventilation, and supplemental oxygen are required. Conventional mechanical ventilation is used initially and high-frequency ventilation often deployed when near-injurious conventional ventilator settings are required or when air leaks occur.[18] Adjunct therapies, including surfactant replacement therapy and inhaled nitric oxide (iNO), are also used.[19,20] The physiology and clinical management of these conditions are well described in Chapter 14 Surfactant Replacement Therapy and Chapter 18 Administration of Gas Mixtures.

The majority of these neonates can be managed with pharmacological and mechanical ventilation—conventional or high frequency. A small percentage are unresponsive to conventional measures manifested in varying degrees of respiratory acidosis, hypoxemia, pre- and postductal shunting, right ventricular dysfunction associated with pulmonary hypertension, and overall poor perfusion and organ function.[21] Before the availability of ECMO, many of these babies died. Using ECMO aids in interrupting the cycle of pulmonary hypertension, improves perfusion and organ function, and allows the use of lung-protective mechanical ventilation.[21]

One particularly challenging disease, occurring in approximately 1 in 2200 births, is congenital diaphragmatic hernia (CDH).[22] The physiology of this disease, well described in Chapter 22 Neonatal Complications and Pulmonary Disorders is characterized by the incomplete formation of the fetal diaphragm and migration of the abdominal contents into the thoracic cavity, which disrupts fetal lung development and causes lung hypoplasia and pulmonary hypertension. Although conventional measures, including lung-protective ventilation, iNO, high-frequency ventilation, and delayed surgical repair, have improved survival, a portion of these infants continue to be supported with ECMO.[23] However, the role of ECMO is unclear and somewhat controversial because the degree of lung hypoplasia and pulmonary hypertension is difficult to predict.[23] Some centers have adopted a philosophy that if conventional interventions fail, the degree of lung hypoplasia and subsequent pulmonary hypertension is considered non–life sustaining and ECMO is felt to be futile.[24] Nonetheless, ECMO continues to be used as somewhat of a rescue modality, but the ELSO survival rates have remained stagnant at around 50% since the availability of ECMO.[17]

Selection Criteria

An important aspect guiding the decision to use ECMO, because it is associated with a number of risks, is the reversible nature of the neonate's underlying condition and the timing of the decision.[25] During the early ECMO era, this decision was made subjectively until more objective criteria were later developed.

Bartlett and colleagues suggested the use of the neonatal pulmonary insufficiency index, which plotted pH and FIO_2 over time to a point at which the risk of mortality exceeded 80%.[13] However, the index was deemed unsuitable for patients who had pharmacologically induced alkalosis as a treatment for pulmonary hypertension.

Krummel and colleagues reported that an alveolar–arterial oxygen gradient (PAO_2–PaO_2; also $(A-a)DO_2$) greater than 620 mm Hg for 6 to 12 hours was indicative of an 80% risk of mortality. However, this criterion was not useful in the neonate who rapidly deteriorated.[26]

Ortega and colleagues proposed the **oxygenation index** (OI), a calculation based on mean airway pressure ($P\overline{aw}$), FIO_2, and arterial oxygenation (PaO_2), as follows:

$OI = P\overline{aw} \times (FIO_2/PaO_2) \times 100$.[27] The authors found that when the OI exceeded 40 during conventional mechanical ventilation, the risk of mortality exceeded 80%. Their results have been reproduced by other institutions, and the OI remains a widely accepted predictor of mortality in neonates with respiratory failure and is used as part of the selection criteria for using ECMO.

The introduction of high-frequency oscillatory ventilation (HFOV) decreased the need for ECMO and is a standard of care in the management of hypoxemic respiratory failure.[28] Because HFOV uses higher mean airway pressure than CMV, an OI of 60 has been considered a more realistic threshold for identifying mortality risk and the need for ECMO when this form of ventilation is used.[29,30]

ECMO use declined further in the late 1990s with the discovery of the selective pulmonary vasodilator properties of iNO and its subsequent approval by the Food and Drug Administration.[19] During the iNO clinical trials, it became apparent that HFOV combined with iNO was optimal and further reduced the need for ECMO by nearly 35%.[20]

HFOV and iNO are no longer limited to specialty centers that have ECMO capabilities and are commonly used in most newborn intensive care units (ICUs). This paradigm shift initially led to concerns that there may be increased mortality in patients who do not respond well to treatment and become too unstable to transfer to an ECMO center.[29] Thus timing is an important factor in determining the use of ECMO. The OI trend, level of support, ability to transport with iNO, and distance to an ECMO center need to be factored into the decision process.[29] A few studies have suggested that mortality has not increased when advanced therapies have been employed and that these therapies lessen the severity of illness at the point of ECMO initiation and do not prolong the time to ECMO.[30]

Contraindications to ECMO in the newborn have become less clear. In the early ECMO epoch, prolonged positive-pressure ventilation was felt to be injurious, thus creating an irreversible condition.[31] With a greater understanding of lung-protective ventilation techniques, there is less concern that chronic lung disease will develop, assuming true lung-protective strategies have been employed. Typically the need for ECMO is identified within the first couple of days. The need for ECMO after a prolonged period of mechanical ventilation, such as 7 to 10 days, may suggest an atypical, potentially irreversible pathological lung condition.[32]

Another consideration for deciding not to use ECMO is the patient's size and gestational age. There are ECMO catheter size limitations for newborns less than 2 kg, and newborns younger than 32 weeks of gestation may be at greater risk for developing intracranial hemorrhage when exposed to anticoagulants. The presence of preexisting intracranial bleeds staged beyond I or II is an added risk with ECMO because anticoagulation may worsen the bleed and result in poor neurological outcomes. The use of antifibrinolytic therapy may help abate the progression of bleeding.[33] Additional relative contraindications include the presence of known fatal congenital anomalies and bleeding disorders. Box 19-1 summarizes patient selection criteria.

Respiratory Failure in Infants and Children

More than 5500 pediatric respiratory ECMO cases have been reported in the ELSO registry, with patients ranging in age from 1 month to 18 years.[17] This group of ECMO cases consists of a less homogeneous group of diagnoses compared with the newborn experience. The broad categories include infectious and aspiration pneumonias and ARDS associated with trauma, surgery, or medical conditions. The role of ECMO in the treatment of severe respiratory failure in infants and children is not well defined because there have been few studies aimed at trying to make this determination.[34]

Box 19-1	ECMO Selection Criteria for Newborns with Hypoxemic Respiratory Failure

- Diagnoses
  - Persistent pulmonary hypertension of the newborn
  - Meconium aspiration syndrome
  - Respiratory distress syndrome
  - Neonatal sepsis
  - Congenital diaphragmatic hernia
  - Air leak syndromes
- Oxygen index more than 40 with CMV and more than 60 with HFOV
- Absence of fatal congenital anomalies
- Reversible lung disease
- Age more than 32 weeks of gestation
- No major intraventricular hemorrhage

CMV, Conventional mechanical ventilation; *HFOV,* high-frequency oscillatory ventilation.

The Pediatric Study Group compared ECMO and non-ECMO groups based on the Pediatric Risk of Mortality (PRISM) score, with the ECMO cohort demonstrating improved survival.[35] Thirty-two centers participated in this study, which included 331 patients. However, only 50% of the centers had ECMO capabilities and only 38 patients were supported with ECMO. This research project was to be the impetus for a randomized controlled trial but none was ever conducted.

The use of ECMO in children with severe septicemia has been described in case series with survival rates of up to 55%.[36,37] ECMO has also been used to support patients with swine-origin influenza A, trauma, and multiorgan systems failure.[38] Creech et al. described the use of ECMO in children with life-threatening methicillin-resistant *Staphylococcus aureus*.[39] In this retrospective review of 45 children, survival rates varied depending on age, with children in the 1- to 4-year group having the best survival at 65%. There were no common pre-ECMO assessments identified to be associated with an increased risk of death.

There is no definitive consensus on when ECMO should be initiated in pediatric respiratory failure. Single-center reviews have attempted to identify pre-ECMO factors that may help predict outcome. Mehta and colleagues suggested that an OI greater than 35 or a pre-ECMO pH of less than 7.20 may result in higher mortality.[40] In a case series by Turner et al., it was suggested that there are no true contraindications to using ECMO in pediatric patients with refractory respiratory failure. They further commented that ECMO is appropriate if patients are transferred to an ECMO center early, if lung-protective ventilation is used, and if severe neurological injury is not present.[38] A PaO_2/FIO_2 ratio of less than 200 mm Hg is one criteria used to identify patients with ARDS, and in severe cases the PaO_2/FIO_2 ratio may be less than 75 and mortality risk exceeds 80%, a point when ECMO is considered.[41]

The decision to initiate ECMO in pediatric patients with refractory respiratory failure may mean the difference between life and death.[42] Once advance treatments fail, ECMO is often the only remaining option. Pre-ECMO management, the reversible nature of the patient's underlying problem, and the potential to exacerbate complications with ECMO are fundamental to formulating a decision. Ideally, the patient will have been transferred to an ECMO center early, managed with lung-protective ventilation, and does not have any known incurable co-morbidities. Monitoring the trajectory of illness with indicators such as the OI, PRISM score, PaO_2/FIO_2 ratio, and pH may aid the decision process.[43]

Cardiac Applications

The development of mechanical circulatory support devices, from implantable artificial hearts to external ventricular assist devices, continues to be a burgeoning field, and ECMO continues to play an important role as these devices move from experimentation to approved applications.[44]

The availability of ECMO is an important facet in the medical-surgical management of congenital heart disease (CHD).[45] In the preoperative period, ECMO is used to augment cardiac output and support organ function until palliative or corrective surgery is undertaken.[46,47] ECMO is also used in the postoperative period, particularly in complex CHD, as more challenging surgical repairs are attempted. ECMO has also been used during interventional procedures.[48]

Patients with cardiac muscle disease, such as fulminant myocarditis or cardiomyopathy, may have such poor heart function that mechanical support with ECMO is necessary.[49] Although other mechanical circulatory support devices can provide equivalent support, ECMO systems are more readily available and can be implemented in the ICU. When cardiac function fails to recover, ECMO becomes a key support device while heart transplantation options or other support devices are considered.[44]

The use of ECMO for cardiac support continues to grow annually particularly as an aid to resuscitation, or ECMO during cardiopulmonary resuscitation, referred to as ECPR.[50] In this scenario ECMO and the associated surgical infrastructure are rapidly deployed to the bedside of a patient who is not responding to conventional resuscitative measures. Skilled teams with organized systems can accomplish cannulation and full ECMO support within 30 minutes.[51] Presuming quality cardiopulmonary resuscitation (CPR) is employed, patient outcomes are favorable, with survival rates around 40%,[17]considering that death would have been the alternative outcome. This approach is somewhat controversial because any patient who has a cardiopulmonary arrest is potentially a candidate for ECPR; however, survival without disability is dependent on the quality of the CPR, expeditious deployment, and an understanding of the patient's underlying condition.[52,53]

MODES OF ECMO SUPPORT

Venoarterial

ECMO support begins by accessing the vasculature in order to establish drainage and reinfusion sites. In newborns and infants, perfusion cannulas are surgically placed in a vein—commonly the right internal jugular—and an artery—usually the right common carotid. This is the classic **venoarterial** (VA) configuration in which deoxygenated venous blood is drained from the patient and blood that is fully saturated with oxygen is artificially pumped and returned to the arterial system (Figure 19-1, *A*).[54] This method provides support of lung and heart function. VA ECMO may also be established by accessing femoral arteries and veins or the heart directly by a transthoracic access, which is commonly used in postoperative cardiac patients.[55] This is referred to as central cannulation and has also been used in patients with profound septic shock.[35]

Oxygen delivery is provided by a combination of blood flow generated by the ECMO system and by the patient's own cardiopulmonary system.[54] The delivery of oxygen is a function of the oxygen content of the blood and the cardiac output, both of which can be augmented during VA ECMO. When the ECMO pump speed is increased, the blood flow rate increases and more of the patient's output is handled by the ECMO system. At maximal performance, about 80% of the patient's cardiac output is supported by ECMO. Oxygenated blood is reinfused to the patient and combines with the patient's native circulation. The oxygen content of the patient's blood therefore depends on the relative contributions of each system. For example, take a neonate with severe lung disease: As more blood is handled by the ECMO system, less is circulated through the native lungs, and gas exchange improves. Because of this parallel circulation, an increase in systemic PaO_2 during ECMO may reflect improving lung function, meaning an increased PaO_2 in the native circulation, or decreasing native cardiac output. Changes in tissue oxygen consumption and hemoglobin concentration will also alter oxygen content.[54]

Similarly CO_2 elimination is also a reflection of the combined blood flow of the ECMO system and the native cardiac output. As more blood is shunted—increased ECMO flow rate—the artificial membrane is the principal route by which CO_2 is removed. As lung function improves and pulmonary blood increases, the native functions of the lung assume more responsibility in CO_2 elimination.

The VA route, although effective in supporting heart and lung functions, does so in a nonpulsatile manner unlike native cardiac function.[56] The diversion of blood away from the native cardiopulmonary system results in less pulsatile flow to the organs and disruption of the normal blood flow patterns. Additionally, because of the combination of the reinfusion cannula orientation in the distant aortic arch and poorly oxygenated blood leaving the left ventricle, lower oxygen delivery to the coronary arteries may occurr.[57] Another potential disadvantage to venoarterial

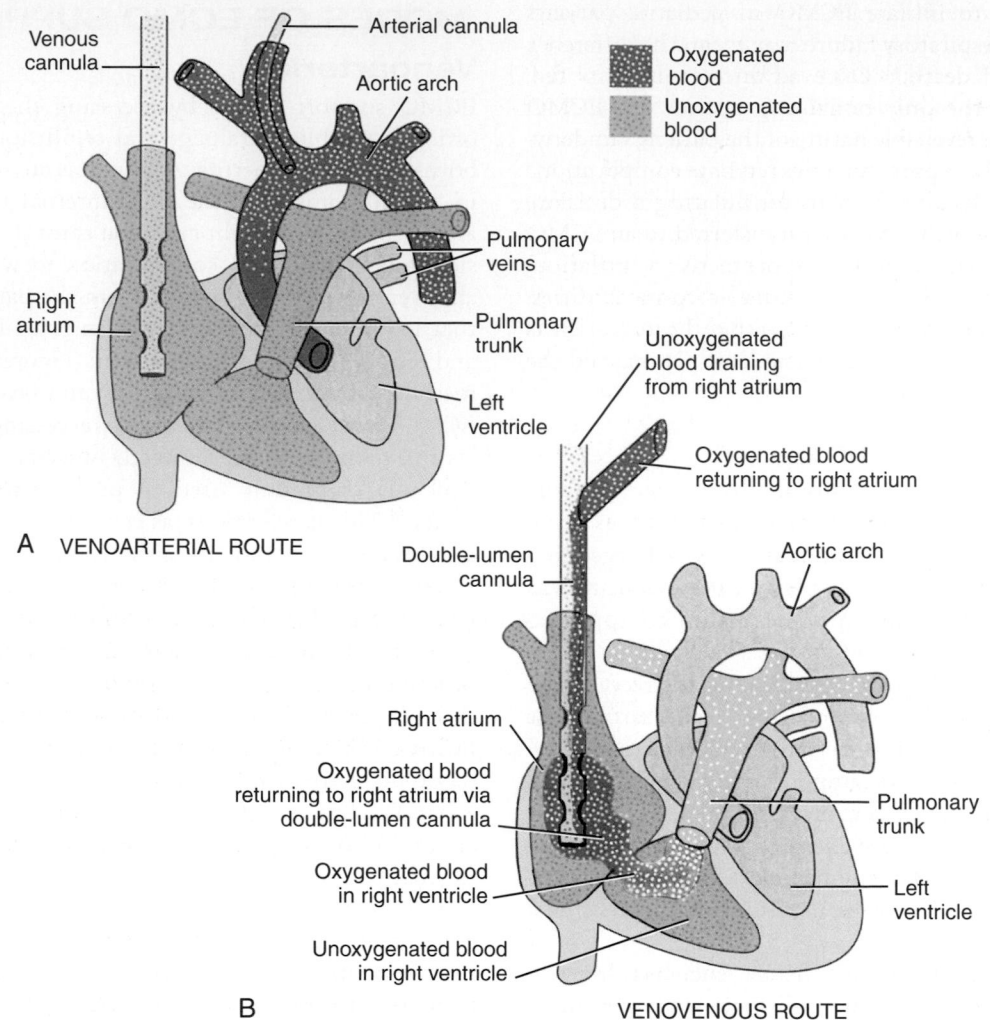

FIGURE 19-1 Mechanisms of blood flow during extracorporeal membrane oxygenation (ECMO). **A,** In the venoarterial route, blood is removed from the right atrium via a cannula inserted in the right internal jugular vein. Oxygenated blood is returned to the aortic arch via a cannula in the right common carotid artery. The shaded area indicates unoxygenated blood. **B,** In the venovenous route, blood is also removed from the right atrium via a cannula inserted in the right internal jugular vein, but the oxygenated blood is returned to the venous circulation. The shaded area indicates unoxygenated blood. Blood in the pulmonary trunk has been oxygenated via the cardiopulmonary bypass machine.

support is that any particle or bubble in the circuit may be directly infused into the arterial circulation and may lead to embolus formation.[58]

Venovenous

In **venovenous** (VV) support, blood is both drained and reinfused back into the venous circulation at the same rate, thereby providing only pulmonary support.[59] The oxygenated blood mixes with the venous blood in the right atrium, raising the oxygen content and lowering carbon dioxide. Because both the drainage and reinfusion cannulas are in the venous system, some of the oxygenated blood returns to the circuit. This phenomenon, known as recirculation, decreases the efficiency of gas transfer between circuit and patient. The degree of recirculation is monitored by comparing the oxygen saturation of the venous drainage ($S\bar{v}O_2$)

with the patient's arterial oxygen saturation (SaO_2).[60,61] If $S\bar{v}O_2$ is greater than SaO_2, the recirculation is excessive, which would require either an adjustment in cannula position or change in blood flow rate. VV ECMO does not provide the same level of oxygenation as VA, and the maximal SaO_2 achievable can be as low as 85% until lung function improves. Because VV ECMO is essentially operating in series with the native circulation, alterations in cardiac output will not have a significant effect on oxygenation. The volume of blood removed is equal to the volume reinfused, so there is also no effect on the patient's hemodynamics.

One advantage of VV support is that carotid artery ligation is not required, full pulsatile native blood flow is maintained, and the potential for air or particulate emboli from the circuit is less.[62] A disadvantage is the lack of cardiovascular support. However, the presence of mild to moderate myocardial dysfunction should not discourage the use of the VV approach as the improved oxygenation and lower airway pressures achieved with implementation of VV ECMO often improve cardiac function.[56] If myocardial dysfunction does not improve or worsens, however, conversion to VA support generally remains an option.[59]

VV is the preferred mode of ECMO support in infants and children with respiratory failure and is accomplished through either a two-cannula approach (VV),[61] a double-lumen cannula (VVDL),[62] or a bicaval dual-lumen cannula.[63] In the two-cannula method, blood is drained from a femoral vein and reinfused through the right internal jugular vein.[64] Although the femoral vein could serve as the reinfusion site, return to the right side of the heart helps lessen recirculation and improve systemic oxygenation. In the larger patient, a second drainage cannula, established through the opposite femoral vein, may be needed to improve drainage in order to increase ECMO pump flow rate, hence VVV—two femoral venous drainage cannulas and one reinfusion.[61]

Another approach to establishing VV support is the use of a single cannula that has two channels or lumens—one for drainage and one for reinfusion—with the drainage lumen representing two thirds of the diameter and the reinfusion one third.[62] The cannula is placed in the right internal jugular vein and is oriented with the reinfusion lumen superiorly so that the oxygenated blood returning to the right atrium is predominantly directed toward the tricuspid valve and subsequently the pulmonary circulation, which helps minimize recirculation (Figure 19-1, *B*). These cannulas had been limited to patients 10 kg or less until bicaval dual-lumen cannulas were developed. Bicaval dual-lumen cannulas provide concurrent drainage and reinfusion similar to the infant VVDL cannulas, with the difference being the presence of two drainage ports—one situated in the superior vena cava and one in the inferior vena cava.[65] Proper orientation of this cannula is critical so that arterialized blood is streamlined in the right atrium.[66,67]

ECMO SYSTEMS

ECMO systems consist of durable components, including the pump, monitoring modules, gas metering devices, and water pump, and the ECMO circuit consisting of customized tubing kits, membrane oxygenator, and heater exchanger. Although there are institution-specific circuit designs and durable component preferences, the mechanics are fairly universal and are best comprehended by considering the path of blood from drainage to reinfusion.

Blood is always drained from the venous system, by gravity or actively through tubing connected to the venous cannula. Blood then flows to the pump and, in many designs, passes through a venous chamber or reservoir that serves as a safety mechanism and a place to monitor venous drainage. The blood path proceeds to the pump, which is either a peristaltic roller design or centrifugal.

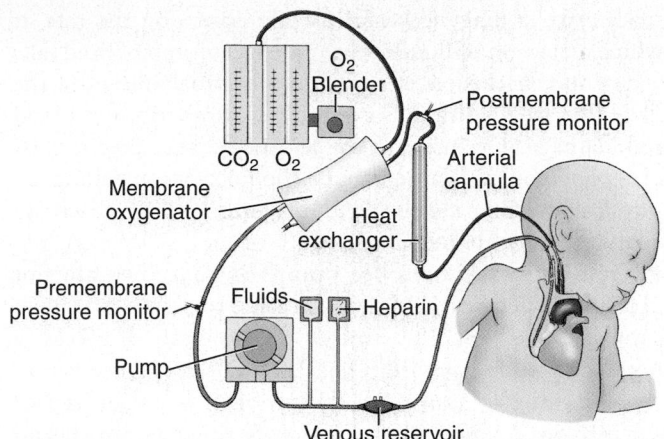

FIGURE 19-2 Circuit for extracorporeal life support. Classic ECMO circuit—infant, VA mode, roller pump, and silicone membrane.

At this point the blood is still deoxygenated until it traverses the artificial lung or membrane oxygenator where gas exchange occurs. Blood, fully saturated with oxygen, exits the membrane and is pumped into the reinfusion limb of the circuit where it is warmed in a heat exchanger and is then returned to the patient, thus completing the loop. Along the ECMO circuit there are ports for monitoring various pressures and for obtaining blood samples.[54] Figure 19-2 depicts the classic ECMO circuit arrangement.

Pumps

Pumps used for ECMO are either occlusive roller pumps or nonocclusive centrifugal pumps. The purpose of the pump is to propel the blood through the contiguous ECMO circuit from the patient to the membrane oxygenator and back to the patient. There is some debate as to which pump is more beneficial. ECMO centers established in the earlier years used roller pumps primarily because of availability and ease of use. In the present ECMO era centrifugal pumps are becoming predominant as pump head design and streamlined systems have been developed.[68]

Roller Pumps

Roller pumps are positive displacement devices that operate on the principle of compression and displacement, with flow being achieved by the compression of a tubing segment between the pump's wall and two roller heads that are spaced 180 degrees apart. The second roller begins compressing the tubing as the first roller is finishing; therefore the raceway is always being compressed. The tubing in the pump housing is referred to as the raceway. The output depends on the size of the tubing, the rotations per minute (RPMs), and the tension or occlusion of the rollers on the raceway.

Evaluating raceway occlusion is essential; too much roller tension—overoccluding—may cause tubing damage and hemolysis, and too little roller tension—underoccluding—may result in inadequate flow. Occlusion adjustments are usually made with a dial mechanism while observing the rate at which a column of fluid drops. When a column of fluid falls 1 cm/min, occlusion is considered optimal—meaning the ideal flow rate with the least amount of raceway and blood cell damage. Occlusion may be judged less precisely by observing the peristaltic kick of the post-pump tubing, by physically feeling a pulse in the tubing, and by observing changes in membrane pressures.

One drawback to roller pumps is that they are not pressure dependent and will continue to pump to deliver preset RPMs, which determines the flow rate. If excessive pressure builds up within the ECMO circuit, the pump will continue to spin until the problem is recognized or rupture occurs. For safe operation, a roller pump should incorporate a venous servoregulation system that consists of a compliant venous reservoir or bladder that resides in a stand placed close to the floor. This aids gravity drainage, which is the principal mechanism by which blood is introduced into a roller pump system. When venous return is sufficient to meet the demands of the flow rate, the venous reservoir is full and the roller pump spins freely at the set speed. As venous drainage decreases, the reservoir becomes less full and may even collapse completely, and either a mechanical switch in the bladder stand or pressure monitoring relays this change in drainage volume to the pump, which will in turn slow its speed or stop all together. Without this servoregulation, the pump will continue to operate and eventually generate significant negative pressure and cause air entrainment. The classic venous reservoir is oriented horizontally and is prone to clot formation because of stagnant areas. A more vertically designed reservoir known as "the better bladder" eliminates stagnant zones and clotting potential and allows it to be positioned off the floor and closer to the patient. Pressure monitoring of venous reservoir is the more common approach to providing servoregulation for roller pumps.

Roller pumps are set to deliver a particular flow rate by adjusting RPMs. This results in the delivery of a consistent flow rate despite changes in patients' hemodynamics. However, there is constant wear and tear on the raceway tubing and a raceway rupture is possible. This risk can be lessened if highly durable tubing with a larger diameter is used, allowing for fewer RPMs along with periodic shifting of the raceway to distribute wear and tear across the length of the raceway.

Centrifugal Pumps

Centrifugal pumps are nonocclusive devices; energy is transferred to the blood by a rapidly rotating cone-shaped pump head that creates a constrained vortex.[69] Blood is actively pulled inward and propelled outward by the energy created by the vortex; thus drainage is considered active. Because this type of pump is nonocclusive it is dependent on the patient's preload and afterload. As preload decreases, such as decreased venous drainage, or if afterload increases because of increased systemic vascular resistance,

flow will decrease. Typically RPMs are set and the patient's preload and afterload influence the amount of flow delivered. In contrast to roller pumps, excessive pressurization will not occur, but flow delivery to the patient will be more variable.

One feature of this type of pump is that shorter ECMO circuits can be used because a venous reservoir is not needed. Earlier centrifugal pump head designs caused more hemolysis because blood came in contact with the rotating parts. Modern centrifugal pump heads use a more floating head design so that blood passes over impellers that move the blood along with less contact.[69]

Artificial Gas Exchange Devices

Artificial gas exchange devices, also known as membrane oxygenators or diffusion membranes, substitute the oxygen and carbon dioxide exchange mechanism of the native lung. These devices are separated into gas and blood compartments and are highly efficient. There are two general types of membranes, silicone and microporous.

Silicone Membrane

Most of the experience in ECMO has been with the silicone rubber membrane originally designed by Kolobow and Bowman.[8] This membrane consists of a flat silicone membrane envelope wound in a spiral coil around a polycarbonate spool[70] (Figure 19-3). The blood path and gas channel are separated by the semipermeable silicone membrane. While the blood is pumped through its compartment, a ventilating gas, known as the **sweep gas,** flows countercurrent through the gas compartment. The sweep gas provides a constant fresh source of oxygen and provides rapid removal of carbon dioxide by the creation of a gradient or driving pressure. Silicone membranes come in various sizes and surface areas. These devices are somewhat time consuming to prepare because meticulous deairing by physical tapping is required to ensure that air embolisms do not occur once connected to the patient.

Gas transfer across the membrane depends on the composition of the gas, the thickness of the membrane, the surface area, and the difference in the partial pressure of the gases on each side of the membrane. This partial-pressure difference is referred to as the driving pressure or the transmembrane pressure.

The driving pressure is different for each gas. For example, if the concentration of the sweep gas is 100% O_2, the P_{O_2} in the gas channel will be 760 mm Hg, and assuming the venous P_{O_2} entering the blood compartment will be approximately 30 mm Hg to 40 mm Hg, there will be an O_2 driving pressure of 730 mm Hg (760 − 30 mm Hg), moving oxygen into the blood (Figure 19-4). The driving pressure of CO_2 is significantly less—0 on the gas side and 48 mm Hg in the blood, so only a 48 mm Hg force moves CO_2 into the gas compartment. Despite this small driving pressure, however, CO_2 exchange is efficient because silicone rubber is six times more permeable to CO_2 than to O_2. Because of this efficiency,

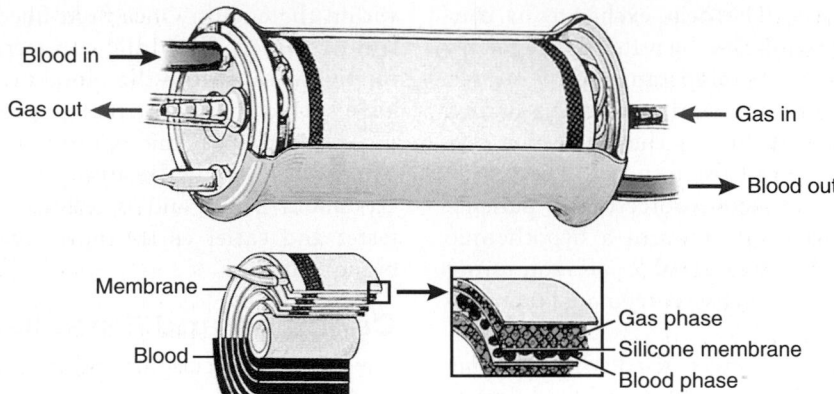

FIGURE 19-3 Diagram of membrane oxygenator (*top*) and the membrane unwound (*bottom*) to demonstrate the large surface area used for gas exchange.

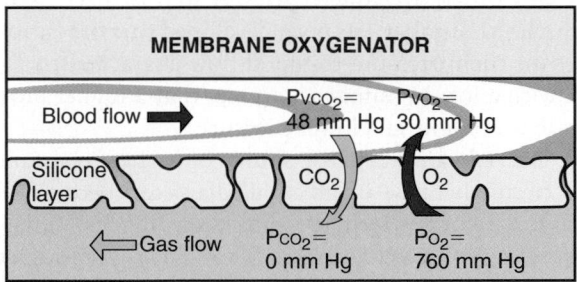

FIGURE 19-4 Schematic drawing of the membrane oxygenator, illustrating separation of blood and gas compartments, with transfer of gases across the silicone membrane because of a pressure gradient. Pco_2, Carbon dioxide partial pressure; Po_2, oxygen partial pressure; $Pvco_2$, mixed venous carbon dioxide pressure; Pvo_2, mixed venous oxygen pressure.

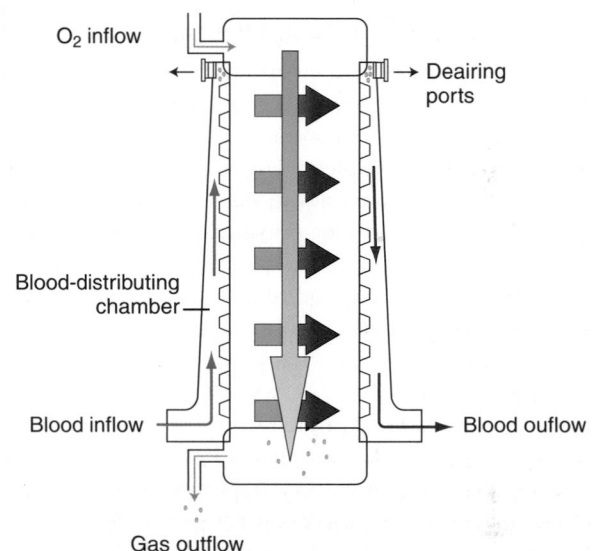

FIGURE 19-5 Diagram of a microporous membrane oxygenator. (From Meyer A, Struber M, Fischer S. Advances in extracoporeal ventilation. *Anesthesiol Clin* 2008;26:381.)

sweep gas composition is typically a combination of O_2 and CO_2, commonly referred to carbogen. The transfer rate of O_2 is also limited by the thickness of the blood film between the membrane layers. As the blood film becomes thicker, the oxygenating efficiency decreases.

Carbon dioxide clearance decreases as water accumulates in the gas compartment of the membrane, because of the temperature difference between the two sides of the membrane. The warm blood and the cooler gas allow condensation to occur. A minimal fresh gas flow is required for continuous flushing of these water droplets. Unfortunately, the minimal flow rate required to remove condensation usually results in excessive elimination of carbon dioxide as well. To compensate for this, sweep gas is often blended with a carbogen mixture, which reduces the driving pressure across the membrane and maintains normocarbia.

Microporous Membrane

Microporous or hollow-fiber membranes are made of woven capillaries of microporous plastic. Gas passes through the capillaries while blood flows around them[71] (Figure 19-5). The microporous membrane has excellent gas exchange capabilities and low resistance and is easy to prime and deair. Older versions were prone to condensation or wetability,

and plasma leakage occurred over long durations, which made it less desirable for long-term use.[72] However, advances have been made in microporous technology with the introduction of polymethylpentene-sealed fibers, which resists the wetting-out or leaking phenomenon.[70]

Gas exchange in this type of membrane occurs by simple diffusion, which is influenced by the composition of sweep gas and the blood flow rate.

Temperature Regulation

As blood travels through the ECMO circuit, heat is continually lost from the exposed surface of the tubing and through the oxygenator because of the cooling effects of the sweep gas and water evaporation. Therefore the ECMO system has to have the capability of providing temperature regulation. This is accomplished by either the addition of a separate heat exchanger, such as used with a silicone membrane, or with an integral heat exchanger common to most microporous devices. The heat exchanger is connected to a water pump that heats the water and regulates the temperature. The patient's temperature is monitored and the temperature of the water is adjusted to maintain a target temperature range. Although the water pump is mainly used for warming, it can also be used for cooling, a strategy employed to aid in neuroprotection of patients after resuscitation, or to slowly rewarm a hypothermic patient. Water pumps are also capable of monitoring blood temperature and providing servoregulated temperature control.[72]

In the add-on heat exchanger used with silicone membranes, water flow is countercurrent to blood flow to improve heat transfer. In microporous membranes the water flows through integral fibers adjacent to blood fibers for maximum heating.

Circuits and Circuit Preparation

ECMO circuits consist of a contiguous loop of polyvinyl chloride tubing arranged in a sterile pack that contains all the necessary disposable components to easily and sometimes rapidly prepare a system for patient use. Most institutions have designed configurations based on the type of pump used and the patient population. The ideal ECMO circuit should be as streamlined as possible, contain minimal access points, and be long enough to have a safe distance between pump and patient while minimizing overall circuit volume. Another attribute that is somewhat debatable is use of components that are coated with biocompatible substances composed of protein- and heparin-based compounds, which may make the circuit less thrombogenic and trigger less of an inflammatory response—the circuit being less foreign as blood comes in contact with it.[73,74]

Circuits designed for infants are mainly ¼ inch in diameter, with the exception of the raceway if a roller pump is used, in which case the raceway may be ⅜ inch so that lower RPMs may be used. Large-diameter tubing is used for larger patients who require higher flow rates—for instance, pediatric circuits usually contain ⅜-inch diameter tubing. ECMO circuits contain a small section of tubing between drainage and reinfusion limbs, referred to as a bridge. The purpose of the bridge is to maintain flow through the circuit while the patient is isolated from ECMO support during troubleshooting procedures or elective weaning trials.

Once a circuit is inspected and arranged on the ECMO system, a sequential priming procedure is performed; for a silicone membrane this includes flushing the circuit with CO_2, applying vacuum to the gas ports, fluid priming with a crystalloid solution, deairing, and finally blood priming. During the first step, the air-filled circuit is replaced with CO_2, which is highly soluble in blood and decreases the risk of microbubbles. Vacuum is applied to the gas ports of the membrane to help expand the blood compartment. This is followed by the introduction of the crystalloid solution, which completely fills all spaces

within the circuit. Once fluid filled, all access points are fluid primed and all connections double-checked for tightness. Before the blood-priming step, albumin is added, which provides a more biocompatible protein coating. Circuits with microporous membranes can be prepared more rapidly because the process begins with the crystalloid prime and is followed by deairing, which is faster and easier as air moves readily across the membrane's fibers.

Cannulas and Establishing Support

The ECLS circuit begins and ends with the cannulas. The cannulas chosen influence the maximal flow rate that the system can achieve. The ideal cannula should be thin walled to achieve the largest internal diameter possible, kink resistant, and radiopaque. Wire-reinforced cannulas have many of these characteristics. A standardized rating system, the M number, has been developed to score various devices on their pressure-to-blood flow characteristic.[75] A device with a low M number indicates that a higher blood flow rate is possible at a lower pressure.

The arterial cannula is the source of highest resistance in the circuit because of its small diameter. Because hemolysis can occur at system pressures exceeding 350 mm Hg, it is important to select an arterial cannula large enough to handle the anticipated flow rates for a given patient.[60] The major differences between the venous and arterial cannulas are that the lower portion of the venous cannula has multiple side ports for optimal drainage, whereas the arterial cannula is shorter to reduce resistance. In addition to the diameter of the venous cannula, drainage depends on cannula position, right atrial pressure, and the height of the patient in a gravity-dependent roller pump system. Subtle manipulations of these variables may be necessary to optimize flow. The most common causes of a decrease in venous return include malpositioning of the venous cannula, kinking of the cannula, shifting of the mediastinum, and a hypovolemic state.

The cannulation procedure begins with the deployment of a surgical team, applicable instruments, and related equipment to the patient's bedside. While the patient is prepped, the ECMO specialist prepares the ECMO system and circuit. Establishing ECMO, although critical, is considered either elective, in which case the circuit is primed with blood, or emergent such as an ECPR application, when there is generally insufficient time to complete the full blood prime step. The surgeon and ECMO specialist confer on the mode of support, type of cannula, and alternatives if cannulation becomes difficult. Once the cannulas are surgically placed and secured, the ECMO circuit is connected to the patient with verification that drainage and reinfusion lines are connected to the correct cannulas. The ECMO pump is activated and several simultaneous observations are made, including hemodynamics, oxygen saturation, venous return, ability to achieve desired flow rates, ECMO circuit pressures, and patient temperature.

Once the ECMO flow is established and the patient has been stabilized, a chest radiograph is obtained to confirm cannula position, and on occasion echocardiography is used to further verify cannula position and flow patterns, particularly with VVDL.

Hemofiltration

It is not uncommon for patients requiring ECMO to develop renal insufficiency from pre-ECMO fluid resuscitation, acute renal dysfunction, and blood product replacement.[76] To augment renal function and remove larger quantities of fluid, a semipermeable membrane or **hemofilter** can be added to the ECMO circuit.[77] The semipermeable membrane, similar to hemodialysis filters, uses hydrostatic pressure to move plasma water from the high-pressure blood side across the low-pressure filter. This results in the removal of plasma water and medium-sized solutes but preserves large cell elements and protein in the blood.

The hemofilter is commonly positioned after the ECMO pump with the return occurring on the prepump side of the circuit—a postpump to prepump shunt. Filter effluence can be regulated by restricting the hemofilter outlet or using a secondary pump in order to achieve a specific output. Standalone renal replacement therapy systems are also used in series with the ECMO system. There are two approaches to using these filters, hemoconcentration and ultrafiltration. Hemoconcentration is the rapid removal of plasma water to reverse hemodilution associated with crystalloid priming. Ultrafiltration is a more gradual removal of fluid.[77]

CLINICAL MANAGEMENT

Anticoagulation

As blood comes in contact with the ECMO circuit, a layer of protein adheres to the foreign surfaces and ultimately a thrombus is formed. For blood to flow through the ECMO circuit, anticoagulation must be established and closely monitored. This is accomplished by the continuous infusion of heparin.[78]

Heparin has no direct anticoagulant effect on the blood by itself but combines with a cofactor, antithrombin III (ATIII), to prevent thrombi from forming. This stops the conversion of fibrinogen to fibrin and ultimately prevents blood from clotting. A deficiency in ATIII can cause heparin to be ineffective, resulting in use of excessive amounts of heparin. If excessive clotting in the circuit is noted, a deficiency in ATIII is a possible cause.[79]

The classic method for monitoring anticoagulation is by measuring the activated clotting time (ACT) with a point-of-care device. The heparin dose is titrated to achieve an ACT range of typically 160 to 180 seconds.[80] Although the ACT is a simple bedside test, it does not fully monitor the complex of the clotting system, and other laboratory tests, including monitoring anti-factor Xa activity in conjunction with ATIII, provide a more complete assessment.[81]

Monitoring Circuit Function

ECMO systems are equipped with integrated safety systems and adjunct components that provide continuous monitoring of various circuit functions.[82] The water pump previously described can be autoregulated with the use of a blood temperature probe placed within the membrane oxygenator. A particular temperature is targeted, and the water temperature is cooled or warmed accordingly.

There are adjunct devices that continuously monitor blood gases, chemistry values, and hematological parameters such as hemoglobin and hematocrit. These provide the ECMO specialist with early warning signs of physiological changes. Additional monitored parameters include venous saturation, which is mainly used to gauge the degree of recirculation during VV ECMO.

The O_2–CO_2 concentration of the sweep gas is regulated by flow meters from oxygen air blenders and standalone CO_2 cylinders. The sweep gas lines can contain an oxygen analyzer equipped with alarms that provide the user with warnings of low CO_2 cylinder pressure or inadvertent changes in sweep gas flow rate.

Circuit integrity is monitored by visually inspecting the circuit and components for thrombus and air, and by continuously monitoring pre- and postmembrane pressures. As circuit or membrane resistance changes, as is common with clot formation, the pressures will change. As an example, a membrane that has been used for a fairly prolonged duration will tend to develop clots and increased resistance, which would be identified by an increase in premembrane pressure.

Membrane function is also evaluated by periodically measuring pre-and postmembrane blood gases. Gas exchange across the membrane may become less efficient over prolonged ECMO duration, which may be diagnosed by changes in the pre- and post–blood gas values. For instance, a narrower pre- and postmembrane P_{CO_2} gradient is suggestive of a decrease in CO_2 elimination.

Another commonly used adjunct monitor measures the blood flow rate by an externally applied ultrasonic probe on the reinfusion limb of the circuit. This displays the true flow rate and is particularly important to observe when there are built-in shunts in the circuit such as used when adding hemofiltration.

An additional commonly used safety device is an air or bubble detector, which consists of a probe clipped onto the external aspect of the circuit and can be placed on either the drainage or reinfusion line. The purpose of the bubble detector is for blood flow to cease in the presence of an air bubble so that the bubble does not reinfuse into the patient and cause an air embolism, particularly concerning during VA ECMO because there is direct communication with the arterial system. Bubble-sensing devices are programmed to directly communicate with the pump so that if a bubble or microbubble is sensed, the pump immediately stops and a warning alarm signals. In some centrifugal pumps the air detection and flow measurement

Box 19-2	Circuit Integrity and Safety

- Circuit inspection
  - Air
  - Clots
- Adjunct monitoring
  - $S_{v}O_2$
  - Hemoglobin
  - Hematocrit
  - Blood flow rate
- Membrane function
  - Pre- and postmembrane pressures
  - Pre- and postmembrane blood gases
- Thermal regulation
  - Normothermia
  - Induced hypothermia
- Sweep gas adjustments
  - O_2-CO_2 combinations
- Safety features
  - Bubble detector
  - Drainage pressure
  - Membrane pressure alarms
  - Temperature alarms

occur with the same sensing mechanism integrated into the pump drive (Box 19-2).

Hemodynamics

Hemodynamic parameters are continuously monitored during ECMO and at a minimum heart rate and blood pressure. In the cardiac patient additional heart pressures, such as central venous, left atrial, and pulmonary artery pressures, may be also monitored. Observing changes in blood pressure is imperative during ECMO, particularly in newborns because anticoagulation combined with hypertensive periods may result in an intracranial hemorrhage. Causes of hypertension include discomfort, increase in afterload, changes in neurological status, and sudden or inadvertent increases in ECMO pump flow rate. Hypotension is associated with increases in urine output, bleeding, decrease in afterload, cardiac tamponade, tension pneumothorax, or sudden or inadvertent decreases in pump flow rate. Additionally, roller pump occlusion that has loosened will cause a lower actual flow delivered to the patient even though the same RPMs are being used; this would result in a decrease in blood pressure.

During VV ECMO, blood pressure support may be needed initially until the patient's condition moves from the acute phase to a more stable period. Blood pressure is supported with the use of vasoactive agents and fluid replacement. As previously noted, VA ECMO supports cardiac function; therefore, blood pressure lability is not usually an issue unless the patient develops a capillary leak, in which fluid moves from the intravascular compartment to the extravascular space. The patient develops total body edema and preload falls to a point where drainage decreases and ECMO pump flows need to be reduced. When using centrifugal pumps, changes in preload and afterload affect pump flow rate, which in turn influences blood pressure.

In cardiac patients, particularly in the postoperative period, additional parameters including central venous pressure and left atrial pressure—the filling pressures of the heart—provide useful information on heart function. In the failing heart, high filling pressures are a sign the heart is not effectively ejecting. This can be remedied by increasing the mechanical support to relieve the heart's work. Occasionally an additional drainage cannula may be placed in the left atrium to help further unload the heart.

Organ Perfusion

Preserving end-organ perfusion by providing sufficient oxygen delivery to the tissues is the fundamental goal of supporting the patient with ECMO. This can be monitored by observing routine laboratory indices of hepatic, renal, and cardiac function and by also monitoring $S\overline{v}O_2$ and the patient's acid-base status. Tissue perfusion is dependent on adequate blood oxygen content and the delivery of that oxygen, which is influenced by the native cardiac output and the ECMO pump flow rate. In a high oxygen demand state the $S\overline{v}O_2$ may decrease from the usual normal of 75%; assuming the oxygen content of the blood is adequate— meaning sufficient hemoglobin—the delivery can be enhanced by increasing the ECMO flow rate.

During the acute postcannulation phase, the patient may require ECMO pump flow rates on the order of 100 to 150 ml/kg, which represents approximately 70% to 80% of the patient's cardiac output. The patient acid-base status may correct slowly or quickly depending on the disease and severity of illness in the pre-ECMO period. For instance, a patient with severe sepsis and profound metabolic acidosis will take longer to stabilize than a newborn with a primary respiratory problem. The septic patient may require higher ECMO flow rates, chemical buffering, and blood transfusions in order to clear or correct the acidemia.

Laboratory Tests

A series of laboratory tests are routinely monitored during an ECMO course and include blood and platelet counts, hemoglobin and hematocrit, blood gases, and also coagulation studies. The interaction of blood with the foreign surface of the ECMO circuit affects platelets the most. Platelets have a tendency to attach to areas in which fibrinogen is present, which causes a platelet consumption phenomenon, requiring the platelets to be transfused, generally on a daily basis. As previously noted, adequate hemoglobin levels are necessary to ensure sufficient oxygen content. Because periodic blood tests are required, the patient's hematocrit and therefore hemoglobin tend to fall but are easily corrected with periodic transfusions of packed red blood cells. In the bleeding patient, hematocrit is monitored more frequently so that transfusions are expedited. Coagulation studies, including prothrombin time and fibrinogen levels, are monitored and replaced with fresh frozen plasma and cryoprecipitate, respectively.

Neurological Assessment

Ensuring adequate perfusion to the brain is vital and is evaluated by physical examination and bedside imaging. To prevent inadvertent dislodgement of cannulas, patients requiring ECMO are kept sedated or, in very tenuous circumstances, chemically paralyzed, somewhat limiting the clinical neurological examination. In newborns, serial head ultrasounds are obtained to identify any development of intracranial bleeding.[83] Continuous near-infrared spectrometry may be used to gauge brain perfusion, and the availability of portable head CT scans is another welcome advancement.

In the early ECMO epoch it was not uncommon to maintain paralysis throughout the entire duration of ECMO.[84] As the learning curve tapered, clinicians became more comfortable with the conscious patient as long as the ECMO circuit and cannulas were secure and stable. Because ECMO was primarily used in newborns and carotid ligation and anticoagulation were unavoidable, intracranial hemorrhage became a primary concern and continues to be one of the greatest risks to the procedure.[85] However, the use of antifibrinolytic medications has allayed this concern somewhat because these medications can help minimize the progression of an intracranial hemorrhage so that the ECMO course can continue, and ECMO can be offered to the newborn with a preexisting but minor intracranial bleed.[86]

A recent paradigm shift has occurred with ECMO being used to support patients with more chronic conditions, such as cystic fibrosis, and as a bridge to lung transplantation.[87] Recognizing the waiting period for donor lungs could be long, ECMO centers are managing patients with minimal sedation, liberation from mechanical ventilation, and even ambulation. This aids in optimizing the patient's physical condition and permits the ability of the patient to interact, which enables a more complete neurological assessment.[88]

Respiratory Support

The goals of respiratory support vary depending on the reason for ECMO—primary cardiac versus primary respiratory. Regardless, because of the ability of an artificially manipulated gas exchange, a lung-protective approach is generally strived for. The patient requiring ECMO for a primary cardiac reason is not likely to have significant pulmonary issues, in which case the ventilator strategy is to maintain lung function as near normal. In this scenario the ECMO ventilator settings are minimized to achieve a tidal volume of around 5 to 7 ml/kg and PEEP to maintain sufficient end-expiratory lung volume—typical settings would be PCV-SIMV (pressure controlled ventilation – synchronized

intermittent mandatory ventilation), 10 to 12 breaths per minute, PIP/PEEP 25 to 27/5 to 7 cm H_2O. In the cardiac patient who has significant pre-ECMO pulmonary edema from heart failure, higher levels of PEEP may be applied until the heart is fully supported and the edema clears.

In patients with a primary respiratory indication for ECMO, the approach is to achieve what is commonly referred to as "lung rest." In these patients the pre-ECMO scenario likely would have necessitated the use of high mean airway pressures and advanced modes that would be near injurious, hence the need for ECMO. Once ECMO is established, the ventilator is adjusted to achieve a strict lung-protective approach.

In the classic ECMO case of a newborn with MAS and PPHN, ventilator settings would be PCV-SIMV, 12 to 15 breaths per minute, PIP/PEEP 25/5 cm H_2O with an FIO_2 of 0.40. Periodic chest radiographs would be obtained to gauge improvements in the disease process—the lung fields would have gradually and steadily improved aeration—and progressive increase in tidal volume would indicate improved lung compliance. After 5 to 7 days the patient would be ready to be assessed for a trial separation from ECMO. An infant or child with viral pneumonia would likely have a more prolonged ECMO course because the reversal process would take significantly longer. In this setting, resting settings may be similar to the newborn with MAS and PPHN, or a high level of CPAP such as 10 to 12 cm H_2O may be used to try to maintain some alveolar recruitment.[89] In contrast, the patient requiring ECMO for a primary air leak is maintained on very low ventilator settings to promote complete healing of the leak, and for the most recalcitrant air leaks, apneic oxygenation may be employed. Other respiratory support includes routine artificial airway care.

In VA support the ventilator FIO_2 is usually maintained at 0.40 to ensure that the coronary arteries receive oxygenated blood because reinfused blood preferentially streams to the descending aorta, whereas coronary perfusion is predominately from the ascending limb. Therefore blood returning to the left atrium will have a higher PaO_2 with the ventilator set to 0.40 as opposed to 0.21.

Fluid and Nutrition

Maintaining a neutral fluid balance is challenging during ECMO because in the pre-ECMO period patients typically receive large amounts of fluid, for blood pressure and cardiac output support, and resuscitation. Once ECMO is established, patients require periodic replacement of blood components, daily fluid associated with medication infusions, and nutrition. The patient who has near-normal renal function can typically handle the increase in fluid and with supplemental diuretics can achieve a neutral balance. Renal function may be impaired and worsen during ECMO in the patient who has experienced prolonged periods of hypoxemia and hypoperfusion in the period before ECMO.[76]

Preserving renal function is vital during ECMO and is hindered by the nonpulsatile nature of ECMO flow.

The longer the ECMO duration, the more likely that renal insufficiency will develop. If renal insufficiency persists despite diuretic therapy, it can be managed with the use of an inline hemofilter, as previously described, or a standalone continuous renal replacement therapy device. Dependence on artificial means of fluid removal is not recommended because renal insufficiency can lead to renal failure, in which case hemodialysis is required and complicates the post-ECMO transition.[76]

There is no consensus on the approach to nutrition during ECMO. One concern is that gastric motility is impaired with the use of sedation and paralytics. Hyperalimentation is commonly used, but more and more centers are becoming more liberal with the volume and caloric makeup of gastric feedings. Certainly a fully awake patient who is extubated but being maintained on long-term ECMO support may better tolerate gastric feeding than a heavy sedated neonate. Nonetheless, a nutrition plan has to be established and advanced as tolerated.

Box 19-3 describes general clinical management guidelines.

Box 19-3	General Clinical Management Guidelines

ANTICOAGULATION WITH CONTINUOUS HEPARIN INFUSION
- Ensure safe and therapeutic dose
  - Activated clotting time 180 to 200 seconds
  - Anti-factor Xa activity 0.3 to 0.7
  - Antithrombin III more than 70%

HEMODYNAMIC MONITORING
- Heart rate
- Blood pressure
- Filling pressures
- Temperature
- SpO_2

ORGAN PERFUSION
- Renal function
- Liver function tests

LABORATORY TESTS
- Gas exchange
  - Arterial blood gases
  - Lactic acid
  - Hematological

NEUROLOGICAL ASSESSMENTS
- Pupillary reflexes
- Pain and comfort
- Imaging

RESPIRATORY SUPPORT
- Lung-protective ventilation
- Airway clearance

FLUID AND NUTRITION
- Balance intakes and outputs
- Assess gastric motility

LIBERATION FROM ECMO

Once ECMO support is established and the patient is stable, much of the care, ongoing assessments, and procedures are routine and driven by standardized prescriber orders and treatment algorithms. As the patient's condition improves, the focus is directed toward assessing the patient's ability to be separated from ECMO support. There are two approaches, weaning and periodic testing, and these fundamental approaches apply to both cardiac and respiratory applications.

With respect to ECMO, weaning is considered the gradual reduction of ECMO flow rates with concomitant gradual increases in ventilator support. This approach, amendable to the respiratory patient, theoretically parallels the improvement in lung function. Once ECMO flow rates are weaned to around 20 to 30 ml/kg, ECMO support is considered minimal. At this point if reasonable ventilator settings result in adequate gas exchange, the patient is isolated from the ECMO circuit.

An alternative approach is to maintain ECMO support and lung rest until evidence exists that the patient may be able to be supported without ECMO. This evidence may be serial lung compliance checks, chest radiograph appearance, and the need to add more CO_2 into the sweep gas as more native CO_2 removal has occurred.[90] The next step is to increase the ventilator settings to clinically safe and acceptable levels and then to perform a trial separation from ECMO. During the separation, serial blood gases are obtained to assess gas exchange on the chosen ventilator settings. A set of decannulation criteria are established, and if the patient meets these requirements, ECMO is discontinued.

Each approach has its merits, and neither has been shown to have any significant advantages over the other. Weaning gradually returns the work of the lungs while the periodic test imposes more work in a shorter period. During weaning there may be less time spent at true lung rest settings, and the ECMO circuit is at lower flows for longer duration, which may lead to more stagnation and clotting.

In the cardiac patient, return of heart function is the focus and both weaning and periodic testing can be used. Weaning is used to gradually "reload" the heart and to allow it to gradually assume all the pumping for the body. Quite often an echocardiogram is used to assess ventricular function while ECMO flows are reduced. The periodic testing is also used and the patient's hemodynamic profile used as the evidence for a trial separation.

The goal of assessing a patient's readiness to be liberated from ECMO is to verify that the ventilator support or hemodynamic support needed to keep the patient stable without ECMO is not too extreme. For instance, if high mean airway pressures are required to achieve desired clinical targets in a patient with respiratory failure, the underlying condition may not have fully reversed and ECMO should be continued. Similarly, if high doses of vasoactive agents are required to maintain the blood pressure of a patient with cardiac failure, the heart may not be ready to assume most of the work.

Although a subsequent ECMO course is possible, it is technically challenging and has added risk.[91] Therefore, parameters for weaning and trialing off ECMO need to provide the clinician with optimal information in order to make the decision to discontinue ECMO without added morbidity. Once the decision to discontinue ECMO is made, a surgical team is assembled and the cannulas are removed.

COMPLICATIONS

Complications associated with ECMO are generally related to equipment and technical issues or are more physiological in nature and can be attributed to the patient's blood coming into contact with the foreign surface of the ECMO circuit. There is a balance of achieving anticoagulation to abate thrombus formation and maintaining circuit integrity while minimizing the risks of bleeding.

Technical

One of the duties of an ECMO specialist is to monitor the functions of the ECMO system and employ troubleshooting procedures to address circuit malfunctions.[92] One important aspect is to assess the patient's ability to remain stable without ECMO support should the patient need to be isolated so that a repair or circuit change can be executed. Few ECMO circuit problems arise that require the patient to be acutely removed from support, with the rare exception of a sudden, unplanned decannulation, tubing or component rupture, or a witnessed air embolism. Most circuit interventions can be executed in a logical and methodical manner and with minimal interruption in support. Troubleshooting procedures are developed for the replacement of the entire circuit or components such as the roller pump tubing, membrane oxygenators, heat exchangers, and hemofilters.[93]

The durable components of an ECMO system such as the pump, water bath, and adjunct monitors are subject to mechanical failure and may need to be replaced, and standby equipment is maintained as a precaution. The ECMO pump typically has a battery backup in the event of power failure. Manual cranking devices are also available and can substitute the mechanical action of the pump if a sudden failure occurred and battery backup malfunctioned. The water pump can cease to pump water and cause the patient to become hypothermic, which would be remedied by replacing the water pump. Other monitoring devices are not as critical and will not cause potential patient harm if they malfunction.

Physiological

The most concerning patient complication that can occur, particularly in the newborn, is an intracranial hemorrhage (ICH). The use of ECMO in newborns has greater risks because of anticoagulation requirements and cerebral blood flow changes associated with the ligation of the right internal jugular vein and the right common carotid artery. As previously mentioned, during the ECMO course newborns receive serial head ultrasounds to identify the presence of ICH and to gauge the progression of the ICH. The slightly premature newborn who experiences periods of hypoxemia and acidosis is even more susceptible. Strategies to minimize the risk of an ICH include continuous blood pressure monitoring and avoidance of hypertensive periods and strict anticoagulation parameters.

In the early ECMO era, infants born at less than 35 weeks of gestation seemed to have a higher incidence of ICH, which led to the recommendation that ECMO be limited to infants born at more than 36 weeks of gestation.[85] Although this seemed to be a prudent approach, it eliminated potentially lifesaving treatment to a wider range of newborns. To address this concern and be able to offer ECMO to more neonates, Wilson and colleagues investigated the use of aminocaproic acid, an antifibrinolytic drug that prevents the degradation of thrombus formation.[33] The use of this medication greatly reduced the incidence of ICH, allowed the use ECMO in infants born before 36 weeks of gestation, and also decreased the incidence of postoperative bleeding in patients with CDH. One drawback to the use of amnicaproic acid is that it did result in increased thrombus formation in the ECMO circuit, which required more circuit interventions.

Bleeding is the predominant complication associated with ECMO. In addition to ICH, bleeding can occur at the cannula site; at surgical incisions; and at oropaharyngeal, pleural, and any other intravenous or access points in the patient. Bleeding usually can be controlled by closely monitoring coagulation studies, maintaining strict anticoagulation parameters, and repleting blood components.

OUTCOMES

Surviving an ECMO course without added morbidity and surviving to hospital discharge without any disability are the main objectives of ECMO. As previously stated, the bulk of the ECMO experience initially was in newborns with hypoxemic respiratory failure, who responded well to a relatively brief ECMO duration. However, concerns about the long-term well-being of these infants were raised and prompted longitudinal studies on their neurodevelopmental outcomes.

The neonatal brain is highly adaptive and responds well to the collateral circulation established in the presence of carotid artery and jugular vein ligation.[94] Early follow-up studies of children who required ECMO support in their neonatal period have been favorable and indicate few long-term deficits.[95] These studies have failed to identify any specific risk factors, such as pre-ECMO severity of illness, or modes and timing of support. The largest and most comprehensive follow-up studies have been conducted in the United Kingdom and have shown that ECMO is clearly beneficial for newborns with severe respiratory failure and that the risks are well balanced with strong survivability and without significant disability.[96,97]

The ELSO registry describes a survival to discharge rate of more than 65% in 27,000 infants and children supported with ECMO over a 24-year period.[17] This likely represents a significant number of patients who would have otherwise died.

CLINICAL HIGHLIGHT

Background
A 3.5-kg male infant was transferred to the newborn ICU with severe respiratory failure associated with PPHN. The patient was intubated and transitioned from CMV to HFOV at 12 hours of life. The patient required $\overline{Paw}$ of 35 cm H_2O, amplitude of 56 cm H_2O, FIO_2 0.95, with 20 ppm iNO. The OI increased from 42 to 50 over a 6-hour period, at which point the decision to use ECMO was made. The venovenous route was selected because the patient had good cardiac function and required little blood pressure support. A VVDL cannula was surgically inserted into the patient's right internal jugular vein and subsequently connected to a blood-primed ECMO circuit consisting of a centrifugal pump and microporous membrane. The blood flow rate was adjusted to 100 ml/kg/min and sweep gases consisting of O_2 and CO_2 were titrated to clinically acceptable blood gases. The patient was stabilized over several hours and iNO was discontinued. Over the next 5 days the patient was made comfortable with sedatives and analgesics, and a head ultrasound was periodically obtained, revealing no abnormalities and no hemorrhage. Anticoagulation was maintained, hemostasis achieved, and ECMO circuit integrity and function closely monitored. The patient's lung compliance improved by day 5 and there was no more evidence of pulmonary hypertension as determined by echocardiography. The patient was successfully separated from ECMO and transitioned to CMV on day 8 of life and subsequently extubated to 6 cm H_2O nasal CPAP, which was discontinued after 3 days. The patient continued to gain weight, and neurodevelopment indicators were within normal limits.

Discussion
This is a fairly typical use of ECMO in a neonate born with PPHN who failed conventional measures including HFOV and iNO. The patient was supported with ECMO while lung recovery occurred and was successfully weaned from ECMO without any associated sequelae.

Why Was ECMO Used in This Patient, and What Were the Clinical Goals?
The OI suggested that the severity of illness was high and could have potentially resulted in death. ECMO was appropriately applied and allowed lung-protective ventilation strategies to be used, the preservation of good organ perfusion, and the time for the reversal of the pulmonary hypertension and improvement in cardiopulmonary function.

KEY POINTS

- The ECMO system is a modified form of cardiopulmonary bypass designed for long-term use. It consists of a contiguous loop of tubing with a drainage and reinfusion limb. Blood is mechanically pumped through an artificial lung that augments gas exchange.
- ECMO is used to support newborns, infants, and children without respiratory or cardiac failure who do not respond to conventional treatment options.
- There are two modes of ECMO support, venous–venous and venous–arterial. Venous–venous is primarily used to support lung function, whereas venous–arterial supports both heart and lung function.
- Monitoring ECMO entails the usual critical care parameters such as hemodynamics, laboratory and radiological studies, and patient comfort; the mechanical aspects of the ECMO system; and anticoagulation.
- ECMO is associated with mechanical or technical complications as well as patient-related complications such as bleeding.

ASSESSMENT QUESTIONS

1. Which of the following patients meets criteria for ECMO?
   A. Male born at 25 weeks of gestation with RDS and receiving CPAP
   B. Full-term male with an OI of 15 and requiring HFOV
   C. Female born at 27 weeks with BPD and requiring CMV
   D. Full-term female with an OI of 34 requiring iNO
2. Which of the following correctly describes the path that a red blood cell travels through an ECMO circuit?
   A. Membrane oxygenator, pump, venous cannula
   B. Arterial cannula, pump, membrane oxygenator
   C. Pump, membrane oxygenator, venous cannula
   D. Venous cannula, pump, membrane oxygenator
3. Which of the following is an advantage of using a VV double-lumen cannula in an infant with PPHN?
   A. Carotid artery ligation is not needed.
   B. Cardiac function is supported.
   C. Higher ECMO flow rates can be used.
   D. Anticoagulation is easier to achieve.
4. Which of the following best describes the difference between a roller pump and a centrifugal pump?
   A. Centrifugal pumps are gravity dependent.
   B. Roller pumps are nonocclusive.
   C. Centrifugal pumps require additional blood.
   D. Roller pumps operate by compression and displacement.
5. Which of the following best describes the difference between silicone membranes and microporous membranes?
   A. Microporous membranes provide better gas exchange.
   B. Silicone membranes have an integral heat exchanger.
   C. Microporous membranes have lower resistance.
   D. Silicone membranes are easier to prime and deair.

6. Which of the following best describes the essential components of an ECMO system?
   A. Roller pump, high-frequency ventilator, membrane oxygenator
   B. Microporous membrane, centrifugal pump, circuit, cannulas
   C. Silicone membrane, circuit, ACT point-of-care device
   D. SvO_2 monitor, centrifugal pump, heparin infusion

7. Which of the following is used to monitor anticoagulation?
   A. Activated clotting time
   B. Hematocrit and hemoglobin levels
   C. Platelet count
   D. Arterial blood gases

8. Which of the following best describes the modes of ECMO support?
   A. VV provides only cardiac support.
   B. VA supports both lung and heart function.
   C. VA is only for patients with cardiac failure.
   D. VV provides better oxygenation.

9. Which of the following is the main objective for using ECMO in a patient with viral pneumonia?
   A. To provide lung protective ventilation
   B. To use high mean airway pressures
   C. To provide lung recruitment maneuvers
   D. To improve the $PaCO_2$

10. Which of the following is the main goal of ECMO?
    A. To support cardiac function
    B. To support lung function
    C. To provide adequate tissue oxygen delivery
    D. To remove carbon dioxide

References

1. Betit P: Extracorporeal membrane oxygenation—quo vadis, *Respir Care* 54:948, 2009.
2. Gibbon JH: Application of a mechanical heart lung apparatus to cardiac surgery, *Minn Med* 37:171, 1954.
3. Gibbon JH: Artificial maintenance of circulation during experimental occlusion of pulmonary artery, *Arch Surg* 34:1105, 1937.
4. Lillehei CW, Cohen M, Warden HE, Ziegler NR, Varco RL: The results of direct vision closure of ventricular septal defects in eight patients by means of controlled cross-circulation, *Surg Gynecol Obstet* 101:446, 1955.
5. Lillehei CW, Dewall RA, Read RC, Warden HE, Varco RL: Direct vision intracardiac surgery in a man using a simple, disposable artificial oxygenator, *Dis Chest* 29:1, 1956.
6. Kolff WJ, Berk HT: Artificial kidney: a dialyzer with a great area, *Acta Med Scand* 117:121, 1944.
7. Clowes GH, Hopkins AL, Neville WE: An artificial lung dependent upon diffusion of oxygen and carbon dioxide through plastic membranes, *J Thorac Surg* 32:630, 1956.
8. Kolobow T, Bowman RL: Construction and elimination of an alveolar membrane artificial heart–lung, *Trans Am Soc Artif Intern Organs* 9:238, 1963.
9. Kolobow T, Zapol W, Pierce J: High survival and minimal blood damage in lambs exposed to long term venovenous pumping with a polyurethane chamber roller pump with and without a membrane oxygenator, *Trans Am Soc Artif Intern Organs* 15:172, 1969.
10. Hill JD, O'Brien TG, Murray JJ, et al: Prolonged extracorporeal oxygenation for acute post-traumatic respiratory failure: use of the Bramson membrane lung, *N Engl J Med* 286:629, 1972.
11. Zapol WM, Snider MT, Hill JD, et al: Extracorporeal membrane oxygenation in severe respiratory failure: a randomized prospective study, *JAMA* 242:2193, 1979.
12. Bartlett RH, Harkin DE: Instrumentation for cardiopulmonary bypass: past, present, and future, *Med Instrum* 10:119, 1976.
13. Bartlett RH, Gazzaniga AB, Huztable RF, Schippers HC, O'Connor MJ, Jefferies MR: Extracorporeal circulation (ECMO) in neonatal respiratory failure, *J Thorac Cardiovasc Surg* 74:826, 1977.
14. Bartlett RH, Roloff DW, Cornell RG, Andrews AF, Dillon PW, Zwischenberger JB: Extracorporeal circulation in neonatal respiratory failure: a prospective randomized study, *Pediatrics* 76:479, 1985.
15. O'Rourke PP, Crone RK, Vacanti JP, et al: Extracorporeal membrane oxygenation and conventional medical therapy in neonates with persistent pulmonary hypertension of the newborn: a prospective randomized study, *Pediatrics* 84:957, 1989.
16. UK Collaborative ECMO Trial Group: The report of the UK collaborative randomized trial of neonatal extracorporeal membrane oxygenation, *Lancet* 348:75, 1996.
17. Extracorporeal Life Support Organization: International Registry. Retrieved from: http://www.elsonet.org. Accessed July 2012.
18. Henderson-Smart DJ, De Paoli AG, Clark RH, Bhuta T: High frequency oscillatory ventilation versus conventional ventilation for infants with severe pulmonary dysfunction born at or near term, *Cochrane Database Syst Rev* Vol. 3 CD002974, 2009.
19. Konduri JP, Solimino A, Singer J, et al: Neonatal Inhaled Nitric Oxide Group, *Pediatrics* 113:559, 2004.
20. Kinsella JP, Abman SH: Inhaled nitric oxide and high frequency oscillatory ventilation on persistent pulmonary hypertension of the newborn, *Eur J Pediatr* 157(Suppl 1):S28, 1998.
21. Farrow KN, Fliman P, Steinhorn RH: The disease treated with ECMO: focus on PPHN, *Semin Perinatol* 29:8, 2005.
22. Waag K-L, Loff S, Zahn K, et al: Congenital diaphragmatic hernia: a modern day approach, *Sem Pediatr Surgery* 17:244, 2008.
23. Betit P, Craig N: Extracorporeal membrane oxygenation for neonatal respiratory failure, *Respir Care* 54:1244, 2009.
24. Stevens TP, van Wijngaarden E, Ackerman KG, Lally PA, Lally KP, Congenital Diaphragmatic Hernia Study Group. Timing of delivery and survival rates of for infants with prenatal diagnosis of congenital diaphragmatic hernia, *Pediatrics* 123:494, 2009.
25. Haile DT, Schears GJ: Optimal time for initiating extracorporeal membrane oxygenation, *Sem Cardiothorac Vasc Anesth* 13:146, 2009.
26. Krummel TM, Greenfield LJ, Kirkpatrick BV, et al: Alveolar–arterial oxygen gradients versus the neonatal pulmonary insufficiency index for prediction of mortality in ECMO candidates, *J Pediatr Surg* 19:380, 1984.
27. Ortega M: Oxygenation index can predict outcome in neonates who are candidates for extracorporeal membrane oxygenation, *Pediatr Res* 22:462A, 1987.
28. Hui TT, Danielson PD, Anderson KD, Stein JE: The impact of changing neonatal respiratory management on extracorporeal membrane oxygenation utilization, *J Pediatr Surg* 37:703, 2002.
29. Fliman PJ, De Regnier RO, Kinsella J, Reynolds M, Rankin LL, Steinhorn RH: Neonatal extracorporeal life support: impact of new therapies on survival, *J Pediatr* 148:595, 2006.

30. Tiruvoipati R, Pandya H, Manktelow B, et al: Referral pattern of neonates with severe respiratory failure for extracorporeal membrane oxygenation, *Arch Dis Child Fetal Ed* 93:F104, 2008.

31. Carey WA, Colby CE: Extracorporeal membrane oxygenation for the treatment of neonatal respiratory failure, *Sem Cardiothorac Vasc Anesth* 13:192, 2009.

32. Mugford M, Elbourne D, Field D: Extracorporeal membrane oxygenation for severe respiratory failure in the newborn infants, *Cochrane Data Sys Rev* 3:CD001340, 2008. doi:10.1002/14651858.

33. Wilson JM, Bower LK, Fackler JC, Beals DA, Bergus BO, Kevy SV: Aminocaproic acid decreases the incidence of intracranial hemorrhage and other hemorrhagic complications of ECMO, *J Pediatr Surg* 28:536, 1993.

34. Brogan TV, Zabrocki L, Thiagarajan RR, Rycus TT, Bratton SL: Prolonged extracorporeal membrane oxygenation for children with respiratory failure, *Pediatr Crit Care Med* 13:e249, 2012.

35. Green TP, Timmons OD, Fackler JC, Moler FW, Thompson AE, Sweeney MF: The impact of extracorporeal membrane oxygenation on survival in pediatric patients with acute respiratory failure, *Crit Care Med* 24:323, 1996.

36. MacLaren G, Butt W, Best D, Donath S: Central extracorporeal membrane oxygenation for refractory pediatric septic shock, *Pediatr Crit Care Med* 12:133, 2011.

37. Luyt DK, Pridgeon J, Brown J, Peek G, Firmin R, Pandya HC: Extracorporeal life support for children with meningococcal septicaemia, *Acta Pediatr* 93:1608, 2004.

38. Turner DA, Rehder KJ, Peterson-Carmichael SL, et al: Extracorporeal membrane oxygenation for severe refractory respiratory failure secondary to 2009. H1N1 influenza A, *Respir Care* 56:941, 2011.

39. Creech BC, Johnson GB, Bartilson RE, Young E, Barr FE: Increasing use of extracorporeal life support in methicillin-resistant *Staphylococcus aureus* in children, *Pediatr Crit Care* 8:231, 2007.

40. Mehta N, Turner D, Walsh B, et al: Factors associated with survival in pediatric extracorporeal membrane oxygenation, *J Pediatr Surg* 45:1995, 2010.

41. Hemmila MR, Napolitano LM: Severe respiratory failure: advanced treatment options, *Crit Care Med* 34:S278, 2006.

42. Betit P: Are indications to ECMO slowly vanishing? *Respir Care* 56:1054, 2011.

43. Swaniker F, Kolla S, Moler F, et al: Extracorporeal life support outcome for 128 pediatric patients with respiratory failure, *J Pediatr Surg* 35:197, 2000.

44. Almond CS, Singh TP, Gavreau K, et al: Extracorporeal membrane oxygenation for bridge to heart transplantation among children in the United States, *Circulation* 123:2975, 2011.

45. Thourani VH, Kirshbom PM, Kanter KR, et al: Venoarterial extracorporeal membrane oxygenation (VA-ECMO) in pediatric cardiac support, *Ann Thorac Surg* 82:138, 2006.

46. Sherwin ED, Gavreau K, Scheurer MA, et al. Extracorporeal membrane oxygenation after stage-1 palliation for hypoplastic left heart syndrome, *J Thorac Cardiovasc Surg* 1, 144(6) 1337-1343, 2012.

47. Duncan B: Mechanical circulatory support for infants and children with cardiac disease, *Ann Thorac Surg* 73:1670, 2002.

48. Allan CK, Thiagarajan RR, Armsby LR, delNido PJ, Laussen PC: Emergent use of extracorporeal membrane oxygenation during pediatric cardiac catheterization, *Pediatr Crit Care Med* 17:212, 2006.

49. Rajagopal SK, Almond CS, Laussen PC, Rycus PT, Wypij DW, Thiagarajan RR: Extracorporeal membrane oxygenation for support of infants, children, and young adults with acute myocarditis: a review of the extracorporeal life support organization registry, *Crit Care Med* 38:382, 2010.

50. Kane DA, Thiagarajan RR, Wypij D, et al: Rapid-response extracorporeal membrane oxygenation to support cardiopulmonary resuscitation in children with cardiac disease, *Circulation* 122(suppl 1):S241, 2010.

51. Thiagarajan RR, Laussen PC, Rycus PT, Bartlett RH, Bratton SL: Extracorporeal membrane oxygenation to aid cardiopulmonary resuscitation in infants and children, *Circulation* 116:1693, 2007.

52. Barrett CS, Bratton SL, Salvin JW, Laussen PC, Rycus PT, Thiagarajan RR: Neurologic injury after extracorporeal membrane oxygenation use to aid pediatric cardiopulmonary resuscitation, *Pediatr Crit Care Med* 10:445, 2009.

53. Cooper DS, Jacobs JP, Moore L, et al: Cardiac extracorporeal life support: state of the art in 2007, *Cardiol Young* 17:104, 2007.

54. Skinner SC, Hirschl RB, Bartlett RH: Extracorporeal life support, *Sem Pediatr Surg* 15(4) 242-250 NOV 2006.

55. Klein MD, Andrews AF, Wesley JR, et al: Venovenous perfusion in ECMO for newborn respiratory insufficiency: a clinical comparison with venoarterial perfusion, *Ann Surg* 201:520, 1985.

56. Hickey PR, Buckley MJ, Philbin DM: Pulsatile and nonpulsatile cardiopulmonary bypass: review of a counterproductive controversy, *Ann Thorac Surg* 36:720, 1983.

57. Gerstmann D: Left carotid artery and coronary arterial flow partitioning during neonatal ECMO, *Pediatr Res* 25:37A, 1989.

58. Somme S, Liu DC: New trends in extracorporeal membrane oxygenation in newborn pulmonary disease, *Artif Organs* 25:633, 2001.

59. Anderson HL 3rd, Otsu T, Chapman RA, Bartlett RH: Venovenous extracorporeal life support in neonates using a double lumen catheter, *ASAIO Trans* 35:650, 1989.

60. Foley DS, Swaniker F, Pranikoff T, Bartlett RH, Hirschl RB: Percutaneous cannulation for pediatric venovenous extracorporeal life support, *J Pediatr Surg* 35:943, 2000.

61. Pettigano R, Fortenberry JD, Heard ML, et al: Primary use of the venovenous approach for extracorporeal membrane oxygenation in pediatric acute respiratory failure, *Pediatr Crit Care Med* 4:291, 2003.

62. Otsu T, Merz SL, Hulquist KA, et al: Laboratory evaluation of a double lumen catheter for venovenous neonatal ECMO, *ASAIO Trans* 35:647, 1989.

63. Abrams D, Brodie D, Javidar J, et al: Insertion of bicaval dual-lumen cannula via the left internal jugular vein for extracorporeal membrane oxygenation, *ASAIO J* 58(6) 636-637, 2012.

64. Mathis CA, Powell AE, Holloway RD, Sha S, Goldberg SP, Boston US: Alternative cannulation strategy for pediatric ECMO, *J Card Surg* 26:444, 2011.

65. Stulak JM, Dearini JA, Burkhart HM, Barnes RD, Scott PD, Schears GJ: ECMO cannulation controversies and complications, *Sem Cardiothorac Vasc Anesth* 13:176, 2009.

66. de Bucourt M, Teichgräber UK: Image guided placement of extracorporeal life support through bi-caval dual lumen venovenous membrane oxygenation an interventional radiology setting—initial experience, *J Vasc Access* 13:221, 2012.

67. Thomas TH, Proce R, Ramaciotti C, Thompson M, Megison S, Lemler MS: Echocardiography, not just chest radiography, for evaluation of cannula placement during pediatric extracorporeal membrane oxygenation, *Pediatr Crit Care* 10:56, 2009.

68. Palanzo D, Qui F, Baer L, Clark JB, Myers JL, Undar A: Evolution of the extracorporeal life support circuitry, *Artif Organs* 34:869, 2010.

69. Ichikawa S, Nosé Y: Centrifugal blood pumps for various clinical needs, *Artif Organs* 26:916, 2002.

70. Thiara APS, Noel TN, Kristiansen F, Karlsen HM, Fiane AE, Svennevig JL: Evaluation of oxygenators and centrifugal pumps for long-term pediatric extracorporeal membrane oxygenation, *Perfusion* 22:323, 2007.

71. Khoshbin E, Westrope C, Pooboni S, et al: Performance of polymethyl pentene oxygenators for neonatal extracorporeal membrane oxygenation: a comparison with silicone oxygenators, *Perfusion* 20:129, 2005.

72. Taylor J, Yee S, Rider A, Kunselman AR, Guan Y, Undar A: Comparison of perfusion quality in hollow-fiber membrane oxygenators for neonatal extracorporeal life support, *Artif Organs* 34:E110, 2010.

73. Thiara AS, Andersen VY, Videm V, et al: Comparable biocompatibility of phisio- and bioline-coated cardiopulmonary bypass circuits indicated by the inflammatory response, *Perfusion* 25:9, 2010.

74. Jacobs S, De Somer F, Vandenplas G, Belleghem YV, Taeymans Y, Van Nooten G: Active or passive bio-coating: does it matter in extracorporeal circulation? *Perfusion* 26:496, 2011.

75. VanMeurs KP, Mikesell G, Seale W, et al: Maximum blood flow rates for arterial cannulae used for neonatal ECMO. *ASAIO* 34:4, 1991.

76. Smith AH, Hardison DC, Worden CR, Fleming GM, Taylor MB: Acute renal failure during extracorporeal support in the pediatric cardiac patient, *ASAIO J* 55:412, 2009.

77. Selewski DT, Cornell TT, Blatt NB, et al: Fluid overload and fluid removal on extracorporeal membrane oxygenation requiring continuous renal replacement therapy, *Crit Care Med* 40:2694, 2012.

78. Baird CW, Zurakowski D, Robinson B, et al: Anticoagulation and pediatric extracorporeal membrane oxygenation: impact of activated clotting time and heparin dose on survival, *Ann Thorac Surg* 83:912, 2007.

79. Oliver WC: Anticoagulation and coagulation management for ECMO, *Sem Cardiothorac Vasc Anesth* 13:154, 2009.

80. VanCott EM: Point-of-care testing in coagulation, *Clin Lab Med* 29:543, 2009.

81. Nankervis CA, Preston TJ, Dysart KC, et al: Assessing heparin dosing in neonates on venoarterial extracorporeal membrane oxygenation, *ASAIO J* 53:111, 2007.

82. Riley JB, Scott PD, Schears GJ: Update on safety equipment for extracorporeal life support (ECLS) circuits, *Sem Cardiothorac Vasc Anesth* 13:138, 2009.

83. Hervey-Jumper SL, Annich GM, Yancon AR, et al: Neurologic complications of extracorporeal membrane oxygenation in children, *J Neurosurg Pediatr* 7:338, 2011.

84. DeBerry BB, Lynch JE, Chernin JM, Zwischenberger JB, Chung DH: A survey for pain and sedation medications in pediatric patients during extracorporeal membrane oxygenation, *Perfusion* 20:139, 2005.

85. Cilley RE, Zwischenberger JB, Andrews AF, Bowerman RA, Roloff DW, Bartlett RH: Intracranial hemorrhage during extracorporeal membrane oxygenation in neonates, *Pediatrics* 78:699, 1986.

86. Downard CD, Betit P, Chang RW, Garza JJ, Arnold JA, Wilson JM: Impact of amicar on hemorrhagic complications of ECMO: a ten year review, *J Pediatr* 38:1212, 2003.

87. Nosotti M, Rosso L, Tosi D, et al: Extracorporeal membrane oxygenation with spontaneous breathing as a bridge to lung transplantation, *Interac Cardiovasc Thorac Surg* 16:55–59, 2012.

88. Schmidt F, Sasse M, Boehne M, et al: Concept of "awake venovenous extracorporeal membrane oxygenation" in pediatric patients awaiting lung transplantation, *Pediatr Transplant* 17(3) 224-230, 2012. doi: 10.1111/petr.12001

89. Keszler M, Rykman, FC, McDonald JV Jr, et al: A prospective multicenter randomized study of high to low positive end-expiratory pressure during extracorporeal membrane oxygenation, *J Pediatr* 120:107, 1992.

90. Lotze A, Short BL, Taylor GA: The use of lung compliance as a parameter for improvement in lung function in newborns with respiratory failure requiring extracorporeal membrane oxygenation, *Crit Care Med* 15:226, 1987.

91. Fisher JC, Stolar CJ, Cowles RA: Extracorporeal membrane oxygenation for cardiopulmonary failure in pediatric patients: is a second course justified? *J Surg Res* 148:100, 2008.

92. Fleming GM, Gurney JG, Donohue JE, Remenapp RT, Annich GM: Mechanical component failures in 28,171 neonatal and pediatric extracorporeal membrane oxygenation course from 1987 to 2006, *Pediatr Crit Care Med* 10:439, 2009.

93. Darling E, Searles B: Oxygenator change-out times: the value of a written protocol and simulation exercise, *Perfusion* 25:141, 2010.

94. Short BL: The effect of extracorporeal life support on the brain: a focus on ECMO, *Semin Perinatol* 29:45, 2005.

95. Nield TA, Langenbacher D, Poulsen MK, Platzker AC: Neurodevelopmental outcome at 3.5 years of age in children treated with of extracorporeal life support: relationship to primary diagnosis, *J Pediatr* 136:338, 2000.

96. Bennett CC, Johnson A, Field DJ, Elbourne D, UK Collaborative ECMO Trial Group: UK Collaborative randomized trial of neonatal extracorporeal membrane oxygenation: follow-up to age 4 years, *Lancet* 357:1094, 2001.

97. McNally H, Bennett CC, Elbourne D, Field DJ, UK Collaborative ECMO Trial Group: United Kingdom Collaborative randomized trial of neonatal extracorporeal membrane oxygenation: follow-up to age 7 years, *Pediatrics* 117:e845, 2006.

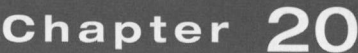

Pharmacology

SEAN T. NGUYEN

LEARNING OBJECTIVES

After reading this chapter the reader will be able to:

1. Identify pharmacokinetic parameters that differ between pediatric and adult patients
2. Discuss the place in therapy of β_2-adrenergic agonists in the treatment of asthma, chronic obstructive pulmonary disease (COPD), and exercise-induced bronchospasms
3. Identify potential adverse events observed with the use of inhaled short-acting β-adrenergic agonists
4. Explain the place in therapy of inhaled long-acting β_2-adrenergic agonists
5. Explain administration issues after inhalation of corticosteroids
6. Discuss the place in therapy of the leukotriene modifiers
7. Discuss the mechanism of action of the mucolytic agents
8. Discuss the place in therapy of antiviral and immunomodulatory agents commonly used in the treatment of pediatric viral infections
9. Discuss the place in therapy of aerosolized antimicrobials used in the treatment of infectious respiratory diseases

The purpose of this chapter is to introduce concepts of developmental pharmacology and to review pharmacological agents commonly used in pediatric airway diseases. The mechanism of action, side effect profiles, dosage ranges, place in therapy, and specific administration techniques will also be reviewed where appropriate.

Before the Pediatric Research Equity Act (PREA) and exclusivity provision of the Best Pharmaceuticals for Children Act (BPCA), approximately 20% of drugs approved by the Food and Drug Administration (FDA) were labeled for pediatric use.[1] Since passed into law in 2003, the PREA grants the FDA authority to require pediatric studies of a new drug if the FDA determines the product is likely to be used in a substantial number of pediatric patients. They can also require pediatric studies if the product can potentially provide a meaningful benefit in the pediatric population over existing treatments. On the other hand, the BPCA is a voluntary pediatric exclusivity provision of the FDA Modernization Act of 1997 that has done more to spur pediatric studies than any other regulatory initiative. This provision allows pharmaceutical companies to qualify for an additional 6 months of marketing exclusivity or patent protection if they perform studies in children as requested by the FDA. As a result, there have been significant advances in pediatric research that have provided new information about pediatric clinical pharmacology, drug safety, and effectiveness.

DEVELOPMENTAL PHARMACOLOGY

Advances in pediatric clinical pharmacology stem from the influence of physiological and **pharmacokinetic** differences between children and adults. Pediatric dosage regimens cannot be simply extrapolated from adult data and corrected for body weight because of significant age-related differences in pharmacokinetic principles specific to children. Human growth is not a linear process because age-associated changes in body composition and organ function are dynamic and can be discordant during the first decade of life.[2]

Drug absorption, distribution, and metabolism vary greatly in neonatal and pediatric patients. Developmental changes in absorptive surfaces such as the gastrointestinal (GI) tract, skin, and pulmonary tree can affect the absorption rate and bioavailability of a drug. Changes in intraluminal pH in different segments of the GI tract can influence the relative amount of the drug available for absorption. Gastric pH is increased in neonates, infants, and young children and will reach adult pH values by 2 years of age. Gastric motility is the primary determinant for the rate of drug to be dispersed along the small intestine, which is decreased in neonates and reaches adult levels in infants and children.[1-3] After a drug is absorbed, it is distributed to a variety of body compartments depending on its physiochemical properties. In neonates and infants, an increase in total body water–to–fat ratio contributes to a higher volume of distribution for hydrophilic drugs (i.e., propofol), thus requiring larger weight-based doses to achieve therapeutic concentrations.[2,4,5] Furthermore, delayed maturation of drug-metabolizing enzyme activity may account for the marked toxicity of drugs in the very young. The metabolic enzyme that is involved in the metabolism of more than 50% of medications is called cytochrome (CYP) 3A4. Although it accounts for approximately 30% of total hepatic CYP, its activity is very low at birth and will increase to nearly 20% of adult values at 1 month of age and approximately 75% of adult values at 1 year of age.[4-6] Disease states such as cystic fibrosis have also been shown to alter drug absorption and have unique pharmacokinetic characteristics that would warrant different dosing regimens.

β-ADRENERGIC AGONISTS

Mechanism of Action

Norepinephrine is a potent α and β_1 **agonist** that has relatively little action on β_2 receptors. However, structural changes and additions to the parent structure of norepinephrine result in compounds with a higher affinity for either α or β receptors and a prolonged duration of action. Therefore, norepinephrine is the parent compound of all the β_2-agonists because additions and substitutions of molecular entities on the terminal amine group will alter the β-receptor activity.[7]

Activation of β-adrenergic receptor sites on airway smooth muscle results in activation of adenylcyclase, which increases the production of cyclic adenosine monophosphate (cAMP) resulting in bronchial smooth muscle relaxation and skeletal muscle stimulation. β agonists can also inhibit the release of inflammatory mediators through stabilization of the mast cell membrane which will slow the progression of the inflammatory cascade. (Figure 20-1).

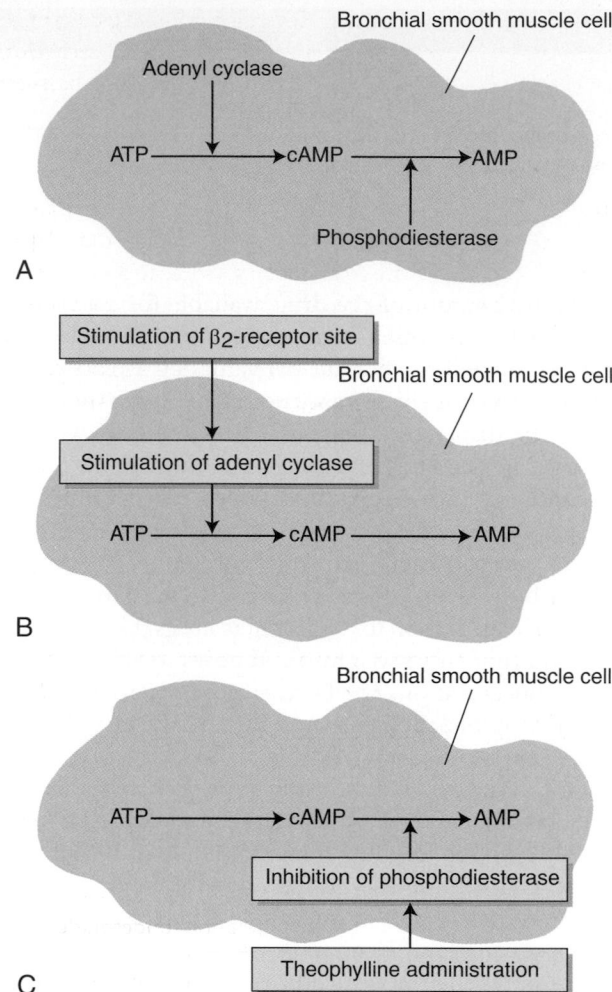

FIGURE 20-1 **A,** Sympathetic mechanisms controlling bronchial muscle tone. The enzyme adenylcyclase is the catalyst for the conversion of adenosine triphosphate (ATP) to cyclic adenosine monophosphate (cAMP). The enzyme phosphodiesterase breaks down cAMP into adenosine monophosphate (AMP). Increased levels of cAMP result in relaxation of bronchial smooth muscle. Decreased levels of cAMP lead to spasm of susceptible bronchial smooth muscle. **B,** Bronchial muscle receptors are called β_2 receptor sites. Stimulation of these sites results in stimulation of the enzyme adenylcyclase, which produces an increased level of cAMP, resulting in bronchodilation. **C,** Administration of the methylxanthine theophylline inhibits the enzyme phosphodiesterase, which inhibits the breakdown of cAMP and results in increased levels of cAMP and bronchodilation.

Place in Therapy

β_2-adrenergic agonists are the cornerstone treatment of bronchoconstriction in asthma, chronic obstructive pulmonary disease (COPD), and exercise-induced bronchospasms. Fast- and short-acting agents are best used for rescue of symptoms, whereas long-acting agents are best used for maintenance therapy. Expert guidelines recommend standard treatment of acute episodes of bronchospasms, and exacerbations of asthma should include short-acting β_2-agonists (i.e., albuterol, levalbuterol).[8] Administration using a handheld metered-dose inhaler

(MDI) with a spacer device is at least equivalent to nebulized β_2-agonist therapy in children and adults.[9-11] Long-acting β_2-agonists (i.e., salmeterol, formoterol) are used concomitantly with glucocorticoids for children who fail to achieve adequate asthma control with a medium-dose inhaled glucocorticoid.[8] The addition of systemic therapy to inhaled β_2-agonist therapy has been used with some success; however, there is no evidence to support the isolated use of a **parenteral** β_2-agonist to treat severe asthma exacerbations.[12,13]

In 2010 the FDA announced that in accordance with long-standing U.S. obligations under the Montreal Protocol on Substances that Deplete the Ozone Layer, MDIs that contain chlorofluorocarbons (CFCs) as a propellant could no longer be manufactured or sold as of 2013.[14] Because of this mandate, manufacturers of short-acting β_2-agonists have since switched to hydrofluoroalkane (HFA)–propelled MDIs. Lung deposition of drug particles with HFA-propelled inhalers may be greater than or at least equivalent to CFC-propelled inhalers.[15,16]

Adverse Events

At recommended doses, aerosol administrations are selective β_2 receptors with minimal systemic adverse events. Adverse events occur through excessive activation of β-adrenergic receptors when high doses of aerosolized selective β_2-adrenergic agonists are used or with the use of nonselective β-adrenergic agonists.

The most common adverse effect observed with the use of selective agents are tremors caused by stimulation of the β_2 receptors in skeletal muscle, which is less likely with inhalational therapy than parenteral or oral therapy.[17,18] Tachycardia and vasodilation are observed when β receptors are stimulated on the heart and peripheral vasculature. Upon initiation and with high-dose treatment, a reduction of serum potassium concentrations can be seen.[19] Hypokalemia is caused by a transient activation of the Na^+/K^+ pump and the transport of K^+ intracellularly, which may predispose the heart to toxic effects such as arrhythmias.[19,20] Headache, nervousness, dizziness, palpitations, cough, nausea, vomiting, and throat irritation may also occur.

Regular β_2-agonist use in patients with asthma may potentially result in **tolerance** to the drug's bronchodilating effects, which can be associated with poorer disease control.[21,22] Chronic administration of selective β_2-adrenergic agonists will create tolerance by reducing the density of β_2 receptors and the binding affinity to the receptors.[22] Tolerance primarily reduces duration of bronchodilation as opposed to peak response.

Overuse of inhaled β_2-agonists has been associated with increased risk of mortality from asthma specifically in those patients using two or more canisters of rescue inhaler each month.[8] The cardiotoxic potential of β_2-agonists may increase the risk of mortality, as may overreliance on medication and the patient's comfort level with β_2-agonist use. Control of symptoms may cause the patient to postpone obtaining adequate medical care in the presence of worsening asthma. With the use of a powerful bronchodilator, the perceived need for corticosteroid therapy may not be realized.[23] Concerns about overuse have led to the recommendation that β agonists be used only on an "as needed" basis in the treatment of acute episodes.[8,24,25] In addition, the association of development of serious adverse events is greater in children who regularly use long-acting β-agonists.[26-28]

Selective Agents

Selective agents have a higher specific affinity for β_2 receptors, with minimal effect on β_1 receptors, so less stimulation of the heart rate is observed. Several β-adrenergic agonists are available for the management of airway obstruction; they differ in β_2 selectivity, potency, elimination half-life, and availability of dosage formulations.

Dosage and Administration

Table 20-1 lists the bronchodilators available in inhalation form that are commonly used in pediatric patients. Generally, weight-based dosing of inhaled medications may not be appropriate for young children because of the low deposition of medication in the lungs. Standard doses, such as 2.5 mg of nebulized albuterol for children who weigh less than 30 kg and 5 mg for children who weigh more than 30 kg, may be used.

TABLE 20-1

Inhaled Bronchodilators[8]

Available Formulations	Pediatric Dose	Adverse Events	Administration Comments
Short-Acting β_2-Agonists			
Albuterol HFA 90 µg/puff (ProAir, Proventil, Ventolin)	Asthma exacerbations: 4-8 puffs q 20 min for 3 doses, then q 1-4 h; or 1-2 puffs q 4-6 h (max, 12 puffs/d) As needed for symptoms: 2 puffs q 4-6 h	Tachycardia, tremor, nervousness, hypokalemia, headache, palpitations, dizziness, nausea, vomiting	Drug of choice for acute bronchospasms. MDI requires periodic cleaning. Use large volume nebulizers for continuous administration.
Albuterol nebulizer solution (AccuNeb) 0.63 mg/3 ml, 1.25 mg/3 ml, 2.5 mg/3 ml, 5 mg/ml	Asthma exacerbations: 0.15 mg/kg (min, 2.5 mg) every 20 min for 3 doses, then 0.15-0.3 mg/kg (max, 10 mg) q 1-4 h PRN As needed for symptoms: <5 years: 0.63-2.5 mg in 3 ml of NS q 4-6 h >5 years: 1.25-55 mg in 3 ml of NS q 4-6 h		May mix with cromolyn solution, budesonide inhalant suspension, or ipratropium nebulizer solution.
Levalbuterol HFA 45 µg/puff (Xopenex HFA)	Asthma exacerbations: 4-8 puffs q 20 min for 3 doses, then q 1-4 h; or 1-2 puffs q 4-6 h (max, 12 puffs/day) PRN for symptoms: 2 puffs q 4-6 h		
Levalbuterol nebulizer solution (Xopenex) 0.31 mg/3 ml, 0.63 mg/ 3 ml, 1.25 mg/ 3 ml, 1.25 mg/0.5 ml	Asthma exacerbations: 0.075 mg/kg (min dose 1.25 mg) q 20 min for 3 doses, then 0.075-0.15 mg/kg (max, 5 mg) q 1-4 h PRN for symptoms: <5 years: 0.31-1.25 mg in 3 ml q 4-6 h 5-11 years: 0.31-0.63 mg q 8 h >12 years: 0.63-1.25 mg q 8 h		
Long-Acting β_2-Agonists			
Salmeterol (Serevent) Pwd for inh: 50 µg/puff	Maintenance: 1 puff q 12 h Prevention of EIB: 1 puff 30 min before exercise. Next dose in 12 h	Prolonged QT interval, tachycardia, palpitations, dizziness, nausea, vomiting	Do not blow into inhaler after dose is activated.

Continued

TABLE 20-1

Inhaled Bronchodilators—cont'd

Available Formulations	Pediatric Dose	Adverse Events	Administration Comments
Formoterol (Foradil) Dry powder inhaler (capsules): 12 µg	Maintenance: 1 capsule q 12 h (max, 2 doses daily) Prevention of EIB: 1 capsule 30 min before exercise. Next dose in 12 h	Tachycardia, tremor, nervousness, nausea, vomiting, headache, hypertension, dizziness, viral chest infection, fatigue tonsillitis	Do not blow into inhaler after dose is activated. Each capsule is for single use only and should not be taken orally.
Formoterol Nebulizer solution (Perforomist) 20 µg/2 ml	Maintenance: 20 µg twice daily (max daily dose: 40 µg)		Dilution is not required before administration.
Racemic epinephrine (Asthmaneffrin) Nebulizer solution: 2.25% (0.5 ml)	0.5 ml diluted with 3-5 ml of NS; administer over ~15 minutes q 3-4 h PRN	Tachycardia, tremor, dizziness, nausea, vomiting, headache, nervousness, palpitations	Not recommended for routine management and treatment of asthma. Protect from light. Solution should be discarded if it contains a precipitate or is discolored.
Anticholinergics Ipratropium bromide (Atrovent) Nebulizer solution: 0.2% (2.5 ml) Intranasal: 0.03% and 0.06%	Asthma exacerbations: 0.25-0.5 mg q 20 min for 3 doses, then as needed Maintenance: 0.25 mg q 6 h	Dry mouth, headache, dizziness, cough, blurred vision, drying of secretions	Protect from light. May mix in same nebulizer with albuterol. Multiple doses in the emergency department provide additive benefit when administered with albuterol.
Ipratropium bromide (Atrovent HFA) HFA: 17 µg/puff	Asthma exacerbations: 4-8 puffs PRN Maintenance: 1-2 puffs q 6 h (max, 12 puffs/day)		
Systemic β₂-Agonists Terbutaline (Brethine, Brethaire) Aqueous 1 mg/ml	Nebulization: 0.01-0.03 ml/kg (min, 0.1 ml; max, 2.5 ml) every 4-6 h Subcutaneous: 0.01 mg/kg (max, 0.25 mg) q 20 min for 3 doses then q 2-6 h PRN	Tachycardia, tremor, dizziness, nausea, vomiting, headache, nervousness, palpitations	No proven advantage of systemic therapy over aerosol.
Epinephrine 1:1000 (1 mg/ml)	Subcutaneous: 0.01 mg/kg up to 0.3-0.5 mg q 20 min for 3 doses		Protect from light. Solution should be discarded if it contains a precipitate or is discolored.

HFA, Hydrofluoroalkane; *MDI,* metered-dose inhaler; *PRN,* as needed; *pwd,* powder; *soln,* solution.

For asthma exacerbations, inhaled β₂-agonists, most commonly albuterol, can be administered continuously or intermittently, via a nebulizer or an MDI with a spacer. Children with moderate exacerbations usually require inhaled short-acting agents every 1 to 3 hours; however, patients who require treatments more frequently should be considered for continuous albuterol nebulization. Patients with a lack of response or worsening of respiratory parameters will require more frequent treatments. Those who display improvement should have the interval between the treatments increased. In addition to the regularly scheduled β₂-agonist treatment, "as needed" treatments should be available for episodes of acute bronchospasm or worsening respiratory distress.[8] Long-acting agents can provide bronchodilation for up to 12 hours when administered as an aerosol.

Albuterol

Although the name suggested by the World Health Organization (WHO, Geneva, Switzerland) is *salbutamol,* albuterol is the official generic name in the United States. Albuterol is indicated for the treatment and prevention of bronchospasms and is available in a variety of dosage forms. The most common reported adverse reactions to aerosolized albuterol are upper respiratory infections, rhinitis, pharyngitis, nausea, throat irritation, cough, and anxiety.[29,30]

Levalbuterol (Xopenex)

Albuterol is composed of both (R)- and (S)-isomers of albuterol. Levalbuterol is the active isomer of albuterol (R-albuterol) and is indicated for the treatment or prevention of bronchospasms in adults and children.[31,32] In studies of asthma treatment in the pediatric patient, levalbuterol has been compared with both racemic albuterol and placebo.[33] In doses of 0.31 and 0.63 mg, levalbuterol produced an equipotent degree of bronchodilation, as measured by percent change from predose forced expiratory volume at 1 second (FEV$_1$), as comparable doses of 1.25 and 2.5 mg of racemic albuterol. This same study found that 0.63 mg of levalbuterol was equipotent to 1.25 mg of racemic albuterol, and 1.25 mg of levalbuterol was equipotent to 2.5 mg of racemic albuterol. Therefore, there is no demonstrable difference in terms of safety or effectiveness between levalbuterol and albuterol.[34,35]

Levalbuterol is supplied as an MDI or in concentrated solution for nebulization that does not require dilution before administration. Each actuation of the MDI delivers 59 μg levalbuterol tartrate (equivalent to 45 μg of levalbuterol free base) from the actuator mouthpiece. The recommended MDI dose for treatment of acute bronchospasms or prevention of asthmatic symptoms is 2 inhalations (90 μg) repeated every 4 to 6 hours; however, in some patients 1 inhalation every 4 hours may be sufficient.[32] The suggested nebulization dosage for children on an "as needed" basis is dependent on their age. The solution should be stored in a protective foil pouch and discarded if the solution is not colorless.[31]

Adverse events in patients receiving levalbuterol are similar to those observed with racemic albuterol. Despite administration of larger equipotent albuterol doses, there is no clinically significant difference between levalbuterol and racemic albuterol in the effect on heart rate.[36] However, the incidence of tremor and nervousness has been reported to be slightly less when using 0.63 mg of levalbuterol.[37]

Terbutaline (Brethine, Brethaire)

Terbutaline is the only selective β$_2$-agonist available in parenteral form for the emergency treatment of status asthmaticus in critically ill children.[38] Its structural formula differs from that of albuterol in that it has a dihydroxybenzene group instead of a benzene ring, with etahydroxymethyl and parahydroxyl groups. It is available as an oral tablet and a sterile aqueous solution for parenteral (subcutaneous and intravenous) administration. Effects are observed rapidly after inhalation or parenteral administration and can persist for up to 3 to 4 hours after inhalation.

In most institutions, terbutaline is reserved for the management of acute episodes of severe asthma or in critically ill children. Although the manufacturer does not recommend use of inhaled terbutaline, in patients younger than 12 years of age doses of 0.2 mg/kg of terbutaline solution given by compressed air–powered nebulizer have resulted in a mean 55% improvement in FEV$_1$ at 1 hour.[39] Continuously nebulized terbutaline has also been reported to be safely administered to children in a pulmonary intensive care setting.[40] Terbutaline administered intravenously

as a continuous infusion or repeated subcutaneous injections have been reported effective in the treatment of refractory status asthmaticus in pediatric patients refractory to more conventional treatments.[41,42] The aqueous solution is supplied in a 2-ml clear glass ampule containing 1 mg of terbutaline sulfate per 1 ml of solution. The ampules must be protected from light and stored at room temperature. Parenteral terbutaline loses much of its β$_2$ selectivity; therefore, cardiovascular effects are often observed. Tachycardia is a common dose-limiting adverse effect and is mostly observed when using doses in the upper range of normal.[39]

Inhaled Long-Acting β$_2$-Agonists

Long-acting β$_2$-agonists (LABA) have a duration of action of at least 12 hours and have an onset of action that occurs approximately 30 minutes after intake.[43] Salmeterol and formoterol are the agents of choice for nocturnal asthma in patients who remain symptomatic despite standard management. Furthermore, studies in adolescents indicate that LABA have the potential of improving overall asthma control when added to corticosteroids in patients who are inadequately controlled with inhaled corticosteroids alone.[43-50] LABA should not be used for acute symptom relief. It is imperative that, when beginning treatment with LABA, patients should be counseled to discontinue any regular use of a short-acting β$_2$-agonist and to use the shorter acting agent for symptomatic, quick relief during acute episodes only.

Adverse reactions to LABAs include tremor, tachycardia, arrhythmias, palpitation, nervousness, agitation, headache, muscle cramps, dizziness, fatigue, insomnia, dry mouth, nausea, hypokalemia, hyperglycemia, and metabolic acidosis.[51] Although uncommon after administration at recommended doses, LABA can produce a clinically significant cardiovascular effect in some patients. Changes in the electrocardiogram include flattening of the T wave, prolongation of the QT interval, and ST-segment depression. Adverse events occur more often in children (ages 5 to 12 years) in need of daily bronchodilator and anti-inflammatory treatment that include viral infection, rhinitis, tonsillitis, gastroenteritis, abdominal pain, nausea, and dyspepsia.

Salmeterol (Serevent)

Salmeterol is indicated for long-term maintenance treatment of asthma and prevention of bronchospasm, including exercise-induced bronchospasm (EIB), in patients 4 years of age and older. It is generally used as an adjunct to inhaled corticosteroid therapy for long-term control of asthma symptoms, nocturnal asthma symptoms, and EIB.[8] Pediatric patients should use a combined product that contains both an inhaled corticosteroid and a LABA to treat the multiple mechanisms that produce airway disease.

Salmeterol is available as a single agent in the form of a dry powder inhaler (DPI) or in fixed-dose combinations with fluticasone as a DPI and MDI.[51] Studies suggest that for patients with inadequate symptom control who are receiving low to medium doses of inhaled corticosteroids, it may be more beneficial to add salmeterol than to increase the dose of inhaled corticosteroid.[52,53]

Formoterol (Foradil)

Formoterol is indicated for long-term, twice-daily (morning and evening) administration in the maintenance treatment of asthma and prevention of bronchospasm in adults and children 5 years of age and older.[54,55] Formoterol is also indicated for the acute prevention of EIB in adults and adolescents 12 years of age and older. Formoterol is available as a single agent in a hard gelatin capsule containing a dry powder blend of 12 µg of formoterol and 25 mg of lactose that is intended for oral inhalation only.[56] Formoterol is also available in a solution for nebulization and in an MDI in combination with budesonide approved for use in those 12 years of age and older.[57]

Formoterol is a highly selective β_2-agonist, whereas salmeterol is a partial agonist. In single-dose studies, when compared with salmeterol, formoterol had a shorter onset of action but similar duration of action.[54,55] In the treatment of asthma, differences between formoterol and salmeterol are not likely to produce clinically significant differences if used in combination with inhaled corticosteroids. However, in a randomized, placebo-controlled trial of patients with COPD receiving twice-daily formoterol, an increase of FEV_1 was significantly inferior to patients receiving once daily indacaterol.[58] Currently indicated for adults with COPD, indacaterol is a promising once-daily LABA currently being studied in pediatric patients with moderate to severe asthma.[59]

Nonselective Agents

Epinephrine

Epinephrine (adrenaline) is a potent **sympathomimetic** that acts on both α- and β-adrenergic receptors. Effects of epinephrine reproduce adrenal medullary stimulation and can be described by the term *flight or flight*. Its effects on target organs, including the heart, and the vascular system and respiratory tract are diverse and extremely complex. Stimulation of the α receptors results in vasoconstriction and a reduction of mucosal and submucosal congestion and edema. The β-adrenergic effects result from stimulation of adenylcyclase and increased cAMP production, which results in reduction of airway smooth muscle spasms (see Figure 20-1).

Parenteral epinephrine plays a vital role in cardiopulmonary resuscitation and reversal of hypersensitivity reactions.[60-64] Epinephrine is ineffective after oral administration because it is quickly metabolized, and absorption is rapid after parenteral and inhaled administration. Acting at β_2 receptors on bronchial smooth muscle, effects after nebulized administrations are restricted to the respiratory tract, thus making it useful in the treatment of postintubation

and infectious croup.[65-67] In children with an acute asthma exacerbation, a meta-analysis of randomized trials failed to show a benefit of nebulized epinephrine over albuterol or terbutaline in an emergency setting.[68]

Epinephrine for injection is available in 1 mg/ml (1:1000), 0.1 mg/ml (1:10,000), and 0.5 mg/ml (1:2000). However, the solution for inhalation of racemic epinephrine is 2.5 mg/ml (2.25%). Every precaution must be taken not to confuse the solution designed for parenteral administration because inadvertent injection can be fatal. A plastic or glass dropper should be used to prepare the dose because the solution reacts on contact with metals. Epinephrine should be protected from light because oxidation will turn the drug pink, then brown in color. Common adverse effects include tachycardia, palpitations, nervousness, tremor, insomnia, headache, loss of appetite, and nausea.[69]

Isoproterenol (Isuprel)

Isoproterenol is a highly potent nonselective β agonist that causes relaxation of bronchial smooth muscle, cardiac stimulation, and peripheral vasodilation in skeletal muscle and mesenteric vascular beds. Common adverse events include palpitations, tachycardia, headache, nervousness, dizziness, nausea, vomiting, tremor, and cutaneous flushing.[61] Use of isoproterenol has dramatically decreased with the introduction of more selective agents, and it is no longer recommended for the treatment of asthma because of the potential for adverse cardiac events.[8]

ANTICHOLINERGICS

Mechanism of Action

The parasympathetic nervous system plays a major role in regulating airway homeostasis and bronchomotor tone. Various noxious stimuli have been demonstrated to increase parasympathetic activity, resulting in bronchoconstriction. Anticholinergics inhibit parasympathetic nerve impulses by selectively blocking the binding of the neurotransmitter acetylcholine to its receptor site in nerve cells. The nerve fibers of the parasympathetic system are responsible for the involuntary movements of smooth muscles present in the gastrointestinal tract, urinary tract, and lungs[70] (Figure 20-2).

Place in Therapy

Anticholinergics are used to treat a variety of respiratory disorders in children, including asthma and chronic bronchitis.[8] Oral and parenteral administration of anticholinergics can be used to inhibit salivation and excessive secretions of the respiratory tract and treat chronic drooling associated with neurological conditions. Inhaled anticholinergics are effective bronchodilators, but not as effective as β_2-agonists, and only attenuate allergen-induced asthma and EIB. Inhaled ipratropium is indicated only as adjunctive therapy in severe acute asthma not completely responsive to β_2-agonists alone, whereas tiotropium is indicated for bronchospasms associated with COPD in adults.

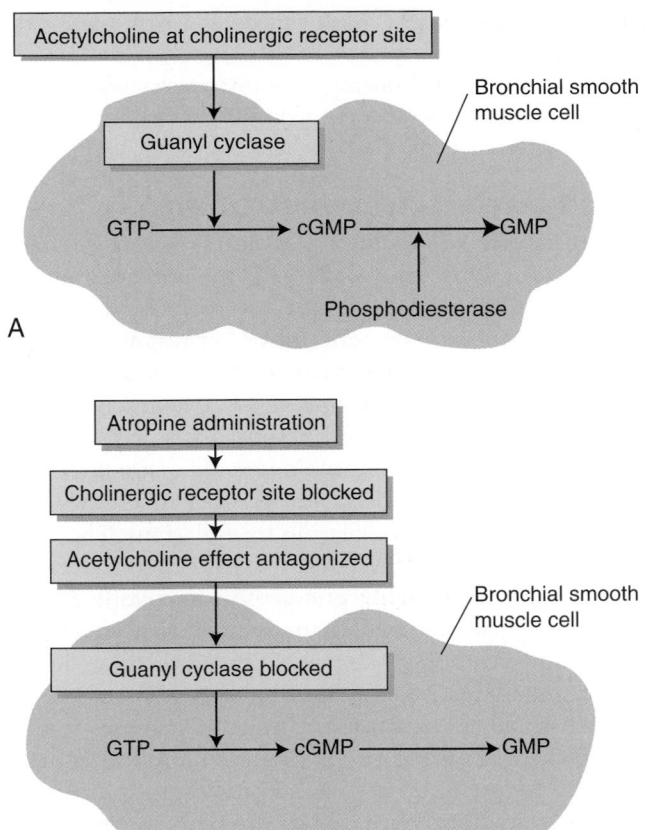

A, Parasympathetic mechanisms controlling bronchial smooth muscle tone. Stimulation of the parasympathetic system causes the release of acetylcholine at the cholinergic receptor site. Acetylcholine stimulates the enzyme guanylcyclase to convert guanosine triphosphate (GTP) to cyclic guanosine monophosphate (cGMP). Phosphodiesterase then breaks down cGMP to guanosine monophosphate (GMP). High cGMP levels result in bronchoconstriction. **B,** Administration of an anticholinergic (atropine) antagonizes the acetylcholinergic effect and prevents cGMP from forming. This relieves the bronchoconstriction.

Ipratropium Bromide (Atrovent)

Aerosolized ipratropium is not sufficiently effective to be used as a single agent in the treatment of acute bronchospasms. When administered to children with severe asthma exacerbations, multiple doses of ipratropium and a β agonist reduced the number of hospitalizations and improved overall lung function.[71] Although the addition of inhaled ipratropium bromide to inhaled β agonist therapy has proven effective in the emergency department setting, studies during hospital admissions have not revealed added benefit.[72,73] Therefore, ipratropium bromide is not recommended as standard therapy during hospitalizations for asthma exacerbations.

Dosage and Administration

Ipratropium bromide is available in a variety of dosage forms including a nasal spray, an MDI, and a nebulizer solution. Concentrations of the nasal spray are 0.03% and 0.06%. The dose for the nasal spray is 2 sprays in each nostril two or three times daily. The nasal spray is used only for symptomatic relief of rhinorrhea associated with allergic and nonallergic rhinitis; it does not relieve nasal congestion, sneezing, or postnasal drip.[74] The nebulizer solution vials are packaged in a foil pouch and must be protected from light. The inhalation solution can be mixed in the nebulizer with albuterol if used within 1 hour. Recommended dosing and administration comments regarding inhaled anticholinergics are listed in Table 20-1.

Ipratropium is also available premixed with albuterol in a solution for nebulization (DuoNeb) and as an MDI (Combivent). Each 3-ml vial of nebulizer solution contains 0.5 mg ipratropium bromide and 2.5 mg albuterol.[75] The recommended pediatric dose for asthma exacerbations is 1.5 to 3 ml every 20 minutes for 3 doses, then as needed. It is important to note that the recommended dose is based on the ipratropium component.[8] The MDI contains soya lecithin and should not be used in patients allergic to soya lecithin or related food products such as soybeans and peanuts.[76] Each actuation of the MDI contains 18 μg ipratropium bromide and 90 μg of albuterol.[75]

Adverse Events

Ipratropium bromide is an anticholinergic agent that is a quaternary ammonium derivative of atropine. Quaternary compounds are poorly absorbed across mucosal membranes and the blood–brain barrier; therefore, inhalation of ipratropium results in opening of the bronchi with minimal systemic effects.[77] The most common adverse reactions are dry mouth, cough, headache, nausea, dizziness, blurred vision, and drying of secretions. Skin flushing, tachycardia, acute angle–closure glaucoma, and palpitations have also been reported.

Glycopyrrolate (Robinul, Cuvposa)
Dosage and Administration

Glycopyrrolate belongs to a class of drugs known as the antimuscarinics that function by blocking muscarinic receptors and inhibiting cholinergic transmission. Glycopyrrolate is available in an oral and parenteral formulation used specifically to inhibit salivation and excessive secretions of the respiratory tract. The dose for control of secretions in children is 40 to 100 μg/kg three or four times daily. The intramuscular and intravenous dosage is 4 to 10 μg/kg every 3 to 4 hours. Glycopyrrolate is also used to counter the muscarinic effects of neostigmine and pyridostigmine during reversal of neuromuscular blockade. Contraindications to glycopyrrolate are similar to other anticholinergics medications, including narrow-angle glaucoma, severe ulcerative colitis, tachycardia, paralytic ileus, and myasthenia gravis.

Adverse Events

The parenteral formulation of glycopyrrolate contains benzyl alcohol, which has been associated with "gasping syndrome" (the quick inhalation and exhalation of breaths—much like gulping for air) in neonates after administration of large amounts of benzyl alcohol (more than 99 mg/kg/day).[78,79] Adverse reactions include thickening of bronchial secretions, tachycardia, behavioral changes, palpitations, drowsiness, headache, and ataxia. Extreme caution should be used in infants, patients with Down syndrome, and children with spastic paralysis or brain damage because of the potential hypersensitivity to the antimuscarinic effects.

CORTICOSTEROIDS

Mechanism of Action

Although the term *corticosteroids* is used for most endogenous steroids, it is the general term that includes both glucocorticoids and mineralocorticoids. Glucocorticoids (i.e., cortisol) control carbohydrate, fat, and protein metabolism and also have anti-inflammatory properties. Mineralocorticoids (i.e., aldosterone) control electrolyte and water levels, primarily by promoting sodium retention in the kidney.

Pharmacology of the corticosteroids is extremely complex and can ultimately affect almost all body systems. Corticosteroids are highly lipophilic and readily cross cell membranes to combine with glucocorticoid receptors found in the cytoplasm of most cells throughout the body. Corticosteroids act by controlling the rate of protein synthesis, depress the migration of polymorphonuclear leukocytes and fibroblasts, reverse capillary permeability, and stabilize lysomal membranes to prevent or control inflammation processes. Corticosteroids also increase the number and responsiveness of β_2-adrenergic receptors to β_2-adrenergic stimulation, therefore reducing hypersecretion, airway edema, and exudation. Cellular effects of corticosteroids are immediate but may require 4 to 12 hours before any clinical response is noted.[80]

Place in Therapy

Corticosteroids are potent anti-inflammatory agents used in a variety of disease states including the management of asthma in pediatric and adult patients. Inhaled corticosteroids have a high anti-inflammatory potency, approximately 1000-fold greater than endogenous cortisol.[81] Inhalation therapy allows the topical administration of the potent anti-inflammatory directly at the site of action, which reduces the risk of adverse events observed with systemic corticosteroid therapy. The Expert Panel Report 3 (EPR-3) on asthma states that inhaled corticosteroids are the most effective anti-inflammatory agents available for persistent asthma, and inhaled corticosteroids are the only therapy proven to reduce the risk of death from asthma.[8] Of note, inhaled corticosteroids are not as effective as systemic therapy for severe asthma exacerbations and should not be used as a substitute for systemic corticosteroid therapy.

Systemic corticosteroids are a vital component in the treatment of exacerbations of asthma because of their ability to decrease airway inflammation and secretions. In the emergency department, intravenous and oral corticosteroids are first-line therapy.[8,82,83] There is no added benefit of using intravenous dosing in a pediatric patient if the patient is able to tolerate oral dosing; thus oral administration is preferred.[84]

Dosage and Administration

Corticosteroids are available in a variety of dosage forms and listed in Table 20-2 along with the potential adverse events. Inhalational dosages are often increased depending on the age of the patient and his or her response to therapy. Once asthma symptoms are under control, the starting dose is adjusted to the lowest effective dose to reduce the possibility of side effects. Maximal benefit may not be achieved for 1 to 2 weeks or longer after starting treatment. There are significant differences in efficacy and safety of the available inhalation formulations. These differences result from differences in the chemical entity, potency, and pharmacokinetic profile. It is important to counsel the patient to rinse the mouth with water after each administration to decrease drug deposition in the mouth and local adverse events (e.g., thrush).

For asthma exacerbations, dosages of systemic corticosteroid therapy vary from 1 to 2 mg/kg/day with a maximum daily dose of 60 mg/day of prednisone.[8] The most commonly used intravenous agent is methylprednisolone; oral forms of hydrocortisone, dexamethasone, prednisone, and prednisolone are also available. Pharmacological and adverse effects of corticosteroids are dependent on the dose and duration of therapy. There is minimal risk of long-term adverse events if systemic agents are used for short periods (4 to 5 days). Because of potential suppression of the **hypothalamic-pituitary-adrenal (HPA) axis,** systemic doses should be tapered in patients who require a course longer than 10 days.[8,80] The lowest effective dose should be used in patients requiring chronic corticosteroid therapy.

Adverse Events

As stated earlier, the likelihood of systemic side effects increases when corticosteroids are used at high doses and/or for a long duration. Chronic use of corticosteroids produces a dose-dependent suppression of adrenal axis steroid production and may potentially impair growth in pediatric patients into adulthood.

The effects of inhaled corticosteroids on linear growth have extensively been described in literature.[85-88] Treatment with inhaled beclomethasone was associated with prepubertal growth impairment but suppression was limited to 1.5 cm/year in children treated with beclomethasone at 400 µg/day. Subsequent studies have shown that inhaled corticosteroid therapy combined with systemic corticosteroid therapy does not clinically affect final adult height.[88,89] Many studies to determine the effects on growth have significant design limitations. Delayed or impaired growth may be a result of the disease itself; the

TABLE 20-2

Corticosteroid Agents

Agent	Available Formulations	Adverse Events	Administration Comments
Inhaled Corticosteroids			
Beclomethasone dipropionate (Qvar)	MDI: 40 µg/puff, 80 µg/puff	Hoarseness, dry throat, dysphonia, cough, oropharyngeal candidiasis (thrush)	Patients should be instructed to rinse mouth with water after administration.
Budesonide (Pulmicort)	Flexhaler DPI: 90 µg/puff, 180 µg/puff Susp for nebulization: 0.25 mg/2 ml, 0.5 mg/2 ml		Most children younger than 4 years cannot provide sufficient inspiratory flow for adequate lung deliver of DPI.
Fluticasone (Flovent Diskus, Flovent HFA)	DPI: 50 µg/blister, 100 µg/blister, 250 µg/blister HFA: 44 µg/puff, 110 µg/puff, 220 µg/puff		
Combined Inhaled Corticosteroid and Long-Acting β₂-Agonist			
Fluticasone/Salmeterol (Advair HFA, Advair Diskus)	HFA (MDI): 45 µg/21 µg, 115 µg/21 µg, 230 µg/21 µg Diskus (DPI): 100 µg/50 µg, 250 µg/50 µg, 500 µg/50 µg,	See individual ingredients	Should not be used for acute symptom relief or asthma exacerbations.
Budesonide/Formoterol (Symbicort)	HFA (MDI): 80 µg/4.5 µg, 160 µg/4.5 µg		Most children younger than 4 years cannot provide sufficient inspiratory flow for adequate lung delivery of the DPI.
Oral Systemic Corticosteroids*			
Prednisone	Tablets: 1 mg, 2.5 mg, 5 mg, 10 mg, 20 mg, 50 mg Solution: 5 mg/5 ml, 5 mg/ml	Short-term use: reversible glucose metabolism, fluid retention, weight gain, mood alteration, hypertension, peptic ulcer	Children on low-dose therapy experience fewer behavioral side effects.
Prednisolone	Tablets: 5 mg Solution: 5 mg/5 ml, 15 mg/5 ml		Other systemic corticosteroids such as hydrocortisone and dexamethasone given in equipotent daily doses are likely to be as effective.
Methylprednisolone	Tablets: 2 mg, 4 mg, 8 mg, 16 mg, 32 mg, 50 mg Solution: 5 mg/5 ml, 5 mg/ml	Long-term use: HPA axis suppression, growth suppression, hypertension, Cushing syndrome	

*Recommended dosing is equivalent for all listed preparations.
DPI, Dry powder inhaler; *HFA,* hydrofluoroalkane; *HPA,* hypothalamic–pituitary–adrenal; *inh,* inhaled; *max,* maximum; *MDI,* metered-dose inhaler; *neb,* nebulization; *soln,* solution.

question remains as to whether the treatment or the underlying disease is the true determinant of linear growth reduction. Further studies have proved that even with this initial reduction in linear growth, the long-term effects do not last. In long-term follow-up, patients with a history of inhaled corticosteroid use achieved a height that fell within the expectation based on hereditary models.[84]

A majority of side effects attributed to corticosteroids are primarily seen with systemic therapy and not inhalational therapy. After corticosteroid inhalation, local adverse events include oropharyngeal candidiasis, **dysphonia,** cough, wheezing, and dry throat. The dysphonia appears to be the result of a direct effect of the steroid on the musculature that controls the vocal cords. Proper inhalation technique such as using a holding chamber device (i.e., spacer) or rinsing the mouth after each inhalation may help decrease the risk of local adverse events.

Major limitations to the long-term use of systemic corticosteroids include HPA axis suppression, Cushing syndrome, osteoporosis, myopathies, glaucoma, cataracts, gastritis, hypertension, **hirsutism,** electrolyte imbalances, glucose intolerance, skin atrophy, and immunosuppression, increasing the risk of opportunistic infections. Varicella infection (chickenpox) or measles may lead to serious or even fatal complications in children taking chronic systemic corticosteroids. If long-term systemic therapy is warranted, considerable care must be taken to avoid exposure to potential infectious diseases.

LEUKOTRIENE MODIFIERS

Mechanism of Action

Release of histamine and leukotrienes is triggered by exposure of allergens from mast cells, which are located throughout the walls of the respiratory tract. The synthesis of leukotrienes is dependent on lipoxygenation of arachidonic acid, a fatty acid found in cell membranes, by 5-lipoxygenase.[90,91] The leukotrienes work to constrict airway smooth muscle and increase vascular permeability, leading to airway edema, mucus production, and activation of inflammatory cells in the airways of patients with asthma.[92] Mast cell degranulation and leukotrienes are believed to be integral causes of exercise-induced bronchospasms after either drying or cooling of the airways.[93]

Current U.S. FDA-approved oral leukotriene-modifying agents are listed in Table 20-3. Classes of leukotriene modifiers are based on their site of action: leukotriene receptor antagonists (zafirlukast, montelukast) and leukotriene synthesis inhibitors (zileuton). Zafirlukast and montelukast act by selectively antagonizing leukotriene binding to its cellular receptor, cysteinyl leukotriene receptor (CysLT$_1$), which prevents a cascade that leads to constriction of bronchial smooth muscle. Zileuton acts as a potent and selective inhibitor of leukotriene formation by inhibiting 5-lipoxygenase, the enzyme responsible for converting arachidonic acid to the cysteinyl leukotrienes.[94-96]

Place in Therapy

Treatment with leukotriene modifiers is associated with improved asthma symptoms and pulmonary function, including improvement in FEV$_1$.[20] Pediatric studies demonstrate the usefulness of leukotriene modifiers in mild asthma and attenuation of exercise-induced bronchoconstriction. Leukotriene receptor antagonists are not an alternative to using β-adrenergic agonists during an asthma exacerbation but are recommended to be continued during an asthma exacerbation.[8]

Zileuton is approved for use in children older than 12 years and is used less commonly than other leukotriene modifiers because of a need to regularly monitor liver enzymes and drug–drug interactions. It is the only leukotriene synthesis inhibitor currently approved for use. Zileuton is effective in the treatment of cold air–induced, aspirin-intolerant, exercise-induced, and nocturnal asthma.[97] Zileuton reduces asthma symptoms, and the supplemental use of β agonists improves FEV$_1$ values and may have an additive effect with inhaled steroids.[98]

Leukotriene receptor antagonists montelukast and zafirlukast are useful as steroid-sparing agents for patients with difficult-to-control asthma. Although an inhaled corticosteroid has been shown to provide better control in patients with persistent asthma, leukotriene receptor antagonists are viable alternatives secondary to their ease of use and better adherence.[99] The most widely used leukotriene inhibitor, montelukast, is FDA approved for control of asthma in children 12 months of age or older and treatment of rhinitis in children 6 months of age or older. Zafirlukast is administered twice daily and approved for children older than 5 years. Use of montelukast or zafirlukast can reduce asthma symptoms and bronchial hyperreactivity and potentially decrease use of β agonists and systemic corticosteroids in children with intermittent or persistent asthma.[100-103] Recent pediatric studies of montelukast use in respiratory syncytial virus (RSV) bronchiolitis have shown promising results. Patients with RSV-positive bronchiolitis receiving daily montelukast demonstrated fewer daytime coughs and a delay in exacerbation when compared with placebo-treated controls.[104]

Zileuton (Zyflo)
Dosage and Administration

Zileuton is available as a 600-mg tablet and an extended-release 600-mg tablet. The recommended dosage in adults and children 12 years and older is 600-mg four times per day for a total daily dose of 2400 mg, or 1200 mg twice daily with an extended-release tablet. Zileuton should be taken with meals and at bedtime but can be taken with or without food. The extended-release tablet should not be crushed, cut, or chewed. Zileuton is a cytochrome P-450 enzyme substrate and as such will affect the plasma concentration of other substrates metabolized by the P-450 system such as theophylline, propranolol, and warfarin.

Adverse Events

The most common side effects are abdominal pain, upset stomach, and nausea. Zileuton is associated with threefold or greater elevations of liver enzymes (serum aminotransferase) in 2% to 4% of patients.[105] The elevations usually occur during the first 3 months of treatment and return to normal when zileuton is discontinued. Therefore liver function should be evaluated before starting zileuton, monthly for the first 3 months of treatment, then every 3 months for the first year, and periodically thereafter.

TABLE 20-3			
Leukotriene-Modifying Agents			
Agent	**Available Formulations**	**Adverse Events**	**Administration Comments**
Zileuton (Zyflo)	600-mg tablet, 600-mg 12-hour extended release tablet	Elevated liver enzymes, reversible hepatitis, and hyperbilirubinemia	Extended-release tablet should not be crushed, cut, or chewed. Zileuton increases serum theophylline and warfarin concentrations.
Zafirlukast (Accolate)	10-mg chewable tablet, 20-mg tablet	Headache, elevated liver enzymes, reversible hepatitis	Administer at least 1 hour before or 2 hours after a meal.
Montelukast (Singulair)	4-mg or 5-mg chewable tablet, 10-mg tablet, 4-mg granule packet	NOTE: Rare cases of eosinophilic vasculitis (Churg-Strauss) have been reported.	Patients with both asthma and allergic rhinitis should take their dose in the evening. Montelukast granules are not intended to be dissolved in liquid and must be administered within 15 minutes of opening the packet.

Montelukast (Singulair) and Zafirlukast (Accolate)
Dosage and Administration

Montelukast is available as both a 4-mg and 5-mg chewable cherry-flavored tablet, as well as a 10-mg film-coated tablet. The dose for children 2 to 5 years old is one 4-mg tablet daily. The dose for children 6 to 14 years old is one 5-mg tablet daily. The dose for adolescents (15 years and older) and adults is one 10-mg tablet daily. Montelukast is dosed once daily in the evening as 4-mg or 5-mg chewable tablets for ages 2 to 5 years and 6 to 14 years, respectively. A 10-mg tablet is available for adolescents older than 15 years. The initial response after a single dose of montelukast occurs in 3 to 4 hours with a duration of action up to 24 hours. Montelukast has also been shown to improve symptoms when used in combination with loratadine for the treatment of seasonal allergic rhinitis.

Zafirlukast is rapidly absorbed after oral administration, with a response in approximately 3 hours. The duration of action is approximately 10 hours. Clinical trials demonstrated that zafirlukast improved daytime asthma symptoms, nighttime awakenings, rescue β agonist use, FEV_1, and morning peak expiratory flow rate.[92] Zafirlukast is not a bronchodilator and is not used to treat acute episodes of asthma. Because food reduces the bioavailability, zafirlukast should be taken on an empty stomach or approximately 1 hour before or 2 hours after meals. Zafirlukast can inhibit the metabolism of warfarin; therefore, patients receiving warfarin anticoagulant therapy concomitantly with zafirlukast should have their prothrombin time closely monitored and adjusted accordingly.

Adverse Events

Leukotriene modifiers are appealing because of their excellent safety profile for long-term control of mild persistent asthma in children. The most common side effect is headache. Other side effects of leukotriene receptor antagonists include mild fatigue, fever, abdominal pain, gastroenteritis, heartburn, dizziness, and rash.

Elevation of liver enzymes, progressing to hepatitis and hepatic failure, has occurred in patients using zafirlukast. Most incidents occurred while using doses four times higher than the recommend dose; however, similar cases have occurred in patients receiving the recommended daily dose.

In rare cases, patients may present with clinical features of vasculitis consistent with **Churg-Strauss syndrome,** which typically have been reported in patients undergoing a reduction in oral corticosteroid medication. Resolution of symptoms occurred when the agent was discontinued and corticosteroid therapy resumed.[106-109] Although further studies are needed to determine the extent of the association, many believe that the syndrome is unmasked after withdrawal of the corticosteroid.[110]

METHYLXANTHINES

Theophylline
Mechanism of Action

The chemical structure of theophylline is similar to dietary caffeine with a mechanism of action that is not completely understood. Theophylline is thought to competitively inhibit phosphodiesterase, the enzyme that degrades cAMP. Increased concentrations of cAMP may mediate the observed bronchodilation (see Figure 20-1). Other proposed mechanisms of action include inhibition of the release of intracellular calcium and competitive antagonism of the bronchoconstrictor adenosine. As a result, theophylline relaxes smooth muscle, stimulates the central nervous system and cardiac muscle, increases mucociliary transport and diaphragmatic contractility, and acts on the kidneys to promote diuresis.[7]

Place in Therapy

Theophylline has both bronchodilatory and anti-inflammatory properties, with potential steroid-sparing and immunomodulatory effects.[111,112] The role of theophylline in the management of childhood asthma has been decreasing because of serious adverse affects. Theophylline is not recommended for acute asthma exacerbations but can be used as an alternative to inhaled corticosteroids for children with mild persistent asthma.[8]

Dosage and Administration

Theophylline is available in a multitude of dosage formulations and strengths, with great variation in the recommended dosing guidelines based on patient age. Sustained-release preparations generally provide more consistent drug levels and allow dosing once, twice, or three times daily, favoring patient compliance. Theophylline is rapidly absorbed, with wide variations in clearance because of differences in hepatic metabolism. Multiple factors increase the clearance rate of theophylline and result in higher dose requirements, including smoking, hyperthyroidism, and concurrent use of medications such as phenobarbital and rifampin. Factors that can decrease clearance and lead to toxicity include hypothyroidism, congestive heart failure, liver failure, and the use of oral contraceptives and various antibiotics, including ciprofloxacin and erythromycin.

Because of the wide interpatient variability of theophylline clearance, routine serum theophylline level monitoring is vital. Doses are adjusted based on serum concentrations, with a goal of 5 to 15 μg/ml when drug concentrations approach steady state. Steady state occurs approximately 48 hours after the administration of the same dose of theophylline.[8]

Adverse Events

The use of theophylline to treat chronic childhood asthma is problematic because of potentially serious short-term and long-term adverse events. Dose-related acute toxicities include tachycardia, nausea, vomiting, supraventricular tachycardia, central nervous system stimulation, seizures, headache, and electrolyte disturbances. Adverse events seen at therapeutic serum concentrations include insomnia, gastric upset, and hyperactivity.[8,113]

MAST CELL STABILIZERS

Cromolyn Sodium (Gastrocrom)
Mechanism of Action

Although the complete mechanism of action of cromolyn is unknown, it does inhibit mast cell degranulation after exposure to antigens, therefore blocking the release of histamine and leukotrienes. These actions serve to inhibit the early asthmatic response through stabilization of the mast cell membrane. Cromolyn has no intrinsic bronchodilator, antihistaminic, anticholinergic, or vasoconstrictor activity.[7]

Place in Therapy

The EPR-3 on asthma recommends cromolyn sodium for treatment of mild and moderate persistent asthma.[8] Inhaled corticosteroids are superior to cromolyn as controller therapy for mild persistent asthma in children. Although there are some studies in which cromolyn compared favorably to other therapies, a systematic review of trials of cromolyn versus placebo found no clear therapeutic effect.[114,115]

Dosage, Administration, and Adverse Events

Cromolyn sodium is only available as a nebulizer solution. The recommended dosage of the solution for nebulization in children older than 2 years is 20 mg (one 2-ml ampule) four times daily. The ampule must be protected from light and should not be used it if it contains a precipitate or becomes discolored. Serious adverse events after cromolyn administration are relatively rare; however, the most commonly reported include cough, nasal congestion, nausea, throat irritation, and sneezing.[116]

MAGNESIUM SULFATE

Mechanism of Action

Magnesium is an abundant intracellular **cation** and a cofactor in more than 300 enzymatic and cellular reactions in the body. Magnesium relaxes smooth muscle and can cause depression of the central nervous system. When given intravenously, magnesium promotes bronchodilation by competing for binding sites with calcium ions, essentially acting as a competitive calcium channel blocker.[117]

Place in Therapy

Magnesium sulfate is generally reserved for patients in the emergency department or those having life-threatening exacerbations who remain in the severe category after 1 hour of intensive conventional therapy.[8] Clinical studies have proven safe improvements of spirometric indices during severe asthma exacerbations when magnesium sulfate is used in addition to standard therapy in the ED.[118-120] Nebulized magnesium sulfate has also been used successfully with and without β_2-agonists in the treatment of acute asthma.[121,122]

Dosage, Administration, and Adverse Events

The intravenous dose of $MgSO_4$ for bronchodilation as adjunctive treatment in an acute severe asthma exacerbation is 25 to 75 mg/kg, with a maximum of 2 g given as a single dose.[8] Oral administrations are not commonly used for asthma exacerbations; however, it is important to note that a 1-g dose of magnesium sulfate is equivalent to 98.6 mg (8.12 mEq) of elemental magnesium if $MgSO_4$ is used to treat hypomagnesemia.

Dose-related facial flushing and vasodilation can occur, as well as infusion-related hypotension and vasodilation. Other adverse events of $MgSO_4$ include fatigue, somnolence, respiratory depression, and blunting of deep tendon reflexes. As the magnesium serum level diminishes, deep tendon reflexes return in reverse order of attenuation.

MUCOLYTIC AND HYDRATING AGENTS

N-Acetylcysteine (Mucomyst)
Mechanism of Action

The viscosity of mucous secretions in the lungs depends on the concentrations of mucoprotein and the presence of disulfide bonds between these macromolecules and DNA. N-acetylcysteine (NAC) acts to split the sulfide bonds in the macromolecules, thereby decreasing viscosity and elasticity of airway mucus, allowing for removal by normal chest physiotherapy.[123] The action of N-acetylcysteine is pH dependent, with mucolytic action significant at pH ranges of 7.0 to 9.0.[124]

Place in Therapy

Oral and aerosolized NAC is indicated as a **mucolytic** agent used as adjunctive therapy for pulmonary complications involving abnormal or viscid mucous secretions such as bronchopulmonary disease, pulmonary complications of surgery, and cystic fibrosis (CF).[125] Use of mucolytics in clearing secretions in patients with non–cystic fibrosis bronchiectasis is controversial and uncertain.[126,127] Intravenous and oral formulations of acetylcysteine are used as emergent antidotes in acetaminophen overdose to prevent or lessen hepatic injury after ingestion of a hepatotoxic quantity of acetaminophen.[128]

Dosage, Administration and Adverse Events

N-acetylcysteine is available as either a 10% or 20% solution. The recommended aerosolized dose of N-acetylcysteine in children is 3 to 5 ml of the 20% solution. The 20% solution should be diluted with an equal volume of water or normal saline and administered by nebulizer three or four times per day. The 10% solution may be used undiluted. The aerosolized solution should be administered separately as it is incompatible with several other medications. A slight color change (light purple) may occur with opened vials but does not affect the safety or efficacy of the solution.[129]

Adverse events reported with *N*-acetylcysteine include stomatitis, vomiting, hemoptysis, bronchospasm, and severe rhinorrhea. It has an unpleasant, pungent odor that may lead to an increased incidence of nausea.[124]

Dornase Alfa (Pulmozyme)
Mechanism of Action

An additional factor that contributes to viscous mucus in patients with CF is extracellular DNA. Bacterial cell death and subsequent cell lysis release DNA into the extracellular environment, which works to thicken airway secretions. Dornase alfa is a highly purified solution of recombinant human deoxyribonuclease I (rhDNase), an enzyme that selectively cleaves DNA, facilitating mucus clearance in the lung.[130]

Place in Therapy

By decreasing the size and viscosity of DNA in sputum, dornase alfa has been demonstrated to reduce mucous obstruction and improve pulmonary function in patients with CF. Studies have shown that daily administration of dornase alfa results in a definite improvement in the FEV_1 above baseline.[131] Furthermore, administration of dornase alfa in CF patients also resulted in a significant reduction in the number of patients experiencing respiratory tract infections requiring parenteral antibiotics.[132-134]

Dosage, Administration, and Adverse Events

Dornase alfa is indicated as an adjunct to standard therapies to improve pulmonary function in the management of patients 5 years of age and older with CF. The recommended dose for most patients with CF is 2.5 mg by nebulizer once daily; however, some patients may benefit from twice-daily treatments. Although dornase alfa is not approved in children younger than 5 years, there are small studies in children as young as 3 months of age with similar reported efficacy and adverse events.[135,136] Because of inactivation, dornase alfa ampules should be kept refrigerated and not diluted or mixed with other medications in the nebulizer.[137]

Common adverse events have included voice alteration, pharyngitis, laryngitis, rash, and chest pain. Other less common adverse events include respiratory symptoms, flu syndrome, malaise, hypoxia, and weight loss.[137] Interestingly, when aerosolized dornase alfa is administered in healthy subjects and CF patients, a lack of an allergic response or serum antibodies has been demonstrated.[138]

Hypertonic Saline
Mechanism of Action

Several hypotheses have been postulated to explain the mechanism by which hypertonic saline works in pulmonary diseases. Proposed mechanisms include alteration of mucus viscosity by osmotic absorption of water from the submucosa, restoration of airway surface liquid, and irritant properties that stimulate cough and mucociliary clearance of mucociliary secretions.[139]

Place in Therapy

Hypertonic saline is considered a hydrator and not a mucolytic agent. Hypertonic saline has been studied in several chronic lung disease states as a means of mobilizing secretions, with most of the literature supporting use in CF patients. Ultrasonic nebulization of 7% hypertonic saline in patients with CF with moderate obstructive lung disease has been shown to increase mucociliary clearance.[140,141] On the other hand, studies in non-CF bronchiectasis have been unclear. A recent Cochrane review found no papers worthy of analysis; however, some studies have shown benefit if added to other mucus-clearance technologies.[142,143] Further studies on the long-term efficacy of hypertonic saline therapy and optimal hypertonic saline concentration are warranted.

Dosage, Administration, and Adverse Events

A variety of hypertonic saline concentrations has been used in conjunction with inspiratory positive ventilation, with a usual dose of 3 to 4 ml via nebulizer every 4 hours up to twice daily. The 3% and 5% nebulized solutions are often used if the 7% hypertonic saline solution is not tolerated. Studies administering hypertonic saline used various types of nebulizers, including jet and ultrasonic nebulizers.[140,145,146] Hypertonic saline should not be mixed with any of the standard bronchodilators or adjunctive agents. The most commonly reported side effect is cough; however, bronchospasms and pulmonary edema have also been reported. Prophylactic bronchodilator administration is recommended to prevent the potential bronchospasms.[140]

ANESTHETICS
Ketamine
Mechanism of Action

The mechanism of action for ketamine appears to be a selective interruption of the association pathways of the brain. The resulting bronchodilation may be of sympathetic origin. There is also a parasympathetic limb of action whereby ketamine diminishes acetylcholine activity on bronchial smooth muscle, resulting in bronchodilation.[147,148]

Place in Therapy

Ketamine is an anesthetic agent that produces anesthesia, sedation, and amnesia without significant respiratory depression. Because of its bronchodilating effects, ketamine has been used as part of rapid-sequence intubation in pediatric patients with status asthmaticus. It has also been used as a combined bronchodilator and sedative in patients with asthma requiring mechanical ventilation. In the setting of quickly deteriorating asthma, ketamine may be one of several last-resort medications to prevent placing the patient on mechanical ventilation. In general, the use of ketamine should be viewed as third- or fourth-line therapy.[149]

Dosage, Administration, and Adverse Events

Ketamine is given through a central venous catheter as a continuous infusion with a normal dose for sedation of 5 to 20 µg/kg/min. For bronchodilation, the starting dose may be as small as 2 µg/kg/min and titrated to effect.[150,151] For sedation or minor procedures, the dose is 0.5 to 1 mg/kg. The duration of action of a single dose can last up to 10 to 20 minutes. Parenteral administrations should not exceed 0.5 mg/kg/min and be given no faster than 60 seconds.[152]

Adverse events seen with ketamine include increased sympathomimetic activity, seizures, delirium, increased laryngeal secretions, and respiratory depression. During the recovery phase, unusual dreams and hallucinations have been reported. Premedication with midazolam (less than 0.1 mg/kg) can attenuate this effect. Intubation equipment must be readily available before administering ketamine, because the sedative effects may result in respiratory failure and the need for emergency intubation. Epinephrine should also be available for possible bradycardia.

AEROSOLIZED ANTIMICROBIALS

The delivery of aerosolized antibiotics is a vital component of treatment for several respiratory disorders, including CF, non-CF bronchiectasis, and pneumonia.[144] Aerosol delivery of antibiotics reduces the likelihood of systemic adverse events and is often used for targeted antimicrobial delivery to a site of infection.[153] However, the delivery of aerosolized antimicrobials to infants and children is complicated by several anatomical and physiological differences in their respiratory systems in comparison to adults.

Several factors influence the ultimate amount of drug delivered to the appropriate anatomical region within the lung, including properties of the delivery device, aerosol particles, disease state, administration technique, and the drug's specific pharmacological properties. The pharmacological effect of a drug is dependent on the site of deposition within the lung, the rate of drug clearance from the airway, and the site of infection.[154] To be effective, drug particles must withstand the forces required to generate the aerosol and often must penetrate a mucus layer (i.e., biofilm) and airway mucosa to reach their target receptor sites or cells.

Pulmonary manifestations as a result of colonization of *Pseudomonas aeruginosa* in CF patients have independently been associated with a decline in lung function and death.[155]

Therapies, including aerosolized antimicrobials, can potentially decrease organism burden or eliminate colonization, improving clinical outcomes of patients with CF.[153,156] Strategies for optimal use of aerosolized antimicrobials differ depending on the status of the patient. Eradication of airway pathogens is most likely early in the disease; once the patient has been colonized, suppressive therapy is unlikely to eradicate the organism but may potentially reduce disease complications. Chronic suppressive therapy cycles between 28-days-on and 28-days-off therapy designed to suppress bacterial burden, which has been shown to improve lung function, quality of life, and hospitalization rates.[157]

Addition of inhaled antimicrobials to the armamentarium of antibiotics may help address the problematic increase in antimicrobial resistance. Antimicrobial classes such as aminoglycosides, β-lactams, and antivirals have all been aerosolized with various degrees of efficacy; however, only a few commercial formulations currently exist for this route of administration.[153] Usual doses and administration comments for nebulized antimicrobials are listed in Table 20-4.

Tobramycin (Tobi, Tobi Podhaler)
Mechanism, Place in Therapy, and Adverse Events

Tobramycin is an aminoglycoside antibiotic typically used to treat gram-negative infections, including *Pseudomonas aeruginosa*. Tobramycin is bactericidal by binding to ribosomal subunits, which in turn inhibits bacterial protein synthesis. An inhalation formulation of tobramycin solution (Tobi) was approved by the U.S. FDA in 1998 primarily for chronic suppressive therapy in CF patients. Use of nebulized tobramycin can improve FEV_1 by 7.8% to 12% in CF patients and potentially eradicate *P. aeruginosa* from the respiratory tract in early colonization and in young patients.[157-159] Several clinical studies have also shown a reduction in hospitalizations for acute exacerbations as well as in the parenteral use of antipseudomonal antibiotics in CF patients with varying degrees of disease severity.[157-159] Tobramycin inhalation solution is indicated for CF patients older than 6 years with *P. aeruginosa* infection and an FEV_1 between 25% and 75% of predicted values.[160] Aerosolized tobramycin has also played a role in the treatment of hospital-acquired pneumonia and treatment of acute exacerbations and suppression for non-CF bronchiectasis.[153] (TOBI PODHALER [tobramycin] capsule [package insert]. Novartis Pharmaceuticals Corporation, East Hanover, NJ, 2013)

Peak sputum levels of aerosolized tobramycin can exceed 10 to 25 times the **minimum inhibitory concentration** (MIC) of bacterial pathogens; however, systemic exposure and incidence of systemic adverse events are relatively low. Cough, pharyngitis, increased sputum production, rhinitis, and dyspnea are the most commonly reported adverse effects.[161]

A tobramycin inhalation powder (TIP) has recently been approved by the FDA designed to relieve the high treatment burden and improve patient adherence in patients with CF with chronic pulmonary *P. aeruginosa* infections. The

TABLE 20-4

Aerosolized Antimicrobial Agents

Antimicrobial	Antimicrobial Class	Usual Dosage	Administration Comments
Tobramycin inhalational solution (Tobi)	Aminoglycoside	300 mg every 12 hours in repeated cycles of 28 days on followed by 28 days off with Pari LC Plus	Doses should be administered at least 6 hours apart. Ampules should be kept in the refrigerator and protected from light.
Tobramycin inhalation powder (Tobi Podhaler)	Aminoglycoside	Inhalation of the contents of four 28 mg capsules twice-daily for 28 days on followed by 28 days off using the Podhaler device	Capsules must not be swallowed and should always be stored in the blister and removed immediately before use.
Aztreonam lysine (Cayston)	Monobactam	75 mg three times daily in repeated cycles of 28 days on followed by 28 days off with Altera nebulizer system	Use of a bronchodilator before administration is recommended. Incompatible with other nebulizer medications.
Colistimethate (Coly-Mycin M)	Polymixin	80-160 mg twice daily	Solution should be used promptly after reconstitution.
Pentamidine (NebuPent)	Antiprotozoal	300 mg every 4 weeks with Respirgard II nebulizer	Safety and efficacy dependent on appropriately sized face mask. Do not mix with other nebulizer solutions.
Ribavirin	Antiviral	Continuous: 12-18 hours/day × 3 days. Intermittent: 2 g over 2 hours three times daily with Viratek small particle aerosol generator	Contraindicated in pregnancy. Incompatible with other nebulizer medications.

inhalation powder formulation is a light, porous particle using PulmoSphere technology designed to deliver the tobramycin in a capsule-based dry powder inhaler over 5 minutes without the need for any device cleaning.[188] Clinical studies in patients older than 6 years have shown that systemic exposure to TIP is comparable with the tobramycin inhalation solution, as is efficacy, and TIP had higher treatment satisfaction scores, a shorter duration of administration, and a higher rate of cough.[189,190]

Aztreonam Lysine (Cayston)
Mechanism, Place in Therapy, and Adverse Events

Aztreonam is a relatively old monobactam antibiotic that historically has been used intravenously to treat gram-negative bacteria by binding to the cell wall penicillin-binding proteins leading to cell wall destruction. The parenteral formulation contains arginine to stabilize the formulation's pH; however, repeated exposure to arginine has been shown to cause airway inflammation and coughing.[162,163] The nebulized aztreonam solution (Cayston) is a newly formulated lyophilized lysine salt approved for chronic suppressive therapy of respiratory symptoms in CF patients. Aztreonam lysine is indicated for patients 7 years and older with FEV_1 between 25% and 75% of predicted values not colonized with *Burkholderia cepacia*. The inhaled formulation of aztreonam is only administered using the Altera nebulizer system, which is designed to produce appropriate-sized particles to achieve high sputum and low systemic concentrations over a treatment period of 2 to 3 minutes. Nebulized aztreonam is dosed three times a day, consistent with other antibiotics that require multiple daily doses secondary to the time-dependent killing.[164] Interestingly, patients with mild lung impairment treated for 4 weeks with inhaled aztreonam did not demonstrate significant improvement in respiratory symptoms; however, patients with an FEV_1 lower than 90% experienced a greater response.[165] Open-label studies of eradication of early *P. aeruginosa* in pediatric patients are currently under way.

Because nebulized aztreonam is fairly new to U.S. markets, the majority of adverse events reported are based on observations from clinical trials and may not reflect the rates observed in a clinical setting. The most common adverse reactions reported were cough, nasal congestion, wheezing, and pharyngolaryngeal pain. Short-acting bronchodilators provides a greater reduction in *P. aeruginosa* density as well as improved FEV_1 and sputum drug concentrations when administered between 15 minutes and 4 hours before each dose.[166,167]

Colistimethate (Coly-Mycin M)
Mechanism, Place in Therapy, and Adverse Events

Colistimethate sodium is a polymyxin antibiotic that acts as a cationic detergent damaging bacterial cytoplasmic membranes of gram-negative organisms, causing leakage of intracellular substances and eventually cell death. Colistin has been aerosolized for several years for eradication and chronic suppression of *P. aeruginosa*. Coincidently, there is a paucity of large, randomized, controlled studies, but colistin has been reported to be used therapeutically in prevention or eradication of bacteria in CF, treatment of hospital-acquired pneumonia, and suppressive therapy in non-CF bronchiectasis.[153] The Cystic Fibrosis Foundation Pulmonary Guidelines Committee found insufficient evidence to recommend for or against the use of colistin for chronic *P. aeruginosa* infection, but the agent was included in the European guidelines on inhaled medications in CF.[160,168]

As compared with other nebulized antimicrobials, colistin has a higher rate and severity of pulmonary adverse events, nephrotoxicity, and bronchospasms. After reconstitution of colistimethate, the drug molecule is hydrolyzed into two active components, polymyxin E1 and polymyxin E2. In animal models, polymyxin E1 can cause localized inflammation of the airway epithelia and eosinophilic infiltration. When colistimethate is used for inhalational therapy, the colistimethate solution should be used promptly after reconstitution to limit the potential risk of lung toxicity.

Pentamidine (NebuPent)
Mechanism, Place in Therapy, and Adverse Events

Pneumocystis jirovecii (formerly known as *Pneumocystis carinii*) pneumonia is an opportunistic infection that historically had a high rate of mortality, which has since decreased because of the routine use of prophylaxis. *P. carinii* is an animal commensal, whereas *P. jirovecii* is the human commensal and pathogen. PCP as an acronym for *Pneumocystis* pneumonia has been retained since the change in nomenclature.[169,170] In severe cases of PCP, such as adult patients requiring mechanical ventilation, mortality can approach up to 50%; PCP is associated with an even higher rate of mortality in children.[171] Disease states associated with immunosuppression are typical candidates for *Pneumocystis* prophylaxis, including patients with human immunodeficiency virus (HIV), solid organ transplant recipients, and patients with hematological malignancies.

Pentamidine is categorized as an antiprotozoal and acts by interfering with protein synthesis by inhibiting oxidative phosphorylation of nucleotides and nucleic acids into protozoa RNA and DNA.[172] Clinical trials have proven a slight inferiority of aerosolized pentamidine compared with trimethoprim-sulfamethoxazole, which has led to the Infectious Disease Society of America (Arlington, VA), Centers for Disease Control and Prevention (CDC, Atlanta, GA), and American Academy of Pediatrics (Elk Grove, IL) to recommend aerosolized pentamidine as a secondary alternative for prevention of PCP in patients with HIV infection.[173] Aerosolized pentamidine is not recommended for the treatment of PCP because of limited efficacy and more frequent relapses.[173]

Aerosol administration of pentamidine is associated with fewer systemic adverse events than oral administration of prophylactic agents. Respiratory symptoms include cough, wheezing, shortness of breath, and reversible bronchospasms Other effects include fatigue, dizziness or lightheadedness, fever, throat irritation, conjunctivitis,

decreased appetite, nephrotoxicity, glucose intolerance, and allergic reactions.[172] Nebulized pentamidine should be administered in a negative pressure room and through a Respigard II, which routes exhaled breaths through a microfilter to avoid potential adverse events to health care workers in the immediate treatment area.

ANTIVIRAL AGENTS

Ribavirin (Virazole)
Mechanism, Place in Therapy, and Adverse Events

Ribavirin is a synthetic nucleoside analogue that disrupts viral protein synthesis through inhibition of messenger ribonucleic acid (mRNA) expression. Oral ribavirin is used in combination with parenteral pegylated interferon alfa-2a for treatment of chronic hepatitis C. Nebulized ribavirin is the only FDA-approved agent for the treatment of hospitalized infants and children with respiratory syncytial virus (RSV) lower respiratory tract infections (see Chapter 26).[174] However, routine use is not recommended and should be reserved for life-threatening RSV infections because of lack of consistent efficacy data and potential risks to health care workers administering the aerosol.[175-177] Nebulized ribavirin has also been used in treating severe influenza virus infections; however, it does not appear to be beneficial other than reducing the duration of fever in hospitalized children.[178]

In nonmechanically ventilated infants, aerosolized ribavirin should be administered in an oxygen hood from the small particle aerosol generator (SPAG-2). Special precautions are essential with mechanically ventilated patients to prevent complications and to reduce the risk of crystalline precipitation in the circuit. The use of one-way valves in the inspiratory lines, a breathing circuit filter in the expiratory line, and frequent monitoring and filter placement are effective in preventing these complications and subsequent ventilator dysfunction.

Adverse events attributed to nebulized ribavirin are infrequent but can include sudden deterioration and adverse cardiovascular effects. The most common reported adverse events include conjunctival irritation, rash, and transient wheezing. Techniques to reduce environmental exposure are highly recommended to reduce risk of toxicity to the health care provider and surrounding staff. Ribavirin is FDA pregnancy category X; thus pregnant women should not directly care for patients receiving aerosolized ribavirin. Because aerosolized particles of ribavirin can precipitate on contact lenses, the use of protective goggles or glasses is recommended.[174]

IMMUNOMODULATORS

Palivizumab (Synagis)
Mechanism, Place in Therapy, and Adverse Events

Palivizumab is a humanized monoclonal antibody with neutralizing activity against the F protein of RSV. It is given intramuscularly on a monthly basis at a dose of 15 mg/kg/dose throughout the annual RSV season. Typically, RSV activity is between November and March with a peak in January or February. Communities in the southern United States, particularly Florida, tend to experience earlier onsets of RSV. Palivizumab has demonstrated benefit in protecting against RSV hospitalization in premature infants with underlying prematurity, chronic lung disease of infancy, and congenital heart disease.[179-181] Five monthly doses of palivizumab provides more than 20 weeks of protective serum antibody concentrations.[182] However, cost considerations have lead to restrictive guideline recommendations for high-risk infants from the American Academy of Pediatrics (Elk Grove, IL), including full-term and premature infants with either chronic lung disease, congenital heart disease, or congenital abnormalities of the airway [175]

Adverse reactions to palivizumab are extremely rare. The most common reported reactions include rash, fever, local injection site reactions, and, rarely, anaphylaxis.[182]

Omalizumab (Xolair)
Mechanism, Place in Therapy, and Adverse Events
Omalizumab is a recombinant humanized monoclonal anti-IgE antibody that binds to the same receptor of the IgE molecule on basophils and mast cells. In turn, omalizumab inhibits the release of free IgE from mast cells in response to an allergen exposure and has been shown to decrease the incidence of asthma exacerbations.[183] Subcutaneous omalizumab is recommended as adjunctive therapy in patients 12 years and older who have allergies and severe persistent asthma that is inadequately controlled with the combination of high-dose inhaled corticosteroids and long-acting β agonists.[8] There is no indication for the use of omalizumab in the treatment of other allergic conditions, including the relief of acute bronchospasms or status asthmaticus.[183]

Adverse reactions include headache, dizziness, fatigue, and local injection site reactions. Although rare, anaphylactic reactions have occurred after the first and subsequent doses in patients who presented no identifiable triggers. Patients should be monitored and medications for treatment of severe allergic reactions should be readily available.[183]

INVESTIGATIONAL AGENTS

Bronchodilators

Simplifying pharmacological regimens to bronchodilating agents is fundamental to increasing patient compliance and controlling symptoms of asthma and COPD. The potential of a single drug with a long duration of action or with a bifunctional mechanism of action presents a new approach to the treatment of restrictive respiratory diseases.

Aclidinium bromide (Tudorza, Forest Pharmaceuticals Inc., St. Louis, MO) is a novel long-acting anticholinergic agent that recently obtained FDA approval for long-term maintenance treatment of bronchospasms associated with

COPD.[184] When compared with other bronchodilatory agents in vitro, aclidinium demonstrated potent anticholinergic activity comparable to both tiotropium and ipratropium. Aclidium displayed a faster onset of action than tiotropium and a significantly longer duration of action versus ipratropium, allowing for a 24-hour duration of action.[185] Clinical studies evaluating dose efficacy and safety have resulted in improvements in bronchodilation, health status, and dyspnea in patients with COPD with a relatively low incidence of adverse events when compared with placebo.[186]

Secondary to the proven clinical efficacy of inhaled anticholinergics and β$_2$-agonists, there has been recent interest in the development of combining both pharmacological agents for the treatment of asthma and COPD. GSK-961081 is a novel long-acting muscarinic receptor antagonist/β$_2$-adrenergic receptor agonist (MABA) bronchodilator that is currently in clinical studies. GSK-961081 has a dual mechanism of action that covalently links a muscarinic antagonist and a β$_2$-agonist within a single drug molecule. In phase I randomized double-blind, placebo-controlled studies of healthy volunteers, GSK961081 was generally well tolerated and demonstrated evidence of bronchodilation more than 24 hours after a single dose and after seven consecutive daily doses.[187] Phase 2 studies with GSK-96108 is currently under way.

Antimicrobials

The emerging recognition of aerosol antibiotics' role as an integral part of treatment regimens in patients with chronic airway infections has stimulated several efforts in drug development research. There have been significant advances in the development of novel aerosolized antibiotic formulations including a liposomal aminoglycoside and fluoroquinolone inhalation solution that are in various stages of clinical development.

Amikacin is an aminoglycoside antibiotic with a similar mechanism of action to tobramycin; it is currently in phase III studies. Liposomal amikacin (Arikace, Transave Incorporated, Monmouth Junction, NJ) is being developed as an inhaled treatment option for gram-negative infections aerosolized with an eFlow nebulizer. Theoretically this novel formulation is advantageous because the liposomes have been shown to penetrate biofilms in vitro, which would allow for sustained high drug concentrations in the lung and potentially improve compliance and clinical outcomes.[191] Once-daily doses of the liposomal amikacin have been shown to be equivalent as twice-daily tobramycin in rat lung models, and a sustained effect in FEV$_1$ versus placebo has been observed in human clinical studies.[191,192]

Inhalational levofloxacin (Aeroquin [MP-376], Mpex Pharmaceuticals, San Diego, CA) is a fluoroquinolone antibiotic that acts by inhibiting DNA gyrase of bacterial pathogens and promoting breakage of bacterial DNA strains. In contrast to other antimicrobials, in vitro studies of aerosolized levofloxacin in patients with CF demonstrated effectiveness against *P. aeruginosa* in the presence of sputum and biofilm and in anaerobic environments.[193,194] Further clinical studies have also demonstrated promising results in CF patients with reductions in *P. aeruginosa* density and patient's need for additional antipseudomonal antibiotics, as well as improvements in FEV_1.[195,196]

CASE STUDY

A 50-kg, 15-year-old boy with a history of asthma presents to the emergency department (ED) with dyspnea with audible wheezing and tachypnea. Patient has taken his prescribed medications of albuterol and montelukast at home with no relief of symptoms before presenting to the ED.

A physical examination revealed a heart rate of 110 beats per minute and a respiratory rate of 40 breaths per minute with signs of accessory muscle use. Auscultation revealed decreased breath sounds with inspiratory and expiratory wheezing. SaO_2 was 83% on room air. An arterial blood gas (ABG) was ordered with the following results: pH 7.5; $PaCO_2$ 27 mm Hg; PaO_2 75 mm Hg.

Which of the following is the best treatment regimen for this patient's asthma exacerbation? (NOTE: More than one answer may be acceptable.)

1. Oxygen to achieve SaO_2 90% or higher
2. Levalbuterol 3.75 mg via nebulizer every 20 minutes for 3 doses
3. Salmeterol 1 puff (50 μg) every 30 minutes
4. Ipratropium 25 mg via nebulizer every 20 minutes for 3 doses

See Evolve Resources for answers.

KEY POINTS

- Adult dosage regimens are not always appropriate for pediatric patients because there are several pharmacokinetic differences between children and adults, such as the gastric motility, volume of distribution, and age-dependent activity of drug-metabolizing enzymes.
- β-adrenergic agonists are the cornerstone treatment of bronchoconstrictions in pediatric asthma, COPD, and exercise-induced bronchospasms. Short-acting selective agents are used for acute relief of symptoms and asthma exacerbations. There is no evidence to support the isolated use of parenteral $β_2$-agonist to treat severe asthma exacerbations.
- The most common adverse effect observed with the use of β-adrenergic agonists is tremors through excessive activation of $β_2$ receptors in skeletal muscle. Tachycardia and vasodilation are also observed when β receptors are stimulated on the heart and peripheral vasculature. Hypokalemia can occur by transient activation of the Na^+/K^+ pump and transport of K^+ intracellularly. Headache, nervousness, dizziness, palpitations, cough, nausea, vomiting, and throat irritation may also occur.

- Long-acting $β_2$-agonists (LABA) have a duration of action of at least 12 hours, with an onset of action that occurs approximately 30 minutes after administration. Aerosolized LABAs, anticholinergics, leukotriene modifiers, and corticosteroids are used for maintenance of asthma symptoms and should not be used for acute symptom relief.
- Oropharyngeal candidiasis is often an adverse effect in patients receiving corticosteroids by inhalation. It is important to counsel patients to rinse their mouth with water after each administration to help reduce the chance of local adverse events.
- Montelukast is the most widely used leukotriene modifier and is indicated for treatment in children 6 months or older. Zileuton has been shown to be effective in the treatment of cold air–induced, aspirin-intolerant, exercise-induced bronchospasms and nocturnal asthma. Zafirlukast and montelukast are effective in improving asthma symptoms and treating allergic rhinitis and should be considered in patients with poor inhaler technique and those who are noncompliant with inhaled corticosteroid therapy.
- *N*-acetylcysteine acts by splitting sulfide bonds in DNA that leads to a reduction in viscosity and elasticity of airway mucus. Dornase alfa is an enzyme that selective cleaves DNA facilitating mucus clearance in the lung.
- Nebulized ribavirin is the only FDA-approved agent for the treatment of hospitalized infants and children with respiratory syncytial virus (RSV) lower respiratory tract infections. Palivizumab and omalizumab are monoclonal antibodies used for RSV prophylaxis and treatment of asthma, respectively. Palivizumab is indicated for infants at high risk for an RSV infection including those with chronic lung disease, congenital heart disease, or congenital abnormalities of the airway. Subcutaneous omalizumab is recommended as adjunctive therapy in patients who have allergies and severe persistent asthma that is not adequately controlled with conventional therapy.
- Tobramycin and aztreonam are typically used for chronic suppressive therapy in CF patients colonized with *Pseudomonas aeruginosa*. Chronic suppressive therapy cycles between 28-days-on and 28-days-off therapy to suppress bacterial burden. Pentamidine is used for prophylaxis for PCP pneumonia caused by *Pneumocystis jirovecii*, most commonly for patients with a suppressed immune system.

ASSESSMENT QUESTIONS

See Evolve Resources for answers.

1. Which of the following is a *true* statement?
    I. Fast- and short-acting β-adrenergic agents are best used for rescue of symptoms, whereas long-acting agents are best used for maintenance therapy.
    II. Levalbuterol is more safe and efficacious than albuterol for the treatment of bronchospasms in adults and children.
    III. Administration using a handheld metered-dose inhaler (MDI) with a spacer device is equivalent to nebulized β_2-agonist therapy in children and adults.
    IV. For an acute asthma exacerbation, albuterol is not recommended to be administered continuously through a nebulizer.
    A. I, II, and III are correct
    B. I and III are correct
    C. II and IV are correct
    D. Only III is correct

2. Overuse of short-acting inhaled β_2-agonists has been associated with increased mortality from asthma. Which of the following are considered short-acting β_2-agonists?
    A. Racemic epinephrine, formoterol, albuterol
    B. Formoterol, salmeterol, levalbuterol
    C. Albuterol, levalbuterol, salbutamol
    D. Formoterol, salmeterol, salbutamol, levalbuterol

3. Which of the following is a *true* statement?
    I. Gastric pH is increased in neonates than in adults.
    II. Larger weight-based doses are sometimes required in pediatrics because of a higher volume of distribution.
    III. Metabolic enzymes involved in metabolizing medications will reach close to adult values at 1 year of age.
    IV. Disease states such as cystic fibrosis have unique pharmacokinetic characteristics that warrant different dosing regimens.
    A. I is correct
    B. II is correct
    C. III is correct
    D. I, II, and III are correct

4. JF is a 15-year-old girl with mild persistent asthma who is being discharged from the hospital with a prescription of Advair (salmeterol/fluticasone). Which of the following is important to counsel the patient on before initiating treatment?
    I. Long-term use may lead to HPA axis suppression
    II. Rinse the mouth with water after each administration
    III. Should not be used for acute symptoms of asthma
    A. I and II are correct
    B. II and III are correct
    C. Only III is correct
    D. All choices are correct

5. Which of the following is a *true* statement regarding leukotriene modifiers?
    A. Zafirlukast prevents bronconstriction by antagonizing leukotriene binding to the $CysLT_1$ receptor.
    B. Theophylline and warfarin are contraindicated with zileuton.
    C. Leukotriene modifiers are efficacious in short-term control of mild persistent asthma in children.
    D. Zafirlukast should be administered with food to increase bioavailability.

6. Which of the following is commonly used to increase mucociliary clearance in patients with bronchiolitis and cystic fibrosis by absorbing water from the submucosa of the airway wall lining, which allows thick mucus to be expectorated more easily?
    A. *N*-acetylcysteine
    B. Albuterol
    C. 3% hypertonic sodium chloride
    D. Dornase alpha

7. JW, a 12-year-old boy with a history of poorly controlled asthma, presents to the emergency department in acute respiratory distress. Which of the following combinations of inhalation solution is safe to mix together in the nebulizer?
    I. Albuterol and ipratropium
    II. Hypertonic saline and cromolyn
    III. Levalbuterol and budesonide
    A. I and II are correct
    B. II and III are correct
    C. I and III is correct
    D. All choices are correct

8. BM is a premature neonate born at 23 weeks with bronchopulmonary dysplasia who qualifies for immunoprophylaxis of a lower respiratory tract infection. _____ is the monoclonal antibody indicated for immunoprophylaxis of premature infants for _____respiratory virus.
    A. Omalizumab, metapneumovirus
    B. Dornase alfa, rotavirus
    C. Palivizumab, respiratory syncytial virus
    D. Cromolyn, herpes simplex virus

9. Which of the following is a *true* statement?
    A. Drug absorption is the primary determinant for the rate of drug to be dispersed along the small intestine in infants and children.
    B. Patients requiring 3 or more canisters of a short-acting β_2-agonist per month are at a higher risk of mortality from asthma as a result of tolerance and lessened bronchodilatory effects.
    C. The parenteral form of aztreonam contains lysine and should not be used for aerosolization because repeated exposure has been shown to cause airway inflammation.
    D. Hypertonic saline is a hydrating agent used as adjunctive therapy for pulmonary complications involving viscid mucus secretions.

10. Which of the following is the mechanism of action for amikacin?
   A. Inhibits DNA gyrase of bacterial pathogens and promotes breakage of bacterial DNA strains
   B. Binds to bacterial ribosomal subunits, which inhibits protein synthesis
   C. Disrupts protein synthesis through inhibition of messenger ribonucleic acid (mRNA) expression
   D. Inhibits oxidative phosphorylation of nucleotides and nucleic acids into RNA and DNA

References

1. U.S. Food and Drug Administration: *Pediatric Product Development*, 2012. Available from: http://www.fda.gov/Drugs/DevelopmentApprovalProcess/DevelopmentResources/ucm049867.htm. Accessed September 5th, 2012.

2. Kearns GL, Abdel-Rahman SM, Alander SW, et al: Developmental pharmacology—drug disposition, action, and therapy in infants and children, *N Engl J Med* 349(12):1157–1167, 2003.

3. Gupta M, Brans YW: Gastric retention in neonates, *Pediatrics*. 62(1):26–29, 1978.

4. Shimada T, Yamazaki H, Mimura M, et al: Interindividual variations in human liver cytochrome P-450 enzymes involved in the oxidation of drugs, carcinogens and toxic chemicals: studies with liver microsomes of 30 Japanese and 30 Caucasians, *J Pharmacol Exp Ther*. 270(1):414–423, 1994.

5. Wrighton SA, Stevens JC: The human hepatic cytochromes P450 involved in drug metabolism, *Crit Rev Toxicol* 22(1):1–21, 1992.

6. Johnson TN, Tucker GT, Rostami-Hodjegan A: Development of CYP2D6 and CYP3A4 in the first year of life, *Clin Pharmacol Ther* 83(5):670–671, 2008.

7. Cazzola M, Page CP, Calzetta L, et al: Pharmacology and therapeutics of bronchodilators, *Pharmacol Rev* 64(3):450–504, 2012.

8. Expert Panel Report 3 (EPR-3): Guidelines for the Diagnosis and Management of Asthma-Summary Report 2007. S94–138, 2007.

9. Leversha AM, Campanella SG, Aickin RP, et al: Costs and effectiveness of spacer versus nebulizer in young children with moderate and severe acute asthma, *J Pediatr* 136(4):497–502, 2000.

10. Pollart SM, Compton RM, Elward KS: Management of acute asthma exacerbations, *Am Fam Physician* 84(1):40–47, 2011.

11. Cates CJ, Crilly JA, Rowe BH: Holding chambers (spacers) versus nebulisers for beta-agonist treatment of acute asthma, *Cochrane Database Syst Rev* (2):CD000052, 2006.

12. Browne GJ, Lam LT: Single-dose intravenous salbutamol bolus for managing children with acute severe asthma in the emergency department: reanalysis of data, *Pediatr Crit Care Med* 3(2):117–123, 2002.

13. Gao Smith F, Perkins GD, Gates S, et al: Effect of intravenous beta-2 agonist treatment on clinical outcomes in acute respiratory distress syndrome (BALTI-2): a multicentre, randomised controlled trial, *Lancet* 379(9812):229–235, 2012.

14. U.S. Food and Drug Administration: *Asthma and COPD Inhalers That Contain Ozone-depleting CFCs to be Phased Out; Alternative Treatments Available*, 2010. Available from: http://www.fda.gov/NewsEvents/Newsroom/PressAnnouncements/ucm208302.htm. Accessed September 5th, 2012

15. Leach CL, Colice GL: A pilot study to assess lung deposition of HFA-beclomethasone and CFC-beclomethasone from a pressurized metered dose inhaler with and without add-on spacers and using varying breathhold times, *J Aerosol Med Pulm Drug Deliv* 23(6):355–361, 2010.

16. Leach CL, Davidson PJ, Hasselquist BE, et al: Lung deposition of hydrofluoroalkane-134a beclomethasone is greater than that of chlorofluorocarbon fluticasone and chlorofluorocarbon beclomethasone: a cross-over study in healthy volunteers, *Chest* 122(2):510–516, 2002.

17. Cockcroft DW: Inhaled beta2-agonists and airway responses to allergen, *J Allergy Clin Immunol* 102(5):S96–99, Nov 1998.

18. Dolovich M: Aerosol delivery to children: what to use, how to choose, *Pediatr Pulmonol Suppl* 18:79–82, 1999.

19. Salpeter SR, Ormiston TM, Salpeter EE: Cardiovascular effects of beta-agonists in patients with asthma and COPD: a meta-analysis, *Chest* 125(6):2309–2321, 2004.

20. Leikin JB, Linowiecki KA, Soglin DF, et al: Hypokalemia after pediatric albuterol overdose: a case series, *Am J Emerg Med* 12(1):64–66, Jan 1994.

21. Carroll WD, Jones PW, Boit P, et al: Childhood evaluation of salmeterol tolerance—a double-blind randomized controlled trial, *Pediatr Allergy Immunol* 21(2 Pt 1):336–344, Mar 2010.

22. Salpeter SR, Ormiston TM, Salpeter EE: Meta-analysis: respiratory tolerance to regular beta2-agonist use in patients with asthma, *Ann Intern Med* 140(10):802–813, 2004.

23. Spitzer WO, Suissa S, Ernst P, et al: The use of beta-agonists and the risk of death and near death from asthma, *N Engl J Med* 326(8):501–506, 1992.

24. Smith L: Childhood asthma: diagnosis and treatment, *Curr Probl Pediatr* 23(7):271–305, 1993.

25. Kornecki A, Shemie SD: Bronchodilators and RSV-induced respiratory failure: agonizing about beta2 agonists, *Pediatr Pulmonol* 26(1):4–5, 1998.

26. Cates CJ, Lasserson TJ, Jaeschke R: Regular treatment with formoterol and inhaled steroids for chronic asthma: serious adverse events, *Cochrane Database Syst Rev* (2):CD006924, 2009.

27. Cates CJ, Cates MJ: Regular treatment with salmeterol for chronic asthma: serious adverse events, *Cochrane Database Syst Rev* (3):CD006363, 2008.

28. Rodrigo GJ, Moral VP, Marcos LG, et al: Safety of regular use of long-acting beta agonists as monotherapy or added to inhaled corticosteroids in asthma. A systematic review, *Pulm Pharmacol Ther* 22(1):9–19, 2009.

29. *PROVENTIL Oral inhalation solution, albuterol sulfate oral inhalation solution* [package insert], Kenilworth, N.J, 2002, Schering Corporation.

30. *PROAIR HFA Oral inhalation aerosol, albuterol sulfate oral inhalation aerosol* [package insert], Horsham, Penn, 2010, L. Teva Respiratory.

31. *XOPENEX Inhalation solution, levalbuterol hydrochloride inhalation solution* [package insert], Marlborough, Mass, 2004, Sepracor Inc.

32. *XOPENEX HFA Oral inhalation aerosol, levalbuterol tartrate oral inhalation aerosol* [package insert], Marlborough, Mass, 2005, Sepracor Inc.

33. Gawchik SM, Saccar CL, Noonan M, et al: The safety and efficacy of nebulized levalbuterol compared with racemic albuterol and placebo in the treatment of asthma in pediatric patients, *J Allergy Clin Immunol* 103(4):615–621, 1999.

34. Qureshi F, Zaritsky A, Welch C, et al: Clinical efficacy of racemic albuterol versus levalbuterol for the treatment of acute pediatric asthma, *Ann Emerg Med* 46(1):29–36, 2005.

35. Berger WE: Levalbuterol: pharmacologic properties and use in the treatment of pediatric and adult asthma, *Ann Allergy Asthma Immunol* 90(6):583–591; quiz 591–592, 659, 2003.

36. Bio LL, Willey VJ, Poon CY: Comparison of levalbuterol and racemic albuterol based on cardiac adverse effects in children, *J Pediatr Pharmacol Ther* 16(3):191–198, 2011.

37. Scott VL, Frazee LA: Retrospective comparison of nebulized levalbuterol and albuterol for adverse events in patients with acute airflow obstruction, *Am J Ther* 10(5):341–347, 2003.

38. Wheeler DS, Jacobs BR, Kenreigh CA, et al: Theophylline versus terbutaline in treating critically ill children with status asthmaticus: a prospective, randomized, controlled trial, *Pediatr Crit Care Med* 6(2):142–147, 2005.

39. *Terbutaline sulfate injection* [package insert], Bedford, Ohio, 2004, B.V. Laboratories.

40. Kelly HW, McWilliams BC, Katz R, et al: Safety of frequent high dose nebulized terbutaline in children with acute severe asthma, *Ann Allergy* 64(2 Pt 2):229–233, 1990.

41. Tipton WR, Nelson HS: Frequent parenteral terbutaline in the treatment of status asthmaticus in children, *Ann Allergy* 58(4):252–256, 1987.

42. Fuglsang G, Pedersen S, Borgstrom L: Dose-response relationships of intravenously administered terbutaline in children with asthma, *J Pediatr* 114(2):315–320, 1989.

43. Pearlman DS, Chervinsky P, LaForce C, et al: A comparison of salmeterol with albuterol in the treatment of mild-to-moderate asthma, *N Engl J Med* 327(20):1420–1425, 1992.

44. Greening AP, Ind PW, Northfield M, et al: Added salmeterol versus higher-dose corticosteroid in asthma patients with symptoms on existing inhaled corticosteroid. Allen & Hanburys Limited UK Study Group, *Lancet* 344(8917):219–224, 1994.

45. Woolcock A, Lundback B, Ringdal N, et al: Comparison of addition of salmeterol to inhaled steroids with doubling of the dose of inhaled steroids, *Am J Respir Crit Care Med* 153(5):1481–1488, 1996.

46. Pauwels RA, Lofdahl CG, Postma DS, et al: Effect of inhaled formoterol and budesonide on exacerbations of asthma. Formoterol and Corticosteroids Establishing Therapy (FACET) International Study Group, *N Engl J Med* 337(20):1405–1411, 1997.

47. Lazarus SC, Boushey HA, Fahy JV, et al: Long-acting beta2-agonist monotherapy vs continued therapy with inhaled corticosteroids in patients with persistent asthma: a randomized controlled trial, *JAMA* 285(20):2583–2593, 2001.

48. Gappa M, Zachgo W, von Berg A, et al: Add-on salmeterol compared to double dose fluticasone in pediatric asthma: a double-blind, randomized trial (VIAPAED), *Pediatr Pulmonol* 44(11):1132–1142, 2009.

49. Ni Chroinin M, Lasserson TJ, Greenstone I, et al: Addition of long-acting beta-agonists to inhaled corticosteroids for chronic asthma in children, *Cochrane Database Syst Rev* (3):CD007949, 2009.

50. Lemanske RF, Jr, Mauger DT, Sorkness CA, et al: Step-up therapy for children with uncontrolled asthma receiving inhaled corticosteroids, *N Engl J Med* 362(11):975–985, 2010.

51. *SEREVENT Inhalation aerosol, salmeterol xinafoate inhalation aerosol* [package insert], Research Triangle Park, N.C, 2004, GlaxoSmithKline.

52. Condemi JJ, Goldstein S, Kalberg C, et al: The addition of salmeterol to fluticasone propionate versus increasing the dose of fluticasone propionate in patients with persistent asthma. Salmeterol Study Group, *Ann Allergy Asthma Immunol* 82(4):383–389, 1999.

53. Murray JJ, Church NL, Anderson WH, et al: Concurrent use of salmeterol with inhaled corticosteroids is more effective than inhaled corticosteroid dose increases, *Allergy Asthma Proc* 20(3):173–180, 1999.

54. Bartow RA, Brogden RN. Formoterol: An update of its pharmacological properties and therapeutic efficacy in the management of asthma, *Drugs* 55(2):303–322, 1998.

55. Pohunek P, Matulka M, Rybnicek O, et al: Dose-related efficacy and safety of formoterol (Oxis) Turbuhaler compared with salmeterol Diskhaler in children with asthma, *Pediatr Allergy Immunol* 15(1):32–39, 2004.

56. *FORADIL AEROLIZER Inhalation powder, formoterol fumarate inhalation powder* [package insert], Kenilworth, N.J, 2006, S. Corporation.

57. *PERFOROMIST Inhalation solution, formoterol fumarate inhalation solution* [package insert], Napa, Calif, 2007, Dey.

58. Dahl R, Chung KF, Buhl R, et al: Efficacy of a new once-daily long-acting inhaled beta2-agonist indacaterol versus twice-daily formoterol in COPD, *Thorax* 65(6):473–479, 2010.

59. LaForce C, Alexander M, Deckelmann R, et al: Indacaterol provides sustained 24 h bronchodilation on once-daily dosing in asthma: a 7-day dose-ranging study, *Allergy* 63(1):103–111, 2008.

60. Neumar RW, Otto CW, Link MS, et al: Part 8: adult advanced cardiovascular life support: 2010 American Heart Association Guidelines for Cardiopulmonary Resuscitation and Emergency Cardiovascular Care, *Circulation* 122(18 Suppl 3): S729–767, 2010.

61. *ISUPREL IV Injection, isoproterenol hcl IV injection* [package insert], Lake Forest, Ill, 2004, Hospira.

62. Kleinman ME, Chameides L, Schexnayder SM, et al: Part 14: pediatric advanced life support: 2010 American Heart Association Guidelines for Cardiopulmonary Resuscitation and Emergency Cardiovascular Care, *Circulation* 122(18 Suppl 3): S876–908, 2010.

63. Lieberman P, Nicklas RA, Oppenheimer J, et al: The diagnosis and management of anaphylaxis practice parameter: 2010 update, *J Allergy Clin Immunol* 126(3):477–480 e471–442, 2010.

64. Kattwinkel J, Perlman JM, Aziz K, et al: Neonatal resuscitation: 2010 American Heart Association Guidelines for Cardiopulmonary Resuscitation and Emergency Cardiovascular Care, *Pediatrics* 126(5):e1400–1413, 2010.

65. Hegenbarth MA: Preparing for pediatric emergencies: drugs to consider, *Pediatrics* 121(2):433–443, 2008.

66. Rosekrans JA: Viral croup: current diagnosis and treatment, *Mayo Clin Proc* 73(11):1102–1106; discussion 1107, 1998.

67. Wright RB, Pomerantz WJ, Luria JW: New approaches to respiratory infections in children. Bronchiolitis and croup, *Emerg Med Clin North Am* 20(1):93–114, 2002.

68. Rodrigo GJ, Nannini LJ: Comparison between nebulized adrenaline and beta2 agonists for the treatment of acute asthma. A meta-analysis of randomized trials, *Am J Emerg Med* 24(2):217–222, 2006.

69. *Epinephrine oral inhalation aerosol* [package insert], West Roxbury, Mass, 2004, Armstrong Pharmaceuticals.

70. Brunton L: *Manual of Pharmacology and Therapeutics*, New York, 2008, McGraw-Hill.

71. Rodrigo GJ, Rodrigo C: The role of anticholinergics in acute asthma treatment: an evidence-based evaluation, *Chest* 121(6):1977–1987, 2002.

72. Craven D, Kercsmar CM, Myers TR, et al: Ipratropium bromide plus nebulized albuterol for the treatment of hospitalized children with acute asthma, *J Pediatr* 138(1):51–58, 2001.

73. Goggin N, Macarthur C, Parkin PC: Randomized trial of the addition of ipratropium bromide to albuterol and corticosteroid therapy in children hospitalized because of an acute asthma exacerbation, *Arch Pediatr Adolesc Med* 155(12):1329–1334, 2001.

74. *ATROVENT HFA Oral inhalation aerosol, ipratropium bromide HFA oral inhalation aerosol* [package insert], Ridgefield, Conn, 2004, Boehringer Ingelheim Pharmaceuticals.

75. *DUONEB Inhalation solution, albuterol sulfate and ipratropium bromide inhalation solution* [package insert], Napa, Calif, 2005, Dey.

76. *COMBIVENT Inhalation aerosol, albuterol sulfate and ipratropium bromide inhalation aerosol* [package insert], Ridgefield, Conn, 2005, Boehringer Ingelheim Pharmaceutical.

77. Baigelman W, Chodosh S: Bronchodilator action of the anticholinergic drug, ipratropium bromide (Sch 1000), as an aerosol in chronic bronchitis and asthma, *Chest* 71(3):324–328, 1977.

78. American Academy of Pediatrics Committee on Drugs: "Inactive" ingredients in pharmaceutical products: update (subject review), *Pediatrics* 99(2):268–278, 1997.

79. *CUVPOSA Oral solution, glycopyrrolate oral solution* [package insert], Atlanta, Ga, 2010, Shionogi Pharma Inc.

80. Kelly HW, Murphy S: Corticosteroids for acute, severe asthma, *DICP* 25(1):72–79, 1991.

81. Pedersen S, O'Byrne P: A comparison of the efficacy and safety of inhaled corticosteroids in asthma, *Allergy* 52 (39 Suppl):1–34, 1997.

82. Edmonds ML, Camargo CA, Pollack CV, et al: Early use of inhaled corticosteroids in the emergency department treatment of acute asthma, *Cochrane Database Syst Rev* (1):CD002308, 2001.

83. Rowe BH, Spooner C, Ducharme FM, et al: Early emergency department treatment of acute asthma with systemic corticosteroids, *Cochrane Database Syst Rev* (1):CD002178, 2001.

84. Becker JM, Arora A, Scarfone RJ, et al: Oral versus intravenous corticosteroids in children hospitalized with asthma, *J Allergy Clin Immunol* 103(4):586–590, 1999.

85. Allen DB, Bielory L, Derendorf H, et al: Inhaled corticosteroids: past lessons and future issues, *J Allergy Clin Immunol* 112(3 Suppl):S1–40, 2003.

86. Kelly HW, Sternberg AL, Lescher R, et al: Effect of inhaled glucocorticoids in childhood on adult height, *N Engl J Med* 367(10):904–912, 2012.

87. Irwin RS, Richardson ND: Side effects with inhaled corticosteroids: the physician's perception, *Chest* 130(1 Suppl): 41S–53S, 2006.

88. Agertoft L, Pedersen S: Effect of long-term treatment with inhaled budesonide on adult height in children with asthma, *N Engl J Med* 343(15):1064–1069, 2000.

89. Erceg D, Nenadic N, Plavec D, et al: Inhaled corticosteroids used for the control of asthma in a "real-life" setting do not affect linear growth velocity in prepubertal children, *Med Sci Monit* 18(9):CR564–568, 2012.

90. Wenzel SE: New approaches to anti-inflammatory therapy for asthma, *Am J Med* 104(3):287–300, 1998.

91. Leff JA, Busse WW, Pearlman D, et al: Montelukast, a leukotriene-receptor antagonist, for the treatment of mild asthma and exercise-induced bronchoconstriction, *N Engl J Med* 339(3):147–152, 1998.

92. Drazen J: Clinical pharmacology of leukotriene receptor antagonists and 5-lipoxygenase inhibitors, *Am J Respir Crit Care Med* 157(6 Pt 2):S233–237; discussion S247–238, 1998.

93. McFadden ER, Jr, Gilbert IA: Exercise-induced asthma, *N Engl J Med* 330(19):1362–1367, 1994.

94. Bernstein PR: Chemistry and structure-activity relationships of leukotriene receptor antagonists, *Am J Respir Crit Care Med* 157(6 Pt 1):S220–226, 1998.

95. Aharony D: Pharmacology of leukotriene receptor antagonists, *Am J Respir Crit Care Med* 157(6 Pt 2):S214–218; discussion S218–219, S247–248, 1998.

96. Aharony D: Pharmacology of leukotriene receptor antagonists, *Am J Respir Crit Care Med* 157(6 Pt 1):S214–219, 1998.

97. Chung KF: Leukotriene receptor antagonists and biosynthesis inhibitors: potential breakthrough in asthma therapy, *Eur Respir J* 8(7):1203–1213, 1995.

98. Liu MC, Dube LM, Lancaster J: Acute and chronic effects of a 5-lipoxygenase inhibitor in asthma: a 6-month randomized multicenter trial. Zileuton Study Group, *J Allergy Clin Immunol* 98(5 Pt 1):859–871, 1996.

99. Courtney AU, McCarter DF, Pollart SM: Childhood asthma: treatment update, *Am Fam Physician* 71(10):1959–1968, 2005.

100. Hakim F, Vilozni D, Adler A, et al: The effect of montelukast on bronchial hyperreactivity in preschool children, *Chest* 131(1):180–186, 2007.

101. Knorr B, Nguyen HH, Kearns GL, et al: Montelukast dose selection in children ages 2 to 5 years: comparison of population pharmacokinetics between children and adults, *J Clin Pharmacol* 41(6):612–619, 2001.

102. Moeller A, Lehmann A, Knauer N, et al: Effects of montelukast on subjective and objective outcome measures in preschool asthmatic children, *Pediatr Pulmonol* 43(2):179–186, 2008.

103. Horwitz RJ, McGill KA, Busse WW: The role of leukotriene modifiers in the treatment of asthma, *Am J Respir Crit Care Med* 157(5 Pt 1):1363–1371, 1998.

104. Bisgaard H: A randomized trial of montelukast in respiratory syncytial virus postbronchiolitis, *Am J Respir Crit Care Med* 167(3):379–383, 2003.

105. *ZYFLO Oral tablets, zileuton oral tablets* [package insert], Lexington, Mass, 2005, Critical Therapeutics.

106. Holloway J, Ferriss J, Groff J, et al: Churg-Strauss syndrome associated with zafirlukast, *J Am Osteopath Assoc* 98(5): 275–278, 1998.

107. Knoell DL, Lucas J, Allen JN: Churg-Strauss syndrome associated with zafirlukast, *Chest* 114(1):332–334, 1998.

108. Wechsler ME, Garpestad E, Flier SR, et al: Pulmonary infiltrates, eosinophilia, and cardiomyopathy following corticosteroid withdrawal in patients with asthma receiving zafirlukast, *JAMA* 279(6):455–457, 1998.

109. Kaliterna DM, Perkovic D, Radic M: Churg-Strauss syndrome associated with montelukast therapy, *J Asthma* 46(6):604–605, 2009.

110. Keogh KA, Specks U: Churg-Strauss syndrome: clinical presentation, antineutrophil cytoplasmic antibodies, and leukotriene receptor antagonists, *Am J Med* 115(4):284–290, 2003.

111. Nassif EG, Weinberger M, Thompson R, et al: The value of maintenance theophylline in steroid-dependent asthma, *N Engl J Med* 304(2):71–75, 1981.

112. Magnussen H, Reuss G, Jorres R: Theophylline has a dose-related effect on the airway response to inhaled histamine and methacholine in asthmatics, *Am Rev Respir Dis* 136(5):1163–1167, 1987.

113. *ELIXOPHYLLIN Oral elixir, theophylline anhydrous oral elixir* [package insert], St. Louis, Mo, 2004, Forest Pharmaceuticals.

114. van der Wouden JC, Tasche MJ, Bernsen RM, Uijen JH, et al: Inhaled sodium cromoglycate for asthma in children, *Cochrane Database Syst Rev* (3):CD002173, 2003.

115. Shapiro GG, Sharpe M, DeRouen TA, et al: Cromolyn versus triamcinolone acetonide for youngsters with moderate asthma, *J Allergy Clin Immunol* 88(5):742–748, 1991.

116. *INTAL Inhalation aerosol, cromolyn sodium inhalation aerosol* [package insert], Bristol, Tenn, 2005, King Pharmaceuticals.

117. Spivey WH, Skobeloff EM, Levin RM: Effect of magnesium chloride on rabbit bronchial smooth muscle, *Ann Emerg Med* 19(10):1107–1112, 1990.

118. Rowe BH, Bretzlaff JA, Bourdon C, et al: Magnesium sulfate for treating exacerbations of acute asthma in the emergency department, *Cochrane Database Syst Rev* (2):CD001490, 2000.

119. Rowe BH, Bretzlaff JA, Bourdon C, et al: Intravenous magnesium sulfate treatment for acute asthma in the emergency department: a systematic review of the literature, *Ann Emerg Med* 36(3):181–190, 2000.

120. Cheuk DK, Chau TC, Lee SL: A meta-analysis on intravenous magnesium sulphate for treating acute asthma, *Arch Dis Child* 90(1):74–77, 2005.

121. Blitz M, Blitz S, Hughes R, et al: Aerosolized magnesium sulfate for acute asthma: a systematic review, *Chest* 128(1):337–344, 2005.

122. Blitz M, Blitz S, Beasely R, et al: Inhaled magnesium sulfate in the treatment of acute asthma, *Cochrane Database Syst Rev* (4):CD003898, 2005.

123. Rogers DF: Mucoactive agents for airway mucus hypersecretory diseases, *Respir Care* 52(9):1176–1193; discussion 1193–1197, 2007.

124. *MUCOMYST Inhalation solution, acetylcysteine inhalation solution* [package insert], Princeton, N.J, 2001, Bristol-Myers Squibb Company.

125. Nair GB, Ilowite JS: Pharmacologic agents for mucus clearance in bronchiectasis, *Clin Chest Med* 33(2):363–370, 2012.

126. Grandjean EM, Berthet P, Ruffmann R, et al: Efficacy of oral long-term N-acetylcysteine in chronic bronchopulmonary disease: a meta-analysis of published double-blind, placebo-controlled clinical trials, *Clin Ther* 22(2):209–221, 2000.

127. Decramer M, Rutten-van Molken M, Dekhuijzen PN, et al: Effects of N-acetylcysteine on outcomes in chronic obstructive pulmonary disease (Bronchitis Randomized on NAC Cost-Utility Study, BRONCUS): a randomised placebo-controlled trial, *Lancet* 365(9470):1552–1560, 2005.

128. Wolf SJ, Heard K, Sloan EP, et al: Clinical policy: critical issues in the management of patients presenting to the emergency department with acetaminophen overdose, *Ann Emerg Med* 50(3):292–313, 2007.

129. *Acetylcysteine oral solution, solution for inhalation, acetylcysteine oral solution, solution for inhalation* [package insert], Roxane Laboratories, editor: Columbus, OH, 2007.

130. Konstan MW, Ratjen F: Effect of dornase alfa on inflammation and lung function: potential role in the early treatment of cystic fibrosis, *J Cyst Fibros* 11(2):78–83, 2012.

131. McCoy K, Hamilton S, Johnson C: Effects of 12-week administration of dornase alfa in patients with advanced cystic fibrosis lung disease. Pulmozyme Study Group, *Chest* 110(4):889–895, 1996.

132. Fuchs HJ, Borowitz DS, Christiansen DH, et al: Effect of aerosolized recombinant human DNase on exacerbations of respiratory symptoms and on pulmonary function in patients with cystic fibrosis. The Pulmozyme Study Group, *N Engl J Med* 331(10):637–642, 1994.

133. Wilmott RW, Amin RS, Colin AA, et al: Aerosolized recombinant human DNase in hospitalized cystic fibrosis patients with acute pulmonary exacerbations, *Am J Respir Crit Care Med* 153(6 Pt 1):1914–1917, 1996.

134. Quan JM, Tiddens HA, Sy JP, et al: A two-year randomized, placebo-controlled trial of dornase alfa in young patients with cystic fibrosis with mild lung function abnormalities, *J Pediatr* 139(6):813–820, 2001.

135. Shah PL, Scott SF, Knight RA, et al: In vivo effects of recombinant human DNase I on sputum in patients with cystic fibrosis, *Thorax* 51(2):119–125, 1996.

136. Geller DE: Aerosolized dornase alfa in cystic fibrosis: is there a role in the management of patients with early obstructive lung disease? *Pediatr Pulmonol* 24(2):155–158; discussion 159–161, 1997.

137. *PULMOZYME inhalation solution, dornase alfa inhalation solution* [package insert], South San Francisco, Calif, 2005, Genentech, Inc.

138. Aitken ML, Burke W, McDonald G, Shak S, Montgomery AB, Smith A: Recombinant human DNase inhalation in normal subjects and patients with cystic fibrosis. A phase 1 study, *JAMA* 267(14):1947–1951, 1992.

139. Elkins MR, Bye PT: Inhaled hypertonic saline as a therapy for cystic fibrosis, *Curr Opin Pulm Med* 12(6):445–452, 2006.

140. Robinson M, Regnis JA, Bailey DL, King M, Bautovich GJ, Bye PT: Effect of hypertonic saline, amiloride, and cough on mucociliary clearance in patients with cystic fibrosis, *Am J Respir Crit Care Med* 153(5):1503–1509, 1996.

141. Rosenfeld M, Ratjen F, Brumback L, et al: Inhaled hypertonic saline in infants and children younger than 6 years with cystic fibrosis: the ISIS randomized controlled trial, *JAMA* 307(21):2269–2277, 2012.

142. Wills P, Greenstone M: Inhaled hyperosmolar agents for bronchiectasis, *Cochrane Database Syst Rev* (2):CD002996, 2006.

143. Kellett F, Redfern J, Niven RM: Evaluation of nebulised hypertonic saline (7%) as an adjunct to physiotherapy in patients with stable bronchiectasis, *Respir Med* 99(1):27–31, 2005.

144. Gibson RL, Burns JL, Ramsey BW: Pathophysiology and management of pulmonary infections in cystic fibrosis, *Am J Respir Crit Care Med* 168(8):918–951, 2003.

145. Dellon EP, Donaldson SH, Johnson R, et al: Safety and tolerability of inhaled hypertonic saline in young children with cystic fibrosis, *Pediatr Pulmonol* 43(11):1100–1106, 2008.

146. Elkins MR, Robinson M, Rose BR, et al: A controlled trial of long-term inhaled hypertonic saline in patients with cystic fibrosis, *N Engl J Med* 354(3):229–240, 2006.

147. Strube PJ, Hallam PL: Ketamine by continuous infusion in status asthmaticus, *Anaesthesia* 41(10):1017–1019, 1986.

148. Sarma VJ: Use of ketamine in acute severe asthma, *Acta Anaesthesiol Scand* 36(1):106–107, 1992.

149. Allen JY, Macias CG: The efficacy of ketamine in pediatric emergency department patients who present with acute severe asthma, *Ann Emerg Med* 46(1):43–50, 2005.

150. Howton JC, Rose J, Duffy S, et al: Randomized, double-blind, placebo-controlled trial of intravenous ketamine in acute asthma, *Ann Emerg Med* 27(2):170–175, 1996.

151. Hemming A, MacKenzie I, Finfer S: Response to ketamine in status asthmaticus resistant to maximal medical treatment, *Thorax* 49(1):90–91, 1994.

152. *KETALAR, ketamine hydrochloride* [package insert], Bristol, Tenn, 2004, Monarch Pharmaceuticals.

153. Le J, Ashley ED, Neuhauser MM, et al: Consensus summary of aerosolized antimicrobial agents: application of guideline criteria. Insights from the Society of Infectious Diseases Pharmacists, *Pharmacotherapy* 30(6):562–584, 2010.

154. Le Souef P: The meaning of lung dose, *Allergy* 54 Suppl 49:93–96, 1999.

155. Langton Hewer SC, Smyth AR: Antibiotic strategies for eradicating Pseudomonas aeruginosa in people with cystic fibrosis, *Cochrane Database Syst Rev* (4):CD004197, 2009.

156. Ryan G, Singh M, Dwan K: Inhaled antibiotics for long-term therapy in cystic fibrosis, *Cochrane Database Syst Rev* (3):CD001021, 2011.

157. Ramsey BW, Pepe MS, Quan JM, et al: Intermittent administration of inhaled tobramycin in patients with cystic fibrosis. Cystic Fibrosis Inhaled Tobramycin Study Group, *N Engl J Med* 340(1):23–30, 1999.

158. Wiesemann HG, Steinkamp G, Ratjen F, et al: Placebo-controlled, double-blind, randomized study of aerosolized tobramycin for early treatment of Pseudomonas aeruginosa colonization in cystic fibrosis, *Pediatr Pulmonol* 25(2):88–92, 1998.

159. Douglas TA, Brennan S, Gard S, et al: Acquisition and eradication of P. aeruginosa in young children with cystic fibrosis, *Eur Respir J* 33(2):305–311, 2009.

160. Flume PA, O'Sullivan BP, Robinson KA, et al: Cystic fibrosis pulmonary guidelines: chronic medications for maintenance of lung health, *Am J Respir Crit Care Med* 176(10):957–969, 2007.

161. *TOBI inhalation solution, tobramycin inhalation solution* [package insert], East Hanover, N.J, 2011, Novartis Pharmaceuticals Corporation.

162. Dietzsch HJ, Gottschalk B, Heyne K, et al: Cystic fibrosis: comparison of two mucolytic drugs for inhalation treatment (acetylcysteine and arginine hydrochloride), *Pediatrics* 55(1):96–100, 1975.

163. *AZACTAM IV, IM injection, aztreonam IV, IM injection* [package insert], Princeton, N.J., 2007, Bristol-Myers Squibb Company.

164. Oermann CM, Retsch-Bogart GZ, Quittner AL, et al: An 18-month study of the safety and efficacy of repeated courses of inhaled aztreonam lysine in cystic fibrosis, *Pediatr Pulmonol* 45(11):1121–1134, 2010.

165. Retsch-Bogart GZ, Quittner AL, Gibson RL, et al: Efficacy and safety of inhaled aztreonam lysine for airway pseudomonas in cystic fibrosis, *Chest* 135(5):1223–1232, 2009.

166. Retsch-Bogart GZ, Burns JL, Otto KL, et al: A phase 2 study of aztreonam lysine for inhalation to treat patients with cystic fibrosis and Pseudomonas aeruginosa infection, *Pediatr Pulmonol* 43(1):47–58, 2008.

167. *CAYSTON inhalation solution, aztreonam inhalation solution* [package insert], Foster City, Calif, 2012, Gilead Sciences.

168. Heijerman H, Westerman E, Conway S, et al: Inhaled medication and inhalation devices for lung disease in patients with cystic fibrosis: a European consensus, *J Cyst Fibros* 8(5):295–315, 2009.

169. Sheldon WH: Pulmonary Pneumocystis carinii infection, *J Pediatr* 61:780–791, 1962.

170. Long SS: 50 Years Ago in The Journal of Pediatrics: Pulmonary Pneumocystis carinii Infection, *J Pediatr* 161(5):798, 2012.

171. Cohen DE, Mayer KH: Primary care issues for HIV-infected patients, *Infect Dis Clin North Am* 21(1):49–70, viii, 2007.

172. *NebuPent, pentamidine isethionate* [package insert], Schaumburg, Ill, 2002, American Pharmaceutical Partners.

173. Mofenson LM, Brady MT, Danner SP, et al: Guidelines for the Prevention and Treatment of Opportunistic Infections among HIV-exposed and HIV-infected children: recommendations from CDC, the National Institutes of Health, the HIV Medicine Association of the Infectious Diseases Society of America, the Pediatric Infectious Diseases Society, and the American Academy of Pediatrics, *MMWR Recomm Rep* 58(RR-11):1–166, 2009.

174. *Virazole, ribavirin* [package insert], Costa Mesa, Calif, 1996, Valeant Pharmaceuticals.

175. Committee on Infectious Diseases, American Academy of Pediatrics, Pickering LK, Baker CJ, et al: Red Book(R): 2012 Report of the Committee on Infectious Diseases, ed 29, Elk Grove Village, IL, 2012, American Academy of Pediatrics.

176. Englund JA, Piedra PA, Ahn YM, et al: High-dose, short-duration ribavirin aerosol therapy compared with standard ribavirin therapy in children with suspected respiratory syncytial virus infection, *J Pediatr* 125(4):635–641, 1994.

177. Meert KL, Sarnaik AP, Gelmini MJ, et al: Aerosolized ribavirin in mechanically ventilated children with respiratory syncytial virus lower respiratory tract disease: a prospective, double-blind, randomized trial, *Crit Care Med* 22(4):566–572, 1994.

178. Rodriguez WJ, Hall CB, Welliver R, et al: Efficacy and safety of aerosolized ribavirin in young children hospitalized with influenza: a double-blind, multicenter, placebo-controlled trial, *J Pediatr* 125(1):129–135, 1994.

179. The IMpact-RSV Study Gorup, a Humanized Respiratory Syncytial Virus Monoclonal Antibody, Reduces Hospitalization From Respiratory Syncytial Virus Infection in High-risk Infants, *Pediatrics* 102(3):531–537, 1998.

180. Feltes TF, Cabalka AK, Meissner HC, et al: Palivizumab prophylaxis reduces hospitalization due to respiratory syncytial virus in young children with hemodynamically significant congenital heart disease, *J Pediatr* 143(4):532–540, 2003.

181. Lacaze-Masmonteil T, Truffert P, Pinquier D, et al: Lower respiratory tract illness and RSV prophylaxis in very premature infants, *Arch Dis Child* 89(6):562–567, 2004.

182. *SYNAGIS IM injection, palivizumab IM injection* [package insert], Gaithersburg, Md, 2011, MedImmune.

183. *XOLAIR subcutaneous solution, omalizumab subcutaneous solution* [package insert], South San Francisco, Calif, 2007, Genetech Inc.

184. *TUDORZA PRESSAIR oral inhalation powder, aclidinium bromide oral inhalation powder*, St Louis, Mo, 2012, Forest Pharmaceuticals.

185. Cazzola M: Aclidinium bromide, a novel long-acting muscarinic M3 antagonist for the treatment of COPD, *Curr Opin Investig Drugs* 10(5):482–490, 2009.

186. Jones PW, Singh D, Bateman ED, et al: Efficacy and safety of twice-daily aclidinium bromide in COPD patients: the ATTAIN study, *Eur Respir J* 40(4):830–836, 2012.

187. Fitzgerald MF, Fox JC: Emerging trends in the therapy of COPD: novel anti-inflammatory agents in clinical development, *Drug Discov Today* 12(11–12):479–486, 2007.

188. Geller DE, Weers J, Heuerding S: Development of an inhaled dry-powder formulation of tobramycin using PulmoSphere technology, *J Aerosol Med Pulm Drug Deliv* 24(4):175–182, 2011.

189. Konstan MW, Flume PA, Kappler M, et al: Safety, efficacy and convenience of tobramycin inhalation powder in cystic fibrosis patients: The EAGER trial, *J Cyst Fibros* 10(1):54–61, 2011.

190. Geller DE, Konstan MW, Smith J, et al: Novel tobramycin inhalation powder in cystic fibrosis subjects: pharmacokinetics and safety, *Pediatr Pulmonol* 42(4):307–313, 2007.

191. Meers P, Neville M, Malinin V, et al: Biofilm penetration, triggered release and in vivo activity of inhaled liposomal amikacin in chronic Pseudomonas aeruginosa lung infections, *J Antimicrob Chemother* 61(4):859–868, 2008.

192. Okusanya OO, Bhavnani SM, Hammel J, et al: Pharmacokinetic and pharmacodynamic evaluation of liposomal amikacin for inhalation in cystic fibrosis patients with chronic pseudomonal infection, *Antimicrob Agents Chemother* 53(9):3847–3854, 2009.

193. King P, Lomovskaya O, Griffith DC, et al: In vitro pharmacodynamics of levofloxacin and other aerosolized antibiotics under multiple conditions relevant to chronic pulmonary infection in cystic fibrosis, *Antimicrob Agents Chemother* 54(1):143–148, 2010.

194. King P, Citron DM, Griffith DC, et al: Effect of oxygen limitation on the in vitro activity of levofloxacin and other antibiotics administered by the aerosol route against Pseudomonas aeruginosa from cystic fibrosis patients, *Diagn Microbiol Infect Dis* 66(2):181–186, 2010.

195. Geller DE, Flume PA, Staab D, et al: Levofloxacin inhalation solution (MP-376) in patients with cystic fibrosis with Pseudomonas aeruginosa, *Am J Respir Crit Care Med* 183(11):1510–1516, 2011.

196. Geller DE, Flume PA, Griffith DC, et al: Pharmacokinetics and safety of MP-376 (levofloxacin inhalation solution) in cystic fibrosis subjects, *Antimicrob Agents Chemother* 55(6):2636–2640, 2011.

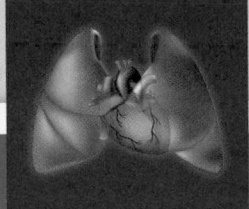

Chapter 21

Thoracic Organ Transplantation*

GEORGE B. MALLORY, JR, MARC G. SCHECTER

OUTLINE

Heart Transplantation
Heart–Lung Transplantation
Lung Transplantation
Immunosuppressive Regimens
Complications
    Respiratory Problems
    Organ Rejection

Infection
Bronchiolitis Obliterans
Drug Toxicity
Other Complications
Survival and Quality of Life
Role of the Respiratory Therapist

LEARNING OBJECTIVES

After reading this chapter the reader will be able to:

1. Recognize clinical indications for heart and lung transplantation in childhood
2. Describe important respiratory complications after heart and lung transplantation
3. Explain reasons why children can have more complications than adults after thoracic transplantation

4. Identify the reasons for increased susceptibility of children after lung transplantation to respiratory infections and their complications

KEY TERMS

Allograft rejection
Bronchiolitis obliterans
Cardiomyopathy

Congenital heart disease
Cystic fibrosis
Heart–lung transplantation

Heart transplantation
Lung transplantation
Pulmonary hypertension

Thoracic organ transplantation dates back to the 1960s for the first heart transplant in South Africa, and for the first lung transplant in Mississippi. In each case, the recipients survived only a few weeks. Despite the development of improved surgical techniques for thoracic organ transplantation in the 1980s, it was not until effective immunosuppressive regimens became available that there was a significant increase in the number of thoracic organ transplantations (Figure 21-1).[1,2]

*This work was supported in part by Health Resources and Services Administration contract 234-2005-37011C. The content is the responsibility of the authors alone and does not necessarily reflect the views or policies of the Department of Health and Human Services, nor does mention of trade names, commercial products, or organizations imply endorsement by the U.S. Government.

In 1982 and 1983, less than a dozen pediatric heart transplants were performed worldwide each year; by 1990, the number had increased to 325 and since then, the worldwide total has slowly increased to more than 500 by 2010.[1,3] In contrast, fewer than 10 pediatric lung transplants were performed in 1986 through 1989.[1] Since 1991, the number of pediatric lung transplants worldwide has also increased and reached 126 in 2010, the vast majority of which were in the adolescent age group.[1,3] In sharp contrast, heart–lung transplantation, which was employed for end-stage pulmonary disease because of the relative easy availability of heart–lung blocks, peaked in 1989 at 61 pediatric transplants per year.[1] Since then, the number of pediatric heart–lung transplants has dwindled, reaching 10 or fewer since 2007.[3]

397

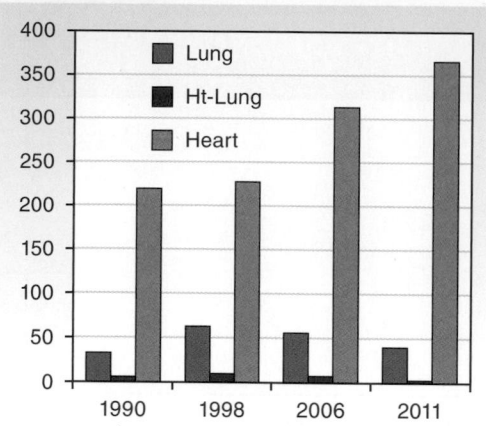

FIGURE 21-1　Relative volume of lung, heart, and heart–lung transplants performed in the United States from 1990 to 2010. (Data from http://optn.transplant.hrsa.gov.)

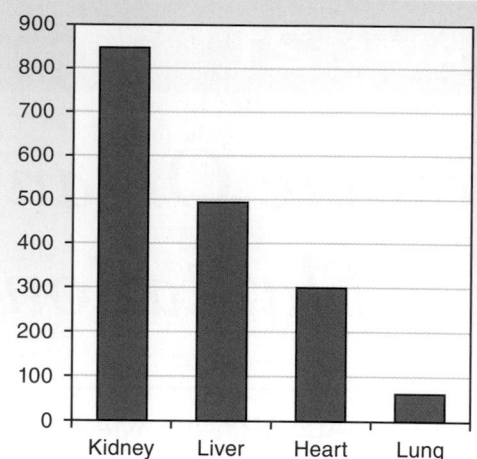

FIGURE 21-2　Number of children in the United States awaiting solid organ transplantation by organ type as of February 2013. (Data from http://optn.transplant.hrsa.gov.)

With the advances in surgical technique pioneered by Cooper in Toronto in the 1980s, lung transplantation became the procedure of choice for most forms of end-stage lung disease. It is now rare to consider heart–lung transplantation for isolated pulmonary disease.[4] In the twenty-first century, heart transplantation is indicated for inoperable congenital heart defects or end-stage myocardial failure. Single or bilateral lung transplantation is used for end-stage pulmonary and pulmonary vascular disease. Heart–lung transplantation is reserved for the infrequent circumstance of combined left ventricular heart failure with pulmonary disease or combined congenital defects of both the heart and lung (Table 21-1).[3,4] In 2010, fewer than 100 heart–lung transplants were performed worldwide, compared with 3500 lung and nearly 4000 heart transplants in all ages[5] Of the 74 heart–lung transplants performed around the world in 2010, only 7 were performed in individuals under the age of 18 years.[3,5]

TABLE 21-1

Pediatric Thoracic Organ Transplantation: Primary Indications

Transplant Type	Clinical Indication
Heart	Cardiomyopathy
	Congenital heart disease
Bilateral lung	Cystic fibrosis
	Pulmonary hypertension
	Interstitial lung disease
	Pulmonary growth abnormalities
	Bronchiolitis obliterans
Lung with heart repair	Congenital heart disease with pulmonary hypertension but preserved left ventricular function
Heart–lung	End-stage lung disease with left ventricular failure
	Irreparable congenital heart disease with pulmonary hypertension or other intrinsic lung disease

Significantly fewer children wait for thoracic organ transplantation compared with those who wait for kidney or liver transplantation (Figure 21-2). Since the late 1990s, there has been a steady increase in the number of pediatric candidates for solid organ transplantation but until recently there has been no increase in the number of donors.

In 2003 the Organ Donation Breakthrough Collaborative was formed under public auspices in the United States to enhance organ donation.[6] The average conversion rate—that is, the rate at which families of brain-dead individuals consent to organ donation—was 46% at that time. Examination of best practices suggested that 75% conversion rate was achievable and this goal was formally set in the final report of the Collaborative in September 2003. Since that time, there has been a significant increase in donors.

In 2005 the Organ Transplantation Breakthrough Collaborative was formed to increase the number of organs harvested from each donor. In the majority of donors historically, the liver and kidneys were deemed suitable for transplant, but only approximately 25% of the hearts and 10% to 15% of the lungs were deemed healthy enough to be transplanted. Myocardial dysfunction is a common response to the dramatic events related to brain death. In most previously healthy donors, modern donor management, given enough time, results in return to near normal cardiac function in the vast majority. On the other hand, lungs are often infected or atelectatic, injured during prolonged intubation and ventilation, or unsuitable because of pulmonary edema, trauma, or aspiration.[7] By the application of best practices, aggressive donor management can increase both heart and lung donation, although it may take longer to manage the donor until the time of recovery.[8,9] In addition, the number of abdominal organs can also be increased by this approach.

It was the goal of the Collaboratives to extend the use of aggressive donor management protocols across the

United States to increase the yield of transplanted organs. One of the mandates of the Organ Transplantation Collaborative was to treat every donor as a thoracic organ donor with early emphasis after declaration of brain death on evaluating and resuscitating the lungs and heart.

Another innovative approach to the donor shortage has included the use of living donor lobar donation (LDLT) for lung transplantation (using a single lobe from two taller individuals, commonly but not always a parent or relative).[10] Starnes popularized this surgical approach in the 1990s.[10] In this approach, two healthy biologically related or unrelated older and taller individuals donate a lower lobe to replace the recipient's native lungs. Despite relative early success, peak volume of living donor lobar transplantation was in 1998 and 1999 with 29 recipients in the United States each year. From 2010 until the present, there has been no more than one reported LDLT surgery per year, according to data from the United Network for Organ Sharing (UNOS).[3,5]

Donation after cardiac death (DCD) has been a rare source of donor organs until recent years.[11] In this clinical scenario, physicians recommend discontinuation of life-sustaining therapy from a terminally ill patient. In some of these patients, especially if there has been a recent central nervous system injury, families sometimes ask about the possibility of organ and tissue donation. If circulatory arrest is anticipated within minutes of withdrawal of ventilatory support, organ donation may be possible. In that situation, the organ procurement center is contacted and recovery surgeons are notified and present in a nearby operating room at the time of extubation. If circulatory arrest occurs within 30 to 60 minutes, kidneys, livers and most recently lungs may be procured for transplantation. In 2009, UNOS documented 33 lung transplants performed in the United States after DCD recovery (Figure 21-3).[12] Rarely, infant heart transplantation has been performed in the DCD setting.[13]

For most children who undergo thoracic organ transplantation, quality of life returns to normal.[14,15] Within weeks after the operation, depending on their pretransplant nutritional and physical state, most patients are able to resume age-appropriate activities with improving exercise tolerance. Cardiac function is generally normal in heart transplant patients.[16] Gas exchange and pulmonary function rapidly return to near normal in the first months after lung transplantation.[14,15] Minor childhood illnesses appear to be well tolerated, although in its initial stage it is often difficult to ascertain whether a febrile illness represents a minor infection, graft rejection, or a life-threatening infection in the immunocompromised host. Somatic growth delay can be a problem, at least in part resulting from the administration of prednisone, which is continued lifelong in almost all lung and a subset of heart recipients. However, subsequent growth of the patient as well as of the allograft is possible, and it is unlikely that the subject will outgrow the transplanted organ.[17]

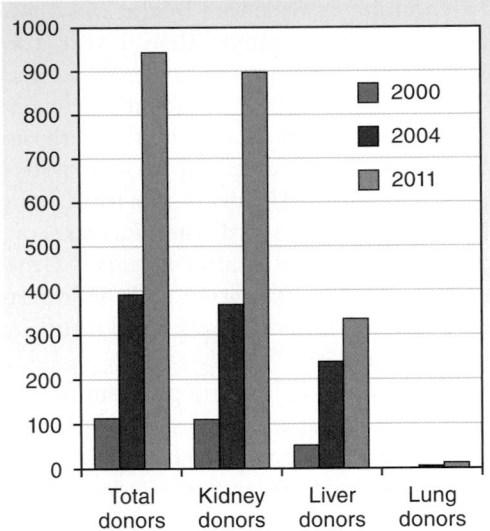

FIGURE 21-3 Volume of kidney, liver, and lung transplants from donors after cardiac death from 2000 until 2009, demonstrating increasing volume in each organ. (Data from http://optn.transplant .hrsa.gov.)

HEART TRANSPLANTATION

In the 1980s the primary indication for heart transplantation was cardiomyopathy. However, in more recent years the proportion of transplantations for congenital heart defects has been increasing (Table 21-2).[1] Congenital lesions are the indication for heart transplantation in 40% of patients younger than 1 year, especially in the United States, but in only 25% of older children.[18] The operative approach in heart transplantation involves a sternotomy with surgical anastomoses to the venae cavae and aorta. Early postoperative mortality arises from graft failure and, less commonly, cardiac rhythm disorders. The newly denervated implanted heart often has an initial intrinsic rhythm too slow to produce an adequate cardiac output. Thus a temporary external pacemaker is attached to the heart at the end of each heart transplant operation. Infectious complications, graft rejection, and central nervous system hemorrhage or embolism occur with lower incidence. Early mortality rate after transplantation is higher

TABLE 21-2

Indications for Heart Transplantation in North America by Age

	1 Year	1-10 Years	11-17 Years
Cardiomyopathy	55%	55%	63%
Congenital heart defects	40%	37%	25%
Other	4%	3%	3%
Retransplantation	1%	5%	9%

Modified from Benden C, Edwards LB, Kucheryavaya AY, et al. The registry of the International Society for Heart and Lung Transplantation: fifteenth pediatric lung and heart–lung transplantation report—2012. *J Heart Lung Transplant* 2012;31:1087.

in younger children, as evidenced by the 25% 1-year mortality rate in recipients younger than 1 year, compared with 10% for the 11- to 18-year age group.[18] Late deaths are caused primarily by coronary vasculopathy (chronic rejection). A small number of deaths in the early and late groups have been related to central nervous system complications such as stroke. The death rate from malignancy (primarily lymphoproliferative disease) increases over time and represents 10% of deaths after 5 years.[18] Other morbidities from heart transplantation include hypertension in approximately 40% of individuals, renal insufficiency in 20%, and seizures in 25%.[19-21]

A troublesome and life-limiting problem in long-term heart transplant survivors, regardless of age, is the development of premature coronary artery disease or coronary vasculopathy, also known as *graft atherosclerosis*.[18,19,21] This condition may be asymptomatic and may be discovered only at the time of surveillance coronary angiography, performed annually in most centers. In some patients the disease can be significant enough to cause myocardial ischemia and may contribute to arrhythmias or sudden death. There is general consensus that premature coronary artery disease is immunologically mediated as a manifestation of chronic graft rejection and therefore may decrease in prevalence with improvements in immunosuppressive regimens.

Neonatal heart transplantation has been successful at some centers. This has been used almost exclusively for hypoplastic left-heart syndrome, which is uniformly fatal if surgical correction or transplantation is not offered. The current experience with either surgical correction (the Norwood procedure) or transplantation does not clearly indicate which is more appropriate to optimize survival.[20] Although once considered promising, anencephalic infants have not proven to be suitable donors for other neonates.[22] Young infants are less sophisticated hosts by virtue of their relatively immature immune response and therefore might tolerate the immunological challenge of transplantation more readily than older subjects. In fact, many pediatric candidates younger than 18 months can receive hearts across the ABO group barriers with long-term success. The survival rate and duration of survival with good cardiac function appear to be the same for children as for adult heart transplant recipients.[18,21]

HEART–LUNG TRANSPLANTATION

Before the surgical technique for successful lung transplantation was developed, heart–lung transplantation was offered for end-stage pulmonary disease. Heart–lung transplantation involves a sternotomy and surgical anastomoses of the trachea, superior and inferior venae cavae, and aorta and is a technically less challenging operation compared with lung transplantation. With the ability to successfully transplant a single lung or two lungs, the use

of heart–lung transplantation for pulmonary disease has dramatically decreased.[1,3] There are multiple reasons for this, including the following:

· The limited availability of satisfactory coupled heart–lung donations from a single donor (governed in part by the distribution algorithm unique to each country)
· The practical advantage of using the heart–lung block for three separate donations (one heart and two single lungs)
· The decreased risk of cardiac rejection if isolated lung transplantation is performed
· The decreased risk of premature coronary artery disease
· The high demand for donor hearts by very ill heart transplant candidates with ventricular assist devices or artificial hearts in place.

Despite concerns about the impact of right ventricular dysfunction commonly associated with chronic pulmonary disease or severe pulmonary hypertension in the immediate postoperative period, improvement in right ventricular function with lung transplantation leads to good outcomes after recovery from surgery.[3,14] For patients with congenital heart defects such as atrial septal defect, ventricular septal defect, or patent ductus arteriosus, as well as pulmonary hypertension from Eisenmenger syndrome, lung transplantation with repair of the congenital heart defect is generally the procedure of choice.[23]

The volume of heart–lung transplantation has decreased by more than half since the late 1990s, from a peak of 240 transplants per year in 1989 to fewer than 100 per year in 2010.[1,3,5] The decrease in use of heart–lung transplantation has been most dramatic in the United States.

LUNG TRANSPLANTATION

A common and severe complication of lung transplantation before 1983 was tracheal and bronchial anastomosis failure. When Cooper developed techniques to overcome this problem in the late 1980s,[2] single- and double-lung transplantation became the preferred options for adult patients with chronic pulmonary disease. Table 21-1 lists the diseases appropriate for bilateral lung transplantation. Single-lung transplantation now is rarely performed in children. Figure 21-4 shows the most common chronic lung diseases that, in children, lead to transplantation. Cystic fibrosis is the most common indication for bilateral lung transplantation, almost exclusively in children older than 6 years.[3]

Enthusiasm for lung transplantation has been tempered by a relatively low survival rate; the initial 1-year survival rate was only slightly more than 50%. This compares with early survival rates after heart–lung or double-lung transplants in patients with cystic fibrosis of 60% to 70% at 1 year in the 1990s.[24,25] As overall experience has increased, survival after lung transplantation has improved; the most recent actuarial survival at 1 year after

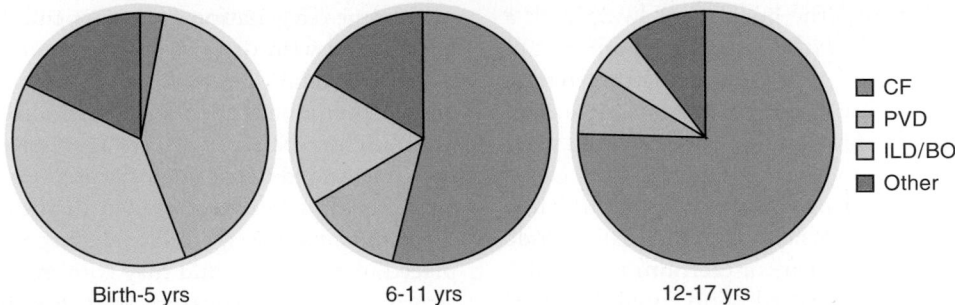

| Birth-5 yrs | 6-11 yrs | 12-17 yrs |

FIGURE 21-4 Frequency of primary diseases leading to lung transplantation in children by age. **A,** Diagnoses from birth through age 5 years. **B,** Diagnoses from birth through age 6 to 11 years. **C,** Diagnoses age 12 through 17 years. *BO,* Bronchiolitis obliterans; *CF,* cystic fibrosis; *PVD,* pulmonary vascular disease; *ILD,* interstitial lung disease; *ReTxp,* retransplantation. (Data from http://optn.transplant.hrsa.gov; and Benden C, Edwards LB, Kucheryavaya AY, et al. The registry of the International Society for Heart and Lung Transplantation: fifteenth pediatric lung and heart–lung transplantation report—2012. *J Heart Lung Transplant* 2012;31:1087.)

transplant is approximately 85%.[3] Longer term survival rates remain disappointing, however, with a 5-year survival in the most recent era less than 50%. Post–lung transplant survival rates have a long way to go to be comparable with the successes of kidney, heart, pancreas, and liver transplantation (Figure 21-5).[123]

Deaths within the first 90 days after lung transplantation (early deaths) result most commonly from graft failure caused by ischemia–reperfusion injury. Less common are surgical problems such as airway anastomotic dehiscence or massive hemorrhage. Even less common are overwhelming infection, either systemic or pulmonary; multiple organ failure; or acute graft rejection. Late deaths are generally related to infection or bronchiolitis obliterans, usually a manifestation of chronic rejection.[4,5]

A particular concern in pediatric lung transplantation is the problem of donor–recipient size matching. In addition to the problems of donor availability among all transplantation candidates, the thoracic dimensions of infants and small children add another obstacle, so that size-appropriate donors are even less commonly available than for adolescents or adults.[27]

A potential solution to this problem is reduced-size transplantation, often from a living donor (e.g., transplanting an adult lower lobe to a pediatric patient to replace the recipient's entire lung[28]). Although initial attempts at living-related donation were disappointing, more recent experience suggests that LDLT can be successful with a 1-year survival of 60% to 80% with only minimal risk to the donor.[29] Therefore LDLT might, in theory, help overcome the obstacles of donor waiting time, size limitation, and organ availability for the urgently ill transplant candidate. The lung allocation score system, which took effect in the United States in 2005, now lists patients according to a computed score of urgency, reducing the need for LDLT.[30]

IMMUNOSUPPRESSIVE REGIMENS

Although children commonly resume normal activity within weeks of transplantation, the medical regimen, including medications and testing, after thoracic transplantation is extensive, especially in the first year. In addition to an intense pharmacological program, there are frequent office visits, multiple blood tests, repeated radiographs, serial echocardiograms in heart recipients and, in most centers, surveillance biopsies. Even a minor illness can lead to hospitalization to rule out graft rejection or serious infection. With increasing time after transplantation and successful graft function, there are fewer impositions on the lives of the child and family.

When children are referred to centers distant from their home communities, their families usually have to spend months before and often months after transplant in the transplant center community. There are considerable financial and psychosocial costs to this dislocation of children and parents from their homes. The transplant patient

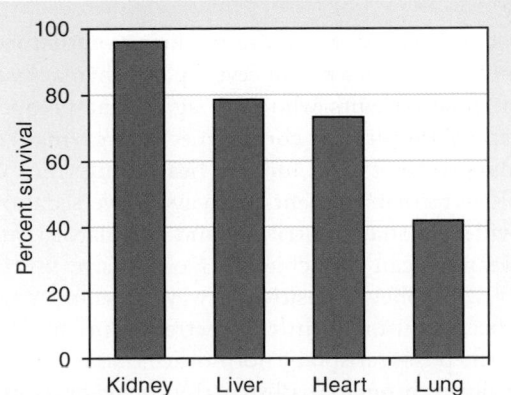

FIGURE 21-5 Five-year survival of patients younger than 18 years after kidney, liver, heart, and lung transplants in the United States. Because of the availability of renal dialysis, patient survival exceeds graft survival by more 20% at 5 years for kidney transplant recipients. (Data from http://optn.transplant.hrsa.gov.)

trades one set of problems (the burdens of living with a terminal disease) for another (the long-term immunosuppression and lifelong risk of potential life-threatening complications). Because the quality of life is dramatically better in most survivors, few families express regret after transplantation.

Most immunosuppressive regimens for organ transplantations (thoracic and other solid organs) include the combined use of cyclosporine or tacrolimus, azathioprine or mycophenolate mofetil, and prednisone.[3,18] Tacrolimus and mycophenolate mofetil are now the most commonly used immunosuppressants and are generally needed for the life of the transplant recipient.[3] There has been an increasing trend to embrace a corticosteroid-free immunosuppressant program in pediatric heart transplant centers.[18] Many transplant cardiologists wean or attempt to discontinue prednisone within weeks to months after the transplantation. Because lung allografts are more susceptible to both acute and chronic rejection, immunosuppressant dosing is generally higher and more prolonged compared with that in heart transplant recipients. Few lung transplant pulmonologists attempt to wean patients from prednisone; at most, some patients can be weaned to alternate-day dosing.

COMPLICATIONS

The complications of thoracic organ transplantation can be grouped into the following categories:
· Respiratory failure and related problems
· Acute rejection
· Infection
· Chronic rejection or bronchiolitis obliterans
· Drug toxicity
· Other complications

Respiratory Problems

All thoracic transplantation patients arrive in the intensive care unit after transplantation and receive mechanical ventilatory support via endotracheal tube. Most well-conditioned heart transplant patients with good myocardial contractility in the immediate postoperative period can be weaned from mechanical ventilation within the first hours to days. The surgical incision and thoracostomy tubes will result in reduced thoracic compliance, and both deep inspiration and cough will likely be compromised. With the judicious use of intravenous analgesics, chest physiotherapy, and, occasionally, regional nerve block or epidural anesthesia, most heart transplant patients, like their counterparts who undergo other cardiac surgical procedures, do well. With the increasingly common use of left ventricular assist devices, there are a growing number of severely deconditioned pediatric cardiac transplant recipients who may require longer periods of ventilator support. A subset of recipients experiences severe myocardial failure postoperatively. Extracorporeal

membrane oxygenation or a ventricular assist device may be required with or without mechanical ventilatory support for several days. With myocardial failure, some degree of pulmonary edema with reduced lung compliance occurs. These patients require aggressive intravenous cardiotonic and diuretic medications. Oxygen supplementation is almost always needed in these patients. Under some circumstances, a relatively large heart graft that is placed in a smaller child may compress the intrathoracic airways, the left mainstem bronchus being particularly vulnerable to such compression. With compression, consolidation with absent breath sounds over the left lower lobe or low-pitched expiratory wheezing with a variable degree of dyspnea may result. Bronchodilators, vigorous chest physiotherapy and noninvasive positive-pressure ventilation may be needed to maintain maximal airway patency, minimize atelectasis, and mobilize retained secretions.

Heart–lung and lung transplant patients are more vulnerable to respiratory complications than are heart transplant patients. The thoracic incision is usually more extensive when lungs are transplanted. Allograft dysfunction after lung transplantation is common but highly variable. The delicate pulmonary capillary bed appears to be more susceptible to ischemic injury than is the myocardium, liver, or kidney in the context of transplantation. So-called ischemia–reperfusion injury in the lung is manifested as pulmonary capillary leak.

This reperfusion injury, which occurs in 10% to 20% of lung transplants, mimics the acute respiratory distress syndrome clinically and radiographically. On chest radiography, pulmonary edema, either immediately after transplantation or within the first 72 hours, is usually a sign of ischemic injury or reperfusion injury (Figure 21-6).[33,34] Interruption of the pulmonary lymphatics, which are cut during the surgery, also contribute to pleural, alveolar, and interstitial fluid accumulation. Reperfusion injury, now called primary graft dysfunction, affects 5% to 25% of adult and pediatric lung transplant recipients with varying severity.[35]

Subacute respiratory failure requiring ventilatory support for 1 to 2 weeks without severe parenchymal disease is seen in some patients who had significant preoperative hypercapnia. Respiratory control mechanisms may require many days to reset after lung or heart–lung transplantation.[36] Keys to management are to avoid oversedation and to provide adequate nutrition and ventilatory support until weaning can be achieved. Noninvasive ventilatory support with bilevel positive airway pressure may help make the transition from the pretransplant hypercarbic state to the post-transplant normocarbic state.

Significant bronchial obstruction may develop after lung or heart–lung transplantation because of stricture or dehiscence at or just beyond the sites of bronchial anastomosis. Most airway complications will present within 3 months of transplantation, and although a few can be

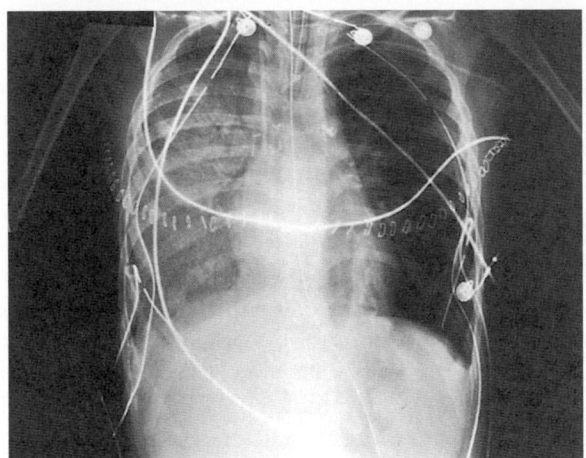

FIGURE 21-6 This chest radiograph demonstrates reperfusion injury to the right lung immediately after double-lung transplantation in an 11-year-old girl with cystic fibrosis. There is a ground-glass haziness with air bronchograms over the right lung field. The staples across the chest are external and used for surgical skin closure. There are surgical clips in each hilar region where the vascular anastomoses were performed. There is also an endotracheal tube, a nasogastric tube, a left subclavian vein catheter, a right internal jugular vein catheter, bilateral chest tubes, and surface electrodes.

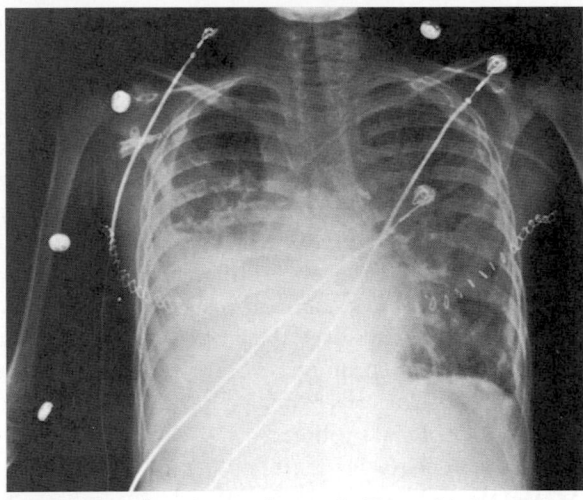

FIGURE 21-7 The same patient as in Figure 21-6, seen 3 weeks later during an episode of acute lung rejection. A large right pleural effusion obscures the right hemidiaphragm and the border of the right side of the heart. There is extensive increase in peribronchial markings in both lungs and a blunted left costophrenic angle. All chest tubes and the endotracheal tube have been removed. A right subclavian vein catheter has been added.

fatal if severe and early, most are treatable with bronchoscopic dilation, laser resection of granulation tissue, or the placement of airway stents.[37,38]

Organ Rejection

The clinical signs and symptoms of organ rejection may be minimal or subtle. Acute rejection of the transplanted heart, if clinically apparent, results in decreased cardiac contractility with signs and symptoms of congestive heart failure. Tachycardia, tachypnea, and malaise may be noted. Echocardiography is the noninvasive diagnostic mode of choice to ascertain the physiological signs of cardiac rejection. In the lung transplant patient, tachypnea, bibasilar inspiratory crackles on auscultation, increased interstitial infiltrates on chest radiography, and hypoxemia by pulse oximetry are often associated with acute rejection (Figure 21-7). For older patients who can perform spirometry, a drop in pulmonary function, either restrictive or obstructive, is often the most sensitive indicator of acute rejection.

Many transplant centers perform routine surveillance biopsies of the transplanted tissue in an effort to identify and treat early rejection before permanent organ damage occurs.[21,39] When clinically suspected, the diagnosis of rejection is also usually confirmed by biopsy.[4,21] Endomyocardial biopsy by means of biopsy forceps passed through a vascular-accessed catheter is the method of choice in heart transplant patients. Flexible bronchoscopy with transbronchial biopsy in children and adolescents is used to obtain multiple pieces of tissue for histopathological examination in lung transplant patients. For infants and young children, rigid bronchoscopy or open-lung biopsy may be required, although tiny biopsy forceps may allow biopsy through the flexible bronchoscope even in very small children. Most transplantation physicians are uncomfortable augmenting immunosuppression without tissue confirmation of graft rejection.

Infection

It can be difficult to separate rejection from infection, especially on a clinical diagnostic basis, and in some cases they may coexist.[34] Although pulmonary infections are common because of the immunosuppression required with any solid organ transplant, the pulmonary infection rate for lung transplantation appears to be high.[39] This may be partially explained by the fact that the lung is the only solid organ that after transplantation is regularly in direct contact with the external environment and multiple potential pathogens. Many pulmonary bacterial infections are readily identified but often require bronchoalveolar lavage for accurate diagnosis and easily treated with antibiotics. Pulmonary viral infections are less frequent but more often fatal, especially if cytomegalovirus is involved.[39] Fungal infections are particularly troublesome in terms of both accurate diagnosis and treatment. Because the transplant patient with cystic fibrosis retains the native trachea and sinuses, there is a potential increase in infections from chronic colonization of the respiratory epithelia in the trachea and from frank infection within the paranasal sinuses.[40] This can be particularly serious if the resident organisms have resistance to multiple antibiotics.[40,41] In fact, some centers consider infection with *Pseudomonas* species with no antibiotic sensitivity a contraindication to transplantation.[4] The highly antibiotic-resistant *Burkholderia cepacia* complex organisms have been associated with significant morbidity and mortality in patients with cystic fibrosis.[39,40] These resistant organisms are found most often in the older patient with advanced lung disease, and this is the patient with cystic fibrosis who most likely needs transplantation. Of concern is the report that *Burkholderia* species can be particularly lethal to transplant patients with cystic fibrosis who acquire it after transplantation.[40] The role of antibiotic prophylaxis in patients with cystic fibrosis who undergo lung transplantation remains to be clarified. A common and potentially effective prophylaxis for transplant patients with cystic fibrosis involves inhaled antibiotics, usually an aminoglycoside such as tobramycin.

Bronchiolitis Obliterans

Bronchiolitis obliterans is unfortunately a common late complication in both heart–lung and lung transplant recipients.[4,5,31] The exact cause in an individual case is sometimes unknown, but it most likely represents the common pathway for different insults such as chronic rejection, infection, and aspiration. Bronchiolitis obliterans can be initially identified by a decrease in flow rates at low lung volumes during surveillance pulmonary function testing and can be confirmed sometimes by transbronchial biopsy but more definitively by open-lung biopsy. Because of the high frequency of false-negative transbronchial biopsies, most clinicians use the clinical definition of "bronchiolitis obliterans syndrome" for both diagnosis and treatment decisions.[44] In the majority of patients, bronchiolitis obliterans is a progressive disease manifested by increasing dyspnea, increased coughing with sputum production, colonization or infection with *Pseudomonas* species, and eventual respiratory failure and death. A small minority of patients responds favorably to augmented immunosuppression, with reversal or stabilization of their airway dysfunction.[32] Bronchiolitis obliterans remains a major obstacle to the success of lung and heart–lung transplantation.

Drug Toxicity

All immunosuppressive regimens place the patient at risk for infection. In addition, each arm of the regimen may cause other complications from side effects or drug toxicity. Cyclosporine and tacrolimus have the highest potential toxicity. Hypertension and nephrotoxicity are most common, but, fortunately, are usually manageable. The major complication from both azathioprine and mycophenolate mofetil is a decreased white blood cell count caused by bone marrow suppression, which usually improves with temporary discontinuation of the medicine or a decrease in dose. There may be more symptoms of gastrointestinal disturbance with mycophenolate mofetil compared with azathioprine. Complications of prednisone are common in the immediate posttransplantation period when high doses are used, but complications lessen with

decreasing doses after several months. Prednisone is usually decreased to low daily doses (0.1 to 0.15 mg/kg/d) or to an alternate-day dosage schedule by 1 year after transplant. Because of the combined effects of tacrolimus and prednisone, some patients become glucose intolerant, particularly patients with cystic fibrosis, and may require long-term insulin therapy.

Other Complications

A broad spectrum of other complications occurs less commonly after transplantation. For patients receiving heart or heart–lung transplants, accelerated coronary artery disease is a potentially serious problem.[18,19,21] Like bronchiolitis obliterans, it is a form of chronic graft rejection and is usually progressive. Other potential complications include obstructive sleep apnea, cerebrovascular accidents, and aspiration of gastric contents. Epstein-Barr virus–related lymphoproliferative disease is a neoplastic disorder that occurs in relation to the intensity and duration of immunosuppression. The incidence in pediatric thoracic transplantation varies from 1% to 10%.[16,45] It may regress with decreased levels of immunosuppression and/or chemotherapy but can occasionally progress to fatal malignancy. Other fairly common medical complications include generalized seizures, aggravated acne, and mild suppression of maximal exercise performance. Up to 25% of lung transplant recipients may experience unilateral vocal cord or hemidiaphragm paralysis, which may recover 3 to 6 months after transplant. Equally important are the psychosocial adjustments to the emotional "roller coaster" of thoracic organ transplantation.[46] Although almost all patients can benefit from extensive psychosocial support, occasionally some will require pharmacological assistance to deal with either anxiety or depression.[46,47] These psychological or psychiatric complications are quite common, and they are potentially serious. Nonadherence to the medical regimen is often fatal. The entire transplantation team must be alert for any psychological or psychiatric complications in the hope of either their prevention or their early detection and treatment.

SURVIVAL AND QUALITY OF LIFE

Survival after pediatric heart transplantation in the most recent era exceeds 60% at 10 years and has shown significant incremental improvement over time.[18] Survival after pediatric lung transplantation is less than 40% at 10 years in the most recent era and there seems to be detectable but less impressive improvement in survival over time.[3] On the other hand, lung transplant recipients appear to have a higher functional status with more than 85% of survivors without any limitations, in contrast to approximately 60% of heart transplant survivors.[3,18] Quality-of-life assessment in pediatric heart transplant recipients shows that overall health-related quality of life is lower than healthy peers but comparable to other chronic disease groups.[48] Furthermore, a significant minority of these children have cognitive or behavioral issues.[49] There is less published information on the quality of life in pediatric lung transplant recipients. The authors' experience is that significant disability or neurodevelopmental deficits are uncommon. There is ongoing research in our own center, which will be published in the near future.

ROLE OF THE RESPIRATORY THERAPIST

There are multiple areas of interaction between the respiratory therapist (RT) and the transplant patient. Care of the patient who undergoes thoracic transplantation always involves the teamwork of a variety of health care professionals. The child who receives a lung or heart–lung transplant is especially likely to require an RT on the team. Familiarity with the diseases leading to transplantation, as well as the transplantation process, will help the practitioner provide more comprehensive care to the patient as well as improve interaction with the health care team. The RT may already be familiar with the transplant candidate because of his/her role in providing routine care for the primary disease process, particularly for chronic pulmonary diseases such as cystic fibrosis. The RT may become a key contact with the transplant candidate in the initial evaluation process or during pulmonary function testing. After the patient has been accepted to the transplantation list, the RT may be involved in providing an exercise evaluation and rehabilitation program in an effort to optimize the patient's condition while he or she is awaiting transplantation. Immediately after the transplantation procedure, the RT will be involved with the patient in the intensive care unit, primarily providing mechanical ventilatory support and maintenance of the artificial airway. Because of the temporary interruption of ciliary function, the RT may be asked to provide aerosolized bronchodilators, mechanical aids to assist full inflation and cough, and bronchopulmonary hygiene. For most patients, this therapy is not required on a long-term basis. Shortly after the patient is taken off mechanical ventilation, the RT may be involved in additional mucus clearance measures. Exercise and rehabilitation should be resumed as soon as possible after extubation.

Over the intermediate and long-term posttransplant period, patients and families often forget the importance of bronchial denervation in masking symptoms of significant lower respiratory tract disease. Lung transplant recipients can develop airway obstruction related to purulent bronchitis with surprisingly little cough. We have emphasized the importance of monitoring lung function at home as the single most sensitive indicator of lung health. We usually teach our lung transplant recipients how to use either the Flutter device (Cardinal Health, Dublin, OH) or the Acapella Vibratory PEP Therapy System (Smiths Medical ASD, Rockland, MA) as a tool

to aid in cough with mucus clearance. Refresher sessions are important during the extended period of follow-up. Lastly, the RT may be involved in the transplant patient's care by assisting with follow-up pulmonary function tests, instructing the patient in the use of home spirometry, and assisting with bronchoscopies.

CASE STUDY 1

An 18-month-old infant with a dilated cardiomyopathy undergoes heart transplantation, receiving a heart from a 3-year-old child weighing twice his weight. The early posttransplant recovery goes well, and he weans from cardiac pressor agents and is extubated. He has a mediastinal drainage tube in place. As the respiratory therapist, you are called because the chest radiograph shows left lower lobe consolidation and auscultation reveals a monophonic expiratory wheeze. SaO$_2$ is 95% on 1 lpm oxygen supplementation. There is a mild increase in work of breathing.

Which intervention would you recommend?
1. Reintubation with positive pressure breathing
2. Nebulized albuterol
3. Trial of nasal continuous positive airway pressure
4. Urgent flexible bronchoscopy
5. Chest computed tomography (CT) scan

See Evolve Resources for answers.

CASE STUDY 2

A 16-year-old girl with cystic fibrosis and advanced lung disease undergoes a successful bilateral lung transplant. She is transferred out of the intensive care unit on the fourth postoperative day with two chest tubes with SaO$_2$ 96% on room air. You are called into her room by her nurse because she is complaining of dyspnea and her SaO$_2$ is 79%. You note a significant air leak in one of the atria connected to the left chest tube.

Which of the following is the correct action after calling for a physician?
1. Clamp the chest tube.
2. Administer oxygen by nonrebreather mask.
3. Order an urgent chest radiograph.
4. Urgent return to the operating room.
5. Order a chest CT scan.

See Evolve Resources for answers.

KEY POINTS

- Pediatric heart transplantation dates to the early 1980s, whereas pediatric lung transplantation really began in the 1990s.
- Heart–lung transplantations have dramatically decreased over the past two decades.

- Survival after transplantation is significantly longer with heart transplantation compared with lung transplantation, which is related to the increased susceptibility of lung transplant recipients to both infection and allograft rejection.
- Lung transplant recipients require higher doses of immunosuppressant medications and have more frequent complications than heart transplant recipients.
- The most common immunosuppressive agents in the current era are tacrolimus and mycophenolate.
- Respiratory complications are common in thoracic organ transplant recipients and often require the input of an informed, well-trained respiratory care practitioner.

ASSESSMENT QUESTIONS

See Evolve Resources for the answers.

1. What is the frequency of transplantations performed in the pediatric age group, in order from most to least?
   A. Lung > heart–lung > heart
   B. Heart > heart–lung > lung
   C. Lung > heart > heart–lung
   D. Heart > lung > heart–lung
2. What is the major reason why fewer lungs are transplanted per donor compared with heart transplants in childhood?
   A. There are fewer lung transplant candidates than heart transplant candidates in childhood.
   B. There are fewer lung transplant programs than heart transplant programs.
   C. The lungs are more likely than the heart to be injured or infected in the brain-dead donor.
   D. The size of lungs is less adaptable to children of different ages than is the size of the heart.
3. What is the major medical problem in the immediate posttransplantation period for pediatric heart transplant patients?
   A. Graft failure
   B. Weaning patients from mechanical ventilatory support
   C. Cardiac arrhythmias
   D. Graft rejection
4. What is the most common serious medical problem in the immediate posttransplantation period for pediatric lung transplant recipients?
   A. Graft failure
   B. Weaning patients from ventilator support
   C. Pneumonia from the donor
   D. Graft rejection
5. For what condition is heart–lung transplant surgery most commonly performed in pediatric patients?
   A. Cystic fibrosis
   B. Pulmonary hypertension
   C. Infants with lung disease as a result of technical difficulties in isolated lung transplantation
   D. Pulmonary hypertension with congenital heart disease

6. Donation after cardiac death most commonly has provided organs for:
   A. Heart transplantation
   B. Heart–lung transplantation
   C. Lung transplantation
   D. All of the above
7. How long is immunosuppression used in lung, heart, and heart–lung transplantation?
   A. Only during the critical 6 months after transplantation; the patient is then weaned.
   B. Lifelong immunosuppression is needed.
   C. Lifelong only in lung and heart–lung transplantation because of the higher incidence of graft rejection.
   D. Lifelong only in heart and heart–lung transplantation because lung infections become a greater risk to survival after the first year because of immunosuppression.
8. Among the most important risks for pulmonary complications after lung transplantation in children are all of the following *except:*
   A. Dangers of childhood vaccines
   B. Absence of cough reflex because of interruption of the nerve supply to the transplanted lungs
   C. Immunosuppression
   D. Frequency of inevitable exposure to community respiratory viruses and other pathogens
9. Organ rejection is:
   A. A problem only in lung and heart–lung transplantation
   B. A problem only in the critical first 6 months after thoracic transplants
   C. The most common cause of late death in heart and lung transplantation
   D. Receding as a common problem because of advances in early detection and better immunosuppression
10. What is the role of the respiratory therapist in transplantation?
    A. Unimportant after isolated heart transplantation because the native lungs are, by definition, healthy
    B. Important only in the postoperative period in heart, heart–lung, and lung transplantation, during the variable period of weaning from mechanical ventilatory support
    C. Needed with many intercurrent respiratory infections after lung or heart–lung transplantation because of the blunting of the cough reflex
    D. Critical in evaluating oxygen saturation trends for cardiologists who are unfamiliar with this technology

References

1. Hosenpud JD, et al: The registry of the International Society for Heart and Lung Transplantation: eighteenth official report—2001, *J Heart Lung Transplant* 20:805, 2001.
2. Cooper JD: The evolution of techniques and indications for lung transplantation, *Ann Surg* 212:249, 1990.

3. Benden C, Edwards LB, Kucheryavaya AY, et al: The registry of the International Society for Heart and Lung Transplantation: fifteenth pediatric lung and heart–lung transplantation report—2012, *J Heart Lung Transplant* 31:1087, 2012.

4. Trulock EP: Lung transplantation, *Am J Respir Crit Care Med* 155:789, 1997.

5. Christie JD, Edwards LB, Kucheryavaya AY, et al: The Registry of the International Society for Heart and Lung Transplantation: twenty ninth adult lung and heart–lung transplantation report—2012, *J Heart Lung Transplant* 31:1073, 2012.

6. Marks WH, et al: Organ donation and utilization, 1995–2004: entering the collaborative era, *Am J Transplant* 6:1101, 2006.

7. de Perrot M, et al: Strategies to optimize the use of current available lung donors, *J Heart Lung Transplant* 23:1127, 2004.

8. Kutsogiannis DJ, et al: Medical management to optimize donor organ potential: review of the literature, *Can J Anesth* 53:820, 2006.

9. Cooper DK, et al: Report of the Xenotransplantation Advisory Committee of the International Society for Heart and Lung Transplantation: potential role in the treatment of end-stage cardiac and pulmonary diseases, *J Heart Lung Transplant* 19:1125, 2000.

10. Starnes VA, et al: Living-donor lobar lung transplantation experience: immediate results, *J Thorac Cardiovasc Surg* 112:1284, 1996.

11. Detry O, Dinh HL, Noterdaeme T, et al: Categories of donation after cardiocirculatory death, *Transplant Proc* 44:1189, 2012.

12. Based on OPTN data as of February 1, 2013. http://optn.transplant.hrsa.gov.

13. Boucek MM, Mashburn C, Dunn SM, et al: Pediatric heart transplantation after declaration of cardiocirculatory arrest, *N Engl J Med* 359:709, 2008.

14. Sweet SC, et al: Pediatric lung transplantation at St Louis Children's Hospital, 1990–1995, *Am J Respir Crit Care Med* 155:1027, 1997.

15. Noyes BE, Kurland G, Orenstein DM: Lung and heart–lung transplantation in children, *Pediatr Pulmonol* 23:39, 1997.

16. Baum D, et al: Pediatric heart transplantation at Stanford: results of a 15 year experience, *Pediatrics* 88:203, 1991.

17. Cohen AH, et al: Growth of lungs after transplantation in infants and in children younger than age, *Am J Respir Crit Care Med* 159:1747, 1999.

18. Kirk R, Dipchand AI, Edwards LB, et al: The registry of the International Society of Heart and Lung Transplantation: fifteenth official pediatric heart transplantation report—2012, *J Heart Lung Transplant* 31:1065, 2012.

19. Pahl E, et al: Coronary arteriosclerosis in pediatric heart transplant survivors: limitation of long-term survival, *J Pediatr* 116:177, 1990.

20. Boucek MM, et al: Cardiac transplantation in infancy: donors and recipients, *J Pediatr* 116:171, 1990.

21. Ross M, et al: Ten- and 20-year survivors of pediatric orthotopic heart transplantation, *J Heart Lung Transplant* 25:261, 2006.

22. Shewmon DA, et al: The use of anencephalic infants as organ sources: a critique, *JAMA* 261:1173, 1989.

23. Spray TL, et al: Pediatric lung transplantation for pulmonary hypertension and congenital heart disease, *Ann Thorac Surg* 54:216, 1992.

24. Ramirez JC, et al: Bilateral lung transplantation for cystic fibrosis, *J Thorac Cardiovasc Surg* 103:287, 1991.

25. Mendeloff EM, et al: Pediatric and adult lung transplantation for cystic fibrosis, *J Thorac Cardiovasc Surg* 115:404, 1998.

26. U.S. Organ Procurement and Transplantation Network and The Scientific Registry of Transplant Recipients. Website: http://www.optn.org. Retrieved October 2008.

27. Noirclerc M, et al: Size matching in lung transplantation, *J Heart Lung Transplant* 11:S203, 1992.

28. Starnes VA, et al: Current trends in lung transplantation: lobar transplantation and expanded use of single lungs, *J Thorac Cardiovasc Surg* 104:1060, 1992.

29. Starnes VA, et al: Comparison of outcomes between living donor and cadaveric lung transplant children, *Ann Thorac Surg* 68:2279, 1999.

30. Egan T, et al: Development of the new lung allocation system in the United States, *Am J Transplant* 6:1212, 2006.

31. Boehler A, et al: Bronchiolitis obliterans after lung transplantation: a review, *Chest* 114:1411, 1998.

32. Date H, et al: The impact of cytolytic therapy on bronchiolitis obliterans syndrome, *J Heart Lung Transplant* 17:869, 1998.

33. Jurmann MJ, et al: Pulmonary reperfusion injury: evidence for oxygen-derived free radical mediated damage and effects of different free radical scavengers, *Eur J Cardiothorac Surg* 4:665, 1990.

34. Paradis IL, et al: Distinguishing between infection, rejection, and the adult respiratory distress syndrome after human lung transplantation, *J Heart Lung Transplant* 11:S232, 1992.

35. Meyers BF, et al: Primary graft dysfunction and other selected complications of lung transplantation: a single center experience, *J Thorac Cardiovasc Surg* 129:1421, 2005.

36. Trachiotis GD, et al: Carbon dioxide response in lung transplant recipients [abstract], *Am Rev Respir Dis* 145:A702, 1992.

37. Patterson GA, et al: Airway complications after double lung transplantation, *J Thorac Cardiovasc Surg* 99:14, 1990.

38. Kaditis AG, et al: Airway complications following pediatric lung and heart–lung transplantation, *Am J Respir Crit Care Med* 162:301, 2000.

39. Trulock EP, et al: The role of trans-bronchial lung biopsy in the treatment of lung transplant recipients: an analysis of 200 consecutive procedures, *Chest* 102:1049, 1992.

40. Mauer JR, et al: Infectious complications following isolated lung transplantation, *Chest* 101:1056, 1992.

41. Nunley DR, et al: Allograft colonization and infections with Pseudomonas in cystic fibrosis lung transplant recipients, *Chest* 113:1235, 1998.

42. Chaparro C, et al: Infection with *Burkholderia cepacia* in cystic fibrosis: outcome following lung transplantation, *Am J Respir Crit Care Med* 163:43, 2001.

43. Snell GI, et al: Pseudomonas cepacia in lung transplant recipients with cystic fibrosis, *Chest* 103:466, 1993.

44. Cooper JD, et al: A working formulation for the standardization of nomenclature and for clinical staging of chronic dysfunction in lung allografts: International Society for Heart and Lung Transplantation, *J Heart Lung Transplant* 12:713, 1993.

45. Cohen AH, et al: High incidence of posttransplant lymphoproliferative disease in pediatric patients with cystic fibrosis, *Am J Respir Crit Care Med* 161:1252, 2000.

46. Kurland G, Orenstein DM: Lung transplantation and cystic fibrosis: the psychosocial toll, *Pediatrics* 107:1419, 2001.

47. Craven JL, Bright J, Dear CL: Psychiatric, psychosocial and rehabilitative aspects of lung transplantation, *Clin Chest Med* 11:247, 1990.

48. Uzark K, et al: Quality of life in pediatric heart transplant recipients: a comparison with children with and without heart disease, *J Heart Lung Transplant* 31:571, 2012.

49. Wray J, et al: Beyond the first year after pediatric heart or heart-lung transplantation: changes in cognitive function and behavior, *Pediatr Transplant* 9:170, 2005.

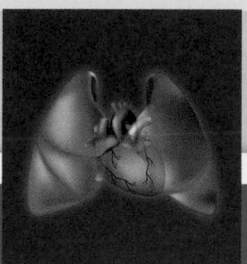

Chapter **22**

Neonatal Pulmonary Disorders

RANIA A. EL-FARRASH

LEARNING OBJECTIVES

After reading this chapter the reader will be able to:

1. Identify and differentiate the causes of neonatal respiratory distress and understand the underlying pathophysiology of each one
2. Discuss the factors in prenatal and postnatal life that may increase the risks for developing respiratory distress
3. Recognize the clinical features of common pulmonary disorders in neonates, differentiate among various diagnostic entities, and identify those that are life threatening
4. Describe preventive and therapeutic approach for various forms of neonatal pulmonary diseases to optimize outcome and minimize morbidity

KEY TERMS

Acute life-threatening event
Amnioinfusion
Apnea
Apnea of infancy
Apnea of prematurity
Atypical or new bronchopulmonary dysplasia
Chronic pulmonary insufficiency of prematurity
Classic bronchopulmonary dysplasia
Extremely low birth weight infant

Gentle ventilation
Low birth weight infant
Meconium
New or atypical bronchopulmonary dysplasia
Oxygenation index
Periodic breathing
Permissive hypercapnia
Pneumomediastinum
Pneumopericardium
Pneumoperitoneum
Pneumoretroperitoneum

Pneumothorax
Postductal
Precipitous delivery
Preductal
Pulmonary interstitial emphysema
Reduced alveolar recruitment
Subcutaneous emphysema
Sudden infant death syndrome
Very low birth weight infant
Volutrauma
Wilson-Mikity syndrome

Disorders that result in respiratory distress remain a major reason for morbidity and mortality among neonates.[1] The more premature the neonate is, the more likely that respiratory complications will exist at presentation. However, term and postterm infants can also experience respiratory difficulty resulting from pulmonary as well as nonpulmonary conditions (Table 22-1). The most common neonatal pulmonary disorders are addressed in this chapter.

RESPIRATORY DISTRESS SYNDROME

Incidence

In the United States, respiratory distress syndrome (RDS) has been estimated to occur in 20,000 to 30,000 newborn infants each year and it is a complication in about 1% of pregnancies.[2]

Its incidence is inversely related to gestational age and birth weight. RDS occurs in 60% to 80% of infants less than 28 weeks of gestational age, in 15% to 30% of those between 32 and 36 weeks, and rarely in those more than 37 weeks.[3] In a report from the National Institute of Child Health and Human Development (NICHD) Neonatal Research Network, the incidence rate of RDS was 44% in infants weighing 501 to 1500 g (Box 22-1).[4]

In 1979, RDS was the second-ranking cause of death in infants but because of the progress made in prenatal care, it has dropped to eighth place in 2007. In 2007, 17 deaths per 100,000 live births, were due to RDS.[5]

The risk of RDS is increased with maternal diabetes, multiple births, cesarean delivery, **precipitous delivery** (unintended delivery of infant anywhere), fetal asphyxia, cold stress, and a maternal history of previously affected infants.[6,7] The incidence is highest in preterm male or white infants.[8]

The risk of RDS is reduced in pregnancies with chronic or pregnancy-associated hypertension, maternal heroin use, prolonged premature rupture of membranes (PROM), and antenatal corticosteroid prophylaxis.[3]

Etiology and Pathophysiology

In 1959, Avery and Mead reported that RDS was associated with a deficiency of pulmonary surfactant and abnormal lung surface tension properties.[9] Since that time, it has been widely accepted that the pathophysiology of RDS is the result of an insufficient amount of surfactant as well as immature cellular and vascular development of the lungs.[10]

At approximately 16 weeks of gestation, the alveolar type II cells synthesize and store surfactant. Increasing amounts are produced as the fetus approaches term. Between 28 and 38 weeks of gestation, surfactant is secreted into the alveoli and eventually migrates into the amniotic fluid through the trachea. With its release into the alveoli, surfactant reduces the surface tension and helps to maintain alveolar stability when the lung transitions to a gas-filled organ at birth[11] (see Chapters 1 and 14). Primitive alveoli developed between 27 and 35 weeks of gestation, with true alveoli developed between 30 and 36 weeks of gestation.[12] Infants born before 28 weeks of gestation have structural underdevelopment of the terminal air spaces with little or no surfactant, leading to a susceptibility to RDS.

Deficient surfactant production or deficient release of surfactant into the immature respiratory alveoli results in an increase in surface forces and lung elastic recoil. Coupled

TABLE 22-1 Neonatal Disorders That May Present as Respiratory Distress

Condition	Gestational Age	History	Examination[a]	Gases[b]	Presentation[c] <6h	Presentation[c] 6h	Chest X-ray	Comments
Respiratory distress syndrome	PT				+++	N	Diagnostic	Working diagnosis in all preterm neonates unless chest radiograph suggests alternative. Always consider infection
Transient tachypnea	FT >PT[d]	Often CS delivery	Mild hypoxemia needing 40% O_2		+++	R	Diagnostic	Commonest cause of "breathlessness" in term babies. By definition, a mild disease
Meconium aspiration	FT[e]	Meconium-stained liquor at resuscitation. Post-maturity	Meconium-stained baby. Meconium in larynx		+++	N	Streaky	Diagnosis obvious based on history. Infection may coexist
Pneumothorax or pneumomediastinum	FT >PT	May be excessive resuscitation at birth	Crepitations; usually marked pallor. Blood in larynx or in endotracheal tube. PDA after presentation		++	R[f]	Diagnostic	Diagnosis based on clinical findings
Massive pulmonary hemorrhage	PT >FT	Asphyxia or other cause of heart failure, bleeding tendency. Use of artificial surfactant			+	+++	Unhelpful; usually a white-out	
After severe asphyxia	FT[g]	Severe asphyxia Low Apgar	Other features of asphyxia (pp. 485-486)	Marked metabolic acidemia	++	N	Unhelpful	Tachypnea driven by acidemia
Infection (pneumonia)	Any	May be helpful	Rarely differentiates this from other causes of dyspnea	Often severe acidemia and easy to reduce CO_2 without increasing Pao_2	++	+++	Unhelpful in most cases though may show patchy changes	Impossible to exclude in any baby. This is the working diagnosis in the absence of specific chest radiograph findings in neonates >6 hours old with respiratory disease. WBC. CRP may be helpful
Congenital malformations	FT >PT	Usually normal delivery. May have been detected on antenatal ultrasound	Rarely helpful	May be profound hypoxemia with raised CO_2	+++	+	Virtually always diagnostic	Diaphragmatic hernia, cysts, effusions, agenesis all present this way. TOF should not present this way

Condition	Gestation[d]	Clinical features other than cardinal features of respiratory disease[a]	Blood gases[b]	[c]	[c]	Chest radiograph	Comments
Congenital heart disease	FT >PT	Murmurs, heart size, signs of heart failure	CO$_2$ normal or reduced. In cyanotic CHD Pao$_2$ rarely >6–7 kPa even in oxygen with IPPV	R	+++	May be helpful or diagnostic	The alternative common diagnosis in infants presenting after 6 hours and particularly after 24 hours of age ECG and echocardiogram usually diagnostic
Pulmonary hypoplasia	Any	Prolonged rupture of membranes	Profound hypoxemia and hypercapnia	+++	N	Diagnostic; very small lungs	Virtually always rapidly fatal
Persistent pulmonary hypertension	FT >PT	May have had mild asphyxia	Gases like cyanotic CHD, i.e., marked hypoxemia with normal or reduced CO$_2$	+++	+	Usually normal or nearly so	Can be difficult to exclude cyanotic CHD unless echocardiogram available
Inhalation of feed	Any	Obvious		R	+++	Unhelpful	Should not happen in well-run units. Normal term babies rarely inhale, so always seek alternative diagnosis, especially infection
Inborn errors of metabolism	FT >PT	No evidence of lung disease Tachypnea driven by acidemia	Severe metabolic acidemia, normal Pao$_2$; low Paco$_2$	R, ++	+++	Often normal	Diagnosis based on blood changes plus ketonemia in many cases
Primary neurological or muscle disease	FT >PT	May be positive FH or history of unexplained NND or infant death Polyhydramnios may occur	Marked hypotonia Areflexia, odd face, deformities No evidence of lung disease	++	++	Often normal	Usually easy to identify as a group
Upper airway obstruction	FT >PT	May be typical in choanal atresia	Gases normal when intubated; CO$_2$ may be raised beforehand	++	++	Often normal	Stridor present Problems resolve on intubation, laryngoscopy be diagnostic

a Mentioning features other than cardinal features of respiratory disease.
b Most conditions cause hypoxemia and hypercapnia; only if the blood gas patterns differ from this is it noted here.
c Frequency of presentation graded + to +++; N = never, R = rarely.
d Full term greater than premature. This means that the condition can occur at any gestation but because full-term babies are more common than preterm ones, there are more cases in full-term neonates.
e If preterm, consider *Listeria*.
f Usually as a complication of preexisting and severe lung disease, especially HMD.
g Severely asphyxiated preterm babies will get RDS.
From Greenough A, Milner AD: Acute respiratory disease. JM Rennie [ed.], In *Rennie & Roberton's textbook of neonatology*, ed 5, Philadelphia, 2012, Elsevier Saunders.

Box 22-1	Incidence of RDS by Birth Weight	
Birth Weight (g)	Incidence of RDS	
501-750	71%	
751-1000	55%	
1001-1250	37%	
1251-1500	23%	

From Fanaroff AA, Stoll BJ, Wright LL, et al. Trends in neonatal morbidity and mortality for very low birth weight infants. *Am J Obst Gynecol* 2007;196:147.e1.

with the extremely compliant chest wall of the preterm infant, this leads to a **reduction in alveolar recruitment** (known as atelectasis). This condition is characterized by decreased functional residual capacity (FRC), decreased pulmonary compliance, increased pulmonary resistance, and ventilation-perfusion mismatch.[13]

The resulting hypoxia, hypercapnia, and respiratory acidosis constrict the pulmonary arteries and reduce pulmonary blood flow. This results in damage to the cells lining the alveoli.[14] The pulmonary hypertension can lead to increased right-to-left shunting through a patent ductus arteriosus (PDA) and the foramen ovale (extrapulmonary), as well as within the lung itself (intrapulmonary).[15] Shunting of blood results in greater hypoxemia and possibly metabolic acidosis, which increases the pulmonary vascular resistance (PVR) even more. This vicious cycle continues and may even lead to further suppression of surfactant synthesis.

Other pathophysiological processes that contribute to the clinical picture include poor gas exchange secondary to inadequate surface area, compliant chest wall that reduces effectiveness of ventilation, thickened alveolar-capillary membrane and insufficient vascularization, and poor clearance of lung fluid that can result in pulmonary edema.[16]

Though rare, genetic disorders of surfactant proteins may contribute to RDS. Abnormalities in surfactant protein B and C genes as well as a gene responsible for transporting surfactant across membranes (ABC transporter 3 [*ABCA3*])[17] are associated with severe and often lethal familial respiratory disease. Other familial causes include alveolar capillary dysplasia, acinar dysplasia, pulmonary lymphangiectasia, and mucopolysaccharidosis. These rare genetic forms lead to neonatal respiratory distress (not RDS) and are not associated with premature birth and can occur in full-term babies.[18]

Chronic stress seems to protect infants at risk for the development of RDS by stimulating surfactant synthesis. Conditions associated with chronic stress including maternal heroin addiction, maternal toxemia, and PROM for a duration of more than 18 hours preceding birth. Histological chorioamnionitis was associated with a decreased incidence of RDS, and in experimental models, bacterial endotoxin or the proinflammatory cytokine IL-1 induces lung maturation when given by intra-amniotic injection.[19] Fetal proinflammatory exposures induce striking increases in surfactant and improvements in postnatal lung function after preterm delivery of lambs without increasing fetal cortisol levels.[20]

Clinical Presentation and Diagnosis
Clinical Presentation

A constant feature of RDS is the early onset of clinical signs of the disease. Most infants present with signs and symptoms either in the delivery room or within the first 6 hours after birth.[21] Infants with RDS are usually preterm and exhibit tachypnea or labored breathing, or both. A decrease in the respiratory rate may indicate impending respiratory failure. A characteristic grunt during expiration (which is an attempt to maintain the FRC) and nasal flaring are also present.[22] Intercostal and subcostal retractions are apparent and occur when the negative intrathoracic inspiratory pressures distort the chest wall instead of inflating the stiff lungs. The retractions may have a "see-saw" appearance, with the abdomen protruding as the chest pulls in. Infants often look distressed, and the very premature infant may be hypotonic and unresponsive. Chest auscultation reveals diminished air in the alveoli in spite of the increased work of breathing.

Without stabilization of the alveoli, infants with RDS have increasing cyanosis that is relatively unresponsive to oxygen therapy. Larger infants may need minimal oxygen initially but require more as atelectasis becomes progressively worse. Some may have decreased oxygen requirements as acidosis and hypothermia (a result of delivery) are corrected but then have an increased need after 3 to 6 hours of life.

Investigations

1. Arterial blood gas (ABG) analysis: reveals moderate to severe hypoxemia, varying degrees of hypercapnia, and mixed acidosis (as a result of respiratory failure and lactic acid accumulation). The partial arterial carbon dioxide pressure ($Paco_2$) may initially be normal or low, but as the work of breathing increases and the infant begins to fail, there is resulting hypercapnia.

2. Chest X-ray (CXR): typically reveals diffuse, fine, granular (reticulogranular) densities, which give a ground-glass appearance. The heart may be slightly enlarged, and the thymus is nearly always present radiographically. The appearance of the CXR in RDS can be described as stages representing increasing severity of the disease (Figure 22-1). The disease may progress from one stage to the next, but the severity of the disease is initially described as the stage of RDS on the first chest film.[23]

3. Lecithin-to-sphingomyelin ratio (L:S) introduced by Gluck and associates in 1971 remains the standard test against which other tests are compared.[24] Lecithin, also known as dipalmitoylphosphatidylcholine, is the most abundant phospholipid found in surfactant. RDS is unlikely if the L:S ratio is 2.0 or greater.[25] The L:S ratio is unreliable in pregnancies characterized by diabetes and Rh isoimmunization.[23]

4. Levels of phosphatidylglycerol (PG), the second most abundant phospholipid in surfactant, increase toward term. The presence of PG in amniotic fluid indicates a low risk for RDS. A patient with an L:S ratio less than 2 and a lack of PG, has more than 80% risk of RDS.[26]

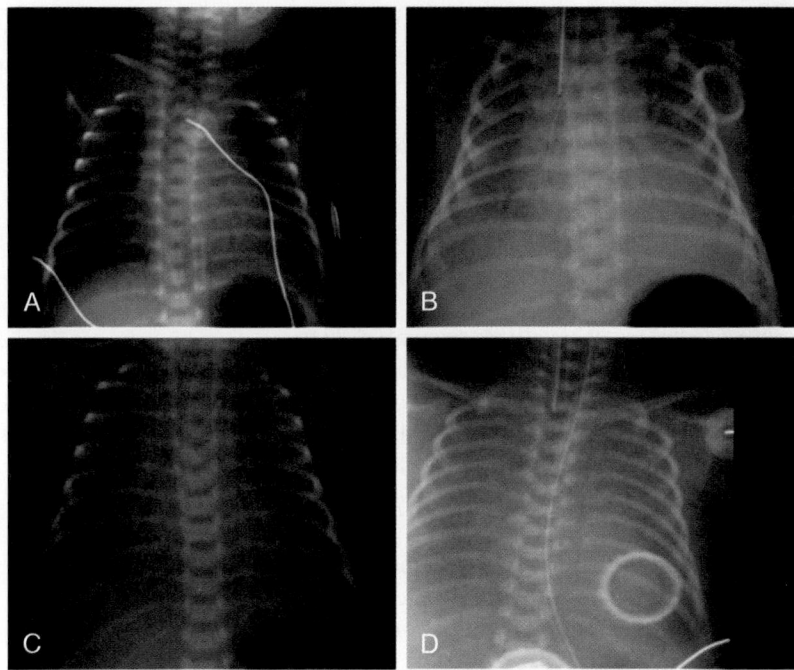

FIGURE 22-1 The images shown here were obtained from various premature infants of the twenty-fifth to the twenty-ninth weeks of gestational age. **A,** Stage I RDS with fine, diffuse reticulogranular pattern over the lung fields. **B,** Stage II RDS reveals a denser lung, with the presence of air bronchograms within the heart border. **C,** Stage III RDS shows increased density and the presence of air bronchograms beyond the heart border. **D,** Stage IV RDS, termed "whiteout," infant with severe disease complicated by pulmonary edema. The view of the heart border and edge of the diaphragm is obliterated. (From Paetzel M. *Respiratory distress syndrome (grade 1-4) of the premature and newborn.* Available at: http://www.radiologyteacher.com/index.cgi?&nav=view&DatID=127. Accessed January 1, 2013.)

5. The foam stability test (shake test) done by mixing amniotic fluid with different volumes of 95% ethanol. When this mixture is shaken with air, a foam develops that can be seen for several hours at room temperature. If no surfactant is present, the foam will not appear or will appear only briefly, indicating the strong possibility of immature lungs. This test is not as specific as a low L:S ratio.[27]

Prevention

1. Prevention of prematurity: Because RDS is associated with incomplete development of the lung at birth, the first line of treatment is prevention. Avoidance of unnecessary or poorly timed elective cesarean section, appropriate management of high-risk pregnancy and labor, and prediction of pulmonary immaturity with possible in utero acceleration of maturation are important preventive strategies.

2. Prevention of fetal/neonatal asphyxia: Since asphyxia is associated with an increased incidence and severity of RDS, antenatal and intrapartum fetal monitoring may similarly decrease the risk of fetal asphyxia. Compliance with consensus neonatal resuscitation techniques outlined by the American Academy of Pediatrics and American Heart Association is critical.[28]

3. Antenatal steroid therapy: Clinical trials have shown that maternal corticosteroid treatments decrease the incidence of RDS by about 50%, and the infants who do develop RDS tend to have less severe disease.[29]

Antenatal steroids also reduce (1) the need for and duration of ventilatory support and admission to a neonatal intensive care unit (NICU) and (2) the incidence of severe intraventricular hemorrhage (IVH), necrotizing enterocolitis (NEC), early-onset sepsis, and developmental delay. Postnatal growth is not adversely affected. Antenatal steroids do not increase the risk of maternal death, chorioamnionitis, or puerperal sepsis.[30]

Guidelines for antenatal steroid usage have been produced by the Royal College of Obstetricians and Gynaecologists,[31] the British Association of Perinatal Medicine,[32] and the U.S. National Institutes of Health.[33] Their recommendations include the following:

• Antenatal treatment with corticosteroids should be considered for all women at risk of preterm labor between 24 and 36 weeks. Treatment should consist of two doses of betamethasone given intramuscularly 24 hours apart or four doses of dexamethasone given 12 hours apart. Betamethasone, however, is now preferred because it was associated with a lower risk of periventricular leukomalacia (PVL) in an observational study.[34] Moreover, In a nonrandomized comparison, betamethasone compared with dexamethasone was associated with lower rates of RDS and bronchopulmonary dysplasia (BPD).[35]

• Treatment for less than 24 hours is associated with significant improvement in outcome; thus, corticosteroids should be given unless immediate delivery is anticipated.

- In the absence of chorioamnionitis, antenatal corticosteroids are recommended in pregnancies complicated by PROM.
- Unless there is evidence that corticosteroids will have an adverse effect on the mother, they are also recommended in other complicated pregnancies.

Treatment

The keys to the management of infants with RDS are as follows[36]:

1. To prevent hypoxemia and acidosis (this allows normal tissue metabolism, optimizes surfactant production, and prevents right-to-left shunting)
2. To optimize fluid management (avoiding hypovolemia and shock, on the one hand, and edema, particularly pulmonary edema, on the other)
3. To reduce metabolic demands
4. To prevent worsening atelectasis and pulmonary edema
5. To minimize oxidant lung injury
6. To minimize lung injury caused by mechanical ventilation

Surfactant Replacement

Current recommendations based on American Association for Respiratory Care (AARC) clinical practice guidelines for surfactant replacement therapy are detailed in Box 22-2.

Types of Surfactants. Several types of surfactant preparations are licensed for use in babies with RDS (Table 22-2). Exogenous lung surfactant can be either natural or synthetic. Both forms of surfactants are effective at reducing the severity of RDS; however, comparative trials demonstrate greater early improvement in the requirement for ventilatory support and fewer pneumothoraces associated with natural surfactant extract treatment. On clinical grounds, natural surfactant extracts would seem to be the more desirable choice.[37]

Timing of Administration. In the era of noninvasive respiratory support, every effort is made to minimize exposure to sustained mechanical ventilation and supplemental oxygen. Two basic strategies for surfactant replacement have emerged: prophylactic or preventive treatment, in which surfactant is administered at the time of birth or shortly thereafter to infants who are at high risk for developing RDS; and rescue or therapeutic treatment, in which surfactant is

Box 22-2	**Current Guidelines for the Use of Surfactant in Neonatal RDS (Evidence-based)**

1. Administration of surfactant replacement therapy is strongly recommended in a clinical setting where properly trained personnel and equipment for intubation and resuscitation are readily available. (1A)
2. Prophylactic surfactant administration is recommended for neonatal respiratory distress syndrome (RDS) in which surfactant deficiency is suspected. (1B)
3. Rescue or therapeutic administration of surfactant after the initiation of mechanical ventilation in infants with clinically confirmed RDS is strongly recommended. (1A)
4. A multiple surfactant dose strategy is recommended over a single dose strategy. (1B)
5. Natural exogenous surfactant preparations are recommended over laboratory-derived synthetic suspensions at this time. (1B)
6. We suggest that aerosolized delivery of surfactant not be utilized at this time. (1B)

From Walsh BK, Daigle B, Diblasi RM, Restrepo RD. AARC Clinical practice guideline. Surfactant replacement therapy: 2013. *Respir Care* 2013;58(2):367.

administered after the initiation of mechanical ventilation in infants with clinically confirmed RDS.[38]

Prophylactic surfactant administration to infants at risk of developing RDS is associated with lower risk of air leak and mortality, compared to selective use of surfactant in infants with established RDS.[39] Surfactant administration with brief lung-protective ventilation (followed by extubation to nasal continuous positive airway pressure) for premature infants at risk for developing RDS is associated with a lower incidence of mechanical ventilation, air leak syndromes, and chronic lung disease, compared to selective surfactant and continued mechanical ventilation.[40]

Methods of Administration. The surfactant preparation is delivered over a period of a few seconds via the endotracheal tube (ETT), usually through a feeding tube that has been cut to an appropriate length to be at a level just above the carina. The peripheral dispersion of surfactant into the terminal airways is facilitated by intermittent positive-pressure ventilation (IPPV), either manually or using the ventilator.

TABLE 22-2

Currently Available Surfactants

	Trade Name	Source	Manufacturer	Dose	Surfactant Protein B
Poractant alfa	Curosurf	Porcine	Chiesi Farmaceutici	100-200 mg/kg/dose (1.25-2.5 mL/kg)	0.45
Calfactant	Infasurf	Bovine	Ony	105 mg/kg/dose (3 mL/kg)	0.26
Beractant	Survanta	Bovine	Abbott Laboratories	100 mg/kg/dose (4 mL/kg)	<1
Lucinactant	Surfaxin	Synthetic	Discovery Labs	5.8 mL/kg	KL$_4$

From Walsh BK, Daigle B, Diblasi RM, Restrepo RD. AARC clinical practice guideline. Surfactant replacement therapy: 2013. *Respir Care* 2013;58(2):367.

Five methods of surfactant administration without intubation have been employed with varying success. These include antenatal intra-amniotic instillation,[41] pharyngeal instillation,[42] laryngeal mask instillation,[43] direct tracheal instillation without intubation,[44] and surfactant nebulization.[45] However, whether these methods really influence short- and long-term respiratory outcome remains to be proven in well-designed randomized, controlled trials.

Complications. Procedural complications resulting from the administration of surfactant include: plugging of ETT by surfactant, desaturation and increased need for supplemental O_2, bradycardia due to hypoxia, tachycardia due to agitation,[46] pharyngeal deposition of surfactant, administration of surfactant to only one lung (ie, right mainstem intubation) and administration of suboptimal dose.[37]

Physiologic complications of surfactant replacement therapy include: apnea, pulmonary hemorrhage from right to left shunting,[47] increased necessity for treatment for PDA and volutrauma resulting from increase in lung compliance following surfactant replacement with failure to change ventilator settings.[48,37]

Oxygen Therapy

Oxygen therapy begins with delivery of oxygen via an oxygen hood in an attempt to maintain the partial arterial oxygen pressure (PaO_2) between 50 and 80 mm Hg, $PaCO_2$ in the 40 to 55 mm Hg range, and pH at least 7.25. The oxygen is warmed, humidified, and delivered through an air–oxygen blender that allows precise control over the oxygen concentration.[36,49] The fraction of inspired oxygen (FIO_2) may be increased in increments of 0.1 and oxygenation assessed by means of either ABG analysis or pulse oximetry until the appropriate oxygen level is obtained. Use of the oxygen hood as an initial therapy for mild respiratory distress symptoms should be reserved for those larger infants who require above ambient FIO_2. When applying oxygen therapy, care should be taken to minimize the FIO_2 to no more than necessary. Current evidence has reinforced the potential for oxygen to contribute to lung damage, BPD, and retinopathy of prematurity (ROP).[50]

Continuous Positive Airway Pressure (CPAP)

If oxygen saturation cannot be kept more than 85% at FIO_2 of 40% to 70% or greater, CPAP via nasal prongs or nasopharyngeal tube using a continuous-flow ventilator may be instituted.[3] Simpler CPAP delivery using tubing submerged in sterile water to deliver the desired CPAP pressure ("bubble" CPAP) is also used and may have some benefits over use of a continuous-flow ventilator[51] (CPAP; see Chapter 20).

A CPAP of 4 to 6 cm H_2O is the usual starting point in these infants, then adjusting the pressure in increments of 1 to 2 cm H_2O to a maximum of 8 cm H_2O, observing the baby's respiratory rate and effort as well as monitoring oxygen saturation. A nasogastric tube is always placed to decompress swallowed air. As the infant improves, begin by reducing the FIO_2 in decrements of 0.05 to maintain the targeted oxygen saturation. Generally, when FIO_2 is less than 0.30, CPAP can be reduced to 5 cm H_2O, after oxygen saturation. Physical examination will provide evidence of respiratory effort during weaning, and CXR may help estimate lung volume. Lowering of the distending pressure should be attempted with caution if the lung volumes appear low and alveolar atelectasis persists. CPAP generally could be discontinued if there is no distress and the FIO_2 remains less than 0.3.[36]

Early nasal CPAP (NCPAP) in preterm newborn of 28 to 32 weeks of gestation can reduce the need for intubation.[52] Stabilization of the alveoli in this gestational age may allow surfactant production to occur without further intervention. During this time, if the infant requires an FIO_2 of more than 0.40 on NCPAP, it is an indication for intubation and exogenous surfactant treatment. Treatment of the **very low birth weight** (VLBW) **infant** (weighing less than 1500 g) is often more assertive. In the current patient care protocols, early stabilization on CPAP with selective surfactant administration to infants requiring intubation improves clinical outcome in the form of reducing the need for prolonged intubation and mechanical ventilation,[53,54] lower risk of pneumothorax, pulmonary interstitial emphysema (PIE), and mortality[39] (see Chapter 14).

Mechanical Ventilation

Classic indications for endotracheal intubation and mechanical ventilation are infants with respiratory failure or persistent apnea. Reasonable measures of respiratory failure are (1) arterial blood pH less than 7.20, (2) $PaCO_2$ of 60 mm Hg or higher, and (3) oxygen saturation less than 85% at oxygen concentrations of 40% to 70% and CPAP of 5 to 10 cm H_2O.[3]

In the **extremely low birth weight** (ELBW) **infant** (weighing less than 1000 g), intubation and positive-pressure ventilation (PPV) may be necessary immediately after birth.

Generally, once the infant is stabilized and in the NICU, a pressure-limited ventilator using a sinusoidal flow pattern is used. Peak inspiratory pressures (PIPs) generally adjusted at 15 to 25 cm H_2O, depending on the size of the infant and the severity of the disease, to establish a tidal volume (V_T) between 3 and 5 ml/kg. Positive end-expiratory pressure (PEEP) levels of 3 to 6 cm H_2O are used to prevent further alveolar collapse, and rates of 20 to 50 breaths per minute are used to treat hypercapnia. Inspiratory times (Ti) should be initiated at 0.3 to 0.4 second. If a longer Ti is required before surfactant administration, it should be lowered to 0.3 second after surfactant is administered.

Most ventilators today use pressure and flow measurements to produce real-time pulmonary function data. These numeric data and graphical displays can be used to correct V_T to optimize ventilation parameters and pulmonary mechanical parameters.[55] Ventilator modes such as synchronized intermittent mandatory ventilation (SIMV) or assist-control modes can reduce work of breathing and blood pressure fluctuations if sensitivities are set properly.[56] Modes that maintain a consistent VT, reduce the risk of **volu-trauma** (damage to the lung caused by overdistention by a mechanical ventilator set for an excessively high VT) particularly after the administration of surfactant (see Chapter 17). High-frequency ventilation (HFV) may be indicated in infants who cannot be ventilated with the usually effective FIO2 levels, ventilator pressures, and rates (see Chapter 16).

Supportive Care and Monitoring

The general principles for supportive care of any premature infant should be followed, taking into consideration that treatment of acidosis, hypoxia, hypotension, and hypothermia might decrease the severity of RDS.

Use of an incubator is preferable to radiant warmer in VLBW infants because of the high insensible water losses associated with radiant heat. Calories and fluids should initially be provided intravenously. Excessive fluids (more than 140 ml/kg/day) might contribute to the development of patent ductus arteriosus and BPD.[3]

Therapy requires careful and frequent monitoring of heart and respiratory rates, oxygen saturation, ABG status, serum electrolytes, glucose, hematocrit, blood pressure, and temperature. Analysis of continuous inline arterial blood gases and electrolytes has been introduced in NICUs. This promising technology offers advantages over intermittent sampling: less handling of the critically ill patient and continuous evaluation of therapeutic maneuvers.[57] Transcutaneous oxygen and CO2 monitors, end-tidal CO2, pulse oximetry, cardiopulmonary monitors, and Doppler flow studies can be used as noninvasive tools to monitor the infant's progress.

Routine daily CXR may be useful in managing the VLBW infant who is mechanically ventilated. Abnormalities ranging from malposition of the ETT to PIE can occur from one minute to the next.[58]

Complications and Prognosis

In milder cases the signs and symptoms reach a peak within 72 hours, followed by gradual improvement. Spontaneous diuresis and an increased ability to oxygenate the infant are the first signs of improvement.

Severely affected infants may die, usually between days 2 and 7, with death most often associated with pulmonary interstitial emphysema, pneumothorax, or IVH. Extremely premature infants (23 to 25 weeks of gestation) may have an initial "honeymoon" period in which the patient has stable ventilator settings but will exhibit increased oxygen and ventilator demands as time progresses. These ELBW infants not only have immature lungs but their extreme prematurity also presents challenges because metabolic and cardiac functions are affected.[59]

Changes in perinatal care, such as the use of antenatal steroids, exogenous surfactant administration, early NCPAP, and lung protective strategies of mechanical ventilation (patient-triggered modalities, volume-controlled modes, and high-frequency oscillatory ventilation), have led to improvement in survival and outcomes of infants with RDS over the past 30 years.[60]

The clinical outcome in preterm infants surviving RDS is often associated with chronic lung disease in the form of BPD, reactive airway disease, and an increase in and vulnerability to respiratory disorders.[61] Often pulmonary function testing demonstrates increased pulmonary resistance and work of breathing as well as decreased lung compliance and a tendency toward oxygen desaturation.[62] Other complications encountered include IVH, ROP, infection, air leaks, and NEC.

BRONCHOPULMONARY DYSPLASIA

Definitions

Classic bronchopulmonary dysplasia (BPD) was first described by Northway et al. in 1967 as a severe chronic lung injury in premature infants who survived hyaline membrane disease after treatment with mechanical ventilation and oxygen.[63]

In 2001, a workshop conducted by the National Institutes of Health (NIH)[64] proposed a definition that divides BPD into three categories based on the duration and level of oxygen therapy required (Table 22-3). Also, the criteria for administering supplemental oxygen can greatly affect the reported incidence of BPD. A physiological test to standardize the need for supplemental oxygen has been proposed as a way of reducing the variability in diagnostic criteria, with arterial oxygen saturation (SaO2) less 90% considered as the cutoff at which supplemental O2 is required.[65]

Chronic lung disease (CLD) has been used as the diagnosis for all babies who are oxygen dependent beyond 28 days of age with an abnormal CXR. On the basis of the clinical course and CXR appearance, some identify distinct forms of CLD, such as Wilson-Mikity syndrome and chronic pulmonary insufficiency of prematurity, which will be discussed later. Currently, following the NIH consensus, *BPD* rather than *CLD* is used as the umbrella term for all oxygen-dependent babies, because it better distinguishes the neonatal lung process from the CLDs seen in later life.[64]

The classic progressive stages of disease first described by Northway et al. are less common, and the severe form of the disease is often absent now and has been replaced by a milder form of chronic lung damage referred to as **atypical or new bronchopulmonary dysplasia**.[66] In contrast with the past, the "new BPD" often develops in preterm newborns who may have required minimal or even no ventilator support and relatively low FIO2 during the early postnatal days.[67]

It is not uncommon for very prematurely born babies who have had no acute respiratory illness to develop chronic pulmonary illness. These forms of chronic lung diseases include **Wilson-Mikity syndrome** and **chronic**

TABLE 22-3

Definition of Bronchopulmonary Dysplasia: Diagnostic Criteria

	GESTATIONAL AGE	
	<32 weeks	≥32 weeks
Time point of assessment	36 weeks PMA or discharge to home, whichever comes first Treatment with oxygen comes first	>28 days but <56 days postnatal age or discharge to home, whichever comes first
Mild BPD	Breathing room air at 36 weeks PMA or discharge, whichever comes first	Breathing room air by 56 days postnatal age or discharge, whichever comes first
Moderate BPD	Need* for >30% oxygen and/or positive pressure, (PPV or NCPAP) at 36 weeks PMA or discharge, whichever comes first	Need* for >30% oxygen and/or positive pressure age or discharge, whichever comes first
Severe BPD	Need* for 30% oxygen and/or positive pressure, (PPV or NCPAP) at 36 weeks PMA or discharge, whichever comes first	Need* for 30% oxygen and/or positive pressure (PPV or NCPAP) at 56 days postnatal age or discharge, whichever comes first

BPD, Bronchopulmonary dysplasia; *NCPAP*, nasal continuous positive airway pressure; *PMA*, postmenstrual age; *PPV*, positive-pressure ventilation.
*A physiological test confirming that the oxygen requirement at the assessment time point remains to be defined. This assessment may include a pulse oximetry saturation range. BPD usually develops in neonates being treated with oxygen and positive pressure ventilation for respiratory failure, most commonly respiratory distress syndrome. Persistence of clinical features of respiratory disease (tachypnea, retractions, rales) is considered common to the broad description of BPD and has not been included in the diagnostic criteria describing the severity of BPD. Infants treated with oxygen >21% and/or positive pressure for non-respiratory disease (e.g., central apnea or diaphragmatic paralysis) do not have BPD unless they also develop parenchymal lung disease and exhibit clinical features of respiratory distress. A day of treatment with oxygen >21% means that the infant received oxygen >21% for more than 12 hrs on that day. Treatment with oxygen >21% and/or positive pressure at 36 weeks PMA or 56 days postnatal age or discharge should not reflect an "acute" event but should rather reflect the infant's usual daily therapy for several days preceding and following 36 weeks PMA, 56 days postnatal age, or discharge.
From Jobe AH, Bancalari E. Bronchopulmonary dysplasia. *Am J Respir Crit Care Med* 2001;163:1723.

pulmonary insufficiency of prematurity (CPIP). In 1960, Wilson and Mikity described five preterm infants with diffuse lung infiltrates appearing at 10 to 30 days.[68] These preterm infants had respiratory distress in the first days of life, which appeared to resolve. Then, 1 to 5 weeks later, the tachypnea and cyanosis returned. Radiologically there were diffuse pulmonary infiltrates that in some infants changed to a cystic emphysematous pattern. CPIP is diagnosed in very immature babies who have made at least a partial recovery from RDS but then go on to develop apnea and increasing oxygen requirements. They have low lung volumes and respond well to CPAP.[69]

Incidence

The incidence of BPD varies widely among different centers. This is due not only to differences in patient susceptibility and in management but also to discrepancies in the way BPD is defined.[70] Although surfactant treatment has improved overall survival for premature infants, the incidence of BPD ranges between 15% and 50% in infants weighing less than 1500 g at birth and increases with decreasing gestational age.[71] The incidence of "new" BPD is 30% in infants born at or before 28 weeks of gestation, and only 3% in infants born after 28 weeks.[72]

Pathogenesis

Northway et al.[63] proposed four major factors in BPD pathogenesis: (1) lung immaturity, (2) respiratory failure, (3) oxygen supplementation, and (4) positive-pressure mechanical ventilation. Beyond these factors, new knowledge suggests additional complex processes involved in the

pathogenesis of BPD, including inflammation, aberrations in lung growth and lung signaling pathways, derangements in transcription factors and growth factors, new evidence related to oxidant lung injury, and a broader understanding of the genetics of BPD (Figure 22-2).

Prematurity

As mentioned earlier, the incidence of BPD is inversely related to gestational age and birth weight, strongly suggesting that incomplete development of the lungs plays an important role in the pathogenesis of BPD.[72]

Ventilation-Induced Lung Injury (Barotrauma or Volutrauma)

IPPV seemed particularly damaging if PIP above 35 cm H_2O was used.[73] Volutrauma may occur at resuscitation if rapid lung expansion is attempted. Prematurely born lambs given six manual inflations of 35 to 40 ml/kg, compared with those not "bagged" at birth, had poorer lung function at 4 hours of age, as indicated by lower inspiratory capacities.[74] Use of high VT at resuscitation can also compromise the response to surfactant therapy in preterm lambs.[75] Ventilation-induced lung injury contributes to a cascade of inflammation and cytokine release, further amplifying the lung injury process.

Hypoxia/Hyperoxia–Induced Lung Injury. Northway and associates[63] originally proposed that both oxygen exposure and ventilator-induced lung injury may deleteriously affect the lung via inflammatory pathways. New clinical and experimental data suggest that although hyperoxia alone plays an important role in BPD pathogenesis, intermittent

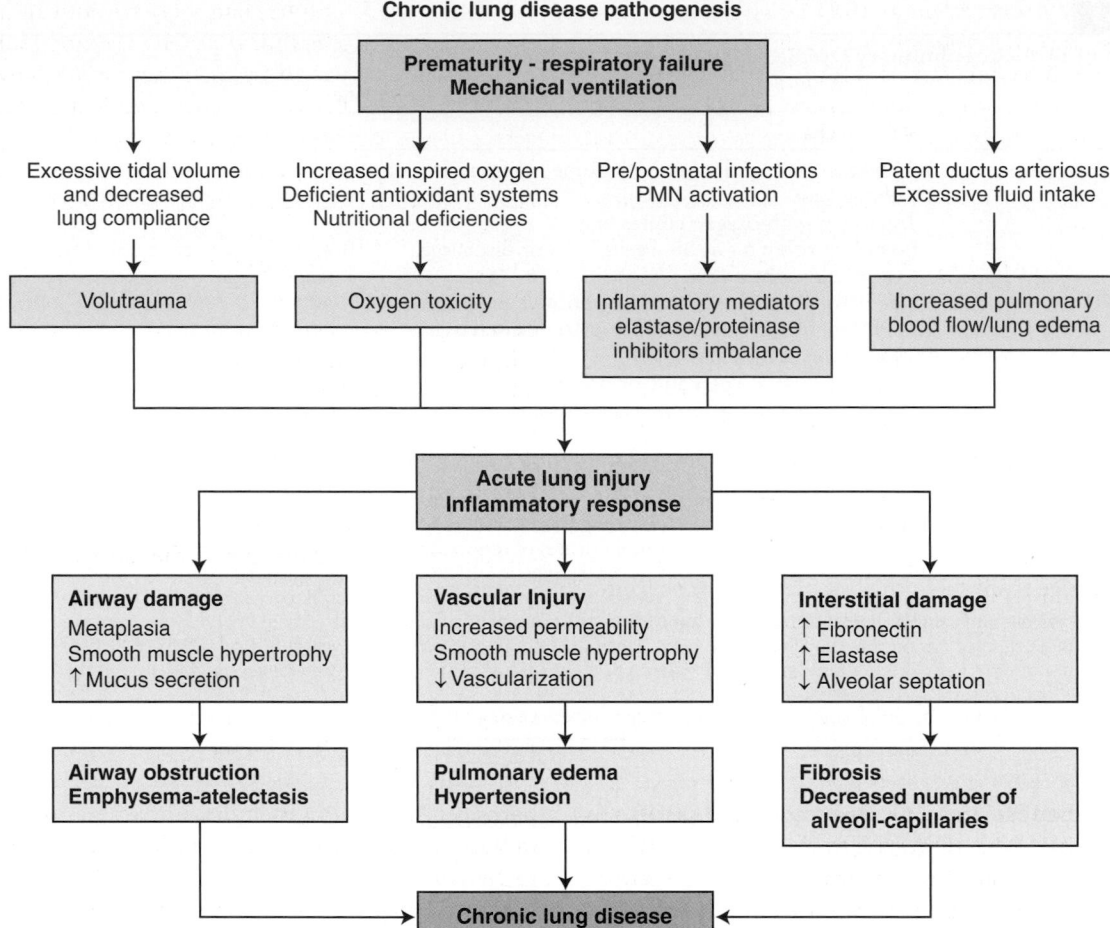

Chronic lung disease pathogenesis

FIGURE 22-2   Algorithm for chronic lung disease pathogenesis in infants. *PMN,* polymorphonucleocytes. (From Bancalari E: Bronchopulmonary dysplasia and neonatal chronic lung disease. In:Fanaroff AA, Martin RJ, editors. *Neonatal-perinatal medicine diseases of the fetus and infant,* ed 9. St Louis: Mosby-Elsevier, 2011.)

hypoxia occurring during exposure to hyperoxia may actually contribute to exacerbation of BPD through worsening of oxidative lung injury.[76,77] Most premature infants requiring supplemental oxygen and/or mechanical ventilation have intermittent spells of hypoxia during their acute course, but those infants in whom BPD develops have more frequent episodes of hypoxemia than those without BPD.[78]

To resist the detrimental effects of oxygen, the body has evolved a number of compensatory antioxidant systems. Antioxidant enzymes such as superoxide dismutase, catalase, and glutathione peroxidase seem to play an important role in preventing the toxic effects of oxygen. Other elements, such as vitamin E, glutathione, and selenium, are also part of the endogenous antioxidant mechanisms. However, preterm infants have lower concentrations of antioxidant enzymes than full-terms.[79]

Inflammation. Evidence suggests that exposure to antenatal inflammation may have a protective effect of reducing the incidence of RDS in premature infants while paradoxically increasing the risk of lung damage and BPD.[80]

The increase in expression of pulmonary proinflammatory cytokines, chemokines, adhesion molecules, proteases, and angiogenic factors in concert with a decreased capacity to downregulate this response in infants who experience BPD suggests that persistent endogenous generation of these factors might contribute to chronic lung injury and inflammation.[81]

Several studies have suggested an association between *Ureaplasma urealyticum* and the development of severe respiratory failure and BPD in VLBW infants.[82-84] Hassanein et al.[85] reported that preterm neonates with positive cord blood polymerase chain reaction (PCR) for *Ureaplasma urealyticum* were more likely to have PROM, chorioamnionitis, earlier gestation, proinflammatory response, and RDS than those with a negative PCR.

Nutrition. Data from experimental animal studies have shown that ability to handle oxidative lung injury is negatively affected by malnutrition, especially protein malnutrition.[86] Undernourishment causes alveolar loss or enlargement, also called nutritional emphysema. This presentation of nutritional emphysema has similarities to the alveolar simplification seen in BPD.[87,88] Slow postnatal growth rates in preterm sheep also result in lower alveolar numbers and reduced surface area for gas exchange in relation to lung or body weight, and this pattern persists into maturity.[89] In preterm humans, the presence of fetal growth restriction independently raises the risk for BPD.[90]

Trace elemental deficiency, especially zinc, copper, selenium, chromium, molybdenum, manganese, iodine, and iron, in preterm neonates may predispose the infant to lung injury, and supplementation may provide protection.[91,92] Vitamins A and E are nutritional antioxidants that may help prevent lipid peroxidation and maintain cell integrity.[93,94]

Patent Ductus Arteriosus. Infants with PDA are exposed to multiple factors that increase the risk of lung injury, and these factors become important confounders in the reported association between PDA and increased risk for BPD.[95]

A retrospective study from the Neonatal Network found that PDA was an independent risk factor associated with the development of BPD, as well as higher fluid intake and lesser weight loss in the first 10 days of life.[96]

Although prophylactic indomethacin decreased the risk of PDA among these preterm infants, it increased the risk of BPD among infants who did not have a PDA, an effect that seemed to be explained by increased oxygen requirements and decreased weight loss in the first week in indomethacin-treated infants. Further, there was an independent association between surgical ligation and the development of BPD among infants who subsequently received treatment for PDA.[97]

Genetics. Bhandari et al.[98] reported that genetic factors accounts for 53% of the susceptibility for BPD. Moreover, genetic factors associated with abnormal airway reactivity may play a role, in that infants with BPD have a stronger family history of asthma than those without BPD.[99] Several specific genetic loci linked to the development of BPD include genes involved in surfactant function,[100] alveologenesis and vascular growth and remodeling,[101] and factors affecting the response to oxidative stress.[102] Polymorphism in the macrophage inhibitory factor (MIF) promoter is associated with BPD; specifically, infants with the MIF-173* allele (predisposing to higher MIF production) were shown to have a lower incidence of BPD.[103]

Vascular Hypothesis. Thébaud and Abman have proposed a "vascular hypothesis" in the pathogenesis of BPD; whereas normal alveolar development progresses in response to the secretion of angiogenic growth factors, such as vascular endothelial growth factor (VEGF) and nitric oxide (NO), lung angiogenic growth factor expression has been found to be decreased in BPD, a finding that may explain the arrest of vascular growth and impairment of alveolar growth.[104] Multiple studies support this "vascular hypothesis" of BPD.[105-107]

Clinical Presentation and Diagnosis

BPD, with rare exceptions, follows the use of mechanical ventilation with IPPV during the first weeks of life. The development of BPD is often suspected when mechanical ventilation and oxygen dependence extend beyond 10 to 14 days.[64] Four distinct clinical stages were described radiographically and pathologically (Table 22-4).[63]

As mentioned earlier, the classic BPD described by Northway et al.[63] is now extremely rare with the advent of antenatal steroids, postnatal surfactant, and ventilator strategies better suited for preterm newborn infants. Instead, the typical picture of the "new BPD" is the one affecting smaller and more immature infants (birth weight 400 to 1000 g) than the original studied population (birth weight more than 1000 g) with milder functional and

---

TABLE 22-4

Radiological Staging of Classic Bronchopulmonary Dysplasia, with Pathological Correlates

Stage	Patient's Age (ds)	Radiologic Description	Pathologic Description
I	2-3	Granular pattern Air bronchograms Small lung volume	Atelectasis Hyaline membranes Lymphatic dilation
II	4-10	Opacification	Necrosis and repair of alveolar epithelium Persistent hyaline membranes Emphysematous coalescence of alveoli and bronchiolar necrosis
III	10-20	Small areas of lucency alternating with areas of irregular density	Resisting airway injury to alveolar epithelium Groups of emphysematous alveoli with atelectasis of surrounding alveoli Interstitial edema and septal thickening Bronchiolar mucosal metaplasia and hyperplasia with marked mucus secretions
IV	Beyond 30 days	Enlargement of lucent areas alternating with thinner strands of radiodensity	Emphysematous

Data from Northway WH et al. Pulmonary disease following respiratory therapy of hyaline membrane disease. *N Engl J Med* 1976;276:357; and Edwards PK, et al. Radiographic-pathologic correlation in bronchopulmonary dysplasia. *J Pediatr* 1979;95:835.

radiographic changes, revealing more diffuse haziness without the marked changes observed in the severe forms of BPD.[64]

Now infants present with milder lung disease, may start out with only minimal or mild RDS, and in fact may receive mechanical ventilation for pneumonia, apnea, or poor respiratory effort. They may require low-pressure ventilatory support with low F_{IO_2} and may already be breathing room air within the first day(s) of life. However, within a few days or weeks after birth, these infants display deteriorating lung function and increased ventilator or oxygen requirements (Figure 22-3). This deterioration in respiratory status may be related to a hemodynamically significant PDA, to inflammation caused by bacterial infection or colonization, or to inflammatory processes triggered by oxygen or mechanical ventilation.[95]

Although infants with "new BPD" may require mechanical ventilation and oxygen for a prolonged period, the majority with this relatively milder form of chronic lung disease are essentially symptom free by discharge.[70] There remains a small minority of infants with "new BPD" who have more severe lung dysfunction, characterized by progressive respiratory failure that may even be associated with persistent pulmonary hypertension of the newborn (PPHN) and cor pulmonale, severe airway damage, bronchomalacia, and airway obstruction, and may result in death.[108] If infants with this more severe form of BPD acquire acute bacterial or viral pulmonary infections, their lung damage may be further exacerbated.[109]

The diagnosis of BPD is based on the clinical and radiographic manifestations, but these are not specific. For this reason specific etiologies that could lead or contribute to the lung damage must be considered before concluding that the infant has BPD. Among these, one must rule out congenital heart disease, pulmonary lymphangiectasia, chemical pneumonitis resulting from recurrent aspiration, cystic fibrosis, and surfactant protein (SP)-B deficiency.[110]

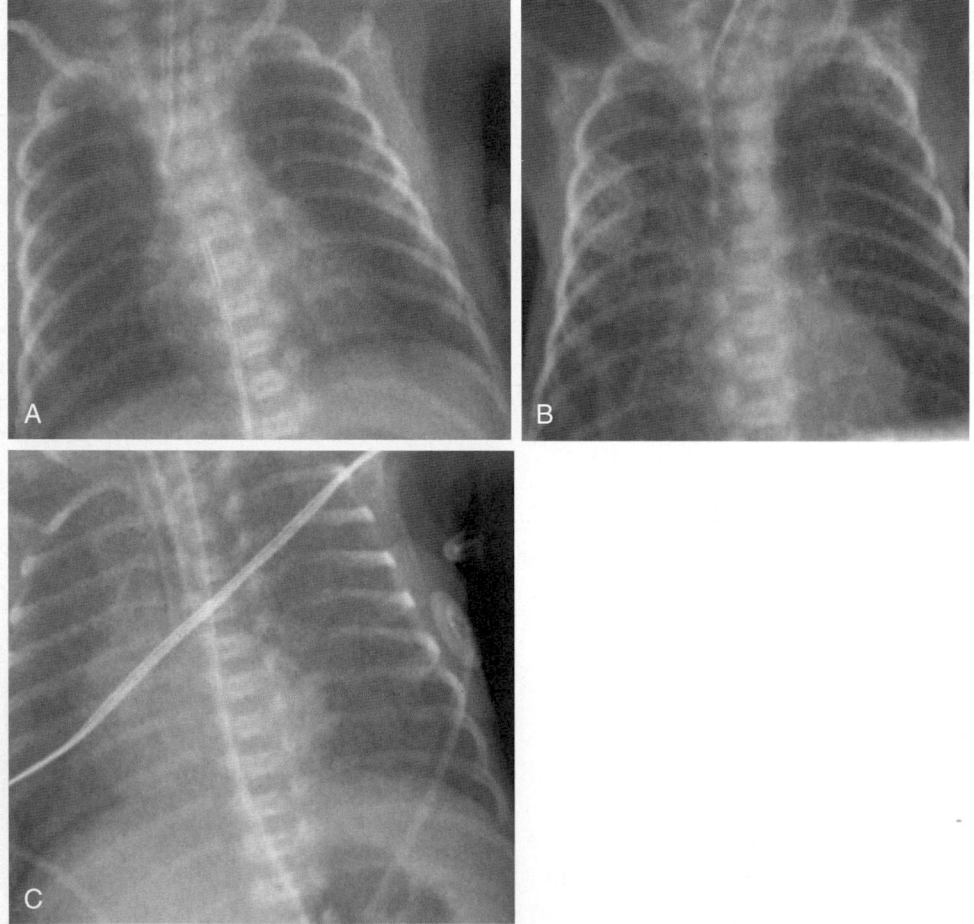

FIGURE 22-3   Chest radiographs of a preterm infant with *Ureaplasma* pneumonitis. **A,** Chest radiograph in the first day of life shows a mild ground-glass appearance consistent with respiratory distress syndrome (RDS). **B,** Chest radiograph at 2 weeks of age with early bronchopulmonary dysplasia (BPD) changes. **C,** Chest radiograph at 1 month of age showing progressive BPD with pulmonary edema or atelectasis. (From Viscardi RM: Prenatal and postnatal microbial colonization and respiratory outcome in preterm infants. In Bancalari E, editor. *The newborn lung: neonatology questions and controversies,* ed 2. Philadelphia: Saunders, 2012.)

Prevention

The cornerstone of management of BPD is prevention by avoiding, as much as possible, factors that predispose to injury.

Lung-Protective Ventilator Strategies

Because of lung immaturity from preterm birth, the majority of premature infants require respiratory assistance to sustain life. As discussed previously, respiratory support can be damaging to the preterm lung, so the therapeutic goal is to provide this lifesaving respiratory support without further compromising the already vulnerable premature lung.

Gentle ventilation is a descriptive term for respiratory support for preterm infants using a low V_T strategy to decrease lung injury, with the acceptance of higher values for $Paco_2$, called **permissive hypercapnia.**[111]

In an attempt to avoid mechanical ventilation via an ETT, newer studies have explored the use of nasal intermittent positive-pressure ventilation (NIPPV) as the primary modality of respiratory support.[112] Several other possible protective modalities of mechanical ventilation have been suggested, including proportional assist ventilation,[113] volume-controlled ventilation,[114] and the addition of pressure-supported ventilation to SIMV,[115] and volume-targeted ventilation.[116] HFV, another approach to potentially limit volutrauma, was not found to be consistently protective in preventing or decreasing BPD.[117]

Oxygen Therapy

Observational studies have shown that those NICUs that set goals of lower oxygen saturation levels for premature infants requiring oxygen therapy had fewer cases of BPD than those using higher oxygen saturation levels.[118]

The SUPPORT study was the only study with an early intervention, comparing target oxygen saturations of 91% to 95% and 85% to 89% within the first 2 hours of life in 1316 infants born at 24 to 28 weeks of gestation. BPD was reduced in the lower oxygen saturation group.[119]

The ability to maintain oxygen saturations within a tightly prescribed range was difficult. Therefore it is likely that tools such as automated regulation of inspired oxygen using a "closed loop" system could potentially improve oxygen stability and perhaps become the standard of clinical care of premature infants.[120]

Antioxidants

Investigators have explored whether exogenous administration of antioxidants could have positive effects on BPD prevention and treatment. Animal studies have found a lung-protective effect of exogenously administered antioxidant enzymes, but human studies have yielded less promising results.[121]

Inhaled Nitric Oxide

Inhaled nitric oxide (iNO) was originally used in critically ill infants to produce vasodilatation in the treatment of PPHN. Since its original clinical application, NO has been extensively investigated in animal models of lung immaturity and lung injury; it has been found to diminish lung inflammation, to reduce lung neutrophil infiltration, and, perhaps more importantly, to enhance lung growth and alveolar development. As a result of these promising experimental findings, investigators have questioned whether iNO might play a role in treating or protecting against BPD.[122]

Nutrition

Early and rigorous provision of adequate calories and protein to premature infants might potentially improve antioxidant capacity and decrease risk for BPD.[123]

Whereas evidence in newborn experimental animals showed protection against oxygen toxicity with increases in both polyunsaturated fatty acid (PUFA) lipid intake and PUFA content of lung lipid,[124] multiple randomized controlled clinical trials in human prematures were unable to affect BPD with early provision of high-PUFA intake in the form of intravenous lipid.[125]

The NICHD Neonatal Research Network trial conducted by Tyson et al.[126] reported a significant reduction in death and BPD in vitamin A–supplemented infants. Moreover, Howlett et al.[127] demonstrated a significant reduction in death and BPD in infants who had received inositol.

Corticosteroids

The anti-inflammatory properties of steroids include inhibition of prostaglandins, leukotrienes, and cyclooxygenases I and II; decrease of neutrophil recruitment in the lung; reduction in vascular permeability; and improvement of pulmonary edema. These properties make their use an effective postnatal strategy to reduce the risk and the severity of BPD.[128]

Methylxanthines

Methylxanthines work as phosphodiesterase inhibitors and play an important role in regulating intracellular levels of second messengers cyclic adenosine monophosphate (cAMP) and cyclic guanosine monophosphate (cGMP), and they may have anti-inflammatory properties as well.[129]

The Caffeine for Apnea of Prematurity (CAP) trial revealed a significant decrease in BPD in infants who received caffeine.[130]

Future Therapies

Pentoxifylline. Pentoxifylline is a methylxanthine that works as a phosphodiesterase inhibitor. Lauterbach et al.[131] reported a significant decrease in the incidence of BPD by day 4 of life after administration of inhaled pentoxifylline in VLBW infants.

Mesenchymal Stem Cells. Bone marrow–derived multipotent mesenchymal stem cells (MSCs) have been found to be efficacious in experimental models of lung injury.[132]

Treatment

The goals of treatment during the NICU course are to minimize further lung injury (e.g., barotrauma and volutrauma, oxygen toxicity, inflammation), maximize nutrition, and diminish oxygen consumption. The big challenge is that the supplemental oxygen and mechanical ventilation needed to maintain gas exchange are the same factors implicated in the pathogenesis of the lung damage.

Optimal care of infants with BPD should be given by a multidisciplinary team, including representatives from neonatology, pulmonology, respiratory therapy, nutrition, occupational therapy, speech therapy, physical therapy, social work, pharmacy, discharge planning, and other services.

Oxygenation

Supplemental oxygen remains a mainstay of therapy for infants with BPD, yet the most appropriate target for oxygen saturation levels remains controversial. Growing concerns regarding the adverse effects of even moderate levels of oxygen therapy have led many neonatologists to accept oxygen saturations below 85% to 90% early after birth of preterm newborns. However, it should also be kept in mind that patients with severe BPD are usually more than 36 weeks postmenstrual age past the time when ROP is a major concern. Currently, most pulmonologists recommend maintaining infants with established BPD at oxygen saturations around 92%, with slightly higher levels (92% to 95%) for infants with BPD and growth failure, recurrent respiratory exacerbations, or PPHN.[133]

Mechanical Ventilation

In most NICUs, NCPAP or high-flow nasal cannula therapy is used to maintain adequate oxygenation and ventilation while avoiding the need for prolonged ventilation or reintubation for ventilator support.[133]

When mechanical ventilation is used, the lowest PIP necessary to obtain adequate ventilation must be applied, using Ti between 0.3 and 0.5 seconds. Shorter Ti and higher flow rates can exaggerate the maldistribution of the inspired gas, and longer Ti can increase the risk of alveolar rupture and cardiovascular side effects. PEEP between 4 and 6 cm H_2O is applied so that the minimum oxygen concentration necessary to keep the PaO_2 above 50 mm Hg is used. In infants with severe airway obstruction, especially those with bronchomalacia, the use of PEEP levels of 5 to 8 cm H_2O can help reduce expiratory airway resistance and improve alveolar ventilation. The duration of mechanical ventilation must be limited as much as possible to reduce the risk of mechanical trauma and infection.

Weaning these patients from the ventilator is difficult and has to be accomplished gradually. When the patient can maintain an acceptable PaO_2 and $PaCO_2$ with low PIP (lower than 15 to 18 cm H_2O) and an FIO_2 lower than 0.3 to 0.4, the ventilator rate is gradually reduced to allow the infant to perform an increasing proportion of the respiratory work. During the process of weaning, it may be necessary to increase the FIO_2. Concurrently, the $PaCO_2$ can rise to values in the 50s or 60s mm Hg. As long as the pH is within acceptable limits, this degree of hypercapnia must be tolerated to wean the patient from the ventilator. In small infants, aminophylline or caffeine can be used as a respiratory stimulant during the weaning phase. When the patient is able to maintain acceptable blood gas levels for several hours on low ventilator rates (10 to 15 breaths per minute), extubation should be attempted.

During the days after the extubation, physiotherapy and increasing the FIO_2 should be the first-line treatments for worsening blood gases, which usually will be because of atelectasis associated with secretions. In smaller infants, the use of nasal CPAP after extubation can stabilize respiratory function and reduce the need to reinstitute mechanical ventilation.[64]

In contrast to an approach to acute RDS using a low VT and high PEEP to minimize acute lung injury, most clinicians favor a strategy of larger VT delivered at slower rates with longer inspiratory and expiratory times in severe BPD (Table 22-5). This strategy is directly related to the striking

TABLE 22-5

Ventilator Strategies in Bronchopulmonary Dysplasia

Early (prevention)	Strategies to prevent acute lung injury:
	  1. Low VT (5-8 mL/kg)
	  2. Short inspiratory times
	  3. Increased PEEP as needed for lung recruitment without overdistention (as reflected by high peak airway pressures)
	  4. Achieve lower FIO_2
	Goals for gas exchange:
	  1. Adjust FIO_2 to target lower O_2 saturations (88%-92%)
	  2. Permissive hypercapnia

Late (established BPD)	Strategies for effective gas exchange:
	  1. Marked regional heterogeneity:
	    · Larger VT (10-12 mL/kg)
	    · Longer inspiratory time ($\geq$0.6 sec)
	  2. Airways obstruction:
	    · Slower rates allow better emptying, especially with larger VT
	    · Complex roles for PEEP with dynamic airway collapse
	  3. Interactive effects of vent strategies:
	    · Changes in rate, VT, inspiratory and expiratory times, and pressure support are highly interdependent
	    · Overdistention can increase agitation and paradoxically worsen ventilation
	  4. Permissive hypercapnia to facilitate weaning

From Abman SH, Nelin LD. Management of infants with severe bronchopulmonary dysplasia. In Bancalari E, editor. *The newborn lung: neonatology questions and controversies*, ed 2. Philadelphia: Elsevier Saunders, 2012.

differences in lung physiology that characterize newborns with acute respiratory failure compared with infants with severe BPD. Dramatic heterogeneity of lung disease, characterized by marked regional variability in time constants, provides the physiological rationale for this strategy in severe BPD, to improve the distribution of ventilation, minimize physiological dead space and gas trapping, and improve gas exchange.[133]

Fluid Management

Infants with BPD tolerate excessive or even normal amounts of fluid intake poorly and, as mentioned earlier, have a marked tendency to accumulate excessive interstitial fluid in the lung. This excess can lead to a deterioration of their pulmonary function, with exaggeration of hypoxemia and hypercapnia and longer ventilator dependency.

To reduce lung fluid in infants with BPD, water and salt intake should be limited to the minimum required to provide the calories necessary for metabolic needs and growth. When increased lung water persists despite fluid restriction, diuretic therapy can be used successfully. Because increased metabolic demands in infants with BPD are associated, in severe cases, with low PaO_2, it is important to maintain a relatively normal blood hemoglobin concentration. This may be accomplished with blood transfusions or by the administration of recombinant erythropoietin.[74]

Drug Therapies

Diuretics. Diuretics improve pulmonary compliance and airway resistance by reducing lung edema. Aerosolized furosemide can acutely improve lung mechanics, but data are lacking regarding its long-term use.[134] The use of alternate-day furosemide may sustain improvements in lung function while minimizing risks for electrolyte imbalance and nephrocalcinosis.[135]

Bronchodilators. Infants with BPD have airway smooth muscle hypertrophy and often have signs of bronchial hyperreactivity that acutely improves with bronchodilator therapy, but response rates are variable.[136]

Aminophylline and caffeine can reduce airway resistance in infants with BPD and may have an additive effect with diuretics. Methylxanthines can improve weaning of infants from mechanical ventilation.[129]

Steroids. Corticosteroid therapy, directed primarily at reducing lung inflammation, is one of the most controversial areas of BPD care.[137] Steroid bursts (e.g., methylprednisolone 1 mg/kg q6h for 2 days, then 1 mg/kg q12h for 2 days, then 1 mg/kg/day for 2 days) may be helpful in the management of infants with severe BPD and acute deteriorations of lung function.[138]

Numerous side effects of steroid therapy have been reported. These include sepsis, NEC, hyperglycemia, hypertension, diabetic ketoacidosis, hypertrophic cardiomyopathy and greater weight loss. Of particular concern is the evidence that prolonged treatment with systemic dexamethasone is associated with increased risk of periventricular leukomalacia and long-term neurological deficits such as cerebral palsy.[139] Thus the use of systemic corticosteroids to prevent BPD early in the course of care of preterm infants is currently discouraged by the American Academy of Pediatrics.[140]

Antireflux Measures. The contribution of gastroesophageal reflux (GER) to severe BPD remains controversial. Patients with severe BPD should be evaluated for GER with radiological studies (barium swallow studies, upper gastrointestinal series), pH or impedance probes, or swallow studies. Many clinicians would also consider gastrostomy and fundoplication in the setting of severe BPD that is failing to improve if clinical suspicion remains high even though results of studies for GER are negative. These findings suggest that medical treatment of GER may improve symptoms in patients with BPD.[141]

Pulmonary Vasodilators. Patients with severe BPD are at high risk for development of PPHN and cor pulmonale. Therefore screening echocardiograms should be performed in patients with severe BPD.

Current therapies used for PPHN therapy in infants with BPD generally include iNO, sildenafil, and endothelin receptor antagonists.[122]

Nutrition

Optimizing both enteral and parenteral nutrition is essential to growth and recovery of preterm infants with BPD. Beginning parenteral nutrition in the first days after birth, as well as the use of aggressive feeding regimens, is crucial to success in these infants.

High-calorie formulas and supplements of protein, calcium, phosphorus, and zinc can be used to maximize the intake of calories while restricting fluid intake to prevent congestive heart failure and pulmonary edema. If for any reason enteral nutrition is precluded for more than 3 or 4 days, parenteral alimentation with glucose, amino acids, and fat should be substituted until the gastrointestinal tract again becomes functional.

Adequacy of nutrition should be closely monitored, and growth charts for weight, head circumference, and height must be kept. Other means of assessment include arm anthropometry to determine muscle mass and fat deposits and measurement of serum levels of albumin. Rib fractures noted on routine CXR together with generalized bone demineralization are often observed in infants with BPD and are usually a manifestation of osteopenia of prematurity.[74]

Social Issues

Dealing with a chronic childhood illness can be frustrating for any parent. Parents must be given all the facts of their baby's status and as much emotional support as possible. Notice must be taken of those parents who might tend toward child abuse.[142]

Outcome

Mortality

The mortality rate among infants with BPD who are discharged on therapy from the hospital is roughly 10%. It reached up to 38% among children with BPD and PPHN.[143]

Long-Term Morbidity

Pulmonary Complications. Tachypnea, retractions, dyspnea, cough, and wheezing can be seen for months to years in seriously affected children. Although complete clinical recovery can occur, underlying pulmonary function, gas exchange, and radiographic abnormalities may persist beyond adolescence. The impact of persistent minor abnormalities of function and growth on long-term morbidity and mortality is not known. Reactive airway disease occurs more often, and infants with BPD are at increased risk for bronchiolitis and pneumonia. The rehospitalization rate for respiratory illness during the first 2 years of life is approximately twice that of matched control infants.[144,145]

Airway problems, such as tonsillar and adenoidal hypertrophy, vocal cord paralysis, subglottic stenosis, and tracheomalacia, are common and may aggravate or cause pulmonary hypertension. Subglottic stenosis may require tracheotomy or an anterior cricoid split procedure to relieve upper airway obstruction.

Cardiac Complications. Cardiac complications include pulmonary hypertension, cor pulmonale, systemic hypertension, left ventricular hypertrophy, and the development of aortopulmonary collateral vessels, which, if large, may cause heart failure.[143,146]

Neurodevelopmental Delays and Neurological Deficits. Delays in development have been reported to be common, with poor developmental outcome correlating positively with prolonged hospitalization and requirement for oxygen in babies with severe BPD. Among children without severe gross motor delays, risk factors for BPD accounted for the association of BPD and developmental delay.[147]

Other Complications. Other complications include growth failure, psychomotor retardation, and parental stress, as well as sequelae of therapy such as nephrolithiasis, osteopenia, and electrolyte imbalance.[148]

TRANSIENT TACHYPNEA OF THE NEWBORN

Incidence

Transient tachypnea of the newborn (TTN) is a relatively benign, typically self-limited disease, first described by Avery and colleagues in 1966.[149] It is also known as RDS type II, wet lung syndrome, or persistent postnatal pulmonary edema. It occurs in approximately 4 to 5.7 per 1000 infants delivered between 37 and 42 weeks of gestation. It is more common after elective cesarean section delivery without labor.[150] Although TTN does appear in infants born prematurely, it occurs more commonly in term infants.

Pathophysiology and Risk Factors

Early theories of lung fluid clearance focused on the role of thoracic compression during vaginal delivery and were supported by the observation that TTN is more common among babies born by elective cesarean section.[151] Current attention has focused on the roles of catecholamines, glucocorticoids, and thyroid hormones in bringing about a permanent change in the lung epithelium phenotype and causing the lung epithelia to switch from lung fluid secretion to absorption.[152] Because resorption of fetal lung fluid is a catecholamine-dependent process, Aslan et al. investigated genetic polymorphisms in β-adrenergic receptor encoding genes and concluded that it is more common in babies with TTN.[153]

Delayed cord clamping or cord milking, is also associated with TTN. This could be explained by the increased placental-fetal transfusion, which might lead to an elevation in the infant's central venous pressure, disrupting lung fluid clearance by the thoracic duct or pulmonary lymphatics, Additional risk factors include male gender and birth to a mother with asthma. The mechanism underlying the gender-associated risk and the increase associated with maternal asthma is unclear, although there is speculation that these infants have an altered sensitivity to catecholamines that may play a role in the delayed clearance of lung fluid.[154]

Macrosomia and multiple gestations also increase the risk of TTN. The associations between TTN and other obstetric factors, such as excessive maternal sedation, prolonged labor, and large amounts of intravenous fluids given to the mother, have been less consistent.

Clinical Presentation and Diagnosis

A term or near-term infant with TTN typically presents with tachypnea (60 to 150 breaths per minute), cyanosis, grunting, retractions, and nasal flaring within the first few hours after birth. ABG analysis reveals mild to moderate hypoxemia, hypercapnia, and respiratory acidosis. CXR may show pulmonary vascular congestion, prominent perihilar streaking, fluid in the interlobular fissures, hyperexpansion, and a flat diaphragm (Figure 22-4). Mild cardiomegaly and pleural effusions may also be present.

Differential Diagnosis

Because TTN is similar in its initial presentation to conditions such as RDS, group B streptococcal pneumonia, and PPHN, TTN is often a diagnosis of exclusion; after these disorders have been ruled out.[155]

TTN also must be distinguished from the clinical syndrome of cerebral hyperventilation. This usually is seen in term infants with a history of birth asphyxia. The infants are

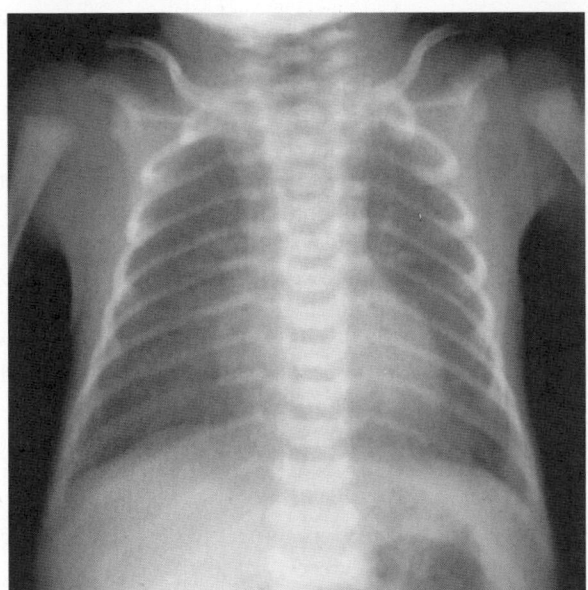

FIGURE 22-4 Transient tachypnea of the newborn with overinflated lungs and increased interstitial streaky markings. (From Arthur R. The neonatal chest x-ray. *Paediatr Respir Rev* 2001;2:311.)

tachypneic without radiographic changes apart from occasional asphyxia-related cardiomegaly. Respiratory alkalosis is typical and is probably the result of respiratory center irritation, although it could be a component of postasphyxial pulmonary edema.[1]

Treatment

Treatment is largely supportive. The objectives of treatment of TTN are to maintain adequate oxygenation and ventilation.[149] Supplemental oxygen via oxygen hood (FIO_2 usually less than 40%) is indicated when signs of respiratory distress are present.[156] CPAP levels of 3 to 5 cm H_2O may be needed when higher FIO_2 levels are required.

Infants with sustained respiratory rates greater than 60 breaths per minute should not be fed orally; therefore, these infants should be maintained either with gavage feedings for respiratory rates between 60 and 80 or nil per os (NPO) with intravenous fluids for more severe tachypnea.[155]

Most infants are initially treated with broad-spectrum antibiotics until the diagnosis of sepsis or pneumonia is excluded. A controlled trial of furosemide administration to accelerate clearance of lung fluid showed no benefit in attenuating the course of TTN.[157]

Complications and Prognosis

The condition is self-limited. The distress, hypoxemia, and mild respiratory acidosis usually resolve within 12 to 24 hours, with the infant frequently breathing room air by 48 hours of age.

Complications are rare, though air leaks may occur, particularly if the baby has required CPAP or IPPV.

NEONATAL PNEUMONIA

Incidence

An estimated 800,000 deaths occur worldwide from respiratory infections in newborn infants.[158] Pneumonia occurs in more than 10% of the infants in a NICU, with premature infants affected more often than term infants. By contrast, at autopsy the incidence of neonatal pneumonia ranges from 20% to 32% of live-born infants and from 15% to 38% of stillborn infants, although the pathological features of inflammation of the lung may not always result from infection.[159] Certain groups of mothers seem to have a higher incidence of infection, including those of lower socioeconomic status, teenagers, and sexually active mothers.

Etiology and Pathophysiology
Causative Organisms

Organisms responsible for infectious pneumonia typically mirror those responsible for early-onset neonatal sepsis. Group B *Streptococcus* (GBS) was the most common bacterial isolate in most locales from the late 1960s to the late 1990s, when the impact of intrapartum chemoprophylaxis in reducing neonatal and maternal infection by this organism became evident. Despite the decreased frequency, GBS remains a common isolate in early-onset (age younger than 3 days) infections in term and near-term infants. Since that time, *Escherichia coli* has become the most common bacterial isolate among VLBW infants.[160] Early-onset pneumonia from GBS may progress rapidly to shock or death, and mortality is high (20% to 50%) regardless of treatment. When the onset of GBS disease is later (2 to 3 weeks after birth), the infant may present with meningitis rather than pneumonia, the pathogen is usually a different strain of the organism, and there is a more optimistic prognosis.[161]

Other bacteria that should be considered when pneumonia is acquired in utero or in the immediate perinatal period include *Klebsiella* spp, group D *streptococci*, *Listeria monocytogenes*, and *Pneumococci*. When neonatal pneumonia develops several days or even weeks after birth, in addition to these organisms, infections from *Staphylococcus* and *Pseudomonas* organisms and Fungi should be considered. Although infection with *Chlamydia trachomatis* does appear to be acquired during parturition, pneumonia caused by this organism typically has a gradual onset of respiratory symptoms beyond 3 weeks of postnatal life.[162] *Ureaplasma urealyticum* is a known cause of maternal chorioamnionitis. This organism has been isolated from the upper and lower respiratory tract of infants with acute respiratory failure or BPD and can contribute to the etiology of these disorders.[163]

Viral pneumonia can be acquired by the fetus from transplacental passage of organisms, as may be the case in the congenital intrauterine infections (TORCH syndrome: *t*oxoplasmosis, *r*ubella, *c*ytomegalovirus, *h*erpes simplex virus). Viruses probably also account for a substantial number of postnatally acquired pneumonias. Viral pneumonia is not usually recognized as such in the neonate, although epidemics resulting from respiratory syncytial virus infection and adenovirus have been associated with significant morbidity and mortality.[164]

Bacterial, viral, and fungal pneumonias of later onset are a cause of considerable morbidity in NICUs, and the risk of a subsequent fatal outcome is small but inversely proportional to birth weight.[162]

Modes of Transmission

Intrauterine (Transplacental). Intrauterine infection is a result of clinical or subclinical maternal infection with a variety of agents (cytomegalovirus [CMV], *Treponema pallidum, Toxoplasma gondii*, rubella virus, varicella virus, parvovirus B19) and hematogenous transplacental transmission to the fetus. Transplacental infection may occur at any time during gestation, with signs and symptoms present at birth or may be delayed for months or years.[161]

Ascending Vertical Transmission. Most pneumonias seen in the newborn are a result of ascending infection from the genital tract before or during labor. The infant can contract pneumonia through contaminated amniotic fluid, which may be aspirated, or by extended exposure to bacteria that may be in the vaginal tract. This type of transmission of bacteria is a result of heavy colonization of the maternal genitourinary tract. Prolonged rupture of membranes greater than 18 hours before delivery creates a significant chance of the infant's contracting bacteria and is thought to be one of the greatest predisposing factors to neonatal pneumonia,[162] although it is possible that bacteria such as GBS could gain access to the fetus by ascent through intact membranes.[1]

Postnatal (Nosocomial or Community Acquired). After birth, neonates are exposed to infectious agents in the nursery or in the community. Postnatal infections, also known as horizontal transmission, may be transmitted by direct contact with hospital personnel, the mother, or other family members; from breast milk (HIV, CMV); or from inanimate sources such as contaminated equipment. Some of the organisms responsible for postnatal pneumonia are airborne, whereas others are spread by contact.[165]

The most common source of postnatal infections in hospitalized newborns is hand contamination of health care personnel.[161] In the treatment of neonates, certain invasive lines (e.g., umbilical catheters, intravenous lines) as well as intubation and respiratory equipment can be avenues for infection. Cross-contamination of bacteria or viruses within the hospital setting is unfortunately a risk with the neonatal patient, especially if there is a large patient-to-caregiver ratio.

Risk Factors

The most important neonatal factors predisposing to infection is prematurity and **low birth weight** (LBW; weighing less than 2500 g). Preterm LBW infants have a 3- to 10-fold higher incidence of infection than full-term, normal-birth-weight infants.[1]

Other risk factors include the following:
· Premature, PROM (more than 18 hours)
· Maternal peripartum fever (38° C/100.4° F) or infection, chorioamnionitis, urinary tract infection (UTI), previous delivery of a neonate with GBS disease
· Perineal colonization with GBS or E. coli
· Amniotic fluid problems; meconium-stained or foul-smelling, cloudy amniotic fluid
· Resuscitation at birth—infants who had fetal distress, were born by traumatic delivery, or were severely depressed at birth and required intubation and resuscitation
· Multiple gestation
· Invasive procedures— invasive monitoring, and respiratory or metabolic support
· Infants with galactosemia (predisposition to E. coli infection), immune defects, or asplenia
· Iron therapy (iron added to serum in vitro enhances the growth of many organisms)

In addition, males are four times more affected than females, and the possibility of a sex-linked genetic basis for host susceptibility is postulated. Variations in immune function may play a role. Neonatal infection is more common in African-American infants than in Caucasian infants, but this may be explained by a higher incidence of PROM, maternal fever, and LBW. Low socioeconomic status is often reported as an additional risk factor, but again this may be explained by LBW. NICU staff and family members are often vectors for the spread of microorganisms, primarily as a result of improper hand washing.[166]

Clinical Presentation and Diagnosis

Early-onset infections are acquired before or during delivery and present before the first week of life; usually less than 72 hours. Late-onset infections develop after the first week of life from organisms acquired in the hospital or the community. The age at onset depends on the timing of exposure and virulence of the infecting organism. The infant may have a history of fetal tachycardia with low Apgar scores and often requires some type of supplemental oxygen or even resuscitation at birth. Very-late-onset infections (onset after 1 month of life) may also occur, particularly in VLBW preterm infants or in term infants requiring prolonged neonatal intensive care.

The nonspecific nature of the clinical signs that are characteristic of neonatal infections makes a high index of suspicion the key to early diagnosis.[1] Early signs and symptoms of pneumonia may be nonspecific; they include poor feeding, lethargy, irritability, cyanosis, temperature instability, and the overall impression that the infant is not well. Respiratory symptoms include grunting, tachypnea, retractions, flaring of the alae nasi, cyanosis, apnea, and progressive respiratory failure. If the infant is premature, signs of progressive respiratory distress may be superimposed upon RDS or BPD. For infants on mechanical ventilation, need for increased ventilating support may indicate infection. Signs of pneumonia on physical examination, such as dullness to percussion, change in breath sounds, and the presence of rales or rhonchi, are very difficult to appreciate in a neonate.[165]

Several factors should alert the health care provider to the possibility of neonatal pneumonia—namely, a history of maternal infection or fever, toxemia, premature labor, PROM, malodorous or stained amniotic fluid, lesions of the vagina or placenta, and frequent digital examinations of the cervix.[61]

Anytime neonatal pneumonia is suspected, appropriate laboratory diagnostic tests should be performed, such as complete blood cell count (CBC), C-reactive protein (CRP), and cultures of blood, urine, and cerebrospinal fluid along with tracheal or gastric aspirates that provide evidence of infection. These test results can help in making a definitive diagnosis of pneumonia.[165]

CXR may show a diffuse granular pattern with widespread bilateral involvement, especially if the infant acquired the infection in utero. If aspiration of contaminated amniotic fluid has occurred, CXR may appear as an aspiration pneumonitis with patchy infiltrates. When an infection is acquired postnatally, the radiographic findings often change from normal to severely abnormal over the first few days. Depending on the severity of the disease process and the causative organism, pleural effusions, pulmonary edema, pneumatoceles, cardiomegaly, and evidence of barotrauma may be seen (Figure 22-5).

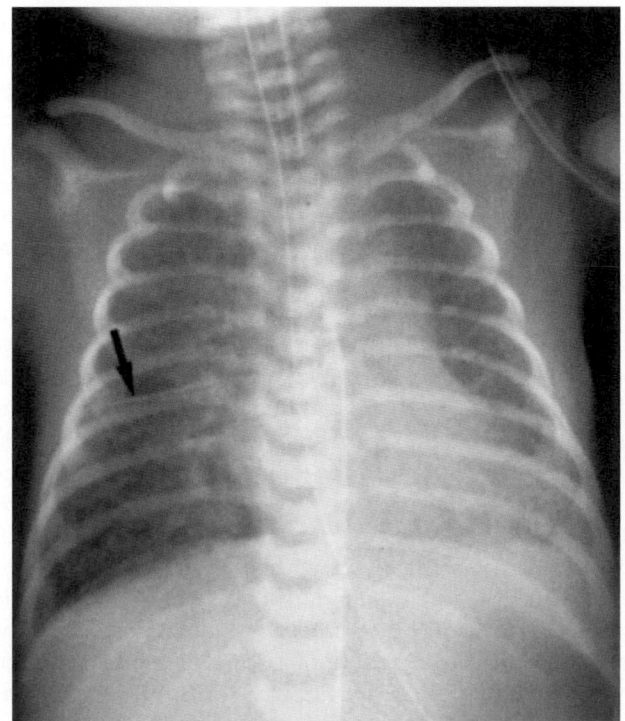

FIGURE 22-5 Group B streptococcal pneumonia. Widespread interstitial shadowing with more confluent alveolar consolidation at the left bases and fluid in the horizontal fissure (*arrow*). (From Arthur R. The neonatal chest x-ray. *Paediatr Respir Rev* 2001;2:311.)

ABG values reveal hypoxemia that is refractory to oxygen therapy and hypercapnia that responds poorly to ventilatory support. Metabolic acidosis may develop as infection becomes more severe.[165]

Prevention

Maternal immunization protects the mother against vaccine-preventable diseases that can cause intrauterine infections (rubella, hepatitis B, varicella) and may also protect the infant via passive transfer of protective maternal antibodies (tetanus). Toxoplasmosis is preventable with appropriate diet and avoidance of exposure to cat feces. Malaria during pregnancy can be minimized with chemoprophylaxis and use of insecticide-treated bed nets. Congenital syphilis is preventable by timely diagnosis and appropriate early treatment of infected pregnant women.

Aggressive management of suspected maternal chorioamnionitis with antibiotic therapy during labor, along with rapid delivery of the infant, reduces the risk of early-onset neonatal sepsis. Vertical transmission of GBS is significantly reduced by selective intrapartum chemoprophylaxis. Neonatal infection with *Chlamydia* can be prevented by identification and treatment of infected pregnant women. Mother-to-child transmission of HIV is significantly reduced by maternal antiretroviral therapy during pregnancy, labor, and delivery, cesarean section delivery before rupture of membranes, and antiretroviral treatment of the infant after birth.[165]

Prevention of Nosocomial Infection

Principles for the prevention of nosocomial infection include adherence to universal precautions with all patients' contacts, avoiding nursery crowding and limiting nurse-to-patient ratios, strict compliance with hand washing, meticulous neonatal skin care, minimizing the risk of catheter contamination, decreasing the number of venipunctures and heelsticks, reducing the duration of catheter and mechanical ventilation days, encouraging appropriate advancement of enteral feedings, providing education and feedback to nursery personnel, and ongoing monitoring and surveillance of nosocomial infection rates in the NICU (Box 22-3).

Treatment

The normal course of treatment in neonatal pneumonia is multifaceted and includes appropriate antibiotic or antiviral therapy, oxygenation, adequate ventilation, and pharmacotherapy. To prevent rapid deterioration, early intervention, aggressive management, and continuous monitoring are required, especially in the infant with early-onset GBS disease.

Pharmacotherapy

Many physicians believe that PROM, or the onset of premature labor by itself, is often the first sign of infection and should be treated as such, with broad-spectrum antibiotic therapy instituted immediately. This has been

Box 22-3	**Principles for the Prevention of Nosocomial Infection in the Neonatal Intensive Care Unit**

Observe recommendations for universal precautions with all patient contact:
- Gloves
- Gowns, mask, and isolation as indicated

Nursery design engineering:
- Appropriate nursing/patient ratio
- Avoid overcrowding and excessive workload
- Readily accessible sinks, antiseptic solutions, soap, and paper towels

Handwashing:
- Improve handwashing compliance
- Wash hands before and after each patient encounter
- Appropriate use of soap, alcohol-based preparations, or antiseptic solutions
- Alcohol-based antiseptic solution at each patient bedside
- Provide emollients for nursery staff
- Education and feedback for nursery staff

Minimizing risk of CVC contamination:
- Maximal sterile barrier precautions during CVC insertion
- Local antisepsis with chlorhexidine gluconate
- Minimize repeated entry into the line for laboratory tests
- Aseptic technique when entering the line
- Minimize CVC days
- Sterile preparation of all fluids to be administered via a CVC

Meticulous skin care

Encourage early and appropriate advancement of enteral feeding

Education and feedback for nursery personnel

Continuous monitoring and surveillance of nosocomial infection rates in the neonatal intensive care unit

CVC, Central venous catheter.
From Adams-Chapman I, Stoll BJ: Prevention of nosocomial infections in the neonatal intensive care unit. *Curr Opin Pediatr* 2002;14:157-164.

shown to be effective in improving the outcome in certain disease processes, especially infection with GBS. Whenever neonatal pneumonia is suspected, broad-spectrum antibiotics are given for at least 72 hours, or until definitive culture results are obtained. If results prove that infection is present, antibiotics are continued for 14 to 21 days.[167]

Antiviral agents (e.g., ribavirin, acyclovir) may be administered in infants with pneumonia of viral origin. In the case of some viral pathogens that are congenitally transmitted, such as CMV and rubella, irreversible damage to the central nervous system (CNS) has already occurred and there is little therapy available to reverse it.

Adequate gas exchange depends not only on alveolar ventilation but also on perfusion and gas transport capacity of the alveolar perfusate (i.e., blood). Preservation of pulmonary and systemic perfusion is essential, using volume expanders, inotropes, afterload reduction, blood products, and other interventions (e.g., iNO) as needed.

Respiratory Support

Assurance of airway patency may be more challenging in neonates with pneumonia because of the often profuse, potentially obstructive secretions and mucopurulent exudates of variable viscosity. Judicious suctioning is warranted. Deep suctioning should be avoided because it can cause airway trauma and swelling, which in turn may cause large airway obstruction.

The infant with cyanosis, hypoxemia, and hypercapnia may require mechanical ventilation to maintain oxygenation. The most critically ill infants may need high ventilatory settings with high PIP, ventilatory rate, and oxygen levels. ABG values and transcutaneous monitors, or pulse oximetry, or both, are used to monitor the patient's respiratory status.[168]

Extracorporeal Membrane Oxygenation

Near-term and term infants who are unresponsive to conventional ventilation and other supportive measures may benefit from extracorporeal membrane oxygenation (ECMO).[169] Improved rates of survival have been reported in this group.

Complications and Prognosis

Morbidity and mortality associated with neonatal pneumonia depend on the causative organism and the ability to successfully treat the infant and keep complications to a minimum.

Careful management requires frequent assessment for signs of complications that may accompany prematurity, sepsis, and treatment interventions. These include the risk of IVH, air leaks, PPHN, and NEC, as well as the development of BPD if mechanical ventilation is required for extended periods. These infants can suffer significant neurological damage and developmental delay, or they may have totally normal capabilities. In some cases, however, the impairment may have occurred in utero and severe neurological problems or even death may be imminent.[170]

The key to treatment in these infants would seem to be early intervention and aggressive therapy; however, the progression of neonatal pneumonia can be variable. Fulminant infection is most commonly associated with pyogenic organisms such as GBS. Onset may occur during the first hours or days of life, with the infant often manifesting rapidly progressive circulatory collapse and respiratory failure. With early-onset pneumonia, the clinical course and CXR may be indistinguishable from those with severe RDS.

In contrast to the rapid progression of pneumonia caused by pyogenic organisms, an indolent course may be seen in nonbacterial infection. The onset can be preceded by upper respiratory tract symptoms or conjunctivitis. The infant may demonstrate a nonproductive cough, and the degree of respiratory compromise is variable. Fever is usually absent, and CXR shows focal or diffuse interstitial pneumonitis. Infection is generally caused by *Chlamydia trachomatis,* CMV, *Ureaplasma urealyticum,* or one of the respiratory viruses. Although *Pneumocystis carinii* was implicated in the original description of this syndrome, its etiological role is now in doubt, except in newborns infected with HIV.[165]

MECONIUM ASPIRATION SYNDROME

Definition

Meconium is the green-tinged bowel content of an infant, which is usually passed within 48 hours after delivery. The term was coined by Aristotle from the Greek words *meconium arion,* meaning "opiumlike," because he believed that the substance induced fetal sleep.[171] Meconium is a sterile substance that is composed of swallowed amniotic fluid, salts, mucus, bile, and other cellular debris. In and of itself, meconium is harmless; however, if in utero the infant passes meconium into the amniotic fluid, it may cause serious airway obstruction, air trapping, and enhanced growth of bacteria. Furthermore, contents of the meconium can compete with surfactant components for adsorption to the alveolar surface, and enzymes in meconium can break down certain surfactant components.[172] Thus it becomes a life-threatening entity that must be dealt with immediately.

Incidence

Despite changing strategies, meconium staining of the amniotic fluid (MSAF) happens in approximately 10% to 15% of childbirths with incidence ranging from 5% to 25%. Meconium aspiration syndrome (MAS) develops in approximately 4% to 10% of the infants born from an MSAF milieu. Of these neonates who develop MAS, one third require ventilatory support, 10% develop air leaks, and in spite of appropriate management strategies, 5% to 10% of them have a fatal outcome. Of the babies who suffer PPHN, 5% to 6% are related to MAS.[173]

Because meconium passage into the amniotic fluid requires strong peristalsis and anal sphincter tone, which is not common in preterm infants, MAS rarely occurs in infants of less than 36 weeks of gestational age.[174] The longer a pregnancy is allowed to continue past 42 weeks, the greater the chances are of the passage of meconium; it may occur in 35% or more of pregnancies 42 weeks of gestation or longer. Aspiration most commonly occurs in utero. Aspiration with the initial postnatal breaths appears to be decidedly less common. The thicker the MSAF consistency, the greater the likelihood of MAS. The more depressed a baby is (as reflected by the need for PPV or low Apgar scores), the greater the likelihood of MAS.[175]

Etiology and Pathophysiology

Fetal passage of meconium has long been accepted as a sign of intrauterine stress or hypoxia. Theoretically, the infant becomes hypoxic in utero (possibly because of cord or fetal head compression or prolonged labor), which exhausts oxygen reserves, causing a vagal response, relaxed anal sphincter tone, and passage of meconium into the amniotic fluid. The normal intrauterine activity of the neonate involves the movement of small amounts (1 to 5 ml) of amniotic fluid into and out of the upper airways. The potential of aspiration is always present, but chances are increased with hypoxia or stress because of greater respiratory effort and possibly gasping respirations in utero. Even more damaging is the aspiration that occurs after delivery of the chest when expansion allows the fluid or meconium, or both, to be dispersed even farther into the infant's lungs.[176]

After delivery, the normal pulmonary mechanisms are hindered and the clinical picture varies drastically. The amount and viscosity or dilution of the meconium present may significantly affect the degree of obstruction that occurs. If the infant has a large amount of thick meconium within the airways at the time of delivery, complete bronchiolar obstruction with subsequent alveolar collapse will result. The more typical picture, however, is that of smaller amounts of meconium within amniotic fluid, causing a ball-valve effect because of partial obstruction of the airways (Figure 22-6).

Inflammation of the airways and secretion production (a normal body response to a foreign substance within the lungs) also occur, and a chemical pneumonitis often develops.[177] Studies have also suggested that meconium hinders surfactant, which may lead to atelectasis and decreased pulmonary compliance.[172,177,178]

It has been suggested that intrauterine hypoxia not only stimulates the passage of meconium but also causes restructuring of the pulmonary vascular bed. The profound hypoxia may result in pulmonary vasoconstriction, which may be the reason that many infants with MAS quickly develop PPHN.[70] Figure 22-7 summarizes the pathophysiological events that occur with the passage of meconium and MAS.

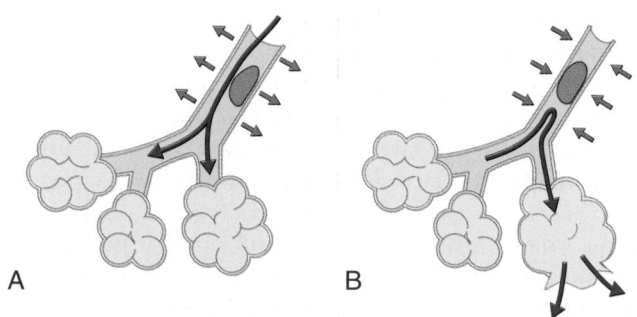

FIGURE 22-6 Air trapping behind particulate matter (i.e., meconium) in an airway, which leads to alveolar overexpansion and rupture. Tidal gas passes the meconium on inspiration when the airway dilates (**A**) but does not exit on expiration when the airways constrict (**B**). (From Harris TR, Herrick BR. *Pneumothorax in the newborn.* Biomedical Communications, Tucson: Arizona Health Sciences Center, 1978.)

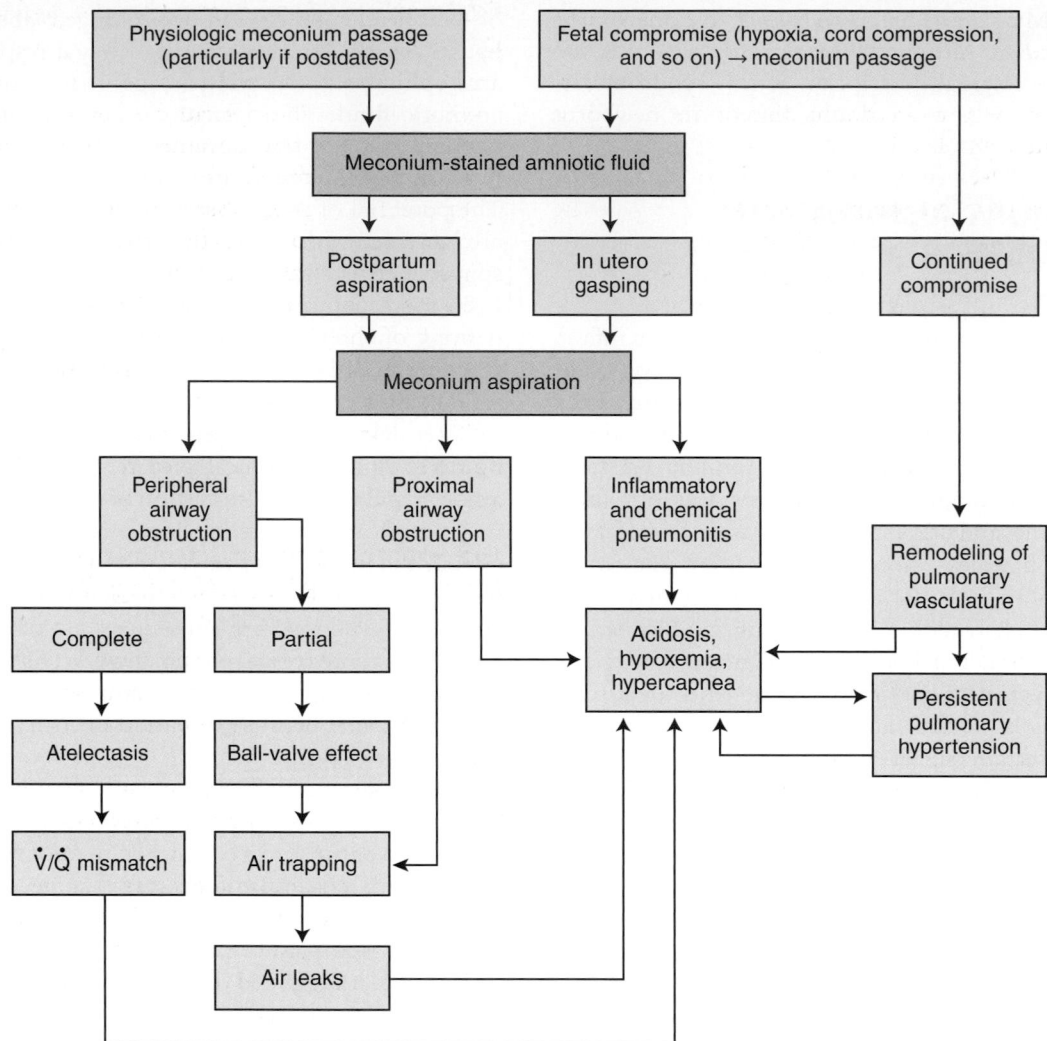

FIGURE 22-7 Pathophysiology of the meconium aspiration syndrome (MAS). (Redrawn from Wiswell TE, Bent RC. Meconium staining and the meconium aspiration syndrome. *Pediatr Clin North Am* 1993;40:957. Modified from Bacsik RD. Meconium aspiration system. *Pediatr Clin North Am* 1977;24:467.)

Clinical Presentation and Diagnosis

Clinical Presentation

The infant with MAS is usually a term or post-term infant who has been delivered through MSAF (often referred to as pea soup) and has already experienced significant intrauterine stress or hypoxia. The history may include prolonged labor, breech delivery, and ominous fetal heart rate monitor tracings such as late decelerations or nonvariability.

On completion of delivery, the physical examination often reveals a mature infant with yellowish skin, nails, and cord, as well as the postmature signs of peeling skin and long fingernails. The umbilical cord may lack or have very little Wharton's jelly. Depending on the extent of stress or hypoxia, the infant is depressed at birth, with low Apgar scores; however, some infants have 1-minute Apgar scores of 5 or more. The infant quickly exhibits signs of respiratory distress, including cyanosis, gasping respirations, grunting, retractions, nasal flaring, and tachypnea. The respiratory distress is often related to the viscosity of the meconium, with a thicker meconium causing more respiratory symptoms.[176] Auscultation of the chest reveals rales as well as areas of significantly diminished aeration, with the anteroposterior diameter of the chest often increased. The infant may or may not need immediate intervention, depending on the severity of the aspiration and the degree of hypoxia.

Investigations

ABG analysis indicates hypoxemia in infants with mild MAS having a normal pH and normal or decreased $Paco_2$ resulting from the increased respiratory effort. The infant may also have significant metabolic acidosis depending on the severity of the hypoxia before birth. The infant with moderate to severe MAS has increasing hypoxemia and hypercapnia. A combination of respiratory and metabolic acidosis eventually develops as the infant is unable to overcome the obstructive and inflammatory processes. This progresses to the point of respiratory failure and severe hypoxemia, alerting the physician to the probability of PPHN, which contributes substantially to morbidity.[179]

The CXR appearance varies according to the severity of the disease and complications. The typical CXR shows patchy areas of atelectasis caused by obstruction, as well as hyperexpansion from air trapping with flattening of the diaphragm sometimes noted on CXR. There is usually widespread involvement, with no particular area of the lungs being more affected (Figure 22-8). CXR of an infant with severe MAS may reveal total bilateral opacity with only large bronchi distinguishable. Pulmonary air leaks, including PIE, pneumothorax, and pneumomediastinum, may also be found. Cardiomegaly also might be detected, possibly as a manifestation of the underlying perinatal hypoxia. A normal CXR in an infant with severe hypoxemia and no cardiac malformation suggests the diagnosis of PPHN.[1]

Prevention
Amnioinfusion (Injection of Normal Saline into the Amniotic Sac)

In the past it was believed that by infusing fluid into the mother's uterus, the uterine fluid volume would either dilute the meconium or alleviate compression of the cord and prevent gasping. However, current evidence proves that aminoinfusion does not reduce the risk of MAS.[180]

Intrapartum Nasopharyngeal and Oropharyngeal Suctioning

Large, international, randomized, controlled trials proved that intrapartum nasopharyngeal and oropharyngeal suctioning does not reduce the incidence of MAS.[181]

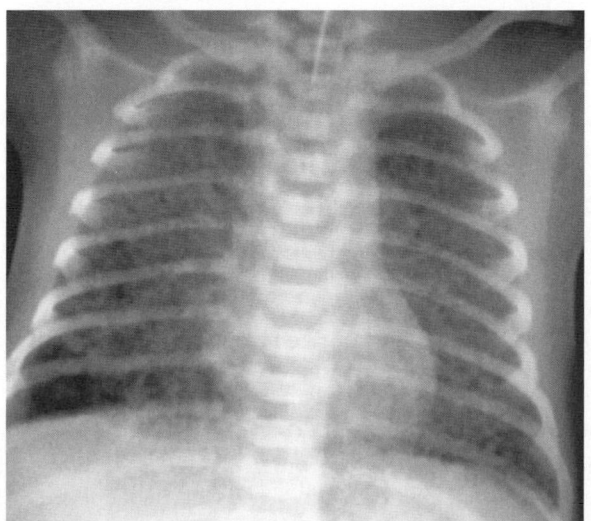

FIGURE 22-8 Meconium aspiration syndrome with heterogeneous pulmonary infiltrates in association with hyperinflated lungs. Note the area of focal hyperinflation in the right costophrenic angle. (From Arthur R. The neonatal chest x-ray. *Paediatr Respir Rev* 2001;2:311.)

Potentially Dangerous Maneuvers of No Proven Benefit

They include the following
- Cricoid pressure: application of pressure to the infant's airway to prevent intratracheal meconium from descending into the lungs
- Epiglottal blockage: insertion of 1 to 3 fingers into the child's airway to manually "close" the epiglottis over the glottis to prevent aspiration
- Thoracic compression: encircling the infant's chest and applying pressure in an attempt to prevent deep inspiration prior to endotracheal cleansing

None of these maneuvers has ever been scientifically validated and all are potentially dangerous (causing trauma, vagal stimulation, or induction of deep inhalation with chest recoil upon removing encircling hands).[182]

Endotracheal Intubation and Intratracheal Suctioning in the Delivery Room

The American Academy of Pediatrics Neonatal Resuscitation Program Steering Committee and the American Heart Association have developed guidelines for management of the baby exposed to meconium.[183] The guidelines are under continuous review and are revised as new evidence-based research becomes available. The current guidelines are as follows:
- If the baby is not vigorous (defined as depressed respiratory effort, poor muscle tone, and/or heart rate less than 100 beats per minute): Use direct laryngoscopy, intubate, and suction the trachea immediately after delivery. Suction for no longer than 5 seconds. If no meconium is retrieved, do not repeat intubation and suction. If meconium is retrieved and no bradycardia is present, reintubate and suction. If the heart rate is low, administer PPV and consider suctioning again later. Once the infant is intubated, the ETT should be used as a suction catheter with 80 to 100 cm H_2O negative pressure applied as the tube is withdrawn. Suction catheters inserted into the ETT are too small to aspirate thick meconium and may become clogged, delaying removal. More than one pass may be needed to clear the trachea of meconium. Saline lavage may be used to dilute the meconium while the infant continues to be intubated. All infants born with MSAF should be closely monitored.
- If the baby is vigorous (defined as normal respiratory effort, normal muscle tone, and heart rate greater than 100 beats per minute): Do not electively intubate. Clear secretions and meconium from the mouth and nose using a bulb syringe or a large-bore suction catheter.
- In both cases, the remainder of the initial resuscitation steps should ensue, including drying, stimulating, repositioning, and administering oxygen as necessary.

Gastric Suctioning

Theoretically, postnatal suctioning of the gastric contents in meconium-stained infants could prevent postnatal reflux or emesis and frank aspiration of MSAF, though routine gastric lavage before feeding did not decrease the incidence of MAS in babies born through MSAF.[184]

Treatment

Supplemental Oxygen Therapy

The goal is to maintain acceptable systemic oxygenation. Generally, this consists of sustaining peripheral oxygen saturation between 92% and 97% or PaO_2 between 60 and 80 mm Hg. Because of the potential for gas trapping and air leaks, some advocate increasing FIO_2 to 1.0 before implementing more aggressive therapy (CPAP, mechanical ventilation, etc.). Typically, however, once FIO_2 requirements exceed 0.60, more aggressive therapy is indicated.

Oxygen is also a pulmonary vasodilator. Because aberrant pulmonary vasoconstriction often accompanies MAS, clinicians often attempt to maintain higher than usual oxygenation early in the course of the disorder (saturation between 98% and 100% or PaO_2 between 100 and 120 mm Hg or even higher).[185]

Mechanical Ventilation

In spite of early intervention with thorough suctioning, some infants will still acquire MAS. The infant who presents with MSAF and progresses to a state of worsening respiratory distress and hypoxemia should be intubated and mechanically ventilated. This infant is a management challenge.

Typically, conventional mechanical ventilation is provided with pressure-limited mechanical ventilators. Some clinicians avoid volume-targeted ventilators because of an unsubstantiated fear of air leaks. Others avoid pressure control because of high flow rates and the propensity for gas trapping.

Multiple strategies have been advocated, including use of ventilatory settings that will maintain arterial blood gases within normal ranges; hyperventilation in order to achieve respiratory alkalosis in an attempt to achieve pulmonary vasodilation; and "gentle" ventilation which allows for higher $PaCO_2$ and lower pH and PaO_2 in an attempt to prevent lung injury (from barotrauma or volutrauma) and to prevent potential side effects from hypocapnia and alkalosis.

To date, there have been no prospective, randomized trials comparing any of the various mechanical ventilator strategies in the management of MAS. Hence, no single approach can be considered optimal.[182]

High-Frequency Ventilation

HFV has been used in MAS in the hope that the lower pressures and higher frequencies will prove advantageous. Benefits may include less barotrauma, increased mobilization of secretions, maintenance of respiratory alkalosis, and fewer chronic changes. High-frequency jet ventilation (HFJV) used with surfactant, but not alone, has been reported to improve oxygenation in MAS.[186] High-frequency oscillatory ventilation (HFOV), particularly when used with iNO, improved oxygenation and outcome in infants with PPHN and MAS.[187] However, the high airway resistance and obstructive nature of MAS may hinder the effectiveness of HFOV. Oxygenation is not necessarily improved with the use of either conventional ventilation or HFV.

Surfactant Therapy

Because surfactant within the lung may be hindered by the presence of meconium, surfactant replacement therapy can be considered as a treatment for MAS.[185] Bolus surfactant administration seems to reduce severity of respiratory symptoms, may reduce the disease progression, and may reduce the need for ECMO.[188]

An alternative approach is the use of dilute surfactant to lavage the lungs of infants with MAS. Two randomized, controlled trial have assessed lung lavage with dilute surfactant. Infants receiving this therapy had more favorable outcomes, such as more rapid and sustained improvement in oxygenation, a shorter ventilator course, and decreased need for ECMO.[188,189]

Inhaled Nitric Oxide

Among MAS babies in the various nitric oxide trials, there has been a slight decrease in the need for ECMO. However, there have been no significant differences in mortality, length of hospitalization, or duration of mechanical ventilation. Currently, iNO should be considered in infants with concomitant PPHN who are not responding to conventional therapy.[190]

Steroid Therapy

Corticosteroids are not recommended. Evidence supporting the use of steroids in the management of MAS is insufficient.[191]

Extracorporeal Membrane Oxygenation

ECMO is the therapy of last resort and is used when mortality is estimated to be very high, 50% to 80%.[192]

Other Therapies

Other therapies used for treatment of neonates with MAS include chest physiotherapy, sedation, alkalosis, paralytic agents, and minimal stimulation.[185] Pressors (dopamine, dobutamine) or fluid boluses have been used to maintain high systemic blood pressure.

Complications and Prognosis

Complications of MAS are widespread and depend on the severity of the disease and the level of treatment necessary for survival. Barotrauma or air leak syndrome is always a risk with PPV, especially in the infant with MAS in whom the ball-valve effect produces air trapping. Because the infant is at significant risk for air leaks, a high index of suspicion is necessary. The patient should be closely monitored for sudden deterioration, which could be indicative of tension pneumothorax. Immediate needle aspiration of the air or insertion of a chest tube, or both, may be indicated.

Another serious complication in MAS is increased intracranial pressure. Because the cranium is a fixed cavity, volume capacity is limited. Venous drainage is inhibited by the increased intrathoracic pressures, creating a potential for elevated intracranial pressure. The neonate with unstable vasculature who is already compromised may be predisposed to a higher incidence of IVH, and frequent ultrasonography of the head is performed to monitor for this complication.

PPHN is associated with MAS in approximately one third of cases and contributes to the mortality associated with this syndrome. Echocardiography should be performed to ascertain the degree of right-to-left shunt and to exclude congenital heart disease as the cause.

The mortality rate of meconium-stained infants is considerably higher than that of unstained infants. The decline in neonatal deaths caused by MAS during the last decades is related to improvements in obstetrical and neonatal care. Residual lung problems are rare but include symptomatic cough, wheezing, and persistent hyperinflation for up to 5 to 10 years. The ultimate prognosis depends on the extent of CNS injury from asphyxia and the presence of associated problems such as PPHN.[182]

PERSISTENT PULMONARY HYPERTENSION OF THE NEWBORN

Definition

PPHN is a clinical syndrome that occurs as a result of disruption in the normal perinatal fetal–neonatal circulatory transition. It is characterized by sustained elevated PVR and alterations in pulmonary vasoreactivity resulting in right-to-left shunting of blood across the foramen ovale or the PDA.[15,193] Although the disorder is also referred to as persistent fetal circulation (PFC), this description is not quite accurate because of the absence of the placenta and onset of air breathing after delivery. Most authors have embraced PPHN as the proper name for this syndrome, with the classic PFC subtype (idiopathic PPHN) representing a relatively small percentage of the cases now commonly encountered.[194]

PPHN is present when an infant with an echocardiographically confirmed structurally normal heart has the following conditions: (1) severe hypoxemia, usually a Pa_{O_2} between 37.5 and 45 mm Hg in an F_{IO_2} of 1.0 and IPPV if necessary; (2) mild lung disease, but the hypoxemia is disproportionately severe for the radiological, clinical, and acid-base abnormalities; (3) evidence of a right-to-left ductal shunt (Pa_{O_2} gradient between a **preductal** (right radial artery) and a **postductal** (umbilical artery) site of blood sampling more than 20 mm Hg). In the absence of a ductal

shunt; a large shunt may be demonstrated echocardiographically at the foramen ovale.[195]

Incidence

PPHN occurs in 1 to 2 per 1000 live births and is most common among full-term and post-term infants and associated with high risk of mortality.[196, 197]

Etiology and Pathophysiology

PPHN can be idiopathic or secondary to different conditions, including intrapartum asphyxia, infection, pulmonary hypoplasia, congenital heart disease, MAS, RDS, or drug therapy.[196,198] Box 22-4 lists factors commonly associated with PPHN.

In fetal life, the placenta functions as the organ for gas exchange. This function is facilitated by both shunting of

---

Box 22-4 | **Factors Associated with Persistent Pulmonary Hypertension of the Newborn**

STRUCTURAL LUNG AND HEART DISEASE
- Congenital diaphragmatic hernia
- Congenital cystic adenomatous malformation
- Alveolar capillary dysplasia
- Pulmonary hypoplasia
- Congenital heart defects
- In utero ductus arteriosus closure

PERINATAL CLINICAL PREDICTORS
- Postmaturity
- Nonvertex presentation
- Fetal distress
- Cesarean section
- Asphyxia
- Twin-twin transfusion
- Placental abruption
- Intrauterine growth restriction

POSTNATAL FACTORS
- Sepsis
- Inflammation
- Oxidative stress
- Antenatal drug exposure
- ASA/NSAIDs
- SSRIs
- Cigarette smoking

MATERNAL HEALTH
- Body mass index
- Asthma
- Diabetes mellitus
- Urinary tract infection
- Preeclampsia

RACE AND GENDER
- Black or Asian
- Male

ASA, Acetylsalicylic acid; *NSAIDs,* nonsteroidal anti-inflammatory drugs; *SSRIs,* selective serotonin reuptake inhibitors.
Adapted from Delaney C, Cornfield DN. Risk factors for persistent pulmonary hypertension of the newborn. *Pulm Circ* 2012;2(1):15.

blood through the foramen ovale and the hypoxic pulmonary arteriole vasoconstriction, which causes the blood to bypass the lungs and move toward the placenta. At birth, the umbilical cord is cut and the lungs make the transition to becoming the organ for gas exchange. With the first postnatal breaths, PVR decreases dramatically. By 24 hours of life, 80% of the total decrease in PVR has occurred, with the remaining reduction taking place over the next 2 weeks of life. The decrease in PVR occurs in response to (1) increase in PaO_2 and pH, (2) air expanding the lung, and (3) release of vasoactive substances, including prostaglandins, bradykinin, and endogenous nitric oxide production.[199]

The fetus prepares for this transition late in gestation by increasing pulmonary vascular expression of nitric oxide synthases and soluble guanylate cyclase. The prostacyclin pathway is another important vasodilatory pathway. Prostacyclin stimulates adenylate cyclase to increase intracellular cAMP levels, which, as with cGMP, lead to vasorelaxation through a decrease in intracellular calcium concentrations (Figure 22-9).

In infants with PPHN, this decrease in PVR either fails to occur or is reversed by pulmonary vascular hyperreactivity to irritating stimuli. PPHN is often characterized as one of three types:
1. Maladaptation: structurally normal but abnormally constricted pulmonary vasculature caused by lung parenchymal diseases such as MAS, RDS, or pneumonia.
2. Excessive muscularization: lung with normal parenchyma but remodeled pulmonary vasculature characterized by increased smooth muscle cell thickness and distal extension of muscle to vessels that are usually nonmuscular.[194] Many factors promote vascular remodeling in PPHN, such as an increase in pulmonary blood flow in utero; hypoxia; hyperoxia; various mediators, including endothelin type 1 (ET-1), platelet activating factor (PAF), reactive oxygen species (ROS), platelet-derived growth factor (PDGF), transforming growth factor β (TGF-β), and other growth factors. On the other hand, some mediators may inhibit vascular remodeling, such as NO/cGMP pathway and vascular endothelial growth factor (VEGF). Thus stimuli suppressing these inhibitory signaling mechanisms may also contribute to pulmonary vascular remodeling.[200,201]
3. Hypoplastic vasculature: associated with underdevelopment of the pulmonary vasculature, as seen in congenital diaphragmatic hernia. This designation is imprecise, however, and high PVR in most patients likely involves overlapping changes among these categories.[194]

Clinical Presentation and Diagnosis
Clinical Presentation
PPHN should be suspected in all term infants who have cyanosis that may occur despite adequate ventilation. The recognition of risk factors for PPHN is one of the major diagnostic tools to differentiate babies with PPHN from those with structural heart disease, keeping in mind that idiopathic PPHN can present without signs of acute perinatal distress. Marked lability in oxygenation is often part of the clinical history.

The infant with PPHN usually presents within the first 12 hours of life with cyanosis, tachypnea, and hypoxia

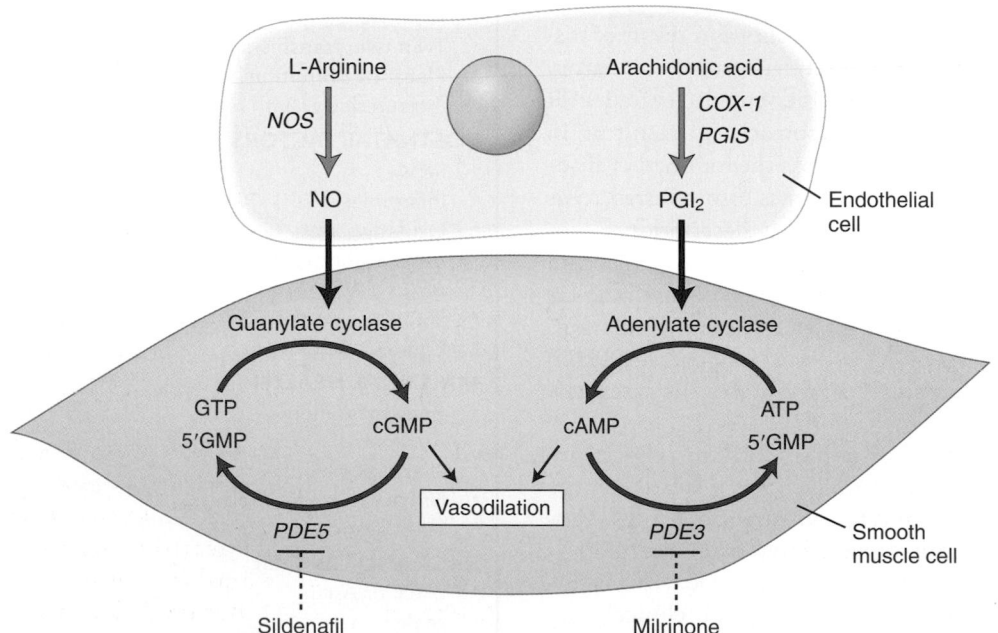

FIGURE 22-9 Nitric oxide (*NO*) and prostacyclin (i.e., prostaglandin I2 [*PGI₂*]) signaling pathways that regulate pulmonary vascular tone in the developing lung. (From Steinhorn RH, Abman SH. Persistent pulmonary hypertension. In Gleason CA, Devaskar SU, editors. *Avery's disease of the newborn*, ed 9. Philadelphia: Saunders, 2012.)

that are refractory to oxygen therapy and signs of respiratory distress, including retractions, grunting, and nasal flaring.[202]

Investigations

CXR appearance varies depending on the associated disorder. Early CXR are often clear, with minimal evidence of respiratory involvement, which is often perplexing in light of the severe cyanosis and respiratory distress the infant exhibits. Idiopathic and asphyxic PPHN may show well-expanded or hyperexpanded lungs with diminished vascularity, whereas PPHN resulting from pulmonary disorders (e.g., MAS, RDS, TTN) reveals abnormal pulmonary findings characteristic of that particular disorder. Cardiomegaly may be evident and develops as a result of the increased right ventricular afterload caused by the pulmonary hypertension.

ABG assessment reveals hypoxemia. Infants may hyperventilate because of the persistent hypoxemia. Hypocalcemia and hypoglycemia may develop rapidly as well.[203]

Classic tests to assess PPHN evaluate the response in PaO_2 to hyperoxia and hyperoxia-hyperventilation. To confirm PPHN, the PaO_2 should not increase appreciably with hyperoxia alone, but PaO_2 will usually rise above 100 mm Hg if the infant is hyperventilated until a $PaCO_2$ of 20 to 25 mm Hg is attained. Now, however, because of the known risk of oxidative injury and the potential for low $PaCO_2$ levels to reduce cerebral blood flow, these tests are no longer considered safe.

A PaO_2 gradient between a preductal (right radial artery) and a postductal (umbilical artery) site of blood sampling more than 20 mm Hg suggests right-to-left shunting through the ductus arteriosus, as does an oxygenation saturation gradient more than 5% between preductal and postductal sites on pulse oximetry. However, a normal test result (difference in preductal and postductal samples less than 20 mm Hg) does not rule out PPHN because a subset of infants with PPHN have hemodynamic shunting only at the level of the foramen ovale. An abnormal test result can also occur in infants with some congenital heart defects.

Real-time echocardiography combined with Doppler flow imaging studies demonstrates right-to-left or bidirectional shunting across a patent foramen ovale and a ductus arteriosus. Deviation of the intra-atrial septum into the left atrium is seen in severe PPHN. Tricuspid or mitral insufficiency may be visualized echocardiographically together with poor contractility when PPHN is associated with myocardial ischemia. The degree of tricuspid regurgitation can be used to estimate pulmonary artery pressure.[193]

Differential Diagnosis

A number of disorders, some of which are associated with secondary pulmonary hypertension, are misdiagnosed as PPHN. Therefore, an important aspect of the evaluation of the infant with presumed PPHN is the effort to rule out competing conditions, including the following:

1. Structural cardiovascular abnormalities associated with right-to-left ductal or atrial shunting, including the following:
   a. Obstruction to pulmonary venous return: infradiaphragmatic total anomalous pulmonary venous return, hypoplastic left heart syndrome, cor triatriatum, congenital mitral stenosis
   b. Myopathic left ventricular (LV) disease: endocardial fibroelastosis, Pompe disease
   c. Obstruction to LV outflow: critical aortic stenosis, supravalvular aortic stenosis, interrupted aortic arch, coarctation of the aorta
   d. Obligatory left-to-right shunt: endocardial cushion defect, arteriovenous malformation, hemitruncus, coronary arteriovenous fistula
   e. Miscellaneous disorders: Ebstein anomaly, transposition of the great arteries
2. LV or right ventricular (RV) dysfunction associated with right-to-left hemodynamic shunting

LV dysfunction as a result of ischemia or obstruction caused by myopathic LV disease or obstruction to LV outflow might present with a right-to-left ductus arteriosus shunt. RV dysfunction may be associated with right-to-left atrial shunting as a result of decreased diastolic compliance and elevated end-diastolic pressure.

These diagnoses must be differentiated from idiopathic PPHN caused by pulmonary vascular remodeling or vasoconstriction. Signs favoring cyanotic congenital cardiac disease over PPHN include cardiomegaly, weak pulses, active precordium, pulse differential between upper and lower extremities, pulmonary edema, grade 3+ murmur, and persistent preductal and postductal PaO_2 at 40 mm Hg or less.[193]

Treatment

PPHN in an infant constitutes a medical emergency in which immediate, appropriate intervention is critical to reverse hypoxemia, improve pulmonary and systemic perfusion, and minimize hypoxic-ischemic end-organ injury.

Adequate respiratory support yields normoxemia and neutral or slightly alkalotic acid-base balance that facilitate the normal perinatal circulatory transition. Once stability is achieved, weaning should be accomplished conservatively with careful attention to the infant's tolerance of each step in tapering cardiorespiratory support.[193]

1. **General management:** Includes maintenance of normal temperature, electrolytes (particularly calcium), glucose, hemoglobin, and intravascular volume.
2. **Minimal handling:** Because infants with PPHN are extremely labile, with significant deterioration after seemingly "minor" stimuli, this aspect of care deserves special mention. ETT suctioning, in particular, should be performed only if indicated and not as a matter of routine.

Noise level and physical manipulation should be kept to a minimum.

3. Mechanical ventilation: Mechanical ventilation is almost always required to improve oxygenation, to achieve normal lung volumes, and to avoid the adverse effects of high or low lung volumes on PVR.[194]

The goal of mechanical ventilation should be to maintain normal FRC by recruiting areas of atelectasis, as well as to avoid overexpansion. Adjust ventilators to maintain adequate oxygenation and mild hyperventilation until stability is achieved for 12 to 24 hours after initially attempting to keep the oxygen saturation above 95%, PaCO$_2$ at 35 to 45 mm Hg, and pH at 7.35 to 7.45.

HFV is an important modality if a newborn has underlying parenchymal lung disease with low lung volumes. This modality is best used in a center with physicians who are experienced in achieving and maintaining optimal lung distention. The response to HFV can be rapid, and care must be taken to prevent hypocarbia and lung overdistention.[204]

Pharmacotherapy

Pulmonary Vasodilator Agents. Guidelines for treatment with vasodilators are as follows:

1. Inhaled nitric oxide (iNO): Nitric oxide (NO) is an endothelially derived gas-signaling molecule that relaxes vascular smooth muscle and that can be delivered to the lung by means of an inhalation device (INOvent; Ikaria, Clinton, NJ).[205] Treatment with iNO is indicated for newborns with an OI of 25 or more. The **oxygenation index (OI;** calculated as [mean airway pressure × FIO$_2$ × 100]/PaO$_2$) is often used to gauge the severity of disease.

2. Intravenous magnesium sulphate (MgSO$_4$) has been used as a vasodilator in the treatment of PPHN in some developing and developed countries. The disadvantage of MgSO$_4$ treatment is that it causes systemic vasodilation, and hypotension is a common side effect.[206]

3. Other agents that are still investigational include the following:
   · Phosphodiesterase inhibitors (sildenafil)[197]
   · Prostacyclin analogues (epoprostenol, treprostinil, beraprost, and iloprost)[207-209]
   · Endothelin receptor antagonists (bosentan and ambrisentan)[210]

Sedation and Analgesia. Because catecholamine release activates pulmonary α-adrenergic receptors, thereby potentially raising PVR, a narcotic analgesic that blocks the stress response, such as fentanyl infusion (2 to 5 μg/kg/hr), is a useful adjunct therapy.

For the full-term baby prone to fight the ventilator, neuromuscular blocking agents should be used; in this situation there are theoretical reasons for preferring D-tubocurarine to pancuronium.[211]

Maintenance of Adequate Cardiac Output and Systemic Blood Pressure. The degree of right-to-left shunting depends on the pulmonary-to-systemic gradient. Avoidance of systemic hypotension is critical. CVP monitoring may be of benefit.

· Correct hypovolemia by administering volume expanders.
· Cardiotonic/vascular agents, such as dopamine, dobutamine, epinephrine, norepineprine, and milrinone, can be used. All have differing effects on PVR, SVR, and contractility.

Antioxidant Therapy. An antioxidant therapeutic approach may have multiple beneficial effects; scavenging superoxide may increase the availability of both endogenous and iNO and may also reduce oxidative stress and limit lung injury.[212]

Extracorporeal Membrane Oxygenation

ECMO is being used in some centers for neonates with severe PPHN who are not responsive to less invasive therapies. ECMO is generally considered for infants with OI greater than 40 (see Chapter 20).

Complications and Prognosis

As recently as the late twentieth century, the mortality rate for PPHN was nearly 40%, and the prevalence of major neurological disability was 15% to 60%.[213] The introduction of ECMO and other new therapies has had a major effect on reducing the mortality rate.[214]

NEONATAL APNEA

Definitions

Apnea is defined as an unexplained episode of cessation of breathing for 20 seconds or longer, or a shorter respiratory pause associated with bradycardia, cyanosis, pallor, and marked hypotonia.

Apnea of prematurity (AOP) is defined as sudden cessation of breathing that lasts for at least 20 seconds or is accompanied by bradycardia or cyanosis in an infant younger than 37 weeks of gestational age.

Apnea of infancy (AOI) generally refers to infants with a gestational age of 37 weeks or more at the onset of apnea.

Acute life-threatening event (ALTE) is defined as an episode that is frightening to the observer and is characterized by some combination of apnea (central or occasionally obstructive), color change (usually cyanotic or pallid but occasionally erythematous or plethoric), marked change in muscle tone (usually marked limpness), choking, or gagging.

Sudden infant death syndrome (SIDS) is defined as sudden death of an infant under 1 year of age that remains unexplained after a thorough case investigation, including performance of a complete autopsy, examination of the death scene, and review of the clinical history.[215]

Periodic breathing (PB) is defined as bursts of respiratory activity of 20 seconds or less, separated by central apneic pauses lasting from 3 to 10 seconds. Periodic breathing is present in almost all preterm babies but is relatively uncommon in term babies. The cause of periodic breathing remains obscure, although the finding that it is absent until 48 hours of age suggests that inactivity of peripheral chemoreceptors at this time might play a role.[216]

Classification

Apnea traditionally is classified into three categories based on the presence or absence of upper airway obstruction:
1. Central apnea is characterized by total cessation of inspiratory efforts with no evidence of obstruction.
2. In obstructive apnea the infant tries to breathe against an obstructed upper airway, resulting in chest wall motion without airflow through the entire apneic episode.
3. Mixed apnea consists of obstructed respiratory efforts, usually after central pauses.[217]

Incidence

Apneic spells occur frequently in premature infants. The incidence of apnea increases with decreasing gestational age. More than 50% of infants weighing less than 1500 g and 90% of infants weighing less than 1000 g will have apnea. Another 30% will have periodic breathing. Mixed apnea accounts for about 50% of all cases of AOP; about 40% are central apneas, and 10% are obstructive apneas.[218]

Apneic spells generally begin at 1 or 2 days after birth; if they do not occur during the first 7 days, they are unlikely to occur later. Apneic spells persist for variable periods postnatally and usually cease by 37 weeks of gestational age. In infants born before 28 weeks of gestation, however, spells often persist beyond term gestational age. The mean time for severe AOP to resolve is approximately 43 weeks after conception, but a prolonged duration of risk is not uncommon.

The incidence of apnea and periodic breathing in the term infant has not been adequately determined. Apneic spells occurring in infants at or near term are always abnormal and are nearly always associated with serious, identifiable causes, such as birth asphyxia, intracranial hemorrhage, seizures, or depression from medication. Failure to breathe at birth in the absence of drug depression or asphyxia is generally caused by irreversible structural abnormalities of the CNS.[219]

Etiology and Pathophysiology

Immaturity and depression of the central respiratory drive to the muscles of respiration have been accepted as key factors in the pathogenesis of AOP.[220] Premature infants are believed to be susceptible to apneic episodes also because of immature afferent input from chemoreceptors and lung and airway receptors.

Sleep-related response may be a factor in apnea and periodic breathing. Nearly 80% of a preterm infant's time is spent sleeping, with approximately 90% of a sleep cycle spent in rapid eye movement (REM) sleep, and the infant often has difficulty making the transition between the sleeping and waking states. This may be associated with an increased risk for apnea. Also, overall muscle weakness (of both the muscles of respiration and the muscles that maintain airway patency) also plays an important role in pathophysiology.[218]

Secondary causes of apnea include the following:
1. Temperature instability: hypothermia and hyperthermia
2. Neurological: birth trauma, drugs, intracranial infections, intracranial hemorrhage, perinatal asphyxia, anesthetic drugs
3. Pulmonary: RDS, pneumonia, BPD, pulmonary hemorrhage, obstructive airway lesion, pneumothorax
4. Cardiac: congenital cyanotic heart disease, hypotension/hypertension, congestive heart failure, PDA
5. Hematological: anemia, polycythemia
6. Infections: sepsis, NEC
7. Metabolic: hypoglycemia, hypocalcemia, hyponatremia, hypernatremia
8. Inborn errors of metabolism
9. Gastrointestinal: GER, esophagitis[221]

GER and apnea are common in preterm infants. Monitoring studies have demonstrated that when a relationship between reflux and apnea is observed, apnea may precede rather than follow reflux. During an apneic episode, loss of respiratory neural output may be accompanied by a decrease in lower esophageal tone, and GER occurs.[222]

Clinical Presentation and Diagnosis
Clinical Presentation

Apnea presents in one of two ways:
1. *Apnea within 24 hours after delivery.* Although apnea may be present at any time during the neonatal period, if it presents within the first 24 hours of life, it is usually not simple AOP. Apnea during this period must be suspected as being associated with infant or maternal pathological conditions (e.g., neonatal sepsis, hypoglycemia, intracranial hemorrhage, maternal antepartum magnesium treatment, or maternal exposure to narcotics).
2. *Apnea after the first 24 hours of life.* When apnea occurs after the first 24 hours of life and is not associated with any other pathological condition, it may be classified as AOP.

Apnea may also occur after weaning from prolonged ventilatory support and may be associated with intermittent hypoxia secondary to hypoventilation or atelectasis.

Diagnosis

A high index of suspicion is necessary to diagnose apnea. If significant apnea is detected, an extensive workup is required to make an accurate diagnosis and develop a logical treatment plan.
1. Monitoring of infants at risk: Close monitoring to evaluate possible causes of apnea should focus on respiratory rate and pattern, heart rate, circumstances preceding the

apneic episode, associated bradycardia, skin color, muscle tone, and termination of the episode (whether spontaneous, with stimulation, or with resuscitation).

2. Detailed history and physical examination: After stabilization, the infant should be evaluated for a possible underlying cause. History should be reviewed for onset of apnea; possible causes of secondary apnea including perinatal asphyxia, maternal drugs, features of neonatal sepsis, and feeding intolerance. The infant should be examined for temperature instability, hypotension, jaundice, pallor, cardiac murmur, and poor perfusion.[221]

3. Evaluation: The diagnostic evaluation is directed by the clinical presentation and the infant's associated findings. It includes sepsis screen, CXR, and serum electrolyte determination. An echocardiogram and a cardiology referral are necessary if the history or physical examination suggests cardiac disease. An electrocardiogram (ECG) is useful when severe unexplained tachycardia or bradycardia exists. Testing of serum ammonia levels as well as urine and serum amino acids and organic acids are indicated if a metabolic disorder is suspected. Intraesophageal pH recording with a multichannel recording should be used if GER is suspected as a precipitating event. An electroencephalogram (EEG) should be considered in infants suspected of having apneic seizures or having persistent pathological central apnea without an identifiable cause. A pneumogram is another tool in the diagnosis of apnea that is especially useful in the infant whose cause of apnea has not yet been identified.[218]

Treatment
General Measures

If an identifiable cause of apnea is determined, it should be treated accordingly.

· Care should be taken to avoid reflexes that may trigger apnea. Suctioning of the pharynx should be done carefully, and oral feedings should be avoided.
· Positions of extreme flexion or extension of the neck should be avoided, to reduce the likelihood of airway obstruction.
· Oxygen saturation should be maintained between 85% and 95%, with supplemental oxygen provided if needed.
· Gentle tactile stimulation is often adequate therapy for mild and intermittent episodes.
· Avoiding swings in environmental temperature may prevent apnea.[219]

CPAP

CPAP at moderate levels (4 to 6 cm H_2O) can reduce the number of mixed and obstructive apneic spells. It is especially useful in infants less than 32 to 34 weeks of gestational age and those with residual lung disease.

Pharmacotherapy

Xanthine Derivatives (Caffeine or Theophylline). Proposed mechanisms for xanthine derivatives include stimulation of skeletal and diaphragmatic muscle contraction, increase in the respiratory center's sensitivity to CO_2, and stimulation of the central respiratory drive. Caffeine appears to be a safer drug, can be given less frequently than theophylline, and is more effective in treating apnea.[223]

Doxapram. Doxapram is a potent respiratory stimulant that has been shown to be effective when theophylline and caffeine have failed. The duration of treatment with doxapram has been limited to 5 days, but the drug may be used longer if indicated. Side effects include abdominal distention, irritability, jitteriness, vomiting, increased blood pressure, and feed intolerance. Although doxapram reduces the number of apneas in the first 48 hours of its administration, there is no evidence to support its use as a first-line agent in the treatment of AOP above methylxanthines in current practice.[224]

Mechanical Ventilation

Some infants continue to have apneic spells despite pharmacotherapy. If the apnea is severe and is associated with hypoxia or significant bradycardia, intubation and mechanical ventilation may be indicated.

Discharge Planning and Follow-up

A major issue in the management of infants with apnea is deciding when to stop administration of methylxanthines and whether or not the infant needs to be discharged on methylxanthines, a home monitor, or both.

The answers to these questions are still under debate. Most neonatologists allow a 5- to 7-day apnea-free period after discontinuing xanthine therapy before sending a premature infant home without a monitor.[225] If home monitoring is recommended for persistent cardiorespiratory events, it can usually be discontinued by 44 weeks of postconceptional age.[226]

Complications and Prognosis

AOP does not alter an infant's prognosis unless it is severe, recurrent, and refractory to therapy. AOP usually resolves by 36 weeks of postconceptional age and does not predict future episodes of SIDS. The associated problems of IVH, BPD, and ROP are critical in determining the prognosis for apneic infants. [215]

AIR LEAK SYNDROMES
Definition

Air leak syndromes include pulmonary interstitial emphysema, pneumothorax, pneumomediastinum, pneumopericardium, pneumoperitoneum, subcutaneous emphysema, and systemic air embolism.[227]

Incidence

The incidence of air leaks in newborns is inversely related to the birth weight of the infants.[227] The incidence in preterm infants is higher. The risk for air leaks is higher in infants with RDS, MAS, and pulmonary hypoplasia and in infants who need resuscitation at birth. CPAP and PPV further increase the incidence of air leaks.[4] Surfactant, use of synchronized or volume ventilation, and high-rate, low VT ventilation decrease the incidence of air leaks.[228]

The incidence of pneumothorax from 1990 to 2002 was 13% in babies weighing less than 750 g and 2% in babies weighing 1251 to 1500 g.[4]

The incidence of PIE, pneumomediastinum, and pneumopericardium in the pre-surfactant era in mechanically ventilated babies weighing less than 1500 g was approximately 20%, 3%, and 2%, respectively.[229]

Etiology and Pathophysiology

Macklin[230] first described the passage of air from a ruptured alveolus in the overdistended cat lung. Air moved up the vascular sheath into the mediastinum and from there into the pleural cavity.

Overdistention of terminal air spaces or airways can result from uneven alveolar ventilation, air trapping, or injudicious use of alveolar distending pressure in infants on ventilatory support.[230] As lung volume exceeds physiological limits, mechanical stresses occur in all planes of the alveolar or respiratory bronchial wall, with eventual tissue rupture.

Air can track through the perivascular adventitia, causing **pulmonary interstitial emphysema,** or dissect along vascular sheaths toward the hilum, causing **pneumomediastinum.** Rupture of the mediastinal pleura results in **pneumothorax. Pneumoretroperitoneum** and **pneumoperitoneum** may occur when mediastinal air tracks downward to the extraperitoneal fascial planes of the abdominal wall, mesentery, and retroperitoneum and eventually ruptures into the peritoneal cavity. Air in the mediastinum can decompress into the fascial planes of the neck and skin, causing **subcutaneous emphysema.**[231]

Clinical Presentation

A high index of suspicion is essential to initiate early diagnosis and aggressive management. Extrapulmonary extravasation of air should be suspected in any infant with respiratory disease whose condition suddenly deteriorates. An increase in respiratory rate might be accompanied by grunting and increasing pallor or cyanosis.

Neonates with spontaneous pneumothorax are usually asymptomatic or have mild signs of tachypnea with increased oxygen requirement. Occasionally, severe respiratory distress (grunting, nasal flaring, and intercostal retractions) may occur. In the ventilated neonate, pneumothorax may result in a rapid clinical deterioration, resulting in cyanosis, hypotension, hypoxemia, hypercapnia, and respiratory acidosis. In unilateral pneumothorax, the cardiac apex can be shifted away from the affected side and breath sounds decreased over that side. Some infants can develop distention of the involved hemithorax or a tensely distended abdomen from downward displacement of the diaphragm. Signs of shock can occur as a result of increased intrathoracic pressure that compromises venous return and decreases cardiac output. In preterm infants with RDS a pneumothorax often develops beyond the first days of life, when the severity of disease is decreasing and lung compliance is increasing.

PIE often presents with a slow, progressive deterioration of the blood gases with the need for increasing ventilatory support. Rarely, the neonate has a sudden deterioration with profound respiratory acidosis and hypoxemia. It may precede the development of a pneumothorax or may occur independently.[232]

Pneumomediastinum occurs in at least 25% of patients with pneumothorax and is usually asymptomatic. The degree of respiratory distress depends on the amount of trapped gas. If it is great, bulging of the midthoracic area is observed, the neck veins are distended, and blood pressure is low. The last two findings are a result of tamponade of the systemic and pulmonary veins. Although often asymptomatic, subcutaneous emphysema, detected by palpation of crepitus in the face, neck, or supraclavicular region, in newborn infants is almost pathognomonic of pneumomediastinum.[233]

Neonatal **pneumopericardium** is almost invariably preceded by other forms of air leak. The clinical signs of pneumopericardium range from asymptomatic to the abrupt onset of cardiovascular compromise from cardiac tamponade, which is a life-threatening complication. The first sign of pneumopericardium may be a decrease in blood pressure or a decrease in pulse pressure. There may also be an increase in heart rate with distant heart sounds.[234]

Usually the pneumoperitoneum is of little clinical importance, but it must be differentiated from intraperitoneal air resulting from a perforated viscus. Rarely, pneumoperitoneum can impair diaphragmatic excursion and compromise ventilation. In these cases, continuous drainage may be necessary.

Systemic air embolism is a rare but usually fatal complication of pulmonary air leak. Air may enter the vasculature either by disruption of the pulmonary venous system or by inadvertent injection through an intravascular catheter. The presence of air bubbles in blood withdrawn from an umbilical artery catheter can be diagnostic.[235]

Diagnosis
Chest Radiograph

CXR remains the gold standard for diagnosis of air leak syndromes. Pneumothorax with anteroposterior (AP) views shows a hyperlucent hemithorax, a separation of the visceral from the parietal pleura, flattening of the diaphragm, and mediastinal shift (Figure 22-10).

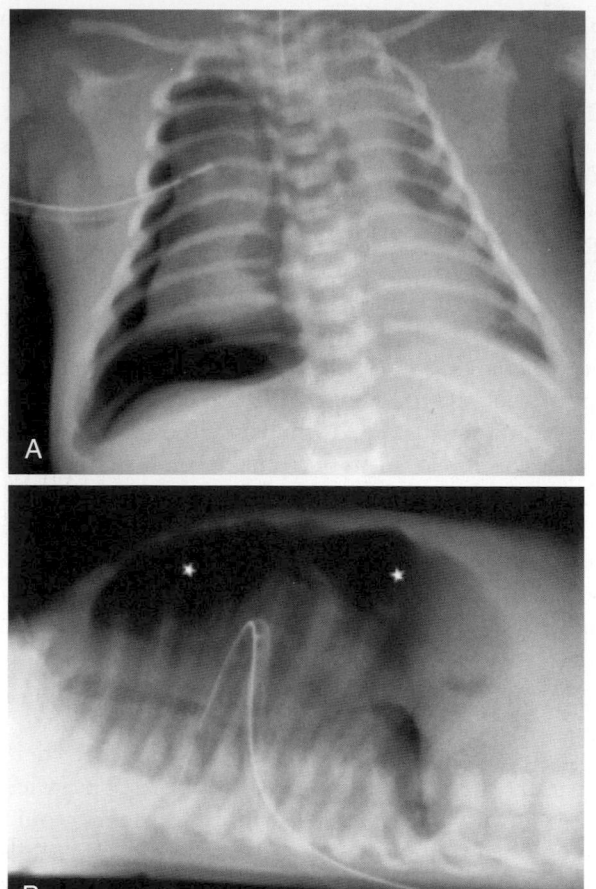

FIGURE 22-10 **A.** Right-sided tension pneumothorax incompletely drained by the intercostal drain. There is flattening of the diaphragm and shift of the midline with compression of the left lung. **B.** Lateral view shows that the chest drain is angulated posteriorly and is not ideally sited to drain the anterior and subpulmonary collection of air leak (*asterisk*). (From Arthur R. The neonatal chest x-ray. *Paediatr Respir Rev* 2001;2:311.)

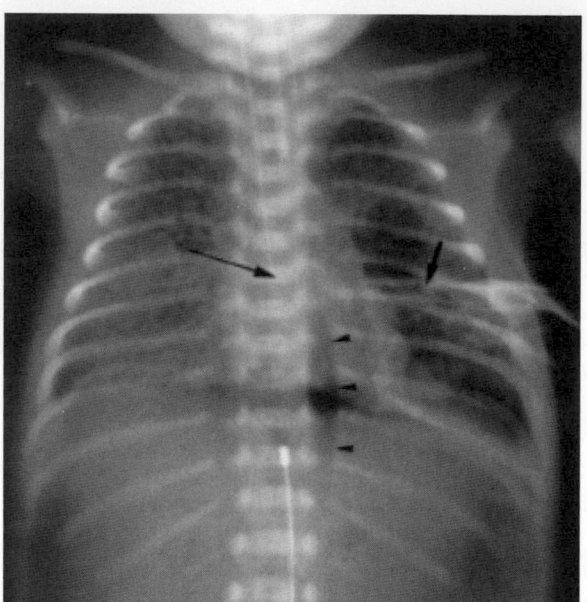

FIGURE 22-11 Severe bilateral pulmonary interstitial emphysema following drainage of left pneumothorax by intercostal drain (*short arrow*). Note mediastinal air to the left of the spine tracking down to the peritoneal cavity (*arrowheads*). The diaphragm is visible throughout its length, and there is increased translucency over the upper abdomen indicating a large pneumopericardium. Note the nasogastric tube is too short with the tip in the mid esophagus (*long arrow*). (From Arthur R. The neonatal chest x-ray. *Paediatr Respir Rev* 2001;2:311.)

Smaller collections of intrapleural air can be detected beneath the anterior chest wall by obtaining a cross-table lateral view; however, an AP view is needed to identify the affected side. The lateral decubitus view, with the side of suspected pneumothorax up, may be helpful in detecting a small pneumothorax and may help differentiate skin folds, congenital lobar emphysema, cystic adenomatoid malformations, and surface blebs that occasionally give the appearance of intrapleural air.[235] The cross-table lateral view permits an optimal evaluation of the relative position of the lung, intrapleural air, and the tip of the chest tube in the supine newborn.[236]

PIE appears as linear or tiny cystic translucencies extending from the hilum to the periphery of the lungs (Figure 22-11). When more severe, the lungs become hyperexpanded and stiff, compressing the heart and mediastinal structures and reducing venous return. PIE generally affects both lungs symmetrically but unilateral and even lobar distribution may be seen.[237]

Typical radiological signs of pneumomediastinum include the continuous diaphragm sign (interposition of air between the pericardium and the diaphragm, which becomes visible in the central mediastinal part) and linear bands of mediastinal air paralleling the left side of the heart and the descending aorta (pleura is shown as a fine opaque line) with extension superiorly along the great vessels into the neck. The "spinnaker sign" or "angel's wings appearance" (an upward and outward deviation of thymic lobes) can be seen when the thymus is raised above the heart by pneumomediastinal air that elevates the thymus and separates it from the cardiac silhouette beneath (Figure 22-12).[238]

In pneumopericardium, AP views show air surrounding the heart. Air under the inferior surface of the heart is diagnostic (Figure 22-13).

In systemic air embolism, gas can be seen in the systemic and pulmonary arteries and veins (Figure 22-14).

Transillumination

A high-intensity fiberoptic light source may demonstrate a pneumothorax. Transillumination of a chest with diffuse

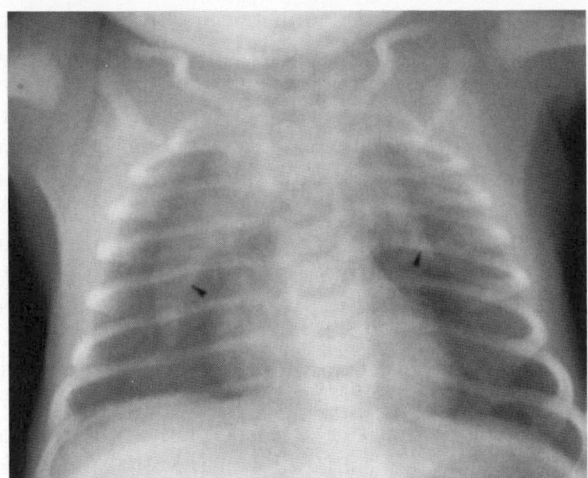

FIGURE 22-12 Neonatal pneumomediastinum. Note the thymus gland outlined by air giving an "angel's wings" appearance (*arrowheads*). (From Arthur R. The neonatal chest x-ray. *Paediatr Respir Rev* 2001;2:311.)

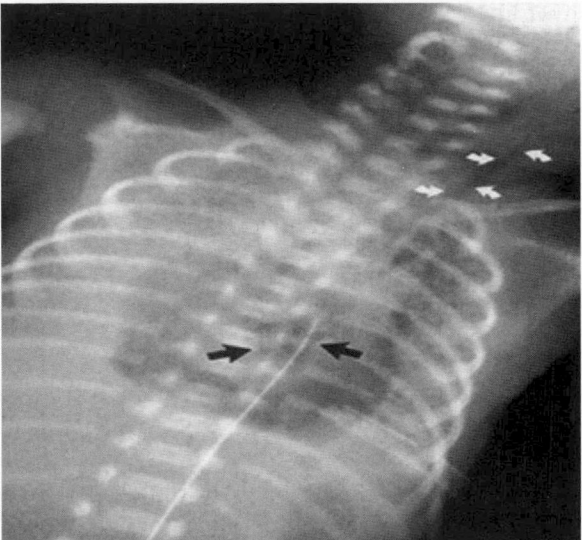

FIGURE 22-14 Postmortem X-ray of a baby who died from systemic air embolism. Gas can be seen (*black arrows*) within the heart and in the great vessels in the neck (*white arrows*). (From Bancalari E: Bronchopulmonary dysplasia and neonatal chronic lung disease. In Fanaroff AA, Martin RJ, editors. *Neonatal-perinatal medicine diseases of the fetus and infant*, ed 9. St Louis: Mosby-Elsevier, 2011.)

Arterial Blood Gases

Changes in ABG measurements are nonspecific and demonstrate a decreased P_{O_2}, increased P_{CO_2}, and decreased pH.

Electrocardiogram

Decreased voltages, manifested by a shrinking QRS complex, are consistent with pneumopericardium.[235]

Prevention

The best mode of treatment for all the air leak syndromes is prevention and judicious use of ventilatory support. Gentle ventilation with low pressure, low V_T, low Ti, high rate, and judicious use of PEEP are the keys to caring for mechanically ventilated infants.[227] The use of surfactant therapy for RDS has been shown to substantially decrease the incidence of pneumothorax and PIE.[228]

Both HFOV and HFJV can provide adequate gas exchange using extremely low V_T and supraphysiological rate in neonates with acute pulmonary dysfunction, and they are considered to have the potential to reduce the risks of air leak syndrome in neonates.[227] Fast rate ventilation (more than 60 beats per minute) may reduce active expiration, a precursor of air leaks. This is done in an attempt to provoke more synchronous respiration.

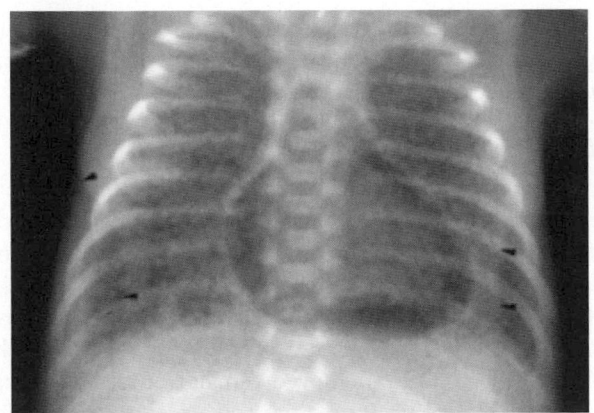

FIGURE 22-13 Pneumopericardium has developed in association with bilateral pulmonary interstitial emphysema. Note bilateral skinfolds at bases simulating a pneumothorax (*arrowheads*). (From Arthur R. The neonatal chest x-ray. *Paediatr Respir Rev* 2001;2:311.)

and widespread PIE will result in increased transmission of light, similar to that seen in a pneumothorax. This technique is less sensitive in infants with chest-wall edema or severe PIE, in extremely small infants with thin chest walls, or in full-term infants with thick chest walls or dark skin. We often obtain a baseline transillumination in infants at high risk for air leak.[239]

Needle Aspiration

In a rapidly deteriorating clinical situation, thoracentesis or pericardiocentesis may confirm the diagnosis and be therapeutic in pneumothorax and pneumopericarium, respectively.

Patient-triggered ventilation reduces the incidence of air leak by synchronizing respiration. Using this mode of ventilation, the infant's respiratory efforts trigger the delivery of the positive pressure inflation. Flow cycling enables complete synchronization, even in expiration.

Providing "routine" paralysis to abolish the baby's respiration does not prevent pneumothorax when compared with synchronous ventilation.[240] Hence, synchronizing the baby's ventilation by increasing the respiratory rate up to 60 to 80 breaths per minute can prevent the need for paralysis. If the baby's oxygenation does not improve and if obvious respiratory effort continues in spite of high rates, paralysis may be beneficial.[228]

Treatment
Conservative Management
Without a continued air leak, asymptomatic and mildly symptomatic small pneumothorax requires only close observation. Conservative management of a pneumothorax is effective even in selected infants requiring ventilatory support. Frequent small feedings may prevent gastric dilation and minimize crying, which can further compromise ventilation and worsen the pneumothorax. Breathing 100% oxygen in term infants accelerates the resorption of free pleural air into blood by reducing the nitrogen tension in blood and producing a resultant nitrogen pressure gradient from the trapped gas in the blood, but the clinical effectiveness is not proven and the benefit must be weighed against the risks of oxygen toxicity.[233]

In generalized PIE, an attempt should be made to decrease ventilatory support and lessen lung trauma. Decreasing the PIP, decreasing the PEEP, or shortening the Ti may be required. All these maneuvers will decrease injury and possibly improve PIE. During this time, some degree of hypercapnia and hypoxia may have to be accepted. In unilateral PIE, positioning the infant with the affected side down minimizes aeration of the affected lung and promotes aeration of the unaffected lung.[241]

Needle Aspiration
Needle aspiration using a "butterfly" needle or intravenous catheter with an inner needle is indicated to treat a patient with symptomatic pneumothorax. Needle aspiration may be curative in infants not receiving mechanical ventilation and is often a temporizing measure in mechanically ventilated infants. In infants with severe hemodynamic compromise, needle aspiration may be a lifesaving procedure.[235]

In pneumoperitoneum, needle aspiration can be used as a temporizing measure or as treatment. Following the general procedure for needle aspiration of pneumothorax, the needle is inserted in the midline approximately 1 cm below the umbilicus. Negative pressure is applied while the needle is advanced through the peritoneum and air is evacuated.[232]

Chest Tube Drainage
In infants with lung disease, the presence of a pneumothorax accentuates the respiratory difficulty and requires prompt, if not urgent, decompression. This consists of the placement of a large-bore, multiple-holed chest tube into the pleural space, anterior to the lung. Anterior placement in the pleural space is best achieved by insertion of the tube into the chest at or just lateral to the anterior axillary line. The tube should then be connected to an underwater seal at a suction pressure of 10 to 20 cm H_2O. The chest tube should be introduced under sterile conditions and secured with a purse-string suture.

Dramatic improvement in color and circulation follows the relief of a tension pneumothorax, which can be confirmed by repeat transillumination. The ease with which the lung can be reexpanded depends to a large extent on the compliance of the underlying pulmonary tissue. Expansion is particularly slow in infants with hypoplastic lungs associated with a congenital diaphragmatic hernia.

Suction should be maintained until fluctuation of air in the tube and active bubbling have ceased. At this time the tube should be clamped and removed within 24 hours if there has been no reaccumulation of air in the pleural cavity.[233]

In pneumopericardium, decompression is essential and requires the placement of a pericardial drain via the subxiphoid route or repeated pericardial taps.[4]

Other Treatments
Severe cases of unilateral PIE may respond to collapse of the affected lung by selective bronchial intubation of the unaffected lung. In cases of severe PIE, surgical lobectomy may be considered.[242]

HFJV is a successful means of ventilation for infants with PIE and with other types of pulmonary air leaks. This mode results in improved ventilation at lower peak and mean airway pressures with more rapid resolution of PIE. The earlier that HFV is initiated after the onset of PIE or pulmonary air leak, the greater the chances for survival.[243]

Complications and Prognosis
The prognosis for the infant in whom an air leak develops depends on the underlying condition. It has been suggested that early recognition and treatment are beneficial to avoid damage as a result of hypoxemia, hypercapnia, and impaired venous return.[244] However, it must be remembered that early-onset PIE (more than 24 hours of age) is associated with a high mortality rate.[245] Severe pulmonary air leak syndromes are associated with an increased risk of IVH, RDS, and death.[246]

PULMONARY HEMORRHAGE
Definition
Pulmonary hemorrhage is an acute, catastrophic event characterized by discharge of bloody fluid from the upper respiratory tract or the ETT. It is a form of fulminant lung

edema with leakage of red blood cells and capillary filtrate into the lungs.[247]

Incidence

About 1.4% of all infants admitted to the NICU have been reported to develop pulmonary hemorrhage; more than 80% have RDS. Such infants are also likely to have been treated with exogenous surfactant and were receiving mechanical ventilatory support at the time of bleeding.

The incidence is inversely proportional to gestational age, especially between 23 and 28 weeks of gestation.[248] In infants with a birth weight less than 1500 g and treated with surfactant, the incidence was reported to be 11.9%.[249] In autopsy studies, pulmonary hemorrhage of any degree is even much more prevalent. Some studies report hemorrhage in up to about 80% of autopsied VLBW neonates. Among infants requiring ECMO therapy, about 6% (range 5% to 10%) of infants have been reported to develop pulmonary hemorrhage either during or after ECMO. [248]

Risk Factors

Risk factors include conditions predisposing the infant to increased left ventricular filling pressures, increased pulmonary blood volume, compromised pulmonary venous drainage, or poor cardiac contractility.

1. *Prematurity, RDS, and exogenous surfactant therapy.* In combination, these three are the most consistent risk factors for pulmonary hemorrhage, especially in infants less than 28 weeks of gestation (or birth weight less than 1000 g). The rate of complication is not influenced by the type of surfactant used or its time of administration (prophylactic, early, or rescue).[21,250]
2. Preterm infants with echocardiographic evidence of *a large left-to-right shunt across a PDA* and a high pulmonary blood flow have a high incidence of pulmonary hemorrhage.[251]
3. *Infants who are small for gestational age* are more likely to suffer a pulmonary hemorrhage, the association being independent of other factors.[252]
4. *Lung complications.* PIE and pneumothorax.
5. *Infections.* Bacterial, viral, or fungal infections, such as *Listeria, Haemophilus influenzae,* and congenital s, have been reported to be associated with pulmonary hemorrhage.[253]
6. *General clinical status.* Metabolic acidosis, especially in infants with RDS; hypothermia; hypoglycemia; shock; and disseminated intravascular coagulation (DIC).
7. *Meconium aspiration syndrome,* especially infants requiring ECMO.
8. *Inherited coagulation disorders.* Although rare, one must consider familial bleeding disorders, such as von Willebrand disease. A report by the Centers for Disease Control and Prevention (CDC) found that von Willebrand disease was the underlying condition in

two of five infants dying from idiopathic pulmonary hemorrhage.[254]
9. *Trauma.* Mechanical injury to the vocal cords, trachea, or other laryngeal and oropharyngeal structures, especially from endotracheal intubation.

Pathophysiology

The underlying mechanisms of pulmonary hemorrhage remain uncertain. The pulmonary effluate has very high protein content, as well as a large number of cellular elements from the blood. Thus the hemorrhage may be a consequence of increased transcapillary pore size. A series of interrelated factors may lead to an eventual bleeding episode.

Some experts consider pulmonary hemorrhage as a manifestation of an exaggerated hemorrhagic pulmonary edema brought about by an acute increase in pulmonary blood flow. The latter can occur from multiple, interrelated causes, including the normal postnatal drop in the pulmonary vascular resistance, improved pulmonary compliance after surfactant therapy, and normal postnatal absorption of lung fluid. These changes may lead to an acute increase in pulmonary blood flow and hemorrhagic pulmonary edema.[247]

Clinical Presentation and Diagnosis
Clinical Presentation

Pulmonary hemorrhage commonly occurs between the second and fourth day of life. Clinically the onset of massive pulmonary hemorrhage is heralded by sudden deterioration of the infant with pallor, cyanosis, bradycardia, or apnea. Pink or red frothy liquid drains from the mouth or can be suctioned through an ETT. The baby usually is hypotensive and is often limp and unresponsive, although term babies may occasionally be active and restless secondary to hypoxemia and fight the ventilator. Occasionally collapse antedates the overt hemorrhage by an hour or two and rarely the baby looks surprisingly well despite the production of copious blood-stained pulmonary edema.[255]

Because the condition is commonly secondary to heart failure, the infant may have a tachycardia and the murmur of a PDA is often heard.[256] Other signs include hepatosplenomegaly, peripheral edema, and a triple rhythm. Auscultation of the chest reveals widespread crepitations with reduction in air entry. In infants who survive the acute episode, widespread pulmonary inflammation from blood in the lung tissues can lead to later complications, such as pneumonia and a prolonged need for assisted ventilation and the development of BPD.[247]

Diagnosis

CXR of infant with massive pulmonary hemorrhage shows a virtual "whiteout" with just an air bronchogram visible (Figure 22-15). As the condition improves with IPPV, the changes may clear or merge into those of BPD. Rarely, a

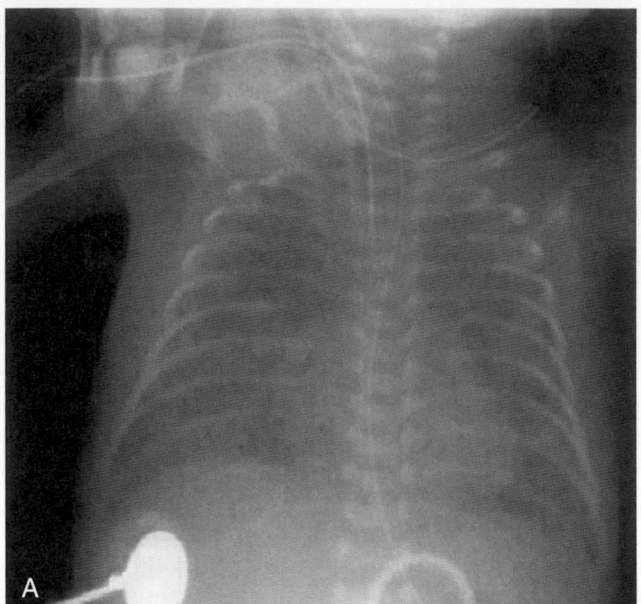

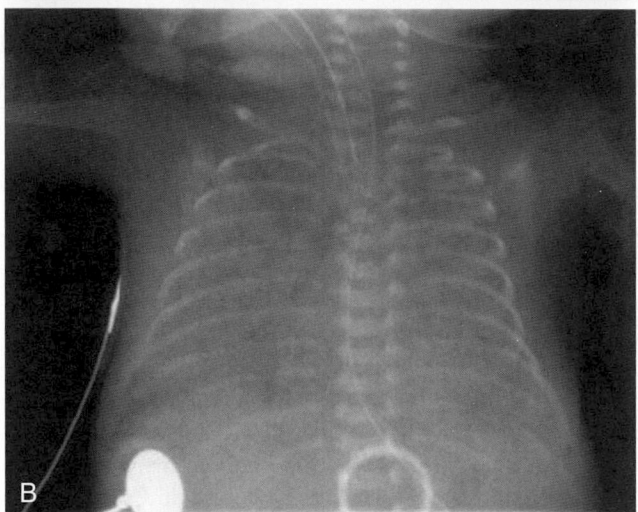

FIGURE 22-15 Chest X-ray of preterm infant (24 weeks of gestational age) with severe respiratory distress syndrome (A) just before and (B) after pulmonary hemorrhage. (From Narasimhan R, Papworth S. Pulmonary hemorrhage in the neonate, *Paediatr Child Health* 2009;19:171.)

lobar pattern of consolidation is found, suggesting that the hemorrhage has just occurred in a part of the lung. A daily CXR should be obtained because of the high ventilator pressures that are often required and the potential complications.[255]

Blood gases should be meticulously supervised. Clotting studies should be done daily until they normalize. All components of the blood gas might deteriorate rapidly with severe hypoxia, hypercapnia, and metabolic acidosis. Although the hematocrit of the edema fluid is usually less than 10%, considerable quantities of blood can be lost, the baby can become severely anemic, and secondary DIC can develop.[257]

Biochemical investigations show that infants with pulmonary hemorrhage usually have the same problems as those with severe RDS, namely hypoglycemia, hypocalcemia, hypoalbuminemia, and renal failure, and these should be sought and remedied.

The possibility of infection should be considered, and the infant should have a sepsis screening.

An echocardiogram is indicated to exclude significant PDA in infants with pulmonary hemorrhage, even in the absence of a typical "PDA murmur," or a wide pulse pressure or hyperdynamic precordium.[248]

Prevention

Antenatal Corticosteroids. Enhancing lung maturity through the use of antenatal corticosteroids may reduce pulmonary hemorrhage through its indirect effect on the lungs and pulmonary vascular bed.

Preventing PDA. Although early indomethacin or ibuprofen therapy has shown a strong effect in reducing the incidence of significant PDA, whether such a strategy will affect pulmonary hemorrhage incidence is unclear. Monitoring for PDA and its prompt therapy should be the mainstay for preventing pulmonary hemorrhage.[248]

HFOV. In a large trial the incidence of pulmonary hemorrhage was 2% in a group of small preterm infants treated with HFOV, compared with 7% in the conventional mechanical ventilation group.[258]

Treatment

Resuscitation

Initial resuscitation is the priority. The airway should be cleared with suction, and the infant should be intubated and ventilated and/or the ventilator pressures increased. The circulatory volume should be restored with boluses of colloid 20 ml/kg, a combination of fresh frozen plasma, blood, and platelets, with regular reassessment.

Ventilation

All babies with massive pulmonary hemorrhage should be intubated and ventilated. They usually have severe lung disease, and a PIP above 30 cm H_2O may be required. A ventilation strategy of high PEEP (up to 6 to 7 cm H_2O) is used with a long Ti (0.4 to 0.5 seconds). Although in experimental studies this does not reduce the total lung water, it redistributes it back into the interstitial space, improving oxygenation and ventilation–perfusion balance. Frequent suctioning may be required to keep the ETT clear.[259,260]

Surfactant

Paradoxically, although surfactant may precipitate pulmonary hemorrhage, after stabilizing the baby on the ventilator a single dose of surfactant has been suggested to improve oxygenation.[261]

Circulation

Intermittent colloid infusions and inotropes are often required to maintain the blood pressure and cardiac contractility. Blood transfusions may be required to correct anemia and fresh frozen plasma for clotting derangements. After the first 24 to 48 hours, when the baby has become stable on IPPV, acid-base disturbances have been corrected, and septicemia (if present) treated, the coagulation problems usually remit and further factor replacement is not usually necessary.

Once the initial circulating volume is restored, the infant must be reassessed for signs of left ventricular failure and pulmonary edema. In such cases, furosemide (1 mg/kg) should be given as soon as possible after the hemorrhage and repeated as necessary, to treat fluid overload.[255]

Fluid input should be restricted to 60 to 80 ml/kg/24 hours, particularly if there is a coexisting PDA. While the baby is critically ill, the use of indomethacin or equivalent for treating PDA is contraindicated, but this should be reconsidered 24 to 48 hours later, once the coagulopathy is controlled and the hypoxia and acid-base disorders corrected.[262]

Other Measures

Other measures that could be taken to stop pulmonary hemorrhage include the following:

- Recombinant factor VIIa , a vitamin K–dependent glycoprotein, structurally similar to the plasma-derived natural factor VII, is considered a universal hemostatic agent. This drug has also been used with success in two isolated cases of neonatal pulmonary hemorrhage at a 50 μg/kg/dose, repeated every 3 hours for 2 to 3 days. More work is needed to establish the dosage and the frequency of its administration, as well as to assess the consistency of response in neonatal pulmonary hemorrhage.[254]
- Nebulized epinephrine with or without 4% cocaine has been found to temporize massive bleeding. Experience using these drugs in newborns is limited.[248]
- Broad-spectrum antibiotics should be started after taking cultures because sepsis is a recognized cause of pulmonary hemorrhage.[247]

Complications and Prognosis

These babies are susceptible to all the major complications of respiratory failure. High-pressure ventilation predisposes to air leaks and BPD is a common sequelae.[249] At the time of their sudden collapse they are susceptible to neurological damage and major IVH0; the occurrence of cerebral bleeds may be doubled in babies who suffer pulmonary hemorrhage,[252] and the occurrence of seizures is increased in infants with pulmonary hemorrhage.[263] In the modern era of intensive care, survival is improved, but affected infants are the sickest and most immature and their mortality rate is of the order of 38%.[252]

CASE STUDY 1

A 3.7-kg male newborn delivered via an elective cesarean section at 41 weeks of gestation. Apgar scores were 7 and 8 at 1 and 5 minutes, respectively. The infant's temperature is 96.4° F (35.8° C), respiratory rate is 92 breaths per minute, and heart rate is 143 beats per minute. He has subcostal and intercostal retractions. The remainder of the examination is normal. CXR is shown in Figure 22-5. Over the next 6 hours she improves and no longer requires oxygen.

What is the diagnosis?

The parents are worried about his prognosis. What would you tell them?

See Evolve Resources for answers.

CASE STUDY 2

A 3.5-kg female infant is vaginally delivered with amniotic fluid stained with thick meconium. She is blue and tachypneic with Apgar scores of 4 and 6 at 1 and 5 minutes, respectively. The infant's temperature is 98.4° F (36.9° C), heart rate is 173 beats per minute, respiratory rate is 110 breaths per minute, and mean blood pressure is 61 mm Hg. She has a barrel-chest with subcostal retractions and poor to fair air entry. Coarse crepitations are audible bilaterally. CXR is shown in Figure 22-8.

What is your provisional diagnosis?

How would you resuscitate this neonate?

See Evolve Resources for answers.

KEY POINTS

- Respiratory distress is encountered often in newborns, typically caused by abnormal respiratory function during the transition from fetal to neonatal life, and represents the most common indication for reevaluation of the young infant.
- Because respiratory distress in the newborn may be a potentially life-threatening condition, physicians are expected to assess and manage affected infants promptly.
- The key to successful management of the infant who has respiratory distress is based on the ability to obtain a complete maternal and newborn history, perform a thorough physical examination, and recognize the common respiratory disorders.
- Therapies for neonatal respiratory diseases are in a constant state of evolution, and both new and old therapies must be continuously reevaluated.

ASSESSMENT QUESTIONS

See Evolve Resources for answers.

1. A newborn with 25 weeks of gestational age appears cyanotic, and ABG analysis indicates hypoxia and hypercapnia. The infant has severe chest wall retractions with inspiratory effort. The amniotic fluid appeared normal at birth. What is most likely the cause of respiratory distress?
   A. Surfactant deficiency
   B. Meconium aspiration syndrome
   C. Pneumonia
   D. Bronchopulmonary dysplasia

2. An infant diagnosed with RDS subsequent to lung prematurity is receiving oxygen therapy with an F_{IO_2} of 0.8 and NCPAP set at 10 cm H_2O. The infant is experiencing progressive hypercapnia, and apneic episodes are appearing prolonged. The next logical course of action is to:
   A. Increase the F_{IO_2} by 0.1 and look for improvements in ABG parameters.
   B. Start iNO therapy to improve the lung V/Q ratio.
   C. Increase NCPAP to 12 cm H_2O and refit the nasal prongs.
   D. Intubate the infant and begin mechanical ventilation.

3. A full-term infant is delivered via cesarean section and demonstrates mild symptoms of respiratory distress, including cyanosis, tachypnea, and nasal flaring. Apgar scores are good, and CXR shows hyperexpansion and perihilar streaking. Which situation most likely fits this case?
   A. This infant is in the "honeymoon" period and is expected to develop more severe RDS.
   B. This infant has TTN and will likely recover completely by 72 hours.
   C. This infant is in the early stages of pneumonia and should be started on broad-spectrum antibiotics.
   D. This infant likely has elevated PVR and a hyperoxia test should be performed to confirm PPHN.

4. A 4-day-old infant, born at 27 weeks of gestational age, develops recurrent symptoms of RDS. The infant had been removed from mechanical ventilation and extubated at day 3 and was receiving NCPAP with an F_{IO_2} of 0.4 when lung function acutely worsened. CXR shows a widespread, diffuse granular pattern, and analysis of arterial blood samples from the umbilical line demonstrates that oxygen saturation is refractory to increases in F_{IO_2}. The most likely cause for these recurrent symptoms of RDS is:
   A. Progressive periods of apnea
   B. Patent ductus arteriosus
   C. Meconium aspiration syndrome
   D. Postnatal pneumonia

5. A newborn infant begins to develop symptoms of respiratory distress at 5 days of life. A cerebrospinal fluid culture test is positive for group B *Streptococcus* infection. Which mode(s) of transmission is most likely the cause of the infection?
   A. Transplacental or perinatal
   B. Transplacental only
   C. Perinatal or postnatal
   D. Postnatal only

6. Which condition would be most critical in leading the caregiver to anticipate MAS?
   A. Desaturation refractory to oxygen therapy
   B. Yellowish-green amniotic fluid
   C. Distinct chest wall retractions with inspiratory efforts
   D. Cyanosis and nasal flaring

7. Which fetal assessments may suggest that, when born, an infant will be at risk for MAS?
   A. Fetal oligohydramnios
   B. Abnormal fetal heart rate tracings
   C. Both A and B
   D. Neither A nor B

8. PPHN can be associated with which underlying pulmonary disorders?
   A. MAS
   B. RDS
   C. None (idiopathic)
   D. All of the above

9. A full-term newborn diagnosed with PPHN is refractory to oxygen therapy and mechanical ventilation. What would be the next logical therapy to try?
   A. High-frequency ventilation
   B. Volume therapy
   C. iNO therapy
   D. All would be have potential benefits

10. A newborn of 34 weeks of gestational age is experiencing brief periods of apnea, which result in bradycardia and cyanosis. Blood and cerebrospinal fluid cultures are negative for infection. Which intervention(s) can help reduce the incidence of apneic episodes?
    A. Upright positioning
    B. Temperature stability
    C. Low F_{IO_2} of 0.23 to 0.25
    D. All of the above

11. A 30-weeks gestational age newborn has been on the ventilator for 9 weeks with Pa_{CO_2} values around 60 and Pa_{O_2} values around 60, despite increased ventilator settings. CXR reveals atelectasis, hyperlucencies, cystic changes, hyperinflation, and mild cardiomegaly. The most likely diagnosis is which of the following?
    A. Cystic fibrosis
    B. Bronchopulmonary dysplasia
    C. Bacterial pneumonitis
    D. Pulmonary interstitial emphysema
    E. Meconium aspiration

12. Among the following, the information that is most helpful in distinguishing cyanotic heart disease from pulmonary parenchymal disease in a newborn who has respiratory distress is:
    A. Decreased P_{O_2} in blood gas analysis
    B. Gestational age less than 32 weeks
    C. Maternal infection during the third trimester
    D. Respiratory rate of 70 breaths per minute
    E. Results of a hyperoxia test

References

1. Miller JM, Fanaroff AA, Martin RJ: Respiratory disorders in preterm and term infants. In Fanaroff AA, Martin RJ, editors: *Neonatal-perinatal medicine diseases of the fetus and infant*, ed 9, St Louis, 2011, Mosby Elsevier.

2. American Lung Association: *American Lung Association State of lung disease in diverse communities 2010*. http://www.lung.org/assets/documents/publications/solddc-chapters/rds.pdf. Accessed December 28, 2012.

3. Carlo WA, Ambalavanan N: Respiratory distress syndrome (hyaline membrane disease). In Kliegman RM, Behrman RE, Jenson HB and Stanton BF, editors: *Nelson textbook of pediatrics*, ed 19, Philadelphia, 2012, Saunders.

4. Fanaroff AA, Stoll BJ, Wright LL, et al: Trends in neonatal morbidity and mortality for very low birthweight infants, *Am J Obst Gynecol* 196:147.e1, 2007.

5. Xu J, Kochanek KD, Tejada-Vera B: Deaths: preliminary data for 2007-2009. Available at: www.cdc.gov/nchs/data/nvsr/nvsr58/nvsr58_01.pdf. Accessed December 28, 2012.

6. Gerten KA, Coonrod DV, Bay RC, et al: Cesarean delivery and respiratory distress syndrome: does labor make a difference? *Am J Obstet Gynecol* 93:1061, 2005.

7. Qiu X, Lee SK, Tan K, et al: Comparison of singleton and multiple-birth outcomes of infants born at or before 32 weeks gestation, *Obstet Gynecol* 11:365, 2008.

8. Anadkat JS, Kuzniewicz MW, Chaudhari BP, et al. Increased risk for respiratory distress among white, male, late preterm and term infants, *J Perinatol* 32:780, 2012.

9. Avery ME, Mead J: Surface properties in relation to atelectasis and hyaline membrane disease, *Am J Dis Child* 97:517, 1959.

10. Rooney SA: The surfactant system and lung phospholipid biochemistry, *Am Rev Respir Dis* 131:439, 1985.

11. Hawgood S, Clements JA: Pulmonary surfactant and its apoproteins, *J Clin Invest* 86:1, 1990.

12. Hislop AA, Wigglesworth JS, Desai R: Alveolar development in the human fetus and infant, *Early Hum Dev* 13:1, 1986.

13. Stark AR, Frantz ID 3rd: Respiratory distress syndrome, *Pediatr Clin North Am* 33:533, 1986.

14. Nelson NM, Prod'hom LS, Cherry RB, et al: Pulmonary function in the newborn infant, the alveolar-arterial oxygen gradient, *J Appl Physiol* 18:534, 1963.

15. Murdock AI, Swyer PR: The contribution to venous admixture by shunting through the ductus arteriosus in infants with respiratory distress syndrome of the newborn, *Biol Neonate* 13:194, 1968.

16. Verma RP. Respiratory distress syndrome of the newborn infant, *Obstet Gynecol Surv* 50:542, 1995.

17. Wert SE, Whitsett JA, Nogee LM: Genetic disorders of surfactant dysfunction, *Pediatr Dev Pathol* 12:253, 2009.

18. Nkadi PO, Merritt TA, Pillers DA: An overview of pulmonary surfactant in the neonate: genetics, metabolism, and the role of surfactant in health and disease, *Mol Genet Metab* 97:95, 2009.

19. Jobe AH: Glucocorticoids, inflammation and the perinatal lung, *Semin Neonatol* 6:331, 2001.

20. Jobe AH, Newnham JP, Willet KE, et al: Endotoxin induced lung maturation in preterm lambs is not mediated by cortisol, *Am J Respir Crit Care Med* 162:1656, 2000.

21. Davis GM, Bureau MA: Pulmonary and chest wall mechanics in the control of respiration in the newborn, *Clin Perinatol* 14:551, 1987.

22. South M, Morley CJ, Hughes G: Expiratory muscle activity in preterm babies, *Arch Dis Child* 62:825, 1987.

23. Whitfield CR, Sproule WD: Prediction of neonatal respiratory distress, *Lancet* 1:382, 1972.

24. Gluck L, Kulovich MV, Borer RC Jr, et al: Diagnosis of the respiratory distress syndrome by amniocentesis, *Am J Ob Gyn* 109:440, 1971.

25. Gluck L, Kulovich MV, Borer RC Jr, et al: The interpretation and significance of the lecithin-sphingomyelin ratio in amniotic fluid, *Am J Obstet Gynecol* 120:142, 1974.

26. Hallman M, Kulovich M, Kirkpatrick E, et al: Phosphatidylinositol and phosphatidylglycerol in amniotic fluid: indices of lung maturity, *Am J Obstet Gynecol* 125:613, 1976.

27. Clements JA, Platzker AC, Tierney DF, et al: Assessment of the risk of the respiratory distress syndrome by a rapid test for surfactant in amniotic fluid, *N Engl J Med* 286:1077, 1972.

28. Kattwinkel J, Perlman JM, Aziz K, et al: Neonatal resuscitation: 2010. American Heart Association guidelines for cardiopulmonary resuscitation and emergency cardiovascular care, *Pediatrics* 126:e1400, 2010.

29. Crowley P: Prophylactic corticosteroids for preterm birth, *Cochrane Database Syst Rev* (2):CD000065, 2000.

30. Brownfoot FC, Crowther CA, Middleton P: Different corticosteroids and regimens for accelerating fetal lung maturation for women at risk of preterm birth, *Cochrane Database Syst Rev* (4):CD006764, 2008.

31. Royal College of Obstetricians and Gynaecologists: *Antenatal corticosteroids to prevent respiratory distress syndrome 1996*. http://www.rcog.org.uk/guidelines/corticosteroids. Accessed October 8, 2011.

32. Feldman DM, Carbone J, Belden L, et al: Betamethasone vs dexamethasone for the prevention of morbidity in very low birthweight neonates, *Am J Obstet Gynecol* 1;97:284, 2007.

33. Baud O, Foix-L'Helias L, Kaminski M, et al: Antenatal glucocorticoid treatment and cystic periventricular leukomalacia in very premature infants, *N Engl J Med* 341:1190, 1999.

34. NIH Consensus Panel Development: Effect of corticosteroids on fetal maturation and perinatal outcomes, *J Am Med Assoc* 273:413, 1995.

35. Sweet D, Bevilacqua G, Carnielli V, et al: European consensus guidelines on the management of neonatal respiratory distress syndrome, *J Perinat Med* 35:175, 2007.

36. Bahakta KY. Respiratory distress syndrome: In Cloherty JP, Eichenwald EC, Hansen AR, Stark AR, editors: *Manual of neonatal care*, ed 7, Philadelphia, 2012, Lippincott Williams and Wilkins.

37. Soll RF, Blanco F: Natural surfactant extract versus synthetic surfactant for neonatal respiratory distress syndrome, *Cochrane Database Syst Rev* (2):CD000144, 2001.

38. Walsh BK, Daigle B, Diblasi RM, et al: AARC Clinical Practice Guideline. Surfactant Replacement Therapy: 2013, *Respir Care* 58:367, 2013.

39. Rojas-Reyes MX, Morley CJ, Soll R: Prophylactic versus selective use of surfactant in preventing morbidity and mortality in preterm infants, *Cochrane Database Syst Rev* (3):CD000510, 2012.

40. Stevens TP, Harrington EW, Blennow M, et al: Early surfactant administration with brief ventilation vs selective surfactant and continued mechanical ventilation for preterm infants with or at risk for respiratory distress syndrome, *Cochrane Database Syst Rev* (4):CD003063, 2007.

41. Zhang JP, Wang YL, Wang YH, et al: Prophylaxis of neonatal respiratory distress syndrome by intra-amniotic administration of pulmonary surfactant, *Chin Med J (Engl)* 117:120, 2004.

42. Kattwinkel J, Robinson M, Bloom BT, et al: Technique for intrapartum administration of surfactant without requirement for an endotracheal tube, *J Perinatol* 24:360, 2004.

43. Trevisanuto D, Grazzina N, Ferrarese P, et al: Laryngeal mask airway used as a delivery conduit for the administration of surfactant to preterm infants with respiratory distress syndrome, *Biol Neonate* 87:217, 2005.

44. Herting E, Kribs A, Roth B, et al: Surfactant via gastric tube in spontaneously breathing very low birth weight infants on nasal CPAP prevents mechanical ventilation, *Neonatology* 97:395, 2010.

45. Finer NN, Merritt TA, Bernstein G, et al: An open label, pilot study of Aerosurf combined with nCPAP to prevent RDS in preterm neonates, *J Aerosol Med Pulm Drug Deliv* 23:303, 2010.

46. Zola EM, Gunkel JH, Chan RK, et al: Comparison of three dosing procedures for administration of bovine surfactant to neonates with respiratory distress syndrome, *J Pediatr* 122:453, 1993.

47. Long W, Corbet A, Cotton R, et al: A controlled trial of synthetic surfactant in infants weighing 1250 g or more with respiratory distress syndrome. The American Exosurf Neonatal Study Group I, and the Canadian Exosurf Neonatal Study Group, *N Engl J Med* 325:1696, 1991.

48. Long W, Thompson T, Sundell H, et al: Effects of two rescue doses of a synthetic surfactant on mortality rate and survival without bronchopulmonary dysplasia in 700- to 1350-gram infants with respiratory distress syndrome. The American Exosurf Neonatal Study Group I, *J Pediatr* 118:595, 1991.

49. SUPPORT Study Group of the Eunice Kennedy Shriver NICHD Neonatal Research Network, Carlo WA, Finer NN, et al: Target ranges of oxygen saturation in extremely preterm infants, *N Engl J Med* May 362:1959, 2010.

50. Davis JM: Role of oxidant injury in the pathogenesis of neonatal lung disease, *Acta Paediatr Suppl* 91:23, 2002.

51. Koti J, Murki S, Gaddam P, Reddy A, Reddy MD: Bubble CPAP for respiratory distress syndrome in preterm infants, *Indian Pediatr* 47:139, 2012.

52. Kamper J: Early nasal continuous positive airway pressure and minimal handling in the treatment of very-low birth-weight infants, *Biol Neonate* 76(suppl 1):22, 1999.

53. Schimmel MS, Hammerman C: Early nasal continuous positive airway pressure with or without prophylactic surfactant therapy in the premature infant with respiratory distress syndrome, *Pediatr Radiol* 30:713, 2000.

54. Rojas-Reyes MX, Morley CJ, Soll R: Prophylactic versus selective use of surfactant in preventing morbidity and mortality in preterm infants, *Cochrane Database Syst Rev* (3):CD000510, 2012.

55. Miller TL, Shaffer TH, Greenspan JS: Pulmonary function evaluation in the critically ill neonate. In DF Askins, editor: *Acute respiratory care of the neonate*, ed 3, Santa Rosa, CA, 2012, NICU INK Book Publishers.

56. Hummler H, Gerhardt T, Gonzalez A, et al: Influence of different methods of synchronized mechanical ventilation on ventilation, gas exchange, patient effort, and blood pressure fluctuations in premature neonates, *Pediatr Pulmonol* 22:305, 1996.

57. Billman GF, Hughes AB, Dudell GG, et al: Clinical performance of an in-line, ex vivo point-of-care monitor: a multicenter study, *Clin Chem* 48:2030, 2002.

58. Greenough A, Dimitriou G, Alvares BR, et al: Routine daily chest radiographs in ventilated, very low birthweight infants, *Eur J Pediatr* 160:147, 2001.

59. Kavvadia V, Greenough A, Dimitriou G, Forsling M: Comparison of respiratory function and fluid balance in very low birthweight infants given artificial or natural surfactant or no surfactant treatment, *J Perinat Med* 26:469, 1998.

60. Levesque BM, Kalish LA, LaPierre J, Welch M, Porter V: Impact of implementing 5 potentially better respiratory practices on neonatal outcomes and costs, *Pediatrics* 128:e218, 2011.

61. Lebourges F, Moriette G, Boulé M, et al: Pulmonary function in infancy and in childhood following mechanical ventilation in the neonatal period, *Pediatr Pulmonol* 9:34, 1990.

62. Costeloe K, Hennessy E, Gibson AT, Marlow N, Wilkinson AR: The EPICure study: outcomes to discharge from hospital for infants born at the threshold of viability, *Pediatrics* 106:659, 2000.

63. Northway WH, Rosan RC, Porter DY: Pulmonary disease following respiratory therapy of hyaline membrane disease, *N Engl J Med* 276:357, 1967.

64. Jobe AH, Bancalari E: Bronchopulmonary dysplasia, *Am J Respir Crit Care Med* 163:1723, 2001.

65. Walsh MC, Wilson-Costello D, Zadell A, et al: Safety, reliability, and validity of a physiologic definition of bronchopulmonary dysplasia, *J Perinatol* 23:451, 2003.

66. Jobe AH: The new BPD: an arrest of lung development, *Pediatr Res* 46:641, 1999.

67. Charafeddine L, D'Angio CT, Phelps DL: Atypical chronic lung disease patterns in neonates, *Pediatrics* 103:759, 1999.

68. Wilson G, Mikity VG: A new form of respiratory disease in premature infants, *Am J Dis Child* 99:489, 1960.

69. Avery GB, Fletcher AB, Kaplan M, et al: Controlled trial of dexamethasone in respiratory-dependent infants with bronchopulmonary dysplasia, *Pediatrics* 75:106, 1985.

70. Bancalari E, Claure N, Sosenko IR: Bronchopulmonary dysplasia: changes in pathogenesis, epidemiology and definition, *Sem Neonatol* 8:63, 2003.

71. Stoll BJ, Hansen NI, Bell EF, et al: Neonatal outcomes of extremely preterm infants from the NICHD Neonatal Research Network, *Pediatrics* 126:443, 2010.

72. Viscardi RM, Muhumuza CK, Rodriguez A, et al: Inflammatory markers in intrauterine and fetal blood and cerebrospinal fluid compartments are associated with adverse pulmonary and neurologic outcomes in preterm infants, *Pediatr Res* 55:1009, 2004.

73. Taghizadeh A, Reynolds EOR: Pathogenesis of bronchopulmonary dysplasia following hyaline membrane disease, *Am J Pathol* 82:241, 1976.

74. Bjorklund LL, Ingimarsson J, Curstedt T, et al: Manual ventilation with a few large breaths at birth compromises the therapeutic effect of subsequent surfactant replacement in immature lambs, *Pediatr Res* 42:348, 1997.

75. Wada K, Jobe AH, Ikegami M: Tidal volume effects on surfactant treatment responses with the initiation of ventilation in preterm lambs, *J Appl Physiol* 83:1054, 1997.

76. Ratner V, Slinko S, Utkina-Sosunova, et al: Hypoxic stress exacerbates hyperoxia-induced lung injury in a neonatal mouse model of bronchopulmonary dysplasia, *Neonatology* 95:299, 2009.

77. Nwajei PO, Young K, Claure N, et al: Impact of intermittent hypoxia on neonatal hyperoxia-induced lung injury, *Soc Pediatr Res E-PAS* 2140:7, 2010.

78. Bolivar JM, Gerhardt T, Gonzalez A, et al: Mechanisms for episodes of hypoxemia in preterm infants undergoing mechanical ventilation, *J Pediatr* 127:767, 1995.

79. Frank L, Sosenko IR: Development of lung antioxidant enzyme system in late gestation: possible implications for the prematurely born infant, *J Pediatr* 110:11, 1987.

80. Watterberg KL, Demers SM, Scott SM, Murphy S: Chorioamnionitis and early lung inflammation in infants in whom bronchopulmonary dysplasia develops, *Pediatrics* 97:210, 1996.

81. Bose CL, Dammann CE, Laughon MM: Bronchopulmonary dysplasia and inflammatory biomarkers in the premature neonate, *Arch Dis Child Fetal Neonatal Ed* 93:F455, 2008.

82. Honma Y, Yada Y, Takahashi N, et al: Certain type of chronic lung disease of newborns is associated with *Ureaplasma urealyticum* infection in utero, *Pediatr Int* 49:479, 2007.

83. Colaizy TT, Morris CD, Lapidus J, et al: Detection of ureaplasma DNA in endotracheal samples is associated with bronchopulmonary dysplasia after adjustment for multiple risk factors, *Pediatr Res* 61:578, 2007.

83. Schelonka RL, Katz B, Waites KB, et al: Critical appraisal of the role of urea plasma in the development of bronchopulmonary dysplasia with metaanalytic techniques, *Pediatr Infect Dis J* 24:1033, 2005.

85. Hassanein SM, El-Farrash RA, Hafez HM, Hassanin OM, Abd El Rahman NA: Cord blood interleukin-6 and neonatal morbidities among preterm infants with PCR-positive *Ureaplasma urealyticum, J Matern Fetal Neonatal Med* 25:2106, 2012.

86. Frank L, Groseclose EE: Oxygen toxicity in newborns: the adverse effects of undernutrition, *J Appl Physiol* 53:1248, 1982.

87. Maritz GS, Cock ML, Louey S, et al: Fetal growth restriction has long-term effects on postnatal lung structure in sheep, *Pediatr Res* 55:287, 2004.

88. Massaro D, Massaro GD, Baras A, et al: Calorie-related rapid onset of alveolar loss, regeneration, and changes in mouse lung gene expression, *Am J Physiol Lung Cell Mol Physiol* 286:L896, 2004.

89. Maritz G, Probyn M, De Matteo R, et al: Lung parenchyma at maturity is influenced by postnatal growth but not by moderate preterm birth in sheep, *Neonatology* 93:28, 2008.

90. Bose C, Van Marter LJ, Laughon M, et al: Fetal growth restriction and chronic lung disease among infants born before the 28th week of gestation, *Pediatrics* 124:e450, 2009.

91. Silvers KM, Sluis KB, Darlow BA, et al: Limiting light-induced lipid peroxidation and vitamin loss in infant parenteral nutrition by adding multivitamin preparations to Intralipid, *Acta Paediatr* 90:242, 2001.

92. Watts JL, Milner R, Zipursky A, et al: Failure of supplementation with vitamin E to prevent bronchopulmonary dysplasia in infants less than 1,500 g birth weight, *Eur Respir J* 4:188, 1991.

93. Darlow BA, Austin NC: Selenium supplementation to prevent short-term morbidity in preterm neonates, *Cochrane Database Syst Rev* (4):CD003312, 2003.

94. Zlotkin SH, Atkinson S, Lockitch G: Trace elements in nutrition for premature infants, *Clin Perinatol* 22:223, 1995.

95. Gonzalez A, Sosenko IR, Chandar J, et al: Influence of infection on patent ductus arteriosus and chronic lung disease in premature infants weighing 1000 grams or less, *J Pediatr* 128:470, 1996.

96. Oh W, Poindexter BB, Perritt R, et al: Association between fluid intake and weight loss during the first ten days of life and risk of bronchopulmonary dysplasia in extremely low birth weight infants, *J Pediatr* 147:786, 2005.

97. Clyman R, Cassady G, Kirklin JK, Collins M, Philips JB 3rd: The role of patent ductus arteriosus ligation in bronchopulmonary dysplasia: reexamining a randomized controlled trial, *J Pediatr* 154:873, 2009.

98. Bhandari V, Bizzarro MJ, Shetty AH, et al: Familial and genetic susceptibility to major neonatal morbidities in preterm twins, *Pediatrics* 117:1901, 2006.

99. Nickerson BG, Taussig LM: Family history of asthma in infants with bronchopulmonary dysplasia, *Pediatrics* 65:1140, 1980.

100. Hallman M, Marttila R, Pertille R, et al: Genes and environment in common neonatal lung disease, *Neonatology* 91:298, 2007.

101. Przemko K, Miroslaw BM, Zofia M, et al: Genetic risk factors of bronchopulmonary dysplasia, *Pediatr Res* 114:e243, 2008.

102. Manar MH, Brown MR, Gauthier TW, et al: Association of glutathione-S-transferase-P1 polymorphisms with bronchopulmonary dysplasia, *J Perinatol* 24:30, 2004.

103. Prencipe G, Auriti C, Inglese RD, Ronchetti MP, et al: A polymorphism in the macrophage inhibitor factor promoter is associated with BPD, *Pediatr Res* 69:142, 2011.

104. Thébaud B, Abman SH: Bronchopulmonary dysplasia: where have all the vessels gone? Roles of angiogenic growth factors in chronic lung disease, *Am J Respir Crit Care Med* 175:978, 2007.

105. Thébaud B, Ladha R, Michelakis ED, et al: VEGF gene therapy increases survival, promotes lung angiogenesis and prevents alveolar damage in hyperoxia induced lung injury, *Circulation* 112:2477, 2005.

106. Fujinaga H, Baker CD, Ryan SL, et al: Hyperoxia disrupts vascular endothelial growth factor-nitric oxide signaling and decreases growth of endothelial colony forming cells from preterm infants, *Am J Physiol Lung Cell Mol Physiol* 297:L1160, 2009.

107. DePaepe ME, Patel C, Tsai A, et al: Endoglin (CD105) up-regulation in pulmonary microvasculature of ventilated preterm infants, *Am J Respir Crit Care Med* 178:180, 2008.

108. McCubbin M, Frey EE, Wagener JS, et al: Large airway collapse in bronchopulmonary dysplasia, *J Pediatr* 114:304, 1989.

109. Groothuis JR, Gutierrez KM, Lauer BA: Respiratory syncytial virus infection in children with bronchopulmonary dysplasia, *Pediatrics* 82:199, 1988.

110. Bancalari E, Sosenko IRS: New developments in the pathogenesis and prevention of BPD. In Bancalari E, editor: *The newborn lung: neonatology questions and controversies*, ed 2, Philadelphia, 2012, Elsevier Saunders.

111. Woodgate PG, Davies MW: Permissive hypercapnia for the prevention of morbidity and mortality in mechanically ventilated newborn infants, *Cochrane Database Syst Rev* (2):CD002061, 2001.

112. Meneses J, Bhandari V, Alves J, Hermann D: Noninvasive ventilation for respiratory distress syndrome: a randomized controlled trial, *Pediatrics* 127:300, 2011.

113. Schulze A, Bancalari E: Proportional assist ventilation in infants, *Clin Perinatol* 28:561, 2001.

114. Cheema I, Ahluwalia J: Feasibility of tidal volume-guided ventilation in newborn infants: a randomized crossover trial using the volume guarantee modality, *Pediatrics* 107:1323, 2001.

115. Reyes ZC, Claure N, Tauscher MK, et al: Randomized controlled trial comparing synchronized intermittent mandatory ventilation and synchronized intermittent mandatory ventilation plus pressure support in preterm infants, *Pediatrics* 118:1409, 2006.

116. Wheeler K, Klingenberg C, McCallion N, Morley CJ, Davis PG: Volume-targeted versus pressure-limited ventilation in the neonate, *Cochrane Database Syst Rev* (11):CD003666, 2010.

117. Johnson AH, Peacock JL, Greenough A, et al: High frequency oscillatory ventilation for the prevention of chronic lung disease of prematurity, *N Engl J Med* 347:633, 2002.

118. Saugstad OK, Aune D: In search of the optimal oxygen saturation for extremely low birth weight infants: a systematic review and meta-analysis, *Neonatology* 100:1, 2011.

119. SUPPORT Study Group of the Eunice Kennedy Shriver NICHD Neonatal Research Network, Carlo WA, Finer NN, et al: Target ranges of oxygen saturation in extremely preterm infants, *N Engl J Med* 362:1959, 2010.

120. Claure N, D'Ugard C, Bancalari E: Automated adjustment of inspired oxygen in preterm infants with frequent fluctuations in oxygenation: a pilot clinical trial, *J Pediatr* 155:640, 2009.

121. Davis JM, Parad RB, Michele T, et al: Pulmonary outcome at one year corrected age in premature infants treated at birth with recombinant human CuZn superoxide dismutase, *Pediatrics* 111:469, 2003.

122. Ballard RA, Truog WE, Cnaan A, et al: Inhaled nitric oxide in preterm infants undergoing mechanical ventilation, *N Engl J Med* 355:343, 2006.

123. Deneke SM, Gershoff SN, Fanberg BL: Potentiation of oxygen toxicity in rats by dietary protein or amino acid deficiency, *J Appl Physiol* 54:147, 1983.

124. Sosenko IRS, Innis SM, Frank L: Intralipid increases lung polyunsaturated fatty acids and protects newborn rats from oxygen toxicity, *Pediatr Res* 30:413, 1991.

125. Sosenko IRS: Polyunsaturated fatty acids: do they protect against or promote oxidant lung injury? *J Nutrition* 125:1652, 1995.

126. Darlow BA, Graham PJ: Vitamin A supplementation for preventing morbidity and mortality in very low birthweight infants, *Cochrane Database Syst Rev* (4):CD000501, 2007.

127. Howlett A, Ohlsson A, Plakkal N: Inositol for respiratory distress syndrome in preterm infants, *Cochrane Database Syst Rev* (3):CD000366, 2012.

128. Rhen T, Cidlowski L: Anti-inflammatory action of glucocorticoids: new mechanisms for old drugs, *N Engl J Med* 353:1711, 2005.

129. Henderson-Smart DJ, Davis PG: Prophylactic methylxanthines for endotracheal extubation in preterm infants, *Cochrane Database Syst Rev* (12):CD000139, 2010.

130. Davis PG, Schmidt B, Roberts RS, et al: Caffeine for apnea of prematurity: benefits may vary in subgroups, *J Pediatr* 156:382, 2010.

131. Lauterbach R, Szymura-Oleksiak J, Pawlik D, et al: Nebulized pentoxifylline for prevention of bronchopulmonary dysplasia in very low birth weight infants: a pilot clinical study, *J Matern Fetal Neonatal Med* 19:433, 2006.

132. Aslam M, Baveja R, Liang OD, et al: Bone marrow stromal cells attenuate lung injury in a murine model of neonatal chronic lung disease, *Am J Resp Crit Care Med* 180:1122, 2009.

133. Abman SH, Nelin LD: Management of infants with severe bronchopulmonary dysplasia. In Bancalari E, editor: *The newborn lung: neonatology questions and controversies*, ed 2, Philadelphia, 2012, Elsevier Saunders.

134. Brion LP, Primhak RA, Yong W: Aerosolized diuretics for preterm infants with (or developing) chronic lung disease, *Cochrane Database Syst Rev* (3):CD001694, 2007.

135. Rush MG, Engelhardt B, Parker RA, Hazinski TA: Double-blind, placebo-controlled trial of alternate-day furosemide in infants with chronic bronchopulmonary dysplasia, *J Pediatr* 117:112, 1990.

136. Wilkie RA, Bryan MH: Effect of bronchodilators on airway resistance in ventilator-dependent neonates with chronic lung disease, *J Pediatr* 111:278, 1987.

137. Halliday HL, Ehrenkranz RA, Doyle LW: Early postnatal (<96 hours) corticosteroids for preventing chronic lung disease in preterm infants, *Cochrane Database Syst Rev* (1):CD001146, 2003.

138. Greir DG, Halliday HL: Management of bronchopulmonary dysplasia in infants: guidelines for corticosteroid use, *Drugs* 65:15, 2005.

139. Yeh TF, Lin YJ, Huang CC, et al: Early postnatal (<12 hrs) dexamethasone therapy for prevention of BPD in preterm infants with RDS—a two-year follow-up study, *Pediatrics* 101:E7, 1998.

140. Watterberg KL: American Academy of Pediatrics. Committee on Fetus and Newborn: Policy statement—postnatal corticosteroids to prevent or treat bronchopulmonary dysplasia, *Pediatrics* 126:800, 2010.

141. Jadcherla SR, Gupta A, Fernandez S, et al: Spatiotemporal characteristics of acid refluxate and relationship to symptoms in premature and term infants with chronic lung disease, *Am J Gastroenterol* 103:720, 2008.

142. ten Bensel R, Paxson C: Child abuse following neonatal separation, *J Pediatr* 90:490, 1977.

143. Khemani E, McElhinney DB, Rhein L, et al: Pulmonary artery hypertension in formerly premature infants with bronchopulmonary dysplasia: clinical features and outcomes in the surfactant era, *Pediatrics* 120:1260, 2007.

144. Howling SJ, Northway WH, Hansell DM, et al: Pulmonary sequelae of bronchopulmonary dysplasia survivors: high-resolution CT findings, *Am J Roentgenol* 174:1323, 2000.

145. Greenough A, Alexander J, Burgess S, et al: Home oxygen status on rehospitalisation and primary care requirements of chronic lung disease infants, *Arch Dis Child* 86:40, 2002.

146. Anderson AH, Warady BA, Daily DK, et al: Systemic hypertension in infants with severe bronchopulmonary dysplasia: associated clinical factors, *Am J Perinatol* 10:190, 1993.

147. Laughon M, O'Shea MT, Allred EN, et al: Chronic lung disease and developmental delay at 2 years of age in children born before 28 weeks' gestation, *Pediatrics* 124:637, 2009.

148. Vrlenich LA, Bozynski MEA, Shyr Y, et al: The effect of bronchopulmonary dysplasia on growth at school age, *Pediatrics* 95:855, 1995.

149. Avery ME, Gatewood OB, Brumley G: Transient tachypnea of the newborn, *Am J Dis Child* 111:380, 1966.

150. Morrison JJ, Rennie JM, Milton PJ: Neonatal respiratory morbidity and mode of delivery at term: influence of timing of elective caesarean section, *Br J Obstet Gynaecol* 102:101, 1995.

151. Milner AD, Saunders RA, Hopkin IE: Effects of delivery by cesarean section on lung mechanics and lung volume in the human neonate, *Arch Dis Child* 53:545, 1978.

152. Barker PM, Olver RE: Clearance of lung liquid during the perinatal period, *J Appl Physiol* 93:1542, 2002.

153. Aslan E, Tutdibi E, Martens S, Han Y, Monz D, Gortner L: Transient tachypnea of the newborn (TTN): a role for polymorphisms in the beta-adrenergic receptor (ADRB) encoding genes? *Acta Paediatr* 97:1346, 2008.

154. Schatz M, Zeiger RS, Hoffman CP, et al: Increased transient tachypnea of the newborn in infants of asthmatic mothers, *Am J Dis Child* 145:156, 1991.

155. Gross TL, Sokol RJ, Kwong MS: Transient tachypnea of the newborn: the relationship to preterm delivery and significant neonatal morbidity, *Am J Obstet Gynecol* 14:236, 1983.

156. Bucciarelli RL, Egan EA, Gessner IH, Eitzman DV: Persistence of fetal cardiopulmonary circulation: manifestation of transient tachypnea of the newborn, *Pediatrics* 58:192, 1976.

157. Kasap B, Duman N, Ozer E, Tatli M, Kumral A, Ozkan H: Transient tachypnea of the newborn: predictive factor for prolonged tachypnea, *Pediatr Int* 50:81, 2008.

158. Garenne M, Ronsmans C, Campbell H: The magnitude of mortality from acute respiratory infections in children under 5 years in developing countries, *World Health Stat Q* 45:180, 1992.

159. Barnett ED, Klein JO: Bacterial infections of the respiratory tract. In Remington JS, Klein JO, Wilson CB, et al, editors: *Infectious diseases of the fetus and the newborn*, ed 7, Philadelphia, 2010, Elsevier Saunders.

160. Stoll BJ, Hansen NI, Higgins RD, et al: Very low birth weight preterm infants with early onset neonatal sepsis: the predominance of gram-negative infections continues in the National Institute of Child Health and Human Development Neonatal Research Network, 2002-2003, *Pediatr Infect Dis J* 24:635, 2005.

161. Stoll BJ, Hansen NI, Sanchez PJ, et al: Early onset neonatal sepsis: the burden of group B streptococcal and E. coli disease continues, *Pediatrics* 127:817, 2011.

162. Stoll BJ, Hansen N, Fanaroff AA, et al: Changes in pathogens causing sepsis in very low birthweight infants, *N Engl J Med* 347:240, 2002.

163. Ollikainen J, Hiekkaniemi H, Korppi M, Sarkkinen H, Heinonen K: *Ureaplasma urealyticum* infection associated with acute respiratory insufficiency and death in premature infants, *J Pediatr* 122:756, 1993.

164. Rocholl C, Gerber K, Daly J, Pavia AT, Byington CL: Adenoviral infections in children: the impact of rapid diagnosis, *Pediatrics* 113:e51, 2004.

165. Stoll BJ: Infections of the neonatal infant. In Kliegman RM, Behrman RE, Jenson HB, Stanton BF, editors: *Nelson textbook of pediatrics*, ed 19, Philadelphia, 2012, Saunders.

166. Naglie R: Infectious diseases. In Gomella TL, Eyal FG, Zenk KG, editors: *Neonatology: management, procedures, on-call problems, diseases, and drugs*, ed %, New York, 2004, McGraw-Hill.

167. Lesprit P, Brun-Buisson C: Hospital antibiotic stewardship, *Curr Opin Infect Dis* 21:344, 2008.

168. Faix RG: *Congenital pneumonia treatment and management.* Available at: http://emedicine.medscape.com/article/978865-treatment, 2009. Accessed March 8, 2013.

169. Hocker JR, Simpson PM, Rabalais GP: Extracorporeal membrane oxygenation and early-onset group B streptococcal sepsis, *Pediatrics* 89:1, 1992.

170. Lahra MM, Beeby PJ, Jeffrey HE: Intrauterine inflammation, neonatal sepsis, and chronic lung disease: a 13-year hospital cohort study, *Pediatrics* 123:1314, 2009.

171. Antonowiez I, Schwachman H: Meconium in health and disease, *Adv Paediatr* 26:275, 1979.

172. Schrama AJ, de Beaufort AJ, Sukul YR, et al: Phospholipase A2 is present in meconium and inhibits the activity of pulmonary surfactant: an in vitro study, *Acta Paediatr* 90:412, 2001.

173. Carbine DN: Meconium aspiration, *Paediatr Rev* 29:212, 2008.

174. Wiswell TE, Bent RC: Meconium staining and the meconium aspiration syndrome, *Pediatr Clin North Am* 40:955, 1993.

175. Rossi EM, Philipson EH, Williams TG, Kalhan SC: Meconium aspiration syndrome: intrapartum and neonatal attributes, *Am J Obstet Gynecol* 161:1106, 1989.

176. Wiswell TE, Foster NH, Slayter MV, Hachey WE: Management of a piglet model of the meconium aspiration syndrome with high frequency or conventional ventilation, *Am J Dis Child* 146:1287, 1992.

177. Moses D, Holm BA, Spitale P, Liu MY, Enhorning G: Inhibition of pulmonary surfactant by meconium, *Am J Obstet Gynecol* 104:758, 1991.

178. Bae CW, Takahashi A, Chida S, et al: Morphology and function of pulmonary surfactant inhibited by meconium, *Pediatr Res* 44:187, 1998.

179. Mitchell J, Schulman H, Fleischer A, Farmakides G, Nadeau D: Meconium aspiration and fetal acidosis, *Obstet Gynecol* 65:352, 1985.

180. Fraser W, Hofmeyr J, Lede R, et al: Amnioinfusion for prevention of the meconium aspiration syndrome, *N Engl J Med* 353:909, 2005.

181. Vain N, Szyld E, Prudent L, Wiswell TE, et al: Oro- and nasopharyngeal suctioning of meconium stained neonates before delivery of their shoulders: results of the international, multicenter, controlled trial, *Lancet* 364:597, 2004.

182. Ambalavanan N, Carlo WA: Meconium aspiration. In Kliegman RM, Behrman RE, Jenson HB, Stanton BF, editors: *Nelson textbook of pediatrics*, ed 19, Philadelphia, 2012, Saunders.

183. Kattwinkel J, Perlman JM, Aziz K, et al: Part 15: neonatal resuscitation: 2010 American Heart Association Guidelines for Cardiopulmonary Resuscitation and Emergency Cardiovascular Care, *Circulation* 122:S909, 2010.

184. Narchi H, Kulaylat N: Is gastric lavage needed in neonates with meconium-stained amniotic fluid? *Eur J Pediatr* 158:315, 1999.

185. Wiswell TE: Advances in the treatment of the meconium aspiration syndrome, *Acta Paediatr Suppl* 436:28, 2001.

186. Wiswell TE, Peabody SS, Davis JM, et al: Surfactant therapy and high-frequency jet ventilation in the management of a piglet model of the meconium aspiration syndrome, *Pediatr Res* 36:494, 1994.

187. Kinsella JP, Truog WE, Walsh WF, et al: Randomised multicentre trial of inhaled nitric oxide and high frequency oscillatory ventilation in severe persistent pulmonary hypertension of the newborn, *J Pediatr* 131:55, 1997.

188. Wiswell TE, Knight GR, Finer NN, et al: A multicenter, randomized, controlled trial comparing Surfaxin (Lucinactant) lavage with standard care for treatment of meconium aspiration syndrome, *Pediatrics* 109:1081, 2002.

189. Dargaville PA, Copnell B, Mills JF, et al: Randomized controlled trial of lung lavage with dilute surfactant for meconium aspiration syndrome, *J Pediatr* 158:383, 2011.

190. The Neonatal Inhaled Nitric Oxide Study Group: Inhaled nitric oxide in full-term and nearly fullterm infants with hypoxic respiratory failure, *N Engl J Med* 336:597, 1997.

191. Ward M, Sinn J: Steroid therapy for meconium aspiration syndrome in newborn infants, *Cochrane Database Syst Rev* CD003485, 2003.

192. Dargaville PA, Copnell B, Australian and New Zealand Neonatal Network: The epidemiology of meconium aspiration syndrome: incidence, risk factors, therapies and outcome, *Pediatrics* 117:1712, 2006.

193. Van Marter LJ: Persistent pulmonary hypertension of the newborn. In Cloherty JP, Eichenwald EC, Hansen AR, Stark AR, editors: *Manual of neonatal care*, ed 7, Philadelphia, 2012, Lippincott Williams and Wilkins.

194. Steinhorn RH, Abman SH: Persistent pulmonary hypertension. In Gleason CA, Devaskar SU, editors: *Avery's disease of the newborn*, ed 9, Philadelphia, 2012, Saunders.

195. Valdes-Cruz LM, Dudell GG, Ferrara A: Utility of M-mode echocardiography for early identification of infants with persistent pulmonary hypertension of the newborn, *Pediatrics* 68:515, 1981.

196. Thérèse P: Persistent pulmonary hypertension of the newborn, *Paediatr Respir Rev* 7: S175, 2006.

197. Steinhorn RH, Kinsella JP, Pierce C, et al: Intravenous sildenafil in the treatment of neonates with persistent pulmonary hypertension, *J Pediatr* 155:841, 2009.

198. Delaney C, Cornfield DN: Risk factors for persistent pulmonary hypertension of the newborn, *Pulm Circ* 2:15, 2012.

199. Loeb AL, Johns RA, Milner P, Peach MJ: Endothelium-derived relaxing factor in cultured cells, *Hypertension* 9:186, 1987.

200. Stenmark KR, Fagan KA, Frid MG: Hypoxia-induced pulmonary vascular remodeling: cellular and molecular mechanisms, *Circ Res* 99:675, 2006.

201. Gao Y, Raj JU: Regulation of the pulmonary circulation in the fetus and newborn, *Physiol Rev* 90:1291, 2010.

202. Drummond WH, Peckham GJ, Fox WW: The clinical profile of the newborn with persistent pulmonary hypertension: observations in 19 affected neonates, *Clin Pediatr* 16:335, 1977.

203. Walsh-Sukys MC: Persistent pulmonary hypertension of the newborn: the black box revisited, *Clin Perinatol* 20:127, 1993.

204. Kinsella JP, Abman SH: Clinical approach to inhaled NO therapy in the newborn, *J Pediatr* 136:717, 2000.

205. Berman Rosenzweig EB, Barst RJ: Pulmonary arterial hypertension: a comprehensive review of pharmacological treatment, *Treat Respir Med* 5:117, 2006.

206. Galli S, Bickle Graz M, Forcada-Guex M, et al: Neurodevelopmental follow-up of neonates treated with magnesium sulphate for persistent pulmonary hypertension, *J Neonat Perinat Med* 1:83, 2008.

207. Nakwan N, Nakwan N, Wannaro J: Persistent pulmonary hypertension of the newborn successfully treated with beraprost sodium: a retrospective chart review, *Neonatology* 99:32, 2011.

208. Khan TA, Schnickel G, Ross D, et al: A prospective, randomized, crossover pilot study of inhaled nitric oxide versus inhaled prostacyclin in heart transplant and lung transplant recipients, *J Thorac Cardiovasc Surg* 138:1417, 2009.

209. Ivy DD, Doran AK, Smith KJ, et al: Short- and long-term effects of inhaled iloprost therapy in children with pulmonary arterial hypertension, *J Am Coll Cardiol* 51:161, 2008.

210. Sitbon O, Beghetti M, Petit J, et al: Bosentan for the treatment of pulmonary arterial hypertension associated with congenital heart defects, *Eur J Clin Invest* 363:25, 2006.

211. Hutchinson AA, Yu VYH: Curare in the treatment of pulmonary hypertension as it occurs in the idiopathic respiratory distress syndrome, *Aust J Paediatr* 16:94, 1980.

212. Firth AL, Yuan JX: Bringing down the ROS: a new therapeutic approach for PPHN, *Am J Physiol Lung Cell Mol Physiol* 295(6):L976, 2008.

213. Rohana J, Boo NY, Chandran V, Sarvananthan R: Neurodevelopmental outcome of newborns with persistent pulmonary hypertension, *Malays J Med Sci* 18:58, 2011.

214. Kattan J, González A, Becker P, et al: Survival of newborn infants with severe respiratory failure before and after establishing an extracorporeal membrane oxygenation program, *Pediatr Crit Care Med* 2013 Jul 16. [Epub ahead of print]

215. American Academy of Pediatrics, Committee on Fetus and Newborn: Apnea, sudden infant death syndrome, and home monitoring, *Pediatrics* 111(4 Pt 1):914, 2003.

216. Barrington KJ, Finer NN: Periodic breathing and apnea in preterm infants, *Pediatr Res* 27:118, 1990.

217. Gauda EB, Martin RJ: Persistent pulmonary hypertension. In Gleason CA, Devaskar SU, editors: *Avery's disease of the newborn*, ed 9, Philadelphia, 2012, Saunders.

218. Ballard H: Apnea and periodic breathing. In Gomella TL, Eyal FG, Zenk KG, editors: *Neonatology: management, procedures, on-call problems, diseases, and drugs*, ed 5, New York, 2004, McGraw-Hill.

219. Stark AR: Apnea. In Cloherty JP, Eichenwald EC, Hansen AR, Stark AR, editors: *Manual of neonatal care*, ed 7, Philadelphia, 2012, Lippincott Williams and Wilkins.

220. Darnall RA, Ariagno RL, Kinney HC: The late preterm infant and the control of breathing, sleep, and brainstem development: a review, *Clin Perinatol* 33:883, 2006.

221. Aggarwal R, Singhal A, Deorari AK, Paul VK: Apnea in the newborn, *Indian J Pediatr* 68:959, 2001.

222. Peter CS, Sprodowski N, Bohnhorst B, et al: Gastroesophageal reflux and apnea of prematurity: no temporal relationship, *Pediatrics* 109:8, 2002.

223. Henderson-Smart DJ, De Paoli AG: Methylxanthine treatment for apnea in preterm infants, *Cochrane Database Syst Rev* (12):CD000140, 2010.

224. Henderson-Smart DJ, Steer P: Doxapram treatment for apnea in preterm infants, *Cochrane Database Syst Rev*(4):CD000074, 2004.

225. Darnall RA, Kattwinkel J, Nattie C, Robinson M: Margin of safety for discharge after apnea in preterm infants, *Pediatrics* 100:795, 1997.

226. Ramanathan R, Corwin MJ, Hunt CE, et al: Cardiorespiratory events recorded on home monitors: comparison of healthy infants with those at increased risk for SIDS, *JAMA* 285:2199, 2001.

227. Jeng MJ, Lee YS, Tsao PC, Soong WJ: Neonatal air leak syndrome and the role of high-frequency ventilation in its prevention, *J Chin Med Assoc* 75:551, 2012.

228. Greenough A, Dimitriou G, Prendergast M, Milner AD: Synchronized mechanical ventilation for respiratory support in newborn infants, *Cochrane Database Syst Rev* 23:CD000456, 2004.

229. Yu VY, Wong PY, Bajuk B, Szymonowicz W: Pulmonary air leak in extremely low birthweight infants, *Arch Dis Child* 61:239, 1986.

230. Macklin CC: Transport of air along sheaths of pulmonic blood vessels from alveoli to mediastinum, *Arch Intern Med* 64:913, 1939.

231. Plenat F, Vert P, Didier F, Ander M: Pulmonary interstitial emphysema, *Clin Perineonatol* 5:351, 1978.

232. Ibrahim CPH, Ganesan K, Mann G, Shaw NJ: Causes and management of pulmonary air leak in newborns, *Ped Child Health* 19:165, 2009.

233. Carlo WA: Extrapulmonary air leaks. In Kliegman RM, Behrman RE, Jenson HB, Stanton BF, editors: *Nelson textbook of pediatrics*, ed 19, Philadelphia, 2012, Saunders.

234. Alpan G, Goder K, Glick B, et al: Pneumopericardium during continuous positive airway pressure in respiratory distress syndrome, *Crit Care Med* 12:1080, 1984.

235. Venkatesh MP: Pulmonary air leak. In Cloherty JP, Eichenwald EC, Hansen AR, Stark AR, editors: *Manual of neonatal care*, ed 7, Philadelphia, 2012, Lippincott Williams and Wilkins.

236. Hoffer FA, Ablow RC: The cross-table lateral view in neonatal pneumothorax, *AJR Am J Roentgenol* 142:1283, 1984.

237. Arthur R: The neonatal chest X-ray, *Paediatr Respir Rev* 2(4):311, 2001. [Review.]

238. Chalumeau M, Le Clainche L, Sayeg N, et al : Spontaneous pneumomediastinum in children, *Pediatr Pulmonol* 31:67, 2001.

239. Kuhns L, Bednarek FJ, Wyman ML, Roloff DW, Borer RC: Diagnosis of pneumothorax or pneumomediastinum in the neonate by transillumination, *Pediatrics* 56:355, 1975.

240. Shaw NJ, Cooke RW, Gill AB, Shaw NJ, Saeed M: Randomized controlled trial of routine versus selective paralysis during ventilation for neonatal respiratory distress syndrome, *Arch Dis Child* 69:479, 1993.

241. Cohen RS, Smith DW, Stevenson DK, et al: Lateral decubitus position as therapy for persistent pulmonary interstitial emphysema in neonates: a preliminary report, *J Pediatr* 104:441, 1984.

242. Al-Nishi N, Dyer D, Sharief N, et al: Selective bronchial occlusion for treatment of bullous interstitial emphysema and bronchopleural fistula, *J Pediatr Surg* 29:1545, 1994.

243. Keszler M, Donn SM, Bucciarrelli RL, et al: Multicenter controlled trial comparing high frequency jet ventilation in preterm infants with pulmonary interstitial emphysema, *J Pediatr* 119:85, 1991.

244. Litmanovitz I, Waldemar AC: Expectant management of pneumothorax in ventilated neonates, *Pediatrics* 122:e975, 2008.

245. Morisot C, Kacet N, Bouchez MC, et al: Risk factors for fatal pulmonary interstitial emphysema in neonates, *Eur J Pediatr* 149:493, 1990.

246. Watkinson M, Tiron I: Events before the diagnosis of a pneumothorax in ventilated neonates, *Arch Dis Child Fetal Neonatal Ed* 85:201, 2001.

247. Narasimhan R, Papworth S: Pulmonary haemorrhage in the neonate, *Paediatr Child Health* 19(4):171, 2009.

248. Raju TNK: Neonatal pulmonary hemorrhage. In Donn SM, Sinha SK, editors: *Manual of neonatal respiratory care*, ed 3, New York, 2012, Springer.

249. Pandit PB, O'Brien K, Asztalos E, et al: Outcome following pulmonary haemorrhage in very low birthweight neonates treated with surfactant, *Arch Dis Child Fetal Neonatal Ed* 81:40, 1999.

250. Fuji AM, Carillo M: Animal-derived surfactant treatment of respiratory distress syndrome in premature neonates: a review, *Drugs Today* 45:697, 2009.

251. Kluckow M, Evans N: Ductal shunting, high pulmonary blood flow, and pulmonary hemorrhage, *J Pediatr* 137:68, 2000.

252. Finlay ER, Subhedar NV: Pulmonary haemorrhage in preterm infants, *Eur J Pediatr* 159:870, 2000.

253. Rao KVS, Michalski L: Intrauterine pulmonary hemorrhage secondary to antenatal Coxsackie B-2 infection, *Pediatr Res* 1:265, 1997.

254. Poralla C, Hertfelder H-J, Oldenburg J, Müller A, Bartmann P, Heep A: Treatment of acute pulmonary haemorrhage in extremely preterm infants with recombinant activated factor VII, *Acta Paediatr* 99:298, 2010.

255. Greenough A, Milner AD: Acute respiratory disease. In Rennie JM, editor: *Rennie & Roberton's textbook of neonatology*, ed 5. London, Elsevier, 2012.

256. Garland J, Buck R, Weinberg M: Pulmonary hemorrhage risk in infants with a clinically diagnosed patent ductus arteriosus. A retrospective cohort study, *Pediatrics* 94:719, 1994.

257. Cole VA, Normand ICS, Reynold EOR, Rivers RPA: Pathogenesis of hemorrhagic pulmonary oedema and massive pulmonary hemorrhage in the newborn, *Pediatrics* 51:175, 1973.

258. Courtney SE, Durand DJ, Asselin M, et al: High-frequency oscillatory ventilation versus conventional ventilation for very-low-birth-weight infants, *N Engl J Med* 347:643, 2002.

259. Malo J, Ali J, Wood LDH: How does positive end expiratory pressure reduce intrapulmonary shunt in canine pulmonary edema? *J Appl Physiol* 57:1002, 1984.

260. Pare PD, Warriner B, Baile EM, et al: Reduction of pulmonary extravascular water with positive end expiratory pressure in canine pulmonary edema, *Am Rev Respir Dis* 127:590, 1983.

261. Pandit PB, Dunn MS, Colucci EA: Surfactant therapy in neonates with respiratory deterioration due to pulmonary hemorrhage, *Pediatrics* 95:32, 1995.

262. Clyman RI: Recommendations for the postnatal use of indomethacin: an analysis of four separate treatment strategies, *J Pediatr* 128:601, 1996.

263. Tomaszcwska M, Stork EK, Friedman HG, et al: Pulmonary haemorrhage in VLBW (<1.5 kg) infants: correlates of death and neonatal and neurodevelopmental outcomes, *Pediatr Res* 43:230A, 1998.

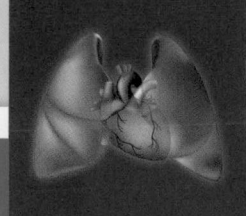

Chapter 23

Surgical Disorders in Childhood That Affect Respiratory Care

ALESSANDRA C. GASIOR, KURT P. SCHROPP

OUTLINE

Choanal Atresia
Macroglossia
Mandibular Hypoplasia
Esophageal Atresia and Tracheoesophageal Fistula
Congenital Diaphragmatic Hernia
Chest Wall Malformations
  Pectus Excavatum
  Pectus Carinatum
  Asphyxiating Thoracic Dystrophy
  Scoliosis and Kyphoscoliosis

Lung Bud Anomalies
  Incidence
  Clinical Correlation
  Bronchogenic Cyst
  Congenital Cystic Adenomatoid Malformation
  Pulmonary Sequestration
  Congenital Lobar Emphysema
  Follow-up
Gastroschisis/Omphalocele
Necrotizing Enterocolitis

LEARNING OBJECTIVES

After reading this chapter the reader will be able to:

1. Discuss the anatomy and pathophysiology of the various congenital anomalies and surgical conditions in newborns and infants
2. Recognize and manage an infant in distress resulting from choanal atresia or other upper airway anomalies
3. Recognize and manage the potential sequelae of upper airway obstruction from upper airway anomalies
4. Discuss the anatomy and pathophysiology of esophageal atresia with or without a tracheal fistula
5. Recognize and manage the signs and symptoms of esophageal atresia with or without a tracheal fistula

6. Discuss the development, anatomy, and pathophysiology of congenital diaphragmatic hernia
7. Recognize and perform the steps related to emergency management of an infant in distress resulting from congenital diaphragmatic hernia
8. Discuss the development, anatomy, and management of the problems associated with chest wall malformations
9. Discuss the anatomy, diagnosis, and management of the infant with lung bud anomalies and pulmonary cystic malformations

KEY TERMS

CHARGE syndrome
Congenital cystic adenomatoid
  malformation
Extracorporeal membrane
  oxygenation

Funnel chest
Gastroschisis
High-frequency oscillatory ventilation

Necrotizing enterocolitis
Omphalocele
VACTERL syndrome

Knowledge of the anatomy and pathophysiology of various congenital anomalies and acquired conditions in childhood is crucial to the proper respiratory care of these patients. Many times the respiratory therapist (RT) is the first caregiver to recognize that a pathological condition exists and may be able to make the preliminary diagnosis. This early knowledge can improve respiratory care, especially in emergent situations.

This chapter focuses on the anatomical and physiological characteristics of the most common congenital anomalies treated by surgery and focuses on the some of the new and sometimes controversial treatments.

CHOANAL ATRESIA

A newborn infant is an obligate nasal breather, so the presence of complete nasal obstruction by choanal atresia results in immediate respiratory distress and possible death by asphyxia. Choanal atresia may be unilateral or bilateral. During the newborn's first breaths, the tongue becomes directly associated with the hard and soft palates, creating a vacuum. An oral airway should be inserted and maintained to relieve the airway obstruction.

The exact embryological malformation causing choanal atresia is unknown; however, certain theories now point to a failure of mesodermal flow to reach preordained positions in the facial process. Any abnormalities in this flow would affect the normal penetration of the nasal pits and the thinning that allows breakthrough at the anterior choana.[1]

Choanal atresia occurs in approximately 1 in 700 live births, with females affected 2:1 over males. Unilateral choanal atresia is twice as common as bilateral choanal atresia. The majority of these atresias are due to bony obstruction or obliteration of the nasal apertures at either the anterior or posterior nasal choana. Fifty percent of patients with choanal atresia have associated congenital anomalies that are either craniofacial or part of a cluster of defects known by the acronym **CHARGE** (colobomas, congenital heart defects, choanal atresia, retarded development, genital hyperplasia, and ear anomalies). Choanal atresia is often associated with isolated congenital heart defects.

The clinical presentation of choanal atresia may be severe, with immediate respiratory distress that requires intubation or an oral airway. Unilateral atresia, which may present as a unilateral mucoid discharge, may not cause acute respiratory distress. Bilateral choanal atresia is a neonatal emergency. At birth, the infant with bilateral choanal atresia will require resuscitation to raise the suspicion of a bilateral defect. Alternatively, bilateral atresia or a secondarily obstructed unilateral atresia may present with a pattern of cyanosis cycling with momentary relief from obstruction. The neonate struggles to breathe normally and creates a vacuum between the tongue and the palate, resulting in obstruction and cyanosis. At the point of complete obstruction there is a cry of distress, and the mouth opens to allow relief.

A no. 8 French catheter is the best diagnostic tool for atresia in the newborn intensive care unit. If the catheter fails to pass through the nose into the oropharynx, choanal atresia should be suspected. The neonate is stabilized by immediately inserting an oral airway. Secondary anomalies should then be sought, and a facial computed tomographic scan with coronal projections, and endoscopy, should be performed to delineate the anomaly. The ultimate management is surgical correction. However, appropriate respiratory care by attending to airway, breathing, and circulation (ABCs) is of utmost importance and must be provided preoperatively to ensure that the oral or orotracheal airway is maintained until the infant can be brought to the operating room.

The surgical procedure addresses the required perforation of the atresia to establish and maintain adequate choanae. The timing and surgical approach depend on coincidental medical problems; however, infants weighing more than 1.5 kg may be operated on by the transnasal route. Recently, endoscopic repair with powered instrumentation has become more popular. However, many feel that this more modern technique is no better than the puncture, dilation, and stenting technique that has been the gold standard.[2] There are risks and benefits with each procedure. The direct visual access afforded by the transpalatal route was once preferred by many surgeons; however, now the transpalatal route is used infrequently because of the adverse risk to palatal and dental growth.[3]

Once the repair is performed, a standard folded endotracheal tube is used to stent the choanae in a U configuration. A 4-mm tube is usually selected for a full-term neonate, and a 3.5-mm tube is used for a premature infant.[4] A suction catheter is measured so that it passes through the end of the stent into the nasopharynx. The catheter is passed through each side of the stent to prevent obstruction. Postoperatively, suction and saline are used to ensure patency in the stent. Prophylactic antibiotics and steroid drops are given, and the stent is usually removed with the patient under general anesthesia. Continuing respiratory problems caused by nasal congestion may be expected for 3 to 4 weeks postoperatively.

The prognosis after reconstruction is excellent and generally without complication; the most significant complication is restenosis of the choanae. This is managed by repeated dilations of the choanae under endoscopic visualization with replacement of the stent. Rarely tracheostomy or long-term intubation may be required when choanal atresia is complicated by reconstructive maneuvers for other craniofacial abnormalities.

MACROGLOSSIA

Macroglossia, or a greatly enlarged tongue, causes respiratory distress by pharyngeal obstruction. Macroglossia can be associated with other disorders, such as Beckwith-Wiedemann and Down syndromes, or it may be due to congenital lymphangioma or hemangioma. The diagnosis is relatively straightforward, and polysomnography (as a result of associated obstructive sleep apnea) and pulse oximetry are used to evaluate the extent to which macroglossia affects respiratory function.

Treatment for macroglossia should be individualized, depending on the severity of respiratory obstruction and etiology. For isolated macroglossia, prone positioning usually relieves mild cases. More severe cases may require one of the many surgical techniques to reduce tongue size.[5] Lymphangiomas and small hemangiomas of the tongue may require excision, and large congenital hemangiomas commonly respond to systemic corticosteroid or interferon therapy. Chronic hypoxia and CO_2 retention are common sequelae of macroglossia and require close follow-up. Immediate intubation may be necessary, along with tracheostomy to temporize for reduction surgery.

MANDIBULAR HYPOPLASIA

Mandibular hypoplasia, or micrognathia, is generally found in conjunction with various other anomalies in conditions such as Pierre Robin syndrome or Treacher Collins syndrome. Pierre Robin syndrome is the most common of these associations, but the pathophysiology of respiratory distress associated with micrognathia is identical in the other disorders.

The primary features of Pierre Robin syndrome include micrognathia, glossoptosis (or posterior displacement of the tongue), and cleft palate. These features result in pharyngeal obstruction and respiratory distress. If left untreated, infants with respiratory complications such as airway obstruction, cor pulmonale, and pulmonary hypertension have a mortality rate approaching 30%. Other complications of Pierre Robin syndrome are failure to thrive, malnutrition, chronic hypoxia, and pneumonia. Recent polysomnographic studies using oximetry have demonstrated that hypoxia and CO_2 retention can occur without overt signs of airway obstruction.[6] Close monitoring and a complete evaluation must be performed before and for a time after therapy has been instituted.

Treatment for patients with micrognathia includes positioning, an intraoral or nasopharyngeal airway, and surgical procedures. Prone positioning combined with supplemental oxygen administration and carefully supervised feedings has been useful in treating mild forms of micrognathia. Intraoral and nasopharyngeal tubes or prostheses have been used in treating mild to moderate forms of micrognathia, but feeding difficulties limit the usefulness of these techniques. Surgical procedures designed to hold the tongue forward have been advocated for symptomatic and severe forms of the disorder. These procedures include suture transfixion, creation of lip-tongue adhesion with sutures, various sling procedures, and mandibular distraction. The most severe cases may require tracheostomy. All these treatments are designed to "buy time," because these disorders gradually improve with facial growth.

Great care must be used in treating these patients, and fiberoptic assistance may be required for intubation. Patients with Treacher Collins syndrome may be extremely difficult not only to intubate but to mask if there are temporomandibular joint abnormalities.[7]

ESOPHAGEAL ATRESIA AND TRACHEOESOPHAGEAL FISTULA

Esophageal atresia and tracheoesophageal fistula represent a clinical spectrum of different malformations. The most essential elements of their pathophysiology are the blockage of the passage of saliva or food by esophageal atresia and the aspiration of either salivary contents or gastric secretions through a fistula between the trachea and esophagus.

Esophageal atresia and associated tracheoesophageal fistula result from an unknown in utero malformation that is one of the better characterized embryological foregut anomalies. Separation of the dorsal foregut from the ventral trachea begins distally at the carinal area and progresses proximally. If these two structures remain fused during this process, tracheoesophageal anomalies occur as atresias, fistulas, or laryngotracheal clefts. Different embryonic studies have focused on the "ingrowth" of the epithelial ridge in this area, which must be uninterrupted for complete tracheoesophageal formation. For unknown reasons, this constellation of tracheal and esophageal abnormalities may be associated with other midline vertebral, anal, cardiac, and renal or peripheral limb anomalies, which are known by the acronym the VACTERL (vertebral, anal, cardiac, tracheal, esophageal, renal, limb) syndrome.[8]

Tracheoesophageal fistula and esophageal atresia have been anatomically classified to describe the presence or absence of esophageal atresia and whether there is an associated fistula (Figure 23-1). This has important management as well as operative significance.[9] The most common combination of lesions is esophageal atresia associated with a distal tracheoesophageal fistula (see Figure 23-1, *A*). More than 85% of patients will present with this form of the anomaly, which results in a blind-ending upper esophageal pouch of variable length associated with a fistula from the lower trachea or mainstem bronchi that leads into the distal esophagus. The second most common anomaly occurs in 5% of patients as isolated esophageal atresia with a proximal blind-ending pouch and a "long gap" of missing esophagus above a small distal esophageal pouch (see Figure 23-1, *B*). In 3% of patients, esophageal atresia may be associated with a proximal and distal tracheoesophageal fistula. In addition, there is the isolated tracheoesophageal fistula that presents without atresia and usually occurs in the lower cervical or upper thoracic area. This is known as the *H*-type fistula.

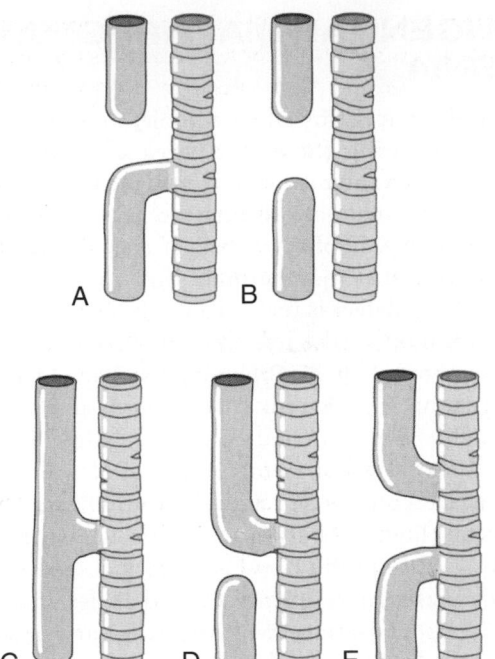

FIGURE 23-1 Five anatomical classifications describing tracheoesophageal fistula and esophageal atresia. **A,** Esophageal atresia with a distal tracheoesophageal fistula. **B,** Isolated esophageal atresia with a long gap of missing esophagus between proximal and distal esophageal pouches. **C,** Tracheoesophageal fistula without esophageal atresia, "*H* type." **D,** Esophageal atresia with proximal fistula. **E,** Esophageal atresia with both proximal and distal tracheoesophageal fistulas.

Finally, the fifth group represents 1% of patients who present with esophageal atresia with an isolated proximal fistula in the same configuration as seen with the isolated *H*-type fistula. In this condition, there is a "long gap" and then a small distal esophageal pouch with no distal tracheoesophageal fistula.

Drooling, along with frothing and bubbling at the nose and mouth, is the first symptom in the majority of newborns with esophageal atresia. The first feedings result in choking, coughing, and episodes of cyanosis. The respiratory distress may be severe and progressive, which should prompt an immediate workup for esophageal atresia. If esophageal atresia is suspected, a stiff nasogastric tube is introduced until resistance is met. The tube is connected to constant suction and irrigated with 1 to 2 ml of saline at frequent intervals.

Esophageal atresia with tracheoesophageal fistula occurs in 1 in 3000 births, with an equal male and female distribution. Because of the obstruction to amniotic fluid during fetal swallowing, polyhydramnios may be part of the perinatal history. The postnatal presentation of each type of anomaly varies significantly with the lesion and consequences of obstruction or aspiration. An isolated tracheoesophageal fistula may present as late as early adulthood with subtle symptoms of wheezing and recurrent respiratory infections often unresponsive to treatment. For infants

with larger fistulas, choking and coughing episodes will be frequent. Significant abdominal distention caused by excessive air moving from the respiratory tract to the gastrointestinal tract through a patent fistula may also be a presenting symptom. Auscultation of the chest may reveal murmurs from concomitant congenital heart disease or decreased breath sounds caused by atelectasis or pneumonitis.

Chest and abdominal radiographs are critical to the diagnosis. Several important radiographic findings are specific for esophageal atresia. The course and end point of the nasogastric tube confirm obstruction of the proximal esophagus by atresia and determine the relative position of the upper esophageal pouch. The lung fields must be examined to determine the presence of parenchymal changes resulting from aspiration. Changes in mediastinal structures give an early indication of congenital heart disease, and a careful search is made for the aortic arch to determine its left- or right-sided position. This is extremely important for surgical management because it directs the surgeon to an operative site away from the arch.

The next most important finding is the presence or absence of a gastric bubble. Proximal atresia with evidence of air in the gastrointestinal tract indicates a distal tracheoesophageal fistula, the most common form of the anomaly. A proximal obstruction without evidence of gas distally most likely indicates the presence of esophageal atresia with or without smaller fistulas. Other studies that aid in the diagnosis of related congenital anomalies include an echocardiogram, a renal ultrasound, and a vertebral spine film. The echocardiogram needs to be done preoperatively not only to identify heart defects but to help identify the aortic arch.

Once the diagnosis is made, the overall clinical condition of the infant dictates the timing of repair.[10] For patients who present with severe respiratory distress and low birth weight, mechanical ventilation is essential.[11] It may be necessary to perform an emergency procedure to divide a persistent distal tracheoesophageal fistula if delivered tidal volume is compromised and respiratory failure progresses. Operative maneuvers that allow placement of balloon catheters in the fistula or stapling of the distal esophagus have been described. The traditional approach is a right thoracotomy with an extrapleural dissection for direct separation and closure of the fistula and trachea. With improved antibiotics many surgeons have changed to a transpleural approach, worrying less about an empyema. Once that is accomplished, a primary anastomosis of the esophagus can be performed in larger, more stable babies.

The last few years has seen a great increase in the number of tracheoesophageal fistula repairs with minimally invasive surgery. It is hypothesized that there will be a better cosmetic result than with thoracotomy and also decreased scoliosis and pain. In a recent multi-institution study of 104 neonates with attempted repair with minimally invasive surgery, only 4.8% were converted to an open surgery. There was an 11.5% leak rate and 31.7% late stricture rate.[12] Long-term follow-up is needed to decide if this difficult surgery will replace the "gold standard" thoracotomy.

In esophageal atresia, the ability to successfully perform esophageal anastomoses has been lifesaving.[13] The most significant complications of primary esophageal anastomosis are stricture or recurrent fistula formation. These complications have important implications for postoperative respiratory care. Even infants with successful anastomoses have persistent respiratory problems. With or without complications, postoperative respiratory symptoms have been noted in up to 50% of patients. Complications range from apnea and bradycardia to aspiration, recurrent pneumonia, and even respiratory arrest.[14] The largest single cause of persistent respiratory disease is gastroesophageal reflux from either esophageal dysmotility or an abnormal lower esophageal sphincter. Infants with reflux have recurrent aspiration pneumonias that must be treated medically; however, many of these infants require further operative management with some form of gastroesophageal fundoplication.

Another large group born with esophageal atresia, with or without tracheoesophageal fistula, has persistent tracheomalacia.[15] This is a much more difficult group of patients to manage. For those with tracheomalacia with even the slightest esophageal stricture formation, however, dilation of the anastomotic stricture may alleviate much of the respiratory compromise. It is possible that recurrent fistulas or an undiscovered proximal fistula may be the source of persistent wheezing and respiratory difficulty. These fistulas can be diagnosed and defined with the use of a barium esophagogram with direct pressure injection at different levels of the esophagus.

With precise preoperative, perioperative, and postoperative management, the survival rate in infants with esophageal atresia has now approached greater than 95%. The respiratory care during each phase must be tailored with an understanding of the pathophysiology of each malformation and its related complications.

Clinical Highlight

A 36-week gestational age baby boy was born by normal spontaneous vaginal delivery. Apgar scores were noted as 1 at 1 minute, 6 at 5 minutes, and 8 at 10 minutes. Patient had continued apnea after deep suctioning and was subsequently endotracheal intubated. On examination, breath sounds revealed inspiratory stridor, a holosystolic murmur was noted, a nasogastric tube was unable to pass 10 cm, and resistance was met. The infant was also seen to have low-set, simple hypoplastic cupped ears. Echocardiogram revealed patent ductus arteriosus (PDA) with intact ventricular septum and hypoplastic right ventricle. The patient was diagnosed with CHARGE syndrome with choanal atresia, heart defect, tracheoesophageal fistula with esophageal atresia, and abnormal ears.

CONGENITAL DIAPHRAGMATIC HERNIA

The diaphragm forms when the pleura and the peritoneum fuse during the eighth week of embryonic life. During closure the pleuroperitoneal canals may remain open. These canals are located on the posteriorlateral portions of the diaphragm, and if they fail to fuse, abdominal contents may herniate into the chest cavity.[16] The resulting defect is termed a Bochdalek hernia and is more common on the left side (90%). The overall incidence is about 1 in 2500 live births. The defect ranges in size from 2 to 3 mm to complete absence of the diaphragm. The herniated contents cause compression of the developing ipsilateral lung bud. The contralateral side may be compressed as well from shift of the mediastinum (Figure 23-2). The lung tissue is hypoplastic, including the pulmonary vasculature, even on the contralateral side. Histological studies demonstrate increased musculature in the media of the arterioles. After birth, hypoxia, hypercapnia, and acidosis develop, causing constriction of the arterioles. This constriction exacerbates pulmonary hypertension and persistent fetal circulation.

The diagnosis of congenital diaphragmatic hernia (CDH) is now easily made on prenatal ultrasound. Clinically, infants with CDH usually develop respiratory distress shortly after birth. The diagnosis of CDH is confirmed by chest radiography but is suggested in a tachypneic newborn with a scaphoid abdomen. Breath sounds are often not heard on the side of the lesion, and heart sounds may be shifted away from the side of the lesion. After diagnosis, resuscitation is immediately begun. The aim is to prevent

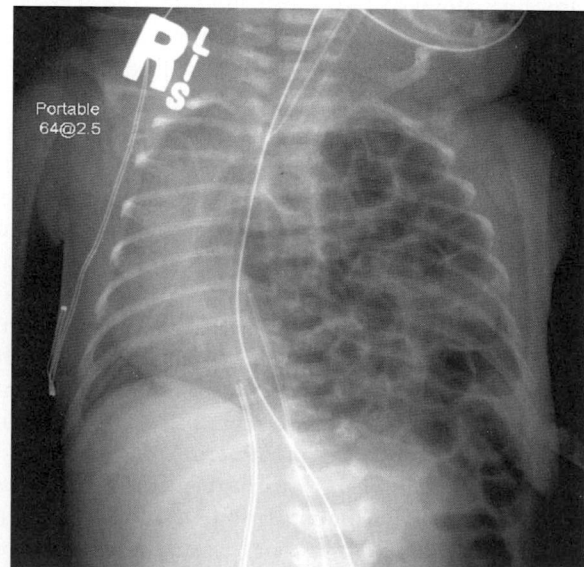

FIGURE 23-2   Radiograph of a left-sided congenital diaphragmatic hernia. Note shift of the mediastinum to the right.

hypoxia, hypercapnia, and acidosis[17] and includes the following steps:

1. A large orogastric tube is placed to decompress the gastrointestinal tract.
2. Bag-mask ventilation is avoided in order to keep the gut in the chest from becoming distended and causing tension pneumothorax physiology.
3. An endotracheal tube is inserted and the infant is placed on mechanical ventilation, avoiding high airway pressures.
4. Barotrauma may be avoided by using high-frequency oscillatory ventilation.
5. Maintaining alkalosis reduces the amount of pulmonary vasospasm. Traditionally $Paco_2$ values were kept between 25 and 30 mm Hg. But a recently developed protocol of "permissive hypercapnia" with increased $Paco_2$ and decreased pH seems to be safe.
6. If a pneumothorax is seen, chest tube placement is indicated. The pneumothorax is seen on the contralateral side and results from excessive ventilation pressures.

Operative repair of the hernia does not reverse pulmonary hypertension or hypoplasia. The timing of operative repair has evolved from immediate repair to delayed repair. Multiple studies have shown better outcomes by allowing the infant to stabilize and adapt to postnatal life.[18] Surgical repair decreases thoracic wall compliance, further strengthening the argument for the delayed operative approach.[19] A transabdominal approach is the standard technique for repair. If small, the defect is repaired with permanent sutures alone. Larger defects may require a prosthetic patch. After surgical repair, air may remain in the ipsilateral pleural cavity. The expanding lung does not completely fill the cavity, so technically a pneumothorax does not exist. The normal placement of a chest tube to suction may be detrimental, so it is used for gravity drainage only. Too rapid a shift of the mediastinum and contralateral lung may cause lung rupture or obstruct the vascular structures.

After operative repair, most infants remain intubated for several days. Low-volume strategies are continued. Elevated pulmonary vascular resistance may develop 8 to 24 hours postoperatively. This elevation will worsen right to left shunting, causing hypoxia and acidosis. Multiple modalities are used to decrease the amount of pulmonary artery vasospasm. Tolazoline, an adrenergic blocker, has been used in the past, but side effects, including fluid retention and hypotension, limit the use. The inotrope dopamine, when used at higher concentrations (10 μg/kg/min), causes vasoconstriction. Raising systemic vascular resistance tends to reverse the right to left shunt. High doses of dopamine also cause vasoconstriction of the gut, which is already at high risk for ischemia. Nitric oxide (NO) is a potent pulmonary vasodilator, and its use in pulmonary hypertension has been established.[20] A large, randomized clinical trial indicated that using inhaled NO for infants with CDH did not reduce mortality or the need

for extracorporeal membrane oxygenation (ECMO).[21] NO may be of benefit further along in the clinical course.

ECMO has probably increased the survival rates in neonates with CDH. This modality is often used to stabilize patients before surgery.[22] In recent years the use of ECMO for patients with CDH has decreased as different ventilator modalities, including high-frequency oscillatory ventilation (HFOV), are increasingly used. The use of ECMO at a large pediatric hospital was analyzed. The number of patients on ECMO had decreased as the number of alternate therapies had increased. Nitric oxide, HFOV, and surfactant were the main alternatives. Although the number of ECMO patients had decreased, the run time for each patient had increased.[23]

Experimental surgical treatments for CDH have been developed as well. Fetal intervention to include in utero repair of CDH was first performed in 1990.[24] Surgical techniques have been refined but survival has not increased. Currently no indications exist for in utero repair of CDH. With improved technique of fetal surgery this modality has been used for another surgical intervention, tracheal occlusion (TO). Experimental studies have shown reduced pulmonary hypoplasia with TO.[22] This procedure is currently performed at a few specialized centers, with long-term results unknown at this time.

CHEST WALL MALFORMATIONS

A wide spectrum of chest wall malformations is seen in children. These can range from mild deformities that have primarily cosmetic implications and the attendant impact on self-esteem to severe deformities with high morbidity and mortality.

Pectus Excavatum

Pectus excavatum is the most common disorder of the chest wall, comprising almost 90% of chest wall deformities. The defect may range for small, deep deformities to large, shallow deformities. The term **funnel chest** has often been applied. Deformity of the cartilaginous ends of the ribs causes an inward curve of the sternum. This inward curve will decrease the anteroposterior diameter of the chest, causing compression of the underlying structures. Familial cases have been reported; however, most are sporadic.[25] A male-to-female ratio of 4:1 is reported in the literature.[26] Connective tissue disorders are also associated with pectus excavatum; Marfan syndrome and Ehlers-Danlos syndrome are seen in 3% and 2.2% of patients, respectively.[27]

Most defects are noted in infancy and progress with the child. Neonates may present with chest wall retraction during respiration as a result of the pliability of the chest wall. This has been termed *pseudopectus excavatum* and often disappears at 6 months of age. During infancy the defect often has no symptoms, but as the chest wall becomes more rigid and activity is increased, symptoms often develop. With a decreased anteroposterior (AP) diameter of the chest, the lungs are not able to fully expand; therefore, exercise capacity decreases. The heart is often displaced, reducing ventricular filling, further decreasing exercise tolerance. Arrhythmias are another sequelae of the altered chest wall diameter. Significant psychosocial effects are seen in these patients. Causative factors of exercise intolerance and embarrassment in front of peers when the shirt is removed contribute to low self-esteem. Surgical repair has been shown to alleviate these effects.[28]

The age to undertake surgical correction has been debated in the literature. Repairing the defect at too early an age may limit chest wall mechanics and growth.[29] As children progress through puberty, cartilage ossifies. The ossification of chest wall cartilage will make more extensive procedures necessary in the future. Secondary scoliosis may also develop if the defect is not repaired. Although a consensus has not been reached, most symptomatic children should undergo surgical repair between 7 to 14 years of age. The standard open approach for repair of pectus excavatum was described in 1912 but was modified in 1949 by Ravitch.[30] This repair involves a transverse incision along the inframammary crease with exposure and resection of the involved cartilages. The sternum is then elevated and a strut is left in place. Within the last 15 years a minimally invasive approach pioneered by Nuss has been developed.[31] Bilateral incisions are made on the lateral chest, and a retrosternal bar is passed between the sternum and the heart. The bar is then rotated 180 degrees, forcing the sternum anteriorly. The bar is left in place, with annual follow-up appointments documenting growth and activity level. Most bars are left in an average of 3 years and then removed. Overall results are excellent and the morbidity of an open repair is avoided. The major disadvantage seems to be that the immediate postoperative pain is worse than with the open procedure.

Pectus Carinatum

Pectus carinatum, a defect that accounts for 5% of chest wall deformities, is the opposite of pectus excavatum. Pectus carinatum is usually seen later in life around a growth spurt. The protrusion is most commonly located on the lower sternum. Because the sternum protrudes, the underlying structures are not compressed. The primary complaint is cosmetic. Surgical repair involves costochondral resection and sternotomy.[32] Results are excellent with rare recurrence.

Asphyxiating Thoracic Dystrophy

Asphyxiating thoracic dystrophy, also known as Jeune syndrome, is a rare genetic disorder with an autosomal recessive inheritance pattern. This disorder is an osteochondrodystrophy that may have mild to severe expressions. The chest cavity is decreased in both the anteroposterior and superior and inferior orientations. Pulmonary development is often

blunted as a result of the decreased cavity size, and in the postpartum period the lungs are not able to fully expand. Multiple associated defects, including polydactyly, hypoplastic iliac wings, and fixed clavicles, may be seen. Heart, renal and airway abnormalities (subglottic stenosis) may also be present.

Recent surgical advances using prosthetic titanium ribs and expansion thoracoplasty have met with success.[34] The technique involves anterior and posterior rib osteotomies in ribs 3 to 9. This creates a mobilized segment that is then attached to the titanium prosthesis, which has been anchored to the second and tenth ribs. The procedure is done in two stages 3 months apart. Every 6 months the devices are expanded. This slowly expands the chest cavity and allows the lungs to grow more normally.

Scoliosis and Kyphoscoliosis

In their most severe forms, scoliosis and kyphoscoliosis may lead to secondary chest wall deformities. Scoliosis is curvature of the spine in a side to side direction. Kyphoscoliosis is curvature in both the coronal and sagittal plane. The resulting chest wall deformity seen with these malformations, especially early in life, often decreases lung capacity.

LUNG BUD ANOMALIES

The term *lung bud anomaly* broadly describes four pathological entities in a spectrum of parenchymal disease: bronchogenic cyst, congenital cystic adenomatoid malformation, pulmonary sequestration, and congenital lobar emphysema. The pathogenesis of these anomalies is poorly understood, but some speculation can be made based on known embryological sequences.[35,36] In early fetal development a tube of endodermal epithelium, the cellular covering of all body cavities, is present along the entire longitudinal axis of the fetus. This tube, the primordial gastrointestinal tract, is referred to as the primitive foregut. At approximately 3 weeks of gestation, a small groove appears in the floor of the primitive foregut, near the oral end of the fetus (Figure 23-3). The groove develops into a ridge, and the ridge branches into two blind pouches at its distal end. This ridge eventually develops into the trachea, and the thickenings are referred to as lung buds; the entire ridge with the lung buds will eventually migrate away from the main epithelial tube, thus separating the early pulmonary system from the esophagus.

As these endodermal structures develop, their blood supply is formed from primitive tributaries to the aorta—the fourth and sixth aortic arches. The lung derives its blood supply from two distinct sources: (1) the pulmonary artery (sixth arch), which brings oxygen-poor blood from systemic veins for oxygenation, and (2) the bronchial arteries (direct branches of the arch), which bring oxygen-rich blood to the parenchyma of the lung for nutritive purposes.

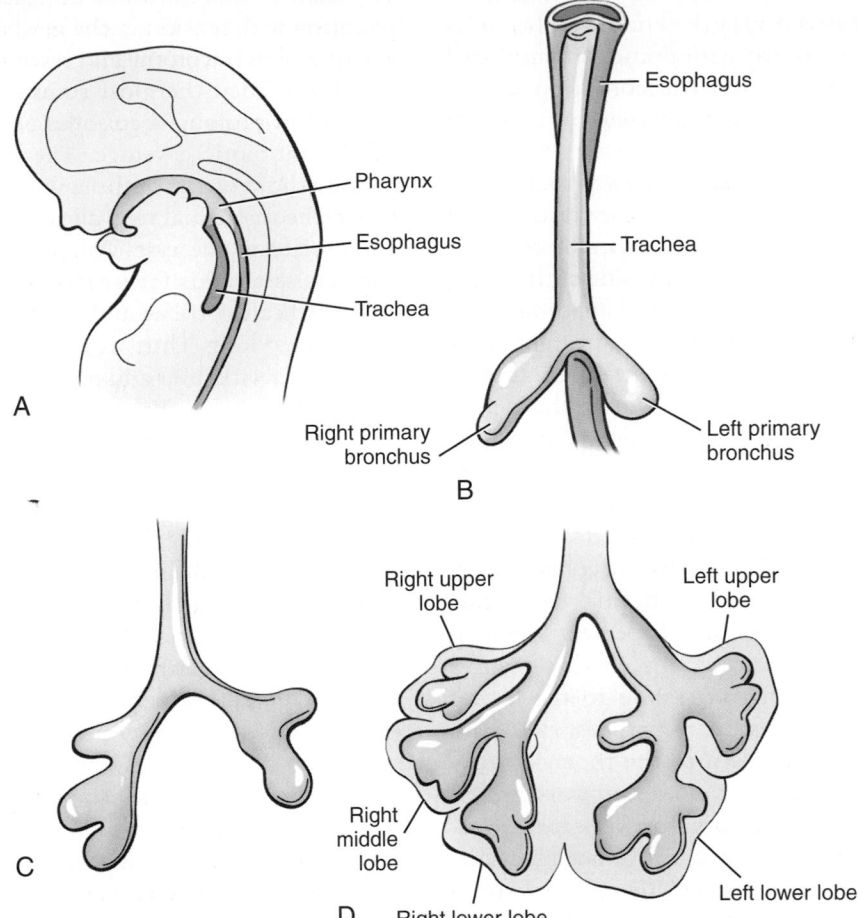

FIGURE 23-3 Developmental anatomy of the lung. **A,** The pulmonary tree develops from a common tube with the esophagus. By 3 weeks of gestation, the trachea (anterior) is separate from the esophagus. **B,** Two blind pouches that represent the left and right lung buds have appeared at the distal end of the primitive pulmonary system. **C** and **D,** Further dichotomous branching of the main bronchi results in the main lobes of each lung.

The budding part of the tube is composed of endoderm, a multipotential tissue in the embryo that forms the "business end" of each organ (e.g., the alveoli of the lungs, the mucosa of the gastrointestinal tract, the nephron of the kidney). The lung buds grow into the mesoderm, which is also a multipotential tissue that forms, in each organ, the connective tissue and the important supporting framework, including the blood vessels.

The interaction between these tissues is important in the development of each organ. In the primitive pulmonary system, the bud-forming endoderm induces important changes in the surrounding mesoderm that lead to a cohesive, functioning organ. Knowledge of these processes may help to explain how each anomaly occurs. For example, if both lung buds fail to form, the fetus would have bilateral pulmonary agenesis, which is incompatible with life; however, unilateral pulmonary agenesis is survivable. If the longitudinal groove with its attached buds fails to completely separate from the epithelial tube, a laryngoesophageal cleft or tracheoesophageal fistula may result.

Although the exact nature of the developmental cause behind each anomaly is unclear, I will speculate as to the embryological defect underlying the four lesions that compose lung bud anomalies as each anomaly is discussed.

Incidence

As a group, these entities are considered uncommon but not rare. Many factors make a precise assessment of the incidence extremely difficult. Some cystic pulmonary disease may result from barotrauma, rather than having a congenital origin. Asymptomatic patients may be uncounted because sequestrations may be silent for many years and become evident only during clinical investigation for unrelated complaints. Congenital lobar emphysema has been thought to resolve spontaneously, which may result in underestimation of its true incidence.

Clinical Correlation

Although these lung bud anomalies have different histopathological patterns, there are patterns in clinical presentation common to all. The presentation seems to follow two distinct patterns: (1) the condition becomes obvious in the early newborn period and is manifested by respiratory distress, and (2) the condition occurs later in childhood and is characterized by repeated infections.

Newborns may be identified in the delivery room if the lesion is so large that immediate respiratory distress and circulatory compromise result. A cyst or emphysematous lobe can obstruct blood flow to the right side of the heart, causing edema that results in a "hydropic" appearance.

In many cases, the distress is not readily apparent but is characterized by a progressive course of intermittent tachypnea over the first few days or weeks. During this period a chest radiograph may be taken and the diagnosis suggested based on location and character of the lesion. In lobar emphysema, there is a hyperlucent lobe with a surrounding zone of atelectasis. The atelectasis may be interpreted as pneumonia, and the hyperlucent abnormal lung is accordingly misinterpreted as normal compensatory hyperinflation. Intubation and hyperventilation in this situation could be disastrous. An emphysematous lobe will expand preferentially according to the law of Laplace. As it enlarges and pressure in the chest rises from the expanding mass, blood return to the thoracic cavity becomes impaired. As the infant's condition worsens, the clinician may mistake the emphysematous lobe for a pneumothorax because of its similar clinical behavior—a shift of the mediastinum to the opposite side and hyperresonance on the affected side. A chest tube inserted into this lobe may considerably worsen the situation.

An important aspect of the differential diagnosis includes a consideration that a "multilocular cyst" may actually be air-filled loops of bowel from a CDH. Auscultation for bowel sounds may help to differentiate these two problems, as will decompression of the bowel loops with a nasogastric tube (pulmonary cysts will not decompress). In some cases, an upper gastrointestinal series may be necessary to differentiate these conditions.

Presentation in the newborn is due to a mass effect in the small thoracic space. Bronchogenic cysts and cystic adenomatoid malformations do not have direct communications with the bronchial tree, but air can still enter these cysts through the pores of Kohn. Some cysts contain tissue so immature that they lack these pores, and air entry is not possible. These lesions, lacking a way for air to enter, are not likely to expand abruptly in the newborn period. Cysts with pores or emphysematous lobes, however, will enlarge with ventilation and can present under tension. Should a cyst rupture, the lesion may present mimicking a pneumothorax. This is rare and less common than a pneumothorax caused by insertion of a chest tube into an intact cyst. As a cyst or lobe enlarges, it may directly compress the trachea, a major bronchus, or the vena cava. Even without direct compression of these structures, the pressure rise within the thorax can cause mediastinal deviation with its attendant consequences of decreased venous return. Presentation with tension in the newborn period may require emergency thoracotomy and resection.

After infancy, the most common presentation is with repeated or prolonged episodes of pneumonia despite adequate antibiotic coverage. The infectious course arises because the contents of the cyst do not communicate with the tracheobronchial tree, allowing bacteria and debris to accumulate in the cyst. This material cannot be cleared and acts as a nidus for infection, which often spreads to adjacent healthy tissue and lymph nodes in the hilum of the involved lung. Thus, a small infected cyst can result in pneumonia with fever and purulent cough. Although antibiotics are helpful, they are not curative, and the underlying cause—that is, the cyst—must be resected to prevent recurrence of pulmonary infections.

The indolent course of this process may result in these children undergoing extensive diagnostic evaluation before the correct diagnosis is reached. There are usually numerous radiographs that, in retrospect, implicate a particular lobe. An ultrasound may have been obtained to evaluate cystic-appearing structures. Computed tomography or magnetic resonance imaging may have been used to elucidate airway anatomy and tissue density in the hope of securing a cause for frequent pneumonias. A child may have also undergone bronchoscopy to rule out aspiration of a foreign body. Bronchoscopy, however, has limited usefulness for the patient whose lung bud anomaly has already been diagnosed and could be dangerous if it causes complete obstruction of a lobe that previously was only partially obstructed. The diagnosis should be suspected when a febrile, septic child has a tube thoracostomy performed for drainage of a postpneumonic empyema and the cavity occupied by the now-drained fluid does not collapse, indicating an infected cyst rather than an empyema. Serial chest radiographs are the most valuable source of information in reaching the diagnosis.

Resection of the infected cyst is curative. Preoperative treatment with antibiotics is important. In patients with severe sepsis, initial simple drainage of the cavity may be required for temporary palliation, allowing time for optimal preparation of the patient before definitive surgery.

As prenatal ultrasound has improved in the last decade, it has become apparent that many of these lesions identified prenatally become smaller or completely disappear. Controversy, therefore, exists regarding the nonemergent treatment of these lesions, especially the small, asymptomatic abnormalities.[37] The correct treatment of these incidentally discovered lesions will evolve as they are more commonly treated at a later stage or nonoperatively.

Bronchogenic Cyst

The bronchogenic cyst may be thought of as a lung bud cyst, with endoderm that differentiates into respiratory epithelium but without normal bronchial components. It is therefore nonfunctional. These cysts can be located

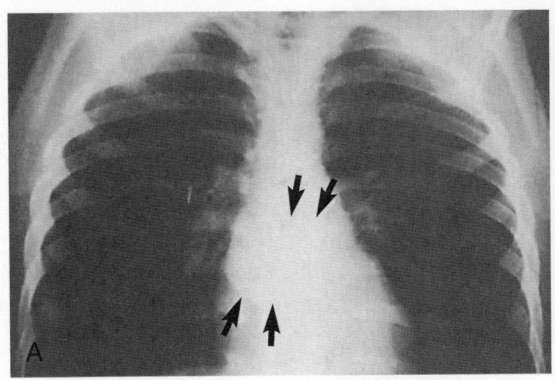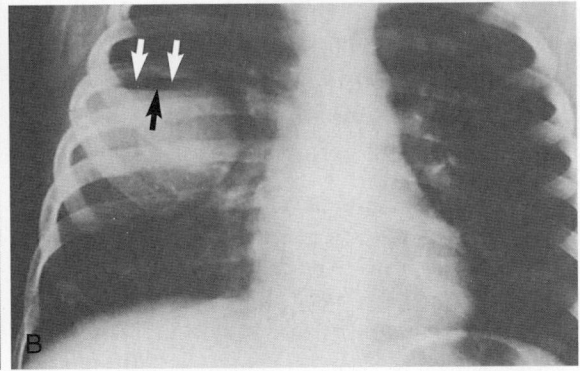

FIGURE 23-4   Bronchogenic cysts. **A,** Note the smooth border of the round, retrocarinal mass on this radiograph (*arrows*). **B,** Chest radiograph demonstrates an intraparenchymal mass that has become infected. Note the air-fluid level (*arrows*). This cyst is located on the right, which is typical of intraparenchymal bronchogenic cysts.

either within the thoracic cavity or outside it. When intrathoracic, the cyst can be in the bronchial wall, the pleura, the mediastinum, or the parenchyma of the lung itself. Ten percent of mediastinal masses are bronchogenic cysts. They are commonly located in the retrocarinal region (Figure 23-4, *A*). When intrapulmonary, they are usually on the right and may be multiple or multilocular (Figure 23-4, *B*).

The diagnosis of a bronchogenic cyst may be apparent radiologically in the newborn with respiratory distress, when the radiograph reveals a circular or ovoid mass with smooth edges. Similarly, the radiograph can suggest the diagnosis in an older child who presents with stridor, wheezing, or recurrent pneumonia.

Treatment of bronchogenic cysts is surgical excision. The extent of resection will depend on the location of the cyst and any associated inflammatory conditions. A unilocular cyst can usually be enucleated or removed by wedge resection and be an ideal case for a minimally invasive thoracoscopy. Lobectomy is performed in the exceptional case. A pneumonectomy is rarely needed.[38]

Congenital Cystic Adenomatoid Malformation

Congenital cystic adenomatoid malformation (CCAM), originally described in 1949,[38] has been recognized more often in recent years. In this lesion, differentiation of mesenchymal tissue appears to stop at the bronchial stage, before cartilage develops. The lesion is a hamartoma—that is, a disorganized overgrowth of embryonal tissue. This lesion reflects a failure of the inductive process, discussed earlier.

The morphological appearance of this lesion may be of a single large cavitary cyst (type I), multiple small cysts (type II), or a solid mass (type III). The CCAM may be multilobular and bilateral, but it is most commonly located in the left lung. The clinical presentation and radiographic diagnosis are similar to those of a bronchogenic

cyst. The surgical treatment usually requires a lobectomy and occasionally a pneumonectomy. Unlike a bronchogenic cyst, this lesion cannot usually be enucleated. Unless there is unusually extensive or bilateral disease, the postoperative course is smooth and the prognosis is excellent. Larger lesions, however, may be associated with pulmonary hypoplasia, hypertension, hydrops fetalis, and myocardiopathy. These features, depending on their magnitude, are associated with a severe prognosis. CCAMs are occasionally severe enough to warrant prenatal intervention ranging from thoracoamniotic shunt to fetal thoracotomy.[39]

Pulmonary Sequestration

Sequestrations are foci of mature lung tissue separate from the rest of the tracheobronchial tree, with concomitant failure of separation of the pulmonary and systemic circulations. The tissue may be either nonaerated or aerated through collateral channels (i.e., pores of Kohn), albeit with poor gas exchange. The sequestration typically has a systemic arterial blood supply (Figure 23-5). In intrapulmonary sequestrations the venous drainage is usually into the pulmonary veins; in extrapulmonary sequestrations the drainage is into systemic veins (azygos or hemiazygos vein, inferior vena cava, or right atrium). The extrapulmonary variety has a separate pleural envelope and may lie below the diaphragm. The defect in development may be caused by migration of an accessory lung bud before separation of the systemic and pulmonary circulations. Sequestrations are most commonly located in the left lower lobe region.

The patient with a sequestration may present with a variety of clinical symptoms, including a large shunt, a heart murmur, and heart failure.[40] A large, nonfunctional intrathoracic mass can present as obstructive respiratory signs such as wheezing and tachypnea. A common presentation is a recurrent febrile course with an occult infected sequestration.

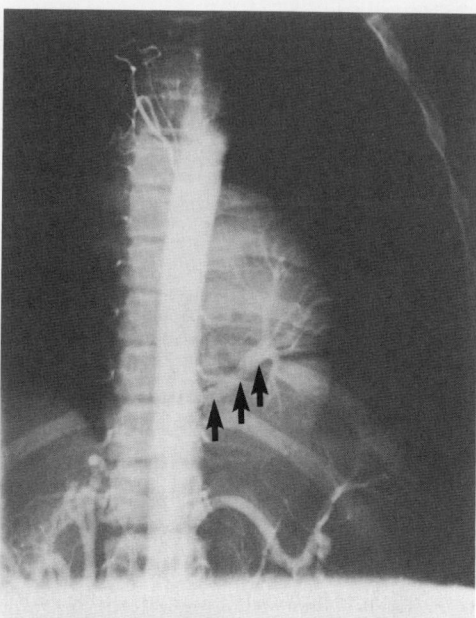

FIGURE 23-5 Sequestration. This aortic angiogram shows the segment of lung above the diaphragm that is supplied by a vessel from below the diaphragm (*arrows*). The splenic and hepatic branches of the celiac axis are seen below.

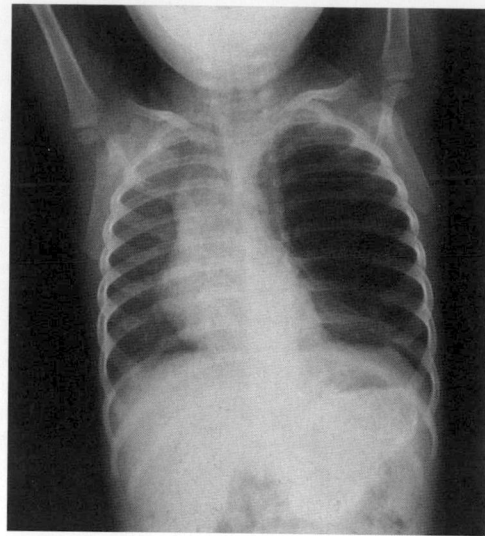

FIGURE 23-6 Radiograph of a newborn child with left-sided congenital lobar emphysema.

The diagnosis of pulmonary sequestration can be elusive. A space-occupying lesion with or without an air–fluid level is often seen on a plain chest radiograph.[41] If a sequestration is suspected, an arteriogram can be diagnostic and help define the arterial anatomy, which is crucial to successful resection. The systemic arterial supply may arise directly from the aorta, at times even through the diaphragm from the intraabdominal aorta. Injury or inadvertent division of this vessel without proper control may result in a hemorrhagic catastrophe. An upper gastrointestinal contrast study may reveal a fistulous connection to the intestinal tract.

Radionuclide lung scanning may reveal an unventilated but perfused mass in the chest. Finally, computed tomography can demonstrate extrathoracic lesions, and magnetic resonance imaging can visualize any abnormal blood supply. Resection of the mass is curative. Resection of the extrapulmonary variety is usually an easy thoracoscopic procedure, with the major risk being losing control of the systemic vessel.

Congenital Lobar Emphysema

Congenital lobar emphysema is an overdistention of one lobe of the lung, usually one of the upper lobes.[42] The lobe becomes distended because air enters but cannot exit, often because of obstruction of a segmental or lobar bronchus. Alternatively, there may be a defect in the cartilage so that increases in parenchymal pressure during expiration cause the bronchus to collapse.[43] This results in airway obstruction and air trapping. Additionally, an aberrant artery or vascular ring may compress the bronchus during

expiration. Regardless of the cause, the lobe becomes progressively more distended, eventually causing obstruction to air entry at the main bronchus or trachea and obstruction of venous return to the right atrium. These two conditions, separately or together, may constitute a surgical emergency.

The radiographic appearance may be confusing. Normal lung in proximity to the diseased lung tissue may be collapsed and appear atelectatic or consolidated (Figure 23-6). Thus, the child with respiratory distress and such a radiograph may be thought to have pneumonia, with the real diagnosis unsuspected. Recognition of this lesion is critical early in the symptomatic course because of the general tendency to hyperventilate a child in respiratory distress. In the case of lobar emphysema, such a maneuver would hasten circulatory collapse by rapidly overdistending the affected lobe. Without a confirmatory radiograph, a chest tube may be inadvertently inserted into the emphysematous lobe with disastrous consequences. Resection of the lobe is curative.

Follow-up

Children tolerate these operations remarkably well. Postoperatively the patient will have a chest tube that is usually removed within a few days of the operation but may have no tubes at all if the procedure was done thoracoscopically. Analgesics are important so that the child will breathe deeply and open atelectatic areas. For children too young to understand the use of incentive spirometry, instructing them to take the kind of deep breath required before blowing soap bubbles or spinning a windmill will achieve the same effect. Patient-controlled anesthesia in the older child, intrapleural or epidural anesthesia, intercostal blocks, and intravenous morphine are all important postoperative pain control strategies. Adequate analgesia also permits chest physical therapy, which is crucial in the recovery process.[44] Recovery is usually rapid, and normal growth is to be expected. When the child has an isolated lung bud anomaly, the prognosis is excellent. For bilateral or extensive disease, or when there are associated cardiac or genetic anomalies, the prognosis may be worse and is related mostly to the degree of parenchymal involvement or the associated anomaly.

GASTROSCHISIS/OMPHALOCELE

The development of the abdominal wall and gastrointestinal tract come from three embryonic folds—cephalic, caudal, and lateral—composed of splanchnic and somatic tissue. If these folds fail to develop normally, a defect is seen in the abdominal wall.[45] The two most common defects are omphalocele and gastroschisis.

When the lateral folds fail to fuse, an omphalocele will develop. This defect is always at the umbilicus and covered by a peritoneal sac, although this sac may rupture to expose the viscera (Figure 23-7). Omphalocele occurs early during fetal development, at the time of organogenesis, so other defects are commonly seen. These defects include cardiac, sternal, hindgut, and bladder defects, with cardiac being the most common. Approximately one third of patients have trisomy 13, 18, or 21. Diagnosis is often made during prenatal visits with ultrasonography. Elevated levels of alpha fetoprotein in the maternal serum and amniotic fluid are oftentimes present.[46] After delivery the gastrointestinal tract should be decompressed with nasogastric suction as well as digital rectal examination to assist with meconium passage. Small to medium defects are often repaired primarily. After reduction and repair, pressure parameters such as airway and intragastric should be monitored. Larger defects may require a staged repair. The first stage uses Silastic sheets or a spring-loaded silo to reduce the size of the sac to the fascial level and thereby permit definitive

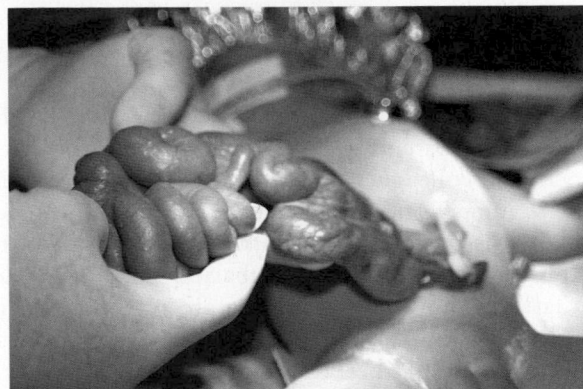

FIGURE 23-8 Typical appearance of bowel in a patient with gastroschisis.

closure.[47] The defect may include the liver, which should be handled with care to prevent liver laceration or hepatic vein injury. The incidence of omphalocele has decreased recently as more of these fetuses are aborted.

Gastroschisis is thought to develop when the umbilical coelom fails to form. The expanding gut cannot be contained in the peritoneal cavity and herniates to the right of the umbilicus[45] (Figure 23-8). The right umbilical vein reabsorbs, leaving a weakness in the abdominal wall allowing herniation. Gastroschisis has been reported on the left side but is extremely rare. This anomaly develops later in gestation than does omphalocele, so associated defects are not usually seen, with the exception of intestinal atresias, which occur in 15% of patients.[48] The herniated viscera are not covered by peritoneum, so this defect should be repaired early. After delivery, the gastrointestinal tract should be decompressed as in the case of omphalocele. Because the viscera are exposed, the infant should be placed in a sterile bowel bag up to the axillae to prevent evaporative fluid losses and to protect the bowel. Operative repair is aimed at reducing the viscera and closing the defect. Often this may be done primarily. In other cases the abdominal contents may be too distended to achieve primary closure. In these instances a Silastic spring-loaded silo is placed over the intestines (Figure 23-9). The spring-loaded portion is placed in the abdominal cavity and sutured to the skin. Sequential tightening

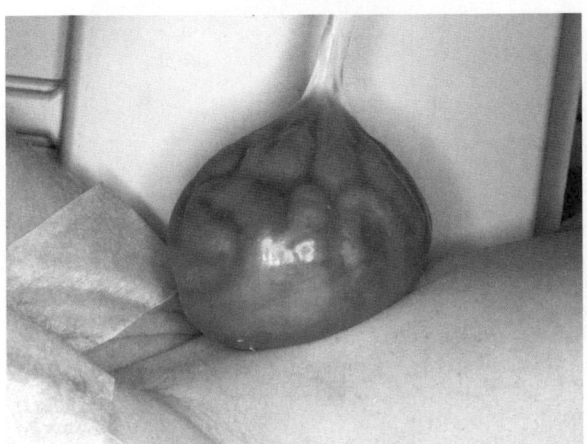

FIGURE 23-7 Baby with moderate-sized omphalocele.

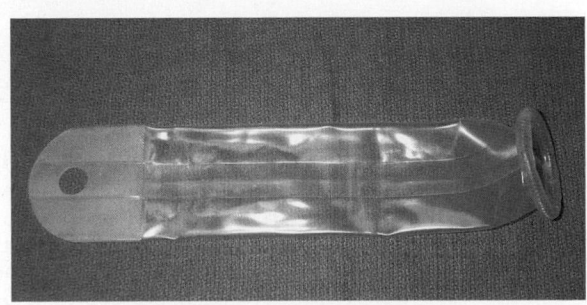

FIGURE 23-9 Spring-loaded silo.

of the sac reduces the viscera until they are contained within the abdominal cavity, which then allows definitive closure.

Recent reports in the literature have described different methods for closure of the abdominal wall defect. Bianchi and colleagues developed a method of reducing the abdominal contents without anesthesia in the neonatal intensive care unit. This technique avoids the complications of tracheal intubation and mechanical ventilation. The extent and the rate of reduction are monitored using the awake infant's reactions.[49] A sutureless closure has been reported by Sandler et al.[50] In this technique the eviscerated contents are reduced until they can be contained within the abdominal cavity and the defect is closed with the umbilical cord. Tegaderm dressings are then applied. The authors report better cosmetic outcome with the umbilicus in the natural position. The technique's simplicity is another advantage because this can be performed at the bedside.

NECROTIZING ENTEROCOLITIS

Necrotizing enterocolitis (NEC) is primarily a disease of premature infants, who account for approximately 90% of cases.[51] The cause of NEC is multifactorial with ischemia and necrotic tissue being the result. The introduction of enteral feeds to the premature gut is thought to be the initial inciting factor. Neutrophils are released, followed by inflammatory mediators that contribute to tissue injury. Specific mediators include platelet-activating factor, tumor necrosis factor, and NO.[52] Inflammatory mediators

also increase the release of acute phase proteins from the liver. Enteral bacteria also play a role, most likely an opportunistic one.

Infants with NEC will present with abdominal distention, intolerance to feeds, rectal bleeding, and abdominal wall erythema. Laboratory values include thrombocytopenia, neutropenia, and metabolic acidosis. Severe acidosis may require intubation and mechanical ventilation. The diagnosis is confirmed radiographically. Distended loops are seen, and pneumatosis intestinalis is pathognomic. Air may be seen in the portal system as well. Pneumoperitoneum confirms a perforated viscus necessitating operation.

Treatment of NEC is nonoperative in the majority of cases. Fluid resuscitation, antibiotics (ampicillin, gentamicin, clindamycin), and nasogastric decompression are the mainstays of therapy. Eighty percent of patients will not require surgery. The management of severe NEC has evolved over the last 20 years. Ein and associates[53] reported their experience with peritoneal drainage using local anesthesia. Their technique involves insertion of a Penrose drain, most often in the right lower quadrant. In 32% of patients this was the definitive management. In this study drainage was used in infants weighing less than 1500 g and provided a stabilizing modality for seriously ill neonates. Peritoneal drainage was used by Morgan et al. for infants weighing less than 1500 g with severe NEC. They reported 62% of patients requiring no laparotomy.[54] Infants with documented perforation and who are stable are taken to surgery for laparotomy (Figure 23-10). The operative approach is to preserve the maximal amount of bowel. Stricture formation is

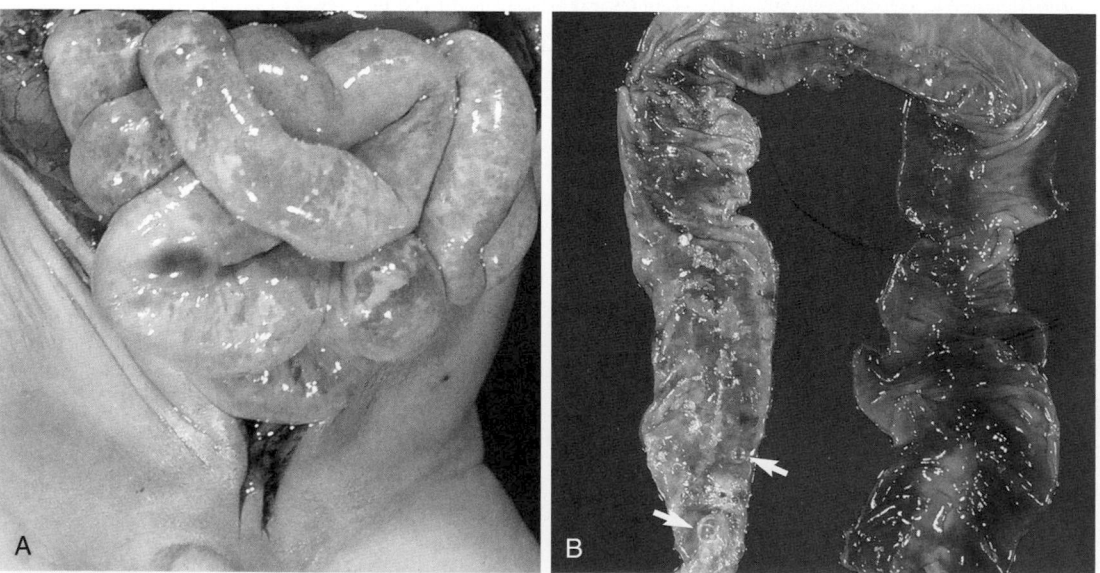

FIGURE 23-10   A, Postmortem examination in a severe case of necrotizing enterocolitis shows the entire small bowel is markedly distended with a perilously thin wall (usually this implies impending perforation). **B,** The congested portion of the ileum corresponds to areas of hemorrhagic infarction and transmural necrosis microscopically. Submucosal gas bubbles can be seen in several areas (*arrows*).

commonly seen in NEC patients, with the colon being the most common site. The overall survival for NEC is between 60% and 70%. Infants with NEC and very low birth weight who require surgery have neurodevelopmental delays when compared with equal-weight infants without NEC.[52]

KEY POINTS

- Infants diagnosed with choanal atresia have immediate respiratory distress and are at risk of death by asphyxia. An oral airway should be inserted and maintained until the infant is taken to the operating room for definitive care.
- Treatment for macroglossia is dependent on the severity of respiratory obstruction and may requirement treatments ranging from simple prone positioning to surgical reduction of tongue.
- Esophageal atresia and tracheoesophageal fistula most commonly present with a blind-ending upper esophageal pouch with an associated fistula from the lower trachea that leads to the distal esophagus.
- Symptoms associated with esophageal atresia with tracheoesophageal fistula include drooling, choking, and cyanosis with feeding and inability to pass a nasogastric tube. Continuous suction of the nasogastric tube with frequent saline irrigations should be initiated to avoid aspiration and respiratory complications.
- The in utero formation of the diaphragm occurs during the eighth month of gestation. Failure of closure is most commonly on the left side, called a Bochdalek hernia. This causes herniation of abdominal contents, subsequent compression of the contralateral side, mediastinal shift, and pulmonary hypoplasia.
- Infants with congenital diaphragmatic hernia present in respiratory distress. Immediate gastric decompression with an orogastric tube, endotracheal tube intubation with avoidance of excessive bag-mask ventilation, and ventilator high airway pressures, as well as permissive alkalosis to prevent pulmonary vasospasm, are necessary to avoid complications.
- Pectus excavatum occurs as a result of deformity of the cartilaginous ends of the rib causing inward curvature of the sternum. Surgical correction includes passing a retrosternal bar between the sternum and heart, then rotating the bar 180 degrees to force the sternum anteriorly. Pectus carinatum is a protrusion of the lower sternum that occurs during the pubertal growth spurt. Surgical correction includes costochondral resection and sternotomy, primarily for cosmetic enhancement.
- Bronchogenic cysts and congenital cystic adenomatoid malformations both may present in the newborn with respiratory distress or in an older child with asthmalike symptoms or recurrent pneumonia. Pulmonary sequestrations present with a large shunt, heart murmur, obstructive respiratory symptoms, or even recurrent fevers. Congenital lobar emphysema may present with airway obstruction at the main bronchus or trachea requiring emergent surgical intervention.

ASSESSMENT QUESTIONS

See Evolve Resources for the answers.

1. An infant brought to the neonatal intensive care unit (NICU) presents with cyanosis and upper airway obstruction relieved by crying with improvement in color. Suspecting choanal atresia, the best action is to:
   A. Insert a no. 8 French suction catheter to verify the diagnosis
   B. Insert an oral airway
   C. Start nasal continuous positive airway pressure
   D. Provide heated humidity
   E. Stimulate the infant to induce crying

2. Complications related to chronic upper airway obstruction from anatomical malformations result in which of the following?
   I. Chronic hypoxia and CO_2 retention
   II. Pulmonary hypertension and cor pulmonale
   III. Hyperventilation and acidosis
   IV. Failure to thrive
   V. Congestive heart failure
      A. I, III
      B. I, II, IV
      C. I, II, III, V
      D. II, III, IV
      E. II, IV, V

3. The most common tracheoesophageal fistula and esophageal atresia lesion is classified as which type?
   A. Esophageal atresia with a long gap
   B. Esophageal atresia with distal tracheoesophageal fistula
   C. *H*-type tracheoesophageal fistula
   D. Esophageal atresia with proximal fistula
   E. Esophageal atresia with proximal and distal tracheoesophageal fistulas

4. A drooling newborn infant with polyhydramnios in utero and suspected kidney and cardiac anomalies is admitted to the NICU and presents with coughing, respiratory distress, and cyanosis during feedings. The most likely diagnosis is:
   A. Gastroschisis
   B. Tetralogy of Fallot
   C. Pulmonary sequestration
   D. Esophageal atresia with tracheoesophageal fistula
   E. Choanal atresia

5. Which of the following are true concerning a congenital diaphragmatic hernia?
   I. Pulmonary hypoplasia is present in both lungs.
   II. Persistent pulmonary hypertension is the main complication.
   III. Surgical correction results in complete reversal of the respiratory distress.
   IV. CDH formation is a defect that occurs very early in gestational age.
   V. The right lung (contralateral side) is not usually affected.
      A. I, II, IV
      B. I, III, IV, V
      C. I, IV, V
      D. II, III, IV, V
      E. II, III, V

6. A 3200-g term infant male is born to a healthy mother. Apgar scores are 7 and 5 with the infant gasping and heart rate decreasing to 90. Physical examination reveals cyanosis, a scaphoid abdomen, and visible tracheal deviation to the right. Considering this information, the *only* appropriate action would be to:
   A. Get a blood gas
   B. Bag-mask ventilate
   C. Suction and stimulate vigorously
   D. Insert an oral suction catheter to vent the stomach
   E. Vigorously stimulate and give 100% O$_2$ blow-by

7. Considering a likely diagnosis of congenital diaphragmatic hernia, which of the following would be an appropriate decision concerning ventilator strategy(s)?
   A. Hypoxic gases
   B. Rapid rate and low pressures
   C. High pressure and long inflation times
   D. Slow rate and short inflation times
   E. Low pressure with high PEEP

8. A female infant was born with a large gastroschisis anomaly. The reduction surgery will most likely affect the respiratory system by causing:
   A. An increase in airway resistance
   B. A decrease in pulmonary compliance
   C. A decrease in transpulmonary pressure
   D. An increase in the respiratory time constant
   E. B and D

9. When comparing gastroschisis and omphalocele, which of the following is true?
   A. They are both full-thickness defects of the abdominal wall.
   B. They are both commonly associated with other anomalies.
   C. Omphalocele is a midline defect, whereas a gastroschisis is a lateral wall defect.
   D. An omphalocele is covered by epidermal tissue.
   E. Gastroschisis requires surgical reductions that often must be performed in several stages, whereas omphalocele is completed in a single surgery.

10. Pectus excavatum may be associated with which of the following?
    A. Secondary scoliosis
    B. Decreased exercise capacity
    C. Ehlers-Danlos syndrome
    D. Decreased self-esteem
    E. All of the above

11. Although the lung bud anomalies have different histopathology, clinical presentation usually:
    A. Becomes obvious in the early newborn period and is manifested by respiratory distress
    B. Becomes obvious in the early newborn period and is manifested by recurrent pulmonary infections
    C. Develops later in childhood and is characterized by severe respiratory distress
    D. Remains undetected until adolescence or early adulthood
    E. Presents as severe respiratory distress requiring mechanical ventilation

References

1. Hengerer AS, Strome M: Choanal atresia: a new embryologic theory and its influence in surgical management, *Laryngoscope* 92:913, 1982.
2. Gujrathi CS, Daniel SJ, James AL: Management of bilateral choanal atresia in the neonate: an institutional review, *Int J Pediatr Otorhinolaryngol* 68:399, 2004.
3. Tneogaray T, Dawson S: Practical management of congenital choanal atresia, *Plast Reconstr Surg* 72:634, 1981.
4. Cotton RT, Stith JA: Choanal atresia in current therapy in otolaryngology. In Gates GA, editor: *Head and neck surgery*, vol 3, Philadelphia, 1987, BC Decker.
5. Wang J, Goodger NM, Pogrel MA: The role of tongue reduction, *Oral Surg Oral Med Oral Pathol Oral Radiol Endod* 95:269, 2003.
6. Freed G, Pearlman MA, Brown AS, et al: Polysomnographic indications for surgical intervention in Pierre Robin sequence: acute airway management and follow-up studies after repair and take-down of tongue-lip adhesion, *Cleft Palate J* 25:151, 1988.
7. Nargozian C: The airway in patients with craniofacial abnormalities, *Pediatic Anesthesia* 14 53, 2004.
8. Quan L, Smith DW, The VATER association: Vertebral defects, anal atresia, T-E fistula with esophageal atresia, radial and renal dysplasia: a spectrum of associated defects, *J Pediatr* 104:7, 1973.
9. Aschcraft KW, Holder TM: The story of esophageal atresia and tracheoesophageal fistula, *Surgery* 65:332, 1969.
10. Weber TR, Smith W, Grosfeld JL: Surgical experience in infants with the VATER association, *J Pediatr Surg* 15:849, 1980.
11. Templeton JM, Templeton JJ, Schnaufer, et al: Management of esophageal atresia and tracheoesophageal fistula in the neonate with severe respiratory distress syndrome, *J Pediatr Surg* 20:394, 1985.
12. Holcomb GW III, Rothenberg SS, Bax KM, et al: Thoracoscopic repair of esophageal atresia and tracheoesophageal fistula: a multi-institutional analysis, *Ann Surg* 242:422, 2005.
13. Randolph JG, Newman KD, Anderson KD: Current results in repair of esophageal atresia with tracheoesophageal fistula using physiologic status as a guide to therapy, *Ann Surg* 209:524, 1989.
14. Delius RE, Wheatly MJ, Coran AG: Etiology and management of respiratory complications after repair of esophageal atresia with tracheoesophageal fistula, *Surgery* 112:527, 1992.
15. Davies MRQ, Cywes S: The flaccid trachea and tracheoesophageal congenital anomalies, *J Pediatr Surg* 13:363, 1978.
16. Skandalakis JE, Gray SW, Ricketts RR: The diaphragm. In Skandalakis JL, Gray SW, editors: *Embryology for surgeons*, ed 2, Baltimore, 1994, Williams and Wilkins, pp 491–493.
17. Cartlidge PH, Mann NP, Kapila L: Preoperative stabilization in congenital diaphragmatic hernia, *Arch Dis Child* 61:1226, 1986.
18. Breaux CW, Rouse TM, Cain WS: Improvement in survival of patients with congenital diaphragmatic hernia utilizing a strategy of delayed repair after medical and/or extracorporeal membrane oxygenation stabilization, *J Pediatr Surg* 26:333, 1991.
19. Sakai H, Tamura M, Hosokawa Y, et al: Effect of surgical repair on respiratory mechanics in congenital diaphragmatic hernia, *J Pediatr* 111:432, 1987.
20. Kinsella JP, Abman SH: Inhaled nitric oxide therapy for persistent pulmonary hypertension of the newborn, *Pediatrics* 91:997, 1993.
21. The Neonatal Inhaled Nitric Oxide Group (NINOS): Inhaled nitric oxide and hypoxic respiratory failure in infants with congenital diaphragmatic hernia, *Pediatrics* 99:838, 1997.

22. Tsao K, Lally KP: Congenital diaphragmatic hernia and eventration. In Holcomb GW III, Murphy JP, editors: *Pediatric surgery*, ed 5, Philadelphia, 2010, Saunders, 2010, pp 304–321.

23. Wilson JM, Bower LK, Thompson JE, et al: ECMO in evolution: the impact of changing patient demographics and alternative therapies on ECMO, *J Pediatr Surg* 31:1116, 1996.

24. Harrison MR, Langer JC, Adzick NS, et al: Correction of congenital diaphragmatic hernia in utero. V: Initial clinical experience, *J Pediatr Surg* 25:47, 1990.

25. Ravitch MM: *Congenital deformities of the chest wall and their operative correction*, Philadelphia, 1977, WB Saunders.

26. Shamberger RC: Congenital chest wall deformities. In Holcomb GW III, Murphy JP, editors: *Pediatric surgery*, ed 5, Philadelphia, 1998, Elsevier, pp 787–817.

27. Nuss D, Kelly RE: Congenital chest wall deformities. In Holcomb GW III, Murphy JP, editors: *Pediatric surgery*, ed 5, Philadelphia, 2010, Saunders, pp 249–265.

28. Lawson ML, et al: A pilot study of the impact of surgical repair on disease-specific quality of life among patients with pectus excavatum, *J Pediatr Surg* 38:916, 2003.

29. Haller JA, Colombani PM, Humphries CT et al: Chest wall constriction after too extensive and too early operations for pectus excavatum, *Ann Thorac Surg* 61:1618, 1996.

30. Ravitch MM: The operative treatment of pectus excavatum, *Ann Surg* 129:429, 1949.

31. Nuss D, et al: A 10-year review of a minimally invasive technique for the correction of pectus excavatum, *J Pediatr Surg* 33:545, 1998.

32. Ravitch MM: The operative correction of pectus carinatum (pigeon breast), *Ann Surg* 151:705, 1960.

33. Oberklaid F, Danks DM, Mayne V, et al: Asphyxiating thoracic dysplasia, *Arch Dis Child* 52:758, 1977.

34. Campbell RM, Hell-Vocke AK: Growth of the thoracic spine in congenital scoliosis after expansion thoracoplasty, *J Bone Joint Surg Am* 85:409, 2003.

35. Ferguson TB. Congenital lesions of the lungs and emphysema. In Sabiston DC, Spencer FC, editors: *Gibbon's surgery of the chest*, ed 4, Philadelphia, 1983, WB Saunders.

36. Skandalakis JE, Gray SW: *Embryology for surgeons: the embryological basis for the treatment of congenital defects*, Baltimore, 1994, Williams & Wilkins.

37. Laberge JM, Puligandla P, Flageole H: Asymptomatic congenital lung malformations, *Semin Pediatr Surg* 14:16, 2005.

38. Haller JA Jr, Gollady ES, Picard LR, et al: Surgical management of lung bud anomalies: lobar emphysema, bronchogenic cyst, cystic adenomatoid malformation, and intralobar pulmonary sequestration, *Ann Thorac Surg* 28:33, 1979.

39. Wilson RD, Hedrick HL, Liechty KW, et al: Cystic adenomatoid malformation of the lung: review of genetics, prenatal diagnosis, and in utero treatment, *Am J Med Genet A* 140:151, 2006.

40. Levine MM, Nudel DB, Gootman N, et al: Pulmonary sequestration causing congestive heart failure in infancy: a report of two cases and review of the literature, *Ann Thorac Surg* 34:581, 1982.

41. John PR, Beasley SW, Mayne V: Pulmonary sequestration and related disorders: a clinico-radiological review of 41 cases, *Pediatr Radiol* 20:4, 1989.

42. Hendren HW, McKee D: Lobar emphysema of infancy, *J Pediatr Surg* 1:24, 1966.

43. Murray GF: Congenital lobar emphysema (collective review), *Surg Gynecol Obstet* 124:611, 1967.

44. McIlvaine WB, Chang JHT, Jones M: The effective use of intrapleural bupivacaine for analgesia after thoracic and subcostal incisions in children, *J Pediatr Surg* 23:1184, 1988.

45. Skandalakis JE, Gray SW, Ricketts R, et al: Anterior body wall. In Skandalakis JL, Gray SW, editors: *Embryology for surgeons*, ed 2, Baltimore, 1994, Williams and Wilkins, pp 540–593.

46. Touloukian RJ, Hobbins JC: Maternal ultrasonography in the antenatal diagnosis of surgically correctable fetal abnormalities, *J Pediatr Surg* 15:373, 1980.

47. Kelleher C, Langer JC: Congenital abdominal wall defects. In Holcomb GW III, Murphy JP, editors: *Pediatric surgery*, ed 5, Philadelphia, 2010, Saunders, pp 625–636.

48. Snyder CL, Miller KA, Sharp RJ, et al: Management of intestinal atresia in patients with gastroschisis, *J Pediatr Surg* 36:1542, 2001.

49. Bianchi A, Dickson AP, Alizai NK: Elective delayed midgut reduction—no anesthesia for gastroschisis: selection and conversion criteria, *J Pediatr Surg* 37:1334, 2002.

50. Sandler A, Lawrence J, Meehan J, et al: A "plastic" sutureless abdominal wall closure in gastroschisis, *J Pediatr Surg* 39:738, 2004.

51. Kliegman RM, Fanaroff AA: Neonatal necrotizing enterocolitis: a nine-year experience, *Am J Dis Child* 135:603, 1981.

52. Henry MC, Moss RL: Necrotizing enterocolitis. In Holcomb GW III, Murphy JP, editors: *Pediatric surgery*, ed 5, Philadelphia, 2010, Saunders, pp 439–455.

53. Ein SH, Shandling B, Wesson D, et al: A 13-year experience with peritoneal drainage under local anesthesia for necrotizing enterocolitis perforation, *J Pediatr Surg* 25:1034, 1990.

54. Morgan LJ, Shochat SJ, Hartman GE: Peritoneal drainage as primary management of perforated NEC in the very low birth weight infant, *J Pediatr Surg* 29:310, 1994.

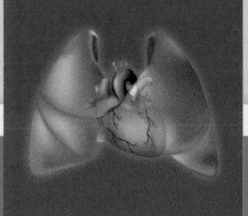

Congenital Cardiac Defects

MICHAEL GREEN

LEARNING OBJECTIVES

After reading this chapter the reader will be able to:

1. Describe normal cardiac anatomy and blood flow in newborns
2. Describe the normal transition from intrauterine to extrauterine blood flow
3. Define *shunt* and understand the different types of shunts seen with congenital heart disease
4. Understand the basic classification schemes for congenital cardiac defects
5. Explain the most common congenital cardiac defects
6. Recognize the various causes of changes in pulmonary vascular resistance
7. Describe the importance of balancing pulmonary and systemic blood flow (Q_P/Q_S) associated with various defects
8. Recommend ventilator strategies commonly used with various congenital cardiac defects
9. Recommend and understand the limitations of various types of physiological monitoring necessary for the care of patients with congenital cardiac defects

KEY TERMS

Atrioventricular septal defect
Coarctation of the aorta
Fontan procedure
Glenn procedure
Hypoplastic left heart syndrome
Left-to-right shunt
Norwood procedure
Patent ductus arteriosus
Right-to-left shunt
Tetralogy of Fallot
Transposition of the great arteries
Truncus arteriosus

More than 40,000 children with congenital heart disease are born each year, making it the most common birth defect in the United States.[1] Major developments in the identification of children with congenital heart disease along with new surgical techniques and improved postoperative care all resulted in significant improvements in mortality over the last two decades of the twentieth century. Mortality has continued to decrease over the last decade, such that many children with congenital heart disease are surviving well into adulthood.[2,3] In fact, recent epidemiological studies have found that there are currently as many adults living with congenital heart disease as there are children.[3,4] The care of all patients with congenital heart disease usually occurs in specialized centers and requires a multidisciplinary team. Respiratory therapists play a key role in the perioperative care of these patients.

CARDIAC ANATOMY AND PHYSIOLOGY

Anatomy and Blood Flow of the Normal Heart

The normal human heart has four chambers: two atria and two ventricles (Figure 24-1). Each "upper chamber," or atrium, is connected to a corresponding "lower chamber," or ventricle, by way of an atrioventricular (AV) valve. The outflow from each ventricle also contains a valve, known as a semilunar valve, which allows blood to flow in only one direction. To understand the normal anatomy of the heart, one can trace the path of blood as it travels through the heart. This begins with deoxygenated venous blood that enters the right atrium (RA) from one of three sources. Venous blood from organs superior to the heart drains to the RA by way of the superior vena cava (SVC). Venous blood from organs inferior to the heart enters the RA via the inferior vena cava (IVC). Finally, venous blood from the heart itself drains into the RA by way of the coronary sinus.

Blood then travels from the RA, through the right AV valve, known as the tricuspid valve, and into the right ventricle (RV). From there, blood travels through the right semilunar valve, known as the pulmonary valve, and into the main pulmonary artery. This artery divides into a right and a left pulmonary artery, each of which carries blood to the lungs. The lungs are the site of gas exchange: carbon dioxide diffuses out of the blood and oxygen diffuses in. This oxygenated blood returns to the heart through four pulmonary veins that empty into the left atrium (LA). Blood then travels through the mitral valve and into the left ventricle (LV). Finally, the blood is pumped out of the LV, through the left semilunar valve, or aortic valve, and into the aorta, the main vessel supplying systemic blood flow to the entire body.

The size and composition of each heart chamber are tailored to the chamber's particular function. For example, because the RA must collect blood coming from nearly all parts of the body, it is slightly larger than the LA, which receives blood only from the lungs. The walls of the atria are thin and compliant, allowing them the ability to expand in the setting of increased blood return from either the body or the lungs. In contrast, the ventricles are muscular, reflecting their essential pump function. The LV is much thicker than the RV because it is responsible for pumping blood throughout the entire body, whereas the RV functions to pump blood through the normally low-resistance lung vessels.

Transition to Extrauterine Life

During the fetal period of development, the fetus depends on the mother's lungs for gas exchange. Because of this,

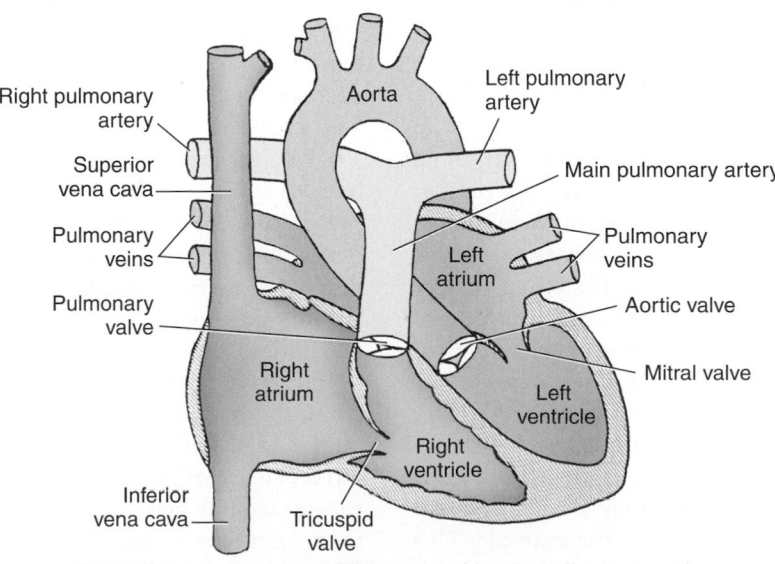

FIGURE 24-1   Anatomy of the normal heart and great vessels.

the fetus has multiple mechanisms to receive oxygenated blood from the mother and to shunt blood away from the fetal lungs, which are not participating in gas exchange (see Chapter 2). Shortly after delivery, a number of anatomical and physiological changes occur in the neonate's body to adapt to extrauterine life. With inflation of the lungs and the beginning of their participation in gas exchange, PaO_2 increases and $PaCO_2$ decreases, both of which contribute to dilation of the pulmonary vasculature and a resultant reduction in pulmonary vascular resistance (PVR). This leads to reduced right ventricular pressures and increased pulmonary blood flow. Another change that occurs in the transition to neonatal life is the decrease and eventual disappearance in shunts present during intrauterine life. The increased fetal blood flow that results from the drop in PVR increases pulmonary venous blood return and therefore increases the left atrial pressure. At the same time, the RA pressure decreases when the umbilical cord is ligated and no longer provides placental blood flow to the IVC. The result of the higher LA pressures and the lower RA pressures is the closure of the foramen ovale. The other large shunt present in fetal life, the ductus arteriosus, also closes shortly after birth. The mechanism behind its closure includes decreased concentrations of circulating prostaglandin E2 and an increase in oxygenation. Usually the ductus arteriosus closes within 48 hours after birth.[5] Several factors can contribute to the ductus arteriosus not closing within the normal period and predisposing neonates to a patent ductus arteriosus (PDA). The ductus arteriosus of premature neonates is less responsive to increased oxygen and decreased PGE2, contributing to a higher incidence of PDA. Other conditions, such as congenital heart disease and persistent pulmonary hypertension, increase blood flow through the ductus arteriosus postnatally and also contribute to a PDA.

CLASSIFICATION OF CARDIAC ANOMALIES

There are numerous ways to classify congenital heart anomalies. Lesions can be categorized by presence or lack of cyanosis, by shunt-type lesions, by lesions that result in obstructed blood flow, and by miscellaneous structural lesions, including those with abnormal valve anatomy or function. There is overlap between several of these categories and there are exceptions to some categories. For example, lesions have often been classified as either *cyanotic* or *acyanotic,* terms that refer to the principal direction of blood shunting. Lesions where shunting is in a right-to-left direction are referred to as cyanotic lesions, whereas lesions where blood flows in a left-to-right direction are categorized as acyanotic. Yet not all patients with right-to-left shunting manifest clinical signs of cyanosis, and some patients with left-to-right shunting may exhibit cyanosis because of inadequate cardiac output, for example. This chapter organizes lesions into shunt lesions, lesions with

left or right ventricular outflow tract obstruction, and miscellaneous lesions. Each section describes the anatomy and physiology, pre and postsurgical management, and surgical care of each lesion.

SHUNT LESIONS

In physiological terms, shunt refers to blood that deviates from the usual flow pattern. The term **right-to-left shunt** refers to desaturated systemic venous blood bypassing the lungs and entering the systemic circulation. **Left-to-right shunting** refers to oxygenated blood mixing with deoxygenated blood. Children with right-to-left shunting often present with central cyanosis, whereas those with left-to-right shunting often appear pink. Deleterious effects of left-to-right shunting often occur later, with prolonged left-to-right shunting leading to increased PVR because of the increase in pulmonary blood flow. Shunting is potentially harmful, either because of prolonged cyanosis and decreased end-organ oxygen delivery or increased PVR over time, but shunting also has an important compensatory effect in patients with obstructed pulmonary or systemic blood flow. In these lesions, referred to as ductal-dependent lesions, the presence of a PDA provides lifesaving blood flow. Lesions with systemic outflow tract obstruction, such as critical coarctation of the aorta or hypoplastic left heart syndrome, rely on the PDA to provide systemic blood flow via a right-to-left shunt; these lesions have ductal-dependent systemic blood flow. Anomalies with obstructed pulmonary blood flow, such as critical pulmonary stenosis, rely on the PDA to provide pulmonary blood flow via a left-to-right shunt; these lesions have ductal-dependent pulmonary blood flow. Infants with undiagnosed ductal-dependent lesions often present with symptoms in the first days to weeks of life when the ductus arteriosus closes.

Patent Ductus Arteriosus

During fetal life the ductus arteriosus functions to shunt blood from the pulmonary artery to the aorta, thus bypassing the lungs. In the first 48 hours after birth, the decrease in PGE2, secreted by the placenta, along with an increase in PaO_2 lead to closure of the ductus arteriosus. A number of conditions predispose infants to having a **patent ductus arteriosus** (PDA), including prematurity, persistent pulmonary hypertension, and respiratory distress syndrome. In these infants, as PVR decreases, aortic pressures exceed pulmonary artery pressures, resulting in a left-to-right shunt and increasing pulmonary blood flow (Figure 24-2). Of the conditions predisposing infants to PDA, prematurity is the most common, making the PDA one of the most commonly seen cardiac defects in neonatal intensive care units. Delayed closure of the ductus arteriosus is inversely related to gestational age, varying from 20% in infants more than 32 weeks of gestation to 60% in infants less than 28 weeks of gestation.[6]

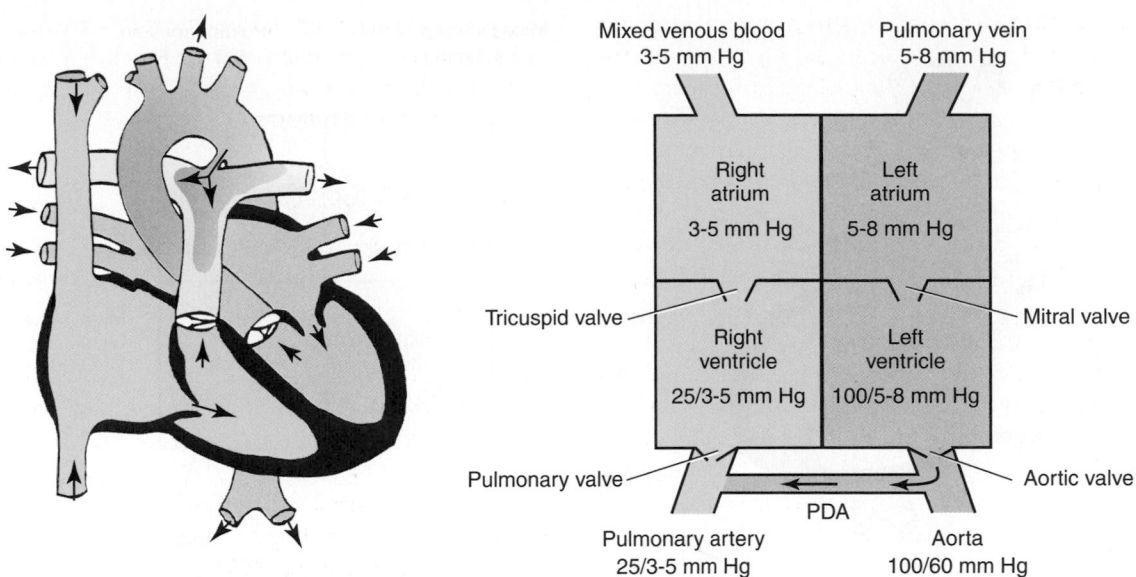

FIGURE 24-2 Patent ductus arteriosus. Communication between the pulmonary artery and the aorta.

Clinical signs of a PDA depend on the degree of left-to-right shunting but may include tachypnea and a continuous murmur. In addition to signs on examination, one can detect the presence of shunting by looking for a difference in oxygenation of preductal and postductal blood. A preductal blood gas should be obtained from the right radial or temporal artery, while a postductal gas may be obtained from the umbilical artery or from a peripheral artery in the lower extremity. A difference in PaO_2 greater than 15 mm Hg is indicative of significant shunting across the PDA.[7,8] Noninvasive measurements of this can be conducted with pulse oximetry. A difference of more than 5% between the preductal saturations, obtained on the right hand, and the postductal saturations, obtained on the left hand or lower extremity indicates possible ductal shunting. Chest radiographs are usually normal, though children with congestive heart failure secondary to PDA may have radiographs with enlarged pulmonary vascular markings. Definitive diagnosis is made by echocardiography.

Over time, the increase in pulmonary blood flow caused by the left-to-right shunting through the PDA can lead to left atrial dilation and left ventricular volume overload, which may result in congestive heart failure. Untreated PDAs may also lead to pulmonary vascular changes and pulmonary hypertension. Increased pulmonary blood flow may delay the ability to wean respiratory support in infants as a result of pulmonary edema and poor lung mechanics. PDAs may spontaneously close at any time, though this is unlikely to occur after 1 year of life.

There are both medical and surgical options for the management of the PDA. Medical management includes maintaining euvolemia and optimizing the hemoglobin to ensure adequate oxygen delivery. In mechanically ventilated patients, increasing positive end-expiratory pressure (PEEP) may serve to decrease the pulmonary blood flow by increasing PVR. In addition, nonsteroidal anti-inflammatory agents such as indomethacin and ibuprofen are often used in the medical management of PDA. Indomethacin may be used prophylactically to prevent PDA and therapeutically to treat a symptomatic PDA. A dose of indomethacin (0.2 mg/kg IV) given in the first 24 hours of life can be effective in preventing a PDA. Therapy later in life is usually given over a 48-hour period. Doses of 0.1 to 0.2 mg/kg IV every 12 to 24 hours are effective. Side effects are uncommon but include oliguria, renal insufficiency, and dilutional hyponatremia. Ibuprofen may also be used, though a recent meta-analysis found that the use of ibuprofen was associated with increased incidence of chronic lung disease when compared with indomethacin.[7]

Typically a trial of medical therapy for a symptomatic PDA is attempted before resorting to surgical management. The surgery, which can often be performed in the intensive care unit, is typically performed via a left thoracotomy. Complications to surgery are rare but include injury to the recurrent laryngeal nerve, which may result in vocal cord paresis. Usually children do not require postoperative ventilator support unless they required it preoperatively. The patients should exhibit normal arterial blood gas and oxygen saturation measurements.

Atrial Septal Defect

An atrial septal defect (ASD) involves a communication between the right and left atria (Figure 24-3). There are several different types of ASDs. The pathophysiology of an ASD involves left-to-right shunting, leading to right atrial enlargement, right ventricular volume overload, and increased pulmonary blood flow. Over time, this may result in right ventricular hypertrophy, congestive heart failure, and pulmonary vascular disease. Infants with ASDs rarely are symptomatic and may remain so well into adulthood.

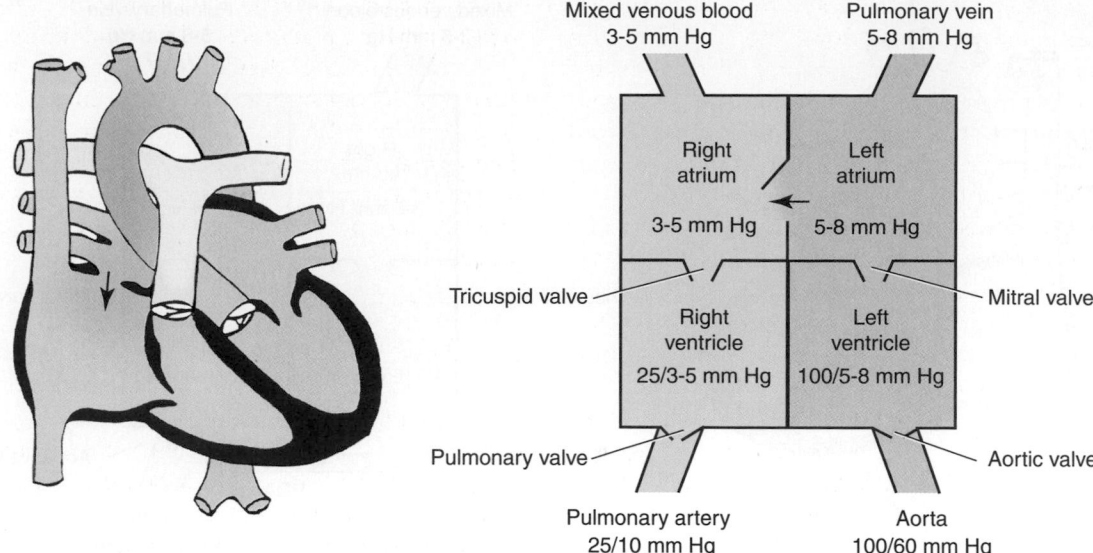

FIGURE 24-3   Atrial septal defect. Communication between the right and left atria through the septum.

Only 8% of children with ASDs develop symptoms before 2 years of age.[8] Chest radiographs are typically normal unless the child has congestive heart failure, which may result in cardiomegaly and prominent pulmonary vascular markings.

Spontaneous closure of small ASDs may occur within the first year of life, so repair is typically delayed until the child is 3 to 5 years of age.[9-11] Surgical repair of an ASD involves a median sternotomy and cardiopulmonary bypass, with closure of the defect obtained with a suture or a patch. After surgery, early extubation is common. Patients should have normal blood gases and oxygen saturations. In recent decades, closure of many ASDs has been achieved in the cardiac catheterization laboratory with transcatheter closure devices, thus avoiding the morbidity of sternotomy and cardiopulmonary bypass.[12,13]

Ventricular Septal Defects

VSDs are the most common congenital heart defect and involve a communication between the right and left ventricles (Figure 24-4). VSDs are described in terms of their location in the ventricular septum and the different types include perimembranous, subpulmonary (also known as outlet, supracristal, conal septal, or subarterial), muscular, and inlet (also known as atrioventricular canal type). The pathophysiology of VSDs involves left-to-right shunting,

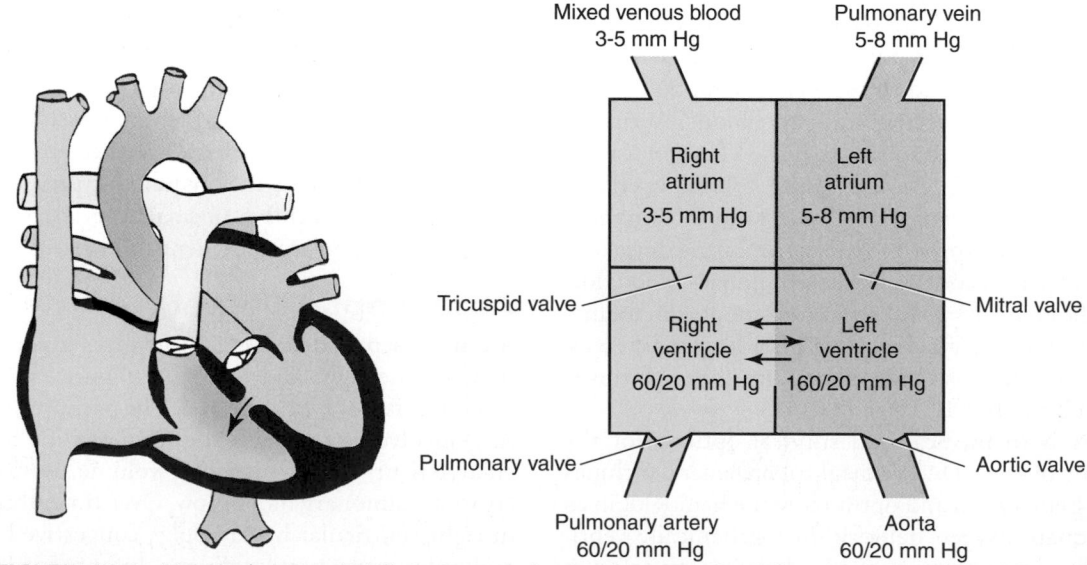

FIGURE 24-4   Ventricular septal defect. Communication between the right and left ventricles through the septum.

left ventricular volume overload, left atrial enlargement, and increased pulmonary blood flow. The size of the defect and the pulmonary vascular resistance determine the amount of shunting, which usually occurs during systole. Large defects may lead to large shunts, sometimes termed nonrestrictive VSDs, and may result in congestive heart failure and pulmonary hypertension. Smaller defects with greater left ventricular pressures than right ventricular pressures are known as restrictive VSDs. Children with restrictive VSDs are often asymptomatic. If a child with a nonrestrictive VSD has a significant left-to-right shunt and resultant increased pulmonary blood flow, over time thickening and fibrosis of the pulmonary vascular bed may develop, which may lead to pulmonary hypertension. If the pulmonary vascular resistance nears that of the systemic vascular resistance, the left-to-right shunt may reverse to a right-to-left shunt, a condition known as Eisenmenger syndrome.

Some types of VSDs, including perimembranous and muscular, commonly close spontaneously in the first 2 years of life. In infants with nonrestrictive VSDs with symptoms of heart failure, medical management includes diuretics and digoxin.[14] If medical therapy is unsuccessful, surgery is typically undertaken. Older children with less severe shunts may be followed for several years before repair is performed. Surgical repair is performed on cardiopulmonary bypass and typically involves patch closure. In rare instances, such as in infants with severe congestive heart failure (CHF), pulmonary artery banding is performed rather than patch repair of the defect in order to limit pulmonary blood flow and to improve symptoms of heart failure. Definitive repair is typically performed later when the child's condition has improved. Recently, percutaneous transcatheter closure of VSDs has been performed

in the cardiac catheterization laboratory. Device closure is typically reserved for older children with muscular VSDs.[15]

Early extubation should be expected in patients after surgical VSD repair, particularly if there is not significant heart failure before repair. Infants or those with heart failure may require a few days of mechanical ventilation and diuresis before extubation. After repair, these patients should have normal arterial blood gases and oxygen saturations.

Atrioventricular Septal Defect

An **atrioventricular septal defect** (AVSD), also known as AV canal or endocardial cushion defect, is an anomaly in which there is absence of the septa between the atria and ventricles. The defect usually involves abnormalities of the AV valves as well. Partial AVSDs are characterized by an ASD and an abnormal mitral valve, most commonly a cleft in the anterior leaflet of the mitral valve. There is no defect in the ventricular septum with partial AVSDs. Complete AVSDs are characterized by absence of the atrial septum, the ventricular septum, and the presence of a common atrioventricular (AV) valve (Figure 24-5). AVSDs occur in approximately 5% of patients with congenital heart disease but it is the most common congenital heart lesion in infants with trisomy 21.[16] The pathophysiology of this defect involves left-to-right shunting between the atria and ventricles along with regurgitation from the common AV valve. If left untreated, this leads to congestive heart failure, increased pulmonary blood flow, and irreversible pulmonary hypertension.[17]

Children with partial AVSD may not have obvious clinical manifestations initially. Those with complete AVSD usually develop signs of heart failure in early life, including respiratory distress, pulmonary edema, and

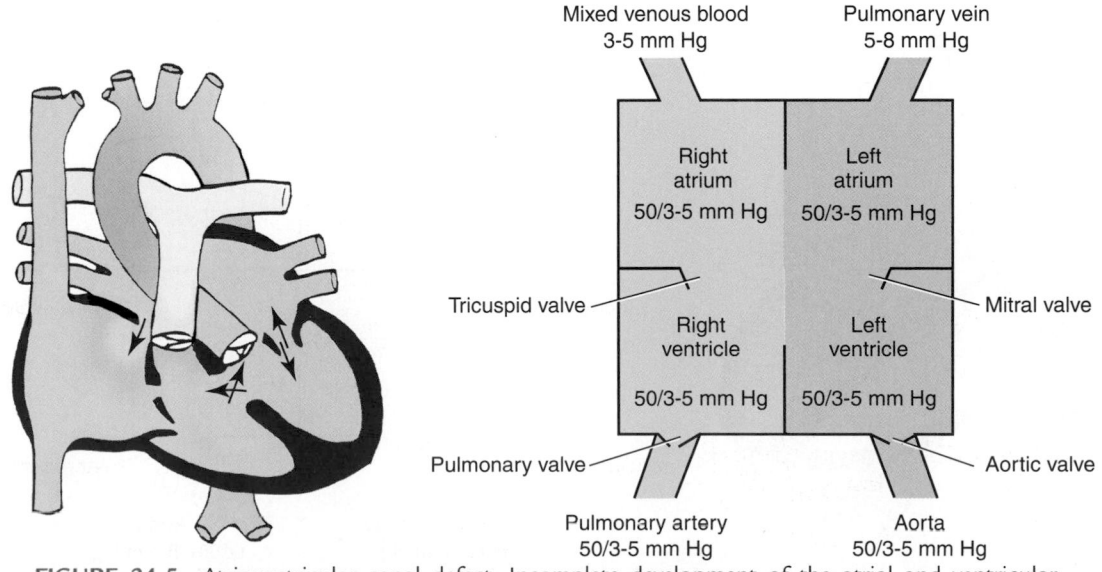

FIGURE 24-5 Atrioventricular canal defect. Incomplete development of the atrial and ventricular septa, which allows complete cardiac mixing of blood.

growth failure. Chest radiography usually reveals cardiomegaly and increased pulmonary vascular markings. Infants without severe heart failure may be managed as outpatients for a time with diuretics and digoxin. Oxygen saturations in these children may be low (75% to 90%) as a result of venous admixing but are tolerated well by most patients. Supplemental oxygen may be given judiciously, given the potential for oxygen to induce pulmonary vascular dilation and increased pulmonary blood flow. Surgical repair of complete AVSD is usually performed before 3 months of age.[18] There are a number of different techniques for repair, including a single-patch technique and a double-patch technique. In addition, the common AV valve is divided into left- and right-sided AV valves.[19] Children with co-morbid conditions who are not good candidates for early complete repair may be managed with banding of the pulmonary arteries in order to stabilize the patient or allow more growth until definitive repair can be performed.

After a complete repair, patients should have normal arterial saturations and arterial blood gases. Arrhythmias or conduction abnormalities are common in the postoperative period, requiring most of these patients to have temporary pacing wires after surgery. Patients without significant heart failure preoperatively may be extubated early after surgery, but infants with significant heart failure or pulmonary hypertension may require a few days of mechanical ventilation before extubation is attempted.

LEFT VENTRICULAR OUTFLOW TRACT OBSTRUCTION

Left ventricular (LV) outflow tract (LVOT) obstructions include several defects that result in obstruction to the ejection of blood from the left ventricle. The obstruction may involve the aortic valve, resulting in aortic stenosis. Lesions that involve the aortic arch, such as aortic coarctation, hypoplastic aortic arch, and interrupted aortic arch, also obstruct systemic blood flow. Finally, hypoplastic left heart syndrome includes LVOT obstruction, both at the levels of the aortic valve and the aortic arch.

Aortic Stenosis

Aortic stenosis (AS) is a narrowing of the aortic valve and is classified by the location of the stenosis. The different locations include subvalvular, valvular, and supravalvular (Figure 24-6). *Subvalvular AS* refers to a discrete ring or membrane below the aortic valve. *Valvular AS* involves abnormalities in the structure of the valve leaflets. *Supravalvular AS* is characterized by narrowing of the aorta immediately distal to the aortic valve. Of the three sites of AS, valvular AS is the most common variety.

The clinical presentation and natural history of aortic stenosis are determined by the time of presentation and the degree of stenosis. Neonates who present with critical aortic stenosis often present in cardiogenic shock with hypotension, poor perfusion, and metabolic acidosis. The chest radiograph often includes cardiomegaly and pulmonary edema. These infants are likely to die unless an intervention is quickly performed on the aortic valve. Infants with less severe stenosis, along with older children and adults with AS, may be asymptomatic, though they are at risk of bacterial endocarditis and the development of left ventricular hypertrophy over time.

As mentioned before, infants with critical AS require emergent therapy. These patients have ductal-dependent systemic blood flow and may develop signs of systemic hypoperfusion as the PDA closes. A mainstay of therapy in these patients is treatment with prostaglandin E1 to maintain ductal patency. Other therapy may include intubation

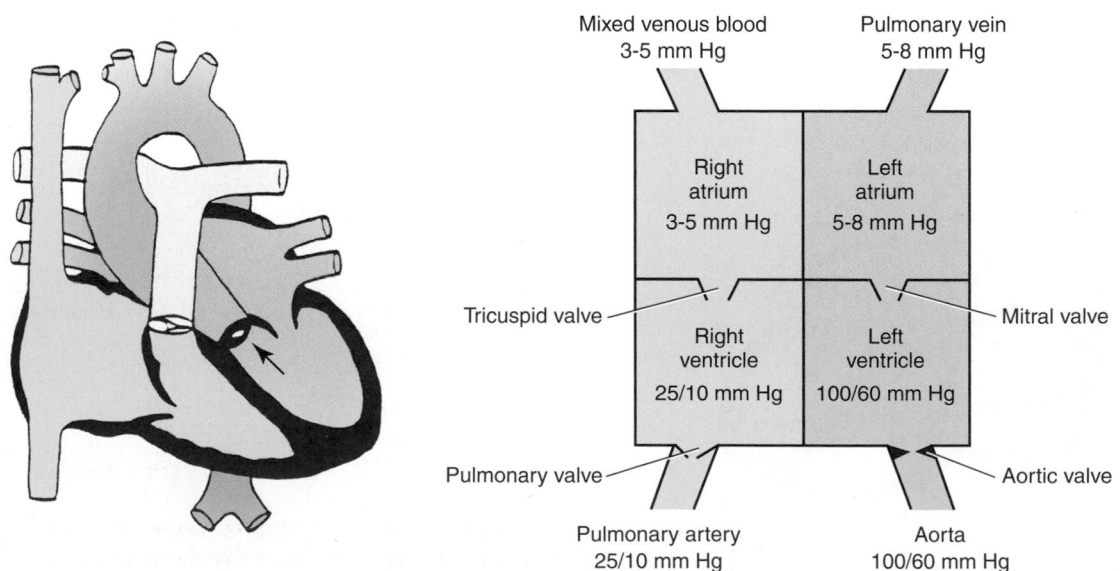

FIGURE 24-6 Aortic stenosis. Outflow obstruction of the aorta, impeding blood flow from the left ventricle.

and mechanical ventilation and inotropic support. Intervention on the stenotic aortic valve is critical and should not be delayed. Currently, options for intervention for critical AS in neonates include catheter balloon valvotomy, performed in the cardiac catheterization laboratory, and surgical valvotomy. The decision to perform a percutaneous intervention versus an open surgical intervention depends on institutional factors and characteristics of the patient. Currently, catheter balloon valvotomy has similarly favorable outcomes to open surgical approaches, though children who have percutaneous interventions often require surgical interventions later in life.[20,21] Surgical procedures for AS vary depending on the anatomy. The options include aortic valvuloplasty, artificial aortic valve replacement, and replacement with a pulmonary valve autograft (Ross procedure). For subvalvular AS, the subaortic membrane is typically resected. For supravalvular AS the stenotic area may be opened up with a synthetic patch. In all these procedures, normal arterial blood gases and pulse oximetry should be expected. Hypertension should be aggressively controlled in these patients to avoid undue stress on the repair site.

Coarctation of the Aorta

Coarctation of the aorta is a severe narrowing of the thoracic aorta in the proximity of the ductus arteriosus. The obstruction, which may occur before, at the site of, or after the ductus (i.e., preductal, juxtaductal, and postductal), may present in the neonatal period or later in infancy or childhood (Figure 24-7). The pathophysiology involves increased afterload to the LV, leading to increased wall tension and myocardial work. In severe coarctation, this may result in myocardial ischemia, pulmonary edema as a result of left atrial hypertension, and congestive heart failure. Systemic blood flow is ductal dependent. A neonate with severe coarctation may present with systemic hypoperfusion caused by the closure of the ductus arteriosus. Older children with less severe coarctation may be asymptomatic, presenting with upper extremity hypertension as the only clue to the underlying lesion. Over time, the increased work of the left ventricle will lead to left ventricular hypertrophy and arterial collateralization around the site of the aortic narrowing.

The chest radiograph of infants with severe coarctation often reveals cardiomegaly and pulmonary congestion. Older children with coarctation have classic findings of cardiomegaly and rib notching, secondary to collateral vessels. Treatment of neonates with severe coarctation includes prostaglandin E1 to restore patency of the ductus arteriosus. These patients may also have significant ventricular dysfunction, congestive heart failure, and acidosis, requiring inotropes, dieresis, and ventilatory support. Surgery for severe coarctation in neonates is usually not delayed, but less severe coarctation in older infants and children may be performed electively.

A number of different surgical techniques are used in aortic coarctation. The most common approaches are (1) resection of the stenotic segment with end-to-end anastomosis of the transected ends; (2) patch aortoplasty, which includes using a synthetic patch to enlarge the area of narrowing; (3) subclavian patch aortoplasty, which uses a flap from the subclavian artery to enlarge the site; and (4) extended resection with primary anastomosis. The most commonly used procedure in neonates is resection with end-to-end anastomosis. Typically, this can be performed via a left thoracotomy. If neonates have significant

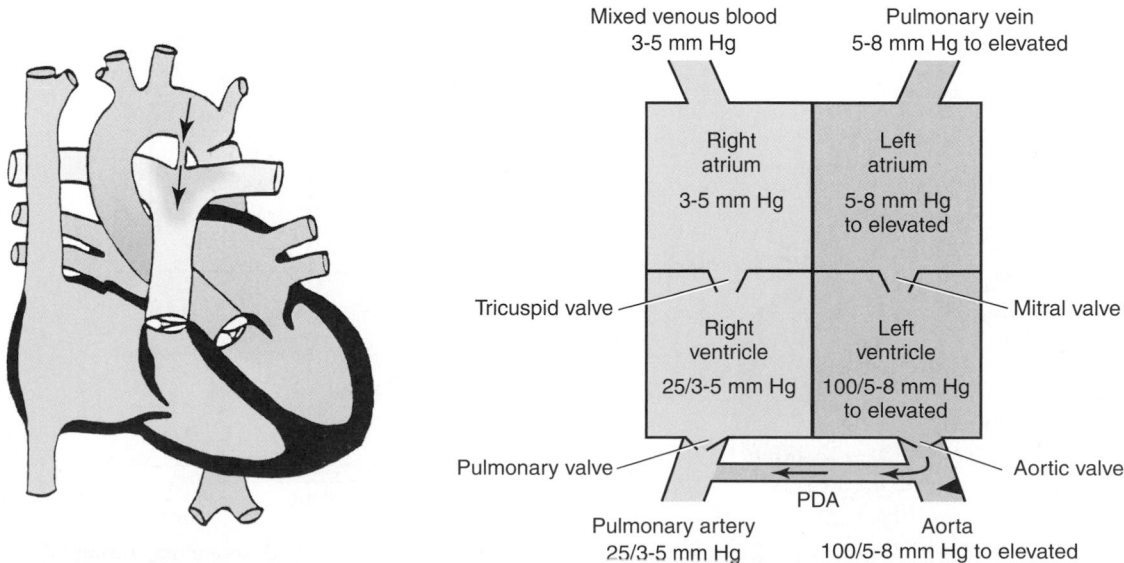

FIGURE 24-7 Coarctation of the aorta. Severe narrowing of the aortic lumen, which decreases blood flow through the aorta. A patent ductus arteriosus is often present to allow pulmonary blood flow when the coarctation is severe. *PDA,* Patent ductus arteriosus.

arch hypoplasia, an extended end-to-end procedure may be performed, which involves an end-to-side connection of the descending aorta to an incision on the underside of the aortic arch proximal to the narrow portion.[22]

Postoperatively, normal blood gas and pulse oximetry values should be expected. A residual coarctation, defined as a gradient between the upper and lower extremity blood pressures, is common postoperatively. Systolic pressure gradients less than 20 mm Hg in the setting of adequate lower body perfusion (including renal perfusion) is generally considered acceptable. After surgery, older children are commonly extubated in the operating room or in the first few hours after surgery. Infants and younger children may require 12 to 24 hours of mechanical ventilation postoperatively. On extubation, caregivers must be on the lookout for signs of stridor, which may be related to intraoperative injury to the recurrent laryngeal nerve, leading to unilateral vocal cord paralysis. Hemidiaphragmatic paralysis from an intraoperative phrenic nerve injury is another potential complication and is diagnosed by an elevated hemidiaphragm on chest radiograph. Finally, injury to the thoracic duct intraoperatively may lead to a chylothorax, which may affect the duration of mechanical ventilation in these patients.

Hypoplastic Left Heart Syndrome

Hypoplastic left heart syndrome (HLHS) describes a spectrum of lesions involving abnormal development of left-sided cardiac structures including the mitral valve, left ventricle, aortic valve, and aortic arch (Figure 24-8). The continuum may include hypoplasia of the LV, atresia or critical stenosis of the aortic or mitral valves, and hypoplasia of the ascending aorta and aortic arch. To maintain systemic blood flow, pulmonary venous blood return must

pass through the foramen ovale to the RA. This oxygenated blood mixes with deoxygenated blood on the right side of the heart before traveling to the pulmonary artery. There, a portion of the blood travels to the lungs and another portion travels through the ductus arteriosus, which is the source of systemic blood flow. With the pulmonary artery supplying both the systemic and the pulmonary circulations, the circulations are said to be in parallel, and the relative blood flow to the respective vascular bed is determined by the balance of the systemic vasculature resistance and the pulmonary vasculature resistance. Adequate systemic perfusion in these infants depends on the presence of a nonrestrictive atrial septal connection, adequate right ventricular function, a patent ductus arteriosus, and a balance between the pulmonary and systemic circulations.

The presentation of infants with HLHS depends on these factors that determine systemic perfusion. Though HLHS is often diagnosed prenatally or shortly after birth, some infants with a PDA and unrestrictive foramen ovale present in the first several weeks of life as the PDA begins to close. In any infant with HLHS, if the ductus closes, hypoperfusion, metabolic acidosis, and circulatory collapse can occur rapidly, leading to death. Adequate interatrial communication is also critical. Babies with intact or restrictive atrial septa not only have inadequate systemic blood flow but also are likely to have high left atrial pressures, which lead to pulmonary edema and elevated pulmonary vascular resistance. Finally, the balance of pulmonary and systemic blood flow (Qp/Qs) is of critical importance. At birth, the normal high PVR of neonates favors adequate systemic blood flow. With the normal drop in PVR that occurs in the first days of life, pulmonary blood flow increases at the expense of systemic blood flow. If this continues unabated,

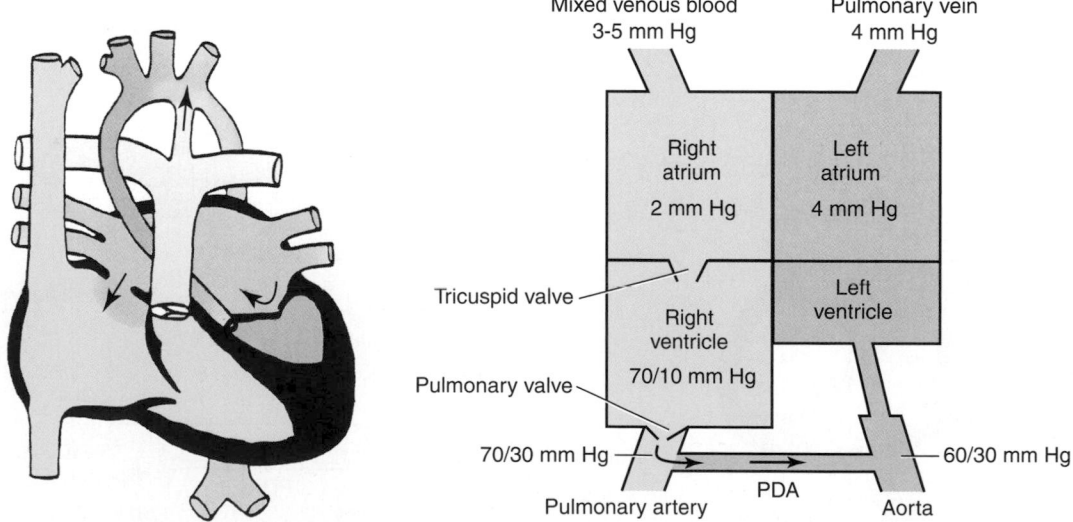

FIGURE 24-8 Hypoplastic left ventricle. Underdeveloped left ventricle and severe narrowing of the ascending aorta. It may include mitral atresia (pictured here), lack of the mitral valve, aortic atresia, lack of the aorta, or a combination. A patent ductus arteriosus is necessary for systemic blood flow. *PDA,* Patent ductus arteriosus.

the baby may develop systemic hypoperfusion and metabolic acidosis because of this phenomenon of relative pulmonary overcirculation.

Preoperatively, therapy for infants with HLHS is targeted at ensuring adequate intracardiac mixing, right-to-left flow at the PDA, and balance between the pulmonary and systemic circulations. If there is evidence of restriction of absence of blood flow across the atrial septum, emergent balloon atrial septostomy is indicated, either in the cardiac catheterization laboratory or at the bedside with echocardiographic guidance. Prostaglandin E1 should be started immediately when the diagnosis of HLHS is confirmed in order to ensure patency of the ductus arteriosus. A number of interventions may be employed to balance the systemic and pulmonary circulations. As the PVR decreases, minimizing the amount of administered oxygen can decrease pulmonary vasodilation and pulmonary blood flow. Occasionally, subambient oxygen concentrations (FIO_2 less than 0.21) are used to increase PVR. Target FIO_2s are usually in the 0.17 to 0.21 range in order to keep systemic oxygen saturations 70% to 80%. Hypercarbia can also be used to elevate PVR. This therapy usually involves intubation and mechanical ventilation with deep sedation or neuromuscular blockade to allow control of $PaCO_2$. Patients are ventilated to a mild respiratory acidosis by decreasing the minute ventilation. In addition to hypoventilation, $PaCO_2$ may be increased by adding CO_2 to the inspired gas in the ventilator circuit. Exhaled CO_2 is usually targeted with an $FICO_2$ of 2% to 5% using an end-tidal CO_2 monitor.[23] Other techniques to balance the systemic and pulmonary circulations include medications such as intravenous vasodilators, which decrease systemic vascular resistance, and transfusion strategies targeting a hemoglobin of 14 to 16 g/dl, which may decrease pulmonary blood flow because of increased blood viscosity.[24]

Before the early 1980s, there were limited surgical options for children with HLHS and long-term outcomes were poor. The advent of the Norwood procedure and staged palliation for HLHS have contributed to much improved outcomes in these patients.[25,26] Typically, patients with HLHS undergo three stages of surgery, with each procedure providing the growing patient with an adequate balance between systemic and pulmonary blood flow.

There are a number of options for the first stage of palliation (Figure 24-9). The usual first stage is the **Norwood procedure** (Figure 24-10), which consists of reconstructing the aorta and adding a shunt to provide pulmonary blood flow. The two main types of shunts employed at the first stage of palliation are the modified Blalock-Taussig (BT) shunt, which connects the subclavian artery to the pulmonary artery with a synthetic shunt, or the right ventricle–pulmonary artery (RV–PA) shunt or conduit, known as the Sano modification (Figure 24-11).

Two other procedures are sometimes employed in neonates with HLHS. In patients who are deemed to be unstable for the risks of the Norwood procedure, pulmonary artery (PA) bands may be applied to limit pulmonary blood flow until the baby is stable enough to undergo the full stage one surgery. The hybrid procedure is another option. It does not require cardiopulmonary bypass and involves PA banding along with catheter-delivered stenting of the ductus arteriosus.[27-29] This procedure is sometimes used in infants thought to be high risk for the Norwood operation. Infants who begin staged palliation with the hybrid procedure must undergo aortic arch reconstruction at the time of the second stage of palliation, significantly increasing the risk of this procedure.

Common postoperative issues after the Norwood procedure include hypoxia, low cardiac output syndrome, and arrhythmias. Infants typically require a period of

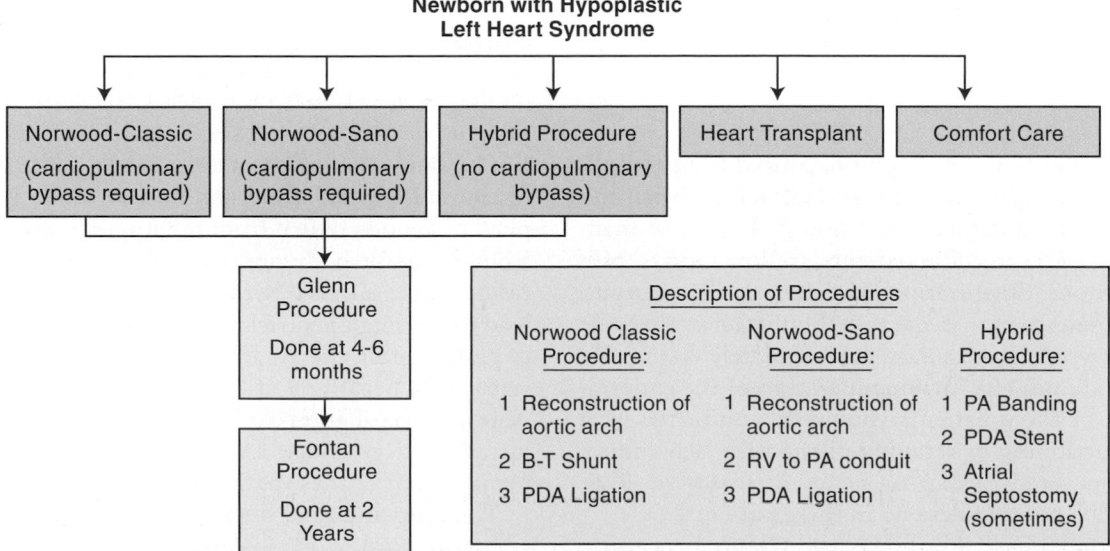

FIGURE 24-9   Sequence of procedures for the treatment of hypoplastic left heart syndrome.

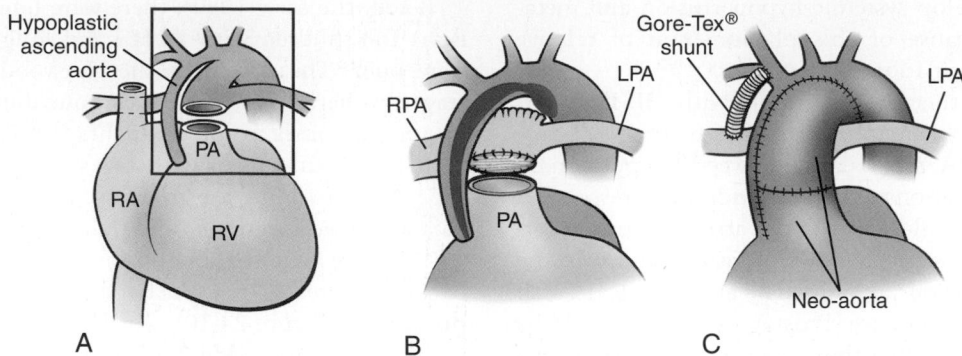

A **B** **C**

FIGURE 24-10 The Norwood procedure. **A,** The heart with aortic atresia and a hypoplastic ascending aorta and aortic arch are shown. The main pulmonary artery (*PA*) is transected. **B,** The distal PA is closed with a patch. An incision that extends around the aortic arch to the level of the ductus is made in the ascending aorta. The ductus is ligated. **C,** A modified right Blalock-Taussig shunt is created between the right subclavian artery and the right PA (*RPA*) as the sole source of pulmonary blood flow. By the use of an aorta or PA allograft (*shaded area*), the main PA is anastomosed to the aorta and the aortic arch to create a large arterial trunk. The procedure to widen the atrial communication is not shown. *LPA,* Left pulmonary artery; *RA,* right atrium; *RV,* right ventricle.

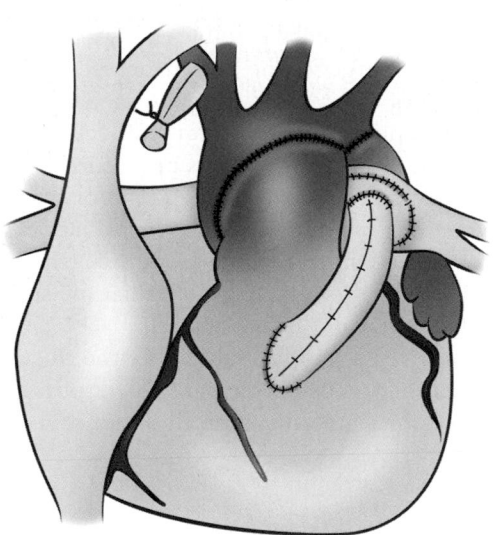

FIGURE 24-11 The Sano shunt.

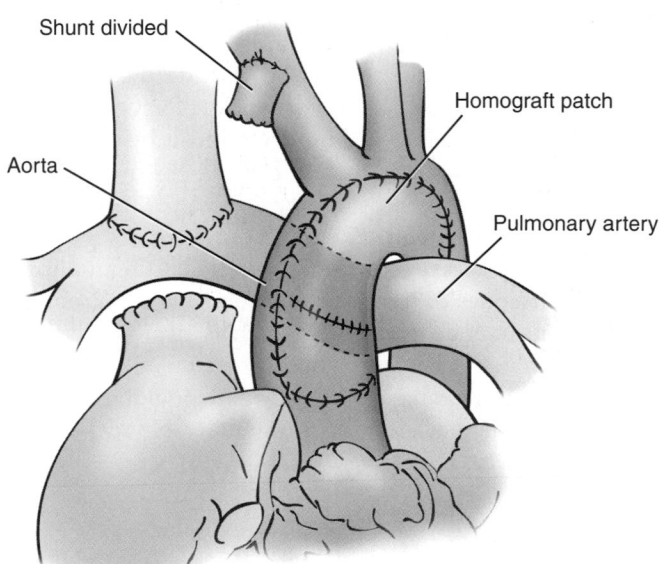

FIGURE 24-12 Bidirectional Glenn shunt. The divided right superior vena cava has been anastomosed at the previous site of the distal anastomosis of the modified right Blalock shunt.

mechanical ventilation because of reduced lung compliance, limited myocardial reserve, and difficulties balancing pulmonary and systemic blood flow.[30] The three main causes of hypoxia in these patients are low Qp/Qs, pulmonary venous desaturation, and low cardiac output. Goal gas exchange in these infants should follow the "rule of forties," which targets PaO_2 approximately 40 mm Hg and $PaCO_2$ 40 mm Hg. Any manipulation of the endotracheal tube in these patients should be conducted with caution. Suctioning or retaping of the tube may induce hypotension, bradycardia, or acute increases in PVR, which may be poorly tolerated in these patients.

The second phase, known as the **Glenn procedure** (Figure 24-12), involves removal of the BT shunt or RV–PA

conduit and connection of the superior vena cava directly to the pulmonary artery. Pulmonary blood flow is supplied by venous return from the upper body, while blood from the lower body returns to the single ventricle. The result of the surgery is removal of some of the volume load to the single ventricle. Because pulmonary blood flow is passive after the stage two surgery, positive-pressure ventilation negatively affects pulmonary blood flow. Expeditious extubation to resume physiological negative intrathoracic pressures is an important component of the management of these patients.

The third and final stage is known as the **Fontan procedure** (Figure 24-13). It consists of connecting the superior vena cava and the inferior vena cava directly to the

Before the 1980s, surgical correction of TGA was achieved with an "atrial switch procedure," such as the Mustard or Senning operation (Figures 24-18 and 24-19). These procedures involved creating an atrial level baffle that directed SVC and IVC blood to the mitral valve and pulmonary venous blood to the tricuspid valve. Long-term complications associated with the atrial switch operation

led to the development of the arterial switch operation (ASO), also known as the Jatene operation (Figure 24-20). This procedure is now the preferred surgical correction for TGA.[41-44] Typically, surgical repair of TGA is performed within the first 2 weeks of life. The ASO is performed via a median sternotomy under cardiopulmonary bypass. The main trunks of the aorta and the pulmonary artery are transected above their respective origins on the heart. The coronary arteries are resected from the aortic sinus area and are ultimately reimplanted into the pulmonary artery. The portion of the pulmonary artery attached to the LV is attached to the cut section of the aorta. The portion of the aorta attached to the RV is attached to the cut section of the pulmonary artery. The result of this procedure is an anatomical repair, with oxygenated blood flowing from the left ventricle and into the aorta and deoxygenated blood flowing from the right ventricle into the pulmonary artery.

After the ASO, infants typically require mechanical ventilation for at least 24 hours. Normal arterial blood gas and pulse oximetry should be expected. Common postoperative issues include low cardiac output syndrome and rhythm disturbances. It is also important to remain on the lookout for signs of coronary artery insufficiency, such as increased left atrial pressures, poor systemic perfusion, or ST changes on the echocardiogram (ECG). Because part of the ASO involves resection and reimplantation of the coronary arteries, coronary artery spasm or occlusion are potential serious complications in the postoperative period.

Pulmonary Atresia with Intact Ventricular Septum

Pulmonary atresia with intact ventricular septum (PA/IVS) is a condition in which blood flow out of the right ventricle

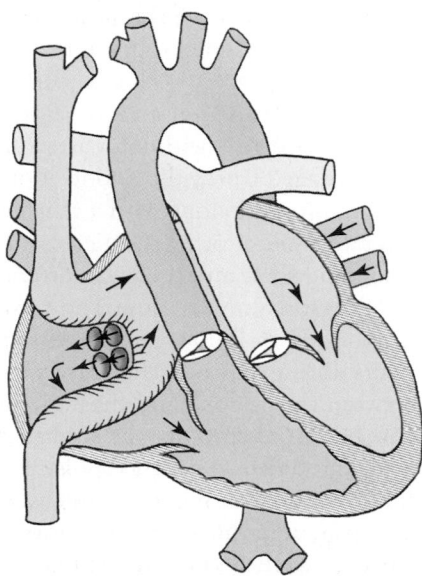

FIGURE 24-18 Mustard procedure. The atrial septum is removed, and a conduit is placed inside the atria. Blood from the right atrium is directed to the mitral valve, into the left ventricle, out the pulmonary artery, and then to the lungs. Blood from the pulmonary veins is directed from the left atrium by a baffle to the tricuspid valve. It then flows into the right ventricle and out the aorta.

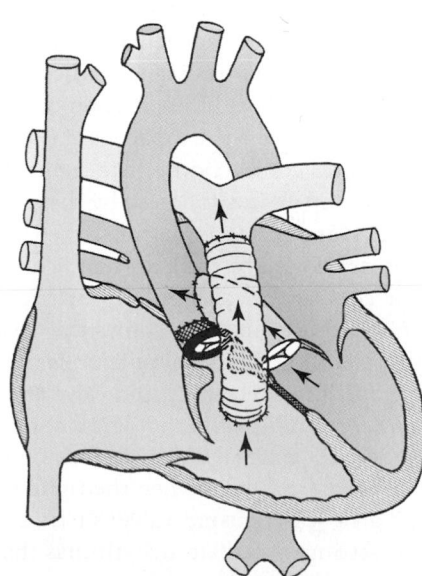

FIGURE 24-19 Rastelli procedure. Blood is routed from the right ventricle to the pulmonary artery through the ventricular septal defect using a conduit. The pulmonary artery is separated and is anastomosed to the aorta

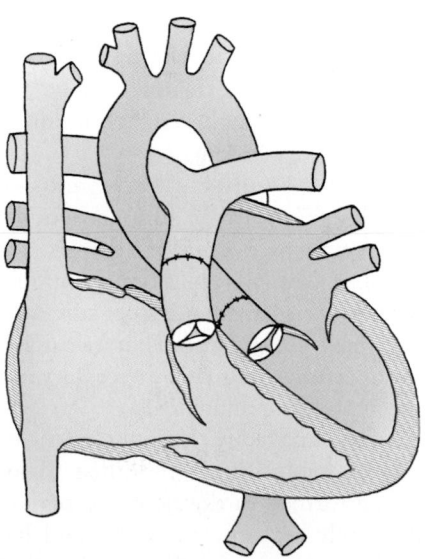

FIGURE 24-20 Arterial switch. The pulmonary artery and aorta are separated from their respective origins and reattached to provide normal pulmonary and aortic blood flow.

is obstructed because of atresia of the pulmonary valve. The RV is typically hypertrophied and the RV cavity is often hypoplastic. The left side of the heart receives blood from the right side via an ASD or patent foramen ovale. Pulmonary blood flow is ductal dependent.

Infants with PA/IVS present early with cyanosis and acidosis. Prostaglandin E1 is necessary to establish pulmonary blood flow via the ductus arteriosus. Patients often require mechanical ventilation as a result of hypoxemia, acidosis, and prostaglandin-induced apnea episodes. Because there is total venous mixing, oxygen therapy should be used judiciously to maintain the balance between pulmonary and systemic blood flow. PaO_2 and $PaCO_2$ should be kept near 40 mm Hg, and goal saturations are approximately 75%.

Treatment of PA/IVS includes both catheter-based and surgical interventions. Catheter-based options include perforation of the atretic valve with radiofrequency catheters or lasers with subsequent balloon dilation.[45-49] There is considerable controversy regarding the efficacy of catheter-based interventions compared with surgical interventions, but typically only infants with mild RV hypoplasia are thought to be candidates for a catheter-based intervention.

Surgical options for PA/IVS also depend on the degree of RV hypoplasia in a given patient. Patients with mild RV hypoplasia may have a biventricular repair, with a surgery to elimination of RVOT obstruction. Children with significant RV hypoplasia typically proceed down the staged single ventricle palliation pathway, with ultimate conversion to the Fontan operation.

Postoperative considerations after the BT shunt, Glenn, and Fontan surgeries were discussed earlier in this chapter.

Tricuspid Atresia

Tricuspid atresia (TA) is a condition in which there is complete obstruction of blood flow between the right atrium and right ventricle. There must be an interatrial connection to supply blood flow to the left side of the heart. Typically the RV is hypoplastic and may be connected to the LV via a VSD. TA is a single ventricle lesion; pulmonary blood flow is ductal dependent.

Most infants with TA present with cyanosis during the first month of life. The cardiac silhouette on chest radiograph may be small or normal if there is not excessive pulmonary blood flow. Before surgery, infants must be maintained on prostaglandin E2 to ensure adequate pulmonary blood flow via the ductus arteriosus. Intubation and mechanical ventilation may be necessary in the setting of significant hypoxemia or acidosis.

TA is typically managed with single ventricle palliation. The first stage is typically the modified Blalock-Taussig shunt that is performed in the neonatal period. Children with TA ultimately require the Glenn and later Fontan procedures. The details of the Blalock-Taussig shunt and Glenn and Fontan procedures, along the postoperative care, were discussed earlier.

CLINICAL MONITORING OF PATIENTS WITH CARDIAC ANOMALIES

Hemodynamic Monitoring

Children with congenital heart disease require close monitoring of their hemodynamic parameters. Both noninvasive and invasive monitoring devices have been developed to aid the clinician in managing these patients. The systemic blood pressure is one of the basic hemodynamic parameters that is followed. Blood pressure may be monitored noninvasively, using an occlusive cuff around an extremity, or invasively, by use of an arterial line, which is a plastic catheter that dwells within an artery. An arterial line has the advantage of providing continuous pressure blood pressure monitoring along with a reliable source of access for laboratory monitoring. Clinicians often follow the systolic blood pressure and the mean arterial pressure as surrogates of end-organ blood flow. The diastolic blood pressure is important to follow because coronary artery perfusion occurs during diastole. The pulse pressure is the difference between the systolic and diastolic blood pressure. A narrow pulse pressure may be seen in conditions such as cardiac tamponade. A widened pulse pressure may be observed during periods of low systemic vascular resistance, such as sepsis, or in the setting of a lesion producing diastolic "run off," such as in the setting of a Blalock-Taussig shunt.

Another frequently measured intravascular pressure is the central venous pressure (CVP). The CVP is measured in the large veins, typically the superior vena cava or the inferior vena cava. The pressure may be transduced continuously through the lumen of a central venous catheter. CVP readings are commonly used as a surrogate of venous blood return to the heart (preload), though elevated CVP values may also reflect poor right ventricular compliance or elevated pulmonary vascular resistance. The normal CVP waveform has a number of different components that reflect different portions of the cardiac cycle (Figure 24-21). The a wave indicates contraction of the right atrium with the tricuspid valve open. It is followed by the c wave, which indicates ventricular contraction against the closed tricuspid valve. This is followed by the x descent, which is caused by ventricular contraction and pulling of tricuspid valve away from the right atrium. Next comes the v wave, which is caused by atrial filling. The final portion is the y descent, which reflects opening of the tricuspid valve and emptying of right atrium. A number of pathological conditions may induce changes in the normal CVP waveform. For example, "cannon a waves" are observed when the right atrium contracts against a closed tricuspid valve, such as one might observe in the setting of cardiac arrhythmias that result in loss of atrioventricular synchrony.

Sometimes, direct measurements of intracardiac pressures provide additional helpful data in the management of children with congenital heart disease. Direct right

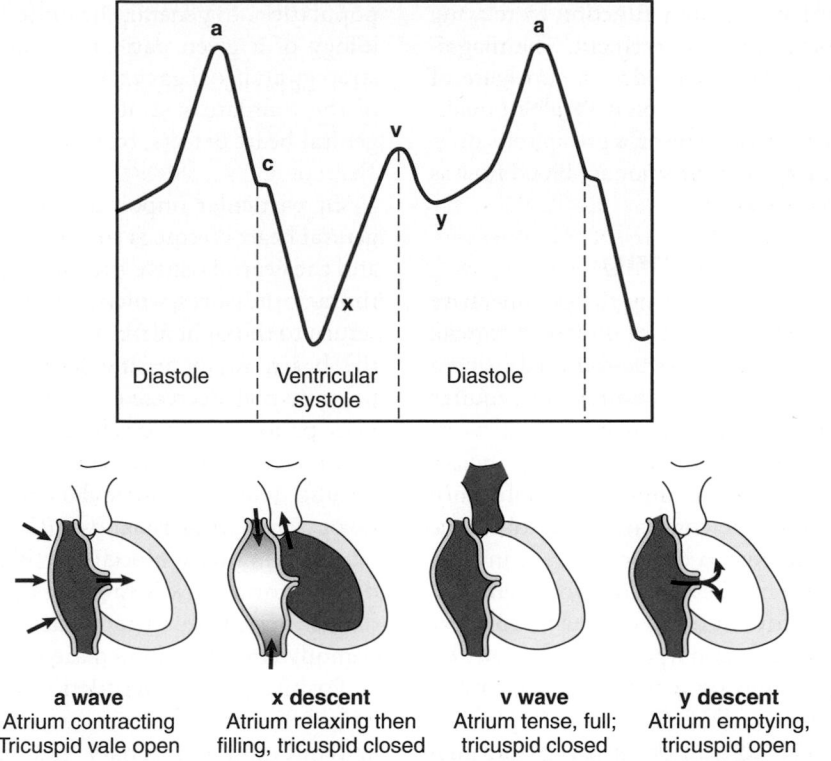

a wave
Atrium contracting
Tricuspid vale open

x descent
Atrium relaxing then
filling, tricuspid closed

v wave
Atrium tense, full;
tricuspid closed

y descent
Atrium emptying,
tricuspid open

FIGURE 24-21   Central venous pressure tracing. Includes *a wave,* caused by contraction of atria; *c wave,* caused by ventricular contraction against closed tricuspid valve; *x descent,* caused by ventricular contraction and pulling of tricuspid valve away from right atrium; *v wave,* caused by atrial filling; *y descent,* caused by opening of tricuspid valve and emptying of right atrium.

atrial pressures or left atrial pressures are measured via catheters placed intraoperatively. Right atrial pressure values often are used as surrogates of right-sided preload. In addition, they may be elevated in the setting of decreased RV function, poor RV compliance, or increased PVR. Left atrial pressure monitoring provides a surrogate of the left ventricular end-diastolic pressure, assuming a competent mitral valve. Elevated left atrial pressures may be seen with left ventricular dysfunction, volume overload, and mitral regurgitation.

Pulse Oximetry

Pulse oximetry is a fundamental monitoring device in children with congenital heart disease. In addition to measuring systemic oxygenation, it can also be used to measure the degree of right-to-left shunting in lesions where this is a possibility. This is done by measuring preductal and postductal saturations. Preductal saturations are measured by placing the pulse oximeter on the right upper extremity. Postductal saturations are reflected by placing the pulse oximeter on any other extremity, though the lower extremities are preferred because pre- and postductal blood may be incompletely mixed at the left upper extremity. If postductal saturations are 5% to 10% lower than preductal saturations, then right-to-left shunting should be suspected. Several conditions may affect the reliability of pulse oximetry readings. At low oxygen saturations

(SaO_2 less than 80%), pulse oximetry has been shown to be less accurate when compared with SaO_2 greater than 90%.[50] Some newer generation pulse oximeters have improved reliability at lower saturations.[51-53] Other factors that may contribute to inaccurate pulse oximeter readings include intravenous methylene blue, excessive ambient light, and patient motion.

Capnography

Capnography, or continuous measurement of end-tidal CO_2 ($ETCO_2$), should be used in all mechanically ventilated children with congenital heart disease. $ETCO_2$ correlates well with $PaCO_2$, with a normal gradient of 2 to 5 mm Hg between the two.[54] Decreased $ETCO_2$ measurements may be caused by endotracheal tube dislodgement or obstruction, air trapping, decreased pulmonary blood flow, low cardiac output, or hyperventilation. Elevated $ETCO_2$ measurements are associated with hypoventilation, fever, or malignant hyperthermia. Increases in the gradient between the $PaCO_2$ and the $ETCO_2$ may be indicative of increased dead space, lower pulmonary blood flow, high airway pressures leading to alveolar overdistention, and pulmonary embolism.

Capnography is useful in a number of specific scenarios when caring for critically ill children. Capnography may be used immediately after intubation to distinguish between endotracheal and esophageal tube placement.[55] Continuous $ETCO_2$ readings allow real-time monitoring of ventilation and serve an important patient safety function by relaying data on proper endotracheal tube placement. The magnitude of the $ETCO_2$ tracing may be used as a surrogate of efficacy of cardiopulmonary resuscitation (CPR).[56,57] Finally, in children with a Blalock-Taussig shunt, a precipitous drop in the $ETCO_2$ may indicate a loss of pulmonary blood flow as a result of shunt thrombosis.

Cardiac Output Monitoring

Monitoring cardiac output (CO) during the perioperative period in patients with congenital heart disease is critical. CO may be measured directly or may be followed using a number of surrogates. Direct CO measurement requires an invasive catheter and typically relies on the indicator-dilution technique. The technique relies on the principle that blood flow is equal to the consumption of a substance divided by the difference in the content of the substance across a vascular bed. A change in dye or a change in temperature (thermodilution) has been used to calculate CO in children. In addition to dye dilution or thermodilution, clinicians can use the change in oxygen across a vascular bed to determine cardiac output, a technique that relies on the Fick principle. To calculate CO, for example, one would measure the oxygen consumption using calorimetry and divide that by the difference in oxygen content in blood between the aorta and the pulmonary artery. Assuming a stable oxygen consumption and a stable arterial oxygen saturation, a drop in the saturations in the pulmonary artery would indicate a drop in CO. Because many patients lack a pulmonary artery catheter, central venous saturations, such as saturations from the SVC, have been used as a mixed venous saturation ($S\bar{v}O_2$). Decreased $S\bar{v}O_2$ has been correlated to low cardiac output in children with congenital heart disease.[58]

To reduce the risks associated with invasive monitoring, clinicians often rely on noninvasive monitors of CO. Near-infrared spectroscopy (NIRS) monitors are a newer technology that measure the venous oxygen saturation in different regions of the body. Several studies have shown that NIRS values correlate well with $S\bar{v}O_2$ and may be used as a real-time indicator to follow cardiac output trends.[59-61] The common sites of regional NIRS monitoring include cerebral, splanchnic, renal, and muscle. Echocardiography is also sometimes used to estimate CO. Other important surrogates of CO to monitor during the perioperative period include serum lactate, urine output, and neurological status.

RESPIRATORY CARE OF PATIENTS WITH CARDIAC ANOMALIES

Ventilator Management

Though the fundamentals of respiratory care for patients with congenital heart anomalies are similar to those for all patients, there are several important considerations in this population. In general, the underlying anatomy and physiology of a given patient should dictate the ventilatory strategy and goal gas exchange for each patient. For details of the ventilatory strategy for each of the common congenital heart defects, refer to the pertinent section in this chapter.

Of particular importance in many patients with congenital heart disease is the interaction between ventilation and the heart. Positive-pressure ventilation increases intrathoracic pressures, which in turn decrease systemic venous return to the right atrium. This is effectively the preload to the heart, so increasing levels of positive intrathoracic pressure may decrease cardiac output by diminishing cardiac preload. Conversely, negative pressure ventilation may increase systemic venous return and therefore cardiac output. This is of particular importance in patients with cavopulmonary anastomoses (Glenn and Fontan surgeries) where pulmonary blood flow is passive and very dependent on intrathoracic pressures. Early extubation to physiological negative intrathoracic pressures improves the hemodynamics in these patients.

Positive-pressure ventilation also has a significant effect on pulmonary vascular resistance and the balance between systemic and pulmonary vascular resistances (Qp/Qs). Normally, the ratio of Qp/Qs is 1. A number of interventions may affect PVR; these are listed in Box 24-2.

Like the ventilatory strategy, the timing of extubation depends on factors such as the underlying physiology, the extent of the surgical procedure, the duration of cardiopulmonary bypass, and the cardiac function, in addition to the parameters one typically assesses in monitoring for extubation readiness in the general population of those who are mechanically ventilated. Many patients with congenital heart disease do not require mechanical ventilation

---

Box 24-2	**Interventions That Affect PVR**

INCREASE
- ↓ pH
    - ↓ Minute ventilation to ↑ $PaCO_2 \geq 45$ mm Hg
    - ↑ Inhaled CO_2 to ↓ pH
- ↓ FIO_2
- ↑ Mean airway pressure
    - ↑ PIP, ↑ PEEP, ↑ Respiratory rate, ↑ I/E ratio

DECREASE
- ↑ pH
    - ↑ Minute ventilation to ↓ $PaCO_2$ to < 45 mm Hg
- ↑ FIO_2
    - ↓ Mean airway pressure

PHARMACOLOGY
- PGE1
- iNO
- Prostacyclin

I/E, Inspiratory to expiratory; *iNO,* inhaled nitric oxide; *PEEP,* positive end-expiratory pressure; *PIP,* peak inspiratory pressure; *PGE1,* prostaglandin E1

preoperatively and are ventilator-dependent only in the immediate postoperative period. Such children may be extubated in the operating room or within the first 4 to 6 hours postoperatively, with good outcomes.[62-64] Other patients may be extubated sooner because of the deleterious effects of positive-pressure ventilation on their cardiac output. For example, children who undergo Glenn or Fontan procedures have pulmonary blood flow that is passive. Physiological negative intrathoracic pressure improves pulmonary blood flow and therefore cardiac output, whereas positive-pressure ventilation may impede pulmonary blood flow.[65]

A number of studies have sought to identify specific predictors of successful extubation of children. Modalities such as daily spontaneous breathing tests, ventilator weaning protocols, and diaphragmatic function have all been used to attempt to assess extubation readiness in children, yet no factor reliably predicts successful extubation.[66,67] No single factor has been identified that reliably predicts extubation failure in children. In general, extubation criteria for most cardiac surgery patients include (1) an intact cough with the ability to clear the airway; (2) adequate oxygenation with the FIO_2 less than or equal to 0.4; (3) normalized $PaCO_2$ in the presence of a normal spontaneous respiratory rate for the patient's age; and (4) adequate cardiac output. The final point is of particular importance in children with myocardial dysfunction. The transition from positive-pressure ventilation to physiological negative-pressure ventilation has the potential to increase afterload on the systemic ventricle. This may negatively affect cardiac output, so the respiratory care practitioner must be attentive to signs of low cardiac output on extubation of patients with marginal cardiac function.

Inhaled Nitric Oxide Therapy

Inhaled nitric oxide is a potent pulmonary vasodilator that has the potential to decrease pulmonary vascular resistance. Though some patients with pulmonary hypertension have PVR that is not responsive to nitric oxide ("fixed" pulmonary hypertension), many others have PVR that is significantly decreased by this drug.

Gas Mixtures to Increase Pulmonary Vascular Resistance

Neonates with single ventricle physiology may develop signs of systemic hypoperfusion as pulmonary vascular resistance drops, favoring more blood flow to the pulmonary vascular bed at the expense of the systemic vascular bed. In addition to other therapies aimed at increasing PVR discussed earlier, clinicians sometimes use gas mixtures to increase PVR.

If a patient has excessive pulmonary blood flow and FIO_2 is 0.21, one may decrease the FIO_2 further by blending amounts of nitrogen in the inhaled gas. Known as subambient or subatmospheric oxygen therapy, this requires the use of a specially modified external blender system in which pure nitrogen is attached to the oxygen inlet of the external blender (Figure 24-22). The outflow of the external blender is then attached to the air inlet of the ventilator. The ventilator FIO_2 control is left at 0.21 and the patient's actual FIO_2 is controlled by the external blender. Turning up the control knob on the external blender *decreases* the FIO_2 delivered to the patient. It is possible to administer pure nitrogen with this setup if the blender control knob is maximally increased. When using this setup, special care must be taken to avoid inadvertent delivery of low oxygen. A continuous oxygen analyzer must

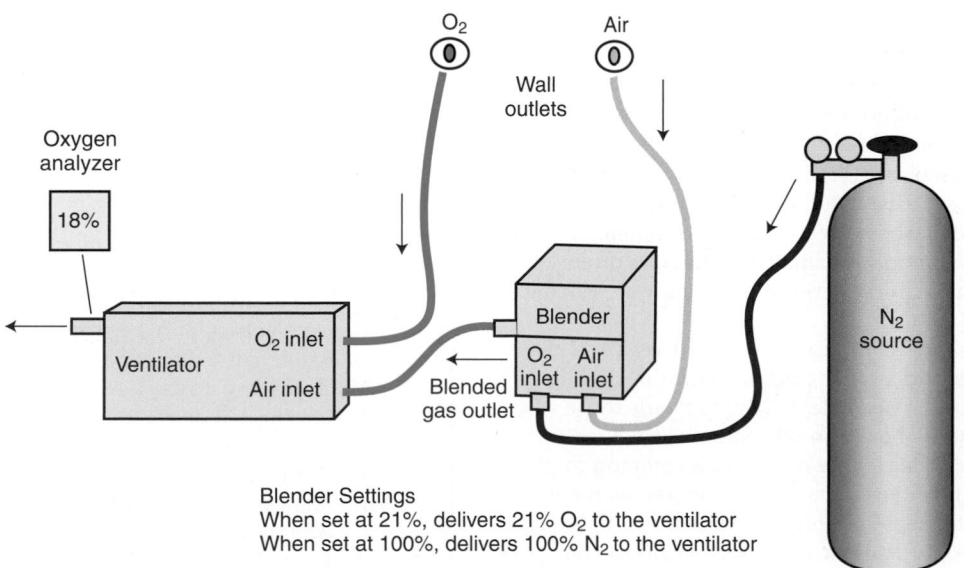

Blender Settings
When set at 21%, delivers 21% O_2 to the ventilator
When set at 100%, delivers 100% N_2 to the ventilator

FIGURE 24-22 Schematic representation of the equipment used for administration of subambient oxygen levels through a ventilator.

be placed in the line with alarms for high and low levels of oxygen. Another safeguard that may be employed is requiring two clinicians to check the setup before applying it to the patient. Typically clinicians target oxygen saturations of 75% to 85%, using an FIO_2 as low as 0.16 to 0.17.

PVR may also be increased by adding CO_2 to the inhaled gas.[23,68-70] This therapy, known as hypercarbic therapy, increases $PaCO_2$ directly by increasing $FICO_2$. Typically 2% to 5% CO_2 is mixed in with the inhaled gas to target an oxygen saturation of 75% to 58%. Adding inhaled CO_2 to the breathing mixture of a spontaneously breathing patient will increase ventilatory drive and precipitate tachypnea. For this reason, this therapy should only be used in patients who are intubated and heavily sedated or under neuromuscular blockade. One method for delivering elevated $FICO_2$ uses a modified air–oxygen mixer that bleeds CO_2 into the ventilator circuit. $FICO_2$ must be closely monitored in the inspiratory portion of the ventilator circuit. One may use a capnometer with high and low $FICO_2$ alarms to safely deliver CO_2 in this manner.

KEY POINTS

- Blood flow in newborns is similar to that in older children and adults, but several intrauterine shunts may persist after birth.
- Shortly after birth several physiological changes occur, including closure of the ductus arteriosus, decrease in pulmonary vascular resistance, and closure of the foramen ovale.
- *Shunt* refers to blood that deviates from its normal flow pattern and may be right to left or left to right in different cardiac defects.
- There are a number of different classification schemes for congenital heart defects including classification by presence or lack of cyanosis, by shunt-type lesions, by lesions that result in obstructed blood flow, and by miscellaneous structural lesions, including those with abnormal valve anatomy or function.
- In understanding the various congenital heart defects, one must understand both the anatomy of each lesion and its underlying physiology.
- Pulmonary vascular resistance may be altered by changes in pH, in oxygenation, and in mean airway pressure.
- In heart lesions where there is mixing of pulmonary and systemic blood, therapeutic maneuvers often target a balance in the ratio of pulmonary to systemic blood flow (Q_P/Q_S).
- Positive-pressure ventilation may negatively affect the pulmonary blood flow or cardiac output in children with a number of heart defects, particularly those who have undergone the Glenn or Fontan procedures.
- In addition to the routine monitoring common to all patients in the intensive care unit, children with congenital heart disease are often monitored with devices that estimate cardiac output or with intravascular devices that provide data on hemodynamics.

ASSESSMENT QUESTIONS

See Evolve Resources for the answers.

1. Normal transition to extrauterine life depends on the pulmonary vascular system:
   A. Remaining in a steady state of balance with the hepatic blood flow
   B. Changing from a low pulmonary vascular resistance to a high pulmonary vascular resistance
   C. Changing from a high pulmonary vascular resistance to a low pulmonary vascular resistance
   D. Maintaining a patent ductus arteriosus
2. Which of the following affects pulmonary vascular resistance?
   A. Changes in PaO_2
   B. Changes in $PaCO_2$
   C. Changes in pH
   D. All of the above
   E. None of the above
3. What are the two categories that have typically been used to classify congenital cardiac defects?
   A. Right sided versus left sided
   B. Atrial versus ventricular
   C. Cyanotic versus acyanotic
   D. Simple versus complex
   E. Above versus below the diaphragm
4. The patent ductus arteriosus connects which two vessels?
   A. Superior vena cava and the pulmonary artery
   B. Aorta to the pulmonary artery
   C. Pulmonary artery and the pulmonary vein
   D. Coronary arteries and the aortic arch
   E. Ductus venosus to the right atrium
5. What is the therapeutic goal of subambient oxygen therapy?
   A. Increase the pulmonary vascular resistance
   B. Balance blood flow between the vena cava and the right atrium
   C. Decrease pulmonary vascular resistance
   D. Increase diastolic blood pressure
6. The purpose of managing pulmonary vascular resistance in the presence of cardiac defects is to ensure the desired balance between systemic and pulmonary blood flow.
   A. True
   B. False
7. Tetralogy of Fallot consists of which four concomitant conditions?
   I. Truncus arteriosus
   II. Left ventricular hypertrophy
   III. Right ventricular hypertrophy
   IV. Overriding aorta
   V. Interrupted aortic arch
   VI. Pulmonary stenosis
   VII. Ventricular septal defect
   VIII. Right ventricular outflow tract obstruction
      A. I, II, III, V
      B. III, IV, VI, VII
      C. V, VI, VII, VIII

8. In complete transposition of the great arteries, the aorta and the pulmonary artery circulation run in series.
   A. True
   B. False

9. For which condition is positive pressure most likely to have a negative impact on pulmonary blood flow and cardiac output?
   A. Unrepaired truncus arteriosus
   B. Total anomalous venous return
   C. Situs inversus
   D. Bidirectional Glenn

10. Increasing gradients between ETCO$_2$ and PaCO$_2$ in patients with congenital cardiac defects are often the result of:
    A. Loss of calibration
    B. Ventilation-perfusion mismatching
    C. Equipment malfunction

References

1. Gilboa SM, Salemi JL, Nembhard WN, Fixler DE, Correa A: Mortality resulting from congenital heart disease among children and adults in the United States, 1999 to 2006, *Circulation* 122(22):2254–2263, 2010.

2. Boneva RS, Botto LD, Moore CA, et al: Mortality associated with congenital heart defects in the United States: trends and racial disparities, 1979–1997, *Circulation* 103(19):2376–2381, 2001.

3. Marelli AJ, Mackie AS, Ionescu-Ittu R, Rahme E, Pilote L: Congenital heart disease in the general population: changing prevalence and age distribution, *Circulation* 115(2):163–172, 2007.

4. Warnes CA, Liberthson R, Danielson GK, et al: Task force 1: the changing profile of congenital heart disease in adult life, *J Am Coll Cardiol* 37(5):1170–1175, 2001.

5. Hermes-DeSantis ER, Clyman RI: Patent ductus arteriosus: pathophysiology and management, *J Perinatol* 26(Suppl 1):S14–18; discussion S22–13, 2006.

6. Wyllie J: Treatment of patent ductus arteriosus, *Semin Neonatol* 8:425, 2003.

7. Jones LJ, Craven PD, Attia J, Thakkinstian A, Wright I: Network meta-analysis of indomethacin versus ibuprofen versus placebo for PDA in preterm infants, *Arch Dis Childhood Fetal Neonatal Ed* 96(1):F45–52, 2011.

8. Holzer R, Hijazi Z: Interventional approach to congenital heart disease, *Curr Opin Cardiol* 19:84, 2004.

9. Cockerham JT, Martin TC, Gutierrez FR, Hartmann AF, Jr., Goldring D, Strauss AW: Spontaneous closure of secundum atrial septal defect in infants and young children, *Am J Cardiol* 52(10):1267–1271, 1983.

10. Mahoney LT, Truesdell SC, Krzmarzick TR, Lauer RM: Atrial septal defects that present in infancy, *Am J Dis Child* 140(11):1115–1118, 1986.

11. Radzik D, Davignon A, van Doesburg N, Fournier A, Marchand T, Ducharme G: Predictive factors for spontaneous closure of atrial septal defects diagnosed in the first 3 months of life, *J Am Coll Cardiol* 22(3):851–853, 1993.

12. Meier B, Lock JE: Contemporary management of patent foramen ovale, *Circulation* 107(1):5–9, 2003.

13. Bartakian S, Fagan TE, Schaffer MS, Darst JR: Device closure of secundum atrial septal defects in children <15 kg: complication rates and indications for referral, *JACC Cardiovasc Intervent* 5(11):1178–1184, 2012.

14. Kimball TR, Daniels SR, Meyer RA, et al: Effect of digoxin on contractility and symptoms in infants with a large ventricular septal defect, *Am J Cardiol* 68(13):1377–1382, 1991.

15. Hijazi ZM, Hakim F, Haweleh AA, et al: Catheter closure of perimembranous ventricular septal defects using the new Amplatzer membranous VSD occluder: initial clinical experience, *Catheter Cardiovasc Interv* 56(4):508–515, 2002.

16. Ghaffar S, Lemler MS, Fixler DE, Ramaciotti C: Trisomy 21 and congenital heart disease: effect of timing of initial echocardiogram, *Clin Ped* 44(1):39–42, 2005.

17. Newfeld EA, Waldman D, Paul MH, et al: Pulmonary vascular disease after systemic-pulmonary arterial shunt operations, *Am J Cardiol* 39(5):715–720, 1977.

18. Stellin G, Vida VL, Milanesi O, et al: Surgical treatment of complete A-V canal defects in children before 3 months of age, *Eur J Cardiothorac Surg* 23(2):187–193, 2003.

19. Setty SP, Shen I: *Atrioventricular septal defects*, ed 2, Philadelphia, 2006, Mosby.

20. McCrindle BW, Blackstone EH, Williams WG, et al: Are outcomes of surgical versus transcatheter balloon valvotomy equivalent in neonatal critical aortic stenosis? *Circulation* 104(12 Suppl 1):I152–158, 2001.

21. Maskatia SA, Ing FF, Justino H, et al: Twenty-five year experience with balloon aortic valvuloplasty for congenital aortic stenosis, *Am J Cardiol* 108(7):1024–1028, 2011.

22. Rajasinghe HA, Reddy VM, Van Son JA, et al: Coarctation repair using end-to-side anastomosis of descending aorta to proximal aortic arch, *Ann Thorac Surg* 61(3):840–844, 1996.

23. Tabbutt S, Ramamoorthy C, Montenegro LM, et al: Impact of inspired gas mixtures on preoperative infants with hypoplastic left heart syndrome during controlled ventilation, *Circulation* 104(12 Suppl 1):I159–164, 2001.

24. Lister G, Hellenbrand WE, Kleinman CS, Talner NS: Physiologic effects of increasing hemoglobin concentration in left-to-right shunting in infants with ventricular septal defects, *N Engl J Med* 306(9):502–506, 1982.

25. Norwood WI, Lang P, Hansen DD: Physiologic repair of aortic atresia-hypoplastic left heart syndrome, *N Engl J Med* 308(1):23–26, 1983.

26. Gaynor JW, Mahle WT, Cohen MI, et al: Risk factors for mortality after the Norwood procedure, *Eur J Cardiothorac Surg* 22(1):82–89, 2002.

27. Akintuerk H, Michel-Behnke I, Valeske K, et al: Stenting of the arterial duct and banding of the pulmonary arteries: basis for combined Norwood stage I and II repair in hypoplastic left heart, *Circulation* 105(9):1099–1103, 2002.

28. Galantowicz M, Cheatham JP: Lessons learned from the development of a new hybrid strategy for the management of hypoplastic left heart syndrome, *Pediatr Cardiol* 26(3):190–199, 2005.

29. Bacha EA, Daves S, Hardin J, et al: Single-ventricle palliation for high-risk neonates: the emergence of an alternative hybrid stage I strategy, *J Thorac Cardiovasc Surg* 131(1):163–171 e162, 2006.

30. DiCarlo JV, Raphaely RC, Steven JM, Norwood WI, Costarino AT: Pulmonary mechanics in infants after cardiac surgery, *Crit Care Med* 20(1):22–27, 1992.

31. Genz T, Locher D, Genz S, Schumacher G, Buhlmeyer K: Chest X-ray film patterns in children with isolated total anomalous pulmonary vein connection, *Eur J Pediatr* 150(1):14–18, 1990.

32. Atz AM, Wessel DL: Inhaled nitric oxide in the neonate with cardiac disease, *Semin Perinatol* 21(5):441–455, 1997.

33. Mitchell SC, Korones SB, Berendes HW: Congenital heart disease in 56,109 births. Incidence and natural history, *Circulation* 43(3):323–332, 1971.

34. Reddy VM, Liddicoat JR, McElhinney DB, Brook MM, Stanger P, Hanley FL: Routine primary repair of tetralogy of Fallot in neonates and infants less than three months of age, *Ann Thorac Surg* 60(6 Suppl):S592–596, 1995.

35. Parry AJ, McElhinney DB, Kung GC, Reddy VM, Brook MM, Hanley FL: Elective primary repair of acyanotic tetralogy of Fallot in early infancy: overall outcome and impact on the pulmonary valve, *J Am Coll Cardiol* 36(7):2279–2283, 2000.

36. Pigula FA, Khalil PN, Mayer JE, del Nido PJ, Jonas RA: Repair of tetralogy of Fallot in neonates and young infants, *Circulation* 100(19 Suppl):II157–161, 1999.

37. Stewart RD, Backer CL, Young L, Mavroudis C: Tetralogy of Fallot: results of a pulmonary valve-sparing strategy, *Ann Thorac Surg* 80(4):1431–1438; discussion 1438–1439, 2005.

38. McFaul RC, Mair DD, Feldt RH, Ritter DG, McGoon DC: Truncus arteriosus and previous pulmonary arterial banding: clinical and hemodynamic assessment, *Am J Cardiol* 38(5):626–632, 1976.

39. Thompson LD, McElhinney DB, Reddy M, Petrossian E, Silverman NH, Hanley FL: Neonatal repair of truncus arteriosus: continuing improvement in outcomes, *Ann Thorac Surg* 72(2):391–395, 2001.

40. Botto LD, Correa A, Erickson JD: Racial and temporal variations in the prevalence of heart defects, *Pediatrics* 107(3):E32, 2001.

41. Backer CL, Ilbawi MN, Ohtake S, et al: Transposition of the great arteries: a comparison of results of the mustard procedure versus the arterial switch, *Ann Thorac Surg* 48(1):10-14, 1989.

42. Hazekamp MG, Ottenkamp J, Quaegebeur JM, et al: Follow-up of arterial switch operation, *Thorac Cardiovasc Surg* 39 (Suppl 2):166–169, 1991.

43. Martin RP, Qureshi SA, Ettedgui JA, et al: An evaluation of right and left ventricular function after anatomical correction and intra-atrial repair operations for complete transposition of the great arteries, *Circulation* 82(3):808–816, 1990.

44. Veelken N, Gravinghoff L, Keck EW, Freitag HJ: Improved neurological outcome following early anatomical correction of transposition of the great arteries, *Clin Cardiol* 15(4):275–279, 1992.

45. Akagi T, Hashino K, Maeno Y, et al: Balloon dilatation of the pulmonary valve in a patient with pulmonary atresia and intact ventricular septum using a commercially available radiofrequency catheter, *Pediatr Cardiol* 18(1):61–63, 1997.

46. Colli AM, Perry SB, Lock JE, Keane JF: Balloon dilation of critical valvar pulmonary stenosis in the first month of life, *Cathet Cardiovasc Diagn* 34(1):23–28, 1995.

47. Gibbs JL, Blackburn ME, Uzun O, Dickinson DF, Parsons JM, Chatrath RR: Laser valvotomy with balloon valvoplasty for pulmonary atresia with intact ventricular septum: five years' experience, *Heart* 77(3):225–228, 1997.

48. Justo RN, Nykanen DG, Williams WG, Freedom RM, Benson LN: Transcatheter perforation of the right ventricular outflow tract as initial therapy for pulmonary valve atresia and intact ventricular septum in the newborn, *Cathet Cardiovasc Diagn* 40(4):408–413, 1997.

49. Agnoletti G, Piechaud JF, Bonhoeffer P, et al: Perforation of the atretic pulmonary valve. Long-term follow-up, *J Am Coll Cardiol* 41(8):1399–1403, 2003.

50. Schmitt HJ, Schuetz WH, Proeschel PA, Jaklin C: Accuracy of pulse oximetry in children with cyanotic congenital heart disease, *J Cardiothorac Vasc Anesth* 7(1):61–65, 1993.

51. Irita K, Kai Y, Akiyoshi K, Tanaka Y, Takahashi S: Performance evaluation of a new pulse oximeter during mild hypothermic cardiopulmonary bypass, *Anesth Analg* 96(1):11–14, 2003.

52. Malviya S, Reynolds PI, Voepel-Lewis T, et al: False alarms and sensitivity of conventional pulse oximetry versus the Masimo SET technology in the pediatric postanesthesia care unit, *Anesth Analg* 90(6):1336–1340, 2000.

53. Torres A, Jr, Skender KM, Wohrley JD, et al: Pulse oximetry in children with congenital heart disease: effects of cardiopulmonary bypass and cyanosis, *J Intensive Care Med* 19(4):229–234, 2004.

54. Hess D: *Capnometry*, New York, 1998, McGraw-Hill.

55. Roberts WA, Maniscalco WM, Cohen AR, Litman RS, Chhibber A: The use of capnography for recognition of esophageal intubation in the neonatal intensive care unit, *Pediatr Pulmonol* 19(5):262–268, 1995.

56. Falk JL, Rackow EC, Weil MH: End-tidal carbon dioxide concentration during cardiopulmonary resuscitation, *N Engl J Med* 318(10):607–611, 1988.

57. Morrison LJ, Deakin CD, Morley PT, et al: Part 8: Advanced life support: 2010. international consensus on cardiopulmonary resuscitation and emergency cardiovascular care science with treatment recommendations, *Circulation* 122(16 Suppl 2):S345–421, 2010.

58. Tweddell JS, Ghanayem NS, Mussatto KA, et al: Mixed venous oxygen saturation monitoring after stage 1 palliation for hypoplastic left heart syndrome, *AnnThorac Surg* 84(4):1301–1310; discussion 1310-1311, 2007.

59. Hoffman GM, Ghanayem NS, Tweddell JS: Noninvasive assessment of cardiac output, *Semin Thorac Cardiovasc Surg Pediatr Cardiac Surg Ann* 12–21, 2005.

60. Li J, Van Arsdell GS, Zhang G, et al: Assessment of the relationship between cerebral and splanchnic oxygen saturations measured by near-infrared spectroscopy and direct measurements of systemic haemodynamic variables and oxygen transport after the Norwood procedure, *Heart* 92(11):1678–1685, 2006.

61. McQuillen PS, Nishimoto MS, Bottrell CL, et al: Regional and central venous oxygen saturation monitoring following pediatric cardiac surgery: concordance and association with clinical variables, *Pediatr Crit Care Med* 8(2):154–160, 2007.

62. Kloth RL, Baum VC: Very early extubation in children after cardiac surgery, *Crit Care Med* 30(4):787–791, 2002.

63. Davis S, Worley S, Mee RB, Harrison AM: Factors associated with early extubation after cardiac surgery in young children, *Pediatr Crit Care Med* 5(1):63–68, 2004.

64. Vricella LA, Dearani JA, Gundry SR, et al: Ultra fast track in elective congenital cardiac surgery, *Ann Thorac Surg* 69(3):865–871, 2000.

65. Shekerdemian L, Bohn D: Cardiovascular effects of mechanical ventilation, *Arch Dis Child* 80(5):475–480, 1999.

66. Wolf GK, Walsh BK, Green ML, Arnold JH: Electrical activity of the diaphragm during extubation readiness testing in critically ill children, *Pediatri Crit Care Med* 12(6):e220–224, 2011.

67. Newth CJ, Venkataraman S, Willson DF, et al: Weaning and extubation readiness in pediatric patients, *Pediatr Crit Care Med* 10(1):1–11, 2009.

68. Jobes DR, Nicolson SC, Steven JM, et al: Carbon dioxide prevents pulmonary overcirculation in hypoplastic left heart syndrome, *Ann Thorac Surg* 54(1):150–151, 1992.

69. Reddy VM, Liddicoat JR, Fineman JR, McElhinney DB, Klein JR, Hanley FL: Fetal model of single ventricle physiology: hemodynamic effects of oxygen, nitric oxide, carbon dioxide, and hypoxia in the early postnatal period, *J Thorac Cardiovasc Surg* 112(2):437–449, 1996.

70. Chang AC, Zucker HA, Hickey PR, Wessel DL: Pulmonary vascular resistance in infants after cardiac surgery: role of carbon dioxide and hydrogen ion, *Crit Care Med* 23(3):568–574, 1995.

Chapter 25

Pediatric Sleep-Disordered Breathing

PETER M. LUCKETT, KAMAL NAQVI

LEARNING OBJECTIVES

After reading this chapter the reader will be able to:

1. Describe normal sleep development
2. Describe normal sleep architecture
3. Describe the difference between central and obstructive apnea
4. Describe the difference between SIDS and ALTE
5. Name the intervention that altered the incidence of SIDS
6. Describe the pathophysiology of obstructive sleep apnea
7. Describe a sleep history and physical examination
8. Describe the basic measurements made during a sleep study
9. Name the most common cause of obstructive sleep apnea in children
10. Name the two most common treatments for obstructive sleep apnea

KEY TERMS

Acute life-threatening event (ALTE)
Apnea of prematurity (AOP)
Central sleep apnea (CSA)
Continuous positive airway pressure (CPAP)

EEG arousal
Electroencephalogram (EEG)
Non–rapid eye movement (NREM) sleep
Obstructive sleep apnea (OSA)

Periodic breathing
Rapid eye movement (REM) sleep
Sleep architecture
Sleep-disordered breathing (SDB)
Sudden infant death syndrome (SIDS)

INTRODUCTION

Sleep may be defined as a neurophysiologically distinct state of awareness that is required for human health. It involves the intersection of developmental, physiological, homeostatic, and behavioral mechanisms. The function of sleep in mammals is not well understood. Nevertheless, sleep deprivation causes serious neurocognitive deficits and is lethal in animals. The association of disordered sleep and daytime function has long been appreciated. Sir William Osler stated that "chronic enlargement of the tissues of the tonsillar ring is an affection of great importance and may influence in an extraordinary way the mental and bodily development of children. . . . *At night the child's sleep is greatly disturbed; the respirations are loud and snorting, and there are sometimes prolonged pauses, followed by deep noisy inspirations.*"[1] The neurodevelopmental and cognitive consequences of disturbed sleep in childhood are now an area of intense study.

NORMAL SLEEP DEVELOPMENT

Sleep patterns progressively change throughout childhood.[2,3] A normal newborn spends 70% of a 24-hour day asleep. The baby typically has 3- to 4-hour sleep periods with 1- to 2-hour awake periods. In the first few months of life, babies have not yet become fully entrained to a day–night cycle, but a circadian rhythm consolidates by about the eighth week. Critical sleep reorganization occurs between 8 to 12 weeks. **Non–rapid eye movement (NREM)** sleep develops by 6 months while **rapid eye movement (REM)**

Box 25-1	Sleep Duration By Age
Full-term Infant	16-18 hours
1 year	15 hours
2 years	13-14 hours
4 years	12 hours
10 years	8-10 hours
Mid-adolescence	8.5 hours
Later adolescence	7-8 hours

sleep amount decreases. At 6 months, total sleep time is 13 to 14 hours and sleep episodes are 6 to 8 hours in duration. Seventy percent of infants are sleeping through the night at 9 months. Toddlers' total sleep time decreases further to about 12 to 14 hours. The sleep cycle length is about 60 minutes. Daytime sleep decreases throughout the first year. In preschool age children the sleep cycle lengthens to about 90 minutes and total sleep time shortens to 11 to 12 hours. Daytime sleep continues to decrease, and most have given up napping by 4 to 5 years. The sleep pattern in school-age children becomes more stable and sleep time continues to decrease. Box 25-1 reviews the sleep duration by age.

The **electroencephalogram (EEG)** is used to characterize sleep.[4] The EEG undergoes maturational changes throughout early childhood. The electrical activity recorded at the surface of the scalp is a summation of electrical activity coming from deep brain structures. As the brain develops, the EEG changes rapidly. In utero the pattern is discontinuous. Three sleep stages are present in the term infant: (1) REM or active sleep, (2) NREM or quiet sleep, and (3) indeterminate sleep. REM sleep predominates in the neonate. During this period REM may be observed at sleep onset, a pattern that is quite abnormal in later life. Quiet sleep (NREM) or slow wave sleep is poorly developed in infants. However, in the first year of life REM sleep duration decreases and NREM sleep duration increases. There is an intermediate EEG pattern that is referred to as indeterminate sleep because it is distinguishable neither as REM nor NREM. As the child develops, REM sleep continues to decrease until the duration of REM stabilizes at approximately 20% to 25% of sleep time sometime after 2 years of age. REM is a period when brain metabolism is the highest and muscle activity is dramatically decreased. NREM sleep has been referred to as regenerative sleep. NREM sleep continues to increase in duration and peaks between 5 and 9 years and then decreases throughout the rest of life. When fully developed, NREM sleep has four distinct stages characterized by four EEG wave patterns. Quantification of these EEG stages provides the basis for a description of **sleep architecture.** In light, or stage 1, sleep, alpha wave activity predominates and slow eye rolling is observed. Stage 1 sleep is approximately 5% of the sleep period. Stage 2 sleep is 45% to 55% of the sleep period. The EEG contains sleep spindles and K complexes, markers of the stage. Stages 3 and 4 sleep together account for approximately 20% of sleep duration. This EEG stage contains slow waves. An additional important pattern is the **EEG arousal.** During an EEG arousal there is disruption of the quality and duration of the sleep stages but no arousal to wakefulness. Disruption of the sleep architecture by EEG arousals causes inefficient and nonrestorative sleep.

DISORDERED BREATHING IN INFANTS

Respiration is under both voluntary and involuntary control. There has been a dramatic increase in our understanding of the anatomical, neurochemical, and genetic basis for the control of the rhythm of respiration. Respiratory control matures as the brain matures. A number of features of this development place babies at increased risk of **sleep-disordered breathing (SDB).** Classically models of control of respiration described central chemoreceptors in the medulla of the brainstem and peripheral chemoreceptors in the carotid body. The central receptors respond to pH and carbon dioxide tension, whereas the peripheral receptors respond to hypoxia. These models are currently undergoing modification as new evidence emerges.[5] Infants have respiratory instability and very commonly have brief apneas up to 10 seconds. These pauses are typically REM related. **Periodic breathing,** a breathing pattern also common in infants, may be defined as a pattern of cycles of rapid breathing followed by pauses longer than 3 seconds. Each cycle may occur 2 to 3 times per minute. Brief apneas and periodic breathing decrease in frequency with increasing age. Apnea is defined as a respiratory pause that is sustained for more than 15 to 20 seconds or as little as 10 seconds if it is associated with bradycardia or cyanosis. Central apnea occurs when respiratory effort ceases; there is no chest movement and hence no air flow. Diagnosis of central apnea must take into account a multitude of factors. Because infants normally have a more rapid baseline respiratory rate and a reduced respiratory reserve, and therefore less protection from hypoxia, shorter central events can be more clinically significant in this age group. Central apnea can yield significant physiological compromise such as bradycardia or color change associated with declining oxyhemoglobin levels.

A number of anatomical and physiological features place the neonate at increased risk for SDB. Infants are near obligate nasal breathers. Nasal obstruction may paradoxically lead to central apnea in neonates or contribute to respiratory obstruction and lead to obstructive apnea. The shape of the chest is more rounded, the diaphragm tends to be flatter, and the rib articulation is less angular. Therefore the rib cage contributes less to overall breathing than in older children. Chest wall compliance is high in the infant. Unlike in the older child and adults in whom functional residual capacity (FRC) is maintained passively by chest wall recoil, FRC in neonates must be maintained actively. FRC is further decreased in REM during the period of decreased muscle activity.

Apnea of prematurity (AOP) is observed in infants born prematurely and is common among infants less than 32 weeks of gestation. The pathophysiology of AOP is not fully understood. Immaturity of neural control of the cardiorespiratory system, often in conjunction with environmental stimuli, seems to be the basis of AOP. AOP is often treated with caffeine, which is thought to stimulate the respiratory centers.

In **central sleep apnea (CSA)** there is an absence of respiratory effort and airflow. The American Academy of Pediatrics (AAP) defines CSA as "an unexplained episode of cessation of breathing for 20 seconds or longer, or a shorter respiratory pause associated with bradycardia, cyanosis, pallor, and/or marked hypotonia."[6] CSA in infants and children is often idiopathic but like AOP, immaturity of the respiratory centers seems to play a role. When significant CSA is present, an underlying cause should be sought because there are many medical conditions associated with CSA (Box 25-2). Central and obstructive apnea may be present at the same time in mixed apnea pattern (Figure 25-1). In some conditions, such as heart disease or obesity, central hypoventilation is due to reduced central chemoreceptor insensitivity.

SIDS AND ALTE

Sudden infant death syndrome (SIDS) is a devastating event that accounted for 2226 infant deaths in 2009.[7] It is the leading cause of death in infants in the first 12 months of life and is the third leading cause of death in infants overall in the United States. It is defined as "the sudden death of an infant less than one year of age, which remains unexplained after a thorough case investigation, including performance of a complete autopsy, *examination of the death scene,* and review of the clinical history."[7]

SIDS almost always takes place when the infant is presumed to have been asleep, either during the day or at night. However, more than 70% of its victims are found in the early morning hours after the nighttime sleep.[8] The incidence peaks in infants from 2 to 4 months of life (Figure 25-2). This period coincides with significant changes known to occur in sleep organization and in the modulation of brainstem centers involved in respiratory and arousal state control. SIDS is uncommon after 6 months of age, with 90% of SIDS victims affected in the first 6 months of life. It is rare after the first birthday.

Many theories have been offered to explain the tragedy of SIDS. Because it is assumed that there must be a cessation of breathing, there has long been a focus on apnea as a proximate event.[9] The apnea hypothesis has driven SIDS research for the last 40 years and led some to catastrophic conclusions.[10,11] Throughout the 1980s an intense search for a predictive model of SIDS was unsuccessful. Abnormalities in cardiac rhythm,[12] control of ventilation,[13] autonomic dysfunction,[14] and faulty arousal[15] have all been a focus of research. More recently it has been suggested that the occurrence of SIDS may not require the susceptible infant to be abnormal but rather is a consequence of normal neonatal development and physiology placed in the proper environmental context. There is now general agreement that the cause of SIDS is multifactorial.

Although a mechanistic explanation of the cause of SIDS has been elusive, significant progress has been made in prevention of SIDS. Risk factors associated with SIDS have been known for decades[16] (Box 25-3). Since the early 1990s numerous epidemiological studies pointed to an increased risk of SIDS in infants who sleep in the prone position.[17,18] It has been estimated that as many as 50% of cases of SIDS may be related to sleep position. In 1992 the American Academy of Pediatrics made official recommendations with respect to sleep position and in 1994 the *Back to Sleep* campaign was initiated in the United States.[19] The movement to aggressively encourage back sleeping has led to a dramatic decrease in the incidence of SIDS worldwide (Figure 25-3).

There are other risk factors that may be modified to reduce the incidence of SIDS. Maternal cigarette smoking during pregnancy has been found to be a major risk factor for SIDS and appears to be dose dependent.[20] Postnatal exposure to cigarette smoke further increases the risk. Some studies have found breastfeeding to be partly protective against SIDS, but this finding has been inconsistent. Overheating and loose bedding have both been associated with SIDS. Bed sharing has been shown to be a hazardous practice. Overlying remains an important cause of unexplained death in infants and should be considered along with other forms of inadvertent suffocation during a death scene investigation. The most effective means of providing a safe sleeping environment is through meticulous risk mitigation.[21]

An **acute life-threatening event (ALTE)** is defined as "an episode that is frightening to the observer and is characterized by some combination of apnea (central and occasionally obstructive), color change (usually cyanotic or

---

Box 25–2	Conditions Associated with CSA

- Arnold-Chiari type II malformation
- Prader-Willi syndrome
- Ondine's curse (congenital central hypoventilation syndrome)
- Central nervous system pathology (intraventricular hemorrhage, brain anomaly, CNS infection, ischemic infarction)
- Drugs
- Sepsis
- Respiratory infections (RSV, pertussis)
- Gastroesophageal reflux
- Metabolic disorder
- Neoplasm
- Hypothermia
- Idiopathic

CNS, Central nervous system; *RSV,* respiratory syncytial virus.

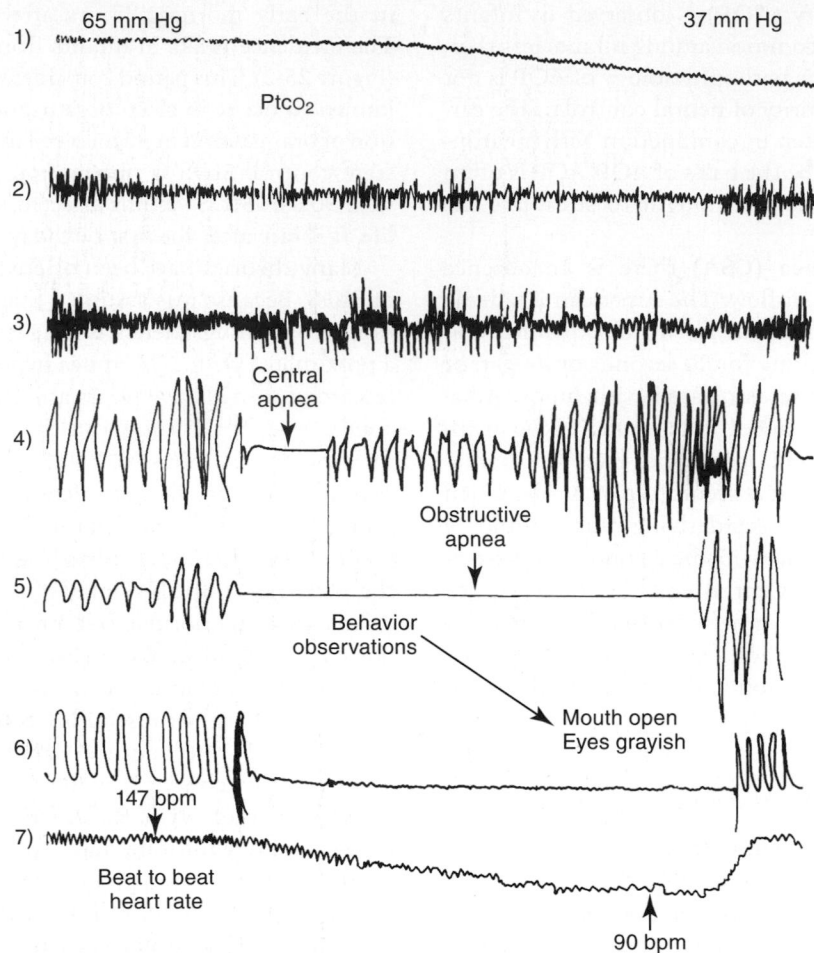

FIGURE 25-1 A 1-minute record from a PSG showing a 37-second mixed apnea. Channel 1 shows a drop in transcutaneous oxygen tension from 65 to 37 mm. Channel 4 shows breathing movements and channels 5 and 6 show airflow. There is an initial cessation of respiratory effort and airflow (central apnea). As effort increases there continues to be no airflow until there is a gasp. Both heart rate and oxygenation fell during this mixed central and obstructive apnea.

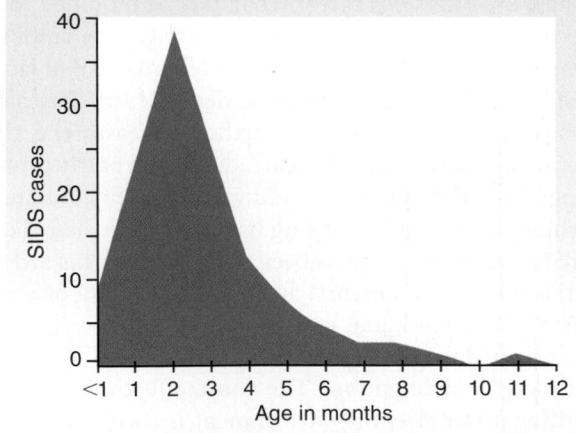

FIGURE 25-2 Sudden infant death syndrome (SIDS) deaths in Maryland in 1985. Note the peak at 2 months of age and a decrease after 6 months of age.

Box 25-3	Risk Factors for Sudden Infant Death Syndrome

EPIDEMIOLOGICAL RISK FACTORS
- Male sex
- African-American race
- Teenage maternal age
- Prematurity
- Winter season
- Low birth weight

MODIFIABLE RISK FACTORS
- Exposure to opioids or cocaine in utero
- Anemia during pregnancy
- Inadequate prenatal care
- Bottle feeding
- Maternal smoking
- Soft bed covers or loose bedding
- Overheating
- Bed sharing
- Prone sleeping position

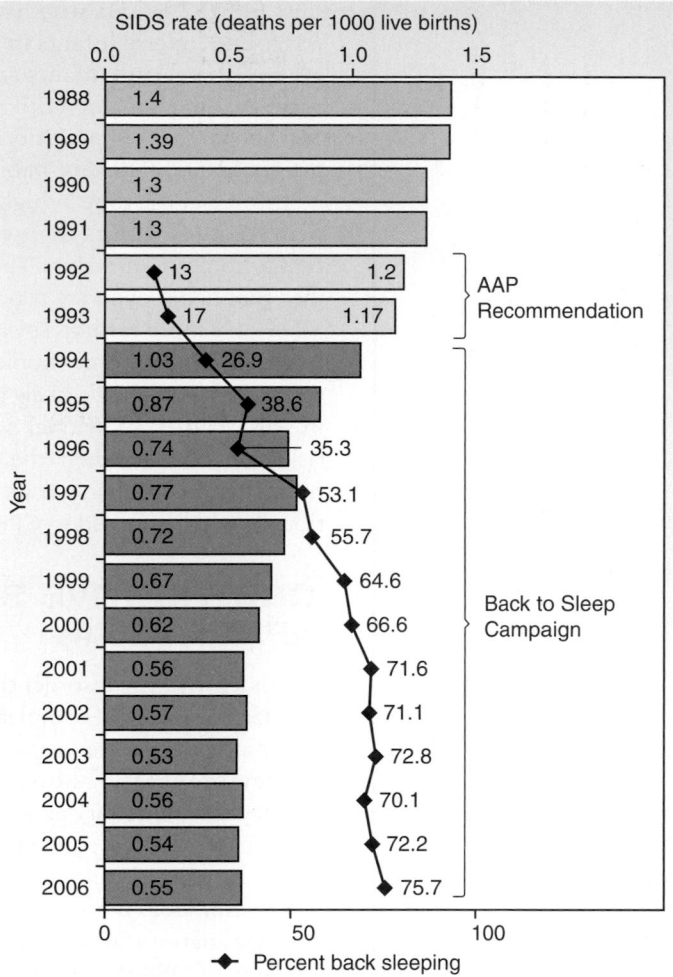

SIDS rate and back sleeping (1988-2006)

FIGURE 25-3   The SIDS rate (deaths per 1000 live births) in the United States from the beginning of the recognition of the importance of sleep position (data from 1988 to 2006). The Back to Sleep campaign began in 1994. The percent back sleeping is also shown. The SIDS death rate fell 60% as back sleeping was rising.

pallid but occasionally erythematous or plethoric), marked change in muscle tone (usually marked limpness), choking, or gagging."[22] The ALTE may be idiopathic or have an underlying cause. The phenomenon of an ALTE is often discussed in relation to SIDS. However, the relationship between ALTE and SIDS is poorly understood and is increasingly controversial. Indeed, the vast majority of infants who die with SIDS have not had an episode of apnea until their terminal event. Parental concern may make getting an accurate account of the event difficult at presentation. With a credible story, especially in the presence of cyanosis or change in heart rate or with a resuscitation effort, an admission to the hospital is warranted. Evaluation must include a thorough history, including a family and social history. An accurate description of the event is crucial. A full review of systems and thorough physical examination should help to narrow the very extensive differential diagnosis.[23] The physical examination should examine carefully for bruising and should include a full

neurological examination including muscle tone and funduscopic examination. The physical examination should include a search for dysmorphic features, and abnormalities of the upper airway, chest, and cardiovascular system should be sought. Basic measurements of head circumference, body weight, length, and blood pressure should be made and compared with norms. The parental concern should be assessed and sensitively addressed. The extent of the workup will be determined by this admission data. A heightened index of suspicion must be maintained throughout because an identifiable cause is found in nearly 50% of cases. Box 25-4 reviews the differential diagnosis of ALTE.

Home monitoring for apnea in infants at risk remains a controversial subject. In the 1980s and 1990s the prevailing sentiment was that home monitoring made sense because some patients who had apnea requiring resuscitation subsequently had a recurrence of this life-threatening event. Furthermore, a small number of patients subsequently died of SIDS. Some centers have had a home

Box 25-4	Differential Diagnosis of ALTE

GASTROINTESTINAL (50%)
Gastroesophageal reflux
Intussusceptions
Volvulus

NEUROLOGICAL (30%)
Seizures
Intracranial hemorrhage
CNS anomaly
Arnold-Chiari malformation
Hydrocephalus
CNS infection
Malignancy

RESPIRATORY (20%)
Viral infection (e.g., pertussis)
Mycoplasma spp. infection
Obstructive sleep apnea
Abnormal respiratory control
  • Breath-holding spells
  • Congenital central hypoventilation
  • Apnea of prematurity

CARDIAC (5%)
Arrhythmia
Long QT syndrome
Wolf-Parkinson-White syndrome
Cardiomyopathy
Myocarditis
Aberrant left coronary artery

METABOLIC (LESS THAN 5%)
Inborn errors of metabolism (fatty acid defects)
Sepsis, all causes
Medication (prescription and nonprescription)
Nonaccidental trauma
Accidental suffocation

CNS, Central nervous system.

for 306 normal term babies, 443 preterm infants, 178 SIDS-sibs, and 152 infants who had an ALTE. No increased risk was found in term infants in the SIDS-sibling or the ALTE groups. Premature infants seemed to be at increased risk of an "extreme" event until 43 weeks postconceptual age but not after. This peak does not coincide with the peak incidence of SIDS. Six babies died but were not being monitored at the time. A high number of obstructed events were recorded, events that would be missed with conventional home monitoring. This study did not support the idea that babies who are thought to be at increased risk of SIDS have more cardiorespiratory events. The AAP has recommended that home monitors not be used as a strategy to prevent SIDS.[26] It is likely that monitoring will continue in select babies. Individual patients thought to be at high risk may benefit when the caretakers are appropriately trained and compliant in its use. Caretakers in this situation should be trained in CPR as well.

OBSTRUCTIVE SLEEP APNEA (OSA)

OSA is a breathing disorder that occurs in sleep and is characterized by repeated complete or partial obstruction of the upper airway such that gas exchange and/or sleep integrity are compromised.[27] Multiple factors influence airway patency including airway geometry, anatomical structures of the upper airway, control of laryngeal muscles, cardiorespiratory control, and neuromuscular factors.[28] Because obstruction does not occur during wakefulness, it is apparent that anatomical features alone do not suffice. The major cause of OSA in children without another predisposing condition (Box 25-5) is adenotonsillar hypertrophy. Anatomical restriction in the airway by the tonsils in combination with altered laryngeal muscle control results in obstruction of the airway. OSA is common and occurs in

monitoring program in place for many years and remain committed to monitoring high-risk infants. These include (1) babies who have had a sibling die of SIDS, (2) premature babies who are known to have had significant apnea, and (3) infants who have had an ALTE. Recently the efficacy of this practice has been called into question. In an editorial accompanying the CHIME study,[24] it was stated that "the physiologic basis for such a practice are more in doubt than ever."[25]

The CHIME study ran from 1994 to 1998 and was published in 2001. It was the first longitudinal study of a large number of infants recording the incidence of cardiorespiratory events before and after "conventional" or "extreme" apnea/bradycardia that were clinically relevant. These investigators enrolled 1079 infants who were either healthy term infants or babies considered to be at risk. The at-risk groups were a SIDS-sibling group, an idiopathic ALTE group, and a preterm group. Using sophisticated monitoring equipment to record events in these babies, more than 29,000 days of monitoring data were obtained

Box 25-5	Conditions with Predisposition for Obstructive Sleep Apnea

Arnold-Chiari malformation
Obesity
Down syndrome
Nasal obstruction caused by septal deviation, polyps, or masses
Achondroplasia
Apert syndrome
Craniofacial syndromes (Pierre Robin syndrome, Treacher Collins syndrome, Crouzon syndrome)
Prader-Willi syndrome
Neuromuscular disease (Duchenne's muscular dystrophy, spinal muscular atrophy)
Adenotonsillar hypertrophy
Sickle cell disease
Macrognathia
Mucopolysaccharide storage disease

approximately 2% of children. In children with a predisposing condition the prevalence is considerably greater than this. It may occur in children of all ages, but the prevalence peaks between 2 and 8 years of age, which coincides with the time at which the size of the tonsils is at their peak relative to the upper airway size.

Narrowing of the airway during respiration is a normal phenomenon. The caliber of the airway oscillates normally with afferent neural activity from the respiratory centers. During sleep, ventilatory drive is decreased. Upper airway muscle tone decreases, especially during REM. Therefore upper airway resistance increases during sleep. The upper airway may be modeled as a Starling resistor. Upstream (nasal) and downstream (tracheal) pressures determine flow only if the upper airway is patent. The collapsible upper airway will remain patent only if the pressure inside is greater than the pressure outside the airway, known as *Pcrit*.[29] Multiple factors may lead to upper airway pressure approaching Pcrit during respiration and collapse of the airway. These include structural narrowing of the airway, abnormal neuromuscular tone, and possibly genetic and hormonal factors. It is likely that multiple factors work in concert. For example, even though adenotonsillar hypertrophy is a common "cause" of OSA in children, it alone is not a sufficient cause.[30]

The variable changes in upper airway resistance and caliber lead to a continuum of clinical syndromes, which range from primary snoring to frank intermittent occlusion of the upper airway.[31] Primary snoring may affect as many as 10% of children but is not typically associated with disturbance of sleep architecture or gas exchange abnormality. Upper airway resistance syndrome (UARS) is characterized by recurrent respiratory effort—related arousals during sleep. These episodes are not typically associated with gas exchange abnormalities but may be associated with significant daytime symptoms. Obstructive hypoventilation (obstructive hypopnea) may occur in the absence of complete obstruction of the airway and cessation of airflow. These sleep-related events lead to disruption of sleep architecture, degradation of sleep quality, and gas exchange abnormalities that may cause significant daytime symptoms.

Unrecognized and untreated upper airway obstruction is a considerable threat to the child's health. It has long been known that chronic obstruction is associated with substantial morbidity. Osler observed over a century ago that in such children during the day, *"The expression is dull, heavy, and apathetic . . . the child responds slowly to questions, and may be sullen and cross. Among other symptoms may be mentioned headache, which is by no means uncommon, general listlessness, and an indisposition for physical or mental exertion."*[1] In 1965 Noonan described two cases of reversible cor pulmonale secondary to tonsillar hypertrophy.[32] Jaffe noted in 1974 that "following adenotonsillectomy in select cases there occurs a period of rapid growth and development."[33] Guilleminault reported sleep apnea in eight children in

1976 and the first large series of children with OSA in 1981.[34,35]

It became clear in the 1980s and 1990s that the childhood syndrome of OSA was distinct from adult OSA. Features that distinguish childhood from adult OSA are shown in Table 25-1. In otherwise normal children, sleep architecture may be relatively preserved in OSA compared with adults and excessive daytime sleepiness is less commonly observed. Children with OSA are not typically obese, though they may be. They may have many fewer true obstructions during the night if any at all. They more typically have intermittent or continuous partial obstruction or UARS. On the other hand, obese children may have a clinical syndrome that is more similar to adult OSA.[36] They may have more excessive daytime sleepiness (EDS), systemic hypertension, left ventricular hypertrophy, insulin resistance, or elevated C-reactive protein (CRP) levels. This form of OSA in children has increased as the incidence of obesity has increased in childhood.

Evaluation of the child for SDB begins with a comprehensive history. Symptoms may be volunteered by an observant parent but must also be actively sought by the clinician. A clear description of sleep habits should be obtained. Both nighttime and daytime symptoms should be recorded. Nighttime symptoms may include snoring, respiratory pauses, snorts, mouth breathing, or abrupt

TABLE 25-1

Features of Childhood and Adult OSA

	Childhood	Adult
Obesity	May be normal or underweight	Common
Snoring	Often continuous	Usually intermittent with respiratory pauses
Excessive daytime sleepiness (EDS)	Infrequent	Common
EEG pattern	UARS or hypopneas common; may not have cortical arousal	Obstructed pattern with EEG arousals
Sleep architecture	Often preserved	Disrupted
Tonsils and adenoids enlarged	Very common	Uncommon
Sleep state abnormality	REM is most common	REM and NREM
Insulin resistance	Absent	Frequent
Cardiovascular effects	Infrequent	Frequent
Prominent symptoms	Behavioral or neurocognitive; enuresis	EDS, work performance, fatigue, morning headache

EEG, Electroencephalogram; *NREM,* non–rapid eye movement; *REM,* rapid eye movement; *UARS,* upper airway resistance syndrome.

awakening. There may also be sweating, restlessness, increased respiratory effort, or extension of the neck. Common medical conditions such as gastrointestinal reflux or asthma may be associated with nighttime symptoms. Upon awakening the patient may describe dry mouth or headache. Enuresis is relatively common in patients with OSA. Parents and children are often reluctant to volunteer the symptom of enuresis because the association with SDB may not be known. Snoring is a very common symptom in children and may not be seen as a symptom. As many as 25% of children may snore occasionally and 10% snore habitually.[5] Snoring does not predict the presence of SDB but itself may be associated with deleterious effects including poor school performance or hypertension.[37] Daytime symptoms include poor school performance, hyperactivity, and inattention or aggressive behavior. Children with the diagnosis of attention deficit/hyperactivity disorder (ADHD) who also snore should have a comprehensive sleep evaluation.

The most common physical findings are limited to upper airway. The most common finding in the child with OSA is tonsillar hypertrophy. Other findings that may be important are mouth breathing, mircrognathia/retrognathia, crowded orophaynx, nasal mucosal edema, nasal septal deviation, and malocclusion. Body weight is important. Obesity is a known risk factor for SDB. However, some children may present with low body weight or even failure to thrive. Other physical findings may be those seen in conditions associated with increased risk for SDB (Box 25-6).

The first line of treatment is adenotonsillectomy.[38] This surgery may be curative in a majority of cases. Patients who are obese or have upper airway abnormalities in addition to tonsillar hypertrophy may have persistent SDB after adenotonsillectomy. In a recent study Guilleminault described a cohort of patients treated surgically in childhood in whom OSA had recurred in adolescence.[29] For these reasons, careful postoperative follow-up is advisable, especially in children with obesity. **Continuous positive airway pressure (CPAP)** is the treatment of choice in patients who either are not suitable candidates for surgery or have persistent SDB.[39] The effective pressure level is usually determined in a titration sleep study. In recent years the selection of interface options for children has dramatically improved. These include nasal masks or pillows and full face masks. Most children will adapt to the use of the device with repetition and the help of a well-trained parent. In some cases bilevel PAP (BPAP) may be better tolerated. Patients who hypoventilate, such as those with neuromuscular disease, should be treated with bilevel PAP. The effectiveness of CPAP is dependent on compliance with its use. The introduction of "smart" CPAP devices has improved the ability to ensure compliance. Indeed, some insurance companies now require a threshold level of documented compliance. Compliance with CPAP use in patients with developmental disability is particularly challenging.

Many medical conditions are associated with increased risk for SDB. Conditions that have decreased oropharyngeal space as a feature include craniopharyngeal syndromes, Down syndrome, mucopolysaccharide storage disease, and Prader-Willi syndrome. Patients with neurological disease, most notably Chiari malformation, may be at increased risk for SDB, and patients with neuromuscular disease have an increased incidence of SDB. These patients are less likely to be "cured" with adenotonsillectomy alone. They may require other surgical procedures (e.g., Chiari malformation decompression, mandibular distraction) or treatment with CPAP, BPAP, or even tracheostomy, depending on the severity of the sleep-related gas exchange abnormalities.[40]

LABORATORY ASSESSMENT OF BREATHING IN SLEEP

Definitive evaluation must include an overnight *polysomnogram* (PSG).[41,42] Pediatric PSG parameters differ in many respects from the adult PSG (Figure 25-4). Box 25-7 lists the channel recordings that are recommended for a diagnostic PSG. Staging of sleep includes the combined measurement of the EEG to record brain activity, the electrooculogram (EOG) to record bilateral eye movements, and the electromyogram (EMG) to record facial and tibial muscle tone. EEG electrode placement for scoring sleep in children is standardized similarly to that used in adults. Electrodes are placed at EEG positions A1, A2, O1, O2, C3, and C4, and sleep stage is determined by the monopolar derivation C3/A2 or C4/A1. In infants less than 6 months old, an extended EEG montage is preferred. This extended montage should include bilateral EEG electrodes using bipolar channels to more accurately evaluate the EEG of the two hemispheres of the brain. In this way, EEG features specific to infants, such as tracé alternant and delta "brushes," as well as certain epileptiform activity, are better seen. This montage may also provide useful information regarding the maturity of the brain or may alert clinicians to potential problems in brain activity. In addition, certain normal features of the infant EEG, such as rudimentary

Box 25-6	Clinical Symptoms of Obstructive Sleep Apnea

NIGHTTIME SYMPTOMS
- Snoring
- Paradoxical breathing
- Enuresis
- Sweating
- Dry mouth

DAYTIME SYMPTOMS
- Hyperactivity
- School performance problems
- Daytime sleepiness

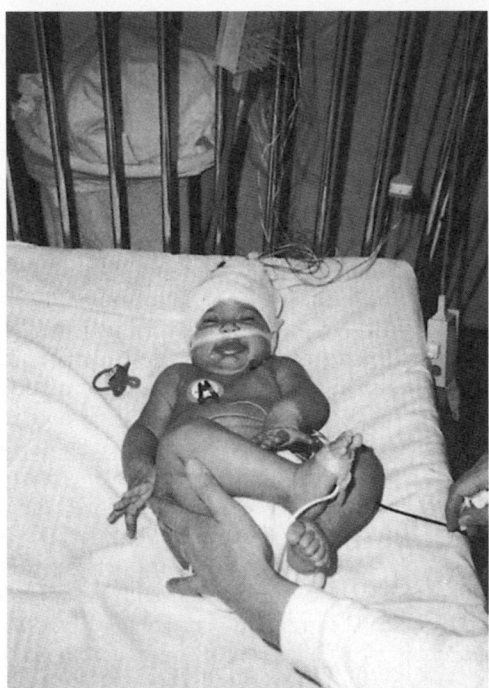

FIGURE 25-4 A baby ready for PSG. The head is wrapped with gauze to protect the scalp EEG electrodes. An electrode to detect eye movement is also covered with gauze. Two eye electrodes are standard. There is a nasal thermistor and CO_2 cannula in place. A strain gauge is attached to the chest to detect breathing movements. A transcutaneous oxygen electrode, ECG electrodes, and oxygen saturation sensor are also attached.

Box 25-7	Recommended Polysomnogram Channels for a Pediatric Sleep Study

- EEG montage to include four to eight channels
- Electrooculogram
- Electrocardiogram
- Oxygen saturation and waveform
- Redundant measure of airflow (nasal pressure and oronasal thermistor)
- End-tidal P_{CO_2} (peak value and waveform)
- Snore volume
- Measure of respiratory effort (chest and abdominal inductance plethysmography)
- Measure of muscle activity (chin and tibial EMG)
- Video and audio recording
- Time-stamped video
- Body position sensor

EEG, Electroencephalogram; *EMG,* electromyography.

sleep spindles, are better seen using an extended EEG montage that includes frontal leads.

The accurate scoring of sleep stages also requires bilateral EOG sensors to monitor the rapid eye movements that normally occur in REM sleep and the slow eye movements that occur with the onset of sleep. An EMG recording of facial muscle tone assists the clinician in more accurately determining the presence of REM sleep when skeletal

muscle tone, particularly the muscles of the face, is normally inhibited.

To comprehensively assess the adequacy of ventilation and differentiate between central and obstructive apnea and its severity, PSGs should also include movements of the chest wall and abdomen, air flow at the nose and mouth, transcutaneous oxygen saturation data (with validating pulse wave from the monitor), and end-tidal carbon dioxide ($ETCO_2$) measures. A pulse waveform is necessary to assess the reliability of oxygenation data because oxygen saturation monitors can yield artifactual data when the infant is feeding or moving. Capnography, a graphic representation of $ETCO_2$, is recommended because it can assess both airflow and ventilation simultaneously. Calibrated $ETCO_2$ measurements can effectively detect possible CO_2 retention associated with apnea or prolonged hypoventilation.

A standard PSG also includes additional parameters that can provide important information relevant to the patient's electrophysiological status. An electrocardiogram (ECG) monitors cardiac rate and rhythm and is useful in evaluating the consequences of breathing disorders on heart rhythm. Inductive plethysmography involving the placement of bands around the rib cage and abdomen detects respiratory effort as well as phase relationship, allowing for differentiation between central versus obstructive apnea. A PSG may include EMG of the anterior tibialis muscles to identify periodic limb leg movement disorders, although these disorders are rare in infants and children. As such, leg EMGs are not routinely monitored in children unless clinically indicated.

To assess for the presence of gastroesophageal reflux and its potential cardiorespiratory consequences, continuous esophageal pH measurement can be done in conjunction with PSG. Video recording with sound is recommended because it provides invaluable information on sleep behavior, snoring, respiratory effort, and sleep positions associated with a particular respiratory pattern. Finally, the PSG must be performed by a trained technologist who ensures the integrity of the recording, provides descriptions regarding unusual events or behaviors, and makes notations on the recording regarding physiological changes such as snoring or color changes such as cyanosis. Polysomnographic technologists working with this age group must be certified in pediatric cardiopulmonary resuscitation (CPR).

CASE STUDY

A 3-month-old female infant is brought to the emergency department by paramedics. They state that they responded to an emergency call and upon arrival found that the mother was distraught and holding the baby. They reported that she had found the baby "not breathing and blue." She had put the baby to bed after a feeding about 1 hour before the event. She could not say how long the episode lasted but she said she blew in the babies' mouth and the baby started to cry. The baby was full term. The baby's examination is now normal. There is no evidence of foul play. What is the differential diagnosis?

    A. Apnea of prematurity
    B. Obstructive sleep apnea
    C. Congenital central hypoventilation syndrome
    D. Near-miss SIDS
    E. Acute life-threatening event (ALTE)

This child was admitted to the hospital and underwent a thorough evaluation. Mother stated that she was afraid of SIDS. There is no family history of SIDS. Further history revealed that the baby often slept with mother in her bed. She stated that the baby was most comfortable "on her tummy." She admitted that she smoked but "only outside." What risk factors must be discussed with this mother?

    A. Co-sleeping
    B. Smoking
    C. Prone position sleeping
    E. All of the above

See Evolve Resources for answers.

KEY POINTS

- *Sleep development:* Infants spend the bulk of their day in sleep. Sleep stages are defined by the EEG. The infant has three stages, referred to as active sleep (REM), quiet sleep (NREM), and indeterminate sleep. REM sleep predominates sleep time in the infant and decreases until about the age of 2. NREM sleep time increases in the child and peaks between 5 and 9 years. NREM sleep has four distinct EEG stages (3 and 4 are now combined). NREM sleep is known as slow wave sleep and has been called restorative sleep. Total sleep time progressively decreases throughout childhood to adult levels in adolescence. The distribution of time spent in each stage is quantified during a sleep study and is referred to as sleep architecture. Disruption of the sleep architecture leads to daytime symptoms.

- *Central sleep apnea:* Central sleep apnea occurs when there is a cessation of airflow and no discernible respiratory effort. In infants this may be due to immaturity of respiratory centers. Later in life it may be due to insensitivity of the chemoreceptors responsible for respiratory drive.

- *Obstructive sleep apnea:* Obstructive sleep apnea occurs when there is cessation or limitation of airflow and continued respiratory effort for more than two respiratory cycles. OSA is due to the collapse of the airway. Multiple factors contribute to this collapse, including anatomical structures limiting airflow, laryngeal muscle control, neuromuscular factors, and cardiorespiratory control. Upper airway obstruction occurs in a continuum from snoring to complete apnea. Partial obstruction leads to limitation of airflow termed hypopnea. The most common cause of OSA in children is adenotonsillar hypertrophy. OSA is most often treated with adenotosillectomy. When this treatment is unsuccessful, CPAP is an effective treatment that maintains airway patency.

- *SIDS and ALTE:* SIDS is defined as "the sudden death of an infant under one year of age which remains unexplained after a thorough case investigation, including performance of a complete autopsy, *examination of the death scene,* and review of the clinical history." It remains the most common cause of death between the ages of 1 month and 1 year. The cause of SIDS remains unknown. Many theories have been advanced. The most important advance arose from epidemiological data demonstrating that back sleeping dramatically decreases the risk of SIDS. The emphasis on back sleeping has decreased the incidence of SIDS worldwide. There is no test that will predict the occurrence of SIDS. The AAP has recommended that home monitors not be used as a strategy to prevent SIDS.

    An ALTE is defined as "an episode that is frightening to the observer and is characterized by some combination of apnea (central and occasionally obstructive), color change (usually cyanotic or pallid but occasionally erythematous or plethoric), marked change in muscle tone (usually marked limpness), choking, or gagging." The relationship of ALTE and SIDS is poorly understood. An identifiable cause may be found in about half of the cases.

- *Laboratory assessment:* The definitive study to assess sleep is the PSG. The diagnostic PSG is performed in an accredited sleep laboratory by trained personnel. Sleep stage is determined using a standard EEG montage that includes bilateral EOG and four EEG leads. Tibial and facial muscle activity is recorded by EMG. In addition, the complete PSG includes the following: nasal airflow, chest and abdominal wall plethysmography, end-tidal CO_2, video and audio recording, snore volume, body position sensor, ECG, and oxygen saturation. Sleep stage scoring allows for quantification of sleep architecture. EEG arousal may not be perceived by the patient as an awakening but may still result in disruption of the sleep architecture and daytime symptoms.

ASSESSMENT QUESTIONS

See Evolve Resources for answers

1. Which of the following statement is true regarding sleep in infants?
    A. Infant neural development is not yet complete and they have not yet developed rapid eye movement sleep.
    B. Infant sleep is dominated by non–rapid eye movement sleep.
    C. Seventy percent of infants sleep through the night by 3 months of age.
    D. The normal newborn spends 70% of a 24-hour day asleep.

2. Which of the following statement is true regarding sleep stages?
   A. During REM sleep in infants, muscle activity is the lowest and therefore metabolic rate is at its lowest.
   B. Newborn infants have immature sleep spindles.
   C. NREM sleep duration peaks between 5 and 9 years of age.
   D. The appearance of REM sleep at sleep onset in the newborn is an abnormal pattern.

3. The mother of a 3-month-old infant arrives at the emergency department with her infant and states that she observed her infant's breathing stop for 8 seconds and then restart. She stated that baby was also breathing fast right before she stopped breathing. The baby has been eating normally, has no other symptoms, and has a normal physical examination. What is your next action?
   A. Order a complete blood cell count (CBC) and a chest radiograph.
   B. Admit the baby for overnight observation.
   C. Reassure the mother that this is a normal infant breathing pattern.
   D. Arrange for the baby to go home with a home monitor.

4. Infants are particularly susceptible to the development of SDB or respiratory failure. What feature of anatomy or physiology places the baby at increased risk?
   A. Nasal breathing
   B. Chest wall compliance
   C. The angle of rib articulation
   D. The shape of the chest
   E. All of the above

5. Which of the following statements is true?
   A. The peak incidence of SIDS occurs at 6 months of age.
   B. Home monitoring should always be prescribed upon discharge for infants who have experienced an ALTE.
   C. SIDS has been called a diagnosis of exclusion. A full investigation should be undertaken including a full autopsy. An examination of the death scene is optional.
   D. The CHIME study demonstrated conclusively that home monitoring prevents SIDS.
   E. The infant who sleeps in the supine position is at decreased risk of SIDS.

6. What percentage of otherwise normal children who have OSA will present with excessive daytime sleepiness?
   A. More than 75%
   B. 50% to 75%
   C. 25% to 50%
   D. Less than 25%

7. Which of the following statements regarding OSA is/are true?
   A. A complete history is a sensitive indicator of the presence of OSA.
   B. School performance is affected when OSA becomes severe.
   C. The prevalence of OSA is approximately 15%, and the peak incidence is between 2 and 8 years.
   D. OSA may be diagnosed without blood gas abnormalities during the sleep study.

8. Which of the following statements regarding OSA is/are false?
   A. Tonsillar hypertrophy is the most common cause of OSA.
   B. Upper airway obstruction occurs along a continuum from snoring through UARS to apnea.
   C. Enuresis may be a presenting symptom of OSA.
   D. A child with ADHD who also snores should be referred to a psychologist.

9. OSA in childhood and adulthood differs in several important ways. Which of the following statements is/are false?
   A. Excessive daytime sleepiness is less common in children than adults.
   B. Adenotonsillectomy is more effective in children than adults.
   C. Sleep architecture is more commonly disrupted in children than in adults.
   D. Obese children with OSA have a phenotype that is similar to adult OSA.
   E. Children tend to have better preservation of REM sleep.

10. The treatment of OSA might include which of the following?
   A. Chiari malformation repair
   B. Tracheostomy
   C. Mandibular distraction
   D. CPAP
   E. All of the above

References

1. Olser W: Chronic tonsillitis. In *The principles and practice of medicine*, New York, Appleton and Co, 1892. 335.
2. Crabtree VM, Williams NA: Normal sleep in children and adolescents, *Child Adolesc Psychiatric Clin N Am* 18:799, 2009.
3. Owens J: Classification and epidemiology of childhood sleep disorders, *Sleep Med Clin* 2:353, 2007.
4. American Thoracic Society: Standards and indications for cardiopulmonary sleep studies in children, *Am J Respir Crit Care Med* 153:866, 1996.
5. Gozal D, Kheirandish-Gozal L: Disorders of breathing during sleep. In Wilmont R et al, editors: *Kendig and Chernick's disorders of the respiratory tract in children*, ed 8, Philadelphia, 2012, Elsevier Saunders.
6. American Academy of Pediatrics, Committee on Fetus and Newborn: Apnea, sudden infant death syndrome, and home monitoring, *Pediatrics* 111(4):914, 2003.
7. Mathews TJ, MacDorman MF: Infant mortality statistics from the 2009 period linked birth/infant death data set, *Natl Vital Stat Rep* 61(8):1, 2013.
8. National Commission on Sleep Disorders Research: *Report of the National Commission on Sleep Disorders*, vol 1. Department of Health and Human Services pub. no. 92, Washington, DC, 1992, US Government Printing Office.
9. Steinschneider A: Prolonged apnea and the sudden infant death syndrome: clinical and laboratory observations, *Pediatrics* 50:646, 1972.
10. Firstman R, Talan J: *The death of innocents: a true story of murder, medicine, and high-stake science*, New York, 1997, Bantam.

11. Hymel KP, National Association of Medical Examiners: distinguishing sudden infant death syndrome from child abuse fatalities, *Pediatrics* 118:421, 2006.

12. Schwartz PJ, Stramba-Badiale M, et al: Prolongation of the QT interval and the sudden infant death syndrome, *N Engl J Med* 338:1709, 1998.

13. Davidson Ward SL, Keens TG, Chan LS, et al: Sudden infant death syndrome in infants evaluated by apnea programs in California, *Pediatrics* 77:451, 1986.

14. Schechtman VL, Raetz SL, Harper RK, et al: Dynamic analysis of cardiac R-R intervals in normal infants and in infants who subsequently succumbed to the sudden infant death syndrome, *Pediatr Res* 31(6):606, 1992.

15. Lijowska AS, Reed NW, Chiodini BA, Thach BT: Sequential arousal and airway-defensive behavior of infants in asphyxial sleep environments, *J Appl Physiol* 83:219, 1997.

16. Valdes-Depena: Sudden infant death syndrome: a review of the medical literature 1974. 1979, *Pediatrics* 66:597, 1980.

17. Tonkin SL: Infant mortality: epidemiology of cot death in Auckland, *N Z Med J* 99:324, 1986.

18. Beal S: Sleeping position and sudden infant death syndrome, *Med J Aust* 149:562, 1988.

19. Wilinger M, Hoffman HJ, Hartford RB: Infant sleep position and risk for sudden infant death syndrome: report of meeting held January 13 and 14, 1994. National Institutes of Health, Bethesda, MD, *Pediatrics* 93(5):814–819, 1994.

20. Haglund B, Cnattingius S: Cigarette smoking as a risk factor for sudden infant death syndrome: a population-based study, *Am J Public Health* 80(1):29, 1990.

21. Trachtenberg FL, Haas EA, Kinney HC, Stanley C, Krous HF: Risk factor changes for sudden infant death syndrome after initiation of Back-to-Sleep campaign, *Pediatrics* 129:630–638, 2012.

22. National Institute of Health, Consensus Conference on Infantile apnea and Home Monitoring. Sept 29 to Oct 1, 1986, *Pediatrics* 79:292–299, 1987.

23. Hall KL, Zalman B: Evaluation and management of apparent life threatening events in children, *Am Fam Physician* 1571. 12):2301–2308, 2005.

24. Ramanathan R, Corwin MJ, Hunt CE, et al: Cardiorespiratory events recorded on home monitors: comparison of healthy infants to those at risk for SIDS, *JAMA* 285(17):2199, 2001.

25. Jobe AH: What do home monitors contribute to the SIDS problem? *JAMA* 285(17):2244, 2001.

26. Committee on Fetus and Newborn: Apnea, sudden infant death syndrome, and home monitoring, *Pediatrics* 111:914, 2003.

27. Arens R: Sleep-disordered breathing in children. In *Pediatric pulmonology: the requisites in pediatrics*, St. Louis, Mosby-Elsevier.

28. Horner RL: Pathophysiology of obstructive sleep apnea, *J Cardiopulm Rehabil Prev* 28:289, 2008.

29. Dempsey JA, Veasey SC, Morgan BJ, O'Donnell P: Pathophysiology of sleep apnea, *Physiol Rev* 90:47, 2010.

30. Guilleminault C, Li KK, Quo S: A prospective study on the surgical outcomes of children with sleep-disordered breathing, *Sleep* 27:95, 2004.

31. Carroll JL: Obstructive sleep-disordered breathing in children: new controversies, new directions, *Clin Chest Med* 24:261, 2003.

32. Noonan JA: Reversible cor pulmonale due to hypertrophied tonsils and adenoids: studies in two cases, *Circulation* 32 (Suppl 2):164, 1965.

33. Jaffe IS: Adenotonsillectomy as the treatment of serious medical conditions: five case reports, *Laryngoscope* 84(7):1135, 1974.

34. Guilleminault C, Eldridge FL, Simmons B, et al: Sleep apnea in eight children, *Pediatrics* 58:23, 1976.

35. Guilleminault C, Korobkin R, Windle R: A review of 50 children with obstructive sleep apnea syndrome, *Lung* 159:275, 1981.

36. Dayyat E, Kheirandish-Gozal L, Gozal D: Childhood obstructive sleep apnea: one or two distinct disease entities? *Sleep Med Clin* 2:433, 2007.

37. Gozal D, Pope DW: Snoring during early childhood and academic performance at ages thirteen to fourteen years, *Pediatrics* 107:1394, 2001.

38. Bhattacharjee R, Kheiandish-Gozal L, Spuyt K, et al: Adenotonsillectomy outcomes in treatment of obstructive sleep apnea in children: a multicenter retrospective study, *Am J Respir Crit Care Med* 182:676, 2010.

39. Marcus CL, Ward SL, Mallory GB, et al: Use of nasal continuous positive airway pressure as treatment of childhood obstructive sleep apnea, *J Pediatr* 127:88, 1995.

40. Halbower AC, McGinley BM, Smith PL: Treatment alternatives for sleep-disordered breathing in the pediatric population, *Curr Opin Pulm Med* 14:551–559, 2008.

41. Beck SE, Marcus CL: Pediatric polysomnography, *Sleep Med Clin* 4(3):396, 2009.

42. American Thoracic Society: Standards and indications for cardiopulmonary sleep studies in children, *Am J Respir Crit Care Med* 153:866, 1996.

Chapter 26

Pediatric Airway Disorders and Parenchymal Lung Diseases

BRIAN K. WALSH

OUTLINE

LEARNING OBJECTIVES

After reading this chapter the reader will be able to:

1. Identify and name upper and lower airway disorders
2. Recognize the signs of severe or complete airway obstructions that require interventions
3. Describe the basic intervention and recommended therapy for each of the airway disorders and parenchymal lung diseases

4. Discuss the different types, and therefore the etiology, of pneumonia

KEY TERMS

Airway obstruction
Aspiration
Choanal atresia
Epiglottitis

Pierre Robin syndrome
Lower airway
Obstructive apnea
Pneumonia

Laryngotracheobronchitis
Tuberculosis
Upper airway

THE PEDIATRIC AIRWAY

Airway disorders may cause severe and at times sudden threats to a child's life. The special susceptibility of children to disorders of the airways stems from several factors. Congenital abnormalities of airway structures tend to cause difficulties early in life. Even when normal anatomy is present, the relatively small size of the pediatric airway puts children at a distinct disadvantage. The inherently narrow trachea, bronchi, and bronchioles can become critically compromised by minimal swelling of the respiratory mucosal lining or by the presence of foreign objects. Children are at increased risk for such narrowing or obstruction because of their susceptibility to respiratory infections and their tendency to engage in risky behaviors, such as placing small objects in their mouths.

In comparison to the adult, once a child's airway becomes narrowed or obstructed, the pediatric respiratory system is less able to cope with the resulting ventilation abnormality. In the event of complete airway obstruction, children undergo rapid onset of hypoxia, with its resultant neurological damage or death. Respiratory events are the major reason for cardiac arrest in children. The rapidity of this oxygen desaturation is in part caused by the child's small functional residual capacity and dependency on dynamic compliance combined with an overall increased metabolic rate. Essentially there is minimal oxygen reserve available to supply the child's oxygen requirement. This combination of increased susceptibility to and decreased ability to cope with airway compromise helps explain why children suffer so frequently from airway disorders.

Upper Airway

Many unique aspects of anatomy must be understood to appropriately support and intervene on behalf of a child during respiratory illness. The **upper airway** consists of all structures connecting the mouth and nose with the glottis. This includes the nose, nasal choanae, nasopharynx, mouth, oropharynx, and structures of the larynx (Figure 26-1). When compared with that of the adult, the anatomy of the infant's airway contains several differences and functional limitations.

The epiglottis is long, floppy, and angled away from the tracheal axis. It shrouds the laryngeal opening because of poor support by the surrounding tissues. Structurally, the infant's larynx is positioned higher in the neck (near C3-4) than is an adult's larynx (at C4-5). Because of this superior location, the tongue base tends to "hide" the larynx from view during direct laryngoscopy. The cricoid cartilage is a nonexpandable cartilaginous ring that is normally the only complete ring of cartilage in the airway. In the pediatric airway, it is the larynx's narrowest portion. With this reduced and fixed dimension, an endotracheal tube may pass through the vocal cords and yet not proceed to the subglottic trachea. This already narrowed portion

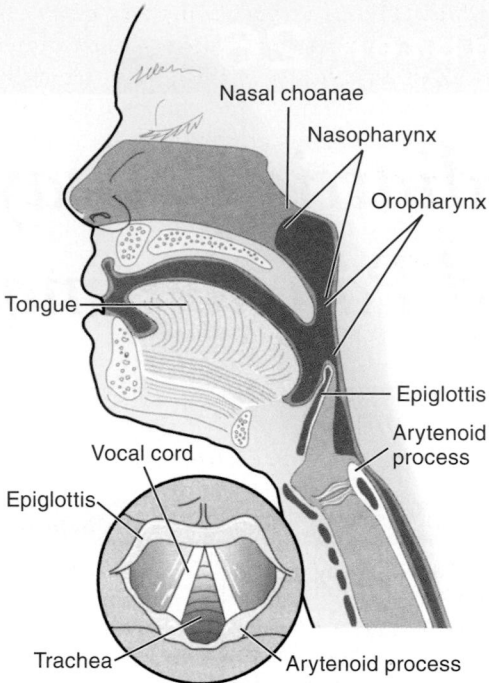

FIGURE 26-1 Normal upper airway structures.

of the airway becomes severely narrowed by even small amounts of edema that develop with diseases such as laryngotracheobronchitis (LTB) or trauma (e.g., endotracheal intubation).

Infants are considered obligate nose breathers until 3 to 6 months of age. Immaturity of coordination between respiration and oropharyngeal motor activity accounts partly for obligate nasal breathing. Also, the infant's tongue is closer to the roof of the mouth and makes mouth breathing difficult. Because the large tongue and small mouth make air passage through the mouth impossible, except when crying, patency of the nasopharynx is critical in an infant.

The upper airway and lung do not complete development until approximately 8 years of age. The immature cartilage found in the infant's trachea and bronchi is soft and highly compressible. When the supporting cartilage is excessively flexible, the diagnosis of laryngomalacia or tracheomalacia is applied.

Lower Airway

The trachea divides into the mainstem bronchi, which in turn divide into smaller divisions called subsegmental bronchi. This repeated division continues in the adult to 23 generations (divisions) of smaller and smaller air passages, creating a huge surface area for gas exchange. At birth, however, the infant has only 16 to 17 generations of airways. The terminal generation of airways, the respiratory bronchioles, is present in relatively small numbers, resulting in a small transectional area for gas exchange in the infant. This is in part compensated for by fetal hemoglobin, which has an oxygen affinity superior to adult hemoglobin. Because of the developmentally small airway cross-sectional area, small amounts of inflammation at the level of the respiratory bronchioles can result in severe respiratory embarrassment. In young children the respiratory bronchioles are commonly attacked by viruses, such as respiratory syncytial virus (RSV), resulting in respiratory failure. The same infection will have little or no respiratory effect on an adult or older child with a larger number of terminal airways.

AIRWAY OBSTRUCTION

Obstruction of the upper or lower airway of a child may lead to life-threatening hypoxia or hypercarbia. With the high risk of morbidity comes the need to identify the etiology, recognize the clinical signs and symptoms, and choose the diagnostic methods for and treatment of the many causes of airway obstruction.

Radiographic evaluation of the upper airways includes both frontal anteroposterior and lateral views of the head and neck. When performed at the proper angle and exposure, these films are helpful in evaluating the site of upper airway obstruction (Figure 26-2).

Fearing the unfamiliar surroundings of a hospital or clinic, a child may wiggle and scream, further increasing respiratory effort. To be successful in what could be a very difficult examination, the practitioner must proceed with slow and deliberate movement in a kind and gentle manner. However, this does not guarantee cooperation from a frightened and ill child.

The narrow airway of the child makes even a small obstruction significant, leading to a marked increase in respiratory effort. Obvious clinical signs of impaired respiratory function are tachypnea, nasal flaring, retractions, cyanosis, and a change in mental state, including a reduced level of consciousness or increased agitation. As a rule, tachypnea and nasal flaring alone suggest a less severe but earlier sign of obstruction than the presence of deep retractions. However, if obstruction is severe, with prolonged respiratory distress, the child may be exhausted and only able to exhibit nasal flaring. In infants the exhaustion of respiratory muscle leads to decreased dynamic compliance and ineffective respiration because they have a relatively soft rib cage leading to increased chest wall compliance. The child's mental state may range from fearful and agitated to lethargic or even unconscious. A child with mild hypoxia tends to have increased levels of agitation, whereas the child with increasing hypoxemia and hypercarbia becomes more lethargic.

Auscultation of the child's upper airway (over the trachea) and the lower airway (over the thorax) is vital to determine the extent of air movement and obstruction. Some sounds, such as stridor, may be so prominent that they are audible from outside the patient's room. Stridor is a coarse, vibrating noise generated by airway soft tissue that typically occurs in the presence of narrowed or obstructed upper airway (extrathoracic). Extrathoracic obstruction of the trachea causes stridor during inspiration. The deeply negative intrathoracic pressure causes the pressure inside the trachea to fall and allows the higher atmospheric pressure (outside the trachea) to collapse the trachea or larynx. This results in the "crowing" sound of stridor. During

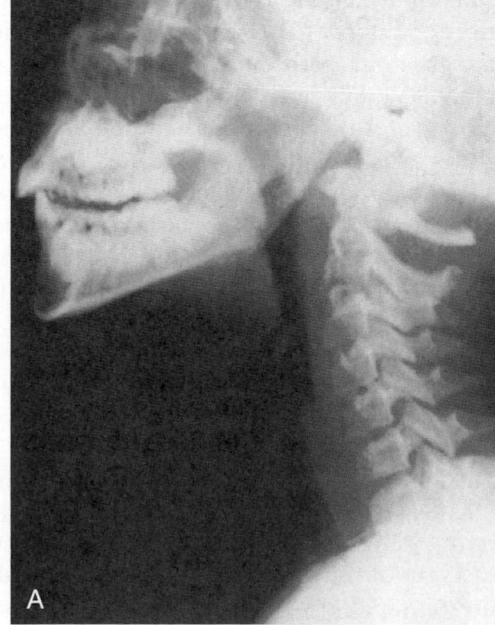
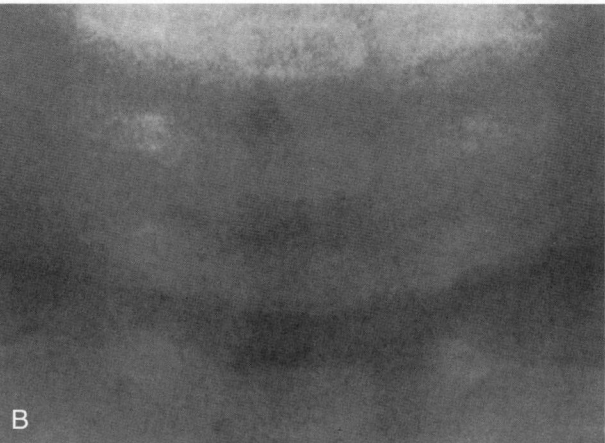

FIGURE 26-2 Normal cervical soft tissue radiographs. **A,** Lateral view shows a thin epiglottis. **B,** Anteroposterior view illustrates the "shoulders" appearance of the subglottic trachea.

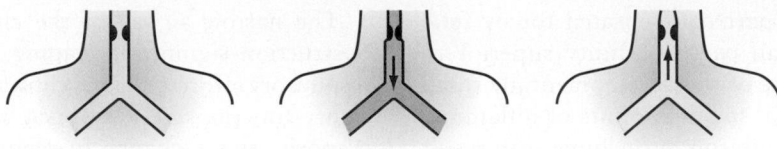

| Resting | Inhaling | Exhaling |

FIGURE 26-3   Obstruction of the upper (extrathoracic) airway. Dynamic motion during the respiratory cycle causes accentuated narrowing during inspiration, resulting in stridor.

exhalation, the positive intraairway pressure forces the airway open and eliminates the stridor (Figure 26-3). When airway narrowing is intrathoracic, stridor is present during a forced exhalation. The positive intrathoracic pressure that occurs with exhalation causes the circumferential tracheal cartilage, and hence the trachea, to collapse. During inspiration, stridor from an intrathoracic airway obstruction is minimized by the radially outward tracheal traction caused by negative intrathoracic pressures.

Auscultation of air movement during inspiration and expiration aids in determining the severity and location of the obstruction. The pitch of the stridor can be used to assess improvement or worsening of the obstruction. Low-pitched sounds signify mild obstruction, whereas a higher pitch indicates that the child is in more distress and is attempting to generate a higher air flow rate. Sounds heard on inspiration but not expiration may indicate a ball-valve obstruction and an accompanying risk for a pneumothorax. Absence of air movement constitutes a true emergency.

UPPER AIRWAY DISORDERS

Supralaryngeal Obstruction

Common causes of obstruction above the larynx include congenital lesions, acute inflammatory disorders, and disorders related to abnormal supralaryngeal tissue or airway tone or both (e.g., obstructive apnea).

Choanal Atresia

Choanal atresia, the stenosis or absence of the nasal passages (choanae), typically occurs in the immediate postnatal period. The infant presents with severe respiratory distress that appears to lessen with crying, when the infant manages to exchange air through the mouth, and is exacerbated again once the crying stops. Occasionally the condition is discovered when, during an attempt to nasally suction the infant, a size 5 or 6 catheter cannot be passed through the nares into the oropharynx for a distance of at least 32 mm. Insertion of an oral airway provides temporary relief of the obstruction but does not preclude early surgical intervention.

Pierre Robin Syndrome

Other congenital anomalies that can appear similar include masses that obstruct the nasopharynx, such as encephaloceles (an outpouching of the brain into the airway) and dermoid cysts. Infants with Pierre Robin syndrome have extremely small mandibles and a small oropharynx that causes the tongue to occlude the airway. The respiratory distress is not relieved by crying. Treatment includes temporary insertion of oral or nasal airways, placement of the infant in a prone position, and surgical repair.

CASE STUDY 1

You are called to the delivery room for a term infant delivery complicated by maternal fever. The infant is delivered via spontaneous vaginal delivery with the umbilical cord around the neck. The obstetrician performs superficial nose and mouth suctioning with a bulb syringe and untangles the umbilical cord from the newborn's neck. The infant is handed to you and no spontaneous respiration is noted under the warmer. You dry the infant and provide stimulation. The infant cries and turns pink. After a few seconds the infant calms down and exhibits respiratory distress relieved by crying.

What is your differential diagnosis, and how do you assess the infant?

See Evolve Resources for answers.

Deep Neck Infections

Deep neck infections are feared complications of upper respiratory and upper gastrointestinal tract infections. Aerobic and anaerobic pathogens are the common cause. They can become rapidly severe, causing airway obstruction and aspiration, and quickly spread to adjoining anatomical structures (such as the mediastinum). Antibiotic treatment, airway protection, and surgical intervention are necessary. Peritonsillar and retropharyngeal abscesses are very common examples of these infections and must be differentiated from simple tonsillar enlargement.

Tonsillar Enlargement

The child with an acute illness characterized by fever and sore throat may develop swelling of the oropharyngeal tissues. Inflammation and swelling can progress to airway obstruction. Tonsillitis, or streptococcal pharyngitis, presents as exudative pharyngitis and cervical adenopathy. However, the presence of a cough and nasal congestion increases the likelihood that the infection is viral. A throat culture or rapid streptococcal antigen test is obtained to identify the causative organism. Therapy is routinely restricted to antibiotics unless the swelling is severe.

Peritonsillar Abscess

This abscess commonly forms unilaterally around the tonsillar tissue. It causes unilateral swelling and protrusion of the affected tonsil into the oropharynx with classical deviation of the uvula to the unaffected side. Patients commonly complain about trismus (difficulty opening their mouth), sore throat, torticollis, and muffled or hoarse voice. The diagnosis is made clinically and by culture; if in doubt, frontal anteroposterior and lateral radiographs of the head and neck can aid in the diagnosis. The most likely causative organisms are *Streptococcus pyogenes* (group A streptococcus) or *Staphylococcus aureus*.

Retropharyngeal Abscess

Retropharyngeal abscess commonly occurs in children younger than 3 years of age and can cause obstruction from forward displacement of the posterior pharyngeal wall. Infectious agents involved are group A streptococcus, *Staphylococcus aureus,* and, occasionally, anaerobic bacteria. The child often presents with a sore throat, fever, dysphagia, and voice changes. The voice sounds as if the child is attempting to speak without moving the tongue while maximally expanding the oropharyngeal airway. This is described as "hot potato voice." A lateral neck radiograph is obtained to determine the tissue thickness surrounding the abscess. Visualization of the posterior pharynx may reveal a displaced retropharynx. Surgical drainage is the preferred treatment, along with administration of appropriate antibiotics based on culture results of the aspirated material.

Obstructive Apnea

Children with a history of chronic noisy snoring and air flow loss, in spite of active chest wall movement, are likely suffering from obstructive apnea. Abnormally large adenoids or tonsils with or without abnormal positioning of the airway tissues are likely causes of obstruction. During sleep, the airway muscular tone is decreased, resulting in more severe airway obstruction. Typically, the child with a neuromuscular disorder, such as cerebral palsy, enlarged tonsils and adenoids, or morbid obesity, is at risk for developing obstructive apnea. An electrocardiogram is obtained if nocturnal hypoxia with right ventricular hypertrophy is suspected. Sedation is usually avoided because it exacerbates airway obstruction. Surgery may relieve the obstruction in a child who has not "outgrown" the obstruction. Weight loss is often beneficial in obese children. In the interim, nasal continuous positive airway pressure can noninvasively ameliorate the disorder.

Periglottic Obstruction

Obstruction of the airway at or just below the level of the glottis typically presents as high-pitched stridor. This region is relatively fixed in diameter because the noncompliant cartilage surrounding the glottis does not "balloon open" to allow air passage around the obstruction, as easily occurs in the more pliable tissues of the supralaryngeal airway. As a result, progressive obstruction of the periglottic area quickly leads to significant distress with both inspiratory and expiratory compromise. The most common causes of periglottic obstruction in the pediatric age group are infectious, with epiglottitis and LTB representing important causes of respiratory morbidity for this patient population.

Congenital lesions that present as periglottic obstruction are rare and include laryngeal webs and cysts and subglottic hemangioma. Vocal cord paralysis may be congenital or iatrogenic, caused by birth trauma or inadvertent surgical injury to the recurrent laryngeal nerve. Subglottic stenosis may also be congenital or acquired secondary to local trauma after intubation. A more common and benign congenital cause of upper airway obstruction is laryngomalacia. In this condition the epiglottis and arytenoid processes are oversized and floppy, causing collapse into the glottis during vigorous breathing. High-pitched stridor is noted during the neonatal period but tends to disappear by the child's first or second birthday.

Epiglottitis

Epiglottitis is a life-threatening infection that affects both children and adults.[1] It results from bacterial invasion of the soft tissues of the larynx, causing inflammation of the supraglottic structures. This leads to sudden, marked swelling of the epiglottis and surrounding tissues and may result in complete airway obstruction and death. Historically, epiglottitis has been a disease of childhood, with little prodrome, and rarely recurs. In contrast, adult symptoms are more nonspecific and often clouded by coexistent diseases.

Incidence and Etiology

The most common organism causing epiglottitis has been *Haemophilus influenzae* type B. Before widespread vaccinations with *H. influenzae* type B vaccine, bacterial epiglottitis was a fairly common pediatric illness, seen most often

---

CASE STUDY 2

A 14-year-old girl presents to the emergency room complaining of sore throat, fever, and dysphagia. She has no prior health issues and no known sick contact. She says she had been well the day before and noticed her symptoms on awakening in the morning. Physical findings include a mild stridor on auscultation over both apical lung fields and over the trachea. Inspection of the retropharynx is complicated by the patient not being able to open her mouth, but you can see that the uvula is being displaced to the left. She also has problems rotating her head to the left.

What is the most likely diagnosis and what would be your next step in diagnosis?

What is the treatment?

See Evolve Resources for answers.

in children younger than 6 years of age. With the advent of widespread vaccination in 1985, the incidence has decreased by more than 95%. Despite the vaccinations and reduced incidence, *H. influenzae* type B still causes 75% of epiglottitis episodes.[2] Although the vaccination program has profoundly reduced the incidence of epiglottitis, multiple isolated cases have occurred in patients with a complete vaccination history.[3] With the initiation of the vaccination program, patients with epiglottitis now tend to be older, with non–*H. influenzae* type B, principally group A β-hemolytic *Streptococcus,* being the infecting organism. Primary group A β-hemolytic streptococcal epiglottitis can develop as a rare complication of varicella in an otherwise normal host. Noninfectious causes of epiglottitis in children include thermal epiglottitis from aspiration of hot liquid and traumatic epiglottitis from repeated intubation attempts or a blind finger sweep to remove a foreign body from the airway.

Signs and Symptoms

Onset of bacterial epiglottitis is usually abrupt and associated with high fever; severe sore throat; dysphagia with drooling; cough, progressing rapidly over a few hours to stridor; muffled ("hot potato") voice without hoarseness; air hunger; and cyanosis. Suprasternal, substernal, and intercostal retractions, along with nasal flaring, bradypnea, and dyspnea, are often displayed. The child assumes a characteristic position of sitting upright with the chin thrust forward and with the neck hyperextended (sniffing position) in a tripod position. The streptococcal variant of epiglottitis may be associated with a longer prodrome lasting more than 24 hours.[4]

Diagnosis

Diagnosis of epiglottitis must be assumed based on the clinical presentation. Table 26-1 lists the clinical characteristics used in the differential diagnoses for epiglottitis and LTB. Because manipulation or agitation of the child with epiglottitis can trigger complete upper airway obstruction, unnecessary diagnostic procedures are avoided (e.g., arterial blood gas analysis, chest radiography) and every attempt made to maintain a nonthreatening atmosphere for the child. Until controlled intubation can be achieved (conducted under general anesthesia with a pediatrician, otolaryngologist, and anesthesiologist present), attempts to directly visualize the epiglottis, draw blood, insert intravenous lines, or lay the child flat for an examination are avoided. Instead, allow the child to assume a position of comfort with "blow-by" oxygen therapy provided if necessary. If the clinical history and physical appearance of the child are only mildly suggestive of epiglottitis, more detailed examination or neck radiographs (Figure 26-4), or both, are helpful in confirming the diagnosis.

Treatment

Establishment of a stable artificial airway is the first priority in the treatment of epiglottitis. Placement of an

TABLE 26-1

Differential Diagnosis of Laryngotracheobronchitis and Epiglottitis

	Laryngotracheobronchitis	Epiglottitis
Age	3 months to 3 years	2 to 6 years
Cause	Viral (parainfluenza, RSV)	Bacterial (*Haemophilus influenzae* type B)
History	Gradual onset (2-3 days)	Acute onset (few hours)
	Previous cold symptoms	Complaint of sore throat
Symptoms	Stridor	Stridor
	Barking cough	Minimal cough
	Fever variable	High fever
	Hoarse voice	Muffled voice
	No position preferred	Prefers sitting upright with chin forward
	Retractions	Retractions
	Irritable	Drooling
	Does not appear acutely ill	Anxiety
		Appears acutely ill
Radiographic findings	Subglottic narrowing	Swollen epiglottis (thumb sign)

RSV, Respiratory syncytial virus.

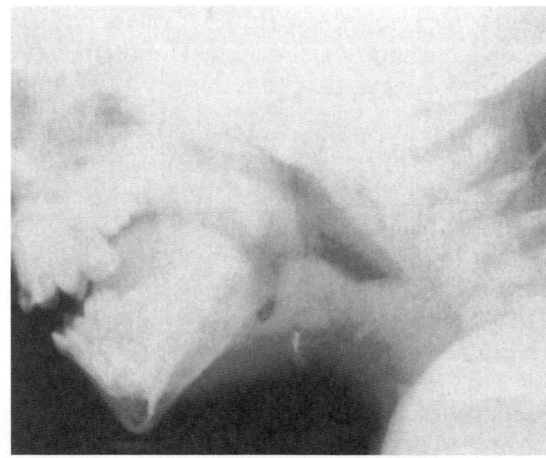

FIGURE 26-4 Epiglottitis. The lateral neck radiograph illustrates the distorted, thumb-shaped epiglottic shadow.

endotracheal tube (ETT) under general anesthesia is a safe way to provide a secure, temporary artificial airway. Because there is considerable swelling to the upper airway structures, an ETT one size smaller than the predicted size (based on age) is typically used. Dramatic improvement in respiratory distress is expected after intubation, which bypasses the site of obstruction. Once the ETT is inserted, it must remain in place during the 12 to 48 hours required for the inflamed tissue to shrink in response to therapy.

Treatment of infectious epiglottitis is relatively short, with a 2-day course of ceftriaxone as effective as 5 days of chloramphenicol. This may be adjusted based on patient response and on the results of culture and sensitivity reports from blood and epiglottis swab specimens taken at the time of intubation. Close nursing supervision, constant use of arm restraints, and continuously infused sedatives may suffice to prevent attempts at self-extubation. Mechanical ventilation may be needed for a short time if heavy sedation is required.

Extubation is usually considered within 24 hours when signs of toxicity (e.g., fever) diminish and when an air leak at 20 cm H_2O pressure develops around the ETT. Traumatic epiglottitis often takes several days longer for complete recovery. The physician may choose to directly visualize the epiglottis (by direct laryngoscopy or bronchoscopy) before attempting extubation to ensure adequate tissue shrinkage has occurred. The child is closely monitored for the return of stridor and other signs of respiratory distress for 12 to 24 hours after extubation.

Laryngotracheobronchitis
Incidence and Etiology
LTB, also known as croup, is the most common cause of airway obstruction in children between 6 months and 6 years of age. Typically it occurs in the fall and winter. Parainfluenza virus 1 is the most common cause, resulting in biennial epidemics in the United States during October through February of odd-numbered years. Other much less common infectious causes include influenza viruses, RSV, herpes simplex virus, and *Mycoplasma pneumoniae.*

The viral infection causes a mucosal edema and exudate formation in the glottic and subglottic areas, involving the airways from the larynx to the bronchus, hence the name *laryngotracheobronchitis.* The edema develops over several days, and the resultant airway narrowing becomes severe enough to cause various degrees of airway obstruction. Obstruction is more severe during inspiration because of the deeply negative airway pressures needed to inspire against the edematous airway. Average hospital admission rate for LTB is more than 40,000 children per year, resulting in an annual cost of $190 million, with approximately 91% of the children younger than 5 years of age.[1]

Signs and Symptoms
The child with LTB presents with a gradual prodrome of low-grade fever, malaise, rhinorrhea, and hoarse voice. Over several days, the illness progresses to inspiratory stridor and a "barky" cough, often described as sounding like the bark of a seal. Physical examination reveals nasal flaring; nasal congestion; use of accessory muscles; and suprasternal, subcostal, and intercostal retractions that, along with the stridor, become worse when the child is agitated.

Estimating the severity of the disease can be difficult. The illness usually occurs during cold seasons. Transporting an ill child in moderate distress in an automobile with cold ambient air commonly results in the child being virtually symptom-free on arrival in the emergency department. Inhalation of the cold air reduces the swelling and rapidly reduces the respiratory distress. More recent attempts to quantify LTB severity have centered around the presence of pulsus paradoxus[5] and the Croup Score developed by Westley (Table 26-2).[6]

Diagnosis
A lateral neck radiograph, sometimes obtained to help differentiate the disease from epiglottitis, demonstrates a large retropharyngeal air shadow without epiglottic swelling. The anteroposterior chest radiograph reveals the classic "steeple sign," a sharply sloped, wedge-shaped, linear narrowing of the trachea. This demonstrates the subglottic tracheal edema that extends from the larynx to the thoracic trachea (Figure 26-5).

Treatment
Treatment of mild cases of LTB is largely supportive—ensuring temperature control, adequate hydration, and humidification of inspired air. Techniques to cool the airway have traditionally used humidified air with water particles large enough to "rain out" onto the upper airway and tracheal mucosa. Cool mist tents (croup tents) were designed to provide continuous humidified air to the trachea. Little, if any, proof of effectiveness exists on the use of this form of humidification, and it has fallen out of favor because of infection control and environment issues associated with its use.

If increasing respiratory effort, irritability, and inability to engage in play or eating develop, hospitalization may be indicated. Hospital care for the child with LTB is largely symptomatic and centers on careful monitoring for advancing

TABLE 26-2

Croup Scoring System

Indicators of Severity	Findings	Croup Score
Inspiratory stridor	None	0
	At rest, with stethoscope	1
	At rest, without stethoscope	2
Retractions	None	0
	Mild	1
	Moderate	2
	Severe	3
Air entry	Normal	0
	Decreased	1
	Severely decreased	2
Cyanosis	None	0
	With agitation	4
	At rest	5
Level of consciousness	Normal	0
	Altered mental status	5

From Westley CR, Cotton EK, Brooks JG. Nebulized racemic epinephrine by IPPB for the treatment of croup: a double-blind study. *Am J Dis Child* 1978;132:484.

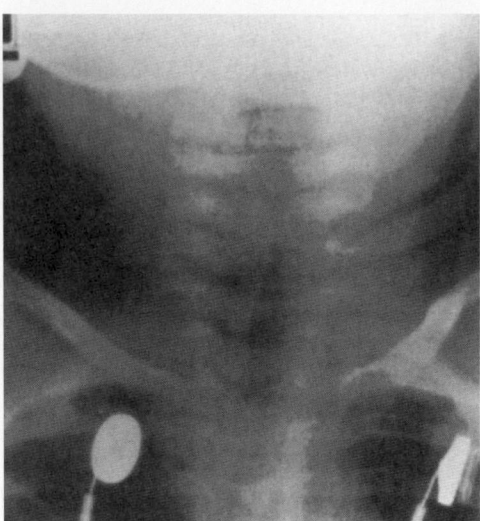

FIGURE 26-5 Laryngotracheobronchitis. The anteroposterior neck radiograph reveals steeply angled subglottic walls ("steeple sign").

respiratory compromise. Regular assessment of the respiratory rate, degree of retractions, mental status, and air exchange is essential. Oxygen saturation monitoring is useful, but generally desaturation is a late finding. Children requiring an FIO$_2$ of more than 0.35 are watched closely for evidence of impending respiratory failure.

Nebulized racemic epinephrine is used to induce vasoconstriction of the upper airway. With the use of a 2.2% solution, 0.5 to 1.0 ml of medication is diluted to a 3.0 ml volume with normal saline and given by inhalation with a face mask over a period of approximately 10 minutes. The aerosols are often begun in an emergency department and the child evaluated for their effectiveness. A reduction in airway edema usually occurs within 10 to 20 minutes, with a gradual reduction of its effect over 2 hours. Although the aerosols may be given as frequently as every 30 minutes, the potential side effects from cardiovascular stimulation and the implied severity of respiratory distress should limit such use to an intensive care unit setting. Reports of a "rebound" effect from persistent use of the racemic epinephrine restricted its use to inpatient settings until recently.[7,8] Today, patients are treated with dexamethasone and racemic epinephrine and discharged from the emergency department to home if they are free of intercostal retractions and stridor after a 2-hour waiting period.[9]

Recommendations for adrenocorticosteroid therapy in patients with LTB have had a long and complicated course. Original proof of effectiveness came with the combined analysis of many studies (meta-analyses) that demonstrated effectiveness of a single dose of dexamethasone at 0.6 mg/kg given intramuscularly. More recent studies have compared inhaled corticosteroids to oral systemic corticosteroids, with and without inhaled racemic epinephrine. Administration of oral dexamethasone at 0.6 mg/kg has been recommended as the least expensive and least invasive means by which to lower hospitalization rates.[7,8]

Endotracheal intubation may be necessary if the child becomes exhausted or severe respiratory distress develops. To avoid traumatizing the inflamed subglottic tissue, the ETT should be at least 1 mm smaller in diameter than that estimated for the child's age. As with epiglottitis, dramatic improvement in respiratory distress is expected after intubation. Attempts at extubation can be made if an air leak develops around the ETT at pressures under 20 to 30 cm H$_2$O. The child is closely monitored in the 4 to 12 hours after extubation for the return of stridor.

Traumatic and Postoperative Laryngotracheobronchitis

Airway obstruction may occur as a sequela of endotracheal intubation. Even the most carefully placed ETT can result in significant injury to the tracheal lining. The cilia in the trachea are easily damaged, especially with aggressive suctioning procedures. Excessively large endotracheal tubes lead to necrosis of the tracheal mucosa. An ETT leak of 20 to 25 cm H$_2$O is recommended to minimize the pressure the ETT applies against the surface of the trachea near the cricoid ring. The value of this leak has been called into question in studies in which the presence of an ETT leak was found to be less predictive of postextubation LTB than the duration of intubation.[10]

Historically, noncuffed endotracheal tubes have been used in children younger than 8 years of age. This practice began several decades ago when low-volume, high-pressure endotracheal tubes used during anesthesia became overdistended when nitrous oxide diffused into the ETT cuff, resulting in pressure-related injury to the trachea. The safety of cuffed endotracheal tubes has since been reevaluated in several studies. In one study when this was done, 99% of the patients

---

CASE STUDY 3

A 2-year-old girl arrives in the emergency room intubated with a 4.0 ETT by EMS. The mother states the toddler had been ill for several days with a runny nose, fever, and a cough. The night before, the mother had noted that the girl was breathing "funny" and had a barking cough. This morning she refused to drink, had increased difficulty breathing, and was very irritable. She has had multiple episodes of vomiting with coughing, but no diarrhea. After consulting her pediatrician by phone, she had been advised to call an ambulance and have the child transported to the hospital. EMS reports to have found the toddler in respiratory distress and in an altered mental state. Marked stridor was audible and the oxygen saturation was measured at 58%. The infant was sedated and paralyzed; the intubation with the 4.0 ETT was extremely difficult and required multiple attempts.

What is your differential diagnosis?

What treatment should you recommend?

What complications should you expect?

See Evolve Resources for answers.

had a minimal leak with no increase in the incidence of postextubation LTB when compared with patients using a noncuffed ETT.[11] Direct airway injury from suctioning induces scar tissue and granuloma development that will result in varying degrees of airway obstruction. Granulomas have developed even after very brief periods of endotracheal intubation in infants.[12] Children who exhibit postextubation moderate stridor are treated with racemic epinephrine inhalation, and dexamethasone. Severe stridor requires reintubation.

LOWER AIRWAY DISORDERS

Bacterial Tracheitis

Bacterial tracheitis is a medical emergency that can result in complete airway obstruction and death. Patients typically have an antecedent upper respiratory infection or LTB-like symptoms for several days before presentation with severe airway obstruction. Although the slow progression of the disease closely resembles LTB, the fever, toxic appearance, and elevated white blood cell count with an increased percentage of premature white cell forms (bands) all suggest the likelihood of a bacterial disease. Neck and chest radiographs reveal narrowing of a subglottic airway with irregular mucosal surface, without evidence of epiglottic swelling.[1]

Bacterial tracheitis responds poorly to racemic epinephrine and typically requires the placement of an artificial airway to manage the copious tracheal secretions. Treatment includes antibiotics to cover for *S. aureus, H. influenzae,* and *S. pneumoniae.* The disease resolves more slowly than epiglottitis, requiring nearly a week before extubation is attempted.

Obstruction of the Trachea and Major Bronchi

Tracheal narrowing produces either expiratory or biphasic (inspiratory and expiratory) wheezing. The degree and flexibility of the airway narrowing will determine the severity of the wheeze. Because the trachea serves as the final conduit for the removal of secretions, lesions in this area may result in pooling of mucus with rhonchi audible during auscultation. The abnormalities are heard radiating throughout the chest but are best appreciated over the sternal area. It is often difficult to discern where the wheezes or rhonchi originate in a small child. Wheezes or rhonchi that remain equal in pitch across all regions of the chest but are heard loudest around the sternum most likely have originated in the trachea. Larger bronchial lesions produce similar manifestations but are more localized to the side of the lesion.

Tracheomalacia

Tracheomalacia is a condition of dynamic tracheal collapse caused by abnormal shape and flexibility of the tracheal cartilage rings. The abnormality can affect either a small section or the entire length of the trachea. Although often idiopathic in origin, there may be identifiable extrinsic causes that have led to tracheal wall softening. Common injurious events include neonatal ventilation with high pressures, chronic trauma to the trachea from a malpositioned ETT or aggressive endotracheal suctioning, and external compressive structures, such as a vascular ring.

In most cases of tracheomalacia the infant or child presents with chronic wheezing that becomes more severe with vigorous breathing. Fortunately, the abnormality tends to improve with time as the child's airway grows, and little intervention is necessary. Severe tracheomalacia may result in complete obstruction and profound episodic hypoxemia, especially during forced exhalation. Repeated airway collapse during exhalation leads to increasingly severe lung hyperinflation. Because exhalation is impaired by airway collapse, once the lung is completely inflated, air movement is no longer possible. This scenario is most often seen in older infants with a history of prolonged positive-pressure ventilation and severe bronchopulmonary dysplasia (BPD). During severe agitation, these infants become cyanotic and even bradycardic, with little or no air movement in spite of increased respiratory effort.

Treatment options are few, mostly unsatisfactory, and include prolonged continuous positive airway pressure (occasionally fairly high pressure of 8 to 12 cm H_2O) or ventilatory support with a tracheostomy tube in place to distend or "splint open" the airways. For milder cases, chronic sedation may avoid the episodic agitation that leads to the airway obstruction.

Congenital Tracheal or Bronchial Stenosis

Like tracheomalacia, congenital tracheal or bronchial stenosis may involve extensive or short lengths of the involved airway. The severity of symptoms depends on the degree and length of the stenosis. A common cause of stenosis in the newborn is the formation of a vascular ring. This occurs in infants with congenital malformation of the great vessels of the heart, usually a double aortic arch. With this malformation, the aorta wraps around both the esophagus and trachea. Infants can present with feeding difficulties and uncontrollable wheezing. Surgical correction of the defect can reduce symptoms, although the residual presence of focal tracheomalacia may cause respiratory symptoms to persist postoperatively.

Tracheal stenosis results from complied or nearly complied rings of cartilage. They present as segmental stenosis anywhere in the tracheobronchial tree or as generalized stenosis/hypoplasia. Funnel-shaped lesions are associated with pulmonary artery sling. This is a very rare anomaly and outcome has recently been improved through new surgical techniques.

Intraluminal Obstruction

An acquired cause of airway narrowing is the development of intraluminal obstruction. In the child, foreign body obstruction is encountered more commonly than the adult problem of endobronchial tumor. Infectious agents (e.g., *Mycobacterium tuberculosis*) or a neoplasm, classically Hodgkin's lymphoma, may cause lymphadenopathy that compresses the airway. The other differential diagnosis to consider is cardiomegaly in patients with congenital heart defects, which especially can compress the left main bronchus because of its anatomical relation to the heart. The diffuse, chronic wheeze associated with these disorders is often confused with asthma. Endobronchial compression is suspected in an infant or child with persistent wheezing who does not respond to bronchodilator therapy. Diagnostic studies to differentiate the cause of wheezing in these patients include barium swallow (for evidence of a vascular ring), bronchoscopy, and computed tomography of the chest. Treatment of intrinsic tracheal and major airway obstruction is often surgical and is directed at widening the narrowed area. Additionally, treatment of the primary cause for the lymphadenopathy, such as Hodgkin's lymphoma, is critical.

Foreign Body Aspiration
Incidence

A leading cause of accidental death in the toddler is foreign body aspiration. The degree of respiratory sequelae depends on the nature of the material aspirated, whereas the severity of neurological sequelae depends on the duration of ventilatory compromise. Mobile infants and toddlers are at particularly high risk by virtue of their tendency to place objects in their mouths. Inappropriate toys for a child's age may have loose parts, and certain foods (e.g., nuts, Vienna sausages, hot dogs) are just the right size to become lodged in a child's airway. The preferred location for small enough objects is the right middle lobe bronchi, which has the most direct and straight connection to the trachea. If the child is neurologically intact, these aspirations commonly occur if the child is straddled or falls while harboring such objects in or near the mouth.

Signs and Symptoms

Signs and symptoms of foreign body aspiration vary with the location of impaction and the degree of airway obstruction. They can range from unilateral wheezing or recurrent pneumonia, as when peanuts or popcorn obstruct the smaller airways, to immediate occlusion of the upper airway with complete absence of air movement and rapid death from suffocation, as seen in hot dog or balloon aspiration fatalities. It is not necessary for the foreign body to be in the trachea: a big enough object stuck in the esophagus can elicit very similar symptoms of respiratory distress.

Diagnosis

The cause of the obstruction and adequacy of ventilation should be quickly determined. A thorough history of the circumstances surrounding the onset of symptoms helps determine whether this is a foreign body aspiration or an infectious process. However, a complete history is often difficult to obtain. Examiners must determine, first and foremost, the adequacy of ventilation, followed by the location of the obstruction. Children with sudden onset of wheezing, particularly if wheezing has never occurred before and is unilateral in nature, raise suspicions of foreign body aspiration.

Anteroposterior and lateral neck and chest radiographs are useful if the object is radiopaque. Although the appearance of a radiopaque foreign body on a radiograph is striking, many aspirated materials, such as peanuts and carrots, cannot be detected in this fashion (Figure 26-6). Foreign body aspiration usually occurs at the laryngeal level. Deviation

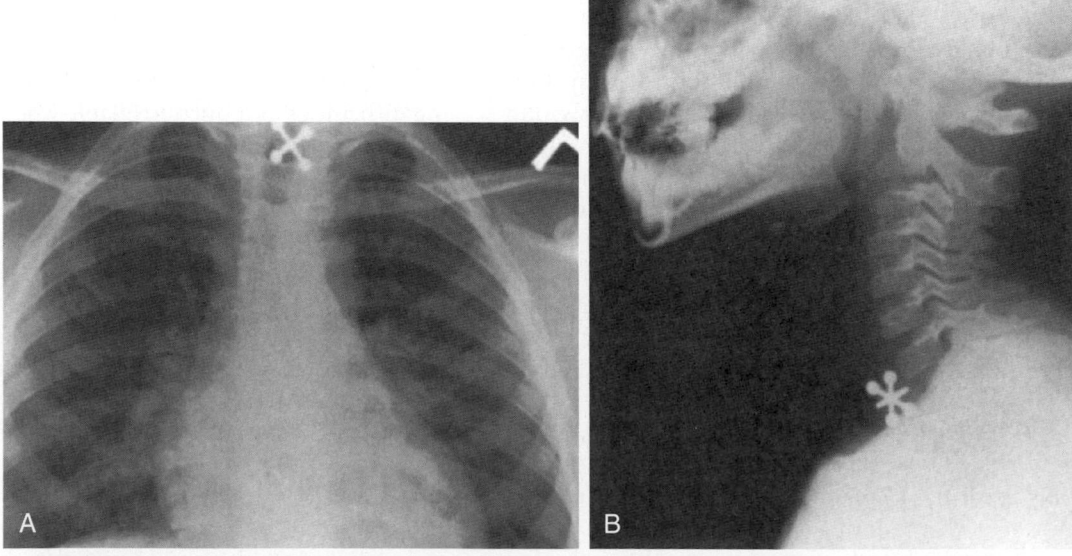

FIGURE 26-6 Foreign body obstruction. Posteroanterior (**A**) and lateral (**B**) chest radiographs reveal an esophageal foreign body that caused respiratory distress from posterior pressure on the trachea.

in the airway shape may indicate a foreign body not otherwise visible. Recurrent pneumonia in the same lobe is also suspicious. Asymmetrical lung hyperinflation can result from a ball-valve effect of foreign material localized in a major bronchus. This defect is most often apparent on an expiratory film (Figure 26-7).[13] Comparison between an expiratory and inspiratory film can also yield the diagnosis but depends greatly on the cooperation of the child.

Fiberoptic laryngoscopy or bronchoscopy is helpful in both finding and retrieving the foreign body. Such procedures are best done in an operating room and with a rigged bronchoscope. Pulse oximetry is used to determine the need for supplemental oxygen. Arterial blood gas analysis is indicated if hypercarbia is suspected in the child with severe obstruction.

Treatment

Therapy employed will vary with the severity of the obstruction. If the child is well oxygenated and ventilated,

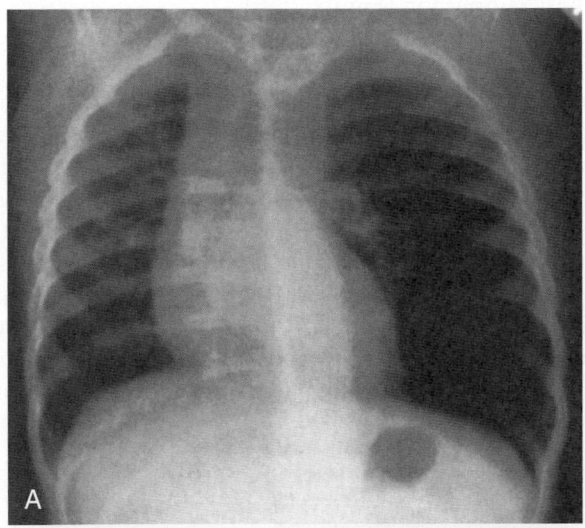

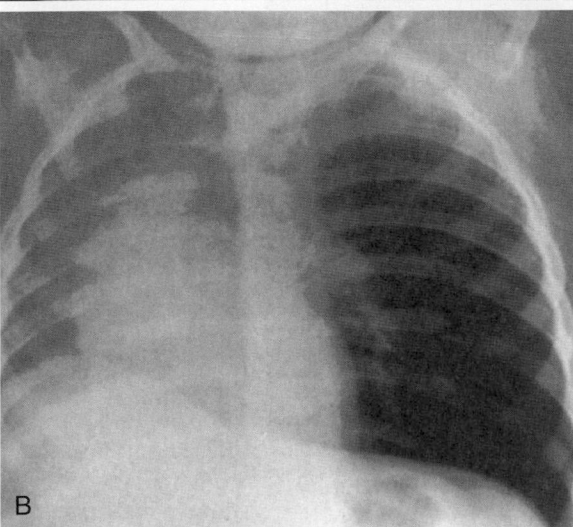

FIGURE 26-7 Foreign body aspiration. Asymmetrical lung volumes (**A**), accentuated during exhalation (**B**), indicate an obstructing ball-valve type of lesion in the left bronchus.

a controlled therapeutic bronchoscopy or laryngoscopy with appropriate anesthesia is preferred. When foreign body aspiration is suspected and respiratory symptoms are acute, urgent bronchoscopy with removal of the object is necessary. Even if the child appears to be stable, movement of the object to a more critical area can result in sudden clinical deterioration. The child with complete obstruction may require emergent cricothyrotomy to establish a patent airway.

Pediatric advanced life support guidelines state that signs of severe or complete airway obstructions that require intervention include the following:

· Inability to speak or cry audibly
· Weak, ineffective cough
· High-pitched sound or no sound during inhalation
· Increased difficulty breathing with distress
· Cyanosis
· Universal choking sign (thumb and index finger clutching neck)

No interventions should be taken if the child can cough forcefully or speak. In this case one should stay with the child monitoring the situation and providing emotional support. The intervention described below addresses the classical, everyday foreign body obstruction scenario. In a hospital setting the situation may be different and more likely related to causes or complications of medical treatment. In those cases troubleshooting equipment and suctioning of the airway should be the first line of action.

Once the obstruction is relieved, some children will be discharged as soon as they recover from anesthesia. In others, resolution of symptoms may be delayed. Airway edema may develop and require corticosteroid therapy along with careful monitoring to ensure that a progressive obstruction does not ensue. Reactive granulation tissue at the site of impaction along with postobstructive infection may take some time to resolve. A second bronchoscopy may be required because of reaccumulation of secretions.

If intubation and mechanical ventilation are indicated, the ventilation strategies often include synchronized intermittent mandatory ventilation (SIMV), pressure support, or volume support. Remembering that these children usually have normal lung function, the FIO_2 and minute ventilation requirements are low and are set to obtain normal arterial blood gas values. Once patency of the airway is ensured, mechanical ventilation is weaned. Secondary infection and prolonged intubation are occasional complications.

Atelectasis
Etiology and Pathophysiology

Atelectasis is collapsed lung parenchyma and is best compared to a wet sponge that fails to reinflate after being compressed. Many processes can cause atelectasis. Internal or parenchymal disorders that are characterized by an inadequate tidal volume, loss of lung compliance (e.g., acute respiratory distress syndrome), airway obstruction (e.g., mucus plugging), and increased elastance of lung tissue can all result in atelectasis. External forces also lead to compression of lung parenchyma, with the reduction in lung volume resulting in atelectasis. These include chest wall disorders (e.g., kyphosis, flail chest), accumulation of pleural fluid, obesity, and abdominal ascites.

The right middle lobe, which has the poorest collateral air circulation and smallest bronchial opening of the major lung segments, is particularly prone to mucus plugging and collapse. Intubated patients, particularly young infants, have a propensity toward right upper lobe collapse. This is most likely related to their supine positioning and tendency toward obstruction of the right upper lobe bronchus (the most proximal of all the lobar bronchi) by a migrating ETT. Postoperative patients are at particular risk of atelectasis because of an ineffective cough, impaired mucus transport, and the effect of anesthesia. Surfactant deficiency may occur in the child after smoke inhalation or lung contusion, resulting in various degrees of lung collapse. Tracheobronchial suctioning has also been related to atelectasis in children and is believed to result from the negative pressure that the airway is exposed to during the suctioning process.

Signs and Symptoms

Clinical presentation will vary with the cause and severity of the lung volume loss. Clinical history may reveal slow regression of activity and deterioration of pulmonary function, as may be seen with a slowly growing pleural tumor. Conversely, the patient may experience rapid-onset dyspnea and cyanosis from a foreign body aspiration that occludes a large bronchus, leading to airway collapse.

Patients with enough atelectasis to create a severe ventilation/perfusion (V/Q) mismatch exhibit clinical symptoms of cyanosis, tachypnea, nasal flaring, retractions, and grunting. The patient may complain of chest pain on deep inspiration if the pleura is inflamed or there is accompanying pneumothorax.[14]

Arterial blood gas analysis reveals low oxygen saturations, manifesting low V/Q ratios. The $Paco_2$ levels often remain normal in the presence of atelectasis, as a result of the rapid diffusion characteristics of CO_2 and close regulation of the $Paco_2$ by an altering respiratory rate.

Diagnosis

Although atelectasis is most often found on a chest radiograph, it may first be suspected during a physical examination. Decreased breath sounds, increased tactile fremitus, tracheal deviation, and an elevated diaphragm may indicate atelectasis; however, many patients with atelectasis are asymptomatic on physical examination. Diagnosis is confirmed with evidence of volume loss on a chest radiograph (Figure 26-8).

Treatment

Treatment of atelectasis is aimed at removing the cause and depends on the individual patient's clinical course. Drainage of pleural fluid or removal of external compressors will allow the lung to reexpand. If the cause is airway obstruction, bronchoscopy or good pulmonary hygiene, including aerosolized bronchodilators and chest physiotherapy, will facilitate returned airway patency. In the intubated patient, the use of continuous distending pressure may reverse and prevent further lung collapse.[15] Early mobilization and position changes in postoperative patients,

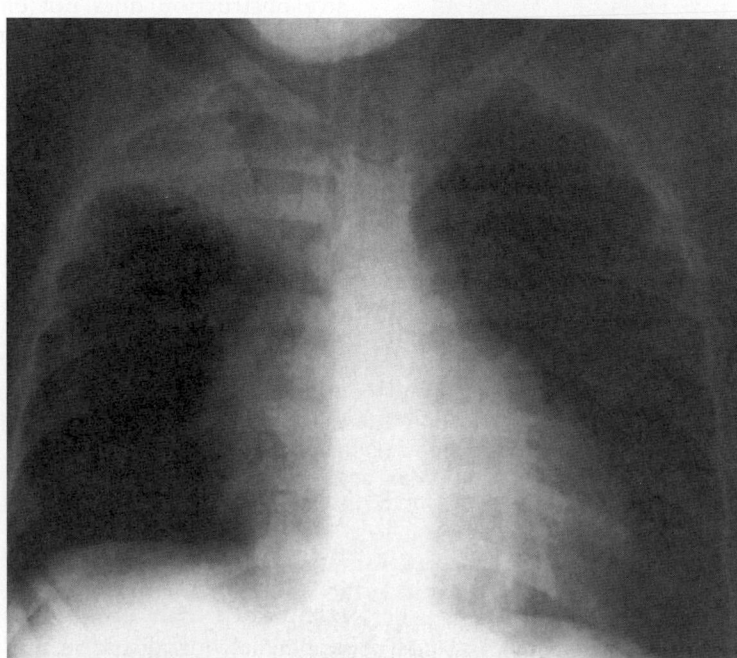

FIGURE 26-8 Anteroposterior chest radiograph with right upper lobe atelectasis.

along with encouragement in coughing and deep breathing (e.g., incentive spirometry), are techniques used to prevent and often treat atelectasis.

Bronchiectasis
Etiology and Pathophysiology

Bronchiectasis is defined as irreversible dilation of the bronchial tree. Typically the segmental and subsegmental bronchi become irregularly shaped and dilated, leading to a loss of the typical funnel configuration that allows smooth central flow of secretions. Additionally, ciliary activity in the area of the dilation is inadequate and further contributes to the difficulty in mobilizing secretions. The secretions become infected as they pool. The lower lobes, particularly the left lower lobe, are most often involved.

A small number of patients may have congenital bronchiectasis in which there is a defect in the development of bronchial cartilage or there is developmental failure of the elastic and muscular tissues of the trachea and main bronchi. Most patients acquire the disease, and bronchiectasis develops as a result of airway obstruction or chronic infection. Causes include bronchial obstruction (e.g., foreign body aspiration, mediastinal mass), infections (e.g., measles, pertussis, pneumonia), Kartagener syndrome, and cystic fibrosis (CF).

Signs and Symptoms

Bronchiectasis may occur acutely after an infection or have a more insidious onset in patients suffering from chronic pulmonary diseases such as CF or reflux and aspiration. Patients experience chronic cough, often productive of copious amounts of thick purulent sputum that has a three-layered appearance if left standing for some time, and only occasional hemoptysis. Pulmonary infections are common, with recurrent fever and foul-smelling breath or sputum. Dyspnea on exertion and clubbing of the digits may manifest in some cases. The lower lobes, particularly the left lower lobe, are most commonly involved.

Diagnosis

Bronchiectasis may be suspected on the basis of the clinical history and physical examination. Plain chest radiographs are seldom normal but alone are not definitive in diagnosing the disease. The abnormal pattern of bronchiectasis is seen most strikingly during bronchography.[16] However, this is rarely performed today. Instead, computed tomographic scanning is used to confirm the diagnosis (Figure 26-9). Pulmonary function may be abnormal, with spirometry demonstrating an obstructive pattern. A combined obstructive and restrictive disease pattern may be present in the more severe cases.[17]

Treatment

Medical management depends on the severity of the disease. Chest physiotherapy, including postural drainage and percussion, along with adequate hydration is performed to improve the mobilization of pulmonary secretions. Newer concepts favor the idea that low mucus salinity rather than underhydration contributes to mucus retention. This may explain the success and increased use of nebulized hypertonic saline in these patients.

Antibiotic therapy is given orally, by nebulization (i.e., tobramycin), or by the intravenous route. The choice of antibiotic is based on the results of the individual patient's sputum culture results. Blind use of broad-spectrum antibiotics in this chronic disease may lead to more resistant colonization.[18] The improved empiric use of intravenous antibiotic and new mucous-clearing medications and treatments in CF patients have improved the outcome in this particular disease.

In those cases in which the child suffers severe illness (i.e., failure to thrive, severe hemoptysis) in spite of antibiotic therapy and chest physiotherapy, surgical resection of the bronchiectatic section of lung may be considered. Patients with the disease localized to only one or two lobes are considered better candidates for surgical intervention.[19,20] (See Case Study 4.)

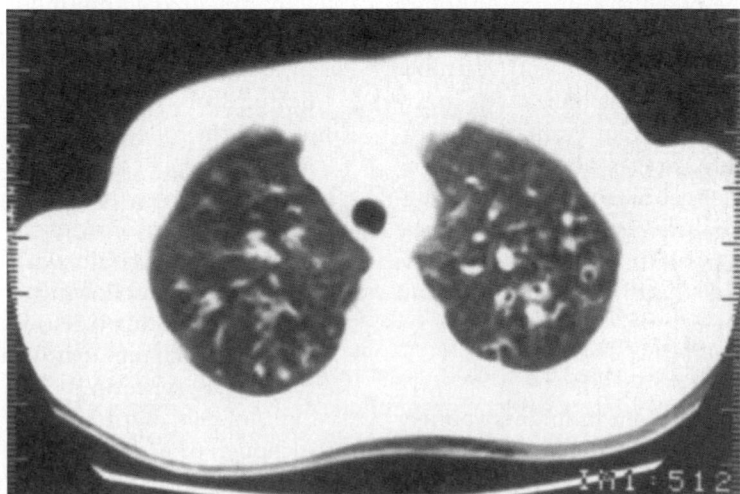

FIGURE 26-9 Widened, thick-walled bronchial tubes (*cut in cross section*) in the peripheral lung zones.

CASE STUDY 4

A 3½-year-old boy is admitted to the intensive care unit (ICU) after heart surgery. He was on cardiopulmonary bypass for 190 minutes and the operation went well. In the ICU he is sedated and ventilated. A chest radiograph and cultures are obtained on postoperative day 1 for fever. The chest radiograph shows consolidation of the left lower lobe, and it remains the same over the next days. All cultures are negative, and he is successfully extubated on postoperative day 4. The chest radiographs remain unchanged, and the decision for bronchoscopy is made. Before the bronchoscopy the plan is to reintubate the child. He is paralyzed, and his baseline oxygen saturation remains at 75% to 79% under bag-mask ventilation. An ETT is placed under good visualization of the vocal cords, but his oxygen saturations fall to 60% to 65% with minimal chest rise and increased resistance to bagging. He is extubated, and it is not possible to bag-mask ventilate him. His oxygen saturations continue to drop, and after a second intubation attempt with good visualization of the vocal cords, he goes into cardiac arrest.

What is your differential diagnosis?

What are your actions?

See Evolve Resources for answers.

Acute Bronchiolitis

Etiology and Pathophysiology

The term *acute bronchiolitis* is applied to a condition in infants in which a viral respiratory tract infection results in clinical symptoms of small airway obstruction.[21,22] In the majority of infants with bronchiolitis, the causative organism is RSV.[23]

RSV is a highly contagious virus and has its greatest impact on young infants. Infants younger than 6 months of age are at particular risk of severe infection, with the peak incidence for hospitalization occurring between 2 and 6 months of age.[24] Bronchiolitis is the number one cause of hospitalization in the United States, and considerable variation exists in the management.[25,26] Although most cases are mild and do not require hospital admission, epidemics of the infection occurring between December and March result in nearly 100,000 hospitalizations in the United States each year.[27] Postmortem evaluation of infants with severe bronchiolitis reveals obstructed airway lumina from impacted cellular debris. In vitro studies suggest that an intense inflammatory response occurs in the infant's airways and may contribute to increased mucus secretion and transudation of fluid into the airways and airway walls.[28]

Incidence

Acute bronchiolitis is seen most often in infants younger than 1 year of age who were born prematurely, live in a crowded environment, attend day care facilities, and are exposed to passive smoke.[26] Bronchiolitis with RSV infection is particularly devastating to infants with certain at-risk conditions, including premature birth, chronic lung disease (e.g., BPD, CF), congenital heart disease (especially those with pulmonary hypertension), and immunodeficiencies.[29] These infants are at risk of respiratory failure and death.

Signs and Symptoms

Physical findings vary considerably with the patient's age. Infants (younger than 1 year of age) develop coryza, cough, respiratory distress, wheezing, and tachypnea. The symptoms of infection usually peak around 48 to 72 hours and a previously healthy infant can progress from what was thought to be a simple cold to severe respiratory distress during that time. In contrast, the principal symptoms in children older than 2 years of age are profound nasal congestion and productive cough. Chest auscultation reveals diffuse, coarse, "sticky" rales ("Velcro" rales), which may be accompanied by wheezes. A chest radiograph typically reveals intense lung hyperinflation with flattened hemidiaphragms (obstructive), with occasional films showing evidence of collapse or consolidation (Figure 26-10).

Severe, life-threatening apnea is a common symptom in the very young infant with bronchiolitis, especially in those with cardiorespiratory disease or a history of premature birth or apnea. An infant may also be agitated and have difficulty feeding as a consequence of hypoxia. This may lead to dehydration as well as respiratory failure. Development of cyanosis usually heralds impending respiratory failure. Arterial P_{CO_2} rising above 45 mm Hg despite tachypnea indicates impending respiratory failure and respiratory support needs to be prepared, including intubation.

Diagnosis

Clinical diagnosis of acute viral bronchiolitis is confirmed by identifying the RSV or other respiratory virus. Nasopharyngeal aspirate or nasal lavage provides samples of the virus. Diagnosis is based on the clinical presentation and the results of viral culture and antigen detection assays (i.e., enzyme-linked immunosorbent assays).[30] Clinical history and physical examination form the basis for a diagnosis of bronchiolitis.

Features of clinical history may include but are not limited to the following:
· Preceding upper respiratory infection or rhinorrhea
· Features of lower respiratory infection
· History of sick contacts

Features of physical examination may include but are not limited to the following:
· Signs of respiratory distress: tachypnea, retraction, hypoxia, color change, nasal flaring, grunting, apnea, head bobbing, or wheezing
· Signs of dehydration

Although the diagnosis of bronchiolitis is clinically evident, the differential diagnosis is broad and always warrants consideration.

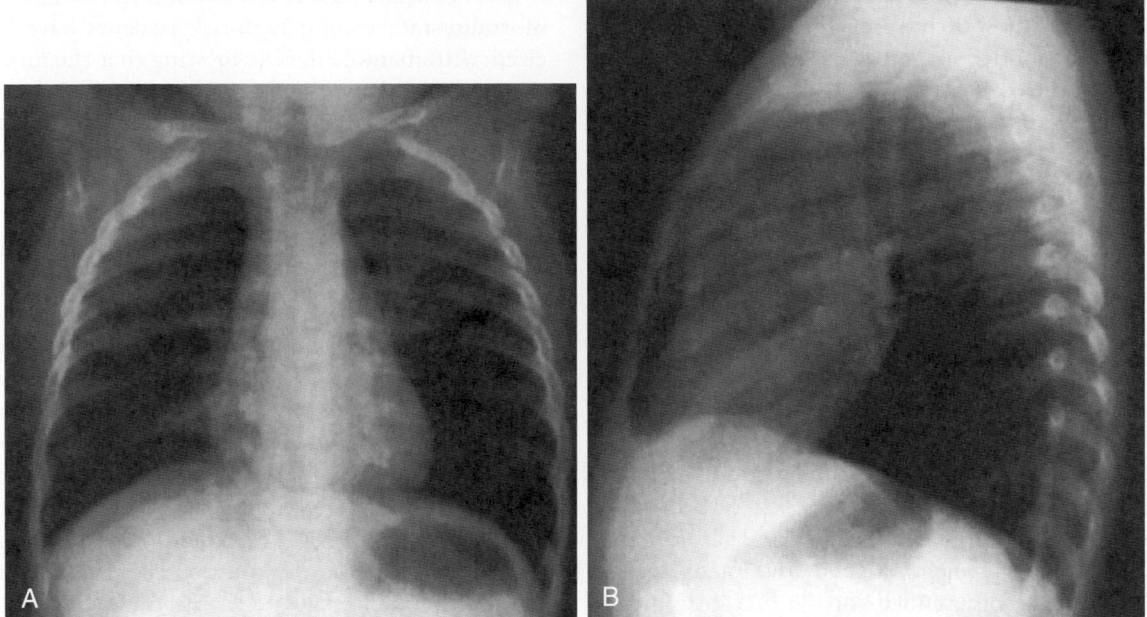

FIGURE 26-10   Severe bronchiolitis. Posterior (**A**) and lateral (**B**) chest radiographs reveal flattening of the diaphragm and widening of the anteroposterior diameter, which is indicative of severe air trapping. Perihilar markings are accentuated.

Treatment

Treatment of bronchiolitis is largely supportive, along with careful monitoring. The infection is self-limiting in many patients, and hospitalization is not necessary if symptoms are mild. The infant is monitored for apnea, hypoxia, and dehydration. Care is taken to provide adequate feedings and prevent further respiratory distress.

The decision to hospitalize a child with bronchiolitis involves a multifactorial assessment of the risk factors, clinical symptoms, age, and familial resources. Supportive care with supplemental oxygen, intravenous hydration if needed, and close clinical monitoring is essential. In most cases, low-flow oxygen therapy (typically nasal cannula) is sufficient to reduce the hypoxia and respiratory distress. Patients with recurrent apnea or respiratory failure may need intubation and mechanical ventilation. Continuous monitoring with pulse oximetry is essential, as well as arterial blood gas analysis for those patients in whom respiratory failure is suspected. Mild yet persistent hypoxia (SpO_2 88% to 92%) despite oxygen therapy can be an ominous sign of impending respiratory failure because the patient could be moving from the obstructive (improved functional residual capacity) to the restrictive (atelectasis) phase of disease. In practice it is very important to ensure patent nares, especially if nasal cannula is used, because RSV typically generates copious amounts of nasal secretions. This is best achieved by frequent and efficient suction of the nares.

Infants with tachypnea, agitation, and cough are at risk of dehydration. In many moderate to severe cases they stop eating because they cannot coordinate the sequence of suck, swallow, and breathe at high respiratory rates. This is a common concern in those patients who experience vomiting with the cough. Intravenous fluids or frequent small-volume feedings are both routes to consider when fluid intake is poor.

Although the role of bronchodilators in the management of bronchiolitis is controversial, there is some evidence that they are effective. In some studies, albuterol brought significant short-term improvement in clinical scores but was not found to reduce admission rates or decrease the length of hospitalization.[31] A single inhalation trial using epinephrine or albuterol can be considered for respiratory distress on an individual basis, such as when there is history of asthma, allergy, or atopy.[32] It is recommended to discontinue inhalation therapy if there is no clinical response such as improved respiratory distress or improved bronchiolitis scores. Nebulized racemic epinephrine demonstrates better short-term improvement in pulmonary physiology and clinical scores but only in the outpatient setting.[33] However, continuation of inhalation therapy despite documented nonresponse exposes the patient to unnecessary therapy and cost.

Ipratropium bromide and theophylline have not proven to be beneficial as bronchodilators in the treatment of bronchiolitis.[34,35] Despite the evidence of airway inflammation, use of systemic or inhaled corticosteroids early in the symptomatic phase of the disease does not tend to improve outcome.[36] However, inhaled corticosteroids are sometimes given to reduce short-term morbidity when there is delayed recovery. It is questionable if these interventions are successful in infants and children with a tendency to have recurrent wheezing or asthma in the future or if the children with treatment success have some other unknown underlying respiratory physiology or chemistry variety.

Nebulized hypertonic saline (3%) is considered an effective and safe treatment for infants with mild to moderate respiratory distress and has been shown to reduce length of stay.[37] The optimal treatment regime for nebulized hypertonic saline in the inpatient setting in acute bronchiolitis remains unclear. A recent randomized controlled trial[37] using hypertonic saline every 2 hours for 3 doses, every 4 hours for 5 doses, and every 6 hours until discharge has shown promising results and is an alternative; however, more evidence is needed on efficacy and dosing regimen. Hypertonic saline therapy significantly reduces bronchiolitis scores (pre/post-hypertonic saline) among patients with mild to moderate bronchiolitis. The first dose of hypertonic saline requires close clinical monitoring for development of acute bronchospasm. A onetime as-needed albuterol order is recommended for the first dose. Acute bronchospasm during or immediately after hypertonic saline therapy is a possible side effect, especially in children with known or unknown asthma. Given the difficulty in distinguishing between asthma and viral bronchiolitis in infants, the first dose should be monitored closely.

Antibiotics. Antibiotics are not recommended in the absence of an identified bacterial focus.[38] Bacterial infections should be treated in the same manner as when in the absence of bronchiolitis. Previously healthy, febrile children 24 months old or younger with bronchiolitis have a low incidence of meningitis, bacteremia, and urinary tract infection. Physician discretion is required when managing infants younger than 60 days old. For infants diagnosed with bronchiolitis and otitis media, please refer to practice guidelines.[32] If using antibiotics without identified bacterial focus, exercise caution and consider potential side effects, such as cost to patient and community and increasing bacterial resistance to antibiotics.

Other Medications. It is recommended that antihistamines, oral decongestants, and over-the-counter (OTC) cough and cold medications not be used for routine therapy because of potential side effects.[39-41] The FDA recommends that OTC cough and cold products not to be used for children younger than 2 years because serious and potentially life-threatening side effects can occur.[41]

Ribavirin, a broad-spectrum virustatic agent, continues to play a contentious role in the treatment of bronchiolitis. It is administered as an aerosol and delivered to the patient, through either an oxygen hood or a ventilator circuit, for 12 to 18 hours per day. Although early studies proclaimed its benefits, concerns remain about its safety, cost, and efficacy. Reported side effects are uncommon; however, precautions are taken to minimize exposure to hospital personnel and family.[42] Ribavirin is expensive to use, and there is no convincing evidence that its use aids in reducing morbidity or mortality.[43-45] Studies that have concluded that there is a reduction in the morbidity and mortality rate among high-risk patients have been criticized, with many centers suggesting that the improvement was caused by improved supportive care rather than the antiviral therapy.[46] For those who support the use of ribavirin, the majority consider it most beneficial in treating extremely ill patients, immune compromised, and those requiring mechanical ventilation. Today the role of ribavirin remains controversial, and its use varies significantly among clinicians.

If the patient requires mechanical ventilation, surfactant replacement therapy may be a consideration. Multicenter trials with animal and synthetic surfactants are being conducted to test this hypothesis. Currently this is an off-label indication and is reserved for the most severe patients.

RSV spreads rapidly and is transmitted through touch, with the virus able to survive on hands and other surfaces (e.g., bed rails, toys). RSV prevention is accomplished by strict avoidance of other infected children and careful attention to hand washing. Disease prevention in high-risk patients (e.g., those with BPD or premature birth) can best be accomplished by passive immunization with immune serum globulin (RSV-IGIV). This passive immunity decreases the incidence of RSV hospitalization by 40% to 65% and decreases the number of hospital days by 50% to 60%.[31,47] Strict avoidance of air pollutants, especially cigarette smoke, assists in the long-term recovery from bronchiolitis.

Prognosis

The mortality rate of infants in high-risk groups is much improved over the past several years. Recurrence of bronchiolitis episodes is seen in some patients; however, subsequent infections are usually much less severe. Studies have indicated that many patients have recurrent cough and wheezing several years after RSV infection. An increase in bronchial responsiveness is often found later in childhood.[23]

Primary Ciliary Dyskinesia
Etiology and Pathophysiology

Normal cilia beat in a coordinated fashion, effectively propelling overlying mucus in one direction out of the airway. The upper and lower respiratory tract is cleared of secretions, inhaled particles, and bacteria. Without the forward thrust of the cilia and coordinated ciliary beating, mucus transport is slowed and there is an accumulation of particles, secretions, and bacteria in the dependent portions of the lungs.

In 1933 Kartagener described a unique clinical triad of situs inversus, chronic sinusitis, and bronchiectasis. This became known as Kartagener syndrome. Subsequent studies found that these patients had defects in the ultrastructure of the cilia that line the mucous membranes of the sinus cavities, lungs, and nose. The syndrome was initially called immotile cilia syndrome. However, further studies have demonstrated that the cilia in patients with this syndrome are not always immotile but often have uncoordinated or ineffective cilia motility.[48] The term *primary ciliary dyskinesia* (PCD) is used increasingly today.

Signs and Symptoms

Chronic cough, often productive, is the most common presenting feature of PCD. It is most apparent early in the morning and with sleep and exercise. Although the mucopurulent sputum initially clears with antibiotic therapy, with age the patient develops increasingly severe airway obstruction. Physical findings include persistent crackles, although wheezing is relatively uncommon. A chest radiograph may reveal lung hyperinflation and changes consistent with bronchiectasis.

Upper respiratory tract infections are common. Persistent nasal congestion, a common presenting feature, may progress to chronic nasal drainage with radiographic evidence of sinusitis. Chronic otitis media, with or without chronic effusions, often occurs and requires prolonged use of transtympanic ventilation tubes.[48]

A right-to-left reversal of the position of the heart and intestinal structures, known as situs inversus, is seen in approximately 50% of the patients with PCD. Isolated dextrocardia may also be found. The accepted explanation for the association of situs inversus with the ciliary defect is that normal rotation of chest and abdominal organs depends on properly functioning embryonic cilia during closure of the thoracic and abdominal cavities. Because similar functional defects are found in both mucosal cilia and sperm flagella, the abnormal cilia motility affects male fertility and males are nearly always sterile.

Diagnosis

Diagnosis can be made rapidly by microscopic evaluation for ciliary motility in specimens taken from paranasal sinuses, nose, or tracheal mucosa. Light and electron microscopy of bronchial mucosal cells reveal abnormal cilia numbers with abnormal ciliary structures. Patients with PCD have defects in the dynein arms, radial spokes, and nexin links. Cilia with an inadequate number of out-dynein arms may be immotile or may have some disorganized rigid movement.[49] Absence of radial spokes and alteration in the figuration of the microtubules in the cilia are other ciliary ultrastructural changes.[50]

Treatment

Treatment of PCD focuses on reducing the volume of pooled respiratory secretions in the lung. Chest physiotherapy for airway clearance is essential and is used with exercise and aerosolized β₂-agonists. Children with PCD have evidence of obstructive pulmonary disease. The obstruction is best minimized by exercise before physiotherapy, instead of relying on β₂ agonist therapy.[51] Because cough is one of the few mechanisms available for removing secretions, antitussive therapy is contraindicated.

Nebulized recombinant human DNase (Pulmozyme) is indicated for treatment of cystic fibrosis. It reduces sputum viscosity, improves pulmonary function, and results in a small reduction in acute respiratory exacerbations. It has been found to be beneficial in the treatment of PCD. Aerosolized or intravenous antibiotics directed by bacterial antibiotic sensitivities, in combination with CPT and Pulmozyme therapy, are believed to reduce the progression of obstructive pulmonary disease. Although rarely necessary, surgical excision of the pulmonary segments is considered when suppurative disease is poorly controlled and localized to a single area.

PNEUMONIA

Lower respiratory tract infections are a leading cause of morbidity and mortality in the pediatric population. They most often affect children younger than 2 years of age. These children typically experience the greatest number of complications. At the University of North Carolina at Chapel Hill, Denny and Clyde monitored the number of patients treated for pneumonia in their outpatient clinic.[52] Their results trace the incidence and cause of pneumonia in specific age groups (Figure 26-11).

Gram-positive cocci, particularly group B streptococcus and *S. aureus,* along with gram-negative enteric bacilli, are the source of most neonatal pneumonias. Children between 1 month and 5 years of age are the most frequent victims of viral pneumonia. RSV and parainfluenza viruses types 1, 2, and 3, along with adenovirus, are the most common infectious viral agents. However, *Chlamydia pneumoniae, H. influenzae, S. pneumoniae,* and *S. aureus* are occasional bacterial agents in this age group. *S. pneumoniae* is the major cause of bacterial pneumonia in children older than 5 years, whereas *M. pneumoniae* and *C. pneumoniae* are more common in school-age children and young adults. Box 26-1 lists the infectious causes of pneumonia in the pediatric population.

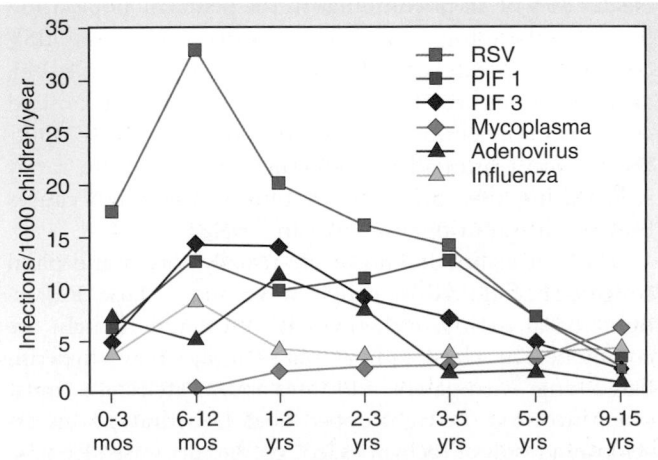

FIGURE 26-11 Etiology of pediatric lower respiratory tract infection in Chapel Hill, NC, by age during an 11-year period.

Box 26-1	Infectious Causes of Pneumonia

VIRUSES
- Respiratory syncytial virus
- Parainfluenza types 1, 2, and 3
- Influenza virus
- Adenovirus
- Rhinovirus
- Cytomegalovirus
- Epstein-Barr virus
- Herpes simplex virus

MYCOPLASMA
- *Mycoplasma pneumoniae*
- *Ureaplasma urealyticum*

BACTERIA
- *Streptococcus pneumoniae*
- *Haemophilus influenzae*
- *Staphylococcus aureus*
- *Streptococcus agalactiae*
- *Legionella pneumophila*
- *Mycobacterium tuberculosis*

PROTOZOA
- *Pneumocystis carinii*

FUNGI
- *Histoplasma capsulatum*
- *Coccidioides immitis*
- *Candida* spp.
- *Blastomyces dermatitidis*
- *Cryptococcus neoformans*

RICKETTSIAE
- *Coxiella burnetii* (Q fever)

CHLAMYDIA
- *Chlamydia pneumoniae*
- *Chlamydia trachomatis*
- *Chlamydia psittaci*

PARASITES
- *Ascaris lumbricoides*

Viral Pneumonia

Respiratory Syncytial Virus

Nearly 80% of all pneumonias in the pediatric population have a viral etiology, with RSV occurring most often. RSV commonly affects children younger than 2 years old, although it has been found in older immunocompromised children or in children with chronic lung disease. Outbreaks occur annually during the winter and are rarely seen during the spring and summer. RSV often causes bronchiolitis, but pneumonia can develop.[53]

The first symptoms noted are usually coryza and nasal congestion, followed by cough, fever, and malaise. Retractions, nasal flaring, tachypnea, wheezes, and rhonchi are common. The chest radiograph typically shows hyperinflated lungs with patchy infiltrates and/or atelectasis (most often involving the right upper lobe). Dehydration can develop as a result of tachypnea, cough, and decreased feeding.

Diagnosis is confirmed with rapid immunofluorescent detection of RSV antigen in nasal washings or enzyme-linked immunosorbent assays of nasal secretions. Test methods are relatively inexpensive.

Aerosolized ribavirin is an antiviral agent that may be used to treat the infection; however, its use remains controversial. Hypoxemia and hypercarbia are complications of RSV pneumonia and may mandate supplemental oxygen for an extended period. Supportive care is aimed at monitoring the severity with pulse oximetry and arterial blood gas analysis. Patients may experience progressive hypoxemia and respiratory failure, necessitating intubation and mechanical ventilation. There may be further progression to advanced respiratory failure, in spite of maximal ventilatory support. Those patients may require extracorporeal membrane oxygenation (ECMO). Patients thought to have a less than 20% chance of survival without ECMO have a nearly 60% chance of survival with ECMO.[54]

Parainfluenza Virus Types 1, 2, and 3

The parainfluenza viruses are the second-most common cause of LTB and pneumonia. Type 3 is the most common cause in children younger than 5 years of age and occurs year round with no seasonal peak. Clinical presentation is similar to that described for RSV. Chest radiographs typically reveal patchy or interstitial infiltrates. Diagnosis is confirmed with rapid antigen testing or viral isolation from a nasal washing. Therapy is supportive, with supplemental oxygen and additional hydration provided as needed. Parainfluenza virus is not to be confused with influenza virus, which has a very narrow seasonal peak.

Influenza Virus

Although influenza virus may cause pneumonia, it occurs predominantly in the very young and very old patient. Yearly epidemics occur during the late winter and early spring. Clinical symptoms consist of rapidly developing fever, malaise, and myalgia. Duration of the illness is usually shorter than that of RSV and the parainfluenza viruses. Although rarely occurring, a rapid pneumonia may result in death within 2 days of onset. Diagnosis and treatment are similar to that of RSV and parainfluenza virus infections. Vaccines are provided annually and are recommended for those high-risk children with chronic cardiopulmonary and immunologic disorders. Chest radiographs typically reveal interstitial or patchy alveolar infiltrates.

Adenovirus

Although it occurs year round, adenoviral pneumonia is most often seen in the late summer and early fall. It occurs most often in children younger than 2 years of age. It is easily confused with bacterial illnesses because it mimics their symptomatology: rapid onset, high fever, leukocytosis, and chest radiograph consistent with pneumonia. Additional findings may include lymphadenopathy and conjunctivitis. A chest radiograph reveals patchy or interstitial infiltrates.

Certain adenoviral types (i.e., 3, 7, 21) are associated with a high mortality rate because of the overwhelming sepsis and cardiovascular collapse that occurs. Diagnosis is confirmed with rapid antigen testing or viral isolation from a nasal washing. Therapy is supportive, and no specific treatment is available. Close monitoring for bacterial superinfection is suggested. New viruses are being isolated, and their implications will become clearer over time. One example is the human metapneumovirus, identified in 2001.

Bacterial Pneumonia

Incidence

Although the incidence of bacterial pneumonia is less than that of viral pneumonia, it has a higher mortality rate. It may occur as a secondary problem to a primary viral pneumonia, as is often seen with pneumonia from influenza virus. Certain other factors known to increase the risk of bacterial pneumonia include compromised immune function, recurrent aspiration from gastroesophageal reflux, malnutrition, day-care attendance or school-aged sibling, exposure to passive cigarette smoke, and congenital abnormalities of the airway (e.g., tracheoesophageal fistula). Bacterial pneumonia is seen throughout the year, with a peak incidence in the winter and early spring.

Etiology

Bacterial agents that cause pneumonia vary considerably throughout the pediatric age group. In the neonatal patient, the offending bacteria are most often contaminants from the mother's genital tract and include group B streptococcus, *Escherichia coli*, *Listeria monocytogenes*, and *Chlamydia trachomatis*.[55] Infants older than 4 to 6 weeks tend to develop pneumonia from *S. pneumoniae*, *H. influenzae*, and *S. aureus*. Less likely organisms include *Bordetella pertussis*, *M. pneumoniae*, and *C. pneumoniae*.

Bacterial pneumonia develops when the intrinsic host defenses are decreased, either by another disease process (e.g., viral infection) or when the anatomical protective mechanisms are destroyed (e.g., primary ciliary dyskinesia). Therefore, any microorganism colonizing the upper respiratory tract has the potential to cause pneumonia if it evades these defenses.

Signs and Symptoms

There are no symptoms that distinguish a bacterial pneumonia from a viral pneumonia in children, although children with bacterial pneumonia tend to present with more severe symptoms of fever and distress. Prodromal symptoms are often nonpulmonary and include headache, fever, malaise, and abdominal pain. Productive cough, with sputum often swallowed, and chest pain during inspiration (pleuritic pain) are common complaints. Physical examination usually reveals nasal flaring, accessory muscle use, intercostal and subcostal retractions, tachypnea, and shallow breathing. Crackles, decreased breath sounds, increased fremitus, and dullness to percussion are often found during auscultation and examination of the chest.[56]

Diagnosis

The chest radiograph is an important diagnostic tool when evaluating a child with suspected bacterial pneumonia. Although bacterial pneumonia is commonly manifested as an alveolar consolidation, lobar and interstitial infiltrates are often found as well as pleural effusion. It has been suggested that certain radiographic findings vary among the various bacterial agents involved and may help determine the etiology.[57,58]

An elevated total band count (>1500 total bands) is common in the presence of bacterial pneumonia. Increased C-reactive protein levels and erythrocyte sedimentation rates provide supporting, albeit not specific, evidence of inflammation. Blood culture is the most helpful test to give absolute confirmation of bacterial disease, but it is only positive in 25% of patients with *S. pneumoniae* pneumonia and 33% of patients with *S. aureus* pneumonia. Similarly, the latex particle agglutination and countercurrent immunoelectrophoresis studies are insensitive in most cases of pneumonia. When pleural fluid is present in significant quantities, sampling for Gram stain and culture will yield specific bacterial diagnosis in 65% to 80% of patients. Bronchoalveolar lavage fluid obtained during a bronchoscopy can be used for atypical presentations. Lung tissue may be obtained for culture through an open-lung biopsy, transthoracic needle aspiration biopsy, or percutaneous lung puncture.

Precise microbiological diagnosis is not always obtained even though bacterial pneumonia is suspected. There are several reasons why clinicians may take an empirical approach to treatment. Many of the diagnostic procedures are much too invasive for any but the sickest patients. Some procedures use instruments (e.g., bronchoscope, suction catheter) that pass through the contaminated pharynx or upper airway. Although it is difficult to obtain a sputum specimen in children younger than 8 years of age, when it is obtained the flora in the upper airway contaminates the sputum, making the diagnosis questionable.

Treatment

Standard initial treatment of bacterial pneumonia varies considerably according to the patient's age and immunological status, time of year, and local antibiotic sensitivity patterns. The need for hospitalization is often determined by the severity of the symptoms. When the cause is identified, antimicrobial therapy is determined and is usually given for 7 to 14 days by the parenteral route, although the clinical symptoms and history of underlying disease often guide empirical therapy. Neonatal pneumonia is routinely treated with intravenous antibiotics. The patient is monitored with pulse oximetry and arterial blood gas analysis when indicated. Supplemental oxygen is provided if hypoxia occurs and mechanical ventilation is provided if there is respiratory failure. The role of chest physiotherapy in the treatment of pneumonia is debated, with some clinicians doubting its efficacy.

Streptococcus pneumoniae

The most common cause of bacterial pneumonia is the pneumococcus.[59] The clinical picture differs with age. The infant presents initially with a sudden fever and diarrhea or vomiting. Signs of respiratory distress, including nasal flaring, tachypnea, grunting, and retractions, appear along with restlessness and cyanosis. The classic clinical presentation of the older child is that of rapid-onset respiratory distress, high fever, shaking chills, headache, pleuritic pain, and cough with rust-colored sputum. The chest radiograph usually reveals lobar or segmental alveolar consolidation, which may be accompanied by a pleural effusion or empyema. Sputum reveals sheets of gram-positive diplococci and many white blood cells. The clinical diagnosis can be made based on these findings. However, in reality the clinical presentation is rarely this clear and treatment of suspected bacterial pneumonia includes pneumococcal coverage.

Pneumococcal pneumonia can be rapidly fatal without appropriate therapy. Penicillin is the antibiotic of choice; erythromycin is used in the penicillin-allergic individual. Although penicillin resistance in the United States is rare, it is increasingly common in Europe and Africa. Therefore treatment should be guided by antibiotic susceptibilities when an organism is recovered. Other antibiotics that have successful activity against *S. pneumoniae* include cephalosporins, chloramphenicol, clindamycin, and vancomycin.

Haemophilus influenzae

Before the use of vaccination against serotype b, this gram-negative rod was a common cause of pneumonia in children. Infection occurs most often in children younger than 5 years of age. The chest radiograph is highly variable and can exhibit any pattern from a bronchiolitic-type picture with hyperinflation to patchy infiltrates to segmental or lobar consolidation. Pleural effusion is present in about one third of the patients. Positive blood culture results or positive results on urine antigen screens confirm diagnosis. Empirical therapy is usually with a cephalosporin. Other potentially therapeutic drugs effective against all *H. influenzae* isolates include trimethoprim-sulfamethoxazole, clarithromycin, azithromycin, chloramphenicol, and amoxicillin/clavulanate.

Staphylococcus aureus

Pneumonia caused by *S. aureus* ("staph") is a virulent, aggressive disease that can be rapidly fatal, particularly in infants younger than 1 year of age. This organism is commonly found on the skin and mucosa, with 20% to 30% of the population carrying bacteria in the nose. Pneumonia is often seen in debilitated patients who often have associated skin infections. It is common to have a history of an antecedent viral infection, particularly influenza.[59]

The severity of clinical symptoms varies, with the typical presentation being an upper respiratory tract infection, fever, cough, and respiratory distress. The clinical course in the neonate is often rapidly progressive and is associated with a high mortality rate shortly after the onset of symptoms. The chest radiograph usually reveals large consolidation that can progress rapidly to a "whiteout" of the lung. Pleural effusion and empyema as well as a pneumothorax often complicate the clinical picture. While resolving, areas of consolidation often progress to pneumatoceles, which are round, air-filled areas of lung destruction that are easily visible on the radiograph. The pneumatoceles may contain fluid and change rapidly in number and size, leading to a mediastinal shift.

Diagnosis is by positive blood, skin abscess, or pleural fluid culture results. Therapy is with antistaphylococcal penicillins such as nafcillin and oxacillin. Susceptibility testing is imperative to exclude the possibility of methicillin-resistant *S. aureus* spreading throughout the general community, which requires treatment with vancomycin.

Atypical Pneumonia

The major pathogens of pneumonia that are commonly missed by the tests listed previously cause atypical pneumonia. In the neonate, those agents include the uncommon viral diseases of rubella, varicella-zoster, and cytomegalovirus and the even rarer nonbacterial agents *Toxoplasma*, *Treponema pallidum*, and *C. trachomatis*. In the older child, *M. pneumoniae*, *C. pneumoniae*, and *M. tuberculosis* cause atypical pneumonia.

Mycoplasma pneumoniae

M. pneumoniae commonly causes a community-acquired pneumonia that is seen year-round but peaks in the late summer and early fall. Although it occurs in all age groups, it is most often a disease of school-aged children and young adults.[60]

The incubation period is 2 to 3 weeks, and it presents as a viral upper respiratory infection. Clinical onset is insidious, with a gradual development of malaise, fever, and cough, which are the most prominent symptoms. Cough is nonproductive or productive with blood-tinged sputum. Chills, pharyngitis, headache, nausea, vomiting, diarrhea, and chest pain are also associated with this infection. Crackles are heard most often during auscultation, with occasional wheezing, although there may be no abnormal findings at the beginning of the illness. The clinical and radiographic findings are often out of proportion with the clinical severity; hence the common lay description of "walking pneumonia" is often applied to this infection. The chest radiograph usually reveals bronchopneumonia with patchy infiltrates.[61,62] The complete blood cell count is usually normal; however, a cold hemagglutinin assay with titers of 1:64 is highly suggestive of infection with *M. pneumoniae*.

Without treatment, the illness resolves in 2 to 4 weeks. Oral erythromycin for 10 to 14 days provides optimal therapy, and the patient usually becomes afebrile within 48 hours. Azithromycin has also shown efficacy and is widely used as a 5-day therapy course.[63]

Chlamydia pneumoniae

Infected respiratory droplets most likely transmit *C. pneumoniae*. Primary infection occurs most often in school-aged children and young adults.[64] Only a small portion of patients infected are clinically symptomatic, yet some patients experience severe illness leading to death. Most infections with *C. pneumoniae* are mild and commonly coincide with other bacterial pathogens. Illness is characterized by pharyngitis, followed several days later with cough. Fever is often present early in the illness but does not persist. Wheezing is often heard on auscultation. In fact, this infection has a strong correlation with recent-onset asthma.[65,66]

Host factors appear to influence the severity of this illness. Immunocompromised patients with the acquired immunodeficiency syndrome, malignancy, primary immune deficits, and sickle cell disease may have severe or frequent infections. *C. pneumoniae* is a common cause of acute chest syndrome in children with sickle cell disease and may also act as a trigger for acute asthma.[67]

C. pneumoniae is difficult to isolate, even in tissue culture, and requires special handling of the culture sample. Because of the long delay in serological diagnosis, empirical antibiotic therapy is commonly employed. Infection with *C. pneumoniae* is treated with tetracycline or erythromycin for 10 to 14 days, although a prolonged course of 21 days is not uncommon.

Ventilator-Associated Pneumonia

A patient who is receiving mechanical ventilatory support is at risk of developing pneumonia. New onset of pulmonary infiltrates can occur, stemming from a multitude of causes including atelectasis, infection, spontaneous or catheter-related pulmonary emboli, or acute lung injury. The pathogenesis appears to involve the microaspiration of oropharyngeal organisms. Clinical and radiographic criteria for diagnosing ventilator-associated pneumonia are unreliable.

The development of ventilator-associated pneumonia (VAP) increases hospitalization stay by 30% but does not change mortality rates. In pediatric patients undergoing mechanical ventilation, polymicrobial aerobic and anaerobic floras are isolated from pulmonary specimens. Predominant aerobic bacteria are *Pseudomonas aeruginosa* and *Klebsiella pneumoniae;* the predominant anaerobic bacteria are *Prevotella, Porphyromonas, Peptostreptococcus, Fusobacterium,* and *Bacteroides fragilis.*[68]

To better establish the diagnosis of VAP, Gram stain of bronchoalveolar lavage fluid is obtained through a fiberoptic bronchoscope. Bronchoalveolar lavage fluid is considered positive for VAP when the following conditions occur:

1. Polymorphonuclear neutrophils are greater than 25 per optic field at a magnification $\times 100$
2. Squamous epithelial cells are less than 1%
3. One or more microorganisms are seen per optic field at a magnification of 1:1000.

Gram stain of bronchoalveolar lavage fluid is 77% sensitive and 87% specific with a positive predictive value of 71% and a negative predictive value of 90%.[69] Although bronchoalveolar lavage samples acquired through bronchoscopy are used to diagnose VAP, quantitative cultures of endotracheal aspirates are easier and less expensive to obtain. Persistence of significant numbers of pathogens in quantitative cultures of endotracheal aspirates occurred in 82% of the samples. This quantitative culture of endotracheal aspirates is reproducible and may be useful in the diagnosis of VAP.[70]

Multiple forms of therapy have been attempted to minimize the risk of developing VAP, including routine hand washing, closed airway suctioning, oral care, and elevating the head of bed. Some studies suggest that the use of heat and moisture exchangers is a cost-effective clinical practice associated with fewer late-onset hospital-acquired VAPs and results in improved resource allocation and utilization.[71] However, other studies conclude their use does not affect the frequency of VAP and could potentially lead to mucus hardening.[72] Decreasing the frequency of ventilator circuit changes from three times per week to once per week had no adverse effect on the overall rate of VAP, thus prompting institutions to change ventilator circuits as needed and convincing the majority of experts that the ventilator has nothing to do with VAP.[73] In fact, some experts are calling for a name change, suggesting that this phenomena be called endotracheal tube–associated pneumonia (EAP) because it appears that the ETT has more to do with VAP than the ventilator. Scheduled changes in antibiotic class for empirical treatment of VAP have been demonstrated to lower the incidence of bacteremia associated with antibiotic-resistant gram-negative bacteria.

TUBERCULOSIS

Incidence and Etiology

Tuberculosis (TB) is the most common infectious cause of death throughout the world. Although the frequency declined in the 1980s and early 1990s, the disease is again increasing in incidence and severity.[74,75] It is a chronic bacterial disease caused by infection with *M. tuberculosis*. This organism is a very hearty and virulent bacterium that resists inactivation by drying, heat, and sunlight. Patients infected with *M. tuberculosis* are usually medically underserved, poverty stricken, or immunocompromised. Most children do not develop clinical disease unless disease resistance declines as a result of malnutrition, fatigue, or chronic illness.[76]

Transmission

Transmission is airborne, occurring through the inhalation of viable respiratory droplets in an enclosed space (e.g., room, hospital). The pathogen is rapidly killed by ultraviolet light in the outside air. The household contact for an infant or child is usually an adult; rarely is there child-to-child transmission. The incubation period lasts from 2 to 10 weeks, at which time a skin test becomes positive, manifesting a delayed-type hypersensitivity (Box 26-2).

Signs and Symptoms

Most infants and children who become infected with *M. tuberculosis* never develop TB and remain asymptomatic. They may continue with few if any clinical symptoms or may manifest nonspecific signs of fever, weight loss, and failure to thrive. Most patients develop cough and wheezing, with crackles and rhonchi heard in some cases. Chest radiography in these individuals reveals focal or diffuse infiltrates. Many cases of pulmonary infection with *M. tuberculosis* are caused by reactivation and are characterized by focal findings on chest radiography in a patient with chronic respiratory and systemic symptoms.

Diagnosis

Diagnosis in the adult is based on identification of stains of gastric or respiratory washings that have bacteria uniquely resistant to acid decoloration ("acid fast"). In children, because of the low number of bacilli, 3 consecutive days of gastric washings may increase the sensitivity of this test. More commonly, the diagnosis of TB is based on a positive skin test (Mantoux skin test) in a patient with an appropriate clinical picture and radiographic findings.[6,76,77] Proper interpretation of these skin tests is critical and is based on the probability of disease using a combination of risk factors, clinical findings, and the size of induration resulting from the skin test (see Box 26-2). Differential diagnosis includes asthma, foreign body aspiration, tumors, sarcoidosis, and all pulmonary pathogens.

Treatment

Treatment of TB in children focuses on early diagnosis, identification of the primary case that spread the disease to the child, and long-term antituberculosis medications. For the patient with active disease, multiple medications are indicated for an extended period. These include isoniazid, rifampin, pyrazinamide, and ethambutol. Corticosteroid therapy can be safely used in conjunction with antituberculosis drug therapy to lower the inflammatory response to the infection, reduce the size of enlarged lymph nodes, and accelerate the resorption of fluid when a large pleural effusion has developed.

CASE STUDY 5

A 13-month-old infant, born premature at 24 weeks of gestation, with resolving BPD is brought to his pediatrician for a 2-day history of decreased appetite, runny nose, and increased cough. It is February. His oxygen saturation, vital signs, and examination are unremarkable and the decision is made to discharge him home with close follow-up. Two days later his oxygen requirement is up to 1 L/min O_2 via nasal cannula (from 0.25 L/min O_2 via nasal cannula), and he exhibits increased respiratory distress. Oxygen saturation is decreased to 80% and he is afebrile. He is admitted to the hospital with decreased oral intake and respiratory distress. A rapid RSV test is positive, and his chest radiograph shows infiltrates in the right middle lobe and the left upper lobe.

What is the likely diagnosis? What therapy would you recommend?

See Evolve Resources for answers.

Box 26-2	Cutoff Size of Induration for Positive Mantoux Tuberculin Skin Test

= 5 MM
- Contacts of infectious cases
- Abnormal chest radiograph
- HIV-infected and other immunosuppressed patients

= 10 MM
- Foreign-born persons from areas of high prevalence
- Low-income populations
- Residents of prisons, nursing homes, institutions
- Intravenous drug users
- Other medical risk factors
- Health care workers
- Locally identified high-risk populations
- Infants

= 15 MM
- No risk factors

HIV, Human immunodeficiency virus.
Modified from Starke JR, Jacobs RF, Jereb J. Resurgence of tuberculosis in children. *J Pediatr* 1992;120:839.

RSV infections demonstrate the difficulty of distinguishing between bacterial and viral pneumonias. In the case of a child with underlying lung disease, such as BPD, this may lead to a more conservative and widespread use of antibiotics. Multiple studies in the recent literature have established the importance of neutrophils in many respiratory diseases, including RSV bronchiolitis,[78,79] and attempted to use bronchoalveolar lavage (BAL) samples and cell count as a clinical marker in conjunction with cultures.[80] They have demonstrated the predominance of neutrophils in viral infections of the airway and other lung diseases.[81,82] More interesting is the observation that neutrophilic inflammation can be correlated to the extent of lung injury.[83] Currently we lack a medical treatment targeting neutrophils in the airway, but the development of such treatments is under way. It remains to be seen how effective they might be in the treatment of RSV, bronchiolitis, and similar pulmonary diseases associated with neutrophilic inflammation and if BAL examination has a future value in the routine testing of pediatric patients with lung diseases.

SICKLE CELL DISEASE

Incidence and Etiology

Sickle cell disease is an autosomal-recessive inherited disorder of the hemoglobin structure and is the most common inherited disease of the African-American population. Defective hemoglobin S converts from a soluble hemoglobin molecule contained in the red cells to a gelatinous state in the presence of low oxygen, low pH, rapid temperature changes, or hypernatremic dehydration. This gelatinous state causes the red cells to "sickle," resulting in a variety of complications, including acute chest syndrome, cardiomegaly and left ventricular failure, splenectomy, and renal disease. Pulmonary complications are the primary cause of illness and death in patients with sickle cell disease.[84,85]

Pathophysiology

A complex interaction between the abnormal cells and vascular endothelium results in a hypercoagulable state. Recent reports indicate that high levels of endothelin-1, an endothelial-derived vasoactive mediator, are present during a vasoactive crisis. An abnormality of the vascular endothelium may contribute to the development of acute chest syndrome. The red blood cells are more rigid, resulting in increased viscosity of blood, which causes plugging of the blood vessels.

The pulmonary effects that occur most often in patients with sickle cell disease include pneumonia, acute chest syndrome, pulmonary vascular injury, pulmonary infarction, and sickle cell chronic lung disease. Bacterial pneumonia is a common cause for hospitalization, and pulmonary vascular injury can cause sudden death if the occlusion is in a large vessel.

Signs and Symptoms

Acute chest syndrome is the leading cause of death in sickle cell disease and presents as pleuritic or chest wall pain and dyspnea. The chest radiograph often reveals pulmonary infiltrates, often located in the lower lobes, as well as atelectasis and pleural effusion. Young children, ages 2 to 4 years old, who present with acute chest syndrome have fever, cough, and a negative physical examination, with little or no pain. Adults are often afebrile, complaining of severe dyspnea, chills, and severe pain along the ribs, sternum, abdomen, and back.[86]

Reports in the 1970s suggested that sickle cell disease was caused by a bacterial infection; however, more recent studies suggest that bacterial infection is found in only 3% to 14% of patients, whereas *Mycoplasma* and/or *Chlamydia* infections are found in approximately 15%. Children younger than 5 years of age tend to have a milder disease course that is usually triggered by infection. Risk of death is four times higher in adults with acute chest syndrome than in children and most likely related to the higher incidence of fat embolism from bone marrow infarction. Aplastic crisis in young children with sickle cell disease is typically associated with acute human parvovirus B19 infection. Infection with this pathogen may also be related to acute chest syndrome.[87]

Pneumonia and pulmonary infarction can occur simultaneously and are sometimes difficult to differentiate. Fever and chills are seen more often with pneumonia, with fever resolving slowly. Acute pulmonary symptoms with tachypnea and pleuritic chest pain are more suggestive of pulmonary infarction. In some cases, pneumonia causes hypoxemia that leads to pulmonary infarction.[88]

Sickle cell chronic lung disease occurs most often during the teenage years and may develop after multiple episodes of acute chest syndrome. Hypoxemia is present as a result of pulmonary fibrosis and a reduction in diffusion and pulmonary perfusion. Parenchymal lung injury and an increase in pulmonary vascular resistance cause progressive dyspnea and cor pulmonale. Diffuse interstitial markings and edema are common findings on the chest radiograph.[85,87,89]

Treatment

Empirical therapy includes antibiotics for gram-positive encapsulated organisms of *Streptococcus*, *Staphylococcus*, and *Salmonella*. Erythromycin is used to provide coverage for the pathogens *M. pneumoniae* and *C. pneumoniae*. Antibiotics are quickly instituted because the infections, especially a pneumococcal pneumonia, can become life threatening.[88]

Adequate hydration is an essential therapeutic modality and is used cautiously to avoid pulmonary edema. Red blood cell transfusions are provided to improve the hemoglobin's ability to transport oxygen and reduce the incidence of acute chest syndrome, myocardial ischemia, and sickle cell chronic lung disease. Aerosolized bronchodilators for bronchiole constriction, incentive spirometry, and adequate pain control can be important adjuvants. Supplemental oxygen is used when indicated, but depending on the case can foster additional sickling. In cases of impending respiratory failure, mechanical ventilation is instituted.[90,91] Successful treatment of acute chest syndrome with venovenous ECMO is reported in patients experiencing life-threatening acute chest syndrome despite maximum conventional ventilation support.[92]

A new experimental approach is to treat acute chest syndrome with inhaled nitric oxide. This idea is based on an abnormality discovered in the nitric oxide metabolism in sickle cell patients. The theory is that the nitiric oxide might prevent the adhesion of sickle erythrocytes to the endothelial. At this time it is under clinical investigation and used only in those settings.

Prevention

Acute Chest Syndrome

The treatment of recurrent acute chest syndrome is aimed at preventing repeated vascular and parenchymal insults, which constitute the greatest risk for the development of sickle cell chronic lung disease. Chronic transfusion programs aim to decrease the sickle cell amount to less than 30%, a level that will prevent recurrence of acute chest syndrome. The risks involved are transfusion-associated infections and iron overload. Hydroxyurea was shown to be clinically effective in reducing acute chest syndrome recurrence and vaso-occlusive crises by 50%, but the long-term effects of this treatment are uncertain and frequent peripheral blood count monitoring is necessary. Antibiotic prophylaxis with penicillin is recommended for patients between 4 months and 3 years of age, as well as routine polyvalent pneumococcal vaccine for children and adults.

RECURRENT ASPIRATION SYNDROME

Etiology

Neurologically impaired patients, those with abnormal anatomy of the gastrointestinal tract or airways, and patients with gastroesophageal reflux are often diagnosed with recurrent aspiration syndrome. The patient aspirates respiratory secretions and/or stomach contents. The low pH of the stomach contents results in a chemical pneumonitis and inflammatory response in the airways. The patients and their families suffer through multiple hospitalizations for pneumonia and airway hyperreactivity. Children who are treated for frequent asthma exacerbations, yet have negative responses to allergens, benefit from evaluation for recurrent aspiration. Infants with gastroesophageal reflux are at particular risk for pneumonia.[93]

Diagnosis

Diagnosis is based on clinical and radiographic findings. Barium swallow may reveal a tracheoesophageal fistula or other malformation that requires surgical intervention. Bronchoscopy with bronchoalveolar lavage can reveal pathogens normally found in the gastrointestinal tract as well as provide visual confirmation of inflamed airways.[94]

Treatment

The cause and severity of the disease determine treatment. Fundoplication, a surgical tightening of the gastroesophageal junction, may alleviate gastroesophageal reflux. Appropriate antibiotic coverage is necessary to control infection. Inhaled corticosteroids are indicated to control and reduce the airway damage that occurs from chronic inflammation. Prevention of recurrent aspiration is paramount to obtaining a long-term, positive outcome. Prognosis in uncontrolled recurrent aspiration syndrome is guarded because of the chronic reinjury of the respiratory parenchyma.[95] Respiratory and cardiac insufficiency may develop over time. Accurate and early diagnosis, prevention, and prophylaxis may reduce the severity of the injury and improve the patient's quality of life.

KEY POINTS

- Establishment of an artificial airway in patients with epiglottitis is the first priority and should be provided in the safest place possible. It is often done in the operating room with surgical assistance on standby.
- Patients with upper airway obstructions tend to have normal lung compliance and function. Improper ventilator management can complicate drastic measures such as intubation or tracheostomy.
- Because crying can cause additional respiratory distress in patients with upper airway disorders, it is imperative that you keep parents involved to reduce stranger anxiety or irritability.
- Most airway disorders and lung diseases can be classified into four pathological categories: obstructive, restrictive, infectious, and vascular. Some patients have a combination of diseases, but understanding the primary culprit can assist with choosing the most appropriate therapy.

ASSESSMENT QUESTIONS

See Evolve Resources for the answers.

1. Where do you find the narrowest portion of the pediatric airway that may compromise endotracheal intubation?
   A. Vocal cords
   B. Oropharynx
   C. Cricoid cartilage
   D. Epiglottis
   E. Trachea
2. What is not a sign of respiratory distress in an infant?
   A. Nasal flaring
   B. Retractions
   C. Irritability
   D. Lethargy
   E. Crying
3. A child presents with high fever; severe sore throat; dysphagia with drooling; cough, progressing rapidly over a few hours to stridor; muffled ("hot potato") voice without hoarseness; air hunger; and cyanosis. Severe intercostal retractions, along with nasal flaring, bradypnea, and dyspnea, are present. The child assumes a characteristic position of sitting upright with the chin thrust forward and the neck hyperextended in a tripod position. Bacterial epiglottitis is suspected. What is the next necessary action?
   A. Visualize the upper airway
   B. Obtain upper airway radiographic imaging
   C. Call supporting services
   D. Lay the child flat and provide flow-by oxygen
   E. Secure an intravenous line for sedation

4. What is the right estimated ETT size for a 6-year-old boy, using a cuffed ETT?
   - **A.** 4
   - **B.** 4.5
   - **C.** 5
   - **D.** 5.5
   - **E.** 6

5. You are in a restaurant and the child at the table next to you starts to cough violently. He is 5 years old and was eating French fries when he suddenly turned red, started to cough, and fell to the floor. His parents are nervously patting his back and try to lift him up from the floor. What intervention needs to be done?
   - **A.** Perform the Heimlich maneuver
   - **B.** Open his airway with the tongue-jaw lift
   - **C.** Finger swipe the oropharynx
   - **D.** Leave the child on the floor and monitor
   - **E.** Push the parents out of the way and perform efficient back blows

6. What is a bronchiectasis?
   - **A.** Irreversible dilation of the bronchial tree
   - **B.** Pus accumulation in the airway
   - **C.** The airway immediately placed before an emphysema
   - **D.** Only found in cystic fibrosis patients
   - **E.** Restrictive lung disease

7. Which infant is especially at risk for severe or life-threatening RSV bronchiolitis infections: an infant with BPD, a premature infant, an infant with congenital cardiac disease, immune-compromised children, or an oncology patient?
   - **A.** Immune-compromised children
   - **B.** Premature infant
   - **C.** Infant with congenital heart disease
   - **D.** Infant with BPD
   - **E.** All of the above

8. What combination of pneumonia to causative pathogen is incorrect?
   - **A.** Viral pneumonia; parainfluenza virus type 3
   - **B.** Bacterial pneumonia; *Escherichia coli*
   - **C.** Atypical pneumonia; *Mycoplasma pneumoniae*
   - **D.** Bacterial pneumonia; *Streptococcus pneumoniae*
   - **E.** Atypical pneumonia; MRSA

9. Which signs suggest acute chest syndrome in a patient with sickle cell disease?
   - **A.** Fever
   - **B.** Rib pain
   - **C.** Pleuritic pain
   - **D.** Tachypnea
   - **E.** All except B

10. The major culprit for ventilator-associated pneumonia (VAP) appears to be what?
    - **A.** Ventilator tubing
    - **B.** Ventilator circuit
    - **C.** Endotracheal tube
    - **D.** Droplet transfection from hospital personnel
    - **E.** Routine antibiotic usage

References

1. Grad R: Acute infections producing upper airway obstruction. In Chernick V, Boat TF, Kendig EL, editors: *Disorders of the respiratory tract in children*, Philadelphia, 1998, WB Saunders, pp 447–461.
2. Frantz TD, Rasgon BM: Acute epiglottitis: changing epidemiologic patterns, *Otolaryngol Head Neck Surg* 109:457, 1993.
3. Breukels MA, et al: Invasive infection with *Haemophilus influenzae* type B in spite of complete vaccination, *Ned Tijdschr Geneeskd* 142:586, 1998.
4. Lacroix J, et al: Group A streptococcal supraglottitis, *J Pediatr* 109:20, 1986.
5. Steele DW, et al: Pulsus paradoxus: an objective measure of severity in croup, *Am J Respir Crit Care Med* 157:331, 1998.
6. Westley CR, Cotton EK, Brooks JG: Nebulized racemic epinephrine by IPPB for the treatment of croup: a double-blind study, *Am J Dis Child* 132:484, 1978.
7. Super DM, et al: A prospective randomized double-blind study to evaluate the effect of dexamethasone in acute laryngotracheitis, *J Pediatr* 115:323, 1989.
8. Kairys SW, Olmstead EM, O'Connor GT: Steroid treatment of laryngotracheitis: a meta-analysis of the evidence from randomized trials, *Pediatrics* 83:683, 1989.
9. Rizos JD, et al: The disposition of children with croup treated with racemic epinephrine and dexamethasone in the emergency department, *J Emerg Med* 16:535, 1998.
10. Khalil SN, et al: Absence or presence of a leak around tracheal tube may not affect postoperative croup in children, *Paediatr Anaesth* 8:393, 1998.
11. Khine HH, et al: Comparison of cuffed and uncuffed endotracheal tubes in young children during general anesthesia, *Anesthesiology* 86:627, 1997.
12. Kelly SM, April MM, Tunkel DE: Obstructing laryngeal granuloma after brief endotracheal intubation in neonates, *Otolaryngol Head Neck Surg* 115:138, 1996.
13. Kenna MA, Bluestone CD: Foreign bodies in the air and food passages, *Pediatr Rev* 10:25, 1988.
14. Johnson NT, Pierson DJ: The spectrum of pulmonary atelectasis: pathophysiology, diagnosis, and therapy, *Respir Care* 31:1107, 1986.
15. Duncan SR, et al: Nasal continuous positive airway pressure in atelectasis, *Chest* 92:621, 1987.
16. Westcott JL: Bronchiectasis, *Radiol Clin North Am* 29:1031, 1991.
17. Ferkol TW, Davis PB: Bronchiectasis and bronchiolitis obliterans. In Taussig LM, Landau LI, editors: *Pediatric respiratory medicine*, St Louis, 1999, Mosby, pp 784–792.
18. Barker AF, Bardana EJ: Bronchiectasis: update of an orphan disease, *Am Rev Respir Dis* 137:969, 1988.
19. Wilson JF, Decker AM: The surgical management of childhood bronchiectasis: a review of 96 consecutive pulmonary resections in children with nontuberculous bronchiectasis, *Ann Surg* 195:354, 1982.
20. Annest LS, Kratz JM, Crawford FA: Current results of treatment of bronchiectasis, *J Thorac Cardiovasc Surg* 83:546, 1982.
21. Balck-Payne C: Bronchiolitis. In Hilman BC, editor: *Pediatric respiratory disease, diagnosis and treatment*, Philadelphia, 1993, WB Saunders, pp 205–217.
22. Wohl MEB: Bronchiolitis. In Chernick V, Boat TF, Kendig EL, editors: *Disorders of the respiratory tract in children*, Philadelphia, 1998, WB Saunders, pp 473–484.
23. Everard ML: Acute bronchiolitis and pneumonia in infancy resulting from the respiratory syncytial virus. In Taussig LM, Landau LI, editors: *Pediatric respiratory medicine*, St Louis, 1999, Mosby, pp 580–595.

24. Sandritter TL, Kraus DM: Respiratory syncytial virus-immunoglobulin intravenous (RSV-IGIV) for respiratory syncytial viral infections, *J Pediatr Health Care* 11:284, 1997.

25. Knapp JF, Hall M, Sharma V: Benchmarks for the emergency department care of children with asthma, bronchiolitis, and croup, *Pediatr Emerg Care* 26(5):364, 2010.

26. Christakis DA, Cowan CA, Garrison MM, Molteni R, Marcuse E, Zerr DM: Variation in inpatient diagnostic testing and management of bronchiolitis, *Pediatrics* 115(4):878, 2005.

27. Levy BT, Graber MA: Respiratory syncytial virus infection in infants and young children, *J Fam Pract* 45:473, 1997.

28. Everard ML, et al: Analysis of cells obtained by bronchial lavage of infants with respiratory syncytial virus infection, *Arch Dis Child* 71:428, 1994.

29. American Academy of Pediatrics Committee on Infectious Disease: Use of ribavirin in the treatment of respiratory syncytial virus infection, *Pediatrics* 92:501, 1993.

30. Hughes JH, Mann DR, Hamparian VV: Detection of respiratory syncytial virus in clinical specimens by viral culture, direct and indirect immunofluorescence and enzyme immunoassay, *J Clin Microbiol* 26:588, 1988.

31. Klassen TP: Recent advances in the treatment of bronchiolitis and laryngitis, *Pediatr Clin North Am* 44:249, 1997.

32. AAP: Subcommittee on Diagnosis and Management of Bronchiolitis, *Pediatrics* 118(4):1774, 2006.

33. Numa AH, Williams GD, Dakin CJ: The effect of nebulized epinephrine on respiratory mechanics and gas exchange in bronchiolitis, *Am J Respir Crit Care Med* 164(1):86, 2001.

34. Wang EEL, et al: Bronchodilators for treatment of mild bronchiolitis: a factorial randomized trial, *Arch Dis Child* 67:289, 1992.

35. Schena JA, Crone RK, Thompson JE: Theophylline therapy in bronchiolitis, *Crit Care Med* 12:225, 1984.

36. Roosevelt G, et al: Dexamethasone in bronchiolitis: a randomised controlled trial, *Lancet* 348:292, 1996.

37. Kuzic et al: Nebulized hypertonic saline in the treatment of bronchiolitis in infants, *J Pediatr* 266-270, 2007.

38. Spurling GKP, Fonseka K, Doust J, Del Mar C: Antibiotics for bronchiolitis in children, *Cochrane Database System Rev* (1), 2009.

39. Vassilev ZP, Chu AF, Ruck B, Adams EH, Marcus SM: Adverse reactions to over-the-counter cough and cold products among children: the cases managed out of hospitals, *J Clin Pharmacy Therapeut* 34(3):313, 2009.

40. Kernan WN, Viscoli CM, Brass LM, et al: Phenylpropanolamine and the risk of hemorrhagic stroke, *N Engl J Med* 343(25):1826, 2000.

41. U.S. Food and Drug Administration: *An important FDA reminder for parents: do not give infants cough and cold products designed for older children.* http://www.fda.gov/Drugs/ResourcesForYou/SpecialFeatures/ucm263948.htm.

42. Fackler JC, et al: Precautions in the use of ribavirin at the Children's Hospital, *N Engl J Med* 322:634, 1990.

43. Moler FW, et al: Effectiveness of ribavirin in otherwise well infants with respiratory syncytial virus-associated respiratory failure, *J Pediatr* 128:422, 1996.

44. De Boeck K, Moens M, Schuddinck L: Early ribavirin treatment did not prevent disease in high-bronchopulmonary dysplasia patients with respiratory syncytial virus infection, *Pediatr Pulmonol* 21:343, 1996.

45. Randolph AG, Wang EE: Ribavirin for respiratory syncytial virus lowers respiratory tract infection, *Arch Pediatr Adolesc Med* 150:942, 1996.

46. Groothuis JR, et al: Early ribavirin treatment of respiratory syncytial viral infection in high-risk children, *J Pediatr* 117:792, 1990.

47. Wandstrat TL: Respiratory syncytial virus immune globulin intravenous, *Ann Pharmacother* 31:83, 1997.

48. Leigh MW: Primary ciliary dyskinesia. In Chernick V, Boat TF, Kendig EL, editors: *Disorders of the respiratory tract in children*, Philadelphia, 1998, WB Saunders, pp 819–826.

49. Pedersen M, Mygind N: Ciliary motility in the "immotile cilia syndrome." *Br J Dis Chest* 74:239, 1980.

50. Boat TF, Carson JL: Ciliary dysmorphology and dysfunction—primary or acquired, *N Engl J Med* 323:1681, 1990.

51. Phillips GE, et al: Airway response of children with primary ciliary dyskinesia to exercise and beta$_2$-agonist challenge, *Eur Respir J* 11:1389, 1998.

52. Denny FW, Clyde WA: Acute lower respiratory tract infections in nonhospitalized children, *J Pediatr* 108:635, 1986.

53. Glezen WP: Viral pneumonia. In Chernick V, Boat TF, Kendig EL, editors: *Disorders of the respiratory tract in children*, Philadelphia, 1998, WB Saunders, pp 518–525.

54. Extracorporeal Life Support Organization (ELSO): *ECMO Registry of the Extracorporeal Life Support Organization (ELSO)*, Ann Arbor, MI, July 1998, ELSO.

55. Correa AG, Starke JR: Bacterial pneumonias. In Chernick V, Boat TF, Kendig EL, editors: *Disorders of the respiratory tract in children*, Philadelphia, 1998, WB Saunders, pp 485–502.

56. Chin TW, Nussbaum E, Marks M: Bacterial pneumonia. In Hilman BC, editor: *Pediatric respiratory disease, diagnosis, and treatment*, Philadelphia, 1993, WB Saunders, pp 271–281.

57. Swischuk LE, Hayden CK Jr: Viral vs. bacterial pulmonary infections in children (is roentgenographic differentiation possible?), *Pediatr Radiol* 16:278, 1986.

58. Overall J: Is it bacterial or viral? Laboratory differentiation, *Pediatr Rev* 14:251, 1993.

59. Miller MA, Ben-Ami T, Daum RS: Bacterial pneumonia in neonates and older children. In Taussig LM, Landau LI, editors: *Pediatric respiratory medicine*, St Louis, 1999, Mosby, pp 595–664.

60. Murphy SM, Florman AL: Lung defenses against infection: a clinical correlation, *Pediatrics* 72:1, 1983.

61. Fernaldl GW: Infections of the respiratory tract due to *Mycoplasma pneumoniae*. In V Chernick, TF Boat, EL Kendig, editors: *Disorders of the respiratory tract in children*, Philadelphia, 1998, WB Saunders, pp 526–531.

62. Hailen M: *Mycoplasma pneumoniae* infections. In Hilman BC, editor: *Pediatric respiratory disease, diagnosis, and treatment*, Philadelphia, 1993, WB Saunders, pp 282–284.

63. Shehab Z: Mycoplasma infections. In Taussig LM, Landau LI, editors: *Pediatric respiratory medicine*, St Louis, 1999, Mosby, pp 737–742.

64. Thom DH, et al: *Chlamydia pneumoniae* strain TWAR. *Mycoplasma pneumoniae* and viral infections in acute respiratory disease in a university student health clinic population, *Am J Epidemiol* 132:248, 1990.

65. Atmar RL, Greenberg SB: Pneumonia caused by *Mycoplasma pneumoniae* and the TWAR agent, *Semin Respir Infect* 4:19, 1989.

66. Hahn DL, Dodge RW, Golubjatnikov R: Association of *Chlamydia pneumoniae* (strain TWAR) infection with wheezing, asthmatic bronchitis, and adult-onset asthma, *JAMA* 266:225, 1991.

67. Hammerschlag MR: *Chlamydia trachomatis* and *Chlamydia pneumoniae* infections. In Chernick V, Boat TF, Kendig EL, editors: *Disorders of the respiratory tract in children*, Philadelphia, 1998, WB Saunders, pp 978–987.

68. Brook I: Pneumonia in mechanically ventilated children, *Scand J Infect Dis* 27:619, 1995.

69. Prekates A, et al: The diagnostic value of Gram stain of bronchoalveolar lavage samples in patients with suspected ventilator-associated pneumonia, *Scand J Infect Dis* 30:43, 1998.

70. Bergmans DC, et al: Reproducibility of quantitative cultures of endotracheal aspirates from mechanically ventilated patients, *J Clin Microbiol* 35:796, 1997.

71. Kirton OC, et al: A prospective, randomized comparison of an in-line heat moisture exchange filter and heated wire humidifiers: rates of ventilator-associated early-onset (community-acquired) or late-onset (hospital-acquired) pneumonia and incidence of endotracheal tube occlusion, *Chest* 112;1055, 1997.

72. Boots RJ, et al: Clinical utility of hygroscopic heat and moisture exchangers in intensive care patients, *Crit Care Med* 25:1707, 1997.

73. Long MN, et al: Prospective, randomized study of ventilator-associated pneumonia in patients with one versus three ventilator circuit changes per week, *Infect Control Hosp Epidemiol* 17:14, 1996.

74. Centers for Disease Control and Prevention: Tuberculosis morbidity—United States, 1997, *Morb Mortal Wkly Rep* 47:253, 1998.

75. Nahmias AJ, et al: Older and newer challenges of tuberculosis in children, *Pediatr Pulmonol Suppl* 11:28, 1995.

76. Inselman LS, Kendig EL: Tuberculosis. In Chernick V, Boat TF, Kendig EL, editors: *Disorders of the respiratory tract in children*, Philadelphia, 1998, WB Saunders, pp 883–919.

77. American Academy of Pediatrics Committee on Infectious Diseases: Update on tuberculosis skin testing of children, *Pediatrics* 97:282, 1996.

78. Emboriadou M, et al: Human neutrophil elastase in RSV bronchiolitis, *Ann Clin Lab Sci* 37:79, 2007.

79. McNamara PS, et al: Bronchoalveolar lavage cellularity in infants with severe respiratory syncytial virus bronchiolitis, *Arch Dis Child* 88:922, 2003.

80. Chang AB, et al: A bronchoscopic scoring system for airway secretions—airway cellularity and microbiological validation, *Pediatr Pulmonol* 41:887, 2006.

81. Simpson JL, et al: Innate immune activation in neutrophilic asthma and bronchiectasis, *Thorax* 62:211, 2007.

82. Sarafidis K, et al: Evidence of early systemic activation and transendothelial migration of neutrophils in neonates with severe respiratory distress syndrome, *Pediatr Pulmonol* 31:214, 2001.

83. Hussain N, et al: Neutrophil apoptosis during the development and resolution of oleic acid-induced acute lung injury in the rat, *Am J Respir Cell Mol Biol* 19:867, 1998.

84. Nickerson BG. The lung in sickle cell disease. In: Chernick V, Boat TF, Kendig EL, editors: *Disorders of the respiratory tract in children*, Philadelphia, 1998, WB Saunders, pp 1117–1122.

85. Smith JA: Cardiopulmonary manifestations of sickle cell disease in childhood, *Semin Roentgenol* 22:160, 1987.

86. Sprinkle RH, et al: Acute chest syndrome in children with sickle cell disease: a retrospective analysis of 100 hospitalized cases, *Am J Pediatr Hematol Oncol* 812:105, 1986.

87. Weil JV, et al: Pathogenesis of lung disease in sickle hemoglobinopathies, *Am Rev Respir Dis* 148:249, 1993.

88. Barrett-Connor E: Pneumonia and pulmonary infarction in sickle cell anemia, *JAMA* 224:997, 1973.

89. Powars D, et al: Sickle cell chronic lung disease: prior morbidity and the risk of pulmonary failure, *Medicine* 67:66, 1988.

90. Bunn HF: Pathogenesis and treatment of sickle cell disease, *N Engl J Med* 337:762, 1997.

91. Collins FS, Orringer EP: Pulmonary hypertension and cor pulmonale in the sickle hemoglobinopathies, *Am J Med* 73:814, 1982.

92. Pelidis MA, et al: Successful treatment of life-threatening acute chest syndrome of sickle cell disease with veno-venous extracorporeal membrane oxygenation, *J Pediatr Hematol Oncol* 19:459, 1997.

93. Orenstein SR, Orenstein DM: Gastroesophageal reflux and respiratory disease in children, *J Pediatr* 112:847, 1988.

94. Meyers WF, et al: Value of tests for evaluation of gastroesophageal reflux in children, *J Pediatr Surg* 20:515, 1985.

95. Blister A, Krespi YP, Oppenheimer RW: Surgical management of aspiration, *Otolaryngol Clin North Am* 2:743, 1988.

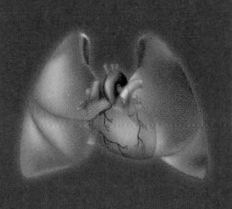

Chapter 27

Asthma

BRIAN K. WALSH

LEARNING OBJECTIVES

After reading this chapter the reader will be able to:

1. Explain the pathophysiology of asthma
2. Treat asthma from an evidence-based approach
3. Identify the five components of asthma
4. Explain how to improve the efficacy of the medications we use to treat asthma

KEY TERMS

Asthma
Asthma action plan
Asthma education

Asthma triggers
β_2 agonist

Corticosteroids
Reactive airway disease

Asthma is the most common chronic childhood disease, affecting more than 20.5 million persons, 6.5 million of whom are children. Approximately 7.7% of children in the United States have asthma. It is the most common reason for pediatric hospitalizations and the most common cause of absence from school. Hospitalization rates have remained stable over the past 10 years, but this has not been consistent through all childhood age groups. The highest incidence of asthma occurs in children 4 years of age or younger.[1] Although the number of asthma patients has climbed, the death rate is decreasing. Improvements in the science behind asthma care have led to increased awareness among patients and physicians about the disease's underlying causes, but widespread misunderstanding still exists. A survey called "Children and Asthma in America" found that most respondents incorrectly believed that only the symptoms of the disease should be treated as opposed to the underlying cause of the disease. Ninety-three percent of the respondents could not correctly identify inflammation as an underlying cause of asthma attacks, and 90% of the respondents were unable to identify airway constriction as the other main cause (visit http://www.asthmainamerica.com/widespread.html for more information).

To improve awareness of the causes and treatments of asthma in America, the National Heart, Lung, and Blood Institute's (NHLBI's) National Asthma Education and Prevention Program (NAEPP) in 1991 released its first set of asthma management guidelines, referred to as the Expert Panel Report.[2] This was followed by Expert Panel Report 2 in 1997[3] and an update of the report on selected items in 2002.[4] In 2007 they released the Expert Panel Report 3, which is available to caregivers and patients. The report provides guidelines for management of asthma based on the expert panel review with an emphasis on evidence-based practice of medicine.[5] There is a wealth of information on the NHLBI as well as the Centers for Disease Control and Prevention,[6] including two videos that demonstrate how to control and prevent asthma exacerbations within a clinic visit[7] and how to control your asthma while you travel.[8] We anticipate new or updated guidelines within the next year or two, so please reference the latest guidelines. Until then, this chapter will reference the 2007 Expert Panel Report 3 as the foundation of this chapter.

PATHOGENESIS OF ASTHMA

Definition

Asthma is a reversible obstructive lung disease created by chronic inflammation of the airways. These inflamed airways often hyperreact (bronchospasm) to various **triggers.** If not properly treated and controlled, asthma can be life threatening. Many cells and cellular elements play a role in the disease—in particular, mast cells, eosinophils, T lymphocytes, immunoglobulin E (IgE), macrophages, neutrophils, and epithelial cells. In susceptible individuals, this inflammation causes recurrent episodes of wheezing, chest tightness, breathlessness, and coughing, especially at night or in the early morning. These episodes are usually associated with widespread but variable airflow obstruction that is often reversible either spontaneously or with treatment. The inflammation also causes an associated increase in the existing bronchial hyperresponsiveness to a variety of stimuli. A number of factors can play a role in the development of inflammation, including exposure to viruses, allergens, and other occupational irritants. The growing awareness that asthma is not a homogeneous disorder has important implications for how asthma will be diagnosed and managed in the future.

Pathophysiology

Asthma is characterized by chronic airway inflammation, bronchial hyperresponsiveness, and hypersecretion of mucus. Airway obstruction is the consequence of these pathological mechanisms. There are six significant components to airway obstruction:

1. Inflammation
2. Acute bronchoconstriction
3. Airway edema
4. Mucous plugging
5. Airway hyperresponsiveness
6. Airway remodeling

The obstruction can result in increasingly difficult air entry, air trapping, atelectasis, ventilation-perfusion abnormalities, hypoxia, and hypercarbia. Approaches to therapy are directed toward blocking the inflammation as well as preventing and relieving airway hyperresponsiveness and remodeling.

Airway Inflammation

Our understanding of the pathogenesis of airway inflammation in asthma continues to grow as the function and interaction of inflammatory mediators are revealed. Inflammation results from the introduction or activation of specific mediators in the airway. In adult asthma there is evidence that inflammatory findings (e.g., eosinophilic airway inflammation, hypergranulation of mast cells, increased IgE levels, and increased allergic response) are due in part to an inappropriate activation of the CD4+ T cells that results in release of inflammatory cytokines.

In some individuals, primarily adults with asthma, neutrophils appear to be the primary mediator of cytokine release and inflammation. These individuals appear to be less responsive to steroids and bronchodilators and are more likely to experience remodeling of their airways. No matter what the underlying pathology is, inflammation and the resulting swelling of airway mucosa can affect the airway caliber and decrease airflow. We now know that airway inflammation is persistent and that early intervention with anti-inflammatory medications may help to slow the course of the disease, but any successful response usually requires weeks to achieve and in some instances may be incomplete.[9]

Following Dr. Hunt and colleagues' discovery in 2000 that exhaled breath condensate (a noninvasive marker of airway lining pH) is acidic during acute exacerbations of asthma,[10] there is an evolving concept that this acidity appears to go hand in hand with inflammatory lung disease such as asthma. Acidification of the airway lining fluid is known to cause important respiratory symptoms. Likewise, bronchoconstriction occurs when the airway lining fluid is acidified.[11] Furthermore, acidification inhibits ciliary motility, increases mucous viscosity, alters nitrogen oxide reactivities and oxidative processes, and enhances eosinophilic and neutrophilic inflammation.[11] These consequences of airway acidification reflect precisely the pathophysiology of acute asthma.[11] A recent publication asserts that nebulized β agonists (discussed later in this chapter) such as albuterol are poorly transported across the alveolar epithelium when the airway lining fluid is acidic,[12] providing one potential explanation for the clinical failure of β agonists in management of chronic bronchitis as well as in many acutely ill asthma patients.

The Path of Inflammation in Allergic Asthma

Asthma has been shown to be predominately allergic in nature, with 80% of children and more than 50% of adults with asthma.[13] IgE has been identified as a key molecule in mediating allergic asthma. Total serum IgE levels have been shown to have a close association with self-reported asthma.[13]

Allergic disease starts with a sensitization phase in which an allergen on the airway mucosa is processed by an antigen-presenting cell (APC), such as a dendritic cell. The dendritic cell travels to regional lymph nodes and acts as a key antigen-presenting cell, causing the release of interleukins that cause the naïve T cell to differentiate into a Th2 cell. The Th2 cell then releases interleukin 4 (IL-4), which enhances the production of IgE by stimulating B cells to differentiate into IgE. IL-4 also stimulates the differentiation of more naïve T cells to Th2 to further this process. IgE binds to high- and low-affinity receptors on mast cells, basophils, and eosinophils. These cells contain inflammatory mediators. The IgE produced is specifically sensitive to the allergen (antigen) that started the process. When the allergen is reintroduced into the system (on mucosa or in the bloodstream), it will bind to the IgE attached to mast cells, eosinophils, and basophils. This will result in cross-linking that causes a calcium influx and resulting degranulation that releases the inflammatory mediators within the cells that cause allergy and asthma symptoms.[14]

There are three phases of inflammation. The first phase involves the preformed mediators that are released with degranulation: histamine, heparin, and tryptase. These mediators result in airway smooth muscle contraction, vasodilation, increased vascular permeability, and mucous secretion. The resulting injury to airway cells attracts other mediators such as cytokines (leukotrienes, IL-4, IL-5, IL-13, tumor necrosis factor (TNF) α, and eosinophils, to name a few), resulting in a late phase that occurs 4 to 8 hours after the immediate response. Persistent inflammation can lead to a remodeling phase that results in airway smooth muscle hypertrophy, hyperplasia, increased angiogenesis, and collagen deposition.[15] This last phase will result in a decline in lung function and irreversible obstructive lung disease.

The Definition and Role of T Cells: The Th1/Th2 Paradigm

T helper cells, Th1 and Th2, cross-regulate each other and regulate immune responses. There continues to be considerable interest in the role of immune responses in airway inflammation. It has become clear that a bias toward the production of Th2 cells results in increased atopy and asthma. Th2 cells produce IL-4, which enhances IgE synthesis; IL-5, which stimulates eosinophil production; IL-9, which increases mast cell production; and IL-13, which increases mucus production and airway hyperresponsiveness. Th1 cells produce interferon-γ and IL-2, which aid in defense of infection. It is believed that a newborn is skewed toward a Th2 response through exposure to infections and other environmental stimuli. When the Th2 response triggers, the Th1 response is activated and a balance between the Th1 and Th2 responses occurs.[16] The "hygiene hypothesis" suggests that because of immunizations and increased use of antibiotics, children are not exposed to the stimuli to drive the Th1 response, and the cytokine pattern then favors the Th2 response in susceptible individuals, which will cause the production of more IgE and thus increase atopy and risk for asthma.

Airway Hyperresponsiveness

Hyperresponsiveness is an exaggerated bronchoconstricting response to stimuli. The level of hyperresponsiveness is often correlated with the severity of constriction created by a bronchoprovocation test (such as a methacholine challenge). Exposure to certain allergens causes an IgE-dependent release of mediators from the mast cell. These mediators include histamine, tryptase, leukotrienes, and prostaglandins. They directly contract airway smooth muscle, giving rise to acute bronchoconstriction or airway hyperresponsiveness. Other "triggers" of airflow obstruction include aspirin and nonsteroidal anti-inflammatory drugs, exercise, cold air, irritants, gastroesophageal reflux, respiratory infections, and psychological stress. When reduction of airway inflammation is achieved, better control of asthma should be expected.

Airway remodeling is the permanent structural change that occurs in the airway. It is associated with progressive loss of lung function and may not be prevented or be fully reversible by current therapeutic interventions.[17] The process of repair and remodeling in the airway are not well understood, but it is certain that these processes are key to explaining why asthma remains persistent and in some cases resistant to therapy. Features of airway remodeling include inflammation, mucous hypersecretion, subepithelial fibrosis, airway smooth muscle hypertrophy, and angiogenesis.[5] Inflammatory mediators stimulate hyperplasia of mucous glands, resulting in more and chronic mucus production. The excessive mucus secretion and plugging of the airway may act to reduce the diameter of the airway and further limit airflow. Activation of inflammatory mediators also results in increased vascular permeability and leakage with activation of structural cells such as epithelial tissue, mucous glands, and blood vessels. Repeated inflammatory episodes result in airway mucosa thickening and eventual fibrosis.

RISK FACTORS FOR DEVELOPMENT OF ASTHMA IN CHILDREN

Asthma is a dynamic disease. Its progression will vary over time regardless of the age of the patient. Although the etiology of asthma is not well defined, there appear to be risk factors associated with its onset and persistence. Asthma is more prevalent in prepubescent boys but more common in girls after puberty. It is more common among inner city and African-American and Hispanic children in the United States; however, there is disagreement as to whether racial and ethnic background is a risk factor or if poverty has the greater impact. Currently available data from genetic studies of asthma suggest a strong genetic component. However, the exact mode of inheritance is unknown. Low-birth-weight infants as well as children born to young mothers or mothers who smoke during pregnancy tend to have an increased incidence of asthma. Other theories have emerged to suggest that asthma develops in children when there is a predominant T2 cell response (as opposed to a predominant T1 cell response) when exposed to various triggers. It has been proposed that this shift results from early exposure to certain viruses or the lack of exposure to early childhood diseases, as well as from the overuse of antibiotics.

Allergic Response—Atopy

Atopy seems to be the strongest identifiable predisposing factor for developing asthma, with atopic dermatitis often preceding its onset. Infants who become sensitized to food allergens early in life have an increased risk for developing asthma. The majority of children with asthma are atopic, but not all atopic children develop asthma. Inhaled allergens are thought to be the most important factor in the onset of asthma in the child predisposed to atopy.

Environmental Triggers

There are several significant indoor environmental triggers. Once an aggravating agent is identified, it is essential that that the household undergo intervention that could remediate or eliminate it. If the child is sensitive to warm-blooded animals, the suggested interventions include the removal of the pet from the home or, if this is not possible, to keep the bedroom door closed so that the animal does not have access to the child's room.

Tobacco smoke is closely linked with increased asthma prevalence and morbidity and therefore it is important that the patient and others who live in the household refrain from smoking. Smoking cessation measures are suggested. If there are smokers in the home, it is important that all smoking take place outside the home.

Cockroach exposure is another concern that impacts patients who live in the inner city.[18] Cockroach antigens are commonly found in the bedrooms of children who are sensitized. It is important that the family practice a routine that includes not leaving food exposed or the garage opened. Poison baits, boric acid, and traps are also important tools that can reduce or eliminate the cockroach problem. Of course in using these interventions it is important to make sure that the child not be able to access baits or poisons.

Molds are another common trigger in the home. Once identified it is essential the mold be cleaned out and the area dried. This can be a particular problem in humid environments or where there are plumbing leaks that are left unattended.

House-dust mites are another trigger. To manage this problem it is recommended that the mattresses and pillow be encased with an allergen-impermeable cover. It also is advisable that the bedding be washed in water that is warmer than 130° F. Other suggested steps would be to reduce humidity in the home to less than 40%, remove carpeting from the bedroom, avoid lying on upholstered furniture, and not carpet over concrete flooring. It is important to not expose stuffed toys to dust but rather keep them covered and consider frequent washing as well. It appears that exposure to any environmental allergen, if it is intense and persistent, may lead to sensitization in atopic children and then be associated with chronic asthma.

Much research has been devoted to the relationship between wheezing illnesses in infants and the development of asthma. Respiratory syncytial virus is the most common viral respiratory tract pathogen isolated from infants who wheeze. Many of these infants with severe infection with respiratory syncytial virus develop recurrent wheezing and asthma later in life.

NATIONAL ASTHMA EDUCATION AND PREVENTION PROGRAM GUIDELINES (REPORT 3)

Purpose

The National Asthma Education and Prevention Program (NAEPP) was formed by the National Institutes of Health in the late 1980s to assist in the promotion of **asthma education** to the public, the health care professional, and the patient. The most significant undertaking of this organization has been the development and dissemination of the *Expert Panel Report 3: Guidelines for the Diagnosis and Management of Asthma,* published in 2007 and also known as "the Asthma Guidelines." Because of ongoing changes in the diagnosis and treatment of asthma, particularly in the pharmacological care, an updated set of guidelines has been published every 5 years. The recommendations in the latest version are also evidence based, which allows for a document that has been under the scrutiny of the Expert Panel. All sets of guidelines have been written by a science-based committee of experts from all medical disciplines, all based in the United States.

The stated purpose of the guidelines is to serve as a comprehensive tool in the diagnosis and management of asthma. The NAEPP states that the report, which is not an official regulatory document, should serve as a guide, and that a patient's specific history must be considered when implementing its guidelines. In spite of massive public promotion directed to the medical community, the response to the report has been mixed. Disagreement by primary care physicians with components of the guidelines has often led to poor compliance, whereas still other physicians remain unfamiliar with the guidelines. Asthma specialists tend to be more familiar with the guidelines and receptive to their use. Getting the guidelines into the hands of all providers who interact with asthma patients and influencing them to use the guidelines to guide therapy remains the goal of the NAEPP. It is also essential that the clinician, patient, and family members understand and abide by the goals of optimal management (Box 27-1).

Box 27-1	**Goals of Asthma Management**

1. Prevent chronic asthma symptoms and minimize asthma exacerbations, using the least aggressive therapy that is sufficient.
2. Maintain normal activity levels including exercise and other physical activities; avoid missing school activities.
3. Maintain normal or near-normal pulmonary function.
4. Prevent recurrent asthma exacerbations and minimize the need for emergency department visits or hospitalizations.
5. Provide optimal pharmacotherapy with minimal or no adverse effects.
6. Meet patient's and family's expectations of and satisfaction with asthma care received.

DIAGNOSIS

Children who present with chronic or episodic cough, wheezing, difficulty breathing, or chest tightness may have asthma. The diagnosis of asthma cannot be established until alternative diagnoses are excluded. There should be evidence of airflow obstruction that is at least partially reversible and episodic symptoms of airflow limitation or airway hyperresponsiveness. The NAEPP guidelines recommend a detailed medical history, physical examination, and spirometry to determine reversible disease. It is also important to determine the severity, control, and responsiveness to therapy to determine the patient's current asthma status. Once a diagnosis has been made, it is important that the clinician use methods (e.g., testing for allergies and determining IgE levels) to identify precipitating factors.

Medical History

A detailed medical history is essential in identifying the symptoms, triggers, and severity of asthma. A diagnostic history includes recurrent wheezing, chest tightness, shortness of breath, and cough, with nocturnal symptoms being common. Symptoms that occur or worsen with various stimuli (e.g., allergens, respiratory infections, emotional expressions, menses, viral infection, exercise, weather changes) or follow a seasonal pattern are highly suggestive of asthma.

A thorough history includes descriptions and frequency of previous exacerbations, hospitalizations, number of emergency department visits or unscheduled office visits, amount of school missed because of symptoms, and response to previous therapy. It is also important to determine if symptoms are episodic or persistent. A history of allergic disorders (including family history), premature birth, and sinus and respiratory infections is often linked to asthma.

Physical Examination

A physical examination of the upper respiratory tract, chest, and skin is essential for the diagnosis of asthma, as well as to rule out another disorder. However, examinations may be completely normal between acute exacerbations, and the medical history is a stronger factor in supporting a diagnosis of asthma. Symptomatic children may present with audible wheezing and prolonged expiration, cough, increased nasal secretions, hyperexpansion of the thorax, retractions, use of accessory muscles, and tachypnea. Examination of the upper airways may show evidence of allergic disease (e.g., allergic shiners, edematous nasal mucosa, postnasal drip). Atopic dermatitis is typical in the presentation of asthma; however, digital clubbing is rarely found in asthma and raises the suspicion of cystic fibrosis. Many physical examination findings lead to consideration of a diagnosis other than asthma.

Pulmonary Function Testing

Pulmonary function testing is used to help confirm the diagnosis of asthma, estimate the severity of airway inflammation, and follow the response to changes in therapy.[19] Because all pulmonary function tests are essentially effort dependent, children must be old enough to correctly perform the test and provide maximum effort. Some children can perform an acceptable expiratory maneuver at 4 years of age, whereas others are unable to accomplish this until they are 7 or 8 years of age. If effort or technique is poor, results are not helpful in diagnosis or treatment of asthma and should not be used.

Typical spirometry measurements in the diagnosis of asthma include the total volume of air exhaled forcefully from a maximal inhalation (forced vital capacity, FVC), the volume of air exhaled during the first second of the FVC (forced expiratory volume in 1 second, FEV_1), and the FEV_1/FVC ratio. Other measurements, including the flow in the middle portion of the FVC (FEF_{25-75}), are often reported. The FEF_{25-75} is also known as the maximum midexpiratory flow. It is sensitive to small changes in airway caliber and also decreases with increasing obstructive disease; however, it is highly variable. Airway obstruction is indicated when the FEV_1 is less than 80% of the predicted value and FEV_1/FVC values are less than 65% (or below the lower limit of normal).

The diagnosis of asthma requires that the airway obstruction be reversible. Spirometry measurements are performed before and after inhalation of a short-acting bronchodilator (e.g., albuterol). Significant reversibility is established when there is a greater than 12% increase in the postbronchodilator FEV_1 measurement.[20]

Pulmonary function tests are performed at the time of initial diagnosis and after treatment has been initiated or changed. It is also performed periodically to document optimal pulmonary function values. If the patient demonstrates deterioration in pulmonary status, additional testing is warranted. It is recommended that children who require long-term control medication for asthma and are capable of performing the tests have pulmonary function tests performed at least annually.

Exhaled Nitric Oxide

Nitric oxide (NO) is known as a biological mediator in humans and is produced by the lungs and presented in exhaled breath. Fraction of exhaled nitric oxide (F_{ENO}) is a quantitative, noninvasive, simple and safe method of measuring airway inflammation in patients with asthma. It is specifically used in the diagnosis and treatment of eosinophilic airway inflammation. Many clinicians today use FENO to determine the eosinophilic response to corticosteroids, unmasking of otherwise unsuspected nonadherence to therapy, and routine monitoring. According to the ATS Clinical Practice Guidelines, a patient with a low FENO level of less than 25 parts per billion (ppb) is considered less likely to respond to corticosteroids than a person with a high FENO level of more than 50 ppb who is symptomatic. Intermediate is considered between 25 and 50 ppb.[21]

Bronchoprovocational Challenges

Airway responsiveness can be assessed using pharmacological (e.g., histamine, methacholine) and nonpharmacological (e.g., exercise, cold air hyperventilation) challenges. Methacholine and histamine are the most common pharmacological agents used for bronchoprovocational challenge. The challenge is performed in a medical facility with a physician and resuscitative equipment present.

Methacholine Challenge

During a methacholine challenge, carefully increased doses of methacholine are nebulized and delivered directly to the patient through a face mask or mouthpiece. The patient's FEV_1 is measured after inhalation of each concentration until there is a 20% decrease in the FEV_1 or until all nine concentrations have been delivered. A 20% decrease in the FEV_1 is considered a positive challenge. This demonstrates the presence of bronchial hyperresponsiveness and is highly associated with asthma. When the test is completed, the bronchoconstriction may be relieved with inhalation of a quick-relief bronchodilator.

Methacholine challenge is safe and reproducible in children. However, it is recommended that the patient's FEV_1 be greater than 70% of predicted before performing the challenge.[22] Patients with well-documented asthma should not be challenged. A negative bronchoprovocational challenge may be useful in ruling out asthma.

Exercise Challenge

Exercise tolerance tests are performed using a variety of forms of exercise, including treadmill running, free running, and bicycle ergometry. Most children are exercised until their heart rate reaches at least 170 beats per minute or more than 85% of the predicted maximum heart rate for their sex and age for 5 to 8 minutes. The FEV_1 is measured immediately after and at 5-minute intervals for 20 to 30 minutes after exercise has stopped. A decrease in the FEV_1 of 15% or more from the pretest baseline indicates a positive response and exercise-induced bronchospasm (EIB).[23] When comparing the results of exercise challenges with the pharmacological challenges, exercise testing has been observed to be less sensitive and a poorer screening test for bronchial hyperresponsiveness.[24]

Differential Diagnosis

Asthma is the most common cause of recurrent or persistent wheezing, cough, and dyspnea in children. However, several diseases and conditions produce similar signs and symptoms and may simulate an asthma exacerbation. Whether it is the first exacerbation for the child or further assessment of the patient with "difficult-to-manage" asthma, other causes of wheezing and airway obstruction must be considered. This is of particular importance in the infant and young child whose small airways are more easily obstructed.[25] The differential diagnosis of conditions that cause wheezing and airway obstruction varies with the age of the child. A thorough history, including response to prior treatment, physical examination, and data from additional tests, can help differentiate other disorders. Box 27-2 lists

---

Box 27-2	**Respiratory Conditions That Mimic Asthma**

- Upper airway disorders
- Allergic rhinitis and sinusitis
- Vocal cord dysfunction
- Tonsillar/adenoid hypertrophy
- Laryngeal web
- Laryngeal papillomatosis
- Laryngotracheomalacia
- Tracheobronchomalacia
- Tracheoesophageal fistula
- Subglottic stenosis
- Tracheal stenosis
- Bronchial stenosis
- Vascular ring
- Enlarged lymph nodes or tumor
- Foreign body aspiration
- Lower airway disorders
- Acute viral bronchiolitis
- Bronchiolitis obliterans
- Bronchopulmonary dysplasia

- Cystic fibrosis
- Primary ciliary dyskinesia
- Mediastinal cysts or tumors
- Pulmonary embolism
- Aspiration syndromes
- Aspiration bronchitis
- Aspiration pneumonia
- Gastroesophageal reflux
- Hypersensitivity pneumonitis
- Allergic bronchopulmonary aspergillosis
- Cardiac disease
- Large left-to-right shunts
- Congestive heart failure
- Cardiomyopathy
- Myocarditis
- Hysterical symptoms
- Psychogenic cough
- Hyperventilation syndrome

respiratory conditions that can produce asthmalike symptoms.

MANAGEMENT OF ASTHMA

After the diagnosis of asthma has been made, the NAEPP guidelines suggest a stepwise approach to classifying the severity of asthma and initiating treatment. For classifications beyond mild asthma, daily control medication is recommended and the amount of medication is increased, described as a "step up," as the need for treatment increases. When the asthma is under control, the amount of medication is decreased and described as a "step down." The treatment prescribed is determined by classification of disease severity. Although asthma morbidity and mortality has increased in the United States, for most children with asthma proper disease management helps to provide a normal lifestyle.

The pharmacological management of asthma requires the use of long-term control and short-term relief medications. Identification, avoidance, and control of factors that worsen asthma symptoms are as essential to asthma management as the use of medication. The regular monitoring and assessment of asthma severity have been proven to aid in control of the disease. Finally, management of a chronic illness such as asthma requires patient and family involvement in developing a treatment plan and in understanding the illness.

Pharmacological Therapy
Long-Term Control Medications

Pharmacological management involves using medications to control and relieve symptoms. Any medication that is taken to provide ongoing control of asthma is classified as a long-term control medication. Long-term control medications are taken daily to achieve and maintain control of persistent asthma.

Anti-inflammatory Agents. Anti-inflammatory agents are still considered the most effective long-term treatment for chronic inflammation in asthma. They block late-phase reaction to allergens, reduce airway hyperresponsiveness, and inhibit anti-inflammatory cell migration and activation.[5] They are considered first-line anti-inflammatory agents for children with mild to moderate asthma. Although the potency of their anti-inflammatory activity is less documented than that of inhaled corticosteroids, they have few adverse effects.[26]

Inhaled **corticosteroids** are the most consistently effective controller medication for asthma and are considered first-line therapy for its treatment. Their advantage over oral corticosteroids is that they are clinically effective without having significant side effects. Oral corticosteroid-dependent patients have been able to decrease or discontinue their use of oral corticosteroids when appropriate inhaled corticosteroid therapy is initiated.

Although there is much less risk of developing adverse events with inhaled compared with systemic corticosteroids, the potential for side effects remains. Dysphonia, voice change, reflex cough, and oral candidiasis occur most often with higher doses, although these manifestations can occur at any dose. Use of spacers or holding chambers along with rinsing after inhalation may reduce these effects. Questions remain about the clinical significance of all side effects, particularly concern regarding growth suppression in children. Until more data are obtained, the NAEPP guidelines recommend that children be maintained on the lowest dose of inhaled corticosteroid tolerated with close monitoring of linear growth and development.

Systemic or oral corticosteroids are often required during an asthma exacerbation. However, daily or every-other-day use, along with high doses of an inhaled corticosteroid, is necessary in some patients with very severe disease. The side effects of long-term, regular use of systemic corticosteroids are significant and are listed in Box 27-3. Once asthma control is achieved, efforts are made to wean the patient from oral corticosteroids.

Long-Acting β_2 Agonists. Salmeterol and formoterol are long-acting inhaled β_2 **agonists** (LABAs) available in the United States. Salmeterol is available alone as a dry-powder discus. It is also available in a dry-powder discus in combination with the corticosteroid fluticasone. Formoterol is available in a dry-powder inhaler device alone and as combination therapy and most recently in a liquid form for nebulization. The biggest difference between the two long-acting bronchodilators is their onset of action. Salmeterol can take from 30 minutes to 90 minutes to have peak effect, whereas formoterol begins to work in 3 to 5 minutes. Evidence on the use of LABAs in asthma has demonstrated that the addition of LABAs to treatment of asthma not well controlled on low- or medium-dose inhaled corticosteroids improves lung function and decreases symptoms more effectively than the use of inhaled corticosteroid (ICS) therapy alone.[5] Concerns were raised regarding the use of these medications when a large clinical trial comparing daily salmeterol with placebo added to

Box 27-3	Side Effects of Long-Term Use of Systemic Corticosteroids

- Adrenal suppression
- Growth suppression
- Muscle myopathy
- Aseptic hip necrosis
- Hyperglycemia
- Increased risk of infection
- Skin atrophy and striae
- Psychological disturbances
- Easy bruising
- Fluid retention
- Hypertension
- Osteoporosis
- Peptic ulcer
- Cataracts
- Acne
- Weight gain
- Obesity
- Hirsutism
- Glaucoma
- "Moon" facies
- "Buffalo hump"

usual asthma therapy demonstrated an increased risk of asthma-related deaths in those on salmeterol.[27] This resulted in the Food and Drug Administration (FDA) placing a black box warning on all asthma medications containing an LABA. These studies resulted in the Expert Panel 3 recommending that the option of increasing the ICS dose be given equal weight to the decision to add an LABA for uncontrolled asthma symptoms. It is also not recommended that LABAs be used in the treatment of acute asthma symptoms or as monotherapy for long-term control.

Methylxanthines. Although theophylline was at one time a prominent component of daily asthma treatment, its role has changed dramatically over the past 10 years. It is listed as an alternative, but not preferred, adjunct therapy to ICS. With the current focus on anti-inflammatory therapy for asthma, along with its narrow therapeutic window and need for close monitoring of serum levels, theophylline has limited use in the pharmacological management of asthma in children.

Leukotriene Modifiers. Leukotrienes are potent pro-inflammatory mediators that promote bronchospasm, mucus production, and airway edema. Leukotriene modifiers are the first new class of medicines for asthma treatment in 20 years. Leukotriene action is modified by agents that either inhibit production of the leukotrienes or block their action. These agents are still relatively new, and studies are needed to determine their role in pediatric asthma care.

Zileuton is the only approved agent that inhibits the production of the leukotrienes; however, suggested dosing is four times daily and there have been reports of elevated results of liver function tests in patients taking the medication. Therefore it has a limited role in pediatric asthma care. The Expert Panel Report recommends that this classification of medication be considered as an alternative but not a preferred therapy in the management of mild persistent asthma. It does recommend its use as an adjunct therapy with inhaled corticosteroids for patients 12 years of age and over.[5]

Cromolyn Sodium and Nedocromil. Stabilized mast cells can interfere with chloride channel function. They are used as an alternative, but not preferred. They can also be used as preventive treatment before exercise or unavoidable exposure to known allergens.[5]

Immunomodulators. Omalizumab, the only drug that specifically binds circulating IgE, is indicated for moderate to severe asthma in patients older than 12 years who have had a positive skin test or positive in vitro test for aeroallergens, a quantitative IgE level between 30 and 700 IU/L, and whose asthma is not controlled on ICS therapy. Omalizumab is dosed based on the quantitative IgE level and the person's weight. Injections of 150 to 375 mg are given subcutaneously 1 to 2 times monthly. Omalizumab can significantly reduce exacerbations in the patient with atopic asthma.[28]

Quick-Relief Medications

Medications in the quick-relief category are short-acting β_2 agonists, anticholinergic agents, and systemic corticosteroids. These medications are used to relieve acute airway obstruction. All patients with asthma need a quick-relief medication, preferably a short-acting β_2 agonist, to take as needed for acute symptoms.

Short-Acting β Agonists. With a rapid onset of action of 5 to 15 minutes and a 4- to 6-hour duration of action, these agents are the treatment of choice for acute episodes of bronchospasm. They are often referred to as "rescue" medications and are most effective when inhaled. They are used only on an as-needed basis and not as part of the regularly scheduled medication regimen. Increased use of these agents, particularly using more than one canister per month, is an indication of inadequate asthma control and increasing severity. The most common side effects are tremor, palpitations, and tachycardia. Although acute respiratory symptoms are relieved, short-acting β_2 agonists have no anti-inflammatory action. They are used to prevent EIB.

Anticholinergics. Ipratropium bromide is the anticholinergic agent approved for use in the United States. It is available alone in a metered-dose inhaler (MDI) and nebulizer formulation. Given alone, it is a less potent bronchodilator than short-acting β_2 agonists. The combination of ipratropium bromide and albuterol is marketed in a metered-dose inhaler and a nebulizer unit-dose preparation.

Systemic Corticosteroids. Patients with acute exacerbations often receive 3- to 10-day bursts of prednisone or methylprednisolone. The bursts are primarily used to hasten recovery and prevent recurrence of symptoms. The dose of corticosteroid is tapered as symptoms resolve. However, if the symptoms return within 1 month or if the bursts are frequently required, changes are likely required in the long-term control medication regimen.

Delivery Systems

Asthma medications are usually given through inhalation in an aerosol form. The medications are administered by a metered-dose inhaler, a dry-powder inhaler, or liquid small-volume nebulization. The majority of propellants that power the metered-dose inhalers use chlorofluorocarbons, chemicals that have been found to contribute to depletion of the ozone. Manufacturers of metered-dose inhalers are actively replacing propellants in accordance with the Montreal Protocol time lines.

Valved holding chambers are simple, inexpensive tools that have been developed to use with metered-dose inhalers. Their purpose is threefold:
1. To slow aerosol velocity
2. To minimize particle impaction in the oropharynx
3. To enhance deposition in the lower respiratory tract

Their use in children is recommended to reduce the problem of coordinating actuation of the metered-dose inhaler with the inhalation. Studies have demonstrated that the decrease in pharyngeal deposition results in improved drug efficacy and reduction in local side effects. It is imperative that patients along with parents or caregivers are instructed in the proper use of all inhalers, nebulizers, masks, and valved holding chambers. See Chapter 11 for more details of delivery devices.

Control of Asthma Triggers

Most children with asthma have an allergic component to their disease. If asthma is to be managed adequately, the allergens and irritants that worsen symptoms must be identified and controlled. The most common allergens implicated in chronic asthma are listed in Box 27-4. Exposure

Box 27-4	Allergens Associated with Asthma
• House dust mite	• Mouse
• Pet allergen	• Cockroach
• Cat	• Indoor mold
• Dog	• *Aspergillus*
• Guinea pig	• *Penicillium*
• Rabbit	• Outdoor mold
• Rodent	• *Alternaria*
• Rat	• *Cladosporium*

to allergens and irritants may significantly increase bronchial hyperresponsiveness, whereas reduced exposure to allergens can decrease asthma symptoms.

Identification of Allergens

Because childhood asthma is often exacerbated by allergen exposure, it is helpful to identify the allergens. Allergy skin testing, along with a thorough history and physical examination, is one method an allergist uses to determine which allergens may be aggravating a child's asthma. Another common test used to determine what allergens are responsible for allergic disease is the radioallergosorbent (RAST) test.

Avoidance and Control Measures

It is nearly impossible for a child with asthma to avoid exposure to all offending allergens and irritants. But it is possible to minimize exposure to them. This begins with teaching the child and family to recognize the triggers and use measures to control and avoid them. Box 27-5 lists control measures for environmental factors that often exacerbate asthma in children.

Role of Immunotherapy

Allergen avoidance can produce changes in asthma disease activity and bronchial hyperresponsiveness, but often there

Box 27-5	Environmental Control Measures

HOUSE DUST MITE
- Kill with hot water (>130° F) and dry cleaning.
- Enforce bedroom dust control.
- Encase pillows, mattresses, and box springs in zippered allergen-impermeable covers.
- Wash sheets and blankets weekly in hot water.
- Replace wool bedding with cotton or synthetics.
- Avoid feather or down bedding.
- Remove stuffed toys, wall hangings, and other "dust-catchers."
- Hot-water wash or freeze stuffed toys weekly.
- Vacuum/dust weekly wearing mask; vacuum with double-thick bag and HEPA filter.
- Keep heat, ventilation, and air conditioner filters clean.
- Remove carpeting; wash rugs; avoid heavy curtains and blinds.
- Keep clothing in closets with doors closed.
- Clean with damp cloths.
- Reduce indoor humidity.
- Replace upholstered furniture with wood, vinyl, or leather.

ANIMAL DANDER
- Remove animal from house or restrict animal to washable area (may take 4 to 6 months to remove cat allergen).
- Banish animal from bedroom.
- Close bedroom door and vents.
- Use HEPA or electrostatic filter in bedroom.
- Remove carpets and minimize upholstered furniture and other allergen reservoirs.

COCKROACH
- Hire professional exterminator.
- Use poison baits.
- Store food and garbage in sealed containers.
- Perform meticulous regular cleaning.
- Eat only in kitchen/dining room.

INDOOR MOLD
- Kitchen, bathroom, and basement are most common sites.
- Leaky pipes, shower curtains, refrigerator drip pans, garbage pails, and window edgings are major sources.
- Wrap plumbing to eliminate condensation.
- Use commercial fungicides and bleach solution.
- Reduce humidity to less than 45% with dehumidifiers, air conditioning, and increased ventilation.
- Avoid humidifiers and vaporizers.
- Close windows, especially in bedroom.
- Remove moldy items.
- Repair water leaks.
- Dry clothing/shoes before placing in closet.
- Limit houseplants and remove them from bedroom.
- Avoid live Christmas trees.

NONALLERGEN IRRITANTS
- Avoid tobacco smoke and passive smoke in the home and closed car.
- Avoid wood stoves, kerosene heaters, cleaning products, and perfumes.

are no practical means for avoiding exposure to all allergens. Allergen immunotherapy, or "allergy shots," should be considered for asthma patients when the following conditions are met:

1. There is clear evidence of a relationship between asthma symptoms and allergen exposure.
2. The patient is symptomatic during a major portion of the year.
3. Symptoms are difficult to control with pharmacological therapy.

The value of immunotherapy in children with asthma remains controversial.[29,30] Evidence suggests that it can be safely given to children with asthma and that life-threatening reactions are uncommon when the process is prescribed and supervised by an appropriately trained physician. However, the risk of anaphylaxis remains and the injections must be administered in a health care facility where personnel, medication, and emergency equipment are immediately available to treat a systemic reaction. The patient waits 20 to 30 minutes after each injection because this is the interval of highest risk for a systemic reaction. It is also suggested that the immunotherapy be delayed when the child has an acute illness or asthma exacerbation. Allergen immunotherapy is typically given every 7 to 28 days for 3 to 5 years, with a positive effect often seen within 1 year of therapy.

Peak Flow Monitoring

Using a peak flow meter to monitor peak expiratory flow rates (PEFR) is an important tool in asthma management when it is accompanied by a written action plan. It can be performed in children as young as 3 to 4 years old. Monitoring assists children and parents or caregivers in recognizing changes in respiratory status, affording them the chance to make necessary interventions. Although lung function measurements such as peak flow or spirometry may be useful in the management of asthma, many children may be unable to do or have difficulties performing maneuvers during an asthma exacerbation.[31] Therefore, the use of peak flow is not as strongly supported in the assessment of hospitalized patients with acute asthma exacerbations.

Peak Flow Meter

The peak flow meter is a comparatively inexpensive monitoring tool that measures the PEFR (Figure 27-1). It is used only for ongoing monitoring and not to diagnose asthma. Different brands of peak flow meters are available, and it is possible to get a slightly different peak flow value when using a different meter. Because there is variation between different brands, it is important to use the same peak flow meter or model for long-term monitoring.[32] Box 27-6 lists the steps in performing a peak flow maneuver. Patients are asked to bring their peak flow meter to their physician's office to check the accuracy of the meter as well as to recheck for proper technique. When a quick-relief medication

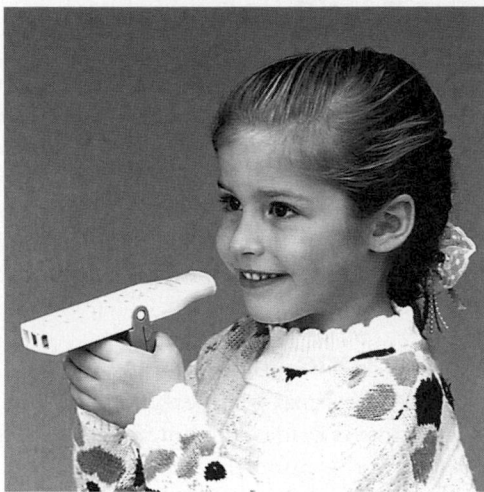

FIGURE 27-1   Child with peak flow meter.

Box 27-6	**How to Use a Peak Flow Meter**

1. Make sure the meter reads zero or the indicator is at the bottom of the numbered scale.
2. Stand up (unless there is a physical disability). Remove any food or gum from your mouth.
3. Take as deep a breath as possible, filling your lungs completely.
4. Place the meter in your mouth, behind your teeth, and close your lips around the mouthpiece. Do not let your tongue block the mouthpiece.
5. Blow out as hard and as fast as you can in a single blow. Do not cough into the meter.
6. The force of your breath moves the indicator on the peak flow meter. The number opposite the indicator is your peak flow.
7. Write down the peak flow number obtained.
8. Repeat the steps two additional times. Record the highest of the three attempts (not the average) in your diary or on your peak flow chart.

is taken because of an increase in asthma symptoms, it is suggested that a peak flow reading be obtained before and after taking the medication.

Peak Flow Diary

Keeping a diary or chart of the readings is for many patients an important part of their treatment plan. Graphs for plotting peak flows are often included with the peak flow meter and can be photocopied for additional use. With daily peak flow monitoring, a patient may see a drop in the peak flow before severe symptoms are felt and may begin early treatment or seek medical help. This may prevent asthma exacerbations from occurring or lessen the seriousness of an episode by medicating at the first sign of low peak flow readings. The physician reviews the peak flow diary at each office visit.

Personal Best Reading

There are predicted "normal" peak flow values that are determined by height, age, gender, and race. However, it is necessary to determine a child's "personal best" peak flow reading. This is defined as simply the highest or best measurement obtained when the patient is free of symptoms and asthma is under control. To determine the personal best reading, the patient records peak flow readings at least once a day for 2 to 3 weeks. The best peak flow reading will usually occur in the early afternoon.

Peak Flow Zone System

Once a patient's personal best peak flow has been established, every effort is made to maintain the peak flow values within 80% of this number. One peak flow monitoring system uses a zone system to indicate asthma severity and to guide a patient to an appropriate response. As illustrated in Box 27-7, green, yellow, and red zones are established. The zones are broad guidelines designed to simplify asthma management.

Asthma Action Plan

The physician provides a written management plan, or **asthma action plan** (Figure 27-2), with information that the patient can immediately refer to should the patient become symptomatic. No action plan should be developed without the physician's input. Based on the patient's current peak flow reading and the personal best number, the plan provides the patient with appropriate actions to take when the peak flow values drop. Included are detailed instructions specifying when to begin quick-relief medications, when to increase daily medications, and when to contact a physician or seek emergency care. Also identified are the specific medications to be given, the route of administration, the dose to be administered, and the frequency of dosing. Reminders to recheck the peak flow reading are included. It is helpful to have the physician's name and phone number on the plan along with the phone number of a close relative or neighbor.

Patients are instructed to take the action plan and peak flow meter with them when traveling. If the patient attends school, a copy of the plan is provided for the school to be used by the teacher or school nurse in the event of an exacerbation or to prevent EIB while at school.

Patient and Family Education

For any asthma disease management program to be successful there must be an active partnership between patients, their families, and health care providers. This partnership is critical when the patient has a chronic disease such as asthma. Patient and family education begins at diagnosis and is a continual process, with the ultimate goal being to improve self-management.

It is unlikely that the patient's physician has the time to devote to a complete and comprehensive regimen of education; therefore, all members of the health care team need to work together to reinforce the same message. A comprehensive asthma education program, which should be provided to patients with asthma, includes a system of well-trained health care providers who specifically address barriers to learning and test comprehension of parent and child; includes the community in which the child lives; and uses age-specific teaching methods (including technology when appropriate) to accomplish the NAEPP objectives (Figure 27-3):

1. Self-monitoring to assess level of asthma control and signs of worsening asthma
2. Using a written asthma action plan
3. Taking medication correctly (proper inhaler technique and use of devices)
4. Avoiding environmental factors that worsen asthma

A successful partnership keeps the lines of communication open. Asking open-ended questions can lead to the patient and family being freer in discussing

---

Box 27-7	Traffic Light Zone System

GREEN ZONE: PEAK EXPIRATORY FLOW IS GREATER THAN 80% OF PERSONAL BEST NUMBER.
• Good control of asthma is indicated.
• Patient is relatively symptom-free.
• Quick-relief medication is not indicated.
• Long-term control medication is the only medication indicated.
• If peak flow is constantly in the Green Zone with minimal variation, the physician may consider changing or decreasing daily medication.

YELLOW ZONE: PEAK EXPIRATORY FLOW IS 50% TO 80% OF PERSONAL BEST NUMBER
• "Cautious" zone; asthma is worsening.
• There is less than optimal control of asthma.
• Asthma symptoms may be increased, with awakening at night.

• Quick-relief medication is needed (usually a short-acting β_2-agonist).
• Increase in daily maintenance therapy may be needed.

RED ZONE: PEAK EXPIRATORY FLOW IS LESS THAN 50% OF PERSONAL BEST NUMBER
• "Danger" zone; exacerbation is severe.
• Asthma is poorly controlled.
• Asthma symptoms are serious and possibly life threatening.
• Immediate intervention is required (usually a short-acting β_2 agonist).
• Depending on physician's direction and patient's response to quick-relief medication, patient may be directed to seek emergency care.

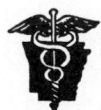

Name: _____ No. _____
Date: _____

ASTHMA ACTION PLAN USING YOUR PEAK FLOW READINGS
Know your zone. Measure your peak flow every _____ and anytime you need to know your zone.

GREEN ZONE: You are in the **GREEN** zone if your reading is at least _____ (>80% personal best).
Green zone means GO. No sign of cough, wheeze, or chest tightness.

Take these medications daily: How much   When to take
1. _____   _____   _____
2. _____   _____   _____
3. _____   _____   _____
4. _____   _____   _____
5. _____   _____   _____

Take ___ puffs of _____ before you exercise, if needed for exercise-induced asthma.

YELLOW ZONES: (50%-80% of personal best). You may have increased asthma symptoms,
awakening at night with asthma, or inability to do your normal activities.
HIGH YELLOW ZONE: Your peak flow is between _____ and _____.
- Take _____ puffs of _____ (quick relief medicine) or an updraft treatment. * Repeat
every _____ hours until in the Green zone.
- Take _____ puffs of _____ (antiinflammatory medicine). Repeat every _____ hours
until in the Green zone. Then return to your Green zone dose.

LOW YELLOW ZONE: Your peak flow is between _____ and _____. Follow this plan if the peak
flow does not reach **High** Yellow Zone within 15 minutes after taking inhaled quick-relief medicine or
updraft treatment, or drops back into Low Yellow Zone within 4 hours.
- Continue _____ puffs of _____ (quick relief medicine) or an updraft
treatment every _____ hours.*
- Add oral steroids** _____. Continue _____ mg/day for _____ days or
till in Green Zone for 24 hours.
- Contact your doctor to report persistent low readings or use of oral steroids.
**If your condition does not improve within 2 days after starting oral steroids, contact your doctor again.

RED ZONE: Your peak flow reading is below _____. (< 50% personal best).
Red zone means STOP. Your asthma symptoms are serious.
- Take _____ puffs of _____ (quick relief medicine) or an updraft
treatment.*
- Take oral steroids _____ mg immediately.
- If your peak flow does **not** reach the **low yellow zone** in 15 minutes after taking your
quick-relief medicine or drops back into the Red zone in 4 hours, contact your doctor
or go to the emergency room.

***Always measure your peak flow 15 minutes after taking your quick-relief medicine.**
FIGURE 27-2   Example of an asthma action plan.

---

concerns, fears, and expectations regarding asthma care. Perception of the disease and beliefs about treatment are influenced by earlier experience with the disease, education, personality characteristics, socioeconomic and cultural background, and the available support systems.[33] It is important to be sensitive to the cultural background of the patient and family. Ethnic beliefs can often affect the way the patient and family view asthma and its treatment. For example, some cultures view an illness as either a "hot" or a "cold" disease. Many in the Hispanic population believe that asthma should be treated with a "hot" remedy such as hot tea. Often there is no harm in the belief; however, there may be

times when the clinician must intercede in the interest of patient safety.

Asthma Disease Process

Key points concerning the disease process include a basic understanding of what asthma is and what can trigger asthma episodes. Often drawings of a normal airway contrasted to that of one with asthma help patients visualize what is occurring in their own lungs.

Medication Skills

It is imperative that patients (depending on age) and families understand the names of their medication, proper

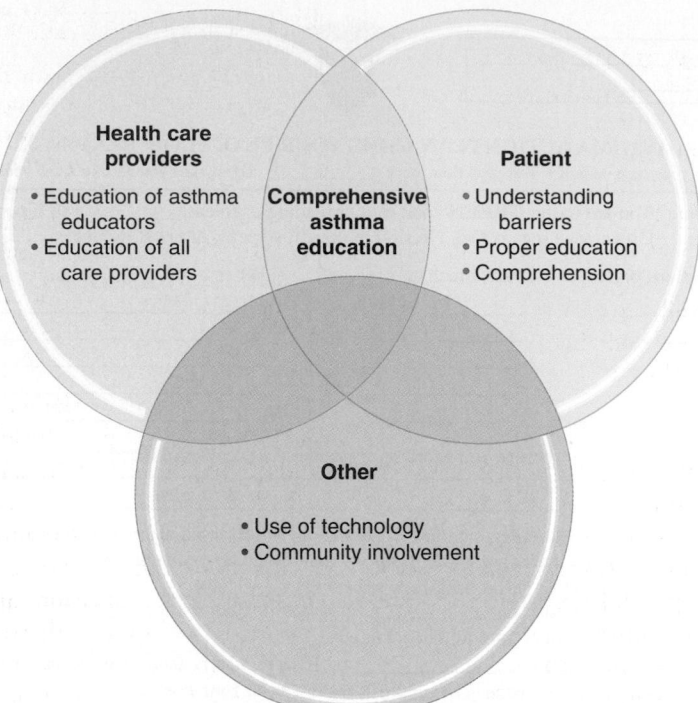

FIGURE 27-3   A comprehensive asthma education program includes all stakeholders in the successful outcome of improved self-management of the patient.

dosing, when and how to take each medication, and the side effects of each. Providing written instructions for each medication assists in understanding and adherence to the treatment regimen. Proper inhaler technique is taught and then reviewed at each subsequent physician visit. It is stressed that the long-term control medications are preventive in nature and are to be taken even if the patient is symptom free. Patients often discontinue use of their controller medications, only to develop an asthma exacerbation within 3 to 4 weeks.

Identification and Control of Triggers

Patients and their families need information to discern what triggers their asthma as well as ways to avoid the triggers. Although all triggers may not be totally avoidable, the patient and family are urged to take all necessary measures to avoid them and learn to monitor which variables influence their symptoms.

Self-Monitoring Techniques

Patients must learn to monitor and recognize signs and symptoms of worsening asthma. Education in the proper use of a peak flow meter and how to follow an asthma action plan is an essential component of asthma education. Reinforcing appropriate behavior includes reviewing peak flow monitoring, inhaler technique, and implementation of the action plan. Review of the action plan at each visit has been shown to improve patient compliance and decrease the chance for confusion.

MANAGING ASTHMA EXACERBATIONS IN THE EMERGENCY DEPARTMENT

Patients presenting to the emergency department have often had previous emergency admissions and hospitalizations for treatment of severe asthma. Often these patients have no primary care physician and rely on symptomatic control and emergency departments as their primary source of medical care. Along with inadequate use of corticosteroids, these characteristics are associated with an increased risk for fatal asthma.[34]

Assessment

The intensity and progression of the asthma exacerbation can vary and will determine the intensity of treatment in the emergency department. It is essential that a primary classification of severity be determined in the emergency department. On admission, a physical examination is performed along with measurement of oxygenation and air flow. A pulse oximeter is used to measure oxygen saturation. Continuous monitoring of oxygen with a pulse oximeter is crucial in order to prevent desaturation.

A peak flow meter or spirometer can provide assessment of the severity of airway obstruction from inflammation and bronchospasm. If a child who normally uses a peak flow meter is unable to perform the maneuver during an attack, severe air flow obstruction is considered and intensive medical therapy is indicated.

β₂ Agonists

One of the first lines of therapy is with β₂ agonist agents, such as albuterol or levalbuterol. The EPR-3 recommends that the patient receive three treatments given every 20 to 30 minutes by either nebulization or MDI. If there is an inadequate response to this, continuous nebulization of albuterol may be initiated. In severe exacerbations the addition of ipratropium bromide to β₂ agonists should be considered. Adverse effects typically seen with the use of β₂ agonists, such as tremor, tachycardia, and nervousness, are often pronounced, and some patients may not want to take the treatment because of this response.[35]

Corticosteroids

It is critical that corticosteroids be given to treat the inflammation that occurs during an acute exacerbation. Early treatment, which may include the use of intravenous corticosteroids, is effective in preventing an increase in the severity of symptoms and may avoid hospitalization and relapses.[36] Because intravenous lines are uncomfortable and can be difficult to place in a child, studies have investigated the use of oral corticosteroids in the emergency setting.[37,38] If the child cannot adequately be given oral corticosteroids, the intravenous route should be considered. Consideration of other adjunct interventions in severe exacerbation should be considered as well. These include intravenous magnesium sulfate or heliox.[5]

CASE STUDY

A 5-year-old previously healthy boy with no medical history is being seen in the emergency department (ED) with wheezing, retractions, and respiratory distress, with an SpO₂ of 99% on room air. You initiate a bronchodilator according to protocol and begin a complete assessment. A chest radiograph reveals hyperinflated lung fields with no concerns for pneumonia or cardiac disease.

What would you want to review before considering asthma as the primary reason for the ED visit?

See Evolve Resources for answers.

HOSPITALIZATION AND RESPIRATORY FAILURE

Regardless of the care given in the emergency department, some children will not respond adequately and will require hospitalization. Criteria for hospitalization vary; however, continuing deterioration or failure to improve with therapy is an indication for intensive monitoring and treatment. Yet the treatment within the inpatient unit is not much different that the emergency department, with the exception of ipratropium bromide, because it is not recommended after admission. Box 27-8 lists criteria considered for hospitalization.

Box 27-8   Criteria for Hospitalization

- Poor response to 4 hours of bronchodilator therapy
- Requires continuous bronchodilator therapy
- Previous visit to emergency department within 24 hours
- Hospitalization with asthma within the past year
- Previous hospitalization with admission to intensive care unit
- History of mechanical ventilation for asthma
- Poor access to medical care
- Recent increase in need for oral corticosteroids

Intubation

If all attempts to reverse bronchospasm and improve air flow are futile, careful consideration is given to intubation and mechanical ventilation. Diligent patient monitoring is essential, and immediate steps are taken once the patient demonstrates respiratory muscle fatigue or failure.

It is best to intubate on a semielective basis rather than in an emergent situation, and the clinician most experienced in managing pediatric airways should perform it. Intubation is attempted only under controlled settings with continuous cardiorespiratory monitoring and resuscitation equipment and medication available. Once intubated and stabilized, the patient is monitored in a pediatric intensive care unit, which may mean transporting the child to another medical facility.

Mechanical Ventilation

After intubation, the child is mechanically ventilated with 6 to 8 ml/kg IBW with low to moderate positive end-expiratory pressure (PEEP) to assist with distal airway collapse and degree of auto-PEEP present. Larger tidal volumes may be required if prolonged expiratory times and low rates are used. The mode of ventilation and set respiratory rate is determined according to the patient's degree of sedation, peak inspiratory pressures generated, oxygenation, and acceptable levels of PaCO₂. Initially the FIO₂ is 1.0, with the goal to decrease the level to 0.5 or less when able. Ventilation with permissive hypercapnia is allowed with an inspiratory-to-expiratory ratio that allows for adequate exhalation. See Chapter 18 for the use of inhaled anesthetics in this patient population.
NOTE: If utilizing noninvasive mechanical ventilation a moderate to high level of PEEP (>8 cmH₂O) may be required to assist with distal airway collapse.

All patients receiving mechanical ventilation are at risk of complications, including auto-PEEP, air trapping, pneumothorax, hypotension, acute respiratory distress syndrome, and death. The child with asthma is especially prone to such problems because of the high degree of airway resistance and the need for high inspiratory pressures.

EXERCISE-INDUCED BRONCHOSPASM

Sometimes referred to as exercise-induced asthma, EIB begins during exercise and tends to reach its peak 5 to

10 minutes after the child has ceased activity. It may take another 20 to 30 minutes for symptoms to spontaneously resolve. EIB is caused by a loss of heat and/or water from the child's airway during exercise. This is often caused by hyperventilation of cool or dry air.

The prevalence of EIB has been reported to vary from 40% to 90% in children with asthma, with greater prevalence in those children with severe asthma. Absenteeism from school and poverty have been associated with findings of EIB. Early detection of EIB in school-aged children through screening could facilitate early treatment, enhance exercise-related activities, and possibly decrease the number of school absences. Notifying day care personnel, schoolteachers, and coaches that a child has EIB can alert them to monitor symptoms and may elicit a more effective response should symptoms occur.

The diagnosis of EIB is based on a history that is compatible with asthma symptoms that occur with or directly after exercise. An exercise challenge can be performed to confirm the diagnosis.

The management of these episodes is generally of a preventive nature. Recommended treatment is inhalation of a β_2 agonist, cromolyn sodium, nedocromil, or salmeterol, given 5 to 60 minutes before exercise, preferably closer to the start of exercise if possible. Providing a 5- to 10-minute "warmup" period before any exercise is recommended as well. An increase or change in long-term control medications may be appropriate in some children with EIB. Outdoor activities may need to be adjusted if conditions are unfavorable. This is particularly important if the pollen, weed, or mold count is elevated. Extreme cold and windy weather are also circumstances that may call for more caution to ensure that asthma symptoms do not develop during the activities. Efforts to prevent EIB require open communication with the schoolteacher and coach to allow premedication by the student athlete under a physician's guidance.

ASTHMA AT SCHOOL

One third of those with asthma in the United States are younger than 18 years of age. Dealing with asthma while at school can present problems for the child, the parent, and the school personnel. Asthma symptoms can interfere with many activities that the school-aged child desires to pursue. It is the leading cause of school absences, with an average of more than 10 days per year missed. The child with severe asthma may miss more than 30 days per year. An obvious conclusion drawn from these statistics is that missing school may result in poor academic achievement, inability to participate in school activities, and low self-esteem. The goal of the school-aged child with asthma is to keep symptoms under control and participate fully in the physical and extracurricular activities the school system may offer.

Various organizations provide resources to aid in the care of children with asthma in the school systems. The American Association for Respiratory Care offers a program that involves direct education of school administrators, teachers, and students. It is called Peak Performance

USA and is available to all members upon request. The educational interventions can address each particular school because not all schools have similar needs or programs. Another similar school intervention is available through the American Lung Association. A child-centered, school-based asthma education program has been associated with an increase in knowledge of asthma, improvement in skills for peak flow meter and inhaler use, and a reduction in the severity of asthma symptoms.[39]

School personnel, including teachers, coaches, and nurses, need to be familiar with the early warning signs of an impending asthma attack and what to do if the symptoms are present. It is recommended that a copy of the child's asthma action plan be kept at the school and that the teacher and school nurse be familiar with the plan. Unfortunately, many school systems do not employ a nurse dedicated to each individual school. Therefore there are occasions when the nurse is not available and other school personnel may need to provide care for the child. It is essential that the asthma action plan, peak flow meter, and rescue medications be readily accessible to school staff.

Parents can take a proactive role by determining how "asthma friendly" the school's environment is for their child. Some key questions to ask are listed in Box 27-9. The school building can present a hostile environment for

---

Box 27-9	**Is Your School Asthma Friendly?**

- Does the school have a "NO SMOKING" policy for all personnel, including teachers and custodial staff?
- Does the school maintain clean indoor air quality? How is this ensured?
- Is there a school nurse available at the school at all times? If not, how often is she/he there? Is she/he trained in pediatric asthma care?
- Can children with asthma take prescribed medications at school? Can they carry their rescue medications on their person? Must the medications be kept in a locked location?
- Does the school have an emergency plan for treating a child with a severe asthma episode?
- Does the school staff know the early warning signs of an asthma episode? Do they know the possible side effects of asthma medications and how they may impact the student's performance at school?
- Are students encouraged to participate in school activities and sports, regardless of having asthma?
- Are less strenuous activities provided if a recent exacerbation precludes full participation?
- Do teachers and coaches understand that exercise, especially in cold air, can trigger asthma?
- Is the school staff provided with opportunities to learn about asthma and allergies?
- Is there a copy of the asthma action plan in each student's classroom?
- Do school personnel understand that asthma is not an emotional or psychological disease but that strong emotions can trigger an acute episode?

children with asthma. There are numerous potential triggers found in most schools, including dust mites, mold, cockroaches, chalk dust, birds, rodents, animal dander, and strong odors (e.g., paint, chemicals, perfumes, pesticides). Therefore it is essential that these irritants be minimized or eliminated so that the child with asthma can attend school without risking further complications.

ASTHMA CAMPS

In recent years we have seen a growth in the number of asthma camps for children. These camps offer children with asthma the opportunity to spend time with other children who have the same disorder. This type of experience can be priceless. The camps are structured to assist children in recognizing symptoms and how to respond to them, with particular attention given to use of an asthma action plan. Identification of triggers and avoidance techniques are discussed as well. The proper use of medication delivery devices and peak flow meters is also reinforced.

Positive effects from attending camp include a reduction in the rate of post-camp hospitalizations, school absenteeism, and emergency department visits.[40,41] The camps are usually operated with a team approach that includes physicians, respiratory therapists, social workers, and nurses.

KEY POINTS

- Asthma is a chronic yet reversible disease if properly maintained and monitored.
- Proper education and ongoing reinforcement of that education are vitally important for the successful self-management of asthma.
- Prolonged expiratory phased ventilation in asthma may be required; however, to maintain an adequate alveolar ventilation a larger tidal volume will be required.
- Long-acting β agonist (LABA) use may mask symptoms of uncontrolled airway inflammation and contribute to asthma-related deaths.
- The use of clinical assessment tools, such as an asthma score, can be helpful; however, some indications of health, such as breath sounds, can be misleading. For example, silent or quiet breath sounds can be an ominous sign or a sign of improvement depending on the remaining factors of your clinical assessment.

ASSESSMENT QUESTIONS

See Evolve Resources for Answers.

1. The incidence of asthma has done what over the past 10 years?
   A. Remained stable
   B. Increased
   C. Decreased
   D. Decreased in incidence but increased in severity

2. When gathering information about a patient's medical history it is essential to include:
   A. Recurrent wheezing or chest tightness
   B. Shortness of breath and cough
   C. Nocturnal symptoms
   D. All of the above

3. Dust mites are better controlled in what environment?
   A. Less relative humidity
   B. When bedding is washed in water hotter than 130° F
   C. When pillows and mattress are enclosed in zippered allergen-impermeable covers
   D. All of the above

4. When educating a patient or family member it is always essential to remember to:
   A. Not ask open-ended questions
   B. Ask open-ended questions
   C. Try not to maintain eye contact for long periods
   D. Avoid questions that deal with a patient's expectations of his or her asthma management

5. The purpose of a spacer is to slow aerosol velocity, to minimize particle impaction in the oropharynx, and to:
   A. Enhance deposition in the lower respiratory tract
   B. Allow for larger particles
   C. Decrease the size of the particles
   D. Change aerosol particles to vapor, thus allowing better delivery of medication

6. Omalizumab is generally dosed for patients with IgE levels between:
   A. 30 and 1500 IU/L
   B. 30 and 700 IU/L
   C. 500 and 1200 IU/L
   D. 3000 and 5500 IU/L

7. What is the best way to manage cockroaches?
   A. Carpet removal
   B. Boric acid
   C. Acetic acid
   D. Bleach

8. Triggers of airflow obstruction include:
   A. Aspirin and nonsteroidal anti-inflammatory drugs, exercise, cold air, irritants, gastroesophageal reflux, respiratory infections, and psychological stress
   B. Aspirin, exercise, cold air, gastroesophageal reflux, respiratory infections, and excessive use of LABA
   C. Respiratory infections, cold or warm air, psychological stress, aspirin, exercise, and anti-inflammatory drugs

9. In adult asthma the inflammatory findings, such as eosinophilic airway inflammation, hypergranulation of mast cells, increased IgE levels, and increased allergic response, are due in part to an inappropriate activation of:
   A. CD4+ T cells
   B. IL-4
   C. T cells
   D. Th2 cells

10. What are the five components of asthma?
   A. Inflammation, acute bronchoconstriction, airway edema, mucous plugging, airway hyperresponsiveness, and wheezing
   B. Inflammation, acute bronchoconstriction, airway edema, mucous plugging, airway hyperresponsiveness, and airway remodeling
   C. Inflammation, acute bronchoconstriction, airway edema, mucous plugging, airway hyperresponsiveness, and increased levels of nitric oxide
   D. Inflammation, acute bronchoconstriction, airway edema, mucous plugging, airway hyperresponsiveness, and an allergic presentation

References

1. National Center for Health Statistics: *Asthma prevalence, health care use and mortality 2003–2005, United States,* Atlanta, GA, Centers for Disease Control and Prevention.
2. National Asthma Education Program: *Guidelines for the diagnosis and management of asthma: expert panel report.* NIH pub. no. 91-3642, Bethesda, MD, 1991, National Institutes of Health; National Heart, Lung, and Blood Institute.
3. National Asthma Education and Prevention Program: *Guidelines for the diagnosis and management of asthma: expert panel report 2.* NIH pub. no. 97-4051, Bethesda, MD, 1997, National Institutes of Health; National Heart, Lung, and Blood Institute.
4. National Asthma Education and Prevention Program: *Expert panel report: guidelines for the diagnosis and management of asthma.* Update on selected topics 2002 (EPR Update 2002). NIH pub. no. 02-5074, Bethesda, MD, 2002, U.S. Department of Health and Human Services; National Institutes of Health; National Heart, Lung, and Blood Institute.
5. National Asthma Education and Prevention Program. *Guidelines for the diagnosis and management of asthma (EPR-3).* NIH pub. no. Bethesda, MD, 2007, U.S. Department of Health and Human Services; National Institutes of Health; National Heart, Lung, and Blood Institute; National Asthma Education and Prevention Program.
6. Centers for Disease Control and Prevention: *National asthma control program.* http://www.cdc.gov/asthma/NACP.htm.
7. Centers for Disease Control and Prevention: *The 15-minute asthma visit,* Medscape. http://www.medscape.com/viewarticle/745863. Accessed August 1, 2011.
8. Centers for Disease Control and Prevention: *Asthma control during travel,* Medscape. http://www.medscape.com/viewarticle/741288. Accessed May 2, 2011.
9. Bateman ED, et al: GOAL Investigators Group: can guideline defined asthma control be achieved? The Gaining Optimal Asthma Control Study, *Am J Respir Crit Care* 170:836, 2004.
10. Hunt JF, Fang K, Malik R, et al: Endogenous airway acidification. Implications for asthma pathophysiology, *Am J Respir Crit Care Med* 161(3 Pt 1):694, 2000.
11. Ricciardolo FL, Gaston B, Hunt J: Acid stress in the pathology of asthma, *J Allergy Clin Immunol* 113(4):610, 2004.
12. Horvath G, Schmid N, Fragoso MA, et al: Epithelial organic cation transporters ensure pH-dependent drug absorption in the airway, *Am J Respir Cell Mol Biol* 36(1):53, 2007.
13. Burrows Johansson and Lundahl: 2001 Curr Allergy Asthma Rep, 1, 89-90 et al., *N Engl J Med* 320:271–277, 1989.
14. Platts-Mills TA: Allergen avoidance in the treatment of asthma and rhinitis, *N Engl J Med* 349:207, 2003.
15. Vignola AM: Effects of inhaled corticosteroids, leukotriene receptor antagonists, or both, plus long-acting beta₂-agonists on asthma pathophysiology: a review of the evidence, *Drugs* 63(Suppl 2):35, 2003.
16. Eder W, Ege MJ, von Mutius E: The "hygiene hypothesis": the asthma epidemic, *N Engl J Med* 355:2226, 2006.
17. Holgate ST, Polosa R: The mechanisms, diagnosis, and management of severe asthma in the development of early childhood asthma, *Pediatrics* 75:859, 1985.
18. Huss K, et al: House dust mite exposure is strong risk factors for positive allergy skin test responses in the Childhood Asthma Management Program, *J Allergy Clin Immunol* 107:48, 2001.
19. Voter KZ, McBride JT: Pulmonary function testing in childhood asthma, *Immunol Allergy Clin North Am* 18:133, 1998.
20. American Thoracic Society: Standardization of spirometry: 1994 update, *Am J Respir Crit Care Med* 152:1107, 1995.
21. Dweik RA, Boggs PB, Erzurum SC, et al: An official ATS clinical practice guideline: interpretation of exhaled nitric oxide levels (FE_NO) for clinical applications, May 2011.
22. Williams PV: Inhalation bronchoprovocation in children, *Immunol Allergy Clin North Am* 18:149, 1998.
23. Custovic A, et al: Exercise testing revisited: the response to exercise in normal and atopic children, *Chest* 105:1127, 1994.
24. Zwiebel AH: Bronchoprovocation testing, *Immunol Allergy Clin North Am* 19:63, 1999.
25. Milgrom H, Wood RP, Ingram D: Respiratory conditions that mimic asthma, *Immunol Allergy Clin North Am* 18:113, 1998.
26. Shapiro GG: Management of pediatric asthma: care by the specialist, *Immunol Allergy Clin North Am* 18:1, 1998.
27. Nelson HS, et al, SMART Study Group: The Salmeterol Multicenter Asthma Research Trial: a comparison of usual pharmacotherapy for asthma or usual pharmacotherapy plus salmeterol, *Chest* 129:15, 2006.
28. Busse WW: Anti-immunoglobulin E (omalizumab) therapy in allergic asthma, *Am J Respir Crit Care Med* 164:S12, 2001.
29. Giovane AL, et al: A three-year double-blind placebo-controlled study with specific oral immunotherapy to Dermatophagoides: evidence of safety and efficacy in paediatric patients, *Clin Exp Allergy* 24:53, 1994.
30. Adkinson NF Jr, et al: A controlled trial of immunotherapy for asthma in allergic children, *N Engl J Med* 336:324, 1997.
31. Gorelick MH, Stevens MW, Schultz TR, Scribano PV: Performance of a novel clinical score the Pediatric Asthma Severity Score (PASS) in the evaluation of acute asthma, *Acad Emerg Med* 11(1):10, 2004.
32. Jackson AC: Accuracy, reproducibility, and variability of portable peak flow meters, *Chest* 107:648, 1995.
33. Ponte CM: Education of the patient with asthma, *Immunol Allergy Clin North Am* 19:161, 1999.
34. Dales RE, et al: Asthma management preceding an emergency department visit, *Arch Intern Med* 152:2041, 1995.
35. White M, Sander N: Asthma from the perspective of the patient, *J Allergy Clin Immunol* 104:S47, 1999.
36. Tal A, Levy N, Bearman JE: Methylprednisolone therapy for acute asthma in infants and toddlers: a controlled clinical trial, *Pediatrics* 86:350, 1990.
37. Barnett PL, Caputo GL, Baskin M: Intravenous vs. oral corticosteroids in the management of acute asthma in children, *Ann Emerg Med* 29:212, 1997.
38. Scarfone RJ, et al: Controlled trial of oral prednisone in the emergency department treatment of children with acute asthma, *Pediatrics* 92:513, 1993.
39. Christianson S, et al: Evaluation of a school-based asthma education program for inner-city children, *J Allergy Clin Immunol* 100:613, 1997.
40. Kelly CS, et al: Outcomes analysis of a summer camp, *J Asthma* 35:165, 1998.
41. Menng A, et al: Asthma day camp, *MCN Am J Matern Child Nurs* 23:300, 1998.

Chapter 28

Cystic Fibrosis

KENSHO IWANAGA

OUTLINE

Introduction
Epidemiology
Genetics and Molecular Biology
Diagnosis
    Sweat Chloride Testing
    CFTR Mutation Analysis
    Nasal Potential Difference
    Newborn Screening
Pulmonary Disease
    Mucus Production and Airway Obstruction
    Bacterial Infection
    Airway Inflammation
    Clinical Manifestations

Treatment of Pulmonary Disease
    Aerosol Therapy
    Airway Clearance Therapy
    Antibiotics
    Anti-inflammatory Agents
    Lung Transplantation
    Small-Molecule CFTR Modulators
Nonpulmonary Manifestations
    Upper Airway Disorders
    Gastrointestinal Disorders
    Hepatobiliary Disorders
Prognosis

LEARNING OBJECTIVES

After reading this chapter the reader will be able to:

1. Describe how the diagnosis of cystic fibrosis is made
2. Understand the pathophysiology of cystic fibrosis
3. List the common pulmonary manifestations of cystic fibrosis
4. List the common nonpulmonary manifestations of cystic fibrosis
5. List the current treatments used to manage cystic fibrosis pulmonary disease
6. Discuss the overall prognosis of patients with cystic fibrosis

KEY TERMS

Autosomal recessive
Bronchiectasis
Carrier
Cystic fibrosis transmembrane
  conductance regulator

Failure to thrive
Genotype
Heterozygote
Homozygote
Immunoreactive trypsinogen

Meconium ileus
Newborn screening
Pancreatic insufficiency
Phenotype
Sweat chloride test

INTRODUCTION

Cystic fibrosis (CF) is a genetic disorder with primary manifestations in the respiratory, digestive, and reproductive systems caused by dysfunction of the **cystic fibrosis transmembrane conductance regulator** (CFTR). It was first described in 1938 when autopsy studies recognized distinct fibrocystic changes of the glandular ducts in the pancreases of severely malnourished infants.[1]

The signs and symptoms of classic CF are related to the overproduction of thick, viscous secretions in multiple organ systems:

- Chronic obstruction, infection, and inflammation of the airways
- Exocrine **pancreatic insufficiency** with malabsorption and small bowel obstruction
- Infertility in males
- Elevated sweat chloride levels

There is considerable variability in the frequency and severity of clinical manifestations and complications, some of which are discussed in this chapter. Successful care of the child with CF therefore requires a multidisciplinary team approach individualized to the needs of the patient.[2]

EPIDEMIOLOGY

CF has an annual incidence between 1 in 3200 to 3700 live births and a prevalence of approximately 30,000 affected individuals in the United States.[3,4] Disease frequency varies in other racial and ethnic groups: 1 in 9200 Hispanics; 1 in 10,900 Native Americans; 1 in 15,000 African Americans; and 1 in 31,000 Asian Americans.[5] It is estimated that 1 in 28 Caucasians and 1 in 60 African Americans in the United States are carriers.[5] In 2010 the median age at diagnosis was 5 months, down from 6 months in 2000.[6]

GENETICS AND MOLECULAR BIOLOGY

CF is caused by a defect in the CFTR gene located on the long arm of chromosome 7. The gene, which is approximately 189,000 base pairs in length, was first cloned in 1989.[7,8] The mature CFTR protein is comprised of 1480 amino acids and functions as a cyclic adenosine monophosphate–regulated chloride channel that mediates the flow of ions and water across the apical membrane of epithelial cells lining the airways, intestines, vas deferens, biliary tree, sweat ducts, and pancreatic ducts.[9] CFTR dysfunction alters sodium, chloride, and water transport, resulting in thickened, viscous secretions that plug the ducts of these organs.

CF is inherited in an **autosomal recessive** manner.[10] An individual with CF is a **homozygote** possessing two abnormal CFTR alleles. Each parent of a child with CF is an obligate **carrier** (or **heterozygote**), possessing one normal CFTR allele and one mutated allele. Each child of two carriers has a 1 in 4 chance of having CF, a 2 in 4 chance of being an asymptomatic carrier, and a 1 in 4 chance of having two normal alleles. Siblings of an individual with CF have about a 7 in 10 chance of being a carrier; there is a family history in only 17% of newly diagnosed patients.[11]

DIAGNOSIS

The diagnosis of CF is based on the presence of one or more distinguishing clinical features with biochemical or genetic confirmation. Box 28-1 lists signs and symptoms that should prompt a clinician to consider an evaluation for CF. Even though the disease occurs most often in the Caucasian population, it should be considered in the differential diagnosis of a patient of any racial background

---

| **Box 28-1** | **Signs and Symptoms That Should Prompt Evaluation for Cystic Fibrosis** |

RESPIRATORY
- Recurrent wheezing
- Chronic cough
- Frequent thick sputum production
- Severe, prolonged, or recurrent sinopulmonary infections
  - Sinusitis
  - Bronchitis
  - Bronchopneumonia
- Respiratory infections with pathogens associated with cystic fibrosis
  - *Staphylococcus aureus*
  - *Pseudomonas aeruginosa*
  - *Haemophilus influenzae*
  - *Burkholderia cepacia* complex
- Persistently abnormal chest radiograph
  - Hyperinflation
  - Persistent atelectasis
  - Bronchiectasis
- Nasal polyps
- Clubbing of the nail beds

GASTROINTESTINAL
- Failure to thrive
- Frequent, greasy, foul-smelling stools
- Rectal prolapse
- Meconium ileus
- Distal intestinal obstruction syndrome
- Pancreatic insufficiency
- Recurrent pancreatitis

HEPATOBILIARY
- Hepatomegaly
- Portal hypertension
- Focal biliary cirrhosis
- Prolonged neonatal jaundice
- Cholestasis
- Cholelithiasis

REPRODUCTIVE
- Obstructive azoospermia
- Congenital bilateral absence of the vas deferens

NUTRITIONAL DEFICITS
- Fat-soluble vitamin deficiency (vitamins A, D, E, K)
- Hypoproteinemia, with or without edema
- Hypochloremic metabolic alkalosis

---

who presents with these features. Box 28-2 summarizes the diagnostic criteria for CF.[12]

Sweat Chloride Testing

The gold standard for the diagnosis of CF is the **sweat chloride test.** Normal secretion and resorption of chloride in the sweat glands are dependent on adequate CFTR function. A sweat chloride concentration 60 mmol/L or greater confirms the diagnosis. A concentration between 40 and 59 mmol/L in infants older than 6 months is considered intermediate and should be repeated along with CFTR mutation analysis. Normal individuals can occasionally

Box 28-2	Diagnostic Criteria for Cystic Fibrosis

At least one item from each of the following categories must be present:

HISTORY OR CONDITION

Clinical signs or symptoms consistent with cystic fibrosis in at least one organ system

or

Sibling with confirmed cystic fibrosis

or

Positive newborn screening result for cystic fibrosis

LABORATORY TESTING

Sweat chloride level ≥ 60 mmol/L

or

Presence of two disease-causing CFTR mutations

or

Abnormal nasal potential difference

CFTR, Cystic fibrosis transmembrane conductance regulator.

have elevated sweat chloride concentrations not related to CFTR dysfunction.[13]

Sweat chloride testing should be performed according to nationally published guidelines at accredited centers.[14] The sweat is obtained by stimulating the skin on the forearm with pilocarpine iontophoresis (Figure 28-1).[15] Technical error can result in false-negative and false-positive results. In addition to inadequate sweat collection, malnutrition, edema, and hypoalbuminemia can also yield false negative results. Therefore, patients with clinical features suggestive of CF but normal or borderline sweat test results should have the test repeated. Conditions that can produce false-positive results include malnutrition, eczema, adrenal insufficiency, pseudohypoaldosteronism, and hypothyroidism.[16]

CFTR Mutation Analysis

A diagnosis of CF can be confirmed with the identification of two disease-causing CFTR mutations. As of this writing, more than 1900 mutations were listed on the Cystic Fibrosis Mutation Database (www.genet.sickkids.on.ca/cftr/). The most common mutation is a deletion of a phenylalanine residue at position 508 (annotated as F508del or ΔF508), which represents 30% to 80% of all mutations depending on the ethnic group.[17] Mutations are categorized into five functional classes based on the type of defect in the formation of the CFTR protein.[18] Generally, class I through III mutations cause more severe disease compared with class IV or V mutations.[19] There are individuals with recognized CFTR mutations (**genotype**) who may not necessarily have the typical clinical manifestations (**phenotype**) of CF. The CF phenotype-genotype correlation is complex and poses many challenges when trying to develop an rational surveillance and care plan.[20]

Nasal Transepithelial Potential Difference

Measuring the difference in voltage potentials across the nasal epithelium is another method used in the diagnosis of CF, particularly when sweat chloride and CFTR mutation analysis results are inconclusive.[21] However, the availability of this test remains limited, and it should only be performed at experienced centers.[22]

Newborn Screening

As of January 2010, all 50 states and the District of Columbia included CF in standard **newborn screening**.[6] The most common method is measurement of **immunoreactive trypsinogen** (IRT) obtained from a dried heel-stick blood sample. Alternatively, many European countries and many states in the United States combine IRT detection with DNA analysis.[23] Evidence from observational studies

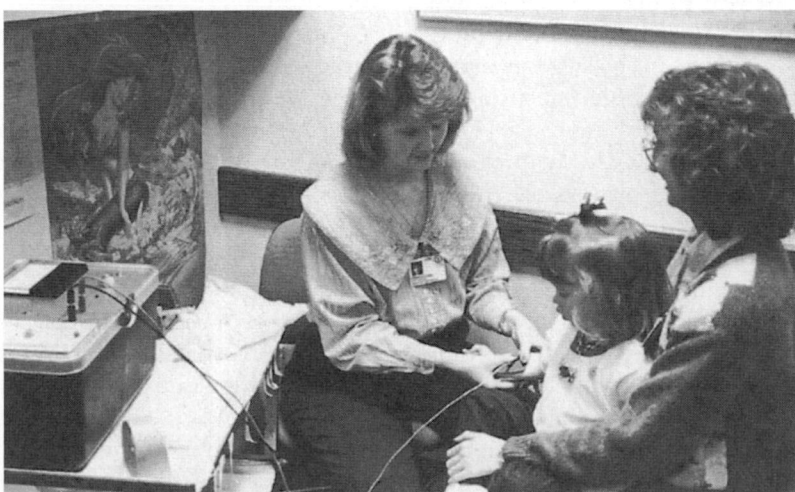

FIGURE 28-1 Sweat test being performed. The child is held in her mother's lap while electrodes are positioned on her forearm to stimulate the skin to produce sweat.

suggest that children with CF identified through newborn screening have benefited from earlier diagnosis and initiation of therapy.[24] Indeed, early diagnosis has helped prevent severe malnutrition and improve long-term growth,[25] and has been associated with reduced therapy.[26]

Not all identified CFTR mutations are associated with clinical disease. There are situations when an infant identified as being at risk for CF with an abnormal newborn screening result does not have a diagnostic sweat chloride value 60 mmol/L or higher or is found to have up to two CFTR mutations, one of which is not recognized as a disease-causing mutation. The term *CFTR-related metabolic syndrome (CRMS)* has recently been proposed as a step toward developing rational guidelines for this unique population of patients with an indeterminate diagnosis.[27] Studies suggest that the course of CRMS may be less severe compared with those with "classic" CF,[28] though long-term prospective data are still lacking.

PULMONARY DISEASE

Although CF is a multisystem disorder, pulmonary disease is the primary cause of morbidity and mortality.[29] As a result of CFTR dysfunction, there is abnormal sodium, chloride, and water transport across the respiratory epithelium. This in turn leads to the production of thick, viscous mucus, with a perpetual cycle of airways obstruction, chronic infection, and airway inflammation.[30] As the disease progresses, there is development of **bronchiectasis,** or abnormal dilation and distortion of the airways. Bronchiectatic airways are more easily collapsible, further perpetuating the cycle of obstruction, infection, and inflammation.

Mucus Production and Airway Obstruction

The lungs of a newborn with CF are histologically normal at birth.[31] However, airway dysfunction appears to begin as early as the first year of life, with the earliest pathological change being thickened mucus and plugging of the submucosal gland ducts in the large airways.[32] These changes appear to precede chronic infection and inflammation.[33]

Goblet cells and submucosal glands are the predominant secretory structures of normal airways. There are an increased number of goblet cells and hypertrophy of submucosal glands in the CF airways,[34] which leads to an increase in secretions and sputum production. Airway secretions are relatively dehydrated and viscous. Thick and viscid mucus is such a common feature that at one time the disease was referred to as "mucoviscidosis".[35]

Mucociliary clearance is variable in CF, with some patients having severe impairment whereas others have normal clearance. The reduction in clearance is believed to be caused by the increased volume of respiratory secretions and the abnormally thick mucus. Studies have shown the cilia from patients with CF to be normal, although chronic inflammation may result in a loss of ciliated cells.[36]

Bacterial Infection

The presence of endobronchial pathogens changes with age. *Staphylococcus aureus* and *Haemophilus influenzae* typically appear early in life, with *S. aureus* reaching maximum prevalence at ages 6 to 17 years and *H. influenzae* peaking at 2 to 5 years of age.[11] A distinctive feature of CF is increased susceptibility to chronic airways colonization and infection with *Pseudomonas aeruginosa*. Median age of acquisition is very early in life, at around 1 year.[37] More than 73% of adults with CF in the United States are chronically infected with *Pseudomonas*.[6] It is strongly associated with accelerated lung function decline and survival.[38,39] Once there is colonization of the airways, *Pseudomonas* is often difficult to eradicate in spite of aggressive antibiotic therapy.[40]

Infection with *Burkholderia cepacia* complex occurs in about 2.5% of patients with CF.[4] It was identified as an important pathogen in CF in the early 1980s.[41] This organism demonstrates in vitro resistance to a number of antibiotics. Infection may result in an acute necrotizing pneumonia and septic shock. Once colonization occurs, there is the possibility of catastrophic deterioration and a poorer prognosis for survival. It is often transmitted either directly or indirectly by person-to-person transmission, with risk factors including hospitalization and having a colonized sibling.[42] The emergence of *B. cepacia* complex has profoundly affected infection control policies and has caused a change in activities and visitation among children with CF.[43] The most common isolates in CF are *B. multivorans* (genomovar II) and *B. cenocepacia* (genomovar III), the latter of which is associated with a more rapid clinical deterioration.[44] The prevalence of methicillin-resistant *S. aureus* (MRSA) has also increased over the last decade[45] and has been associated with poorer outcomes compared with those who have never been culture positive for MRSA.[46]

Patients with CF who do not respond to antimicrobial agents may have colonization of other organisms. These include *Stenotrophomonas maltophilia, Achromobacter xylosoxidans*, nontuberculous mycobacteria (particularly *Mycobacterium avium* complex and *M. abscessus* complex), and *Aspergillus* species.[47]

Airway Inflammation

Inflammation of the airways is a major component of CF and may occur early in the disease process. Recent studies of bronchoalveolar lavage fluid from infants suggest that airway inflammation is present in those as young as 4 weeks old, likely occurring before infection.[48] An abundance of neutrophils and the enzyme neutrophil elastase may be responsible for the airway destruction and inflammatory response found in the lungs of patients with CF.[49]

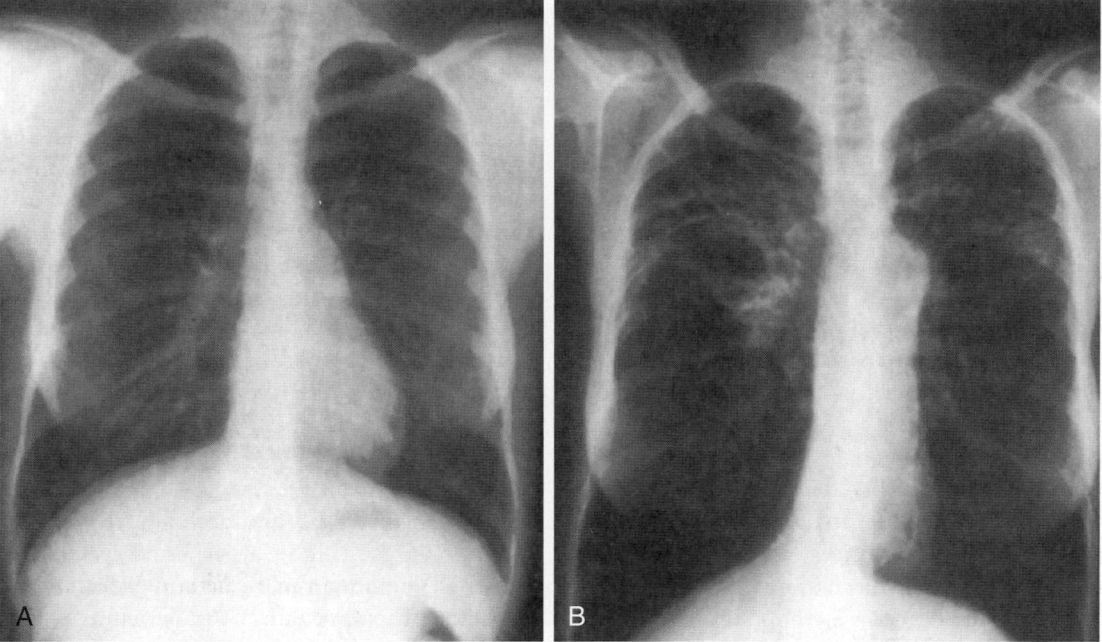

FIGURE 28-2 Cystic fibrosis. Chest radiographs from a patient at ages 14 years (**A**) and 22 years (**B**) illustrating the changes of advancing disease.

Clinical Manifestations

Nearly half of all patients with CF are diagnosed as a result of pulmonary symptoms.[50] The diagnosis of CF should be considered in every patient who presents with chronic or recurrent lower respiratory tract disorders, including bronchitis, bronchiectasis, pneumonia, and refractory asthma. Children with CF have frequent pulmonary exacerbations, with the most consistent feature being a chronic cough. The cough may be dry and hacking, or it can be paroxysmal with the patient gagging, choking, or even vomiting during coughing episodes. Sputum often becomes mucopurulent and difficult to expectorate. Other symptoms include tachypnea, retractions, dyspnea, and use of accessory muscles. Occasionally, patients will present with hemoptysis and fever. Wheezing, crackles, rhonchi, and decreased air exchange are common findings during auscultation of the chest.

The chest radiograph in more advanced disease may show hyperinflation with flattened diaphragms secondary to air trapping (Figure 28-2). Mucus plugging and patchy atelectasis can also be seen. Diffuse fibrosis, bronchial wall thickening, and bronchiectasis are found predominantly in the upper lobes. Over time, however, all of the lung fields become involved. Pneumothorax occurs most often in older patients with more advanced disease and is a result of rupture of subpleural blebs. The recurrence rate is high at 50% to 90%.[51] The progressive lung disease and chronic hypoxemia lead to an increase in pulmonary vascular resistance, pulmonary hypertension, and cor pulmonale. As cor pulmonale progresses, the electrocardiogram shows thickening in the wall and enlargement of the right ventricle.

Pulmonary function testing initially demonstrates air flow obstruction. As the disease progresses, both a restrictive and an obstructive pattern can be seen, along with a decrease in air flow. About 50% of patients with CF have a positive methacholine challenge test, which indicates airway hyperreactivity. Digital clubbing and pulmonary hypertrophic osteoarthropathy are universal findings in CF patients with advanced pulmonary disease. Acute pulmonary exacerbations of CF vary in severity and are usually defined by subjective symptoms. Although there is no clear definition of a CF exacerbation[52,53] most are associated with the characteristics found in Box 28-3.

Box 28-3	**Signs and Symptoms of a Pulmonary Exacerbation in Cystic Fibrosis**

- Increased cough
- Increased sputum production
- Change in sputum appearance
- Hemoptysis
- Dyspnea
- Tachypnea
- Chest pain
- Change in findings of chest physical examination
- Decrease in oxyhemoglobin saturation
- Change in chest radiograph
- Deterioration in pulmonary function
- Fever
- Weight loss
- Decreased appetite
- Increased fatigue
- Decreased exercise tolerance

TREATMENT OF PULMONARY DISEASE

Treatment of the pulmonary manifestations of CF focuses on routine therapy aimed at physically removing thickened mucus from the airways and pharmacological control of infection with the aggressive use of antibiotics.[54] Each of the various components of respiratory care for the child with CF is described in detail.

Aerosol Therapy

Aerosol therapy is an important aspect of CF respiratory care in the hospital and in the home. A number of medications designed to address specific aspects of CF pulmonary disease are used and are described in this section. Put together, a commonly used sequence is as follows: bronchodilator, hypertonic saline, recombinant human DNAse, airway clearance therapy, maintenance medication (inhaled corticosteroid or antibiotic). A more detailed discussion of aerosol therapy can be found in Chapter 11.

Bronchodilators

Airway hyperreactivity is common in the majority of patients with CF.[55] Inhalation of a bronchodilator followed with an airway clearance technique is the most common treatment regimen used routinely between exacerbations. Medications used most often include short-acting β_2 agonists, such as albuterol, and anticholinergic agents such as ipratropium bromide. The medication is delivered with either a metered-dose inhaler or a nebulizer. Although bronchodilators are routinely used, their responsiveness has been shown to be variable in patients with CF.[56,57] Occasionally a patient worsens after bronchodilator therapy.[58] In these patients, treatment with ipratropium bromide has resulted in significant improvement in pulmonary function, especially in adult patients.[59] Some patients respond better to combination therapy using albuterol and/or ipratropium bromide.[60] Finally, it is important to evaluate for allergic bronchopulmonary aspergillosis (ABPA) in situations where there is marked wheezing and deteriorating lung function despite seemingly appropriate medical management.[62]

Mucolytic Agents

The sputum of patients with CF is not only produced in greater abundance but also has abnormal viscosity. This is believed to be caused by increased glycoprotein sulfation and the high concentrations of DNA released from dead neutrophils.[63]

Recombinant human DNAse (rhDNAse) has been developed to reduce the viscosity of purulent CF sputum.[64] The synthetically produced rhDNase breaks up the thickened mucus by disrupting the long, sticky DNA molecules. One study demonstrated significant improvement in lung function of patients with mild pulmonary disease after receiving aerosolized rhDNase.[65a]

Nebulized 7% hypertonic saline is used to facilitate airway clearance by rehydrating airway surface layer. Because hypertonic saline causes bronchospasm in some patients, it is generally recommended to premedicate with a β_2 agonist. In general, it has been found to be an inexpensive, safe, effective additional therapy in CF patients with stable lung function. Its use has been associated with a modest improvement in lung function and reduced frequency of pulmonary exacerbations.[66] A systematic review concluded that incorporation of hypertonic saline is beneficial in the routine care of children with CF more than 6 years of age.[67]

Airway Clearance Therapy

As discussed earlier, the pathophysiology of CF lung disease involves the production of thick, viscous airway secretions resulting in a perpetual cycle of small airways obstruction, inflammation, and infection. Thus airway clearance therapies are a fundamental aspect of routine and acute respiratory care. A more detailed discussion of the various techniques and devices can be found in Chapter 12. There are limited data establishing superiority of any airway clearance therapy modality over others.[68] Thus selection of a particular airway clearance technique or device will largely depend on a combination of factors including patient age, disease severity, tolerance, perceived benefit, feasibility, and personal preference. It is very common for an airway clearance therapy regimen to evolve as the child matures.

Antibiotics

Aerosolized antibiotics such as tobramycin are often used as chronic suppressive therapy to treat patients infected with *P. aeruginosa* to prolong the time between pulmonary exacerbations and to slow the progression of lung function decline. A Cochrane review of inhaled tobramycin for CF concluded that aerosolized antipseudomonal antibiotics improved lung function.[69] A unit dose of 300 mg/5 mL is considered standard. It is given twice a day for 28-day cycles every other month. Additional inhaled antibiotics with antipseudomonal activity include aztreonam and colistin.[70] However, the main focus in the treatment of pulmonary symptoms continues to be secretion removal and antibiotic therapy. Because the airway infection cannot be eradicated, the goal of antibiotic therapy in the treatment of CF is suppression of the infecting organism to a level at which clinical symptoms are minimal.[11]

Antibiotic Selection

Antibiotic therapy is usually given for 2 weeks during pulmonary exacerbations. Antibiotics can be administered orally, by nebulization, or intravenously. The choice of antibiotic is based on results of the individual patient's sputum or throat culture and the in vitro sensitivity profile of the specific organisms. Agents known to be particularly effective against *S. aureus* and *Pseudomonas* species are usually chosen. For patients infected with *P. aeruginosa*, combination therapy with a β-lactam and an aminoglycoside is typically administered. Ciprofloxacin is a common choice for an oral antibiotic. Therapy can be extended to cover *S. aureus* if it is also present in the sputum. Because of abnormal pharmacokinetics of most antibiotics in patients with CF, a higher than normal dose is usually required to achieve therapeutic levels.[11]

Hospitalization

Advances in providing stable long-term vascular access have allowed the intravenous administration of antibiotics at home, with the patient continuing school or work activities.[71] Criteria for proceeding with hospitalization and intravenous therapy include severe illness but also moderate illness that is unresponsive to home therapy or even mild illness complicated by growth failure. If a patient does not respond to outpatient management, hospitalization is recommended with a 10- to 21-day course of intensive antibiotic therapy. Hospitalization for a pulmonary exacerbation also includes aggressive treatment to remove secretions. Despite timely and aggressive medical therapy, one registry study observed that upwards of 25% of patients fail to recover baseline lung function after an exacerbation.[72]

Anti-inflammatory Agents

Because inflammation of the airways is a significant aspect of CF pathophysiology, anti-inflammatory agents are an important part of the treatment regimen.

Macrolide Antibiotics

Macrolide therapy is a relatively recent addition to the list of available anti-inflammatory agents. The specific mechanisms by which they improve CF pulmonary disease is not fully understood but believed in part to be due to its immuno-modulatory effects.[73] Azithromycin is given (in doses of 250 mg or 500 mg for those weighing less than or greater than 40 kg, respectively) three times per week. There are limited data on potential long-term side effects with prolonged therapy, though recent reports have suggested a possible increase in risk for nontuberculous mycobacterial infection.[74]

Corticosteroids

Systemic corticosteroids have been shown in clinical trials to improve lung function; however, side effects are serious and include growth suppression and increased susceptibility to osteoporosis and cataracts.[75] They may, however, play a limited role in the management of acute pulmonary exacerbations.[76] Studies have reported using inhaled corticosteroids in CF with improvement in lung function and respiratory symptoms, but the studies had small sample sizes[77] and they are currently not recommended for routine use unless there is evidence of an asthma component warranting chronic therapy.

Ibuprofen

Ibuprofen has been demonstrated to slow the progression of lung disease over a 2-year period.[78] However, specific dosing and close pharmacokinetic monitoring are required when using this medication.[79]

Lung Transplantation

Lung transplantation is an option for CF patients with severe and end-stage lung disease.[81] There has been no evidence of the redevelopment of CF in the transplanted lungs, but new problems related to lung rejection and opportunistic infection in patients receiving immunosuppressive agents can occur. Although more than 200 patients with CF underwent first-time lung transplantation in 2010,[6] rate of decline of forced expiratory volume in 1 second (FEV_1) as well as worsening of clinical status are key factors in determining the timing of referral for lung transplantation. In addition, the median regional waiting period for donor lungs for patients with CF may assist in the timing of referral. Chapter 21 provides a thorough discussion of lung transplantation.

Small-Molecule CFTR Modulators

With the approval of ivacaftor by the U.S. Food and Drug Administration in January 2012 came a radical shift in the approach to CF care and management. Thus far, all the treatment modalities discussed in this chapter have focused on the downstream effects of CFTR dysfunction. Ivacaftor and other small-molecule CFTR modulators currently in development represent a class of medications specifically designed to reverse the underlying cause of CF-related disease. Ivacaftor is an oral CFTR "potentiator," increasing chloride transport function among individuals with at least one copy of the G551D (class III) mutation.[82] Another class of CFTR modulators are CFTR "correctors," which are designed to facilitate intracellular trafficking of the CFTR protein to the cell surface.[83] The long-term benefits and potential side effects of small-molecule CFTR modulators remain to be seen. Nevertheless, it represents a significant step toward the development of personalized, allele-specific therapy.

NONPULMONARY MANIFESTATIONS

Although pulmonary compromise is the main factor that limits longevity in patients with CF, there are a number of other organ systems affected by the disease. Certain conditions can prompt consideration of the diagnosis of CF. Common conditions include **meconium ileus** (obstruction of the small bowel with meconium in neonates), prolonged neonatal jaundice, rectal prolapse, and **failure to thrive** (global growth failure).

Upper Airway Disorders

Nearly all patients with CF have sinusitis, most often involving the maxillary and ethmoid sinuses. It is often difficult to control in spite of oral and intravenous antibiotic therapy. The abnormally thick mucus that is characteristic of CF occludes the sinus passages and prevents drainage.[84] These patients also have a high incidence of nasal polyps, occurring most often in the older child and adolescent. More than half the patients who require surgical removal of the polyps experience a recurrence. CF should be suspected in children who present with chronic sinusitis and nasal polyposis.

Gastrointestinal Disorders

Pancreatic Insufficiency

More than 90% of patients with CF have pancreatic insufficiency. CFTR dysfunction results in insufficient secretion of pancreatic fluid, which causes plugging and obstruction of the pancreatic ducts. Siblings with CF often share similar degrees of pancreatic insufficiency.[85] Symptoms are controlled with supplementation of pancreatic enzymes. Therapy is individualized to weight and caloric intake, and supplements must be taken at each meal. Formula and breast-feeding infants require supplementation with each feeding, and older children also require supplementation with snacks.

Failure of the pancreas to produce sufficient enzymes results in malabsorption of fat and protein. The presence of steatorrhea, which is excessive loss of fat in the stool, is often the first indication of CF. These children frequently produce bulky, foul-smelling, oily stools and may experience rectal prolapse. Complaints of constipation or stomach cramps, especially after eating, can lead to a decrease in appetite and oral intake. Infants often present with failure to thrive, failing to gain weight in spite of a voracious appetite and meet developmental milestones. Other clinical consequences include hypoproteinemia with or without edema and deficiency of vitamins A, D, E, and K.

The incidence of diabetes mellitus is much greater in children with CF than in the general pediatric population.[88] As fibrosis of the pancreas progresses, endocrine function becomes affected and CF-related diabetes (CFRD) can develop.[86] At 10 years of age, there is an increasing incidence of CFRD and annual screening with an oral glucose tolerance test is recommended.[6] Weight loss is usually the first symptom. Initiation of insulin therapy has been associated with increased body mass and improved lung function.

Meconium Ileus and Distal Intestinal Obstruction Syndrome

Failure to secrete water into the gut is another manifestation of CFTR dysfunction, and abnormal intestinal electrolyte and water transport can lead to a number of disorders. The earliest clinical manifestation of CF may be meconium ileus.[89] Occurring at birth, nearly every full-term infant who has meconium ileus is considered to have CF until proven otherwise. Presentation includes abdominal distention, vomiting, and abdominal radiographs showing distended loops of bowel with gas bubbles trapped among meconium, giving a ground-glass appearance. With an incidence higher in older patients, distal intestinal obstruction syndrome occurs when the thick, sticky stool of the patient with CF adheres to the bowel wall and obstructs the small intestine and colon. Only rarely is this seen in a patient with pancreatic sufficiency.

Rectal Prolapse

Episodes of rectal prolapse are related to malnutrition, abnormal stooling patterns (e.g., diarrhea, constipation), and increased abdominal pressure with frequent coughing. Onset rarely occurs after 5 years of age.[87] The association with CF is so great that a sweat test should be considered in any child presenting with rectal prolapse.

Gastroesophageal Reflux Disease

Patients with CF often experience heartburn and gastric reflux, especially those with advanced pulmonary disease.[90,91] This may be the result of frequent coughing and increased abdominal pressure. Treatment includes dietary restrictions and often long-term acid-suppression therapy with proton pump inhibitors or histamine-2 blockers.

Hepatobiliary Disorders

The hepatobiliary manifestations of CF occur less often than the gastrointestinal disorders. Serious complications are uncommon before adolescence. Cirrhosis and portal hypertension are the most common hepatic disorders that occur in patients with CF, although only 2% to 4% of patients with CF develop any apparent liver disease.[92] Prolonged neonatal jaundice may also occur in neonates and should raise suspicion for CF.

Gallbladder abnormalities are common in patients with CF.[93] Microgallbladder is the most common biliary tract disorder. It is believed that mucus obstruction of the cystic duct results in atrophy of the gallbladder. Most patients are asymptomatic. The incidence of abnormalities increases with age, with gallstones occurring quite commonly in patients with pancreatic insufficiency. Cholecystectomy is considered in patients who are symptomatic with recurrent abdominal pain.

PROGNOSIS

Earlier diagnosis through the recent establishment of nationwide newborn screening and advances in CF care has resulted in continually improving outcomes. In 2010 the median predicted age of survival was 38.3 years, substantially increased from 27 years in 1986.[4] This is a long stride from the life expectancy of less than 1 year when CF was described by Anderson in the late 1930s.[1] Although patients with CF continue to survive longer, some children still succumb to the disease before reaching adulthood in spite of advances in diagnostic techniques and treatment. We know that various factors influence a patient's prognosis, including the progression of pulmonary disease, the involvement of other organ systems, nutritional status, and the home environment. Investigations to better understand and even modify these factors will make a difference in the lives of many children. The respiratory therapist is an essential member of the CF multidisciplinary care team delivering direct care to every patient. In addition, the therapist assesses, teaches, and periodically reviews the most effective airway clearance technique for each patient.

KEY POINTS

- CF is a clinical diagnosis corroborated by laboratory testing (biochemical and/or genetic).
- CFTR dysfunction results in thick and viscous secretions in the airways and other organ systems.
- The majority of CF care and management focuses on the downstream effects of CFTR dysfunction (airway clearance, anti-inflammatory agents, antibiotics, nutrition), though there may soon be an increase in the use of medications that reverse the underlying cause of CF-related disease.
- Though lung disease is the primary cause of morbidity and mortality, there are a number of nonpulmonary manifestations of CF.
- With advancements in many aspects of CF care, overall prognosis continues to improve.

ASSESSMENT QUESTIONS

See Evolve Resources for the answers.

1. Which of the following are true regarding the diagnosis of cystic fibrosis?
   A. The sweat chloride concentration is 60 mmol/L or greater.
   B. CFTR mutation analyses may be helpful when considering a diagnosis of CF.
   C. Nasal transepithelial potential difference measurements may assist in the diagnosis of CF.
   D. There may or may not be a history of CF in a sibling.
   E. All of the above
2. The increased production of thick, viscous airway secretions of a patient with CF are caused by all of the following except:
   A. Abnormal cilia
   B. Increased goblet cells
   C. Hypertrophied submucosal glands
   D. Both A and C

3. CF can present with which of the following signs and symptoms?
   A. Chronic airway obstruction
   B. Pancreatic insufficiency and malnutrition
   C. Male infertility
   D. Clubbing of the nail beds
   E. All of the above
4. Bacterial pathogens commonly encountered in an individual with CF include all of the following except:
   A. *Staphylococcus aureus*
   B. *Pseudomonas aeruginosa*
   C. *Burkholderia cepacia* complex
   D. *Salmonella* species
   E. *Haemophilus influenzae*
5. Which of the following factors influence selection of a particular airway clearance therapy method?
   A. Patient age
   B. Disease severity
   C. Perceived benefit
   D. Personal preference
   E. All of the above
6. Which of the following medications are used in the management of CF pulmonary disease?
   A. Albuterol
   B. Ipratropium bromide
   C. Nebulized antibiotics such as tobramycin
   D. Nebulized 7% hypertonic saline
   E. All of the above
7. The chest radiograph of a patient with cystic fibrosis can have all of the following except:
   A. Hyperinflation with flattened diaphragms
   B. Diffuse fibrosis and bronchiectasis
   C. Blebs and pneumothoraces
   D. Patchy atelectasis
   E. All of the radiographic findings may be seen
8. Which of the following is true regarding small-molecule CFTR modulators?
   A. Ivacaftor, an oral CFTR potentiator, is indicated for all patients with CF.
   B. Unlike other treatments to date, they represent a new class of medications that are designed to reverse the underlying cause of CF-related disease.
   C. Data on the long-term benefits and potential side effects are not yet available.
   D. Both B and C
9. In 2010 the median predicted age of survival among patients with CF was _____ years.
   A. 10
   B. 15
   C. 25
   D. 38
10. The most common upper airway problems encountered by children with CF include:
    A. Nasal polyps
    B. Sinusitis
    C. Croup
    D. Subglottic stenosis
    E. Both A and B

References

1. Anderson DH: Cystic fibrosis of the pancreas and its relation to celiac disease: a clinical and pathological study, *Am J Dis Child* 56:344, 1938.
2. Cohen-Cymberknoh M, Shoseyov D, Kerem E: Managing cystic fibrosis: strategies that increase life expectancy and improve quality of life. *Am J Respir Crit Care Med* 183:1463, 2011.
3. Rosenstein BJ, Cutting GR: The diagnosis of cystic fibrosis: a consensus statement. Cystic Fibrosis Foundation Consensus Panel, *J Pediatr* 132:589, 1998.
4. National Newborn Screening and Genetics Resource Center: *National newborn screening report—2000*, Austin, TX, 2003, NNSGRC.
5. Hamosh A, FitzSimmons SC, Macek M Jr, et al: Comparison of the clinical manifestations of cystic fibrosis in black and white patients, *J Pediatr* 132:255, 1998.
6. *Patient Registry Annual Data Report 2010*. Bethesda, MD, 2011, Cystic Fibrosis Foundation.
7. Cutting GR: Cystic fibrosis. In Rimoin DL, Connor JM, Pyeritz RD, editors: *Emery and Rimoin's principles and practice of medical genetics*, London, 1997, Churchill Livingstone, pp 2685.
8. Kerem B, Rommens JM, Buchanan JA, et al: Identification of the cystic fibrosis gene: genetic analysis, *Science* 245:1073, 1989.
9. Guggino WB, Banks-Schlegel SP: Macromolecular interactions and ion transport in cystic fibrosis, *Am J Respir Crit Care Med* 170:815, 2004.
10. Steen CD: Cystic fibrosis: inheritance, genetics and treatment, *Br J Nurs* 6:192, 1997.
11. Davis PB: Autonomic and airway reactivity in obligate heterozygotes for cystic fibrosis, *Am Rev Respir Dis* 129:911, 1984.
12. LeGrys VA: Sweat testing for the diagnosis of cystic fibrosis: practical consideration, *J Pediatr* 129:892, 1996.
13. Mishra A, Greaves R, Smith K, et al: Diagnosis of cystic fibrosis by sweat testing: age-specific reference intervals, *J Pediatr* 153:758, 2008.
14. LeGrys VA, Yankaskas JR, Quittell LM, et al: Diagnostic sweat testing: the Cystic Fibrosis Foundation guidelines, *J Pediatr* 151:85, 2007.
15. MacLean WC Jr, Tripp RW: Cystic fibrosis with edema and falsely negative sweat test, *J Pediatr* 83:86, 1973.
16. Worldwide survey of the delta F508 mutation—report from the Cystic Fibrosis Genetic Analysis Consortium, *Am J Hum Genet* 47:354, 1990.
17. Moskowitz SM, Chmiel JF, Sternen DL, et al: Clinical practice and genetic counseling for cystic fibrosis and CFTR-related disorders, *Genet Med* 10:851, 2008.
18. Kerem E: Pharmacological induction of CFTR function in patients with cystic fibrosis: mutation-specific therapy, *Pediatr Pulmonol* 40:183, 2005.
19. McKone EF, Emerson SS, Edwards KL, Aitken ML: Effect of genotype on phenotype and mortality in cystic fibrosis: a retrospective cohort study, *Lancet* 361:1671, 2003.
20. Bombieri C, Claustres M, De Boeck K, et al: Recommendations for the classification of diseases as CFTR-related disorders, *J Cyst Fibros* 10:S86, 2011.
21. Sermet-Gaudelus I, Girodon E, Sands D, et al: Clinical phenotype and genotype of children with borderline sweat test and abnormal nasal epithelial chloride transport, *Am J Respir Crit Care Med* 182:929, 2010.
22. Boyle MP, Diener-West M, Milgram L, et al: A multicenter study of the effect of solution temperature on nasal potential difference measurements, *Chest* 124:482, 2003.
23. Farrell PM, Rosenstein BJ, White TB, et al: Guidelines for diagnosis of cystic fibrosis in newborns through older adults: Cystic Fibrosis Foundation consensus report, *J Pediatr* 153:S4, 2008.
24. Balfour-Lynn IM: Newborn screening for cystic fibrosis: evidence for benefit, *Arch Dis Child* 93:7, 2008.
25. Farrell PM, Kosorok MR, Rock MJ, et al: Early diagnosis of cystic fibrosis through neonatal screening prevents severe malnutrition and improves long-term growth. Wisconsin Cystic Fibrosis Neonatal Screening Study Group, *Pediatrics* 107:1, 2001.
26. Sims EJ, Clark A, McCormick J, et al: Cystic fibrosis diagnosed after 2 months of age leads to worse outcomes and requires more therapy, *Pediatrics* 119:19, 2007.
27. Cystic Fibrosis Foundation, Borowitz D, Parad RB, et al: Cystic Fibrosis Foundation practice guidelines for the management of infants with cystic fibrosis transmembrane conductance regulator-related metabolic syndrome during the first two years of life and beyond, *J Pediatr* 155:S106, 2009.
28. Ren CL, Desai H, Platt M, Dixon M: Clinical outcomes in infants with cystic fibrosis transmembrane conductance regulator (CFTR) related metabolic syndrome, *Pediatr Pulmonol* 46:1079, 2011.
29. Rosenfeld M, Emerson J, McNamara S, et al: Risk factors for age at initial *Pseudomonas* acquisition in the cystic fibrosis EPIC observational cohort, *J Cyst Fibros* 11:446, 2012.
30. Ratjen FA: Cystic fibrosis: pathogenesis and future treatment strategies, *Respir Care* 54:595, 2009.
31. Lamb D, Reid L: The tracheobronchial submucosal glands in cystic fibrosis: a qualitative and quantitative histochemical study, *Br J Dis Chest* 66:239, 1972.
32. Zuelzer WW, Newton WA Jr: The pathogenesis of fibrocystic disease of the pancreas: a study of 36 cases with special reference to the pulmonary lesions, *Pediatrics* 4:53, 1949.
33. Katz SM, Holsclaw DS Jr: Ultrastructural features of respiratory cilia in cystic fibrosis, *Am J Clin Pathol* 73:682, 1980.
34. Hays SR, Ferrando RE, Carter R, et al: Structural changes to airway smooth muscle in cystic fibrosis, *Thorax* 60:226, 2005.
35. Farber S: Pancreatic function and disease in early life v. pathologic changes associated with pancreatic insufficiency in early life, *Arch Pathol* 37:238, 1944.
36. Thomassen MJ, Demko CA, Doershuk CF: Cystic fibrosis: a review of pulmonary infections and interventions, *Pediatr Pulmonol* 3:334, 1987.
37. Li Z, Kosorok MR, Farrell PM, et al: Longitudinal development of mucoid *Pseudomonas aeruginosa* infection and lung disease progression in children with cystic fibrosis, *JAMA* 293:581, 2005.
38. Rosenfeld M, Gibson RL, McNamara S, et al: Early pulmonary infection, inflammation, and clinical outcomes in infants with cystic fibrosis, *Pediatr Pulmonol* 32:356, 2001.
39. Emerson J, Rosenfeld M, McNamara S, et al: *Pseudomonas aeruginosa* and other predictors of mortality and morbidity in young children with cystic fibrosis, *Pediatr Pulmonol* 34:91, 2002.
40. Li Z, Kosorok MR, Farrell PM, et al: Longitudinal development of mucoid *Pseudomonas aeruginosa* infection and lung disease progression in children with cystic fibrosis, *JAMA* 293:581, 2005.
41. Isles A, Maclusky I, Corey M, et al: *Pseudomonas cepacia* infection in cystic fibrosis: an emerging problem, *J Pediatr* 104:206, 1984.
42. Khan TZ, Wagener JS, Bost T, et al: Early pulmonary inflammation in infants with cystic fibrosis, *Am J Respir Crit Care Med* 151:1075, 1995.

43. Mahenthiralingam E, Baldwin A, Dowson CG: *Burkholderia cepacia* complex bacteria: opportunistic pathogens with important natural biology, *J Appl Microbiol* 104:1539, 2008.

44. Jones AM, Dodd ME, Govan JR, et al: *Burkholderia cenocepacia* and *Burkholderia multivorans*: influence on survival in cystic fibrosis, *Thorax* 59:948, 2004.

45. Goss CH, Muhlebach MS: Review: *Staphylococcus aureus* and MRSA in cystic fibrosis, *J Cyst Fibrosis* 10:298, 2011.

46. Dasenbrook EC, Checkley W, Merlo CA, et al: Association between respiratory tract methicillin-resistant *Staphylococcus aureus* and survival in cystic fibrosis, *JAMA* 303:2386, 2010.

47. Emerson J, McNamara S, Buccat AM, et al: Changes in cystic fibrosis sputum microbiology in the United States between 1995 and 2008, *Pediatr Pulmonol* 45:363, 2010.

48. Suter S, Schaad UB, Roux L, et al: Granulocyte neutral proteases and *Pseudomonas* elastase as possible causes of airway damage in patients with cystic fibrosis, *J Infect Dis* 149:523, 1984.

49. Wistrak BJ, Meyer CM, Cotton RT: Cystic fibrosis presenting with sinus disease in children, *Am J Dis Child* 147:258, 1993.

50. Spector ML, Stern RC: Pneumothorax in cystic fibrosis: a 26-year experience, *Ann Thorac Surg* 47:204, 1989.

51. Flume PA: Pneumothorax in cystic fibrosis, *Curr Opin Pulm Med* 17:220, 2011.

52. Goss CH, Burns JL: Exacerbations in cystic fibrosis. 1: Epidemiology and pathogenesis, *Thorax* 62:360, 2007.

53. Rosenfeld M, Emerson J, Williams-Warren J, et al: Defining a pulmonary exacerbation in cystic fibrosis, *J Pediatr* 139:359, 2001.

54. Cystic Fibrosis Foundation, Borowitz D, Robinson KA, et al: Cystic Fibrosis Foundation evidence-based guidelines for management of infants with cystic fibrosis, *J Pediatr* 155:S73, 2009.

55. Pattishall EN: Longitudinal response of pulmonary function to bronchodilators in cystic fibrosis, *Pediatr Pulmonol* 9:80, 1990.

56. Kattan M, Mansell A, Levison H, et al: Response to aerosol salbutamol, SCH 1000, and placebo in cystic fibrosis, *Thorax* 35:531, 1980.

57. Hordvik NL, Sammut PH, Judy CG, et al: The effects of albuterol on the lung function of hospitalized patients with cystic fibrosis, *Am J Respir Crit Care Med* 154:156, 1996.

58. Zach MS, Oberwaldner B, Forche G, Polgar G: Bronchodilators increase airway instability in cystic fibrosis, *Am Rev Respir Dis* 131:537, 1985.

59. Weintraub SJ, Eschenbacher WL: The inhaled bronchodilators ipratropium bromide and metaproterenol in adults with CF, *Chest* 95:861, 1989.

60. Sanchez I, Holbrow J, Chernick V: Acute bronchodilator response to a combination of beta-adrenergic and anticholinergic agents in patients with cystic fibrosis, *J Pediatr* 120:486, 1992.

61. Deleted in pages.

62. Stevens DA, Moss RB, Kurup VP, Cystic Fibrosis Foundation Consensus Conference, et al: Allergic bronchopulmonary aspergillosis in cystic fibrosis—state of the art, *Clin Infect Dis* 37:S225, 2003.

63. Shak S, Capon DJ, Hellmiss R, Marsters SA, et al: Recombinant human DNase I reduces the viscosity of cystic fibrosis sputum, *Proc Natl Acad Sci U S A* 87:9188, 1990.

64. Shak S: Aerosolized recombinant human DNAse I for the treatment of cystic fibrosis, *Chest* 107:65S, 1995.

65. Deleted in pages.

65a. Quan JM, Tiddens HA, Sy JP, et al: A two-year randomized, placebo-controlled trial of dornase alfa in young patients with cystic fibrosis with mild lung function abnormalities, *J Pediatr* 139:813, 2001.

66. Donaldson SH, Bennett WD, Zeman KL, et al: Mucus clearance and lung function in cystic fibrosis with hypertonic saline, *N Engl J Med* 354:241, 2006.

67. Wark P, McDonald VM: Nebulised hypertonic saline for cystic fibrosis, *Cochrane Database Syst Rev* CD0011506, 2009.

68. Flume PA, Robinson KA, O'Sullivan BP, et al: Cystic fibrosis pulmonary guidelines: airway clearance therapies, *Respir Care* 54:522, 2009.

69. Ryan G, Mukhopadhyay S, Singh M: Nebulised antipseudomonal antibiotics for cystic fibrosis, *Cochrane Database Syst Rev* CD001021, 2003.

70. Jensen T, Pedersen SS, Garne S, et al: Colistin inhalation therapy in cystic fibrosis patients with chronic *Pseudomonas aeruginosa* lung infection, *J Antimicrob Chemother* 19:831, 1987.

71. Ramsey B, Richardson MA: Impact of sinusitis in cystic fibrosis, *J Allergy Clin Immunol* 90:547, 1992.

72. Sanders DB, Bittner RC, Rosenfeld M, et al: Failure to recover baseline pulmonary function after cystic fibrosis pulmonary exacerbation, *Am J Resp Crit Care Med* 182:627, 2010.

73. Wagner T, Burns JL: Anti-inflammatory properties of macrolides, *Pediatr Infect Dis* 26:75, 2007.

74. Renna M, Schaffner C, Brown K, et al: Azithromycin blocks autophagy and may predispose cystic fibrosis patients to mycobacterial infection, *J Clin Invest* 121:3554, 2011.

75. van Haren EH, Lammers JW, Festen J, et al: The effects of inhaled corticosteroid budesonide on lung function and bronchial hyperresponsiveness in adult patients with cystic fibrosis, *Respir Med* 89:209, 1995.

76. Hester KL, Powell T, Downey DG, et al: Glucocorticoids as an adjuvant treatment to intravenous antibiotics for cystic fibrosis pulmonary exacerbations: a UK Survey, *J Cyst Fibros* 6:311, 2007.

77. Nikolaizik WH, Schoni MH: Pilot study to assess the effect of inhaled corticosteroids on lung function in patients with cystic fibrosis, *J Pediatr* 128:271, 1996.

78. Konstan MW, Byard PJ, Hoppel CL, Davis PB: Effect of high-dose ibuprofen in patients with cystic fibrosis, *N Engl J Med* 332:848, 1995.

79. Konstan MW, Schluchter MD, Xue W, Davis PB: Clinical use of ibuprofen is associated with slower FEV1 decline in children with cystic fibrosis, *Am J Respir Crit Care Med* 176:1084, 2007.

80. Deleted in pages.

81. Braun AT, Merlo CA: Cystic fibrosis lung transplantation, *Curr Opin Pulm Med* 17:467, 2011.

82. Ramsey BW, Davies J, McElvaney NG, et al: A CFTR potentiator in patients with cystic fibrosis and the G551D mutation, *N Engl J Med* 365:1663, 2011.

83. Van Goor F, Hadida S, Grootenhuis PD, et al: Correction of the F508del-CFTR protein processing defect in vitro by the investigational drug VX-809, *Proc Natl Acad Sci U S A* 108:18843, 2011.

84. Drake-Lee AB, Morgan DW: Nasal polyps and sinusitis in children with cystic fibrosis, *J Laryngol Otol* 103:753, 1989.

85. Corey M, Durie P, Moore D, et al: Familial concordance of pancreatic function in cystic fibrosis, *J Pediatr* 115:274, 1989.

86. Moran A, Diem P, Klein DJ, et al: Pancreatic endocrine function in cystic fibrosis, *J Pediatr* 118:715, 1991.

87. Stern RC, Izant RJ Jr, Boat TF, et al: Treatment and prognosis of rectal prolapse in cystic fibrosis, *Gastroenterology* 82:707, 1982.

88. Moran A, Brunzell C, Cohen RC, et al: Clinical care guidelines for cystic fibrosis–related diabetes: a position statement

of the American Diabetes Association and a clinical practice guideline of the Cystic Fibrosis Foundation, endorsed by the Pediatric Endocrine Society, *Diabetes Care* 33:2697, 2010.

89. Riordan JR, Rommens JM, Kerem B, et al: Identification of the cystic fibrosis gene: cloning and characterization of complementary DNA, *Science* 245:1066, 1989.

90. Scott RB, O'Loughlin EV, Gall DG: Gastroesophageal reflux in patients with cystic fibrosis, *J Pediatr* 106:223, 1985.

91. Malfroot A, Dab I: New insights on gastro-oesophageal reflux in cystic fibrosis by longitudinal follow up, *Arch Dis Child* 66:1339, 1991.

92. Colombo C: Liver disease in cystic fibrosis, *Curr Opin Pulm Med* 13:529, 2007.

93. Stern RC, Rothstein FC, Doershuk CF: Treatment and prognosis of symptomatic gallbladder disease in patients with cystic fibrosis, *J Pediatr Gastroenterol Nutr* 5:35, 1986.

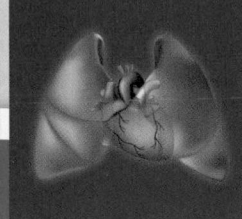

Chapter 29

Acute Respiratory Distress Syndrome

JAN HAU LEE, IRA M. CHEIFETZ

LEARNING OBJECTIVES

After reading this chapter, the reader will be able to:

1. Define the criteria to diagnose acute respiratory distress syndrome
2. Describe the pathological stages of acute respiratory distress syndrome
3. Describe the pathophysiology of acute respiratory distress syndrome
4. Explain the clinical approach to the management of the patient with acute respiratory distress syndrome
5. Apply appropriate ventilator strategies in conventional mechanical ventilation of patients with acute respiratory distress syndrome
6. Outline adjunct therapies in the management in the management of acute respiratory distress syndrome
7. Understand the role of high-frequency ventilation and extracorporeal membrane oxygenation in the management of acute respiratory distress syndrome

KEY TERMS

Acute lung injury
Acute respiratory distress syndrome
Hypoxemia

Inflammatory mediators
Lower inflection point
Low tidal volume ventilation

Open lung strategy
Oxygenation index
Permissive hypercapnia

Acute respiratory distress syndrome (ARDS) represents an acute lung injury characterized by pulmonary edema and alveolar collapse secondary to the disruption of the alveolar-capillary membrane and surfactant dysfunction. Subsequently hypoxemia and widespread infiltrates on chest radiograph can occur after a variety of pulmonary and nonpulmonary insults. Pulmonary edema in the absence of heart failure was initially described almost a century ago. These conditions were originally known by the inciting injury rather than the overall clinical manifestation and included such names as shock lung, noncardiogenic pulmonary edema, and traumatic wet lung.[1] In 1967, Ashbaugh and colleagues[2] recognized ARDS in 12 patients as a constellation of pathophysiological findings that were precipitated by a variety of insults, highlighting ARDS as a final common pathway initiated by local or systemic insults.

DEFINITION

The simplest clinical definition of ARDS is a diffuse, hypoxemic acute lung injury. Radiographically, there are bilateral

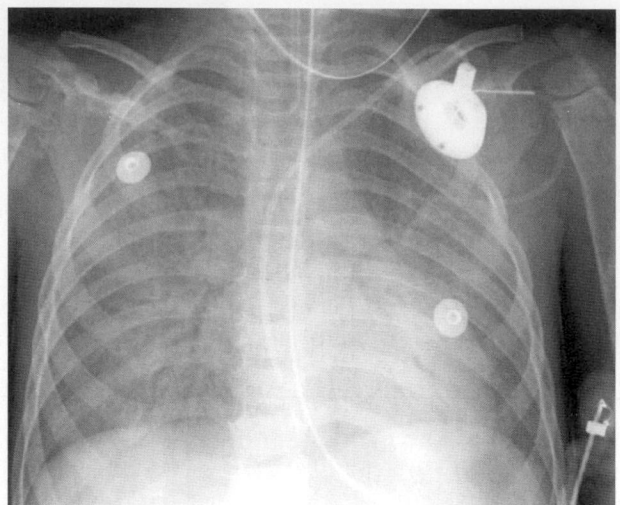

FIGURE 29-1 Chest radiograph of a patient with ARDS. Note the infiltrates in all five lobes, the air bronchograms that appear as a result of areas of consolidation, and the loss of lung volume.

areas of consolidation with air bronchograms that reflect alveolar filling and atelectasis (Figure 29-1). Clinically, the patient demonstrates moderate to severe respiratory failure, hypoxemia, and decreased pulmonary compliance. In 1994 the American-European Consensus Conference on ARDS (AECC) was charged to formally define ARDS, provide uniformity and clarity in diagnosis, and facilitate comparison of clinical investigations (Table 29-1).[3] However, the AECC definition has several limitations. The time frame of "acute onset" was not specifically defined; there was often moderate interobserver variability in defining bilateral infiltrates on chest radiographs, and some patients with ARDS have elevated pulmonary artery wedge pressure because of increased pleural pressure or aggressive fluid resuscitation. Despite these limitations, the AECC definition has facilitated conduct of many landmark trials in ARDS.

To address these limitations, a consensus panel was held in Berlin in 2011 to revise the definition for ARDS (see Table 29-1).[4,5]

In contrast to the AECC definition, the Berlin definition specifies the time frame for the development of ARDS, better defines the nature of infiltrates on radiological investigations, moves away from the need for invasive pulmonary artery measurements if risk factors for ARDS are present, incorporates positive end-expiratory pressure (PEEP) in the definition of severity of hypoxemia, and finally merges the previous term **acute lung injury** (ALI) into the subgroup of mild ARDS.

An alternative objective scoring system used in the clinical setting of ARDS is the **oxygenation index** (OI)[6-9]:

$$OI = (\overline{Paw} \times FIO_2) / PaO_2 \times 100$$

where $\overline{Paw}$ is the mean airway pressure, FIO_2 is the fraction of inspired oxygen, and PaO_2 is the arterial oxygen tension. The OI equation accounts not only for the ratio of administered FIO_2 to arterial oxygenation but also the mean airway pressure during mechanical ventilation support. OI has been correlated with outcome, can be objectively used to define entry or response criteria for clinical studies, and can describe criteria for more highly invasive therapies such as extracorporeal membrane oxygenation (ECMO).[6-9] Whether the degree of hypoxemia as provided by the Berlin definition in determining severity of ARDS correlates well with OI remains to be determined.

ETIOLOGY

ARDS can be caused by numerous insults (risk factors) that both directly and indirectly affect the lung via the generation of **inflammatory mediators.** Direct pulmonary insults include pneumonia, aspiration, chest trauma, and smoke inhalation. Indirect lung injury may be the

TABLE 29-1

Comparison Between the AECC's Definition and the Berlin Definition of ARDS

	AECC Definition 1994[3]	Berlin Definition 2011[4,5]
Time of onset of respiratory symptoms	Acute	Within 1 week of known clinical insult or new/worsening respiratory symptoms.
Radiological findings	Frontal CXR with bilateral infiltrates	Bilateral opacities that are not fully explained by effusions, lobar/lung collapse, or nodules. Can be either on CXR or CT scan.
Degree of hypoxemia	ALI: PaO_2: $FIO_2 < 300$ ARDS: $PaO_2/FIO_2 \leq 200$	With PEEP ≥ 5 Mild ARDS: PaO_2/FIO_2 201-300 Moderate ARDS: $PaO_2/FIO_2 \leq 200$ Severe ARDS: $PaO_2/FIO_2 \leq 100$
Origin of pulmonary edema	No clinical evidence of left atrial hypertension as defined by a pulmonary artery wedge pressure ≤ 18 mm Hg, if measured	Risk factors for ARDS must be present. Respiratory failure that is not fully explained by cardiac failure or fluid overload. If no risk factors are present, objective assessment (e.g., echocardiography) is required to exclude hydrostatic edema.

AECC, American-European Consensus Conference on ARDS; *ALI,* acute lung injury; *ARDS,* acute respiratory distress syndrome; *CXR,* chest radiograph; *CT,* computed tomography; *FIO₂,* fraction of inspired oxygen; *PaO₂,* arterial oxygen tension; *PEEP,* positive end-expiratory pressure.

result of generalized systemic conditions, such as sepsis, closed head injury, multiple trauma, transfusion reactions, and hemorrhagic shock. Although numerous insults may generate an inflammatory response, innate genetic differences regulate the immune responses of the lungs and are important in pathogenesis and determining mortality from ARDS.[10,11]

PREVALENCE

The diversity of underlying etiologies makes it difficult to determine the true prevalence of ARDS. Several studies agree that of all adult intensive care unit (ICU) admissions approximately 7% of patients meet the AECC ARDS diagnosis criteria.[3,8,12,13] A European study (ALIVE) involving 78 ICUs from 9 countries in which all patients (n = 5457) were admitted to one of the participating units for at least 4 hours during a 2-month study period reported that 7.4% had, or developed, ALI/ARDS.[14] However, this study noted considerable variations in the occurrence of ALI/ARDS among countries ranging from 1.7% to 19.5%.[14] This study indicates that although diagnostic criteria may be the same, interpretation and/or true prevalence of ARDS does vary between countries and possibly within countries. Future epidemiological studies in ARDS using the Berlin definition will hopefully give more robust data.

The prevalence of pediatric ARDS appears to be lower than for adults.[15,16] In a large study (n = 6235) conducted in the United States, 828 (13%) patients who required mechanical ventilation had ARDS. This study reported an incidence rate of 16 per 100,000 person-years for patients 15 to 19 years old compared with an incidence rate of 306 per 100,000 person-years for patients 75 to 84 years old.[15] In a follow-up study involving children younger than 18 years, the incidence rate was 12.8 per 100,000 person-years.[16] A more recent study conducted in Europe involving 21 pediatric ICUs (PICUs) showed a much lower incidence rate of 3.9 per 100,000 person-years in children 15 years old or younger.[17] The low incidence of ARDS in children is also reflected by the fact that ARDS accounted for a small proportion (1.4% to 2.7%) of all PICU admissions.[18,19]

CLINICAL COURSE

Respiratory distress and failure are clinical diagnoses of a pulmonary system that is no longer capable of providing normal gas exchange. The term *respiratory distress* indicates that the patient is using compensatory mechanisms to preserve adequate gas exchange. Respiratory failure is a late clinical finding resulting from the failure of these compensatory mechanisms.

Respiratory failure indicates the need for either noninvasive or invasive respiratory support. The main function of the respiratory system is to provide adequate oxygenation and carbon dioxide elimination. In the setting of acute respiratory failure, the lungs are unable to preserve adequate gas exchange. Subsequently, tissue oxygen delivery can be impaired, resulting in anaerobic metabolism and lactic acid formation. Additionally, ventilation can be inadequate resulting in hypercapnia and worsening acidosis. In patients with ARDS, impairment of oxygenation is an early finding, whereas impairment of ventilation occurs much later in the disease process.[20]

Respiratory disease, especially in infants and young children, can rapidly progress from respiratory distress to the acute onset of respiratory failure and significant impairment in gas exchange. Although respiratory failure is classically described by arterial blood gas values (PaO_2 less than 60 mm Hg and/or $PaCO_2$ greater than 50 mm Hg), clinically it is best recognized at the bedside as a syndrome of the progression of the physical signs and symptoms of respiratory distress. Infants and young children are particularly prone to developing respiratory distress and failure because of the following:

- Smaller caliber of airways resulting in a greater resistance to air flow
- Increased chest wall compliance, which can cause paradoxical breathing and restrict lung capacitance as a result of chest wall retractions as may occur with forceful inspiratory effort
- Greater propensity for rapid fatigue of the respiratory muscles and the diaphragm

However, the progression of respiratory failure to ARDS is more likely to occur in adult patients as indicated by the prevalence data as described earlier.[15,16]

Stages of ARDS

The clinical course of ARDS is characterized by distinct clinical, radiographic, and pathological manifestations.[21] The first stage consists of direct or indirect acute injury to the lung tissue. Clinically patients may display mild tachypnea and dyspnea and tend to have normal radiographic findings. The second stage, or latent period, lasts a variable period after the onset of acute injury. During this time the patient may appear clinically stable but begins to develop early signs of pulmonary injury or insufficiency manifested by hyperventilation with hypocarbia and respiratory alkalosis. The chest radiograph may remain clear or may begin to demonstrate a fine reticular pattern related to the development of pulmonary interstitial fluid.[22,23]

The third stage, acute respiratory failure, is heralded by the rapid onset of respiratory failure with hypoxemia refractory to supplemental oxygen. Diffuse pulmonary edema and worsening compliance cause significant atelectasis and intrapulmonary shunting. Clinically patients develop rapid, shallow tachypnea with increased work of breathing. The physical signs of respiratory failure vary with age and include subcostal and supraclavicular retractions, grunting (i.e., an attempt to generate an increased intrinsic PEEP), nasal flaring, and head bobbing. Lung examination usually reveals diffuse crackles on auscultation.

Radiographically there are bilateral areas of consolidation with air bronchograms that reflect alveolar filling and atelectasis (see Figure 29-1).[22,23] A significant percentage of these patients will require endotracheal intubation and mechanical ventilation. However, noninvasive ventilation may be an alternative for a subgroup of patients with mild ARDS.[24,25]

Mortality

Most studies indicate that mortality associated with ARDS is due to nonrespiratory causes (i.e., patients die *with*, rather than *of*, ARDS).[13,26,27] In a cohort study of 416 adult patients with ARDS over a span of 8 years, Stapleton et al. reported that sepsis syndrome with multiple organ failure (MOF) is the most common cause of mortality (30% to 50%), whereas respiratory failure only accounted for a small percentage (13% to 19%) of deaths.[28] The severity of hypoxemia in ARDS is a risk factor for mortality. This is evident from increasing mortality rates in the three different groups under the Berlin definition (mortality rate of 27% [mild] vs. 32% [moderate] vs. 45% [severe]).[4] However, given the fact that most patients with ARDS die from causes other than directly from respiratory failure, other factors also modulate the mortality in patients with ARDS. In adults, these factors include age, severity of disease, and predisposing conditions for ARDS.[29]

Recent published systematic reviews suggest that mortality from ARDS is declining[30,31]; however, the reason behind this overall improvement in outcome is not clear. Except for low tidal volume ventilation, no single intervention for adult ARDS has been clearly shown to decrease mortality.[32] This highlights the pressing need for development of effective management strategies for ARDS.

Mortality rates for pediatric ARDS are generally accepted as lower compared with adults ARDS. A large report of 328 PICU admissions for ARDS indicated a mortality rate of 22%.[33] This prospective evaluation additionally demonstrated that, as in adults, pneumonia, sepsis, and aspiration are the most common causes of ALI and ARDS in children. More recent data, albeit involving a smaller number of children with ARDS, showed a fairly similar mortality rate of 18%.[16]

PATHOLOGY AND ROLE OF IMMUNOMODULATORS

Pathology/Pathophysiology

The clinical stages of ARDS coincide with three pathological stages, namely the exudative stage, the proliferative stage, and the fibrotic stage. The exudative stage is marked by the development of diffuse injury to the alveolar-capillary membrane. Influx of inflammatory cells and mediators destroy type I pneumocytes, resulting in sloughing of these cells and subsequent formation of a protein-rich hyaline membrane on the denuded basement membrane. Furthermore, activation of the endothelium and leukocytes results in barrier

dysfunction and the formation of microthrombi within the vasculature, which contributes to the propagation of acute lung injury and alterations in pulmonary vascular tone. Disruption of both the epithelial and endothelial surfaces of the alveolar-capillary membrane significantly increases permeability and results in flooding of the alveoli with proteinaceous fluid.

The loss of the alveolar-capillary integrity and the subsequent development of pulmonary edema in both the interstitial and alveolar spaces are due to both altered capillary permeability and oncotic gradients early in the disease process and to increases in pulmonary vascular resistance in later stages of ARDS. Pulmonary compliance is significantly worsened by the presence of edema and can result in widespread atelectasis. Pulmonary compliance is further impacted by the inactivation of surfactant that results from the presence of plasma protein, such as fibrin, and inflammatory mediators, such as proteinases, in the alveolar space.[34,35] The development of microthrombi within the pulmonary vasculature together with the release of numerous vasoactive mediators from inflammatory cells and the activated endothelium contributes to the development of pulmonary hypertension and further contributes to the ventilation/perfusion abnormalities characteristic of ARDS. The degree of epithelial injury and the subsequent ability to clear edema fluid, as well as the reversibility of pulmonary hypertension, are important predictors of outcome in ARDS.[36,37]

The proliferative stage occurs 1 to 3 weeks after the initiation of injury and is characterized by an attempt to repair the disrupted epithelium. This involves the proliferation of type II pneumocytes to replace type I cells on the denuded basement membrane and to begin to replace surfactant. Although the turnover of type II cells is typically low, it accelerates after acute lung injury, and these cells may differentiate abnormally.[38,39] Epithelial repair requires not only the close coordination of numerous growth factors but also an intact basement membrane to provide a platform for cell adhesion and migration.[40] Inflammatory cells continue to be recruited to phagocytose hyaline membrane and debris, which provides a framework for the elaboration of fibrous tissue.[41] Alternatively, fibroblasts proliferate to convert hemorrhagic exudates into cellular granulation tissue.

The ability of the lung to recover depends on the presence of functional epithelium to clear the alveolar fluid and the body's ability to attenuate the inflammatory process. If lung injury and inflammation persist, the patient may develop severe physiological abnormalities and may progress to the fibrotic stage of ARDS. This injury can be seen as early as 5 to 7 days after the onset of disease, although this is more definitive after several weeks. Histologically, the alveolar space becomes filled with mesenchymal cells, and lung tissue is replaced by collagenous tissue.[42] In addition, there is increased evidence of angiogenesis (new growth of blood vessels from preexisting ones). Vascular changes occur throughout the later stages of ARDS with obliteration of small precapillary vessels and an increase in the medial thickness of intraacinar pulmonary arteries. Overall, these changes markedly decrease the available surface area for gas exchange and result in intractable respiratory failure or chronic lung disease, potentially requiring prolonged ventilator support. Treatment strategies seek to avoid this final, intractable stage of ARDS.

Inflammatory Mediators

Numerous mediators of inflammation are implicated in the pathogenesis of ARDS.[43,44] It is unclear, however, whether some of these mediators directly cause ARDS or are a secondary product of the inflammation resulting from lung injury. Direct lung injury from aspiration or smoke inhalation, for example, may result in inflammation and the release of inflammatory cytokines that augment microvascular permeability. Regardless of whether inflammatory mediators are primarily or secondarily involved in the pathogenesis of ARDS, they are clearly complex contributors to its development. The effects of mediators and inflammatory cells involved in ARDS, as well as those of their regulatory molecules, are tightly interwoven and ultimately result in a balance between pro- and anti-inflammatory and pro- and antiedematous factors.[45] Although inflammatory mediators could themselves disrupt the capillary-alveolar membrane, they may also create effects that keep the inflammatory response in check. This may account for the lack of success of pharmacological inhibitors to decrease the mortality associated with ARDS. Research efforts continue to investigate potential ways to more effectively modulate the inflammatory response during ARDS.[43,45,46] Ongoing research also focuses on finding novel biomarkers to predict morbidity and mortality of patients with ARDS.[47]

PULMONARY MECHANICS

ARDS alters pulmonary mechanics in several ways. The loss of surfactant function, coupled with the development of edema around and within the alveoli, leads to alveolar collapse. The result is a decreased lung compliance, lung volume, and functional residual capacity. This is associated with a large intrapulmonary shunt fraction that contributes to the significant hypoxemia associated with ARDS.

During ARDS, marked hysteresis of the pressure-volume loop occurs, such that significantly higher transpulmonary pressures are necessary to achieve a given lung volume on inspiration than on expiration. The point on the pressure-volume loop where the shape changes from concave to exponential is known as the **lower inflection point.** It reflects the pressure point at which alveoli begin to open and is located above functional residual capacity (Figure 29-2). This suggests that many gas exchange units will collapse at normal transpulmonary pressures in acutely injured lungs

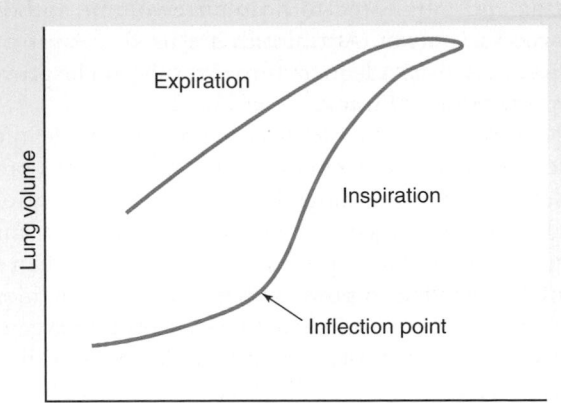

FIGURE 29-2 Representation of the pressure-volume (compliance) loop in ARDS. Below the inflection point is the pressure at which the alveoli begin to collapse, leading to loss of lung volume, or functional residual capacity.

and may need significant PEEP to maintain patency during expiration. The clinical application of recruitment maneuvers followed by maintenance with an appropriate level of PEEP to prevent alveolar collapse is known as the **open lung strategy.**[48,49]

Finally, lung injury and areas of involvement in ARDS are heterogeneous and not uniform through all lung units. Some areas of the lung, typically in the dependent regions, are grossly affected. Other regions of the lung, typically in the nondependent regions, may be relatively unaffected.[50] This creates varying areas of compliance within the lung itself. Dependent regions are generally fluid filled, atelectatic, and noncompliant. Nondependent areas are relatively normal and thus at risk for overdistention (i.e., volutrauma) and barotrauma during mechanical ventilation.

TREATMENT/VENTILATORY SUPPORT

Management of the patient with respiratory distress or failure includes an assessment of airway, breathing, and circulation ("ABCs"). Prompt cardiopulmonary resuscitation is vital to restoring adequate systemic oxygen delivery. Identification and targeted therapy for the underlying etiology and elimination of any potential source for exacerbation of the disease is a critical first step in treatment.

The goal in the treatment of ARDS is to treat the underlying disease (if possible), achieve adequate (but not necessarily optimal) tissue oxygenation, and avoid complications. All ARDS patients require supplemental oxygen, and most require mechanical ventilation. Tissue oxygenation is provided by ensuring adequate cardiac output and hemoglobin levels. Overhydration could augment pulmonary edema, so fluids should be carefully titrated and monitored to normalize volume and maintain cardiac output. Antibiotics are used to treat pneumonia and sepsis. Adequate nutrition should be provided to optimize caloric intake.

Every patient with ARDS is hypoxemic by definition. Prolonged administration of high concentrations of oxygen can damage the lungs because of the formation of highly reactive oxygen free radicals. Human and animal studies suggest that a prolonged FIO_2 greater than 0.60 should be avoided to prevent oxygen-induced pulmonary damage.[51-53] However, the exact FIO_2 cutoff for oxygen toxicity in the ARDS patient remains unknown and may be less than 0.60.

Positive End-Expiratory Pressure

The mainstay in treating ARDS is the administration of PEEP. No gas exchange will occur in atelectatic or fluid-filled alveoli. PEEP helps maintain alveolar patency and restore functional residual capacity. PEEP also maintains the transthoracic pressure above the point at which additional alveoli will collapse during expiration. PEEP is typically increased to a level that allows adequate oxygenation as defined by an arterial oxygen saturation (SaO_2) of 85% or greater at an acceptable FIO_2 of 0.60 or less. It should be noted that the minimal acceptable arterial oxygen saturation remains very controversial.[54] A PEEP level of 10 to 15 cm H_2O, or even higher, may be required to achieve adequate oxygenation. However, as PEEP levels exceed 12 to 15 cm H_2O, the increase in intrathoracic pressure may adversely affect cardiac output, primarily by decreasing systemic venous return.[55] As PEEP is increased, the ARDS patient should be monitored for a decrease in cardiac output with a decrease in peripheral perfusion.[56] In most cases, a decrease in cardiac output can be compensated for by intravascular volume loading and possibly inotropic support.[57]

The ARDS Network investigated the optimal PEEP-FIO_2 strategy for adults with ARDS.[58] The results of this prospective, randomized, multicenter study indicate that in adult ARDS patients who are ventilated with 6 ml/kg tidal volumes and an end-inspiratory plateau pressure of less than 30 cm H_2O, a "moderately high" or "very high" PEEP strategy produced similar survival rates. It must be noted that this study investigated two relatively aggressive PEEP strategies. Subsequent studies performed outside the United States also showed similar results. In a study involving 30 ICUs and 983 adult patients with ARDS, there was no difference in hospital mortality despite the reduction in the need for rescue therapies in the "high" PEEP group.[49] A recent systematic review on the effect of PEEP in ARDS showed that the subgroup of ARDS patients who may stand to benefit most from a "high" PEEP strategy are those with the worst degree of hypoxemia.[59]

The implication of current clinical studies in this area is that once appropriate PEEP is applied to maintain the lungs at an ideal lung volume, a further increase in PEEP in an attempt to reduce the FIO_2 does not lead to an improved outcome.

Low Tidal Volume Ventilation

Ventilation is achieved through a combination of respiratory rate, tidal volume, and inspiratory time. Historically, ventilator tidal volumes between 10 and 15 ml/kg were used for patients with ARDS. Because the remaining compliant lung volume in a patient with ARDS is significantly reduced, these tidal volumes often required inflation pressures that resulted in pulmonary overdistention and progressive secondary lung injury.[60-62]

The ARDS Network reported in the *New England Journal of Medicine* in 2000 that in adult patients with acute lung injury and ARDS, low tidal volume mechanical ventilation (6 ml/kg) decreased mortality by 22% and increased the number of ventilator-free days as compared with a more traditional tidal volume (12 ml/kg).[32] The mortality rate was 31.0% in the low tidal volume group and 39.8% ($p = 0.007$) in the higher tidal volume group. Additionally, the plateau pressure (Pplat) was significantly decreased in the low tidal volume group as compared with the control group.

Although still unproven, the results of this landmark study are likely applicable to infants and children with ARDS. Until a similar large-scale, prospective, randomized trial is accomplished in pediatrics, it seems reasonable to use the low tidal volume guideline. A meta-analysis of **low tidal volume ventilation** in patients without acute lung injury showed that this lung-protective strategy results in less lung injury and mortality.[63] This collective evidence suggests that low tidal volumes should be used in patients with more normal lung function. However, this meta-analysis only included adult patients. It remains uncertain whether larger tidal volumes can be safely applied in children with normal lung function.

Before the ARDS Network's low tidal volume study, several studies offered conflicting results on this topic. Amato et al. concluded that a lung-protective ventilation strategy was associated with a significant decrease in mortality at 28 days but was not associated with a higher rate of survival to hospital discharge.[64] A major limitation in the application of the results of this study is the high mortality rate in the control group (71%). In contrast, the next article in the same issue of the *New England Journal of Medicine* was a report by Stewart et al. that concluded that a low tidal volume strategy does not reduce mortality for adult patients with ARDS.[65]

The apparently conflicting results from the low tidal volume studies by Amato, Stewart, and the ARDS Network become more consistent when considering the plateau pressures used. In the ARDS Network study, the protocol was designed to maintain plateau pressure less than 50 cm H_2O in the control group and less than 30 cm H_2O in the low tidal volume group.[32] The results indicate that in the low tidal volume group Pplat remained 26 cm H_2O

or less throughout the first week of ventilation, whereas in the control group Pplat ranged from 33 ± 9 to 37 ± 9 cm H_2O over the first week. In the Amato study, Pplat remained less than 32 cm H_2O for the protective ventilation group; in the control group Pplat ranged from 34.4 ± 1.9 to 37.8 ± 1.2 cm H_2O over the first 7 days of ventilation.[64] Of interest, the study by Stewart et al. revealed no improvement with mortality with low tidal volume ventilation; however, in both groups the Pplat was maintained at less than 29 cm H_2O throughout the study.[65] This finding is similar to the study by Brochard et al., which also failed to demonstrate improved survival with low tidal volume ventilation.[66] For both groups, Pplat was maintained at less than 32 cm H_2O throughout the first week of ventilation.

Thus the data support the conclusion that for adult patients with ARDS, the Pplat should be limited to less than approximately 32 cm H_2O to improve outcome. The applicability of this conclusion to pediatric ARDS patients requires investigation. It is very possible that the "critical" limit on plateau pressure for infants and children will be less than 32 cm H_2O and may vary with patient age and size.

It must be stressed that although the ARDS Network study indicates that a 6 ml/kg tidal volume led to improved mortality as compared with a 12 ml/kg tidal volume, the tidal volume associated with the least mortality may lie somewhere between 6 and 12 ml/kg, or possibly even less than 6 ml/kg. Lastly, it should be stressed that most previous ARDS trials have been based on a "magic bullet" strategy in which a single intervention is studied. Mortality from ARDS has improved over the past decade without ever truly finding the "magic bullet." Most likely, the improvements in the care of ARDS patients have been multifactorial. Although difficult, future clinical studies should investigate a combination of therapies to further decrease mortality from ARDS.

Multiple modes of mechanical ventilation are currently used in clinical practice to provide respiratory support for patients with ARDS. To date, no data exist to determine the ventilatory mode that provides the greatest benefit and the least risk to an individual patient. Prospective, randomized, multicenter studies of mechanical ventilation and ARDS in pediatrics are limited. For most clinical questions, data are extrapolated from studies in the adult population.

When "toxic" conventional ventilatory support is required to achieve the desired gas exchange goals, clinicians often transition to high-frequency oscillatory ventilation (HFOV). Only one randomized, controlled study of HFOV in the pediatric population has been performed, which showed improved oxygenation and reduced need for supplementation oxygen at 30 days with HFOV.[67] However, it must be noted that the control group was not ventilated with a low tidal volume approach. Despite the paucity of data showing the superiority of HFOV in pediatric ARDS, the use of this alternative mode of ventilation remains

common in PICUs worldwide.[68] Readers are referred to Chapter 17 for a more comprehensive discussion of HFOV.

Current medical evidence does not show that a particular mode of conventional mechanical ventilation (pressure controlled or volume controlled) or alternative modes of ventilation (e.g., airway pressure release ventilation, HFOV) results in a significant difference in mortality in patients with ARDS. Except for low tidal volume strategy, no particular conventional or unconventional mode of ventilation has been demonstrated to improve clinical outcomes in ARDS.

Gas Exchange Goals

Improved oxygenation is not correlated with improved outcomes. This was best demonstrated in the ARDS Network low tidal volume study, in which the control (12 ml/kg) group demonstrated improved oxygenation for the first 72 hours of ventilation.[32] If this study had been designed as an acute gas exchange study, the conclusion would have been false and mortality for ARDS could have increased. This lack of association between oxygenation and survival has been demonstrated in multiple other studies.[69-71] Timmons et al. demonstrated no correlation between oxygenation or ventilation in survivors or nonsurvivors of pediatric ARDS.[72] Dobyns et al. showed that, in acute hypoxic respiratory failure in children, although oxygenation improved with inhaled nitric oxide, there was no difference in mortality.[69] Improved oxygenation without a significant improvement in survival was also demonstrated in a follow-up study of inhaled nitric oxide in combination with high-frequency oscillatory ventilation.[70]

The concept of accepting lower arterial oxygenation saturation is termed permissive hypoxemia.[54,73] Although the acceptable arterial oxygen saturation target remains controversial, ventilatory strategies should aim to provide adequate tissue and organ oxygenation while minimizing oxygen toxicity and ventilator-induced lung injury. It should be noted that long-term neurological effects of permissive hypoxemia have not been studied. Clinicians must weigh the potential benefits and risks of this approach for each individual clinical situation.

Permissive Hypercapnia

A logical consequence of low tidal volume ventilation is hypercapnia. Limiting the peak inspiratory pressure by reducing the tidal volume may decrease minute ventilation and result in hypercapnia. The exact degree of respiratory acidosis that can be safely tolerated remains controversial. However, most undesirable effects are reversible and minor with respiratory acidosis when pH is greater than approximately 7.20.[74] Laboratory studies have suggested that respiratory acidosis may, in fact, be lung protective.[75]

Of note, a Cochrane review of the large, multicenter low tidal volume studies of adult ARDS was unable to reach a firm conclusion on the implications of **permissive hypercapnia**.[76] It should be stressed that these low tidal volume studies were not designed to answer the specific question of hypercapnia. However, the medical literature does support the beneficial role of permissive hypercapnia in ARDS. Limited evidence suggests that low-volume, pressure-limited ventilation with permissive hypercapnia may improve outcome in patients with ARDS.[77,78] In a 10-year study, Milberg et al. reported a positive association between permissive hypercapnia and outcomes.[79] Recent data from a laboratory model of ischemia-reperfusion acute lung injury indicate that hypercapnic acidosis is protective and that buffering of the hypercapnic acidosis attenuates its protective effects.[75] In allowing permissive hypercapnia, the rate at which carbon dioxide rises may be more important than the actual value itself. A rapid regression to normocapnia may be more deleterious to the cardiac system than hypercapnia itself.

It should be noted that permissive hypercapnia is generally not recommended for those patients with intracranial pathology in which increased cerebral blood flow related to hypercapnia may be detrimental or for those with significant pulmonary hypertension in which the elevated carbon dioxide level may further increase pulmonary vascular resistance.

ADJUNCT THERAPIES

Some patients are unable to achieve acceptable therapeutic goals while avoiding oxygen toxicity or an intolerably high peak inspiratory pressure with conventional ventilator strategies. Two of the more commonly used therapeutic modalities for treating patients with ARDS are HFOV and extracorporeal membrane oxygenation.[67,80-83] HFOV has been described briefly in the prior section on Treatment/ Ventilatory Support. We discuss ECMO briefly in this section. The reader is referred to Chapters 17 and 19 (and the Evolve website: https://evolve.elsevier.com) for a more comprehensive discussion of these important topics.

Briefly, ECMO is used in patients with severe ARDS who are unable to achieve acceptable therapeutic goals despite maximal therapies at intolerably high ventilator settings and/or inotropic support. In patients with severe ARDS and preserved cardiac function, venovenous ECMO can be used to minimize oxygen toxicity and minimize ventilator-induced lung injury while achieving acceptable oxygenation and carbon dioxide clearance. Keeping in mind that ECMO is usually implemented in critically ill children with an extremely high mortality rate, the survival data from the Extracorporeal Life Support Organization registry for children with ARDS is fairly good at approximately 65% overall.[83] Experience with the 2009-2010 H1N1 influenza A pandemic suggests that ECMO may be an important management strategy in future viral epidemics/pandemics, with survival rates reported in excessive of 70%.[84,85]

Other potential adjunct therapies include trials of corticosteroids, prone positioning, inhaled nitric oxide,

and surfactant replacement. Meta-analyses of corticosteroid used within the first 2 weeks in adults with established ARDS demonstrated that steroids may reduce mortality and reduce total days of mechanical ventilation.[86,87] Although controversial, there does not seem to be a role for steroids in the prevention of progression of ARDS.[86] Unfortunately, there are no studies of corticosteroids for treatment of ARDS in children.

Prone positioning improves oxygenation in pediatric and adult patients with ARDS through various mechanisms, such as improvements in ventilation-perfusion matching and chest wall mechanics.[88] However, proning is associated with a risk of endotracheal tube obstruction and accidental catheter or tube dislodgment. A meta-analysis has shown that proning improves survival in those with severe ARDS.[89] Unfortunately the only study to date on proning in children with acute lung injury was closed because of futility.[71] This prospective, randomized, multicenter study by Curley et al. revealed no change in mortality with prone positioning.[71]

Studies of inhaled nitric oxide for pediatric ALI/ARDS have demonstrated improved oxygenation acutely, but this improvement in gas exchange has not translated into improved survival.[69,70] Willson et al. reported that exogenous surfactant (calfactant) acutely improved oxygenation and significantly decreased mortality in infants and children with acute lung injury; however, this study revealed no significant decrease in duration of mechanical ventilation, length of PICU admission, or length of hospital stay.[90] Furthermore, the control group had a higher percentage of higher risk, immune-incompetent patients.

CASE STUDY

A 15-year-old boy with a significant medical history of acute lymphoblastic leukemia in remission presented with fever, cough, and shortness of breath. On presentation, he was noted to have bilateral crackles on auscultation and a pulse oximeter reading of 85% on room air. Supplemental oxygen was provided, and he was admitted to the general ward for further management. The patient's oxygen requirement continued to increase with increasing work of breathing. Chest radiograph showed worsening bilateral infiltrates. He was transferred to the PICU and was intubated in view of the rapid progression of illness. Respiratory virus isolation was notable for H1N1 influenza. The patient was supported on conventional mechanical ventilation for 3 days before transitioning to high-frequency ventilation. Before his transition to high-frequency ventilation, his arterial blood gas on conventional mechanical ventilation, with peak inspiratory pressure of 28, PEEP 13, mean airway pressure of 19 and FiO_2 of 90%, was pH 7.33, PaO_2 46 mm Hg, $PaCO_2$ 57 mm Hg, HCO_3 30.0, Base Excess 6. Unfortunately his condition worsened, with refractory hypoxemia (high-frequency ventilation with mean airway pressure of 35, amplitude of 60, frequency of 8 Hz and FiO_2 100%, with an arterial blood gas of pH 7.31, PaO_2

57 mm Hg, $PaCO_2$ 75 mm Hg, HCO_3 32.0, BE 10.6), and he was cannulated for venovenous ECMO with a dual-lumen cannula in the right internal jugular vein. After 3 weeks on ECMO, he was decannulated, weaned, and then extubated. After 8 weeks, he was discharged home without the need for ongoing respiratory support.

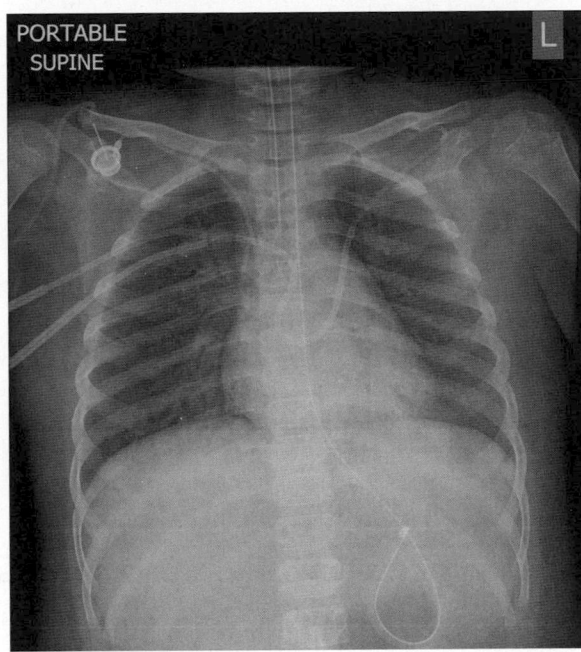

1. Does this case satisfy the Berlin criteria for ARDS? What features of ARDS are present, and what additional information, if any, is required?
2. What conventional mechanical ventilation strategies should be considered in this type of patient?
3. What other adjunct therapies, if any, could have been considered in the management of this case?

See Evolve Resources for answers.

SUMMARY

Acute lung injury and acute respiratory distress syndrome represent a continuum of clinical disease of varying pulmonary (direct) and nonpulmonary (indirect) etiologies. Although much has been learned about the pathophysiology of acute lung injury over the past two decades, the only treatment strategy that has been proven to improve clinical outcome is low tidal volume ventilation. However, the optimal tidal volume remains unclear because it may not be 6 ml/kg. Furthermore, it should be noted that in the years before publication of the low tidal volume ventilation data, overall survival rates for adult and pediatric patients with acute lung injury had been gradually increasing. Future clinical investigations are likely to study combined therapeutic strategies as opposed to focusing on discovering the single "magic bullet."

KEY POINTS

- The Berlin definition for adult ARDS includes the following criteria: timing of onset within 1 week, bilateral infiltrates on chest radiograph or computed tomography (CT) scan, presence of hypoxemia (PaO_2/FIO_2 less than 300), and risk factors (if absent, will require additional investigation to exclude hydrostatic edema).
- Classically, ARDS is divided into three pathological stages: exudative, proliferative, and fibrotic. Neutrophils are central to the pathogenesis of ARDS. Regardless of the inciting event, ARDS begins with inflammatory injury to the alveolar epithelium and endothelium, which results in accumulation of protein-rich edema in the alveoli. Recovery from ARDS depends on the resolution of inflammation, removal of the edema, and reparative processes of the epithelium.
- Mechanical ventilation forms the cornerstone of ARDS management. Mechanical ventilation strategies must aim to minimize ventilator-induced lung injury. Such strategies include low tidal volume ventilation, optimization of PEEP/mean airway pressure, and possibly (based on the clinical scenario) permissive hypoxemia and permissive hypercapnia. High-frequency ventilation, as described elsewhere in this textbook, is often used in pediatric acute lung injury based on tremendous clinical experience; however, this modality has never been studied in comparison to low tidal volume ventilation in pediatrics.
- Beyond mechanical ventilation, other adjunct therapies may be considered in severe cases of acute lung injury/ARDS. Although clinically used, data are lacking to definitely support prone positioning, exogenous surfactant administration, or inhaled nitric oxide for the management of severe hypoxemia. ECMO, as described elsewhere in the textbook, can be lifesaving when refractory hypoxemia develops.
- Meticulous attention to treatment of the precipitating factors, sedation, fluid management, and nutrition is important in the overall management of a child with acute lung injury.

ASSESSMENT QUESTIONS

See Evolve Resources for the answers.

1. A 13-year-old boy is admitted to the PICU with a diagnosis of ARDS. His PaO_2/FIO_2 ratio is 176 with a PEEP of 8. According to the 2011 Berlin consensus definition, what is the severity of his ARDS?
   A. ALI
   B. Mild
   C. Moderate
   D. Severe

2. A patient undergoing mechanical ventilation has a mean airway pressure of 18 cm H_2O, and the blood gas shows a PaO_2 of 90 mm Hg at an FiO_2 of 0.80. What is this patient's oxygenation index (OI)?
   A. 20
   B. 16
   C. 140
   D. 90

3. Which of the following are pathological stages of ARDS?
   I. Exudative
   II. Proliferative
   III. Fibrotic
   IV. Edematous
      A. I, II, III
      B. II, IV
      C. II, III, IV
      D. III, IV

4. A 68-year-old man with a history of chronic alcoholic consumption was admitted to the unit for aspiration pneumonia. His clinical course was complicated by ARDS. Which of the following treatment strategies for acute lung injury in adult patients has been demonstrated to improve mortality in a prospective, randomized clinical trial?
   A. Prone positioning
   B. Inhaled nitric oxide
   C. Low positive end-expiratory pressure
   D. Low tidal volume ventilation

5. A 6-year-old child with a history of acute lymphoblastic leukemia was admitted to the intensive care unit for *Klebsiella pneumoniae* septic shock. He developed ARDS on the third day of septic shock. The overall goal(s) in the treatment of ARDS for this child include:
   I. Treatment of the underlying disease
   II. Achieve adequate tissue oxygenation
   III. Minimize ventilator-induced lung injury
   IV. Ensure normocarbia
      A. I, II
      B. II, III
      C. II, IV
      D. I, II, III

6. The criteria used to define ARDS include:
   I. Hypoxemia
   II. Bilateral pulmonary infiltrates
   III. Presence of risk factors
   IV. Need for invasive mechanical ventilation
      A. I, II, III, IV
      B. I, II
      C. I, IV
      D. I, II, III

7. Which of the following are useful therapies in pediatric patients with acute lung injury?
   I. Permissive hypercapnia
   II. Permissive hypoxemia
   III. Administration of activated protein C for sepsis
   IV. Low tidal volume ventilation
      A. I, II
      B. I, IV
      C. I, II, III
      D. I, II, IV

8. Which of the following characteristics of infants and young children (as compared with older children and adults) causes this population to be particularly prone to respiratory failure?
   I. Small caliber airways
   II. Increased chest wall compliance
   III. Greater propensity for rapid fatigue of respiratory muscles
   IV. Reduced cardiac function in children compared with adults
      A. III, IV
      B. I, II
      C. I, II, III
      D. I, II, III, IV

9. The most common nonpulmonary risk factor in patients with ARDS is:
   A. Multiple trauma
   B. Cardiac failure
   C. Sepsis
   D. Acute pancreatitis

10. Of the choices listed, which is generally the latest clinical finding in pediatric patients with ARDS?
   A. Hypoxemia
   B. Decreased pulmonary compliance
   C. Increased work of breathing
   D. Hypercapnia

References

1. Bernard GR: Acute respiratory distress syndrome: a historical perspective, *Am J Respir Crit Care Med* 172:798, 2005.
2. Ashbaugh DG, Bigelow DB, Petty TL, et al: Acute respiratory distress in adults, *Lancet* 2:319, 1967.
3. Bernard GR, Artigas A, Brigham KL, et al: The American-European Consensus Conference on ARDS. Definitions, mechanisms, relevant outcomes, and clinical trial coordination, *Am J Respir Crit Care Med* 149:818, 1994.
4. Ranieri VM, Rubenfeld GD, Thompson BT, et al: Acute respiratory distress syndrome: the Berlin definition, *JAMA* 307:2526, 2012.
5. Ferguson ND, Fan E, Camporota L, et al: The Berlin definition of ARDS: an expanded rationale, justification, and supplementary material, *Intensive Care Med* 38:1573–1582, 2012.
6. Rivera RA, Butt W, Shann F: Predictors of mortality in children with respiratory failure: possible indications for ECMO, *Anaesth Intensive Care* 18:385, 1990.
7. Durand M, Snyder JR, Gangitano E, et al: Oxygenation index in patients with meconium aspiration: conventional and extracorporeal membrane oxygenation therapy, *Crit Care Med* 18:373, 1990.
8. Monchi M, Bellenfant F, Cariou A, et al: Early predictive factors of survival in the acute respiratory distress syndrome. A multivariate analysis, *Am J Respir Crit Care Med* 158:1076, 1998.
9. Mehta S, Granton J, MacDonald RJ, et al: High-frequency oscillatory ventilation in adults: the Toronto experience, *Chest* 126:518, 2004.
10. Matsuda A, Kishi T, Jacob A, et al: Association between insertion/deletion polymorphism in angiotensin-converting enzyme gene and acute lung injury/acute respiratory distress syndrome: a meta-analysis, *BMC Med Genet* 13:76, 2012.

11. Kangelaris KN, Sapru A, Calfee CS, et al: The association between a Darc gene polymorphism and clinical outcomes in African American patients with acute lung injury, *Chest* 141:1160, 2012.

12. Roupie E, Lepage E, Wysocki M, et al: Prevalence, etiologies and outcome of the acute respiratory distress syndrome among hypoxemic ventilated patients. SRLF Collaborative Group on Mechanical Ventilation. Societe de Reanimation de Langue Francaise, *Intensive Care Med* 25:920, 1999.

13. Bersten AD, Edibam C, Hunt T, et al: Incidence and mortality of acute lung injury and the acute respiratory distress syndrome in three Australian States, *Am J Respir Crit Care Med* 165:443, 2002.

14. Brun-Buisson C, Minelli C, Bertolini G, et al: Epidemiology and outcome of acute lung injury in European intensive care units. Results from the ALIVE study, *Intensive Care Med* 30:51, 2004.

15. Rubenfeld GD, Caldwell E, Peabody E, et al: Incidence and outcomes of acute lung injury, *N Engl J Med* 353:1685, 2005.

16. Zimmerman JJ, Akhtar SR, Caldwell E, et al: Incidence and outcomes of pediatric acute lung injury, *Pediatrics* 124:87, 2009.

17. Lopez-Fernandez Y, Azagra AM, de la Oliva P, et al: Pediatric acute lung injury epidemiology and natural history study: incidence and outcome of the acute respiratory distress syndrome in children, *Crit Care Med* 40:3238, 2012.

18. Yu WL, Lu ZJ, Wang Y, et al: The epidemiology of acute respiratory distress syndrome in pediatric intensive care units in China, *Intensive Care Med* 35:136, 2009.

19. Hu X, Qian S, Xu F, et al: Incidence, management and mortality of acute hypoxemic respiratory failure and acute respiratory distress syndrome from a prospective study of Chinese paediatric intensive care network, *Acta Paediatr* 99:715, 2010.

20. Gattinoni L, Bombino M, Pelosi P, et al: Lung structure and function in different stages of severe adult respiratory distress syndrome, *JAMA* 271:1772, 1994.

21. Ware LB, Matthay MA: The acute respiratory distress syndrome, *N Engl J Med* 342:1334, 2000.

22. Aberle DR, Brown K: Radiologic considerations in the adult respiratory distress syndrome, *Clin Chest Med* 11:737, 1990.

23. Effmann EL, Merten DF, Kirks DR, et al: Adult respiratory distress syndrome in children, *Radiology* 157:69, 1985.

24. Antonelli M, Conti G, Esquinas A, et al: A multiple-center survey on the use in clinical practice of noninvasive ventilation as a first-line intervention for acute respiratory distress syndrome, *Crit Care Med* 35:18, 2007.

25. Piastra M, De Luca D, Marzano L, et al: The number of failing organs predicts non-invasive ventilation failure in children with ALI/ARDS, *Intensive Care Med* 37:1510, 2011.

26. Ferring M, Vincent JL: Is outcome from ARDS related to the severity of respiratory failure? *Eur Respir J* 10:1297, 1997.

27. Estenssoro E, Dubin A, Laffaire E, et al: Incidence, clinical course, and outcome in 217 patients with acute respiratory distress syndrome, *Crit Care Med* 30:2450, 2002.

28. Stapleton RD, Wang BM, Hudson LD, et al: Causes and timing of death in patients with ARDS, *Chest* 128:525, 2005.

29. Walkey AJ, Summer R, Ho V, et al: Acute respiratory distress syndrome: epidemiology and management approaches, *Clin Epidemiol* 4:159, 2012.

30. Phua J, Badia JR, Adhikari NK, et al: Has mortality from acute respiratory distress syndrome decreased over time? A systematic review, *Am J Respir Crit Care Med* 179:220, 2009.

31. Zambon M, Vincent JL: Mortality rates for patients with acute lung injury/ARDS have decreased over time, *Chest* 133:1120, 2008.

32. The Acute Respiratory Distress Syndrome Network. Ventilation with lower tidal volumes as compared with traditional tidal volumes for acute lung injury and the acute respiratory distress syndrome, *N Engl J Med* 342:1301, 2000.

33. Flori HR, Glidden DV, Rutherford GW, et al: Pediatric acute lung injury: prospective evaluation of risk factors associated with mortality, *Am J Respir Crit Care Med* 171:995, 2005.

34. Seeger W, Gunther A, Walmrath HD, et al: Alveolar surfactant and adult respiratory distress syndrome. Pathogenetic role and therapeutic prospects, *Clin Investig* 71:177, 1993.

35. Lewis JF, Veldhuizen R, Possmayer F, et al: Altered alveolar surfactant is an early marker of acute lung injury in septic adult sheep, *Am J Respir Crit Care Med* 150:123, 1994.

36. Matthay MA, Wiener-Kronish JP: Intact epithelial barrier function is critical for the resolution of alveolar edema in humans, *Am Rev Respir Dis* 142:1250, 1990.

37. Ware LB, Matthay MA: Alveolar fluid clearance is impaired in the majority of patients with acute lung injury and the acute respiratory distress syndrome, *Am J Respir Crit Care Med* 163:1376, 2001.

38. Tanswell AK, Byrne PJ, Han RN, et al: Limited division of low-density adult rat type II pneumocytes in serum-free culture, *Am J Physiol* 260:L395, 1991.

39. Berthiaume Y, Lesur O, Dagenais A: Treatment of adult respiratory distress syndrome: plea for rescue therapy of the alveolar epithelium, *Thorax* 54:150, 1999.

40. Piantadosi CA, Schwartz DA: The acute respiratory distress syndrome, *Ann Intern Med* 141:460, 2004.

41. Bitterman PB: Pathogenesis of fibrosis in acute lung injury, *Am J Med* 92:39S, 1992.

42. Kuhn C 3rd, Boldt J, King TE, et al: An immunohistochemical study of architectural remodeling and connective tissue synthesis in pulmonary fibrosis, *Am Rev Respir Dis* 140:1693, 1989.

43. Ranieri VM, Suter PM, Tortorella C, et al: Effect of mechanical ventilation on inflammatory mediators in patients with acute respiratory distress syndrome: a randomized controlled trial, *JAMA* 282:54-61, 1999.

44. Matthay MA, Zemans RL: The acute respiratory distress syndrome: pathogenesis and treatment, *Annu Rev Pathol* 6:147-163, 2011.

45. Matthay MA, Zimmerman GA: Acute lung injury and the acute respiratory distress syndrome: four decades of inquiry into pathogenesis and rational management, *Am J Respir Cell Mol Biol* 33:319-327, 2005.

46. Rinaldo JE, Christman JW: Mechanisms and mediators of the adult respiratory distress syndrome, *Clin Chest Med* 11:621, 1990.

47. Dolinay T, Kim YS, Howrylak J, et al: Inflammasome-regulated cytokines are critical mediators of acute lung injury, *Am J Respir Crit Care Med* 185:1225, 2012.

48. Papadakos PJ, Lachmann B: The open lung concept of mechanical ventilation: the role of recruitment and stabilization, *Crit Care Clin* 23:241, ix-x, 2007.

49. Meade MO, Cook DJ, Guyatt GH, et al: Ventilation strategy using low tidal volumes, recruitment maneuvers, and high positive end-expiratory pressure for acute lung injury and acute respiratory distress syndrome: a randomized controlled trial, *JAMA* 299:637, 2008.

50. Gattinoni L, Caironi P, Pelosi P, et al: What has computed tomography taught us about the acute respiratory distress syndrome? *Am J Respir Crit Care Med* 164:1701, 2001.

51. Thiel M, Chouker A, Ohta A, et al: Oxygenation inhibits the physiological tissue-protecting mechanism and thereby exacerbates acute inflammatory lung injury, *PLoS Biol* 3:e174, 2005.

52. Li LF, Liao SK, Ko YS, et al: Hyperoxia increases ventilator-induced lung injury via mitogen-activated protein kinases: a prospective, controlled animal experiment, *Crit Care* 11:R25, 2007.

53. Altemeier WA, Sinclair SE: Hyperoxia in the intensive care unit: why more is not always better, *Curr Opin Crit Care* 13:73, 2007.

54. Abdelsalam M, Cheifetz IM: Goal-directed therapy for severely hypoxic patients with acute respiratory distress syndrome: permissive hypoxemia, *Respir Care* 55:1483, 2010.

55. Mitaka C, Nagura T, Sakanishi N, et al: Two-dimensional echocardiographic evaluation of inferior vena cava, right ventricle, and left ventricle during positive-pressure ventilation with varying levels of positive end-expiratory pressure, *Crit Care Med* 17:205, 1989.

56. Cheifetz IM, Craig DM, Quick G, et al: Increasing tidal volumes and pulmonary overdistention adversely affect pulmonary vascular mechanics and cardiac output in a pediatric swine model, *Crit Care Med* 26:710, 1998.

57. Pollack MM, Fields AI, Holbrook RP: Cardiopulmonary parameters during high PEEP in children, *Crit Care Med* 8: 372, 1980.

58. Brower RG, Lanken PN, MacIntyre N, et al: Higher versus lower positive end-expiratory pressures in patients with the acute respiratory distress syndrome, *N Engl J Med* 351:327, 2004.

59. Briel M, Meade M, Mercat A, et al: Higher vs lower positive end-expiratory pressure in patients with acute lung injury and acute respiratory distress syndrome: systematic review and meta-analysis, *JAMA* 303:865, 2010.

60. Dreyfuss D, Basset G, Soler P, et al: Intermittent positive-pressure hyperventilation with high inflation pressures produces pulmonary microvascular injury in rats, *Am Rev Respir Dis* 132: 880, 1985.

61. Kolobow T, Moretti MP, Fumagalli R, et al: Severe impairment in lung function induced by high peak airway pressure during mechanical ventilation. An experimental study, *Am Rev Respir Dis* 135:312, 1987.

62. de Prost N, Ricard JD, Saumon G, et al: Ventilator-induced lung injury: historical perspectives and clinical implications, *Ann Intensive Care* 1:28, 2011.

63. Serpa Neto A, Cardoso SO, Manetta JA, et al: Association between use of lung-protective ventilation with lower tidal volumes and clinical outcomes among patients without acute respiratory distress syndrome: a meta-analysis, *JAMA* 308:1651, 2012.

64. Amato MB, Barbas CS, Medeiros DM, et al: Effect of a protective-ventilation strategy on mortality in the acute respiratory distress syndrome, *N Engl J Med* 338:347, 1998.

65. Stewart TE, Meade MO, Cook DJ, et al: Evaluation of a ventilation strategy to prevent barotrauma in patients at high risk for acute respiratory distress syndrome. Pressure- and Volume-Limited Ventilation Strategy Group, *N Engl J Med* 338:355, 1998.

66. Brochard L, Roudot-Thoraval F, Roupie E, et al: Tidal volume reduction for prevention of ventilator-induced lung injury in acute respiratory distress syndrome. The Multicenter Trial Group on Tidal Volume reduction in ARDS, *Am J Respir Crit Care Med* 158:1831, 1998.

67. Arnold JH, Hanson JH, Toro-Figuero LO, et al: Prospective, randomized comparison of high-frequency oscillatory ventilation and conventional mechanical ventilation in pediatric respiratory failure, *Crit Care Med* 22:1530, 1994.

68. Randolph AG, Meert KL, O'Neil ME, et al: The feasibility of conducting clinical trials in infants and children with acute respiratory failure, *Am J Respir Crit Care Med* 167:1334, 2003.

69. Dobyns EL, Cornfield DN, Anas NG, et al: Multicenter randomized controlled trial of the effects of inhaled nitric oxide therapy on gas exchange in children with acute hypoxemic respiratory failure, *J Pediatr* 134:406, 1999.

70. Dobyns EL, Anas NG, Fortenberry JD, et al: Interactive effects of high-frequency oscillatory ventilation and inhaled nitric oxide in acute hypoxemic respiratory failure in pediatrics, *Crit Care Med* 30:425, 2002.

71. Curley MA, Hibberd PL, Fineman LD, et al: Effect of prone positioning on clinical outcomes in children with acute lung injury: a randomized controlled trial, *JAMA* 294:229, 2005.

72. Timmons OD, Havens PL, Fackler JC: Predicting death in pediatric patients with acute respiratory failure. Pediatric Critical Care Study Group. Extracorporeal Life Support Organization, *Chest* 108:789, 1995.

73. Randolph AG: Management of acute lung injury and acute respiratory distress syndrome in children, *Crit Care Med* 37:2448, 2009.

74. Feihl F, Perret C: Permissive hypercapnia. How permissive should we be? *Am J Respir Crit Care Med* 150:1722, 1994.

75. Laffey JG, Engelberts D, Kavanagh BP: Buffering hypercapnic acidosis worsens acute lung injury, *Am J Respir Crit Care Med* 161:141, 2000.

76. Petrucci N, Iacovelli W: Ventilation with lower tidal volumes versus traditional tidal volumes in adults for acute lung injury and acute respiratory distress syndrome, *Cochrane Database Syst Rev* CD003844, 2004.

77. Hickling KG, Henderson SJ, Jackson R: Low mortality associated with low volume pressure limited ventilation with permissive hypercapnia in severe adult respiratory distress syndrome, *Intensive Care Med* 16:372, 1990.

78. Hickling KG, Walsh J, Henderson S, et al: Low mortality rate in adult respiratory distress syndrome using low-volume, pressure-limited ventilation with permissive hypercapnia: a prospective study, *Crit Care Med* 22:1568, 1994.

79. Milberg JA, Davis DR, Steinberg KP, et al: Improved survival of patients with acute respiratory distress syndrome (ARDS): 1983–1993, *JAMA* 273:306, 1995.

80. Green TP, Timmons OD, Fackler JC, et al: The impact of extracorporeal membrane oxygenation on survival in pediatric patients with acute respiratory failure. Pediatric Critical Care Study Group, *Crit Care Med* 24:323, 1996.

81. Arnold JH, Anas NG, Luckett P, et al: High-frequency oscillatory ventilation in pediatric respiratory failure: a multicenter experience, *Crit Care Med* 28:3913, 2000.

82. Brogan TV, Thiagarajan RR, Rycus PT, et al: Extracorporeal membrane oxygenation in adults with severe respiratory failure: a multi-center database, *Intensive Care Med* 35:2105, 2009.

83. Domico MB, Ridout DA, Bronicki R, et al: The impact of mechanical ventilation time before initiation of extracorporeal life support on survival in pediatric respiratory failure: a review of the Extracorporeal Life Support Registry, *Pediatr Crit Care Med* 13:16, 2012.

84. Norfolk SG, Hollingsworth CL, Wolfe CR, et al: Rescue therapy in adult and pediatric patients with pH1N1 influenza infection: a tertiary center intensive care unit experience from April to October 2009. *Crit Care Med* 2103, 2010.

85. Turner DA, Rehder KJ, Peterson-Carmichael SL, et al: Extracorporeal membrane oxygenation for severe refractory respiratory failure secondary to 2009. H1N1 influenza A, *Respir Care* 56:941, 2011.

86. Peter JV, John P, Graham PL, et al: Corticosteroids in the prevention and treatment of acute respiratory distress syndrome (ARDS) in adults: meta-analysis, *BMJ* 336:1006, 2008.

87. Tang BM, Craig JC, Eslick GD, et al: Use of corticosteroids in acute lung injury and acute respiratory distress syndrome: a systematic review and meta-analysis, *Crit Care Med* 37:1594, 2009.

88. Gattinoni L, Tognoni G, Pesenti A, et al: Effect of prone positioning on the survival of patients with acute respiratory failure, *N Engl J Med* 345:568, 2001.

89. Sud S, Friedrich JO, Taccone P, et al: Prone ventilation reduces mortality in patients with acute respiratory failure and severe hypoxemia: systematic review and meta-analysis, *Intensive Care Med* 36:585, 2010.

90. Willson DF, Thomas NJ, Markovitz BP, et al: Effect of exogenous surfactant (calfactant) in pediatric acute lung injury: a randomized controlled trial, *JAMA* 293:470, 2005.

Chapter 30

Shock and Meningitis

ANTHONY D. SLONIN, NANA COLEMAN

OUTLINE

LEARNING OBJECTIVES

After reading this chapter, the reader will be able to:

1. Define *shock* and the key elements of shock pathophysiology
2. Understand the concept of oxygen delivery and consider it in the context of select pediatric clinical cases
3. Recognize the clinical presentation of select shock states—anaphylaxis and sepsis—and describe basic principles of management and treatment
4. Identify the necessary elements of diagnosing and treating pediatric patients with meningitis

KEY TERMS

Anaphylaxis
Meningitis

Oxygen delivery
Sepsis

Shock

SHOCK

Shock represents a disruption of the natural homeostasis that exists within the body to ensure adequate oxygen delivery to all tissues. In this abnormal metabolic state, the body is unable to maintain sufficient supply of oxygen despite often increased demand, resulting in a complex cascade of compensatory mechanisms designed to restore this balance. When untreated, shock is potentially fatal, particularly when the recognition of its onset is delayed. *Cardiac output* is the term typically used to encompass the delivery of blood and thus oxygen to organs and tissues in the body. Thus, in shock, cardiac output is impaired; the nature of this impairment is based on the specific shock state.

Definition and Classification

Formally defined, shock represents an abnormal physiological state characterized by inadequate oxygen delivery or, in particular shock states, impaired oxygen utilization despite appropriate delivery. At a cellular level, these derangements result in less efficient energy metabolism with diversion to secondary metabolic pathways to maintain cellular function. When shock is unchecked, cellular function is severely compromised, with resultant cell death and a refractory shock state. If shock is reversed and tissue oxygenation is restored, organs and organ systems can function better. Although there are common features that characterize shock states, it is of value to discuss the nomenclature of various shock states (Table 30-1).

Typically, shock can be classified in four general states: hypovolemic, cardiogenic, obstructive, and distributive. The first, hypovolemic shock, is most common worldwide among children, most often resulting from severe dehydration. When there is loss of intravascular volume, cardiac output is impaired as stroke volume decreases. In hypovolemic shock, rapid restoration of the vascular volume is paramount. For hemorrhagic shock, a subtype of hypovolemic shock, blood loss causes shock and thus treatment requires replacement of the lost blood volume. Other potential causes of hypovolemic shock include osmolar diuresis such as from diabetic

TABLE 30-1

Pathophysiological and Clinical Shock Classification

Hypovolemic	Low-volume shock state with intravascular volume loss as cause; examples include severe dehydration and hemorrhage leading to hemorrhagic shock
Cardiogenic	Primary heart pump failure with resultant low cardiac output; examples include myocarditis and cardiomyopathy
Obstructive	Physiological or physical impairment to heart pump function resulting in low cardiac output state; examples include cardiac tamponade and pulmonary embolism
Distributive	Low systemic vascular resistance and high cardiac output state resulting in maldistribution of blood flow; examples include septic shock, anaphylaxis, adrenal crisis, and neurogenic shock

ketoacidosis or from infectious enteritis. With timely and aggressive volume resuscitation, this shock state can readily be reversed.

Cardiogenic shock, as its name implies, describes primary failure of the heart pump. In children, cardiogenic shock may be observed after cardiac surgery or from primary diseases processes such as myocarditis or cardiomyopathy. In each of these instances, cardiovascular function is impaired and often vasoactive or mechanical support such as extracorporeal membrane oxygenation is required to prevent cardiac and systemic ischemia. As described in detail later in this chapter, the goal of these therapies is to optimize cardiac output by optimizing the preload, afterload, and contractile function of the heart.

A third classification of shock is obstructive, which characterizes a shock state in which a physical obstruction to blood flow impairs cardiac output and ultimately oxygen delivery. Examples include cardiac tamponade, tension pneumothorax, and pulmonary embolism, and in all cases a functional obstruction to intrathoracic blood flow impedes the heart's ability to pump blood and thus oxygen to the body. The final and perhaps most broad category of shock is distributive, including such shock states as sepsis, anaphylaxis, adrenal crisis, and neurogenic shock. Each of these shock states is characterized by a maldistribution of blood flow with a resultant low systemic vascular resistance state. Whether mitigated by cytokines released by infectious organisms, histamine release secondary to allergen exposure, or loss of sympathetic tone from decreased adrenergic or neuronal control, each of these shock states results in insufficient oxygen delivery and/or utilization to meet the body's metabolic demands. Given the significance of septic shock and anaphylactic shock to morbidity among pediatric patients, we will undertake a more extensive discussion of these shock states.

Sepsis

Sepsis or sepsis syndromes are differentiated by the role of infection in their pathophysiology, although the potential for culture-negative sepsis does exist. As illustrated in Box 30-1, there is a broad but specific spectrum of sepsis syndromes in pediatric patients. Septic shock, which encompasses infection and is specifically distinguished by hypotension, is a common cause for admission to the pediatric intensive care unit. Early septic shock can be managed with volume resuscitation, antimicrobials, and supportive therapy; however, when progressed, it may require vasoactive support as detailed later. Late or refractory septic shock may not respond to fluids and catecholamines and may rapidly progress to multiorgan dysfunction. Gram-positive and gram-negative bacteria may both cause septic shock, with the clinical patterns of shock often distinguishable by organism. Classically described as "cold shock," gram-negative organisms result in severe vasoconstriction, with epinephrine typically the vasoactive of choice. Gram-positive sepsis more often manifests as "warm" or vasodilatory shock, with norepinephrine used to increase systemic vascular resistance and thus cardiac output. In this shock state, the cardiac output is rather increased, reflecting high-output failure; however, given the resultant alterations in systemic vascular resistance, both oxygen delivery and utilization are impaired.

When septic shock is refractory to fluid or catecholamines, consideration must also be given to adrenal insufficiency as a component of the shock state, particularly in patients who are at risk for impairment in their hypothalamic-pituitary-adrenal axis or who have had a

---

Box 30-1   **Definition of Sepsis and Sepsis Syndrome in Pediatric Patients**

Bacteremia: Culture-confirmed presence of live bacteria in blood

Sepsis: Evidence of infection with temperature changes, increased heart rate, increased respiratory rate, and leukocytosis or leukopenia

Sepsis syndrome: Sepsis plus at least one of the following: acute mental changes, decreased PaO_2, increased plasma lactate, or decreased urine output

Septic shock: Sepsis syndrome plus hypotension that responds to fluid therapy and/or drug therapy

Refractory septic shock: Sepsis syndrome plus hypotension for more than 1 hour that is not responsive to fluid and/or drug therapy and necessitates use of vasopressors

Multiple organ system failure: Any combination of disseminated intravascular coagulation, acute respiratory distress syndrome, renal failure, and hepatobiliary dysfunction

From Goldstein B, Giroir B, Randolph A. International Consensus Conference on pediatric sepsis: definitions for sepsis and organ dysfunction in pediatrics. *Pediatr Crit Care Med* 2005 Jan;6(1):2.

history of steroid exposure. In such patients, the clinical status may not improve unless the patient receives "stress-dose" steroids with hydrocortisone.[1]

Select patients with refractory shock who fail conventional therapy may be considered for salvage therapy with extracorporeal membrane oxygenation. For these individuals, ECMO can provide circulatory support until the causative organism is sufficiently treated to allow for potential and gradual organ system recovery. The risk of morbidity and mortality with ECMO for septic shock patients remains high; thus its use is limited. The current algorithm for management of sepsis is best detailed in the *Surviving Sepsis Campaign: Revised 2011 Guidelines* (Figure 30-1).

Anaphylaxis

A second type of distributive shock that results from peripheral vasodilation is anaphylactic shock. **Anaphylaxis** occurs when a foreign antigen interacts with the body and elicits a systemic, immediate hypersensitivity reaction caused by immunoglobulin E–mediated release of mediators from tissue mast cells and circulating basophils.[2] A variety of substances can elicit these reactions.[3,4] There are times, however, when a cause of anaphylaxis may not be found despite an exhaustive search.[5,6]

After the introduction of an antigen into the body, either by an enteral or parenteral route, reaction with the IgE antibody on tissue mast cells or circulating basophils occurs. This evokes the release of a number of chemical

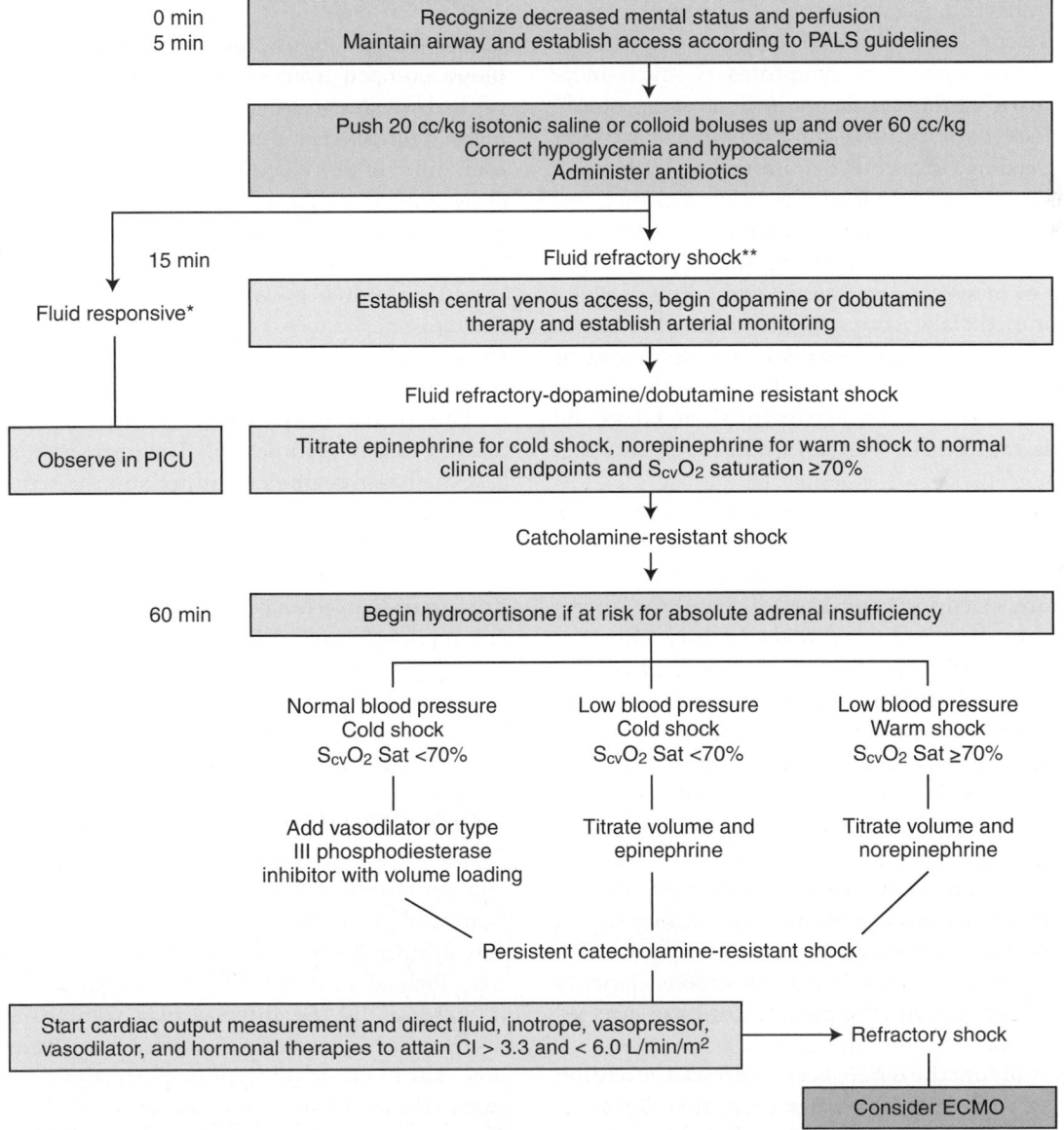

FIGURE 30-1 Algorithm for pediatric shock treatment. (Dellinger RP, Levy MM, Carlet JM, et al. Surviving Sepsis campaign: international guidelines for management of severe sepsis and septic shock: 2008. *Crit Care Med* 2008 Jan;36(1):296-327.)

mediators responsible for the clinical and hemodynamic symptom complex elicited. Histamine is one of the most prominent mediators and is believed to be responsible for the increase in airway resistance and the fall in partial pressure of oxygen as a result of its contractile action on the smooth muscle of the lung.[5] There is vasodilation and increased vascular permeability that produce a rapid loss of intravascular volume, which then stimulates the release of catecholamines. Initially, systemic vascular resistance is reduced and cardiac output is increased; however, with prolonged shock these reverse and the decrease in preload and afterload leads to myocardial depression.

The presentation of the child with anaphylaxis varies depending on the severity of symptoms. Some children may present with only a skin eruption or edema, whereas other patients may present with respiratory compromise or cardiovascular collapse and shock characteristic of an overt anaphylactic episode.[4,5] The presentation with an urticarial rash or respiratory symptoms is much more common than a cardiovascular source of symptoms.[3,6] However, shock and cardiovascular collapse can occur without a preceding cutaneous manifestation.[5] Other presenting symptoms may include gastrointestinal complaints or neurological symptoms such as dizziness, headache, or syncope. Symptoms may begin within minutes of antigen presentation or may be delayed for several hours. If symptoms begin immediately on exposure, the reaction tends to be more severe and can be rapidly fatal. An episode may be biphasic, where symptoms can abate for several hours and then return. Attacks may also persist for several days and have multiple recurrences with asymptomatic periods in between.

The rapid recognition of anaphylaxis and prompt initiation of therapy is essential. The treatment of anaphylactic shock can be divided into two major phases. First, as with any shock state, attention is directed to the ABCs. Airway compromise may be present and takes priority. Once the airway is secure, oxygenation and ventilation are assessed. There is often bronchospasm with concomitant wheezing. Providing oxygen will help ensure adequate oxygenation, and the wheezing often abates with the administration of epinephrine for circulatory support. Epinephrine is the mainstay of therapy. Circulatory dysfunction and shock are the next most pressing issues. For circulatory collapse, large volume infusions, as in other types of shock, help to restore the circulating blood volume. Hypotension can be severe and resistant to therapy. Circulatory support with repeated doses of epinephrine and a continuous epinephrine infusion help support the patient until the directed therapy can begin.[4,5]

Once the vital functions have been addressed, attention should turn to combating the antigen exposure. If the antigen and route are known—for instance, if a blood transfusion is being administered—limitation of the antigen exposure becomes the next priority. Antihistamines should be given to counter the effect of the inciting mediator.

A combination of H1 (diphenhydramine) and H2 (ranitidine) inhibitors is superior to an H1 antagonist alone for resolution of symptoms.[5] Corticosteroids may have a role in anaphylaxis by improving the inflammatory response and may help alleviate late phase reactions. Aerosolized β-adrenergic agents may be useful if the bronchospasm is unresponsive to epinephrine.[5]

Pathophysiology

The key pathophysiological derangement that occurs in shock is the impairment of oxygen delivery and utilization. Without adequate cardiac output, oxygen cannot be effectively delivered to body tissues, and the systemic effects of this substrate-depleted state result in the clinical manifestations of shock.

Cardiac Output

In physiological terms, the cardiac output is the amount of blood pumped from the heart to the organs and tissues of the body. It can be expressed mathematically as liters of blood pumped per minute.[7] Children are different from each other in terms of their size, so all hemodynamic measurements must be corrected for these size differences. When the cardiac output is corrected for size, the cardiac index (cardiac output divided by body surface area) is derived.[8] In children, normal values for the cardiac index are in the range of 3.3 to 6.0 $L/min/m^2$.[1,9] A cardiac index of less than 2.0 $L/min/m^2$ has been associated with an increase in mortality.[1]

The cardiac output is determined by the heart rate and the stroke volume.[1,10,11] The heart rate is simply how fast the heart beats per minute and the stroke volume is the amount of blood pumped out of the heart with each mechanical beat. Three components contribute to the stroke volume: preload, inotropy, and afterload.[10,12] Another representation of cardiac output, which represents "blood flow," can be characterized as the change in pressure (mean arterial pressure [MAP] – central venous pressure [CVP]) divided by resistance (systemic vascular resistance [SVR]). This relationship is mathematically expressed as (MAP − CVP)/SVR.[1,13]

Components of Stroke Volume

Preload is measured as the central venous pressure and is a representation of the amount of volume present in the heart and great vessels at rest. This volume exerts a pressure against the walls of the blood vessels in the vascular tree. Preload is dependent on adequate venous return. It increases as the intravascular volume increases and decreases when there is a reduction in intravascular volume. The Frank-Starling principle relates this central pressure to the initial stretch on the myocardial muscle fibers.[12] The stretch, and the resultant contractile ability, increases as this central pressure increases, up to a threshold limit determined by the individual's myocardial compliance. At this point, the contractile ability cannot increase further.

Inotropy is the term that characterizes the contractile state of the heart muscle. Inotropic problems may occur despite an adequate preload if the contractile state is compromised. Further, problems with contractility increase the susceptibility of the myocardium to increases in afterload.[1]

Afterload is a measure of the resistance or force against which the heart must pump. Resistance to the flow of blood in a vessel is proportional to the length of the vessel and the viscosity of the blood, and inversely proportional to the radius of the vessel to the fourth power.[10] The vessel's cross-sectional area determines the vascular resistance and is highly dependent on the arteriolar tone. The systemic vascular resistance index is expressed mathematically as the difference of the mean arterial pressure and the central venous pressure divided by the cardiac output and multiplied by a factor of 80; $SVRI = [MAP - CVP)/CO] \times 80$. The diastolic blood pressure is a surrogate marker for the basal level of pressure present within the vascular system. As afterload increases, stroke volume decreases. Infants and children have a limited ability to increase stroke volume. As a result, they will attempt to compensate for a reduction in cardiac output by increasing their heart rate.[8] Tachycardia is one of the first signs of decreased peripheral perfusion in children. Hypotension is an unreliable and late finding of shock in children, occurring when the child's compensatory mechanisms have already failed.[13,14]

Shock can be classified based on the adequacy of the cardiac output or by one of its components: heart rate, preload, inotropy, or afterload.[15] This schema also provides for therapeutic interventions targeted to the area of the circulatory system experiencing a problem (Figure 30-2).

In addition, each one of these physiological parameters can be measured clinically in the child with shock, thereby allowing continuous monitoring and assessment of the response to therapeutic interventions.[8,11,13]

Nutrients and Oxygen in Blood

The cardiac output is responsible for transferring blood and nutrients from the heart to the tissues and organs and back again. The nutrients are carried in the blood by two physical methods.[16] First, some nutrients and oxygen are dissolved in the blood, accounting for a relatively small amount of oxygen transport. Second, nutrients and oxygen can be bound to red blood cells or macromolecules and "carried" by the cardiac output to the site of utilization. Oxygen delivery depends significantly on hemoglobin concentration.[13] The amount of oxygen bound to hemoglobin is described by the oxyhemoglobin dissociation curve and is affected by physical properties such as temperature and acidosis.[16] The contribution of each of these components is symbolized in a mathematical formula that represents the arterial oxygen content (Box 30-2).[16-18] The case study features an example that demonstrates how the mathematical formulas shown in Box 30-2 may be used to quantify oxygen transport. Once the oxygen content is calculated, it can be considered within the framework of the cardiac output.

Oxygen Delivery

The concept of oxygen delivery is fundamental to the understanding of shock and is illustrated by the following clinical highlight.

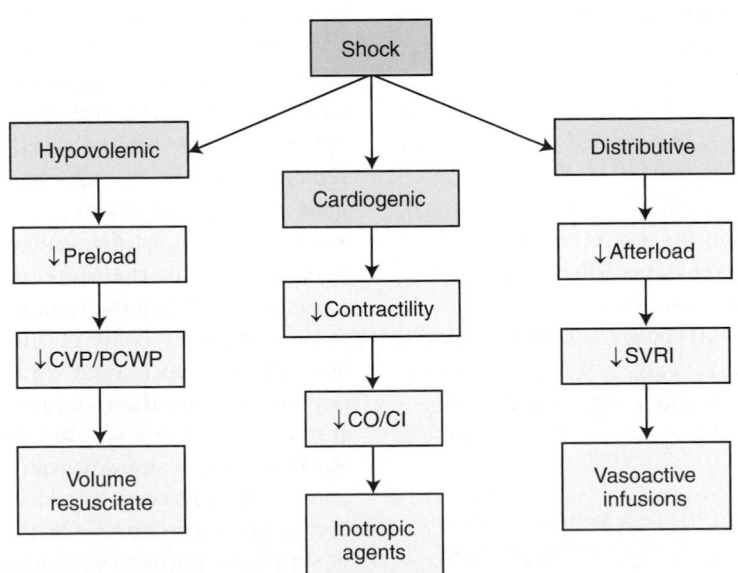

FIGURE 30-2   Diagrammatic representation of shock, its classification, clinical measures of altered stroke volume, and treatment strategies. *CI,* Cardiac index; *CO,* cardiac output; *CVP,* central venous pressure; *PCWP,* pulmonary capillary wedge pressure; *SVRI,* systemic vascular resistance index.

CLINICAL HIGHLIGHT

A 5-year-old girl is in septic shock in the pediatric intensive care unit as a result of an overwhelming infection. She has a hemoglobin level of 10 g/dl, a cardiac output of 4.0 L/min, and arterial blood gas findings of pH 7.35; PCO_2, 36 mm Hg; PaO_2, 85 mm Hg; HCO_3^-, 20 mEq/L; and a corresponding oxygen saturation of 95%. A mixed venous blood sample demonstrates pH, 7.32; PCO_2, 34 mm Hg; PaO_2, 37 mm Hg; and an oxygen saturation of 62%.

Calculate the oxygen content, delivery, and consumption as follows:

ARTERIAL OXYGEN CONTENT

$$CaO_2 = \text{Amount dissolved in blood} + \text{Amount bound to hemoglobin (arterial side)}$$

$$\text{Amount dissolved} = 0.003 \times PaO_2$$

$$\begin{aligned}\text{Amount dissolved} &= 0.003 \times 85 \text{ mm Hg}\\ &= 0.255 \text{ or } 0.255 \text{ ml of } O_2 \text{ in } 100 \text{ ml of blood}\end{aligned}$$

$$\text{Amount bound} = 1.34 \times \text{Hemoglobin} \times \% \, O_2 \text{ saturation}$$

$$\begin{aligned}\text{Amount bound} &= 1.34 \times 10 \times 0.95\\ &= 12.73 \text{ ml of oxygen per } 100 \text{ ml of blood}\end{aligned}$$

$$\begin{aligned}CaO_2 &= 0.255 + 12.73\\ &= 12.99 \text{ ml of } O_2 \text{ per } 100 \text{ ml of blood}\end{aligned}$$

MIXED VENOUS OXYGEN CONTENT

$$C\bar{v}O_2 = \text{Amount dissolved} + \text{Amount bound to hemoglobin (venous side)} = 0.003 \times P\bar{v}O_2$$

$$\text{Amount dissolved} = 0.003 \times P\bar{v}O_2$$

$$\begin{aligned}\text{Amount dissolved} &= 0.003 \times 37 \text{ mm Hg}\\ &= 0.115 \text{ or } 0.115 \text{ ml of } O_2 \text{ in } 100 \text{ ml of blood}\end{aligned}$$

$$\text{Amount bound} = 1.34 \times \text{Hemoglobin} \times \% \, O_2 \text{ saturation}$$

$$\begin{aligned}\text{Amount bound} &= 1.34 \times 10 \times 0.62\\ &= 8.31 \text{ ml of } O_2 \text{ per } 100 \text{ ml of blood}\end{aligned}$$

$$C\bar{v}O_2 = 0.115 + 8.31 = 8.425 \text{ ml of } O_2 \text{ per } 100 \text{ ml of blood}$$

OXYGEN DELIVERY

$$DO_2 = O_2 \text{ content} \times \text{Cardiac output}$$

$$DO_2 = 12.99 \text{ ml of } O_2 \text{ per } 100 \text{ ml of blood} \times 4000 \text{ ml/min}$$

$$\text{Arterial } DO_2 = 519.6 \text{ ml/min}$$

OXYGEN CONSUMPTION

$$\dot{V}O_2 \text{ (ml/min)} = (\text{Arterial} - \text{venous}) \, O_2 \text{ content} \times \text{Cardiac output (ml/min)}$$

$$\begin{aligned}\dot{V}O_2 \text{ (ml/min)} &= (12.99 - 8.425) \text{ ml of } O_2\\ &\text{per } 100 \text{ ml of blood} \times\\ &4000 \text{ ml/min} = 182.6\end{aligned}$$

Delivery of Blood to the Tissues

The cardiac output delivers oxygenated blood to the tissues on a global or systemic level.[12,16,19] Delivery of oxygenated blood, however, is only one part of this complex physiological process. **Oxygen delivery** depends on oxygen carrying capacity (% hemoglobin), oxygen provided (oxygen bound to hemoglobin plus dissolved oxygen), and cardiac output.[1] Once oxygenated and nutrient-rich blood reaches the target organ, the organ must be able to utilize the substrates it receives.[19] There must be uptake of oxygen in the tissues and cells of the organ along with the exchange of organ byproducts that are then transported back to the lungs. A major component of these byproducts is carbon dioxide, which has a higher solubility in the blood than oxygen.[16]

Oxygen consumption is a measure of the amount of oxygen, or substrate, utilized by the organs of the body.[15] Comparing the amount of oxygen being supplied to the organs from the arterial circuit and the amount of oxygen remaining in the venous circuit after removal by the organs provides an estimate of how much is being consumed.[16,20,21] As cardiac output decreases and metabolic demands remain the same, the tissues will extract more oxygen to maintain the same consumption, but the oxygen returning to the heart in the venous circulation will be less.[1] In children oxygen consumption depends more on oxygen delivery than oxygen extraction.[13] Oxygen consumption greater than 200 ml/min/m² has been associated with improved survival.[1,13] The amount of nutrient consumed by the organs relative to delivery is referred to as the oxygen extraction.[19] Oxygen extraction is independent of supply for patients with shock. As shock worsens, organ tissue perfusion decreases and the organ extracts fewer nutrients from the blood. This measure of the severity of shock has been associated with survival.[8] Regardless of the etiology of the shock, alterations in cellular metabolism, mitochondrial dysfunction, abnormal carbohydrate metabolism, and the failure of many energy-dependent enzyme reactions lead to difficulty with utilization of substrate at the cellular level and eventually cell death.[10] These changes in cellular oxygen utilization alter the consumption of oxygen in each of the organs, leading to organ dysfunction. Organ system dysfunction resulting from shock, if left untreated, ultimately leads to failure of multiple organ systems. The term *multiorgan dysfunction syndrome* (MODS) has been applied to this disseminated pathological response.[10]

Metabolic Response

The body's response to poor tissue perfusion results in a number of metabolic reactions. Many of the manifestations of shock represent the body's compensatory mechanisms, which attempt to maintain effective tissue perfusion and correct the abnormalities of shock. These responses attempt to maintain mean circulatory pressure, maximize cardiac output, redistribute perfusion to the most vital organs, and optimize the unloading of oxygen to the tissues.[10] The compensatory mechanisms are designed to autoregulate in the setting of hemodynamic or metabolic dysfunction.

The central nervous system releases adrenocorticotropic hormone in the setting of stress, which stimulates the adrenal glands to release cortisol. Adequate adrenocortical function is essential to survive critical illness, and most critically ill patients will exhibit elevated cortisol levels.[1,22] Many patients, however, exhibit a state of "relative" adrenal insufficiency because of an inadequate production of cortisol.[22] The sympathetic nervous system is regulated by arterial and cardiopulmonary baroreceptors and releases epinephrine and norepinephrine, which increase cardiac output by increasing heart rate and stroke volume. Cortisol assists the actions of these two catecholamines. Intrinsic vasoactive substances are released in response to increased metabolic activity and oxygen tension. The angiotensin/aldosterone–ADH/vasopressin system is activated to preserve intravascular volume.[1] Other vasodilators released locally and systemically include nitric oxide, prostacyclin, and kinins; vasoconstrictors include endothelin, renin, and oxygen free radicals. These substances affect the vascular tone, systemic vascular resistance, and therefore blood pressure.

The inflammatory response is a physiological, homeostatic mechanism designed to respond to injury or infection. Inflammatory mediator release usually provides beneficial effects; however, in shock, the inflammatory response becomes unregulated.[10] The production of immune mediators is triggered by ischemic or hypoxic insults and produces further tissue injury. The systemic inflammatory response syndrome (SIRS) is the term used to describe the nonspecific inflammatory process that accompanies these insults.[14] The immune response leads to changes in T and B lymphocyte responses, activation of the complement cascade, activation of coagulation factors, and cytokine release (tumor necrosis factor [TNF] and interleukin [IL]-6). These mediators exert their influence on the vasculature to produce inadequate perfusion or direct cellular injury.[10] All of these contribute to organ dysfunction and the eventual signs and symptoms the body may experience in shock.

Management and Treatment
General Considerations

The overall goals of treatment for shock are to maintain adequate tissue perfusion, to avoid end-organ damage, and to treat the underlying primary process. Therapeutic strategies should enhance the delivery of oxygen and nutrients to the tissues, reduce the oxygen demand, and correct the metabolic abnormalities. Continuous monitoring of the patient's response to interventions is critical and may lead to redirection of therapies. Early aggressive therapy of shock, focused on maintaining blood pressure and oxygen delivery, improves the outcomes in critically ill children.[1]

Assessment and Evaluation

The approach to the child in shock begins with an evaluation of vital functions as expounded by the ABCs of resuscitation.[23] Maintenance of the airway and attention to oxygenation and ventilation are the initial priorities no matter the type of shock. The circulatory system is evaluated by the presence of a pulse. If a pulse is absent, cardiopulmonary resuscitation needs to be performed and cardiotonic medications consistent with advanced life support need to be administered.[23] The presence and quality of the pulse reflect systemic vascular tone as well as cardiac output. Vascular access should be rapidly obtained, and if there is difficulty with peripheral venous access, an intraosseous or central venous route should be used.[13]

Once the ABCs are established, attention can be directed to measuring vital signs and performing a secondary survey. Normal values for pulse, respiratory rate, and blood pressure are age dependent. The knowledge of these age-related differences is essential to being able to care for any child.[14,27]

A brief and directed patient history and physical examination can be obtained at this point. It should be directed at determining a potential cause of the shock. In addition, obtain essential information regarding medical history, especially a history of congenital heart disease, immunodeficiency, trauma, possible ingestion of toxic substances, medications, and allergies.

After assessment of vital signs, an evaluation of the systemic perfusion as a sign of the effectiveness of the cardiac output is completed. Capillary refill (the process of blanching the skin for several seconds and timing the return of blood flow to the blanched skin) is a quick, useful, and noninvasive test that provides important information regarding perfusion in the acute setting.[23] The normal capillary refill time should be less than 2 seconds and correlates with a cardiac index of more than 2.0 L/min/m[2].[23] Prolongation of the capillary refill is considered a sign of inadequate tissue perfusion and impending shock. Assessment of the perfusion to the skin, the brain, and the kidney is often performed next because they are easy to perform and correlate better with hemodynamic measurements than capillary refill.[25]

Evaluation of the skin color and temperature is easily performed. The skin of children in shock may be pale, cyanotic, or mottled because of poor perfusion. Traditionally, practitioners have described two phases of septic shock.[1,13] In early septic shock the skin appears well perfused, warm, and pink. This occurs from the vasodilation and increased cardiac output. Later in the course of shock, the cardiac output begins to fall. The skin during this period is likely to be cool, cyanotic, or mottled and represents a decrease in the amount of substrate reaching the skin. Further assessment of the skin may reveal petechiae, poor skin turgor, or skin rashes indicative of a coagulopathy, hypovolemia, or an infectious etiology.

Examining the child's level of awareness, orientation, and response to commands can assess perfusion to the child's brain. It is important to ensure that medications that might obscure the examination have not been given. Children in shock may show signs of agitation or restlessness. Alternatively, they may also have a mental status that is stuporous or comatose.

Monitoring urine production assesses perfusion of the child's visceral organs. If the child is making adequate urine (at least 1 ml/kg/hr), then the cardiac output to the kidneys, which produces renal blood flow and drives glomerular filtration, is considered adequate. Both the kidney and the brain have vasomotor autoregulation mechanisms that maintain blood flow and perfusion in shock until a critical point is reached and perfusion pressure falls below the ability of the organ to maintain adequate blood flow.[1,13] At this point, the shock is classified as decompensated shock. In decompensated shock, the blood pressure falls and the perfusion of end organs is compromised.

Laboratory values can often provide useful clues to the proper diagnosis and management of shock. Evaluation of the acid-base status including routine electrolytes and an arterial blood gas with the calculation of the anion gap are important first steps.[26] As shock progresses, a metabolic acidosis and an elevated lactate level may occur. Lactate is a measure of anaerobic metabolism but can also be elevated in many conditions in the absence of shock.[1]

Anemia, thrombocytopenia, and elevation of prothrombin time and partial thromboplastin times (PT/PTT) may identify a coagulopathy or disseminated intravascular coagulation (DIC). An elevated or reduced white blood cell count may indicate the presence of infection or an immunodeficiency. Elevated liver enzymes or creatinine may provide evidence about the extent of hypoperfusion to the liver and kidneys and potential for subsequent dysfunction in these organs. An electrocardiogram and a chest radiograph may offer valuable clues as the etiology of the shock is investigated.

Monitoring

The child in shock requires ongoing assessment, intervention, and reassessment. Attention to the effects of an intervention on vital signs and end organ perfusion must be continually observed. Children with fluid-responsive shock can be monitored with standard noninvasive methods. However, if the child fails to respond to fluid (e.g., more than 60 ml/kg), additional strategies for monitoring and maintaining equilibrium may need to be incorporated. In addition, if a treatment does not have its intended effect on restoring homeostasis, the therapeutic approach and underlying etiology need to be reconsidered.

A number of technologies are available in the pediatric intensive care unit (PICU) for the assessment and monitoring of the child in shock. These techniques augment the information derived from the vital signs and physical examination. The arterial catheter, the CVP monitor, and the pulmonary artery catheter are three of the more common strategies employed to detect physiological changes and to supplement the clinical assessment of the child in shock. Echocardiography can also be an important noninvasive technique that provides valuable information regarding cardiac structure and function as contributors to the shock state.[13]

The placement of a catheter in a peripheral or central artery can be performed for the monitoring of blood pressure on a continuous basis in the intensive care unit. Arterial catheterization can provide beat-to-beat monitoring of the blood pressure.[10] The shape and characteristics of the waveform provide additional information regarding the characteristics of the cardiac output, including volume, afterload, and contractility.

The placement of a catheter in the central venous system allows for an assessment of the volume status of the child with shock. The catheter, when attached to a continuous column of fluid and a pressure transducer, measures the downstream intravascular pressure, or CVP, in the right atrium. This intravascular pressure represents preload, one of the contributors to the stroke volume, which contributes to the cardiac output. Because the left side of the heart receives its blood from the right side of the heart, the measurement of these right-sided heart pressures is accepted as an alternative for the dynamics on the left side of the heart in the patient whose myocardial and pulmonary compliance is normal. If biventricular function is equal and pulmonary artery resistance is low, CVP measurements closely reflect pulmonary artery wedge pressure.[27] This information helps the provider to diagnose and treat the patient in shock. If the CVP is high in the setting of normal myocardial compliance, then the intravascular volume is adequate and may not be accounting for the reduction in cardiac output. The CVP may be elevated if the blood is unable to be ejected because of a failing myocardium. If the CVP is low, additional intravenous fluid needs to be given to improve the intravascular volume deficit being observed. A central venous catheter also provides easy access for blood sampling, measuring mixed venous oxygenation, and providing access for rapid fluid resuscitation and provision of inotropic medications if necessary.

The use of a pulmonary artery (PA) catheter in children has been debated, but in children with fluid refractory and dopamine-resistant shock, the PA catheter may provide additional information to make a more appropriate assessment of the hemodynamic status of the patient.[13,28] The use of PA catheters in children is supported by the American College of Critical Care Medicine for circumstances in which irreversible shock manifesting as poor perfusion, acidosis, and hypotension persists despite the use of therapies directed at the arterial blood pressure, CVP pressure, and oxygen saturation indices.[13] In addition to the measurements obtained directly from the catheter, a number of derived values provide information regarding the homeostatic function of the child, including systemic vascular resistance as a measure of afterload and oxygen consumption and oxygen extraction.

System-Based Treatment Approach

Respiratory. Airway and breathing should be rigorously monitored and maintained for patients in shock. Endotracheal intubation with mechanical ventilation may reduce the work of breathing and optimize oxygen content. During intubation, induction agents, cardiotonic medications, and respiratory support modes must be chosen carefully so as not to worsen an already compromised cardiovascular status.

Vascular Volume. The rapid restoration of an adequate circulating blood volume is essential for a patient in shock regardless of the cause.[27-30] Normal saline or lactated Ringer's solutions are the fluids of choice for initial resuscitation because they maintain intravascular volume.[1,10,13,29,30] The use of colloids, such as albumin or starch, to maintain intravascular volume has not been demonstrated to have a beneficial effect on survival.[1,10,13] If there is evidence of anemia or suspected losses of blood, repletion of the intravascular volume with packed red blood cells should be performed.[1,13,14]

The initial administration of 20 ml/kg of fluid is recommended.[1,13,23,30] Reassessment of the patient's condition based on vital signs and end-organ perfusion helps to determine the need for additional fluid.[13] The administration of intravenous fluid will decrease the heart rate

and increase the MAP and CVP. Carcillo and colleagues demonstrated that when the initial amount of volume resuscitation administered within the first hour was cumulatively greater than 40 ml/kg, the survival rates were improved.[25] Thus both the amount of fluid and the rapidity of administration have outcome benefits. Rapid volume resuscitation restores intravascular volume and reduces the inflammatory response and coagulopathy that often accompany shock.[1] Large fluid deficits typically exist, and initial volume resuscitation usually requires 40 to 60 ml/kg but can be as much as 200 ml/kg in some cases of septic shock.[1,13,31] Continued fluid losses and persistent hypovolemia as a result of capillary leak can persist despite fluid resuscitation. Ongoing fluid replacement is necessary to maintain adequate tissue perfusion, and large volumes may be required because vascular permeability results in peripheral and third space losses.[31] When total administered volumes of 60 ml/kg are reached, intravascular monitoring and initiation of vasoactive support should be considered.

The development of rales, a gallop rhythm, hepatomegaly, and increased work of breathing may all indicate worsening cardiovascular function leading to pulmonary edema because of the relationship to the Frank-Starling principle.[32] Additional aliquots of fluid may be contraindicated at this point.[28,33] In these instances, careful invasive monitoring with pulmonary artery catheters can provide valuable information and help guide further management.

Myocardial Function. Once the intravascular volume is optimized, manipulation of other components of cardiac output should be attempted. Abnormalities in heart rate resulting in poor perfusion and shock should be addressed quickly. An unstable tachycardia manifested with hypotension or signs of shock should be treated with electrical therapy in the form of synchronized cardioversion or defibrillation.[23] Cardioversion synchronizes the delivery of the shock with the QRS complex to prevent deterioration to a more lethal arrhythmia and should be used in patients who have a palpable pulse. Defibrillation delivers a shock regardless of the timing of the cardiac cycle and is indicated in pulseless rhythms that have resulted in cardiovascular collapse.[23]

Inotropic dysfunction can result from an abnormality in any of the structures of the heart or the abnormal contractility of the cardiac myocytes. Initially, adequate preload through the judicious use of fluid resuscitation to maintain stroke volume should be ensured. After preload has been restored, additional fluid may worsen the ability of the myocardium to maintain cardiac output, especially in cardiogenic shock. Hence, the support of the myocardium can then take place with inotropic agents that act by a number of different mechanisms and can be titrated to the appropriate clinical response, including the achievement of appropriate MAP, CVP, and cardiac index to ensure adequate perfusion.[13,33] Inotropic agents are used to increase contractility and cardiac output. Dobutamine is a β_1-adrenergic agonist with chronotropic and inotropic actions, as well as afterload reduction. Dopamine, the most commonly used inotrope, increases renal blood flow but also has vasoconstrictive properties at high doses as a result of release of norepinephrine. Epinephrine is a naturally circulating neurohormone that increases contractility during stress and shock.[1] At low dose it provides inotropy, but at higher doses it increases peripheral vascular tone and acts as a vasopressor. Patients with heart failure and increased systemic vascular resistance may be harmed by these higher doses unless epinephrine is combined with an inodilator or vasodilator.[1] Norepinephrine is another common inotropic agent and is effective for dopamine-resistant shock. It is a strong vasoconstrictor even at low doses but has better inotropic effects when combined with an inodilator.

Inodilators work through a different mechanism. These drugs enhance inotropy while simultaneously vasodilating and reducing afterload, making it easier for the heart to eject blood.[1,32] Phosphodiesterase inhibitors, such as milrinone, mediate inotropy and vasodilation by preventing hydrolysis of cAMP and therefore potentiate the effects of β receptor stimulation in cardiac and vascular tissue.[13] Alone, these improve contractility and diastolic relaxation and also cause vasodilation of pulmonary and systemic arterial vasculature. When combined with inotropes, vasodilators, and vasopressors, the interaction provides even better contractility and relaxation.[1]

If the problem with inadequate cardiac function is related to elevations in afterload, vasodilators should be administered.[33] Vasodilators reduce pulmonary vascular resistance or systemic vascular resistance and thereby improve cardiac output by reducing afterload.[1] Nitroprusside is a systemic and pulmonary vasodilator. Nitroglycerin has dose-dependent effects on coronary artery vasodilation, pulmonary vasodilation, and systemic vasodilation that increase with increasing doses. Prostaglandins can also be used as vasodilators, especially in ductal-dependent congenital heart disease. The use of vasodilators should be titrated to reducing afterload without causing tachycardia or diastolic hypotension. In many circumstances, inotropic agents in combination with vasodilators may be useful.[1,13,23] Conversely, vasopressors such as norepinephrine and epinephrine increase vascular tone, peripheral vascular resistance, and afterload and have inotropic effects. This helps to maintain perfusion to vital organs such as the brain, kidneys, and gastrointestinal tract.

Hematological. In hemorrhagic shock or anemic shock, intravascular volume should be replaced with packed red blood cells. Although there are variable data regarding the ideal hemoglobin for pediatric patients in septic shock, it is known that mortality rates increase when hemoglobin levels are less than 6 mg/dl. Provision of blood improves circulating blood volume and increases the oxygen delivery and substrate to the tissues. Coagulation abnormalities occur in all forms of shock. Activation of the coagulation cascade can lead to disseminated intravascular coagulation, which results in thrombocytopenia, decreased fibrinogen, elevated fibrin split products, and microangiopathic hemolytic anemia.[10] In prolonged states of shock, thrombosis and hypofibrinolysis can occur. The rapid reversal of shock often prevents disseminated intravascular coagulation and bleeding.[1] When resuscitation is inadequate, the replacement of clotting factors may be beneficial. Vitamin K, fresh frozen plasma, cryoprecipitate, and platelet transfusions should correct most coagulopathies. Activated factor VII has been effective in reversing refractory hemorrhagic shock in many situations. Patients with hemophilia or von Willebrand's disease may need specific replacement therapy to control bleeding.

Endocrine. Maintaining metabolic and hormonal homeostasis is important in children with shock. Adrenal insufficiency is common in the intensive care setting and presents with low cardiac output and high systemic vascular resistance or with high cardiac output and low systemic vascular resistance.[1] Adrenal insufficiency should be considered in any child who is unresponsive to catecholamines, and there is a possibility that adrenal dysfunction actually contributes to the development of catecholamine-resistant shock.[22] This insufficiency has been associated with worsening of multiple organ failure and higher mortality.[22,34] Steroid replacement should be considered when a measured cortisol level is less than 18 mg/dl. Hydrocortisone has glucocorticoid and mineralocorticoid effects and should be given at either a "stress" dose of 2 mg/kg/day or a "shock" dose of 50 mg/kg/day during acute shock.[1,31]

Electrolyte abnormalities are common in the ICU, and following their values is an important part of the evaluation and management of the shock patient. As patients are resuscitated with fluid, sodium values may become abnormal and need correcting or they may be part of the presenting signs of dehydration and hypovolemic shock. If kidney dysfunction is present, hyperkalemia may become an issue that contributes to cardiac dysfunction or arrhythmias. Hypocalcemia is a common, reversible contributor to cardiac dysfunction and should be treated to maintain normal ionized calcium levels. Increased intracellular calcium increases contractility, whereas decreased calcium leads to relaxation in cardiac and vascular smooth muscle cells.[1] Correction of electrolyte abnormalities is crucial in maintaining stability.

Hyperglycemia occurs as a result of glycogenolysis and gluconeogenesis mediated by increases in adrenocorticotropic hormone, glucocorticoids, glucagons, and catecholamines as well as decreases in insulin.[10] Hyperglycemia contributes to reduced immune system function and promotes microbial and fungal growth. Although there is now more evidence to suggest that tight glucose control may not be as beneficial as once thought, extremes in either direction are not desirable.

Immunological. Treatment with broad-spectrum antibiotics with activity against gram-positive and gram-negative organisms should be started as soon as septic shock is considered. The choice of antibiotics should be based on the suspected focus of infection,[35] and the first doses should be given during the initial resuscitation. The choice of antibiotic can be narrowed once an organism is identified. In many cases of septic shock, especially in neutropenic patients, cultures are negative. Despite this, antibiotics are typically continued for up to 14 days. Early antifungal therapy should be considered in immunocompromised patients and in those who are unresponsive to antibacterial therapy.

Nutritional Status. Nutritional support of the critically ill child has a role in maintaining stability, promoting healing, and improving the outcome from acute and chronic illness.[2,36] The goals of nutritional support are to promote these end points while simultaneously providing adequate metabolic substrate for the growth and development of the child.[36] The optimal balance is to maintain an anabolic state with positive nitrogen balance. Ideally, enteral or, alternatively, parenteral nutrition should begin as soon as cardiovascular stability is obtained. Early enteral nutrition appears to prevent gut mucosal atrophy and bacterial translocation.[35] Evaluation of vitamins, trace elements, and immune-modifying nutritional agents did not demonstrate clear benefit.

Extracorporeal Membrane Oxygenation. Patients remaining in shock despite the supportive therapies may benefit from mechanical cardiac support, such as extracorporeal membrane oxygenation (ECMO). ECMO is highly effective for cardiogenic shock because it helps support the ailing heart, but it is less successful in septic shock, except possibly refractory low cardiac output septic shock.[1] Patients may still require vasoactive agents (Table 30-2) for persistent hypotension but less inotropic support because the circuit provides inotropy.[13] There is also a potential role for ECMO in patients with other shock states such as septic shock.

TABLE 30-2

Commonly Used Vasoactives and Key Characteristics

Dopamine	Systemic effect determined by dose range; causes splanchnic and renal vasodilation at low to moderate doses; higher doses result in alpha effects
Epinephrine	Causes increase in peripheral vascular resistance; at lower doses, β_2 effects of smooth muscle dilation predominate; useful for anaphylaxis and vasoconstrictive shock states
Norepinephrine	Augments systemic vascular resistance; best in vasodilatory shock states
Vasopressin	Systemic vasoconstriction
Milrinone	Inodilator; causes lusitropy (end-diastolic relaxation)

MENINGITIS

Meningitis describes an inflammation of the overlying membranes of the brain and spinal cord, known as the meninges. The causes of meningitis are varied and include bacterial, viral, and other infectious etiologies; the natural history of the disease is equally diverse, with factors such as organism, age of patient, time to recognition, and other co-morbidities affecting clinical outcome.

Definition and Classification

The common causative agents for meningitis are age specific. For neonates, the primary bacterial agents include *Streptococcus agalactiae*, *Klebsiella* species, *Escherichia coli*, and, uniquely, *Listeria monocytogenes*. In older infants through the early toddler years, *Streptococcus pneumoniae*, *Neisseria meningitides*, and *Haemophilus influenzae* are most likely. Infants are at particular risk for herpes simplex and enteroviral infections. For specific circumstances such as after trauma or subsequent to neurosurgical procedures, staphylococcal species and gram-negative organisms may predominate. Antimicrobial therapy must thus be directed at the most likely causative agents. Universal vaccination programs have helped to substantially decrease the incidence of many types of bacterial meningitis.

Viral meningitis typically follows a more indolent and benign course than bacterial and thus may have delayed diagnosis. With the increased availability of viral and antigen testing, these organisms can now be identified. Although less common, fungal, parasitic, and tuberculous meningitis can occur with fulminant clinical courses.

Pathophysiology

The key pathological derangements of meningitis involve two primary components: disruption of the blood–brain barrier and resultant alternation of cerebral autoregulation. After typically hematogenous spread after nasopharyngeal colonization, the blood–brain barrier becomes disrupted by the pathogen leading to meningeal invasion. Inflammation of the subarachnoid space ensues with an accompanying inflammatory cascade. The presence of these cytokines alters the neural vasoregulation, resulting in abnormal cerebral blood flow and potential alterations in intracranial pressure.

Management and Treatment
General Considerations

Infants and children with meningitis may present with acute alteration in mental status, usually with bacterial meningitis, although especially in older children with viral infections, there may be a nonspecific prodrome before meningeal signs develop. Meningitis caused by bacterial infections such as *N. meningitides* may also present with multi-organ system dysfunction and characteristic signs such as purpura fulminans. If intracranial pressure is elevated, the patient may have vital sign abnormalities consistent with

Cushing's triad. Symptoms such as loss of consciousness and seizures are late signs and may be preceded by headache, photophobia, emesis, meningismus, or alterations in mental status.

Laboratory Testing

Timely recognition and high index of suspicion for meningitis are essential to its successful management and treatment. Even with mere suspicion for meningitis, patients should receive early and aggressive antibiotic treatment given the relative low risk versus potential high value of antimicrobials. Cerebrospinal fluid (CSF) sampling should ideally occur before antibiotics are initiated; however, this should not delay therapy in circumstances when it is not possible. Observed pleocytosis within the CSF and, more recently, antigen testing can reliably aid the diagnosis of meningitis even when antibiotics have been administered beforehand; thus the goal is to treat without delay. Cerebrospinal fluid is commonly analyzed for cell count, presence of organisms by Gram stain, glucose, and protein; additional testing such as bacterial antigen panels, herpes simplex virus (HSV) antigen, and latex agglutination testing may also be sent.

The role of neurological imaging before lumbar puncture is somewhat controversial. When patients have clear signs of intracranial hypertension, imaging is warranted to assess for presence of mass lesion and the associated risk of herniation with spinal tap. There is yet to be a universal recommendation for preimaging in children, especially in consideration of the risks of childhood exposure to ionizing radiation.

In most cases, empiric antibiotic therapy with vancomycin and a third-generation cephalosporin is recommended. When there is concern for HSV, acyclovir is included, and for neonates, ampicillin is routinely added because of the risk of *Listeria* infection. Dexamethasone is recommended as adjunctive therapy in cases of *H. influenzae* meningitis to reduce the incidence of hearing loss.[37] For aseptic meningitis, which typically follows a benign clinical course, supportive care is recommended.

The primary complications of meningitis include lasting neurological impairment, seizures, brain abscess, disorders of sodium homeostasis, and cerebral edema. As discussed, timely diagnosis and therapy may help to mitigate the worst of the possible outcomes.

SUMMARY

Although most children remain healthy, medical conditions such as shock and meningitis still pose a significant risk to their well-being. We have provided an overview of these two disease processes here, with specific attention to septic shock and anaphylaxis as two shock states that account for a substantial amount of pediatric morbidity. Through our discussion of these topics, we hope we have sufficiently underscored the value of thoughtful and timely clinical evaluation coupled with prompt institution of therapy in the care of pediatric patients.

KEY POINTS

- Timely recognition and early treatment of shock can help mitigate the risk of its morbidity and mortality in children.
- The goal of all shock treatment is to optimize oxygen delivery.
- Judicious antimicrobial therapy is the mainstay of managing sepsis syndromes.
- Anaphylaxis should be primarily managed with epinephrine.
- Meningitis is still an important cause of neurological disability in children, but again, timely recognition and early treatment are essential.

ASSESSMENT QUESTIONS

1. All but which of the following describes a shock state?
   A. Hemorrhagic
   B. Obstructive
   C. Hypovolemic
   D. Cardiogenic
   E. Oliguric

2. Cardiac output is determined by all of the following *except*:
   A. Afterload
   B. Inotropy
   C. Preload
   D. Heart rate
   E. Oxygen content

3. Which of the following is a correct statement about oxygen consumption?
   A. It depends on oxygen-carrying capacity.
   B. It can be measured directly from the pulmonary artery catheter.
   C. It is a measure of the oxygen utilized by the body.
   D. Oxygen consumption increases as cardiac output decreases.
   E. Lower oxygen consumption has been associated with improved survival.

4. How would shock from a burn be classified?
   A. Distributive
   B. Obstructive
   C. Cardiogenic
   D. Hypovolemic
   E. Anaphylactic

5. What should initial assessment of a patient in shock include?
   A. Attention to ABCs
   B. Examination of mental status
   C. Brief, directed history
   D. Examination of the skin
   E. All of the above

6. Regardless of etiology, what is the first step in treatment of shock?
   A. Begin rapid fluid infusion.
   B. Establish and maintain an airway.
   C. Place a central line.
   D. Start dopamine.
   E. Give a shock dose of steroids.

7. Which of the following enhances inotropy and vasodilation?
   A. Milrinone
   B. Dopamine
   C. Norepinephrine
   D. Dobutamine
   E. Phenylephrine

8. Which of the following are commonly seen as part of the shock state?
   A. Adrenal insufficiency
   B. Disseminated intravascular coagulation
   C. Electrolyte abnormalities
   D. Hyperglycemia
   E. All of the above

9. What are the major components of sepsis?
   A. Infecting organisms leading to direct tissue damage and organ dysfunction
   B. An excessive host inflammatory response
   C. A failure of counterregulatory mechanisms
   D. All of the above

10. Which of the following is correct regarding the treatment of sepsis?
    A. Limited volume resuscitation improves outcome.
    B. Dopamine is the best initial vasoactive substance for the hypotensive patient.
    C. ECMO is a commonly used form of hemodynamic support.
    D. Activated protein C is recommended for pediatric patients.
    E. Early empiric antimicrobial therapy is critical in the treatment of sepsis.

11. Which patient group(s) have an increased risk of sepsis?
    A. Oncology patients
    B. Transplant patients
    C. Patients with chronic diseases
    D. Patients with indwelling central venous catheters
    E. All of the above

12. Symptoms from anaphylaxis may be:
    A. Immediate
    B. Delayed
    C. Cutaneous
    D. Cardiovascular collapse
    E. All of the above

13. The treatment of anaphylactic shock includes which of the following?
    A. Epinephrine
    B. Antihistamines
    C. Steroids
    D. Limiting antigen exposure
    E. All of the above

14. Which of the following are true regarding meningitis?
    A. Inflammation of the meninges is always due to bacterial infection.
    B. Meningitis does not cause cerebral edema.
    C. Bacterial meningitis is most often the result of hematogenous spread.
    D. There is little risk of chronic morbidity with bacterial meningitis.
    E. Bacteria, the cause of meningitis, are always gram-positive organisms.

15. Which of the following is/are complications of bacterial meningitis?
    A. Vision loss
    B. Hearing loss
    C. Mental retardation
    D. Subdural empyema
    E. All of the above

References

1. Dellinger RP, Levy MM, Carlet JM, et al: Surviving Sepsis campaign: international guidelines for management of severe sepsis and septic shock: 2008, *Crit Care Med* 36(1):296, 2008.
2. Curley MAQ, Castillo L: Nutrition and shock in pediatric patients, *New Horiz* 6:212, 1998.
3. Balk RA, Ely EW, Goyette RE: *Sepsis handbook,* Knoxville, TN, 2004, Thomson Healthcare Advanced Therapeutics Communications.
4. Schears GJ, Deutschman CS: Common nutritional issues in pediatric and adult critical care medicine, *Crit Care Clin* 3:669, 1997.
5. Dibs SD, Baker MD: Anaphylaxis in children: a 5-year experience, *Pediatrics* 99:E7, 1997.
6. Lieberman P: Specific and idiopathic anaphylaxis: pathophysiology and treatment. In Bierman CW, editor: *Allergy, asthma, and immunology from infancy to adulthood*, ed 3, Philadelphia, 1996, WB Saunders, pp 297–319.
7. Gauthier PM, Szerlip HM: Metabolic acidosis in the intensive care unit, *Crit Care Clinics* 18:289, 2002.
8. Ross J, Covell JW: Frameworks for analysis of ventricular and circulatory function: integrated responses. In West JB, editor: *Best and Taylor's physiological basis of medical practice*, ed 12, Baltimore, 1990, Williams & Wilkins.
9. Pollack MM, Fields AI, Ruttimann UE: Sequential cardiopulmonary variables in infants and children in septic shock, *Crit Care Med* 12:554, 1984.
10. Parillo JE: Approach to the patient with shock. In Goldman, editor: *Cecil textbook of medicine*, ed 22, Philadelphia, 2004, WB Saunders, pp 608.
11. Pollack MM, Fields AI, Ruttimann UE: Distributions of cardiopulmonary variables in pediatric survivors and nonsurvivors of septic shock, *Crit Care Med* 13:454, 1985.
12. Hazinski MF: Shock in the pediatric patient, *Crit Care Nurs Clin North Am* 2:309, 1990.
13. Ross J: The cardiac pump. In West JB, editor: *Best and Taylor's physiological basis of medical practice*, ed 12, Williams & Wilkins, 1990, Baltimore.
14. Carcillo JA, Fields AI: Clinical practice parameters for hemodynamic support of pediatric and neonatal patients in septic shock, *Crit Care Med* 30:1365, 2002.

15. Goldstein B, et al: International pediatric sepsis consensus conference: definitions for sepsis and organ dysfunction in pediatrics, *Pediatr Crit Care Med* 28:3–5, 2005.

16. Levy FH, O'Rourke PP: Topics in pediatric critical care. In Barnhart S, Czervinske M, editors: *Perinatal and pediatric respiratory care*, Philadelphia, 1995, WB Saunders.

17. West JB: Gas transport to the periphery. In West JB, editor: *Best and Taylor's physiological basis of medical practice*, ed 12, Baltimore, 1990, Williams & Wilkins.

18. Tobin JR, Wetzel RC: Shock and multi-organ system failure. In Rogers MC, Nichols DG, editors: *Textbook of pediatric intensive care*, ed 3, Baltimore, 1996, Williams & Wilkins.

19. Thomas NJ, Carcillo JA: Hypovolemic shock in pediatric patients, *New Horiz* 6:120, 1998.

20. Ross J: Intracardiac and arterial pressures and the cardiac output: cardiac catheterization. In West JB, editor: *Best and Taylor's physiological basis of medical practice*, ed 12, Baltimore, 1990, Williams & Wilkins.

21. Seear M, Wensley D, MacNab A: Oxygen consumption-oxygen delivery relationship in children, *J Pediatr* 123:208, 1993.

22. Carcillo JA, Cunnion RE: Septic shock, *Crit Care Clin* 13:553, 1997.

23. Feltes TF, Pignatelli R, Kleinert S: Quantitated left ventricular systolic mechanics in children with septic shock utilizing noninvasive wall stress analysis, *Crit Care Med* 22:1647, 1994.

24. Lieberman P: Anaphylaxis and anaphylactoid reactions. In Middleton E, editor: *Allergy: principles and practice*, ed 6, St Louis, 2003, Mosby, pp 1497–1517.

25. In Behrman RE, Kliegman RM, Jenson HB, editors: *Nelson's textbook of pediatrics*, ed 16, Philadelphia, 2000, WB Saunders.

26. Carcillo JA et al: Pediatric shock. In Slonim, Pollack, editors: *Pediatric critical care medicine*, Philadelphia, Lippincott Williams and Wilkins, in press.

27. Tibby SM, Hatherill M, Murdoch IA: Capillary refill and core-peripheral temperature gap as indicators of haemodynamic status in paediatric intensive care patients, *Arch Dis Child* 80:163, 1999.

28. Evans JM, et al: Principles of invasive monitoring. In Fuhrman BP, Zimmerman JJ, editors: *Pediatric critical care*, ed 3, St. Louis, 2006, Mosby-Elsevier, pp 251–264.

29. Ceneviva G, et al: Hemodynamic support in fluid refractory pediatric septic shock, *Pediatrics* 102 E19, 1998.

30. Carcillo JA, Davis AL, Zaritsky A: Role of early fluid resuscitation in pediatric septic shock, *JAMA* 266:1242, 1991.

31. RJ Kallen, JM Lonergan: Fluid resuscitation of acute hypovolemic hypoperfusion states in pediatrics, *Pediatr Clin North Am* 37:287, 1990.

32. Saladino RA: Management of septic shock in the pediatric emergency department in 2004, *Clin Ped Emerg Med* 5:20–27, 2004.

33. Morgan WM, O'Neill JA: Hemorrhagic and obstructive shock in pediatric patients, *New Horiz* 6:150, 1998.

34. Ross J, Schmid-Schoenbein G: Dynamics of the peripheral circulation. In West JB, editor: *Best and Taylor's physiological basis of medical practice*, ed 12, Baltimore, 1991, Williams & Wilkins.

35. Smith L, Hernan L: Shock states. In Fuhrman BP, Zimmerman JJ, editors: *Pediatric critical care*, ed 3, St. Louis, 2006, Mosby-Elsevier, pp 394–410.

36. Burns JP: Septic shock in the pediatric patient: pathogenesis and novel treatments, *Pediatr Emerg Care* 19:112, 2003.

37. Odio CM, Faingezicht I, Paris M, et al: The beneficial effects of early dexamethasone administration in infants and children with bacterial meningitis, *N Engl J Med* 324(22): 1525–1531, 1991.

Chapter 31

Pediatric Trauma

PATRICE JOHNSON, JENNIFER WATTS

OUTLINE

LEARNING OBJECTIVES

After reading this chapter the reader will be able to:

1. Discuss the three general causes of brain damage
2. Recognize the spectrum of thoracic injuries seen in pediatric practice
3. Explain the complications of blunt thoracic trauma in children
4. Recognize the spectrum of penetrating thoracic injuries seen in children
5. Discuss the epidemiology of thermal injury
6. Discuss the basic management of thermal injury
7. Define *drowning* and other terms used to describe submersion injury
8. Discuss strategies for respiratory management of drowning victims
9. Describe various factors that contribute to mortality and morbidity in drowning victims
10. Describe strategies for prevention of unintentional injuries

KEY TERMS

Carboxyhemoglobin
Diplopia
Drowning
Encephalopathy
Escharotomy
Fontanels

Glasgow Coma Scale score
Hypothermia
Intracranial pressure
Mechanism of injury
Nonaccidental trauma
Papilledema

Persistent vegetative state
Plasticity
Rule of nines
Status epilepticus
Strabismus

EPIDEMIOLOGY

Trauma remains the leading cause of death for children ages 1 to 19 years. In the past decade the nation has generally seen a decrease in incidence of pediatric trauma. Child injury, which is preventable, is the number one cause of death in the United States. Death rates as a result of unintentional injuries have dropped by almost 30%. Yet these preventable injuries accounted for more than 9000 pediatric deaths in 2009. Motor vehicle accident (MVA) fatalities have decreased 41% from 2000 to 2009. Unfortunately motor vehicle accidents are the leading cause of death, accounting for nearly half of the deaths. Deaths as a result of drowning, fire/burn, and falls have all decreased, whereas poisoning and suffocation have increased 80% and 30%, respectively.[1] Violent (intentional) deaths accounted for approximately 4900 pediatric deaths in 2009. Homicide and suicide are the leading contributors to intentional deaths among youth in the United States.[2]

ANATOMICAL CONSIDERATIONS

Children are not just small adults. It is important to understand the fundamental differences between adults and children. Notable are the size and shape differences. There is a greater distribution of force per unit body area because of smaller body mass resulting in greater acceleration. The child's body has less fat, elastic connective tissue, and close proximity of multiple organs. This can place the child with a penetrating injury at risk of multiple organ involvement. Children also have a large surface area relative to volume, predisposing them to thermal evaporative loss resulting in hypothermia. A child's skeleton is more pliable because of incomplete calcification. Trauma can result in serious organ injury without overlying skeletal fracture. Children have multiple active growth centers (physes). Injury can result in unique fractures with potential growth arrest or abnormality. The pediatric airway has several features that are unique and challenging. The oral cavities are small with relatively large tongue and tonsils, which can cause obstruction. Infants and children have relatively large occiputs, which can cause an airway obstruction when the neck is flexed while the child is lying in the supine position. The airway is narrow with a floppy, U-shaped epiglottis creating unique challenges for artificial airway placement.

MECHANISM OF INJURY

Knowledge of the **mechanism of injury (MOI)** provides clinicians with information on the traumatic external event and the potential internal injuries. MOI includes the cause or the reason for the injury, the amount of force applied, and the vector or direction of that force. For example, "The patient was the front seat passenger in a two-car motor vehicle accident (MVA). The car in which she was riding was hit on the driver's side at 30 mph while entering an intersection at 5 to 10 mph when the light had just turned green.

Both she and the driver were wearing seat belts." This explanation of the mechanism of the patient's injuries provides information concerning potential pathophysiological impact and helps determine the type and extent of possible injuries.

INITIAL ASSESSMENT AND DIAGNOSIS

The initial assessment is the same for all pediatric patients who have sustained a traumatic injury regardless of mechanism. Always assume cervical spine (C-spine) injury and take necessary precautions during the assessment. The head and neck should be held in line with the body by placing a cervical collar or by assigning an individual to hold the patient in C-spine precautions.

A complete head-to-toe assessment of the patient is desirable but may have to be postponed or abbreviated until the patient's condition is stabilized. The initial assessment, or the primary survey, consists of ABCD:

- **A**irway patency
- **B**reathing support
- adequacy of **C**irculation
- **D**isability (neurological assessment)

Airway Patency

Without a patent (open or clear) airway, other interventions are of little value. A patent airway will help maintain physiological integrity and help ensure oxygenation.

A patent airway can be initiated by means of a jaw-thrust maneuver to open the airway. Maintain the airway with orotracheal intubation, nasotracheal intubation, cricothyrotomy, or tracheostomy. In order to maintain cervical spine stabilizations, *do not use the head-tilt, sniff position, or chin-lift maneuvers because these procedures change the orientation of the spinal column and increase the risk of additional spinal injury. The jaw-thrust technique may be used in these children unless otherwise contraindicated.*

Caution is necessary when moving or positioning the patient to prevent further displacement of any spinal fractures and additional damage to the spine, spinal cord, and cranial or spinal nerves. Therefore the head, neck, spine, and body should be treated as a single entity and moved in unison and in the same plane.

Breathing Support

Breathing support includes providing supplemental oxygen. The patient may require only a nasal cannula or possibly artificial ventilation with bag-valve-mask resuscitators. Breathing support may progress to intubation with bag-valve-tube ventilation and eventually to mechanical ventilation.

Provide for all possible adverse airway events by having the appropriate equipment on hand. Give high concentrations of oxygen, and monitor oxygen saturation with a pulse oximeter (SpO_2) and ventilation with a capnometer ($ETCO_2$). Correlate SpO_2 and $ETCO_2$ with arterial blood gas (ABG) measurements to determine the adequacy of oxygenation and ventilation. If the patient is breathing without difficulty and is not likely to vomit and aspirate, a face mask is appropriate. Remember to protect the airway from aspiration of blood, vomit, and other substances. If respirations deteriorate or the patient's state of consciousness declines, mechanical ventilation should be instituted immediately.

Adequacy of Circulation

Assess pulse rate and pressure at all pulse points and note significant discrepancies. Pulse oximetry is a valuable adjunct for this purpose. Both manual and automatic blood pressure monitors are appropriate.

Assessing capillary refill is a quick and specific method of checking the adequacy of peripheral circulation. One method of determining capillary refill is to depress the patient's thumbnail with moderate force. This will cause the underlying tissue to blanch (turn white or pale pink) by forcing blood from the tissue. Releasing the pressure allows blood to refill the tissue's capillaries. Normal capillary refill time is less than 2 seconds. Inadequate capillary refill on initial assessment may be caused by regional perfusion problems. To rule out this possibility, repeat the capillary refill test on the opposite hand.

Failure of the patient to maintain blood pressure, heart rate, and rhythm indicates the need for vasopressors, fluid administration, or cardiopulmonary resuscitation (CPR).

When assessing pulse rate, remember to differentiate between electrical activity (as measured with electrocardiogram [ECG]) and pulsate beats. ECG measures the electrical activity of the heart, not necessarily the beating of the heart. In this case pulse oximetry, which detects pulsate flow (blood flow caused by the heart's beating action), is a better assessment of perfusion than the ECG.

Disability

Immediate assessment of neurological status is beneficial in acute trauma management. The most common way to perform this assessment is with the **Glasgow Coma Scale (GCS) score.** Patients are scored in three areas: eye opening, verbal response, and motor response. Although the standard GCS is accurate for use in adults, older children, and adolescents, the age-specific GCS combines adult and child forms so it is applicable to all ages. The age-specific GCS is particularly useful in nonverbal children (Table 31-1).

If the GCS is less than or equal to 8, the patient likely does not have the ability to protect his or her airway and a more definitive airway should be established. Intubation is the most common option for a definitive airway, with cricothyroidotomy being a secondary option.

After assessment and stabilization, the secondary survey can be performed. A complete head-to-toe examination will be performed. Diagnostic testing and imaging may be used. Once all injuries are identified, a plan of care can be developed for the patient. All members of the trauma team should be aware of the plan so everyone is working toward the same goals, both short term and long term.

TABLE 31-1

Age-Specific Glasgow Coma Scale*

Points	Infant/Preverbal Child	Verbal Child/Adult
Eye Opening (E)		
4	Spontaneous	Spontaneous
3	To speech	To speech
2	To pain	To pain
1	None	None
Verbal Response (V)		
5	Coos, babbles	Oriented
4	Irritable cries	Confused
3	Cries to pain	Inappropriate words
2	Moans to pain	Incomprehensible sounds
1	None	None
Motor Response (M)		
6	Normal, spontaneous	Obeys commands
5	Withdraws to touch	Localizes pain
4	Withdraws to pain	Withdraws to pain
3	Abnormal flexion	Abnormal flexion
2	Abnormal extension	Abnormal extension
1	None	None

Modified from Laskowsi-Jones L, Salati DS. Responding to pediatric trauma. *Nursing* 2001;31:37.
* Score = E + V + M. Normal, 15 or 16 points; mildly impaired consciousness, 13 or 14 points; moderate impairment, 9 to 12 points; severe impairment, 3 to 8 points.

HEAD INJURIES

Epidemiology

Damage to the brain or skull is among the most potentially serious and handicapping of all traumatic injuries. Head injuries are a primary cause of trauma deaths in both adults and children. A brain injury occurs in the United States every 15 seconds, and more than 1 million people with head injury are seen in emergency departments (EDs) each year. More than 5.3 million Americans are disabled from traumatic brain injury (TBI).[3] An estimated 1.7 million people sustain a TBI annually. Of them, 52,000 die, 275,000 are hospitalized, and 1.35 million, nearly 80%, are treated and released from an emergency department.

The National Center for Injury Prevention and Control estimates that more than 510,000 traumatic[4] brain injuries occur annually in children 0 to 14 years of age in the United States.

· In every age group, TBI rates are higher for males than for females.
· Males age 0 to 4 years have the highest rates of TBI-related emergency department visits, hospitalizations, and deaths combined.
· TBI is a contributing factor to a third (30.5%) of all injury-related deaths in the United States.[5]
· The number of people disabled or killed is even higher when nontraumatic organic causes are factored into the epidemiology of brain injury.

A child's head is large and heavy in relation to the body. Therefore the center of gravity shifts toward the head. In

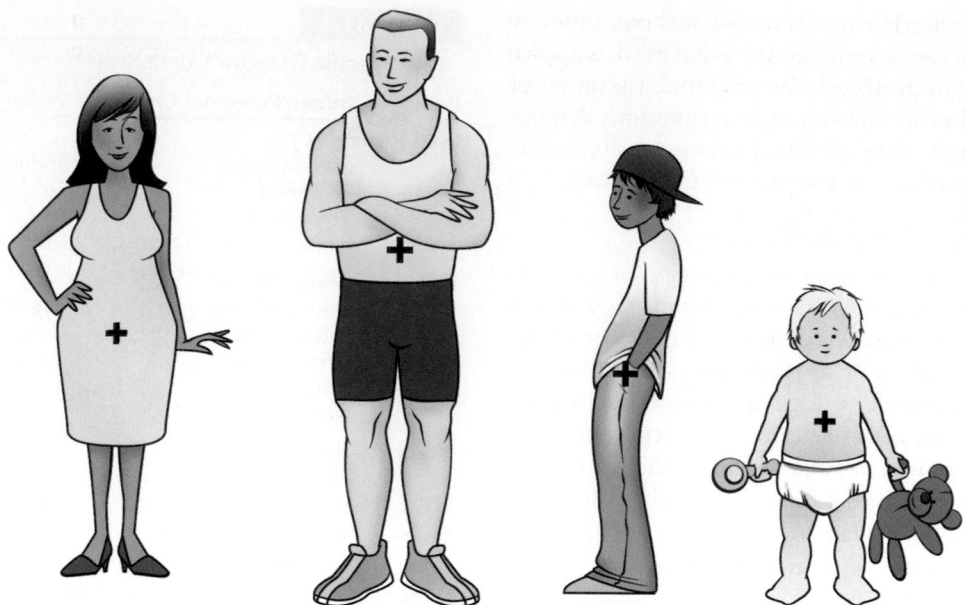

FIGURE 31-1   Centers of gravity by age and gender.

addition, a child's balance, coordination, gait, and judgment are immature, which results in children being especially vulnerable to falls with head injury[6] (Figure 31-1). Because of these factors, children fall more frequently than adults and thus have a higher percentage of head injuries. The size and weight of the head also tend to rotate the child's body into a head-down position, often leading to headfirst impacts.

Inertial injuries, such as what is commonly seen in automobile accidents or shaken baby syndrome (SBS), account for a large number of head and central nervous system (CNS) injuries, especially in infants younger than 1 year of age. Infants have weak neck muscles and struggle to support their relatively heavy head. When a baby is shaken, forceful movement of the head results in brain injury as the brain impacts the sides of the skull with each movement. Health care professionals, including respiratory

therapists, are required by law to report suspected incidents of SBS to legal authorities.

Anatomical Considerations

Injuries from head trauma can fall anywhere on the spectrum from no harm to the worst-case scenario of death or significant disability.

The outcome and potential disability caused by each injury may vary in effect and seriousness based on many factors. Age is a major factor in some cases, allowing infants and young children to compensate for injuries when adults might sustain a permanent injury. Also, repetitive injuries have a cumulative effect, as evidenced by "punch drunk" boxers or football players with multiple concussions.

The brain has functional specificity (Figure 31-2). That is, certain areas of the brain are responsible for certain

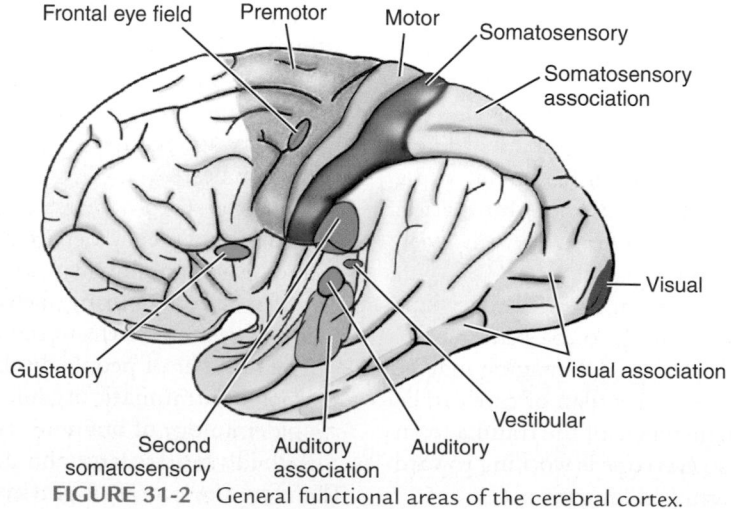

FIGURE 31-2   General functional areas of the cerebral cortex.

functions. However, the brains of infants and children apparently have a large degree of plasticity in redistributing function from a damaged area to an undamaged area. In adults the ability of the brain segments to adapt to new functions seems to be rarely, if ever, present. This flexibility of assigned purpose provides protection and enhances rehabilitative potential for infants and children but decreases with age as the maturing brain becomes patterned and locked into its distribution of functional capacity.

Infants and young children also have malleable skulls because of the large **fontanels** ("soft spots") and the flat bones of the skull, which have not yet fused and still may be cartilaginous before ossification (Figure 31-3). These factors allow for elasticity of the cranial vault and lessen or prevent both fractures and pressure-related brain injuries during passage through the birth canal. Skull malleability also protects against damage from other sources, such as trauma or illness causing increased pressures in the cranial vault. This protection occurs by allowing a degree of expansion of the cranial volume.

The normal newborn brain and spinal cord are immature and not completely myelinated until about 18 months of age. As interbrain connections (synapses) are completed and the integrative functions of the brain begin to mature, more of the brain becomes active and functional. Knowledge of these processes and conditions are crucial when assessing neurological status in infants and children with incomplete CNS development and integration. Their reactions and responses will change as the children age and gain maturity.

Diagnostic Assessment

As in other conditions, the proper diagnosis of the cause, type, and extent of cerebral injury depends on both the subjective and objective data associated with the patient's condition.

Subjective Data

Subjective data cannot be collected by the assessor's senses (e.g., sight, touch, smell) without input from the patient.

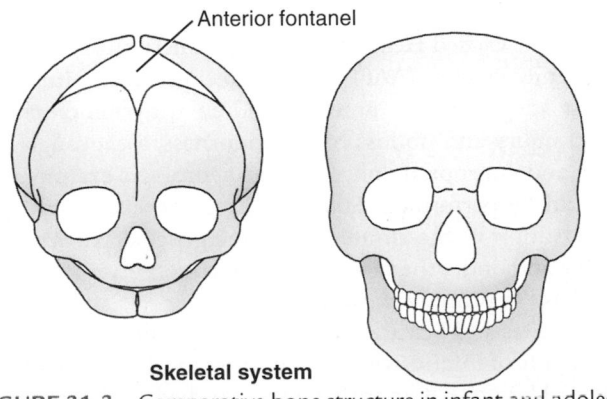

Skeletal system

FIGURE 31-3 Comparative bone structure in infant and adolescent skulls.

The presence, extent, and magnitude of pain and fear status are examples of subjective data that the patient must be asked to reveal. Because infants and young children often cannot effectively verbalize these factors, the assessor must be alert for clues that suggest a problem. For example, an exaggerated response to the examiner's touch may indicate pain.

Parents may be the best sources of information about variations from normal behavior. The exception would be if a high index of suspicion of child neglect or **nonaccidental trauma** (NAT) exists. NAT, or child abuse, should be suspected if the severity of injury does not match the stated mechanism, the child has other injuries consistent with NAT, or the parent or child displays significantly odd behavior. "Accidental falls rarely produce significant head injuries," according to Dr. Karl Johnson. A study of 94 patients ages 4 months to 5 years who had been witnessed falling from heights ranging from 20 cm (8 inches) to more than 3 meters (9.9 feet) found that 89% to 95% had "no significant long-term problems." Severe head injury in patients younger than 5 years of age blamed on falls or household accidents should raise suspicions about the possibility of abuse.[6] Further, head injury, according to Rubin et al., is the leading cause of death in abused children younger than 2 years of age.[7]

In these cases the law requires that, among others, licensed health care professionals, including respiratory therapists (RTs), notify legally designated authorities.

Objective Data

Objective data relate to the mechanism of injury, the patient's medical history (past and present), and the situation that led to injury event. The child's past medical history indicates the body's preinjury state. The present medical history may reveal exposure to harmful substances or activities.

Additional objective data help the clinician track the patient's physiological response to injury and treatment. Objective data are measurable and allow discovery and recording of trends in the treatment and recovery process. Such data include laboratory studies, radiographs, computed tomography (CT) scans, magnetic resonance imaging (MRI), electrocardiograms (ECGs), electroencephalograms (EEGs), and lumbar puncture (LP). Objective data also include pulse, blood pressure, temperature, and respirations. Recently two other "vital signs" have been added to this list. One, pulse oximetry, is objective (measurable and quantifiable) and the other, pain, is considered subjective. Pain, however, is often measured using "pain scales." The use of these scales is a method of objectifying this symptom.

Data Gathering

Age-specific subjective and objective data are gathered simultaneously during the patient assessment process. Children are often poor historians because of age, emotional/psychiatric problems, or the injury itself. It is often necessary to rely on eyewitness accounts of the events or reports or educated guesses of accompanying adults to determine cause and mechanism of injury. Trends and alteration from the norm are particularly important in this and other noncommunicative populations. Cultural or language differences may markedly affect both data gathering and interpretation. Care should be taken to ensure that patients and their families understand what information is needed and what care methods are to be employed during the diagnosis and treatment process. Time spent gathering data may not seem important to parents awaiting focused treatment for their child, but they should be informed that the more knowledge about the child, the child's medical and social history, and the details of the circumstances of the injury the medical staff have, the better and more focused the care for their child.

Stabilization

The initial approach to all traumatic injuries, including head injuries, is with the primary survey, ABCD (Airway, Breathing, Circulation, Disability). This was discussed previously. In this section, a few items specific to head injuries are highlighted.

Airway Patency

The first step should always be to ensure a patent airway. In a child with a head injury, remember to assume cervical spine injury and maintain C-spine stabilization. Therefore the most effective airway maneuver, while in C-spine precautions, is a jaw-thrust.

In patients with direct cranial trauma, avoid nasotracheal intubation, nasotracheal suctioning, or inserting nasogastric tubes because inadvertent cranial intubation may result through open fractures of the cranial vault, especially in patients who may have basilar skull injuries or paranasal fractures. In addition, irritating procedures such as nasopharyngeal or nasotracheal suctioning, insertion of a nasogastric tube, or intubation may result in an exacerbation of an already increased intracranial pressure. If these procedures are necessary, they should be performed with caution.

Breathing Support

Breathing support ensures adequate oxygenation and ventilation. Skull and facial fractures or lacerations may preclude mask ventilation. Remember to protect the airway from aspiration of blood, vomit, and other substances.

If respirations deteriorate or the patient's state of consciousness declines, mechanical ventilation should be instituted immediately. Minimize peak inspiratory pressure (PIP), mean airway pressure (Paw), and select inspiratory and expiratory times that favor prolonged expiration if possible. Decreasing Paw minimizes outflow tract resistance from the cerebral vasculature, enhancing cerebral perfusion by minimizing effects on **intracranial pressure**

(ICP). Remember to minimize suctioning to prevent coughing and gagging on the tracheal tube or suction catheter, which may increase ICP.

Adequacy of Circulation

Circulation should be assessed as part of the primary survey, as explained previously, with pulses and capillary refill being the main focus. Blood pressures will be equally important in head injuries to ensure adequate circulation to the brain taking into consideration increased intracranial pressure. Vasopressors may be necessary to increase systemic blood flow.

Disability (Neurological Assessment)

This is a vital component of the primary survey in patients with head injuries. A quick GCS score will help the provider know if the patient is able to protect his or her own airway, or if a more definitive airway needs to be established. In addition, if a head injury is significant, maintaining lower body temperatures should be considered. (This is discussed further in the increased ICP section.)

Secondary Survey

In the overall head-to-toe examination, there may be some physical findings that can help the provider establish a diagnosis with respect to head injury. Variation in the respiratory pattern can help reveal the location of brain injury and the body's attempt to compensate for physiological change. In some patients the abnormal respiratory patterns are the body's attempt to alter cerebral perfusion pressure and distribution. In other patients these changes in respiration are the direct result of injury to respiratory control centers in the brain. Some classic "signs" are associated with certain head injuries. These signs indicate fractures of the basilar skull. Traumatic head injury may be highlighted by the presence of Battle's sign or "raccoon eyes." Battle's sign represents ecchymosis or bruised areas behind the ear that indicate basilar skull fractures. The self-explanatory term *raccoon eyes* represent bruising discolorations around the orbits. Both Battle's sign and raccoon eyes are the body's attempts to show internal injury with as simple a sign as a small bruise.

As a result of a meta-analysis conducted by Bergman and colleagues and published in *Pediatrics*, a joint Subcommittee on Minor Closed Head Injury of the American Association of Family Practice (AAFP) Committee on Quality Improvement suggests that "among children with minor closed head injury and no loss of consciousness, a thorough history and appropriate physical and neurologic examination should be performed. Subcommittee consensus was that observation in the clinic, office, emergency department or home and under the care of a competent observer should be used as the primary treatment strategy."[8]

Greenes and Schutzman report the results of a prospective study of infants with head injuries in which 608 infants (ages 11.2 ± 6.8 months) were studied. "The authors' findings suggest that radiology screening of head-injured infants should be directed at two groups of patients: those with symptoms and signs of brain injury, and those without symptoms or signs of brain injury but with significant scalp hematomas."[9]

Increased Intracranial Pressure
Anatomical Considerations

The size of a normal infant's skull is determined by its contents. The normal skull contents consist of three substances: brain tissue, blood, and cerebrospinal fluid (CSF). The growing brain causes the skull to increase in size. Normal circumferential head growth in the term newborn is 2 cm per month for the first 3 months, 1 cm per month for the second 3 months, and 0.5 cm per month for the next 6 months. Excessive head growth resulting from separation of the cranial sutures is an important feature of increased ICP throughout the first year of life. When the separation of cranial sutures is no longer sufficient to decompress increased ICP, the infant becomes lethargic, does not take feedings, and vomits.

After infancy or when the suture lines and fontanels close, the skull can no longer increase in size, and the total pressure within the skull is caused by the size of its contents—the brain tissue (80% to 90% of the intracranial content by volume), CSF (5% to 10%), and blood (5% to 9%). The Monro-Kellie doctrine or hypothesis may be paraphrased as follows: In a closed system, such as the skull, an increase in the size of one component requires compression of the other components to maintain a constant ICP.[10] If the internal volume of the skull is 500 ml, for example, and the brain, blood, and CSF volume is 450 ml, then 50 ml of expansion volume remains in the skull. According to the Monroe-Kellie doctrine, if the volume of these three components increases by more than 50 ml, compression of the skull contents occurs.[11] Because CSF and blood are fluids and thus almost incompressible at physiological pressures, the compression will occur in the brain tissue. Compression of the brain tissue inhibits blood flow by reducing cerebral perfusion pressure (CPP) and causes cerebral tissue hypoxia, ischemia, and coma. CPP = mean BP − ICP and averages 85 ± 15 mm Hg.

The patient whose condition has progressed to coma requires testing to determine the presence of increased intracranial pressure. Normal ICP is 130 mm H_2O (10 mm Hg). Computed tomography (CT) scans or magnetic resonance imaging (MRI) are used to evaluate the brain for evidence of fluid buildup, displacement of the brain, or displacement of the ventricles of the brain. Alternatively, direct pressure measurements may be obtained by lumbar puncture or by inserting a needle into the interspinal spaces between L3 and L4 or L4 and L5 and attaching a pressure monitor. Other methods of measuring ICP include using an intracranial pressure monitor (subarachnoid screw) or a cerebral ventricular catheter. Because these direct methods are invasive and potentially dangerous, CT or MRI are the preferred, at least as screening tools.

Increased ICP can be a life-threatening feature of an encephalopathy. CSF and blood acting on the brain and bony structures of the skull generate ICP. In the newborn and infant, measuring the head circumference and palpating the anterior fontanel allow rapid assessment of ICP. Bulging of the fontanels may be a key sign of increased ICP that requires a response by caregivers. Gentle palpation of the fontanels may reveal pulsations of the fontanels that may occur normally at a frequency equal to the pulse rate. It is unusual for these pulsations to be either absent or of bounding force.

Clinical Features

Headache. A common symptom of increased ICP at all ages is headache, primarily caused by traction and displacement of intracranial arteries. When increased ICP is generalized, as from cerebral edema or obstruction of the ventricular system, headache is generalized and is more prominent in the morning on awakening. The pain is constant but varies in intensity. Coughing, sneezing, straining, and other maneuvers that transiently increase ICP exaggerate the headache. The quality of pain is often difficult to describe. Vomiting in the absence of nausea, especially on arising in the morning, is often a concurrent feature. Vomiting itself is, of course, also a source of increased ICP. With knowledge of the MOI, the clinician is able to assess the potential pathophysiological impact on the patient.

Diplopia and Strabismus. Diplopia is characterized by double vision caused by a disruption of the extraocular muscles or the muscle nerves. **Strabismus,** caused by paralysis of one or both abducens nerves so that the eye cannot turn outward, is a relatively common feature of generalized increased ICP. Strabismus may be a more prominent feature than headache in children with increased ICP.

Papilledema. Papilledema is passive swelling of the optic disc caused by increased ICP. Examining the eye with an ophthalmoscope allows visualization of the disc. The edema is usually bilateral; unilateral edema suggests a mass lesion behind the affected eye. Early papilledema is asymptomatic, and the patient experiences transitory disturbances of vision only with advanced disease. Preservation of visual acuity differentiates papilledema from primary optic nerve disturbances, such as optic neuritis, in which blindness occurs early in the course of disease.[12]

As edema progresses, the optic disc swells and is raised above the plane of the retina, causing the disc margin to be obscured. Tortuosity (twisted appearance) of the veins also results. If the process continues, the retina surrounding the disc becomes edematous so that the disc appears greatly enlarged and retinal exudate radiates from the fovea. Eventually the exudate clears; however, optic atrophy ensues and blindness may be permanent. Even if increased ICP is relieved during the early stages of disc edema, 4 to 6 weeks are required before the retina appears normal again.

Herniation. Increased ICP may cause portions of the brain to shift from their normal location into other compartments, compressing structures already occupying that space. Such shifts may occur under the falx cerebri, through the tentorial notch, and through the foramen magnum. Brainstem herniation is an emergency condition that, if not rapidly addressed, will almost surely result in major injury and probable death.

Lumbar puncture is generally contraindicated in patients with increased ICP because of the concern that a change in fluid dynamics will cause brainstem herniation. LP is especially hazardous when pressure between cranial compartments is unequal. This prohibition is relative, and early LP is the rule in infants and children with suspected CNS infections, despite the presence of increased ICP. LP is also used to diagnose and treat increased ICP in pseudotumor cerebri.

Monitoring

Enthusiasm is declining for the continuous monitoring of ICP in children. Despite advances in technology, the effect of pressure monitoring on outcome is questionable. It is not indicated in children with hypoxic-ischemic encephalopathies and has marginal value in children with other types of encephalopathy.[13] Use of LP to obtain CSF pressure readings is a dangerous and risky procedure in infants with disorders such as hydrocephalus—a condition that causes increased production or reduced clearance of cerebral spinal fluid leading to markedly increased ICP as evidenced by a large swollen skull. The symptoms and prognosis of increased ICP depend more on the *cause* than on the level of pressure attained. Systemic arterial blood pressure should be monitored along with ABG values and oxygen saturation.

Treatment
Head Elevation
Elevating the head of the bed 30 to 45 degrees above horizontal decreases ICP by improving jugular venous drainage. The head should also be kept in the midline position so that the vasculature on each side of the neck is not compressed. Systemic blood pressure is not affected, so the overall result is increased CPP.

Hyperventilation
ICP declines within seconds of beginning hyperventilation. The mechanism is vasoconstriction resulting from hypocarbia. The goal is to lower the partial pressure of arterial carbon dioxide ($Paco_2$) from 40 to 25 mm Hg. Further reduction can result in cerebral ischemia and is contraindicated. Vasoconstriction is maintained as long as hyperventilation is continued. When hyperventilation is withdrawn, however, the vessels again dilate and blood flow returns to normal. To prevent a rebound effect, in which blood flow increases above baseline, hyperventilation should be withdrawn gradually. Disponde writes,

"The limits of cerebral autoregulation may be shifted to significantly lower values (mean arterial pressure [MAP] 20 to 60 mm Hg) in the neonates and infants. The 'margin of safety' is narrower as the infant is less able to compensate for acute hypo- or hypertension. Low MAP presents the risk of ischemia while hypertension in infants may present risk of intracranial hemorrhage. Response to hyperventilation (low $Paco_2$) in infants may be brisk, with a risk of inducing cerebral ischemia with extremely low $Paco_2$ (<20 mm Hg)."[14]

Hyperventilation is achieved by endotracheal intubation or tracheostomy and mechanical ventilation. Use of hyperventilation should be limited to the first few hours of care to protect against rebound vasoconstriction and increased ICP. Careful monitoring of ICP and $Paco_2$ should always accompany hyperventilation. Colorimetric end-tidal carbon dioxide monitoring is not appropriate in these cases because that technique does not provide accurate numerical data for use in either monitoring or trending the hyperventilated patient.

Also, be aware that intubation and tracheostomy, in addition to the risks of damage to the tracheal mucosa and development of tracheoesophageal fistula, carry the risk of ventilatory-associated pneumonia (VAP). A strong correlation exists between nosocomial pneumonia and aspiration of oropharyngeal and gastric emesis. These fluids travel down the exterior of the artificial airway into the open airway past the epiglottis, which is propped open by the tracheal tube. In older children with a cuffed tube, these secretions pool between the larynx and the top of the cuff, poised to flow down the airway into the lungs. The use of continuous positive airway pressure (CPAP) may help prevent this type of pneumonia by increasing the pressure gradient between the airway and the oral cavity, thus restraining the fluid flow.[15]

Osmotic Diuretics

Mannitol and hypertonic saline are the two osmotic diuretics most widely used in the United States. Mannitol is given intravenously as a 20% solution. It does not cross the blood–brain barrier and remains in the plasma, creating an osmotic gradient that draws water from the brain into the capillaries, thus reducing cerebral fluid volume and therefore ICP. The effect is short term, and infusions must be given 3 to 6 times each day. Repeated infusions of mannitol also cause dehydration as well as fluid and electrolyte imbalances. Rebound may occur when mannitol is discontinued.

Hypertonic saline is given intravenously as an initial bolus and then continuously. Close monitoring of sodium levels is necessary, as well as monitoring for signs of dehydration.

Corticosteroids

Corticosteroids, such as dexamethasone, are controversial in the treatment of vasogenic edema. Onset of action is

12 to 24 hours, and peak action may be delayed even longer. The mechanism is uncertain, but cerebral blood flow (CBF) is not affected. Corticosteroids are most useful for reducing edema surrounding mass (space-occupying) lesions. These agents are not beneficial in cytotoxic edema, as seen after hypoxic-ischemic injuries. The delay in onset of action limits the usefulness of corticosteroids in patients needing emergent or urgent cerebral volume reduction.

Hypothermia

Hypothermia decreases CBF and is often used concurrently with pentobarbital coma. It is not clear how much improvement is gained by hypothermia in addition to other measures that decrease CBF, such as head elevation, hyperventilation, and pentobarbital coma.

In a recent well-designed study in adults, 392 subjects (16 to 65 years of age), all sustaining closed head trauma, were randomly assigned to a control (normothermic) group or an experimental group (hypothermia within 6 hours of injury to 33° C for 48 hours), with the patients in each group having similar injuries by type and severity and mean age. The outcomes were poor in 57% of each group (resulting in a vegetative state, disability, or death). The death rates were 27% in the normothermic subjects and 28% in the hypothermic group. The hypothermic subjects also had more complications and more hospital days but fewer episodes of increased ICP. The authors concluded that hypothermia was not advantageous in this group of patients.[16-18]

The studies for benefits of hypothermia in children after traumatic brain injuries have not been as positive. Currently the standard of care is to keep the body temperature cool but not hypothermic. However, in neonates, hypothermia has been shown to be extremely beneficial for hypoxic-ischemic encephalopathy after birth trauma.

Pentobarbital Coma

Barbiturates such as pentobarbital reduce CBF, decrease edema formation, and lower the brain's metabolic rate. These effects do not occur at anticonvulsant plasma concentrations but require brain concentrations sufficient to produce a burst-suppression pattern on the EEG. Pentobarbital medically induced coma is particularly useful in patients with increased ICP resulting from disorders of mitochondrial function, such as Reye's syndrome. In adults, medically induced coma is increasingly being seen as a way of "resting the brain" to aid healing of the fragile brain tissue.

Ventilatory Maneuvers

The increase in intrathoracic pressure that occurs during positive-pressure ventilation may impede cerebral venous return and increase ICP. Therefore the patient should be mechanically ventilated with the lowest peak pressures possible. A minimal level of positive end-expiratory pressure (PEEP) should be used to maintain adequate ventilation at low mean airway pressures. Chest physical therapy and postural drainage positioning may also exaggerate the ICP and should be used with caution. Care should be taken to monitor and maintain inflation of newly recruited alveoli. Suctioning may increase the ICP and should be performed minimally and must be preceded with oxygen-supplemented hyperventilation. It is also important to prevent Valsalva maneuvers and coughing, each of which can cause marked increases in ICP.

Treatment

After assessment and stabilization, a plan is developed for definitive treatment and evaluation. Before and throughout treatment, a comprehensive plan should be in place that includes goals, outcomes, and evaluation criteria. Preferably these plans are developed by an interdisciplinary team of acute care and rehabilitation professionals and will be reviewed with the patient's family as care progresses.

As previously discussed, protection of the airway and cervical spine, protection from further injury, and progress toward recovery goals guide the plan of care for the brain injury patient. The plan encompasses three major goals, as follows:

1. Determine the correct diagnosis.
2. Treat the injuries and sequelae in an appropriate, caring, and resource-sparing manner.
3. Develop and implement a rehabilitation plan that is timely, centers on increasing quality of life, and employs strategies that maximize the patient's control of and autonomy in the rehabilitation process.

Evaluation of any plan of care is based on the desired outcomes. This evaluation should result in improvements and should be adaptable to make both the assessment and the plan dynamic processes. Outcomes goals and evaluation objectives should be dynamic guides that are revised as the clinical situation changes with the patient's response to treatment. The evaluation process should be based on achievable and measurable therapeutic goals and objectives. For example, a goal in the brain-injured patient might be to reduce positional hypertension or hypotension. The associated objective might be to reduce blood pressure swings to 10 mm Hg with position changes.

Clearly, all members of the care team, the patient, and family should be aware of the plan, its goals and objectives, and the progress toward fulfillment of the goals. This requires open and honest communications beginning early in the process and maintained throughout the stabilization and rehabilitation phases.

In addition to neurological care, the incapacitated patient needs care for the eyes, the skin, gastrointestinal tract, urinary tract, and pulmonary and cardiovascular systems. Keep the head of the bed elevated to control cerebral edema. In some cases hyperventilation or hypoventilation assists in controlling edema as well as maintaining body integrity. Nutritionally, caloric demands need to be met. Preventing skin and muscle deterioration helps to prevent further injury. Additionally, head of the bed elevation to 30 to 45 degrees helps prevent aspiration and hospital-acquired pneumonia. All these systems must be functional when the patient's brain recovers.

Status Epilepticus

The condition in which seizures are repetitive and do not stop spontaneously is called status epilepticus. Seizures begin with abnormal neurons that discharge repeatedly. Repetitive seizures increase the body's requirements for adenosine triphosphate (ATP), which in turn increases metabolic needs for oxygen and glucose. Apnea, hypoxemia, and hypoglycemia may result, along with increased oxygen consumption and lactic acidosis. Anoxic injury to the brain and other organs, as well as cardiac arrhythmias and traumatic injuries (e.g., tongue laceration, concussion), may also occur.

Status epilepticus is a medical emergency that requires prompt attention. A controlled airway must be established immediately, and supplemental oxygen and mechanical ventilation should be rapidly available. Venous access must be established and blood withdrawn for measurement of glucose and electrolyte levels. Other tests, such as anticonvulsant drug concentrations and toxicology screens, are performed as indicated.

Intranasal midazolam and rectal diazepam can be used initially as anticonvulsants while intravenous (IV) access is being established. Once an IV or an intraosseous line is obtained lorazepam is the most common medication used. Lorazepam is typically given multiple times. If the seizure has not stopped, other IV medications include fosphenytoin, keppra, valproic acid, and phenobarbital. All the anticonvulsants used in the emergency setting can cause some degree of respiratory depression. It is important to note that when the medications are used together there is a compounding effect on respiratory depression. If none of the medications administered is effective in stopping the seizure, a pentobarbital coma may be necessary. For this, the patient should be intubated and mechanically ventilated and vital signs need to be monitored closely.

To achieve pentobarbital coma in the patient with status epilepticus, boluses of pentobarbital are infused until a burst-suppression pattern appears on the ECG monitor, which is continuously recording. Hypotension occurs with large doses, and vasopressor support may be necessary.

The coma can be safely maintained for 3 days; longer coma periods may cause pulmonary edema. The ECG should be checked several times each day for the burst-suppression pattern. The coma can be lifted every 48 to 72 hours to see whether the seizures have stopped. Mechanical ventilation should be continued until the patient regains consciousness and can spontaneously support ventilation and until reflexive airway protection is adequate.

This discussion of head injury is not exhaustive but should serve to illustrate to the reader that these injuries and conditions are potentially life threatening and life altering. The mastery of skills relate to ventilator and airway control are often among the most crucial in the care and survival of these patients.

Specific Considerations

Cerebral disorders are the result of trauma, altered cellular function secondary to drugs, metabolic problems, anoxia, or genetic-developmental disorders. Cerebral disorders range from inconsequential to profoundly debilitating, from not being able to remember a distant relative's phone number to being in a persistent vegetative state (PVS).

The term **encephalopathy** is used to describe a diffuse disorder of the brain with many causes. The prominent features of encephalopathy are a decreased state of consciousness, abnormal response to external stimulus, and seizures. An encephalopathy is called encephalitis when inflammatory cells are found in the CSF. These altered states of consciousness and rationality may be constant or transitory; they may be temporary disabilities or permanent life-altering conditions.

Encephalopathy secondary to oxygen deprivation is called anoxic or hypoxic encephalopathy (anoxic brain damage) and is the cause of many serious brain injuries. The primary goal of management of head injury in children is to prevent secondary injury to the brain. Prevention of hypoxia, ischemia, and increased intracranial pressure is essential.[10]

Lethargy and Coma

A progressive decline in consciousness can be caused by diffuse or multifocal disturbances of the cerebral hemispheres or by focal injury to the brainstem. Specific characteristics are used to describe and delineate various states of decreased consciousness (Table 31-2).

TABLE 31-2

Classifications of Stupor and Coma

| Grade | State of Awareness | Responds Appropriately to | | |
		Name	Light Pain	Deep Pain
1	Drowsy, lethargic, indifferent; does not lapse into sleep	Yes	Yes	Yes
2	Stuporous; lapses into sleep; may be disoriented	No	Yes	Yes
3	Deep stupor; responds to deep pain	No	No	Yes
4	Does not respond to appropriate stimuli; possible decorticate and decerebrate posturing; retains deep tendon reflexes	No	No	No
5	Nonresponsive, flaccid, no deep tendon reflexes, apneic	No	No	No

The GCS, although originally designed for trauma cases, is now used to provide clinicians with a standardized system to assess a patient with an altered level of consciousness. The pediatric coma scale was developed to assess infants and toddlers who are unable to speak or follow commands (Figure 31-4 and Box 31-1).[19] Although pupil diameter and light reactivity are not addressed in the coma scales, they are important indicators of cerebral herniation and should be assessed during a neurological examination.[20] Combining the pediatric and adult GCS scoring method may be helpful in evaluating transitionally aged children or when age is uncertain.

The clinical features that localize the anatomical site of disturbed brain function are state of consciousness, pattern of breathing, pupillary size and reactivity, eye movements,

Box 31-1	Children's Coma Scale*

I. OCULAR RESPONSE
4 = Pursuit
3 = Extraocular movement intact, reactive pupils
2 = Fixed pupils or extraocular movement impaired
1 = Fixed pupil and extraocular movement paralyzed

II. VERBAL RESPONSE
3 = Cries
2 = Spontaneous respirations
1 = Apneic

III. MOTOR RESPONSE
4 = Flexes and extends
3 = Withdraws from painful stimuli
2 = Hypertonic
1 = Flaccid

*Score = I + II + III. Maximum score = 11; minimum score = 3.

and motor responses.[21] Lethargy and obtundation are generally caused by mild depression of the cerebral hemispheres. Stupor and coma occur when hemispheric dysfunction is more extensive or when the diencephalon or upper brainstem is involved. Abnormalities in the dominant hemisphere have a greater effect on consciousness than those in the nondominant hemisphere.

Respiratory Effects

Hypothalamic and midbrain damage results in rapid, sustained, deep hyperventilation (central neurogenic hyperventilation). Injury to the medulla and the pons affects the respiratory centers and produces several different patterns:
1. Apneustic breathing, with a prolonged pause at full inspiration;
2. Ataxic breathing, which consists of random, ineffective, haphazard breaths and pauses without a predictable pattern; and
3. Primary alveolar hypoventilation (Ondine's curse), a failure to breathe while sleeping, which is the failure of automatic breathing centers when asleep.

Cheyne-Stokes respirations, during which periods of hyperpnea alternate with periods of apnea, result from an extensive, usually bilateral, diencephalic disturbance with an intact brainstem.

The most common cerebral causes of respiratory insufficiency are increased ICP and drugs that depress brain function. Barbiturates are often used to put the brain into an inactive state, inducing a coma to treat encephalopathies and intractable seizures (status epilepticus). Intubation and mechanical ventilation must be initiated before barbiturates are given.

Persistent Vegetative State

The terms **persistent vegetative state** (PVS) and *neocortical death* are used interchangeably to describe patients who, after recovery from coma, return to a state of wakefulness

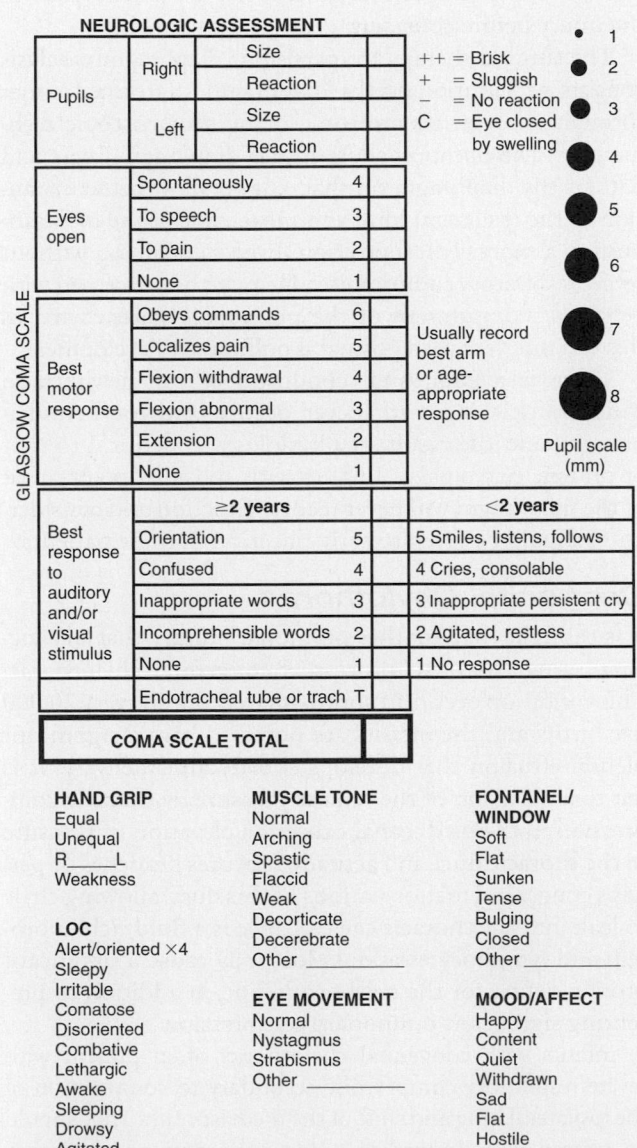

FIGURE 31-4 Pediatric coma scale. (From Hockenberry M, Wilson D: *Nursing care of infants and children,* ed 9. St. Louis: Mosby, 2011.)

without cognition. PVS is "a form of eyes-open permanent unconsciousness in which the patient has periods of wakefulness and physiological sleep/wake cycles, but at no time is the patient aware of him- or herself or the environment."[22] Brainstem functions such as respiration and circulation are intact, and with good nursing care, survival is indefinite. With intensive and aggressive therapy, patients tend to maintain basic vital signs but are usually technology dependent and have an apparent poor quality of life.

PVS occurs in 12% of adults who survive nontraumatic coma but is probably less common in children. The usual causes, in order of frequency, are anoxic and ischemic brain injury, metabolic or encephalitic coma, and head trauma. Recovery is rare when the vegetative state has persisted for 1 month in adults. The prognosis may be better in children, although recovery after 3 months is unlikely.

The American Academy of Neurology has adopted the policy that all medical treatment, including the provision of nutrition and hydration, may be ethically discontinued when the following conditions are met:[23]

1. A patient's condition has been diagnosed as a PVS
2. It is clear that the patient would not want to be maintained in this state
3. The family agrees to discontinue therapy

Recent adult cases have brought these issues to the forefront of public and professional debate without a clear consensus on the discontinuation of medical support technologies and techniques used to accomplish life-sustaining activities.

THORACIC TRAUMA

Thoracic trauma encompasses a broad range of injuries in the pediatric population, from those iatrogenic injuries encountered in the newborn infant through acquired traumatic injuries seen in adolescents. The traumatic thoracic injuries encountered in children generally present in a somewhat different fashion from those encountered in adults and usually are better tolerated, within a background of normal pulmonary function. Overall, thoracic trauma accounts for about 5% to 10% of admissions in pediatric trauma centers.[24] This section covers the more common forms of thoracic birth trauma, acquired blunt and penetrating thoracic trauma, and special forms of iatrogenic thoracic trauma, perhaps seen more commonly in children than adults.

Birth Trauma

The fetus is exposed to considerable compression stresses in passage through the birth canal for vaginal delivery. The flexibility of the fetal thoracic skeleton allows considerable pulmonary compression in this process and occasional pulmonary trauma.[25]

Nerve Injury

Distortion of the axial skeleton during delivery can stretch and damage the nerves involved with the respiratory mechanics of the newborn, particularly the phrenic nerve, which arises from the C4 level in the neck.[26] Flexion and extension of the neck during the delivery process can stretch the origin of the phrenic nerve and cause diaphragmatic paralysis. Depending on the degree of injury, this may be transient or permanent.

The newborn infant, with diminutive extrathoracic musculature, is primarily a diaphragmatic breather. Paralysis of the diaphragm may cause significant respiratory embarrassment. Abdominal pressure is always greater than pleural pressure in the newborn, and the paralyzed diaphragm tends to elevate in the chest, compressing the ipsilateral lung and shifting the mediastinum to compress the contralateral lung. In this setting the infant may have a tidal volume sufficiently restricted to require intubation and mechanical ventilation. In general, one should wait for 3 to 6 weeks to judge if the phrenic nerve will recover from the injury before considering surgical treatment.

The surgical therapy for persistent diaphragm paralysis consists of plication of the diaphragm, performed either through an open thoracotomy or by thoracoscopic techniques.[27] The plication shortens the diaphragm fibers and flattens the diaphragm on that side to allow better expansion of the ipsilateral lung and movement of the mediastinum to a more central position. Even in neonates without severe respiratory compromise, one must be concerned with persistent compression of the pulmonary parenchyma as this can interfere with postnatal pulmonary development.

There is a congenital condition of the newborn in which muscle ingrowth never occurs into the hemidiaphragm, and the resultant physiology is identical to that of phrenic nerve palsy. Infants with so-called eventration of the diaphragm will never recover function and consideration should be given to early plication in these patients.

Congenital Chylothorax

It is thought that another pulmonary injury that may occur during the birth process is congenital chylothorax. This condition occurs in approximately one in every 20,000 live births and the infants are noted to have a significant pleural effusion that develops shortly after delivery. It is felt that elevation of the venous pressure by thoracic compression in the birth canal causes an elevation of pressure in the thoracic duct and actually ruptures branches or perhaps congenital malformations of this duct, allowing chyle to leak into the thoracic cavity. Chyle is a fluid rich in protein and lymphocytes and its loss may cause a significant protein deficit for the newborn infant, in addition to presenting significant pulmonary compression.

Infants with congenital chylothorax often present with severe respiratory compromise secondary to compression of the ipsilateral lung and shift of the mediastinum. They should be treated with immediate chest tube drainage and they should receive nothing by mouth to minimize the formation of thoracic duct lymph. Their nutrition should be supplied by total parenteral nutrition until the chyle leak ceases.

In approximately 30% of these patients the leak will not stop with these measures and surgical treatment will be required, either by placement of a pleuroperitoneal shunt to drain the fluid into the peritoneal cavity, where it can be absorbed, or by thoracotomy with thoracic duct ligation to cease all lymphatic flow through the chest. Both these techniques have approximately an 80% success rate in managing infants with congenital chylothorax.[28,29]

Pneumothorax

Pneumothorax occurring in the newborn infant will be discussed in more detail in the section on iatrogenic trauma because in most cases this is caused by overzealous positive-pressure ventilation of the newborn.

Transition from fetal life—with a fluid-filled, consolidated lung—to newborn life with an expanded and aerated lung is a complicated process. Compression of the thorax in the birth canal can begin to mobilize fluid from the pulmonary parenchyma, but many infants will require positive-pressure assistance to fully expand their lung. This is particularly true in the premature infant in whom pulmonary surfactant levels may be quite low. Positive-pressure ventilation of these small infants must be performed at very low peak inspiratory pressures. If high pressures are employed to rapidly expand regions of consolidated lung, the portions of the lung that are aerated will expand more rapidly. Occasionally this expansion is sufficient to rupture the visceral pleura and cause a pneumothorax, with sudden deterioration in pulmonary function. These infants must be treated with prompt placement of a chest tube and reduction of the peak inspiratory pressures.

Blunt Thoracic Trauma

Pulmonary Contusion

Significant blunt thoracic trauma is relatively less common in the pediatric population than in adults. Overall, blunt chest trauma accounts for 80% of the chest injuries that occur in civilian populations.[30] The child's ribs and cartilage are more flexible than the adult's, and the thorax can be quite significantly compressed without fracturing ribs. This compression causes trauma to the underlying pulmonary parenchyma with resultant edema and occasional hemorrhage into the parenchyma. As children get older and approach adolescence the ribs begin to calcify and stiffen and rib fractures are seen more commonly in this population. If the fractured end of a rib penetrates the visceral pleura of the lung beneath it, a pneumothorax is produced. These patients can present to the emergency room in extreme respiratory distress and improvement in ventilation is often seen immediately with placement of a chest tube.

Flail Chest

When several adjacent ribs are fractured in two areas, a flail segment of the chest wall may be produced. This segment of the chest moves in paradoxical fashion with respiratory effort, collapsing with inspiratory effort and expanding with expiration. This paradoxical motion interferes with tidal ventilation of the ipsilateral lung and, in conjunction with pulmonary parenchymal contusion, may cause serious respiratory embarrassment.

Although in the past attempts had been made to wire the rib ends together to stabilize this segment of the thoracic wall, these were difficult operations requiring multiple incisions and often did not provide sufficient stability. Likewise, merely strapping that segment of the chest wall with stiff bandages may prevent the flail segment from expanding with expiration but will not prevent the collapse and pulmonary compression with inspiration. Children with significant segments of flail chest wall are best treated with intubation and positive-pressure ventilation with paralysis.[31] Over a 5- to 7-day interval, the inflammatory healing process stabilizes the ends of the ribs and minimizes the flail, and these patients can usually be successfully extubated at that point.

Penetrating Thoracic Trauma

Although the majority of thoracic trauma in children occurs from blunt injury, penetrating thoracic trauma carries a significantly higher mortality for these patients. Isolated penetrating trauma, without significant associated injury, carries approximately 5% mortality in pediatric patients, and the mortality with multiple injuries may be as high as 15% to 20%.[32] The range of injuries encountered with penetrating trauma in children varies considerably, depending on the offending object and the axis of injury. In general, stab wounds, particularly those with pocket knives having short blades, cause the least severe injuries, while high-velocity missiles, such as occur in hunting accidents, cause the most severe tissue damage and internal injury.

Incidence

The incidence of penetrating thoracic trauma varies with age, with older children and adolescents having a significantly higher incidence than infants and younger children. A greater proportion of injuries in the older children are associated with handguns or knives used in criminal activity, although a small percentage are secondary to hunting or industrial accidents. The most common injury sustained with penetrating thoracic trauma is a pneumothorax or hemothorax with accumulation of air or blood within the pleural space.

Resuscitation

Often the extent of intrathoracic injury is difficult to predict from the mechanism of injury, particularly in those cases with gunshot wounds, in which the missile may be deflected by bony structures and take a circuitous route. All these patients should be stabilized in the emergency department before any diagnostic studies are obtained.

An adequate airway must be ensured, with many of these children requiring immediate intubation. The adequacy of ventilation should be monitored with transcutaneous oxygen saturation, and mechanical ventilation may be required for those individuals who are hypoxic (SaO_2 less than 80%) or tachypneic (respiratory rate more than 45 breaths/min). Two large-bore IV catheters should be inserted for fluid resuscitation to maintain adequate tissue perfusion. Several clinical studies in the past decade have suggested more favorable clinical outcomes in individuals resuscitated with limited intravenous volume administration before control of the source of bleeding.[33] For most pediatric patients, systolic blood pressures of 80 to 100 mm Hg should be sufficient to maintain adequate tissue perfusion during this interval.

Imaging

Although the diagnosis of penetrating thoracic trauma is usually rapidly evident from the history of the mechanism of injury and the physical examination, specific information with regard to intrathoracic organ injuries will require further radiologic and interventional procedures. Patients presenting with severe respiratory distress should be treated immediately by intubation and ipsilateral tube thoracostomy, before any radiologic studies are obtained. Patients with less severe symptoms and those who have been stabilized are initially investigated with an AP chest radiograph. Although this should ideally be obtained with the patient in a semiupright position, in practice it is usually acquired with the patient supine. Small collections of blood and air may be difficult to appreciate in the supine chest radiograph as blood tends to layer posteriorly and air collections accumulate anteriorly. Subtle changes in the density of the radiograph on the ipsilateral side, compared to the contralateral side, may be the only clue to these injuries. Careful attention to the ribs, cardiac shadow, mediastinal space, and diaphragm contours should be observed on this initial radiograph. The position of the endotracheal tube and nasogastric tube, if present, should also be noted. A chest CT scan may be more sensitive for identifying small pneumothoraces and pneumomediastinum. CT arteriogram may define major vascular injuries, although aortography may be necessary to provide more precise anatomic details in some of these injuries.[34,35] The evacuation of more than 300 cc of blood from the pleural space after placement of a chest tube, or continuous bleeding through the chest tube, should prompt evaluation for a major vessel injury. Patients with penetrating injuries suspected of involving the mediastinum should undergo esophagoscopy or contrast esophagography. These patients also should undergo fiberoptic bronchoscopy. Patients with penetrating injury in whom either entrance wounds or exit wounds are below the level of the nipples should be suspected of having diaphragm and intraabdominal injuries. These patients should undergo abdominal CT scan to assess for that possibility.

Pneumothorax/Hemothorax

The injuries associated with penetrating thoracic trauma include pneumothorax, hemothorax, pulmonary parenchymal injuries, major airway injuries, great vessel injuries, esophageal injuries, and diaphragmatic injuries. Pneumothorax is seen as a consequence of virtually all penetrating thoracic trauma as the pleural space is opened to atmospheric pressure, even if the visceral pleura is not violated (Figure 31-5). The presence of both blood and air in the pleura space is referred to as hemopneumothorax. Air under pressure in the pleural space, as might occur with a ball-valve–type injury of the visceral pleura, is termed a tension pneumothorax.[36]

In any instance in which intubation is considered in the presence of a traumatic thoracic injury, attention should be paid to the possibility of a tension pneumothorax being present, because positive-pressure ventilation may increase the pressure within the chest and further compromise the patient's respiratory and hemodynamic status. Otherwise healthy young individuals can generally tolerate a moderate unilateral pneumothorax but may be quite symptomatic with a tension pneumothorax because of the mobility of the mediastinum in children. Although some patients with a small unilateral pneumothorax may be treated expectantly, most children with pneumothorax as a consequence of penetrating trauma should be treated with a chest tube. Likewise, all children with a significant hemopneumothorax should receive a chest tube for drainage of the pleural blood. Some of these children will not require

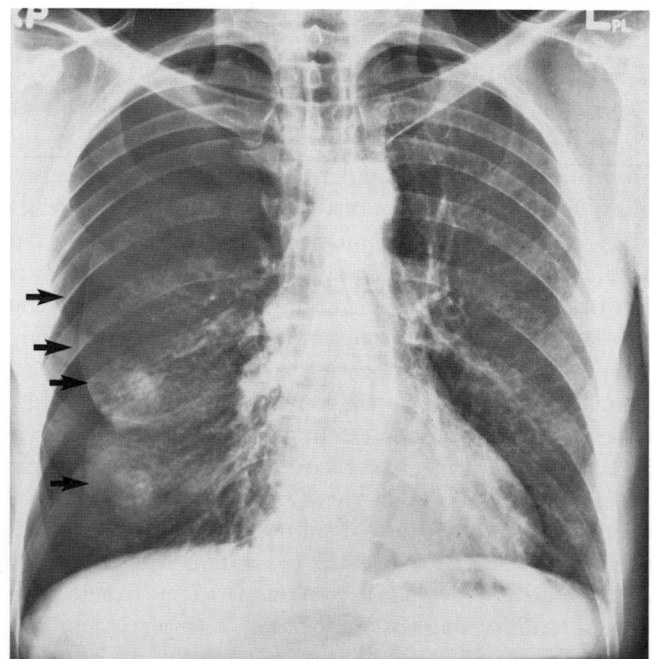

FIGURE 31-5 Pneumothorax involving the right lung. Note the pleural line along the right lateral chest wall where the lung has pulled away from the chest wall as it collapsed toward the hilum. (From Heuer A. *Wilkins' clinical assessment in respiratory care,* ed 7. St. Louis: Mosby, 2014.)

intubation and most will not require thoracotomy for control. On the other hand, children who suffer high-velocity penetrating injuries of the chest wall will require intubation and often thoracotomy to control bleeding and pulmonary parenchymal injuries.

Airway Injury

Patients with penetrating thoracic trauma, presenting with a significant pneumothorax in which there is a continuous air leak through the chest tube, should be suspected of having major airway injuries. The majority of these patients will be found to have a pneumomediastinum on plain chest radiographs or chest CT scans. Airway penetration should be confirmed by bronchoscopy. If the patient has been intubated for respiratory distress, this may be performed with a flexible bronchoscope passed through the endotracheal tube. One must be aware that the injury may be proximal to the level of the end of the endotracheal tube; in some cases the flexible bronchoscope may need to be passed through the larynx, beside the endotracheal tube, to examine for this possibility. Patients who are not intubated may undergo either flexible or rigid bronchoscopy. Most major airway lacerations will require open exploration and repair, although smaller injuries may be stented with the endotracheal tube and may heal without significant stricture.[37]

Vascular Injury

Patients with high-velocity penetrating injuries and significant ongoing blood loss should be suspected of having major vessel injuries. Many of these patients may require urgent thoracotomy for control of the bleeding, although some may be stable enough to obtain a CT angiogram or arteriogram to help localize the area of injury.

Some patients with penetrating thoracic trauma may also have sustained significant intra abdominal injury. In most of the respiratory cycle the apex of the diaphragm is as high as the fourth intercostal space. This is because intra abdominal pressure always exceeds intrapleural pressure, throughout all phases of ventilation. Penetrating injuries at or below this level, the level of the nipples, must be suspected of having diaphragm penetration and potential intra abdominal injuries. These patients should be evaluated with a chest-abdomen CT scan. In otherwise stable individuals, thoracoscopy has been reported to be helpful in diagnosing traumatic diaphragm lacerations.[38]

Children with penetrating thoracic injuries who require intubation may present significant ventilatory difficulties because of a massive air leak. To minimize the air leak, ventilator strategies in these patients generally attempt to reduce peak inspiratory pressures and mean airway pressures. This can often be accomplished by reducing the tidal volume and using a minimal level of PEEP, with an increase in respiratory rate. Patients with very large air leaks may benefit from the use of high-frequency or oscillating ventilators. Further reduction of mean airway pressure is possible using these ventilators, thereby reducing the volumes of air lost across the chest wall. Most children can be successfully ventilated with these strategies, but on rare occasions emergency surgery and control of the pulmonary leak or pulmonary resection may be necessary.

Iatrogenic Thoracic Trauma

Many of the same types of injuries that may be encountered with blunt or penetrating thoracic trauma may be seen as a consequence of iatrogenic trauma. As physicians perform more and more invasive procedures around the chest, the incidence of iatrogenic thoracic trauma has increased.

Pneumomediastinum

Pneumomediastinum, the collection of air in the mediastinal space in the central chest, may be seen as a consequence of sudden Valsalva maneuvers or even asthma. Iatrogenic perforation of the esophagus during esophagoscopy may result in accumulation of mediastinal air and fluid, often rupturing into one of the pleural spaces. Pneumomediastinum may be an isolated clinical finding or it may be associated with a pneumothorax or subcutaneous emphysema. Patients with iatrogenic pneumomediastinum may be asymptomatic, but symptoms of dyspnea, cough, or cervical pain are not uncommon. The primary importance of the finding of pneumomediastinum is that it manifests a significant underlying injury and indicates that appropriate investigation must be undertaken. These investigations may include chest CT scans, contrast studies of the esophagus, or panendoscopy.

Pneumothorax

There are a variety of the iatrogenic causes of pneumothorax. These may include overly deep endotracheal suctioning, laceration of the trachea during intubation, penetration of the airway during endoscopy, high-pressure mechanical ventilation, central venous catheter placement, or thoracentesis.

A small pneumothorax may be asymptomatic, but larger pneumothoraces usually present with ipsilateral chest pain, dyspnea, tachypnea, and oxygen desaturation. The severity of these symptoms will increase as the magnitude of the pneumothorax increases. Breath sounds from the ipsilateral chest will be diminished or absent and, with tension pneumothorax, the trachea will be shifted to the contralateral side in the suprasternal notch. Chest radiographs will show a collapsed lung and may show shift of the mediastinum.

Treatment of symptomatic pneumothorax requires immediate decompression. In the absence of a hemopneumothorax, this can be accomplished with a small pigtail catheter (8 to 12 Fr) placed in the anterior second intercostal space. This catheter is connected to an underwater seal drainage system and may be connected to suction. Patients with a hemopneumothorax should receive a larger chest tube (16 to 24 Fr) to avoid clotting.

Iatrogenic airway injuries are known to occur as a consequence of overzealous endotracheal suctioning in young infants.[39] The suction catheter should be carefully measured and only passed down to the level of the end of the endotracheal tube in order to avoid direct tracheal or bronchial injury. The most common site of injury is in the medial-basal segment of the right lower lobe. This segmental bronchus is on a straight line beyond the end of the endotracheal tube, and catheters that are passed without attention to the depth will puncture the visceral pleura in this segment. A right pneumothorax is a consequence and an infant will develop sudden respiratory compromise. Because most of these patients are intubated and ventilated, air accumulates in the hemithorax quite rapidly. These patients should be treated with prompt placement of a chest tube and reduction in peak inspiratory pressure.

Esophageal-Pharyngeal Injuries

Nasogastric Tube Placement. Esophageal injuries from catheters usually occur during attempts to pass nasogastric tubes but occasionally may be seen with vigorous postpartum suctioning to clear the posterior pharynx.[40] These injuries typically manifest with the finding of pneumomediastinum on chest radiograph, although pneumothorax, pleural effusion, or subcutaneous emphysema may also be present. If the tube has been left in place, it may be noted to be in the pleural space on chest radiograph. These injuries will almost uniformly heal spontaneously if the tube is removed and the patient is kept NPO. A chest tube is placed to evacuate a pneumothorax and intravenous antibiotics are administered.

Central Venous Pressure Catheter Placement. Central venous pressure (CVP) catheters have become a mainstay for pediatric patient care, particularly in young infants. Most of these catheters may be considered "temporary," in that they are expected to be used for only a few days and may be easily removed. More "permanent" central venous catheters may be expected to last for weeks or months if needed. These catheters typically are tunneled before entering the vein and have a Dacron cuff that is placed in midtunnel to allow tissue ingrowth and catheter fixation. Access to the venous system for placement of all these catheters is typically accomplished by percutaneous puncture of one of the subclavian or internal jugular veins. A wire is then threaded through the needle under fluoroscopic control, and the catheters are passed over this wire to ensure intravascular placement.

The vast majority of the iatrogenic injuries of this procedure occur with attempts to percutaneously access the vein, and the most common complication is a pneumothorax.[41,42] Hemothorax can be seen from accidental arterial puncture; rarely, cardiac tamponade may be seen if the right atrium or ventricle is punctured by the catheter or the introducing sheath. Precautions that may minimize the frequency of these complications include an appreciation of the inherent risks of the procedure, familiarization

with the anatomy of the region, and ensuring that the child is under appropriate sedation or anesthesia and does not move during placement. Fluoroscopic assistance in guiding the advancement of the wire is invaluable. Some operators have found real-time ultrasound to be helpful in accessing the vein. The development of hemodynamic or respiratory changes during the placement of a central catheter should prompt an evaluation for possible pneumothorax, hemothorax, hemopneumothorax, or even pericardial tamponade. Because the majority of these procedures are done with fluoroscopic control, immediate fluoroscopy of the chest can be helpful in making these diagnoses.

Intubation. Intubation injuries, although rare, can create life-threatening conditions, particularly in small infants. The predisposing factors include inappropriate use of a stylet, with the rigid stylet extending beyond the end of the endotracheal tube, or multiple attempts at intubation.[43] The injury usually occurs in the vallecula, posterior and lateral to the laryngeal opening, and the endotracheal tube may be advanced into the pleural space. The symptoms include significant respiratory decompensation as well as shift of the trachea to the contralateral side. Treatment should include immediate chest tube placement and withdrawal of the improperly placed endotracheal tube with control of the airway either through placement of a new endotracheal tube or a tracheostomy.

Endoscopy. Injury to the airway or the esophagus may occur as a consequence of bronchoscopy or esophagoscopy, with both rigid and flexible endoscopes. Injuries may be a consequence of penetration of the trachea or esophagus by the endoscope itself or perforation by injudicious use of biopsy or laser therapy.[44] The risks of injury increase if there is already an anatomical distortion of the trachea or esophagus, such as stricture or displacement. The injury may be suspected at the time of the procedure by the presence of unusual bleeding, or, more commonly, may be discovered afterward on a postprocedure radiograph or by the development of postprocedure symptoms. Risk of injury from endoscopic procedures can be reduced by avoiding passage of the instrument when resistance is met and ensuring that the lumen is visualized before the endoscope is advanced. The postprocedural chest radiograph should always be obtained to assess for the presence of pleural, mediastinal, or subcutaneous air.

Ventilator-Induced Injuries

Injuries from mechanical ventilation are not uncommon in the pediatric population. This is particularly true for infants who develop pulmonary disease from prematurity and those who have been ventilated for long periods of time.[45] Acute presentations of pneumothorax, pneumomediastinum, or subcutaneous emphysema may occur. These complications are usually accompanied by oxygen desaturation and possibly hemodynamic compromise. The mechanism of injury is usually secondary to alveolar overdistention, caused by high peak inspiratory pressures or tidal volume. These abnormalities are complicated by patchy areas of consolidation in these infants, allowing the airway pressure to be transmitted to the small volume of ventilated lung. Because tidal volumes are often calculated from body weight, premature babies are particularly prone to injuries secondary to the lower volume of lung and alveoli. Lung injury can be minimized by judicious use of respiratory settings, particularly keeping tidal volumes at the lowest effective level and peak inspiratory pressures low. Inability to safely ventilate with a standard ventilator may prompt the use of the oscillating ventilator to achieve adequate minute ventilation. These injuries are treated by placement of a chest tube and adjustment of ventilator settings to minimize continued injury. Pneumomediastinum and subcutaneous emphysema, if present, should resolve spontaneously and should not require aggressive treatment.

THERMAL INJURY

Epidemiology

According to the Centers for Disease Control and Prevention (CDC), since 1999 an average of 496 children ages 14 and under have died each year because of unintentional fire- or burn-related injury. In 2008 there were a reported 366 children ages 14 and under who died as a result of fire- or burn-related injuries.[46] This number is the lowest in a decade. Burn-related deaths remain the third highest cause of death behind motor vehicle crashes and drowning.[46]

Since 2001 the average number of children ages 14 and under who have sustained nonfatal fire or burn injuries each year is 107,170. In 2009 this number was down to 90,000. Since 2001 an average of 1293 children ages 4 and under were hospitalized for fire- or burn-related injuries each year.[46]

Scald injuries are the most common type of burn resulting from hot liquids, occurring most commonly in children up to 4 years old and often in the presence of an adult. Scalds are the leading cause of burn injury hospitalizations and emergency room visits.[46] Other types of burns include electrical, chemical, and intentional injury. "Mechanisms of injury are often unique to children and involve exploratory behavior without the requisite comprehension of the dangers in their environment."[47]

In 2010 approximately 2500 fireworks-related injuries were reported among children ages 14 and younger. Reportedly, children ages 5 to 14 accounted for approximately 1800 injuries and those younger than age 5 700 injuries. These numbers account for 40% of all fireworks-related injuries. Sparklers accounted for nearly half the 2500 injuries among children ages 14 and younger.

Annual hospitalization costs, in children age 14 and younger, for scald burn–related deaths and injuries is approximately $44 million. Burn center admission charges average $22,700 per case.[46]

Medical advances have had an impact on reducing the mortality rate and outcome in burn and inhalation injury. However, prevention remains the most important aspect of lowering the risk of these injuries to children. Important measures in preventing pediatric thermal-related injuries are having working smoke detectors, keeping matches out of reach, lowering hot water temperatures, covering electrical outlets, and using flame-resistant children's clothing.[48,49]

Independently cited as high mortality risk factors in children are burn injuries exceeding 30% body surface area (Figure 31-6), associated smoke inhalation, and age younger than 4 years.[50] However, with improved treatment of inhalation injury, advancements in early wound repair techniques, effective antibiotics, precise fluid resuscitation and metabolic control, and avoidance of high pulmonary pressure and oxygen concentrations, the pediatric mortality rate and outcomes continue to improve.[51] With these advances, the mortality rate has dropped 53% over 20 years, and the likelihood is that a child will survive even after burn exposure of up to 60% of the body surface area.[4,46,52]

Pathophysiology

The skin provides four essential functions that are necessary for survival:
1. Protecting the body from infection and injury
2. Preventing fluid loss
3. Regulating body temperature
4. Providing sensory input from the environment

It is composed of two layers: the epidermis and the dermis. The epidermis is the thin outer layer. Below it is the dermis, which is a deeper, thicker layer. The dermis contains hair follicles, sweat glands, sebaceous glands, and sensory fibers for touch, pain, pressure, and temperature. Beneath the dermis lies the subcutaneous tissue, which is composed of connective tissue and fat.

Classification of Burn Injury

The depth of the burn injury classifies the degree of burn and depends on the temperature and duration of contact with the skin. Contact with flame, heat, chemicals, or electrical current results in varying degrees of tissue destruction. Burn depths also vary as a result of body position and skin thickness. Very young children and elderly patients are especially vulnerable to more severe, full-thickness burns because of their particularly thin skin.

Superficial burns involve only the epidermis. The skin appears red without blisters and is hypersensitive and painful.[53]

Superficial partial-thickness injuries involve the epidermis and the only the superficial part of the dermis. These burns are usually very painful because nerve endings in the mid and superficial dermal layer survive the injury. Blistering is often present. Healing generally

Area	Birth 1 yr	1-4 yr	5-9 yr	10-14 yr	15 yr	Adult	2°	3°	Total	Donor areas
Head	19	17	13	11	9	7				
Neck	2	2	2	2	2	2				
Ant. trunk	13	13	13	13	13	13				
Post. trunk	13	13	13	13	13	13				
R. buttock	2½	2½	2½	2½	2½	2½				
L. buttock	2½	2½	2½	2½	2½	2½				
Genitalia	1	1	1	1	1	1				
R. U. arm	4	4	4	4	4	4				
L. U. arm	4	4	4	4	4	4				
R. L. arm	3	3	3	3	3	3				
L. L. arm	3	3	3	3	3	3				
R. hand	2½	2½	2½	2½	2½	2½				
L. hand	2½	2½	2½	2½	2½	2½				
R. thigh	5½	6½	8	8½	9	9½				
L. thigh	5½	6½	8	8½	9	9½				
R. leg	5	5	5½	6	6½	7				
L. leg	5	5	5½	6	6½	7				
R. foot	3½	3½	3½	3½	3½	3½				
L. foot	3½	3½	3½	3½	3½	3½				
						Total				

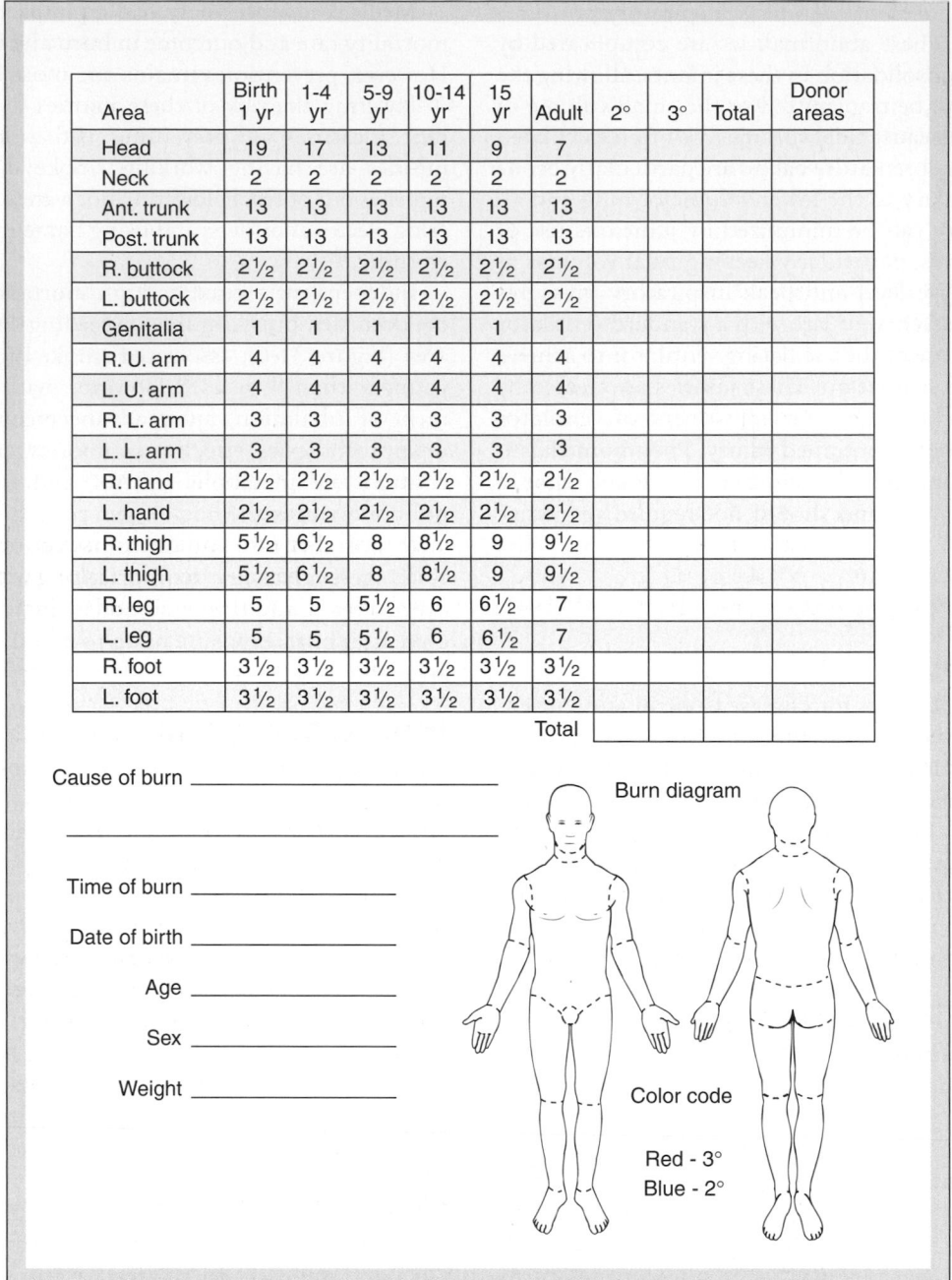

Cause of burn _____

_____

Time of burn _____

Date of birth _____

Age _____

Sex _____

Weight _____

Burn diagram

Color code

Red - 3°
Blue - 2°

FIGURE 31-6 Body surface area estimates of burn size based on age. Note the decrease in the surface area of the head and the increase in the areas of the legs from infant to adult. Using this table provides the most accurate percentage for burn size estimates when calculating fluid and nutritional requirements.

occurs quickly and completely because epithelial cells survive in deeper portions of hair follicles and migrate to the surface.

Deep partial-thickness burns involve the epidermis and the entire dermis. These burns vary in pain because they involve some superficial nerve endings. They also include dermal appendages including hair follicles and sweat glands. These burns do not typically blanch with pressure. They heal by scarring and may take 3 to 4 weeks to heal.

These can be difficult to diagnose upon initial presentation and may need a period of observation to determine the extent of injury.

Full-thickness burns involve injury and necrosis beyond the depths of the hair follicles, through the entire thickness of the skin, and into the subcutaneous tissue. The area swells less rapidly than a second-degree burn and is usually blanched in appearance. Sensory nerves are destroyed, causing local anesthesia.

Percent of Body Surface Area Burn

An estimate of burn size and depth assists in determining the severity, prognosis, and disposition of the patient. Because fluid resuscitation requirements, nutritional support, and surgical interventions are all based on the size of the burn, an accurate assessment of the percent of body surface area burned is critical. The size of the burn wound is described in terms of the percent of total body surface area.

The **rule of nines** is the method most often used to estimate percent body surface area burned. This estimate is based on various anatomical regions representing 9% of body surface area, or a multiple of nine. However, infants and younger children have body proportions different from those of an adult and a modified rule of nines may be used. Figure 31-6 describes the percentages of various anatomical regions as the child ages.[49] In children, the patient's palm size can also be used to measure percent body surface area, with the palmer surface of the child's hand, including to the tips of the fingers, representing 1% total body surface area.

Management

Superficial burns heal spontaneously, usually within 2 weeks, and do not require surgical intervention. Excision and grafting of partial- and full-thickness burns, along with topical antimicrobial therapy, have decreased the incidence of burn wound sepsis. Topical agents most commonly used are sulfadiazine (Silvadene), silver nitrate, and mafenide acetate (Sulfamylon).

After burn injury, the area of deepest burn contains cells that are dead without hope of salvage. The dead skin forms an eschar, which is tough and leathery. Because the eschar layer does not expand well, circumferential burns of the limbs often swell and occlude perfusion to peripheral portions of the extremities. In the same manner, circumferential burns of the thorax can restrict ventilation. An **escharotomy,** which consists of making long incisions into the eschar to allow for wound expansion, relieves the tight, restricting band created by the eschar (Figure 31-7).[49,54] It is important to prevent both early edema and infection that can destroy dermal remnants and convert a burn wound from partial thickness to full thickness.

A crucial component of burn care is initiating accurate fluid resuscitation as soon as possible after the injury. Several formulas for resuscitation are available, with children younger than 10 years of age requiring a modified formula. Delays in resuscitation often lead to increased fluid requirements. Overaggressive fluid resuscitation may result in increased extravascular hydrostatic pressure, pulmonary edema, and soft tissue swelling. Urine output is the usual indicator of adequate resuscitation. Careful hemodynamic monitoring is required, along with intubation for most patients with severe burns. It is important to view the formulas as simply guidelines to fluid resuscitation and not substitutes for diligent monitoring of urine output, electrolytes, and volume status.[55,56]

The metabolic rate can increase as much as two to three times normal after burn injury and is generally related to the size of the burn. This is accompanied by constant hyperthermia. Nutritional support is extremely important and is best accomplished by calculating caloric needs and correcting electrolyte disturbances that are common to burn patients. Pharmacological support of the hypermetabolic response consists of using anabolic agents to alleviate muscle wasting and preserve lean body mass and antiadrenergic drugs to decrease myocardial oxygen consumption and cardiac work.[53]

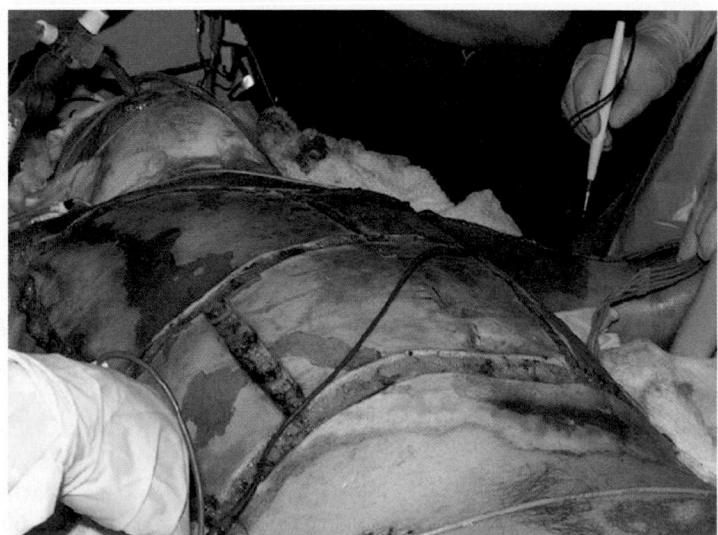

FIGURE 31-7   Escharotomy. (Courtesy University of Michigan Trauma Burn Center, Ann Arbor, MI. From Sole et al. *Introduction to critical care nursing,* ed 6. Philadelphia: Saunders, 2013.)

INHALATION INJURY

Over the past decade there have been many advances in the critical care of burn patients. Burn shock, which in the 1930s and 1940s accounted for nearly 20% of burn deaths, is now treated with early, vigorous fluid resuscitation and rarely leads to loss of life.[52,54] Invasive sepsis originating from the burn wound was at one time found to be the major cause of mortality in 80% of autopsies.[57] Aggressive wound excision and grafting, along with the use of topical antibiotics, have dramatically decreased the incidence of burn wound sepsis. Inhalation injury has now emerged as the most common cause of death in patients with severe burns.[55,58-61]

Although the mortality from smoke inhalation alone is low (0% to 11%), smoke inhalation injury in combination with cutaneous burns is fatal in 30% to 90% of patients.[62] Inhalation injury impairs the mucociliary transport mechanism in the lung, predisposing the patient to retain secretions, which leads to pneumonia and atelectasis. The combination of inhalation injury and pneumonia has been shown to carry a mortality rate of 60%.[63,64] Along with burn size and the patient's age, inhalation injury is one of the most significant predictors of burn-related mortality.[65]

Pathophysiology

Airway injury after smoke inhalation is complex and can occur at any level of the respiratory system, resulting in impaired ventilation and oxygenation. Box 31-2 lists the physiological consequences that accompany smoke inhalation.

Upper Airway Injury

Direct thermal trauma is limited to the upper airway and results in obstruction from edema, hemorrhage, and ulceration of the mucosa. In only a few hours, mild pharyngeal edema can rapidly progress to complete upper airway obstruction with asphyxia.[66,67] The worsening of upper airway edema is most prominent in supraglottic structures. Serial nasopharyngoscopic evaluations demonstrate obliteration of the aryepiglottic folds, arytenoid eminences, and interarytenoid areas created by edematous tissue that prolapses and occludes the airway.[68,69]

Smoke particles vary in size and most often deposit in the upper airway. The type of gas released during combustion depends on the material burned, the temperature, and the amount of oxygen present. Many of the gases, such as ammonia and hydrogen chloride, are chemical irritants and cause intense coughing, bronchospasm, and upper airway edema.[70]

Lung Parenchyma Injury

Direct thermal trauma after inhalation injury is not responsible for the pathophysiological changes in the parenchyma of the lung, and the carbonaceous material present in smoke is not directly responsible for parenchymal damage, although it can serve as a carrier for other agents.[71] Only steam, with a heat-carrying capacity many times that of dry air, is capable of overwhelming the extremely efficient heat-dissipatory capabilities of the upper airways and transmitting heat to the subglottic airways.[72]

The damage to the lung parenchyma is caused by inhalation of incomplete products of combustion. There is direct cellular injury to the respiratory epithelium and pulmonary macrophages, resulting in an inflammatory response. The inflammatory mediators cause bronchoconstriction, an increase in tracheobronchial blood flow with edema formation, and leukocyte infiltration. Bronchoscopic study of the airways in the first 24 hours after inhalation injury shows gradual evolution of an edematous tracheobronchial mucosa.[73] As large portions of the respiratory epithelium slough, necrotic cellular debris accumulates in the airways. Progressive separation of the epithelium with formation of pseudomembranous casts causes partial or complete airway obstruction that can be fatal.[74]

The pulmonary parenchyma surrounding injured airways shows varying degrees of congestion, interstitial and alveolar edema, occasional hyaline membranes, and dense atelectasis. Systemic effects of inhalation injury are manifested by the following:[75,76]

1. An increase in airway resistance, ventilation-perfusion mismatch, and oxygen consumption
2. A decrease in lung compliance, oxygenation, and surfactant production

Carbon Monoxide Poisoning

Carbon monoxide (CO) is a colorless, odorless, tasteless gas produced by the incomplete combustion of carbon-containing compounds. Smoke inhalation from all types of fires often results in significant CO exposure. The majority of immediate deaths that occur at the scene of building fires are caused by CO poisoning. Every patient received from a fire scene should be evaluated for CO poisoning.

Box 31-2	Physiological Consequences of Inhalation Injury

- Hypoxemia
- Bronchospasm
- Airway edema
- Airway obstruction
- Impaired ciliary activity
- Impaired surfactant production
- Increased dead space
- Increased airway resistance
- Increased mucus production
- Increased work of breathing
- Increased oxygen consumption
- Increased intrapulmonary shunting
- Increased ventilation/perfusion mismatch
- Decreased lung and chest wall compliance

The affinity of CO for the binding sites on the hemoglobin molecule is 200 to 280 times that of oxygen. The formation of **carboxyhemoglobin** (COHb) leads to a tremendous reduction in the oxygen-carrying capacity of the blood.[77] This shortage of oxygen is made worse by a concomitant shift of the oxyhemoglobin dissociation curve to the left, reducing the ability of hemoglobin to release oxygen to the tissues.[78-80]

Pulse oximetry measurement does not accurately reflect oxygen saturation in the presence of COHb. The pulse oximeter equates COHb with oxygenated hemoglobin and measures the percentage of saturation of available binding sites, regardless of whether the sites are occupied by CO or oxygen. This causes the pulse oximeter to read falsely elevated oxygen saturation values in the presence of COHb.[81] Direct measurement of COHb using co-oximetry is recommended.

The symptoms of CO poisoning correlate roughly with the percentage of COHb in the blood. Table 31-3 lists the expected symptoms based on CO blood concentrations. The major effects are on organs that are most susceptible to anoxia, such as the brain, heart, and central nervous system.

Evaluation of Injury
Clinical Manifestations
The clinical diagnosis of inhalation injury has traditionally rested on various unreliable observations. Smoke inhalation injury is more likely to be present in those with a history of burn injury in an enclosed space, the appearance of facial burns, singed nasal vibrissae and facial hair, erythema of the oropharynx, and the presence of carbonaceous sputum and debris around the nose, mouth, and pharynx.[82] Rhonchi, crackles, wheezes, stridor, dyspnea, cough, and hoarse voice are seldom present on admission, occurring only in persons with the most severe injury and implying an extremely poor prognosis.[83] The admission

TABLE 31-3	
Symptoms of Carbon Monoxide Poisoning	
Carboxyhemoglobin (%)	**Symptoms**
0–10	None
10–20	Frontal headache, tightness across forehead
20–30	Dyspnea, headache, throbbing temples
30–40	Dizziness, blurred vision, nausea, vomiting, severe headache
40–50	Tachypnea, tachycardia, confusion, collapse
50–70	Depressed consciousness level, seizures, bradycardia
>70	Respiratory failure, death

Modified from Lacey DJ. Neurologic sequelae of acute carbon monoxide intoxication. *Am J Dis Child* 1981;135:145. Copyright 1981, American Medical Association.

chest radiograph is often normal and is a very poor indicator of severity of acute lung injury.[84] However, two thirds of patients develop changes of diffuse or focal infiltrates or pulmonary edema within 5 to 10 days of injury.

Bronchoscopy
The current gold standard for the diagnosis of inhalation injury in most burn centers is fiberoptic bronchoscopy.[85] Direct visualization of the upper airway provides information concerning the extent of upper airway injury. The diagnosis of inhalation injury is confirmed in the presence of soot, charring, mucosal erythema and ulceration, hemorrhage, airway edema, and inflammation.[86] The widespread use of bronchoscopy has led to an approximately twofold increase in diagnosis over that based on the traditional clinical signs.

Xenon Scan
The xenon scan is a safe, rapid test used to evaluate parenchymal damage.[87] Requiring minimal patient cooperation, it involves serial chest scintiphotograms after an initial intravenous injection of radioactive xenon gas. It demonstrates areas of decreased alveolar gas washout, which identifies sites of small airway destruction caused by edema or cast formation. Both false-negative and false-positive results are possible, occurring mainly in patients in whom scanning is delayed for 4 or more days or who have preexisting lung disease. The most important limitation is the logistic problem of transporting the unstable patient to the hospital's nuclear medicine department. Although reported in the literature, few burn centers currently use the xenon scan for diagnosis of inhalation injury.

Spirometry
Although not routinely used for the diagnosis of inhalation injury in children, pulmonary function studies are abnormal after inhalation injury. Reductions in the forced expiratory volume in 1 second (FEV_1) and the ratio of FEV_1 to vital capacity (FEV_1/VC) are seen within 24 hours of injury.[88] Over the next several days, vital capacity and peak flow are reduced and pulmonary resistance is increased.[89,90]

Thermal and Dye Dilution
A more recent method of evaluating inhalation injury is the estimation of extravascular lung water by simultaneous thermal and dye dilution measurements. This procedure has been unable to quantify the severity of injury but has proven useful in separating parenchymal injury from upper airway injury.[91]

Management
The management of any patient with an inhalation injury is determined by the degree of hypoxia, airway obstruction and edema, sepsis, and respiratory failure. Current treatment includes oxygen therapy, adequate airway maintenance,

aggressive bronchial hygiene therapy, pharmacological management, and mechanical ventilatory support.

Oxygen Therapy

The goal of oxygen therapy in a patient with inhalation injury is to increase the oxygen content of the blood. All patients should be given 100% oxygen through a nonrebreathing mask immediately after inhalation injury. Oxygenation is monitored by arterial blood gas analysis, and COHb level is analyzed with co-oximetry. The use of hyperbaric oxygen is widely debated.

Airway Maintenance

Acute upper airway obstruction occurs in one fifth to one third of hospitalized burn victims with inhalation injury. Stridor, hoarseness, wheezing, retractions, and tachypnea are all signs of upper airway compromise and mandate prompt intervention. Whenever airway obstruction is suspected, the most experienced clinician should perform endotracheal intubation. It is better to intubate early than to wait and find that the obstruction has progressed to where visualization of the larynx is reduced.

Securing the endotracheal tube can be difficult because of burn wounds and the rapid airway swelling that occurs within the first 72 hours after the injury. A nasotracheal tube is often more readily secured than an orotracheal tube. Reintubation after an accidental extubation may be difficult if not impossible if facial and oropharyngeal edema is severe. It is important to secure the tube in a manner that avoids trauma to the skin, especially when the face and neck are burned.[89]

Burns of the neck, especially in children, can cause unyielding eschars that externally compress and obstruct the airway. Escharotomies to the neck may be helpful in reducing the tight eschar and therefore decreasing the pressure exerted on the trachea.

Bronchial Hygiene Therapy

Aggressive bronchial hygiene therapy is an essential component of the respiratory management of patients after inhalation injury. Retained secretions may result in life-threatening airway obstruction. They can also lead to atelectasis and ventilation-perfusion mismatch and ultimately contribute to the development of pneumonia, which has been shown to increase mortality after burns and inhalation injury.[92] Early ambulation, therapeutic coughing, positioning, airway suctioning, therapeutic bronchoscopy, and pharmacological agents are used to mobilize and remove retained secretions and fibrin casts.

Early ambulation includes having the patient stand, walk, and sit in a chair. Patients with inhalation injury are routinely gotten out of bed and allowed to sit in a chair to improve lung function. Parents are encouraged to hold and rock their children as a means of therapy and to provide patient comfort.

Tracheobronchial suctioning and lavage are imperative for the removal of secretions and casts in the patient who has an ineffective cough or incapacitated mucociliary apparatus. When secretions or casts become thick and adhere to the airways, bronchial lavage is used as an adjunct to suctioning. Care is taken not to use excessive lavage fluid. Nasotracheal suctioning may be used as a mechanism to stimulate coughing and remove secretions in patients who are not intubated.

Routine repositioning of the patient every 2 hours has been effective in mobilizing secretions. However, positioning is often limited because of the location of fresh skin grafts and donor sites.

When these techniques fail to remove secretions, the use of fiberoptic bronchoscopy has proven effective. Bronchoscopy allows for visualization of the airway and enables meticulous pulmonary toilet for retained secretions. The presence of inspissated secretions and fibrin casts may require repeated bronchoscopy to maintain airway patency and adequate gas exchange.[84,93]

Pharmacological Management

Inhalation injury to the lower airways results in a chemical tracheobronchitis that can cause intense bronchospasm and wheezing. This is best managed with β_2 agonists, especially in patients who also have preexisting asthma or reactive airway disease. Aerosolized bronchodilators are effective by providing bronchial smooth muscle relaxation and stimulating mucociliary clearance. However, when using these agents it is important to remember they are also increase overall metabolic rates in a patient who is already hypermetabolic secondary to thermal injuries.

Racemic epinephrine may be used as an aerosolized vasoconstrictor, bronchodilator, and secretion bond breaker. The vasoconstrictive action of racemic epinephrine is useful in reducing mucosal and submucosal edema within the walls of the pulmonary airways. A secondary bronchodilator action serves to reduce potential spasm of the smooth muscle of the terminal bronchioles. Racemic epinephrine has also been used in the treatment of postextubation stridor.

Investigators have suggested that of corticosteroids may be administered to decrease mucosal edema and bronchospasm, maintain surfactant function, and decrease the inflammatory response that occurs after inhalation injury. Prospective studies showed no benefit in morbidity and mortality in patients who received intravenous corticosteroids after inhalation injury. Some researchers have suggested that there might be an increase in infection-related complications in patients who receive corticosteroid therapy.[94,95]

N-acetylcysteine is a powerful mucolytic agent used in respiratory care. It contains a thiol group, the free sulfhydryl radical of which is a strong reducing agent that ruptures the disulfide bonds that stabilize the mucoprotein network of molecules in mucus. Agents that break down these disulfide bonds produce the most effective mucolysis.[96] N-acetylcysteine has been proven effective in combination with aerosolized heparin for the treatment of inhalation injury in animal studies.[97] Heparin and N-acetylcysteine combinations have been used as scavengers for the oxygen free radicals produced when alveolar macrophages are activated, either directly by chemicals in smoke or by one or more compounds in the arachidonic cascade.[98] Animal studies have shown an increased ratio of PaO_2 to FIO_2, decreased peak inspiratory pressures, and a decreased amount of fibrin cast formation with heparin/N-acetylcysteine combinations.[99] Pediatric patients treated with aerosolized heparin/N-acetylcysteine combinations showed a reduction in the incidence of atelectasis, number of ventilator days, incidence of reintubation for progressive respiratory failure, and mortality.[100]

Although pneumonia occurs in as many as 50% of children with inhalation injury, the prophylactic use of antibiotics is not recommended. Instead, antibiotic therapy is directed by sputum Gram's stain and blood cultures, with culture specimens obtained when infection or pneumonia is suspected.

Mechanical Ventilatory Support

Despite conservative efforts to support unassisted ventilation, patients with moderate or severe inhalation injury may develop respiratory failure and require mechanical ventilation.[101] Patients with severe inhalation injury are at a substantial risk for iatrogenic, ventilator-induced lung damage. Airway resistance is increased secondary to edema and obstruction caused by cast formation. The increased resistance requires higher airway pressures to maintain sufficient flow to support minute ventilation. Ideally, the optimal treatment of any disease should reverse the pathophysiological process without causing further injury. When inhalation injury is severe enough to require conventional mechanical ventilation, such an outcome is rarely achieved.

Conventional Mechanical Ventilation

Conventional mechanical ventilation does not reverse the pathological process, is not characterized by improved clearance of secretions, and may actually compound the existing injury.[102] Conventional volume-limited ventilation in patients with inhalation injury is usually instituted at a tidal volume of 6 to 8 ml/kg.[89] Numerous factors, such as lung/thorax compliance, system resistance, compressive volume loss, oxygenation, ventilation, and barotraumas, must be considered when tidal volumes are selected. PEEP is applied to recruit lung volumes, elevate mean airway pressures, and improve oxygenation. The level of PEEP used varies with the disease process. High levels of PEEP are often required with severe smoke inhalation injury.

Over the past 30 years, and especially in the past decade, there has been an increase in new ventilator techniques that present alternatives for the treatment of patients with inhalation injury. Unfortunately, although the number of options available to the clinician has appeared to increase exponentially, well-controlled prospective trials defining the specific role for each mode of ventilation and then comparing them with other modes of ventilation have not been forthcoming, particularly in the pediatric population.

Other ventilator modes have been employed in both animal models and clinical trials of inhalation injury. Pressure-limited ventilation with and without inverse inspiratory/expiratory ratios has been studied in an ovine smoke inhalation model.[103] Although gas exchange was not significantly improved with this mode, adequate ventilation was achieved at lower mean airway pressures, suggesting that ventilator-induced lung injury may be reduced. Excellent results have been reported using pressure-controlled ventilation in a cohort of pediatric burn patients.[104] Their results suggest that the incidences of barotrauma, pneumonia, and deaths were all considerably less than that expected based on historic controls.

High-Frequency Percussive Ventilation

High-frequency ventilation has also been employed after inhalation injury. This mode provides oxygenation at lower inspired oxygen concentrations and adequate ventilation at lower peak and mean airway pressures. In addition, a few reports have indicated increased secretion clearance with some forms of high-frequency ventilation.[105]

The terms *high-frequency flow interruption* and *high-frequency percussive ventilation (HFPV)* are used to describe a technique in which ventilation is accomplished by a positive-phase percussion delivered at the proximal airway. In clinical trials, HFPV was found to permit adequate ventilation and oxygenation without increasing barotrauma in a small cohort of patients for whom conventional ventilatory support after inhalation injury had failed.[106,107] Studies in adult patients with burns and inhalation injury reported optimal ventilation, decreases in pneumonia, and improved survival with HFPV when compared with conventional volume-limited ventilation.[108] A retrospective study of the effects of HFPV and conventional ventilation in pediatric patients with inhalation injury found that those patients treated with HFPV showed a decrease in the incidence of pneumonia, a lower peak inspiratory pressure, and improvement in the ratio of PaO_2 to FIO_2.[109]

Complications

The most common complications of inhalation injury that lead to increased mortality are infection and respiratory failure. Patients with inhalation injury have a high incidence of pneumonia. Burn-wound infection and sepsis place the patient at extremely high risk for multiple organ system failure.

Early Complications

The reported early complications of inhalation injury are usually mechanical or infectious. Immediate recognition of these complications is imperative so that appropriate treatment can begin and thus decrease the severity of the injury.

Mechanical complications are usually manifestations of barotrauma. Barotrauma can result from a variety of injuries caused by mechanical ventilation, especially when high peak inspiratory pressures are maintained. Patients with inhalation injury often develop sloughing of the tracheobronchial mucosa, which results in a ball-valve–type obstruction. This type of obstruction acts as a one-way valve. The volume from the mechanical ventilator is allowed to enter the lungs; however, expiration is only allowed to partially occur. If this problem is left untreated, further barotrauma may occur and a pneumothorax may result.

Infectious complications may result in tracheobronchitis or pneumonia. The injured trachea is known to be at risk for infections, with respiratory infections being the most common complication after inhalation injury.[110]

The diagnosis of tracheobronchitis or pneumonia can be difficult to establish because of the presence of inhalation injury and bacterial colonization of the airways. The diagnosis of tracheobronchitis rests on the presence of fever, leukocytosis, and productive cough, as well as on organisms and white blood cells on Gram's stain of sputum specimens. Additionally, parenchymal infiltrates must be present on the chest radiograph to make the diagnosis of pneumonia.

Late Complications

Late complications of inhalation injury may be related to mechanical damage or to the consequences of an inflammatory response. Mechanical complications occur most often as a result of iatrogenic injury from endotracheal or tracheostomy tube cuffs. This damage may cause erosion of the tracheal cartilage and result in tracheomalacia. Injuries to the tracheal epithelium may result in fibrosis and stenosis of the trachea, which lead to subglottic stenosis. Cuff erosion into adjacent structures (e.g., innominate artery) may result in exsanguinating hemorrhage. The injuries are difficult to diagnose and often develop slowly. Endotracheal tube instability, high cuff pressures (greater than 20 cm H_2O), and duration of intubation all contribute to airway damage. Meticulous attention to detail regarding tube security and cuff pressures can reduce the incidence of mechanical damage that occurs with artificial airways.

Inflammatory complications, such as bronchiectasis and bronchial stenosis, are thought to occur as a result of neutrophil activation at the site of the airway damaged by inhalation injury. Activated neutrophils produce proteases and oxygen radicals, which may cause severe damage to the already injured bronchial mucosa and extracellular matrix. Although most proteases are produced by neutrophils, other cells—including alveolar macrophages, mast cells, eosinophils, and fibroblasts—all may participate in protease secretion. Normal host defense mechanisms protecting mucosal integrity have been shown to function poorly after inhalation injury.[111] Damage of both smoke-injured and normal tissues by proteases and oxidants may lead to persistent worsening of the inflammatory response, which may prevent healing.

LONG-TERM OUTCOMES

Early reports in the literature indicate that long-term pulmonary parenchyma dysfunction after inhalation injury appears to be uncommon. Patients with inhalation injury alone have significant obstructive defects, whereas those patients with both inhalation and burn injury have a mixed obstructive and restrictive pattern. Although the abnormalities may persist in the early convalescent period, in general most patients have normal lung parenchyma within 5 months of injury.

A study of children with inhalation and burn injury reported pulmonary function changes for up to 8 years after injury. The results indicated the following:[112]
1. Resting lung function showed some degree of residual pulmonary pathology.
2. Altered lung mechanics, impaired gas exchange, chest wall scarring, and respiratory muscle weakness may have contributed to the decrease in lung function.
3. Children with severe thermal injury and smoke inhalation may not regain normal lung function.

Children evaluated with cardiopulmonary stress testing after thermal and inhalation injury showed an increased ratio of physiological dead space to tidal volume during exercise as late as 2 years after the injury.[113] The physiological insults that occur as a result of thermal injury may limit exercise endurance in children.[114] Data from exercise stress testing showed evidence of a respiratory limitation to exercise. This was confirmed by a decrease in maximal heart rate, decreased maximal oxygen consumption, and increased respiratory rate.

Although thermal and inhalation injuries present a challenge to the health care team, an orderly, systematic approach can simplify management. Successful outcome requires careful attention to treatment priorities, protocols, and meticulous attention to details in all areas of care.

DROWNING

Drowning is a significant cause of childhood morbidity and mortality around the globe. In some countries, drowning is the first or second leading cause of death among children.[115] **Drowning** is the process of experiencing respiratory impairment from submersion/immersion in a liquid medium. Drowning outcomes are classified as death, morbidity, and no morbidity. Although historically many terms have been used to describe submersion events and subsequent morbidity, an international consensus conference was convened in 2002 in order to develop guidelines for definitions and reporting of data related to drowning. This definition of drowning was adopted by the World Congress on Drowning and should be widely used.[116] It was also the consensus opinion that drowning without aspiration does not occur. Previously used terminology to describe alternative outcomes, such as *dry, wet, secondary,* and *near-drowning,* have been discouraged in future research and publication.[117] Therefore, for the purposes of this discussion, we use the World Congress consensus term of *drowning* to refer to all forms of submersion injury leading to respiratory impairment, including nonfatal events that previously have been described as *near-drowning.*

A drowning may be classified as "witnessed" when the episode is observed from onset, or "unwitnessed" if the victim is found in the water. *Immersion* means to be covered in water—that is, the face and airway are immersed in order for a drowning to occur. Submersion occurs when the entire body is under water.

Injuries may be further classified as cold-water or warm-water drowning. Warm-water drowning occurs at water temperatures of 20° C (68° F) or higher, and cold-water drowning occurs at water temperatures of less than 20° C (68° F). Some references include very cold water drowning, which refers to submersion in water at temperatures of 5° C (41° F) or less. Additional classification may include the type of water in which the submersion occurred, such as freshwater and saltwater drowning. The distinction between freshwater and saltwater drowning, however, is primarily academic, because initial treatment is not affected by water type.[118-120]

Incidence

Worldwide estimates of drowning incidence indicate that approximately 500,000 such deaths occur yearly. According to the Centers for Disease Control and Prevention, in 2005 there were 3582 fatal unintentional drownings in the United States, averaging 10 deaths per day.[121] More than one in four fatal drowning victims were children 14 years of age and younger. For every child who died of drowning, another four received emergency department care for non-fatal submersion injuries. During this year, males were four times more likely than females to die of an unintentional drowning episode. Reviewers estimate 8000 hospitalizations and more than 31,000 emergency department visits per year because of childhood immersion.[122] Hospitalization costs have been estimated at $23,000 per death and $7000 per survivor. In an extensive review of a national hospital database, total hospital costs for these patients in 2003 alone were close to $10 million.[123]

Many factors affect the exact nature and circumstances surrounding submersion events. The most extensive review of autopsied drowning cases was published in 2005 and covered a 20-year period in Canada.[124] In this review, the most common site of drowning was open water, followed by residential pools and bathtubs. The largest single group affected was male preschoolers. Factors implicated in drowning deaths included intoxication of victim or supervising adult, recreational boating, epilepsy, cervical spine injury after a high-velocity dive, overestimation of swimming abilities, and hypothermia. Inadequate or lapsed supervision of infants and toddlers results in accidental submersion in bathtubs and other small amounts of water. These incidents should always raise suspicion of child abuse and neglect.[125] Drowning in younger children is witnessed in less than 20% of cases, although more than 80% of victims are in the care of a responsible adult. Adolescent submersions have the highest mortality rate at about 70%, despite being witnessed by adolescent peers about 60% of the time.[126-129]

Pathophysiology

The drowning process begins when the victim's airway moves below the surface of the liquid, at which time the victim has a period of voluntary apnea, or breath holding. This is usually followed by an involuntary period of laryngospasm secondary to the presence of liquid in the oropharynx or larynx. If immersion continues, the victim becomes hypercarbic, hypoxemic, and acidotic and begins to swallow large amounts of water. As the victim becomes more hypoxic, the laryngospasm relaxes, and the victim actively breathes in liquid. Aspiration of water leads to destruction of surfactant, impaired alveolar capillary gas exchange, intrapulmonary shunting, and pulmonary edema.[130,131] The ongoing hypoxia quickly produces unconsciousness, apnea, and finally cardiac arrest. The duration of this hypoxia and cardiac arrest is the primary determinant of outcome after a submersion injury.[120] Victims often become hypothermic, which leads to extravascular fluid shifts and renal diuresis resulting in increased fluid losses and decreased systemic perfusion. If the victim is not rescued early on in this continuum, multiple organ dysfunction will ensue and death will result from tissue hypoxia.[128,129]

Central Nervous System Effects

CNS injury remains the major determinant of subsequent survival and long-term morbidity in cases of near drowning.[120,132] Primary CNS injury is initially associated with tissue hypoxia and ischemia. If the period of hypoxia and ischemia is brief or if the person is a very young child who rapidly develops core hypothermia, primary injury may be limited. The patient may actually recover with minimal neurological sequelae.[133] Submersion injuries that are associated with prolonged hypoxia or ischemia, however, are likely to lead to both significant primary injury and secondary injury from reperfusion, sustained acidosis, cerebral edema, hyperglycemia, release of excitatory neurotransmitters, seizures, hypotension, and impaired cerebral autoregulation.[130]

Autonomic instability (diencephalic/hypothalamic storm) is common after severe traumatic, hypoxic, or ischemic brain injury, often presenting with signs and symptoms of hyperstimulation of the sympathetic nervous system (including tachycardia, hypertension, tachypnea, diaphoresis, agitation, and muscle rigidity).[130] CNS infection is an uncommon but serious complication of near drowning. Infection may result from unusual soil and waterborne bacteria and fungi and is usually insidious in onset, typically occurring more than 30 days after the initial submersion injury.[134]

Pulmonary Effects

Fluid aspiration of as little as 1 to 3 ml/kg can result in significantly impaired gas exchange and a decrease in compliance of 10% to 40%, primarily secondary to altered surfactant function.[117,135,136] Aspiration of either freshwater or saltwater can produce surfactant destruction, damage and blockage of alveolar–capillary gas exchange, and increased intrapulmonary shunt. This contributes to atelectasis, lower functional residual capacity, and pulmonary edema and ultimately leads to profound hypoxia. Hypoxia results in decreased cardiac output, arterial hypotension, and increased pulmonary arterial pressure and pulmonary vascular resistance.[133,137]

Acute respiratory distress syndrome (ARDS) from altered surfactant function and neurogenic pulmonary edema is a common complication among survivors of submersion injury.[120] Increased airway resistance secondary to plugging of the patient's airway with debris, as well as release of inflammatory mediators that result in vasoconstriction, also impair gas exchange. Ventilator-associated lung injury can further compromise noncompliant, edematous lung tissue. Pneumonia is a rare consequence of submersion injury and is more common with submersion in stagnant, warm, and fresh water. As with CNS infections, uncommon pathogens, including *Aeromonas, Burkholderia,* and *Pseudallescheria,* cause a disproportionate percentage of cases of pneumonia.[138]

Cardiovascular Effects

During the drowning event, aspiration of water produces a reflex pulmonary vasoconstriction as detailed previously with pulmonary hypertension and impaired cardiac output. Hypoxia and acidosis may lead to cardiac arrhythmias and impaired myocardial function both at the time of the injury and later as the clinical course progresses. In a large review of out-of-hospital pediatric cardiac arrest it was noted that in drowning events asystole is the first recorded rhythm in 61% of patients, ventricular tachycardia or fibrillation in 20%, and bradycardia in 16%.[139] Pulmonary hypertension may result from the release of pulmonary inflammatory mediators, increasing right ventricular afterload and thus decreasing both pulmonary perfusion and left ventricular preload. Hypovolemia is primarily secondary to

fluid losses from increased capillary permeability and hypothermia during the drowning episode. Profound hypotension may occur during and after the initial resuscitation period, especially when vasodilation occurs as the patient is rewarmed. Although cardiovascular effects may be severe, if the victim is rescued during the event, they are usually transient, unlike severe CNS injury.

Other Effects

Differences in the fluid and electrolyte changes seen in saltwater submersion and freshwater submersion have been stressed in the past. The theory was that the hypertonicity of saltwater aspirated into the lung may cause an influx of fluid from the vascular space, resulting in intravascular volume depletion and hemoconcentration with hypernatremia.[116,117] Aspirated freshwater may have the opposite effect on fluid balance, producing volume overload, hyponatremia, and hemolysis caused by decreased serum osmolality. This has been demonstrated in laboratory models experimentally, but more recent studies have shown that the volumes of fluid actually aspirated during human drowning are inadequate to produce these effects.[118,120,134,140,141] Most patients have fluid aspiration of less than 4 ml/kg.[117] Fluid aspiration of at least 11 ml/kg is required for alterations in blood volume to occur, and aspiration of more than 22 ml/kg is required before significant electrolyte changes develop.[140,141] Ingestion, rather than aspiration, is more likely to cause clinically significant electrolyte imbalances, including hyponatremia from ingestion of large volumes of freshwater (especially in children).[116,124,138,139]

The clinical course after a drowning episode may be complicated by multiorgan system failure resulting from prolonged hypoxia, acidosis, rhabdomyolysis, acute tubular necrosis, or infection or from the treatment modalities. Patients may also be at risk of disseminated intravascular coagulation, hepatic and renal insufficiency, metabolic acidosis, and gastrointestinal injuries and should be appropriately managed.[118,124]

Treatment
At the Scene

The most important point in treatment is the quality of resuscitation at the scene of a drowning event. Airway management and rescue breathing should begin before the victim is out of the water, if possible, and cardiopulmonary resuscitation (CPR) should be started as soon as an adequate surface is available. Care should be taken to stabilize the cervical spine if there is any risk of cervical spine injury (i.e., boating or diving accident). If the airway is not patent, standard maneuvers should be used to clear the airway. The Heimlich maneuver, however, should not be used to remove water from the lung.[142] Any efforts to remove water from the lungs, including the Heimlich maneuver, only delay initiation of effective rescue efforts. As soon as trained emergency personnel are available, more advanced techniques should be used, including endotracheal intubation, positive-pressure ventilation, intravenous access, and resuscitation drugs if needed. Hypoxia may be underrecognized, so 100% oxygen should be administered to all victims.

Rapid and appropriate response at the scene may result in the return of spontaneous heart rate and respirations; however, resuscitation is likely to be prolonged if hypoxia has been present for several minutes. Even if spontaneous respiration is restored, the need for continued assisted ventilation should be expected. The presence of hypothermia, hypoxia, and acidosis makes treatment of arrhythmia more difficult and their recurrence more likely until these factors are corrected. Once a perfusing rhythm has been restored, inotrope and pressor therapy may be needed along with volume resuscitation.[128,134] Cardiac monitoring and management of arrhythmia should be priorities. Hypothermia is difficult to reverse in the field, but every effort should be made to prevent further cooling during the resuscitation.

Emergency Department

In the emergency department, stability of the airway and adequacy of ventilation should be assessed. The first priority for managing drowning victims is to reverse hypoxemia by restoring adequate oxygenation and ventilation. All patients should be assumed to be hypoxic, acidotic, and hypothermic. Arterial blood gas sampling reveals critical information regarding oxygenation, ventilation, and the severity of acidosis. An arterial line is often invaluable for management of severely affected victims. Electrolytes, blood urea nitrogen, creatinine, and hemoglobin should also be serially monitored.

Indications for intubation include rising arterial carbon dioxide pressure ($PaCO_2$ greater than 35 mm Hg), a ratio of arterial oxygen pressure to inspired fraction oxygen (PaO_2/FIO_2) less than 300, arterial oxygen saturation (SaO_2) less than 90%, or tachypnea (compared with normal respiratory rate for age). It is also common for drowning victims to have swallowed a large amount of water and therefore be at high risk of vomiting.[143] Unconscious patients or those with respiratory compromise should be intubated by a rapid sequence induction technique using minimal bag-mask ventilation. Mechanical ventilation with the use of a cuffed endotracheal tube is the most effective method for reversing hypoxemia and preventing further aspiration. Aspiration of liquid, development of pulmonary edema, and decreased lung compliance may make effective ventilation difficult. Positive end-expiratory pressure should be initiated at 5 cm H_2O and increased in 2- to 3-cm H_2O increments to 15 cm H_2O as cardiac output and blood pressure allow.[134]

If ventilation is adequate, treatment of metabolic acidosis with tromethamine (THAM) or sodium bicarbonate is advisable. Cardiac arrhythmias should continue to be treated but may be refractory in the presence of significant hypothermia. Tissue perfusion and blood pressure should

be assessed to determine the adequacy of cardiac output. Intravascular volume expansion is often necessary in the presence of postarrest myocardial dysfunction, and inotrope and vasopressor therapy should be used if indicated, often necessitating placement of a central line.

Some degree of **hypothermia** (core temperature less than 35° C) is almost always present after a significant submersion, and severe hypothermia is associated with characteristic physical examination findings (Table 31-4). The goals of management are to prevent a further fall in core temperature and establish a safe and steady rewarming rate while maintaining cardiovascular stability. The health care team should attempt to rewarm the patient 1° C to 2° C per hour to a range of 33° C to 36° C.[144] Aggressive rewarming above this range should be avoided because hyperthermia has been shown to worsen underlying cerebral injury in postcardiac arrest patients.[145] When warming is attempted, cardiac arrhythmia, electrolyte abnormalities, and hypotension caused by vasodilation should be anticipated. Increasing core body temperature is the goal, and simple warming of the skin surface alone should be avoided. Warmed intravenous fluid and ventilator gases should be used. Irrigation of the stomach, urinary bladder, and peritoneal cavity with warmed saline is effective and relatively low risk. Irrigation of the pleural space with warmed saline has the advantage of warming the central circulation but may compromise ventilation and oxygenation. Extracorporeal bypass is the most effective means of increasing body temperature for patients presenting with temperature less than 28° C, and in some cases this technique should be considered early in the course of management, although evidence of success in the pediatric population has not been thoroughly studied to date.[146] An algorithm for initial resuscitation is presented in Figure 31-8.

TABLE 31-4

Key Findings at Various Degrees of Hypothermia

Temperature (°C)*	Clinical Findings
37	Normal oral temperature
36	Metabolic rate increased
35	Maximum shivering seen/impaired judgment
33	Severe clouding of consciousness
32	Most shivering ceases and pupils dilate
31	Blood pressure may no longer be obtainable
28-30	Severe slowing of pulse/respiration
	Increased muscle rigidity
	Loss of consciousness
	Ventricular fibrillation
27	Loss of deep tendon, skin, and capillary reflexes
	Patients appear clinically dead
	Complete cardiac standstill

*As documented by low-registering thermometer.
Data from Weinberg AD. Hypothermia, *Ann Emerg Med* 1993;22:370.

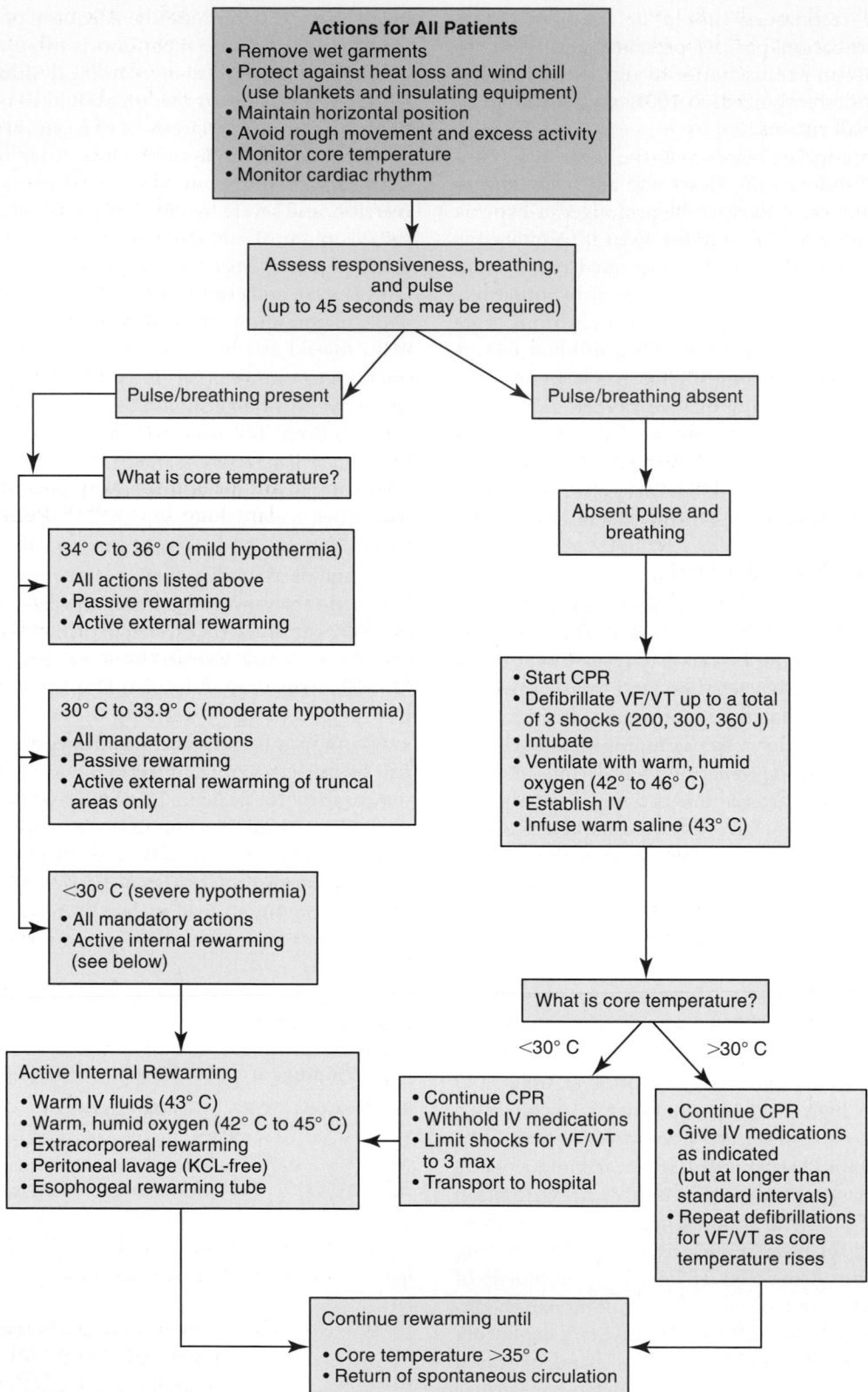

FIGURE 31-8 Algorithm for initial resuscitation. (Data from Weinberg AD. Hypothermia. *Ann Emerg Med* 1993;22 (Pt 2):370-377.)

Patients evaluated in the ED who are minimally affected with no history of loss of consciousness, no altered mental status, and no respiratory signs and symptoms may be observed for a period of hours in the ED and discharged home if no complications arise. Patients with any degree of respiratory compromise, history of need for rescue breathing, or loss of consciousness should be admitted to the hospital even if stable in the ED, because both neurologic injury and lung injury may progress over the first hours to days.[131]

Inpatient

For patients requiring admission to the hospital, intensive care unit (ICU) treatment is primarily supportive. Most ICU patients will require invasive monitoring with a central venous catheter, an arterial line, a nasogastric tube (to prevent further aspiration), and a Foley catheter (to monitor urine output). Neurological injury is the most serious consequence of submersion injury and should be the focus of care. In more severely affected patients, progression of cerebral edema with resultant increased ICP should be anticipated through the first 3 to 5 days. Seizures and fever may occur and should be aggressively treated because both will exacerbate ICP. Although cerebral edema is a common consequence of prolonged submersion (or submersion followed by prolonged circulatory insufficiency), retrospective reviews and animal studies have not demonstrated any benefit from the use of intracranial pressure monitoring with diffuse axonal injury.[147-149] Therefore, as with any hypoxic brain injury, ICP monitoring and aggressive pressure-directed therapy for drowning victims is not recommended.[146,147]

Basic measures to decrease ICP should be employed (Box 31-3). In patients who have a functional recovery, a slow return of neurological function occurs over weeks to months as the cerebral edema resolves.

Fever and chest radiograph changes should be expected early in the chemical course of submersion injury. Lung infiltrates, fever, and leukocytosis are common after submersion injury and do not necessarily indicate an infectious pneumonia. It has been widely studied and accepted that early or prophylactic treatment with antibiotics increases the likelihood of later infection with resistant

organisms and is therefore discouraged.[117,136] If strong evidence of bacterial pneumonia develops, such as persistent fever, evolving focal infiltrates on chest radiograph, or positive bacterial cultures for likely organisms, then antibiotic therapy should be tailored to treat those organisms most likely in this setting or those found in bacterial culture. Foreign bodies should be suspected if lung changes are focal or if segmental air trapping is present. Bronchoscopy may be indicated in order to evaluate and remove foreign bodies.

Pulmonary edema and ARDS may progress rapidly in the first 24 hours and complicate management, but as with most causes of ARDS, the patient usually responds to careful and aggressive respiratory management. Acute respiratory distress in the context of submersion injury is managed as in any other setting. Adequate PEEP is the key element of the ventilator strategy, along with minimizing tidal volume and peak inspiratory pressure to reduce the risk of secondary lung injury.[134,136] PEEP should be increased from 5 cm H_2O with the goal of a PaO_2/FIO_2 ratio of 300 or more. The level of PEEP or continuous positive airway pressure needed to maintain oxygenation should be continued for 24 to 48 hours before attempting to decrease it in order to permit adequate surfactant regeneration. To minimize oxygen toxicity, the delivered FIO_2 should also be reduced to 50% or less as tolerated. Other modes of ventilation, including high-frequency oscillatory ventilation and airway pressure release ventilation, may support ventilation and oxygenation with less risk of ventilator-associated lung injury than is associated with older methods of ventilation. Use of artificial surfactant is usually not indicated in ARDS caused by drowning. Although providing temporary improvement in lung function in many reports, surfactant most likely does not change outcome and is an ongoing focus of investigation.[128] There is also no specific indication for early use of corticosteroids in submersion injury.

Myocardial dysfunction requiring inotropic support may persist for days after a significant hypoxic insult.[114] Recurrent arrhythmia may also occur but is less likely after the initial hypothermia, acidosis, and hypoxia are corrected. Although it is not especially common in submersion injury, acute renal failure and other organ dysfunction may occur after cardiac arrest from any cause and may require any level of support, including hemodialysis or continuous venovenous hemofiltration and dialysis.

As the patient becomes more stable, early involvement of physical and occupational therapy is appropriate. The need for extensive rehabilitation is common. Attention to the emotional and social needs of the parents is also important. Anger and guilt are common because most submersions are preventable accidents. Family dysfunction should be anticipated and appropriate referral made when needed.

Box 31-3	**Initial Strategies to Control Intracranial Hypertension**

1. Elevate the head 15 to 30 degrees.
2. Maintain the head in the midline.
3. Avoid hypercarbia.
4. Ensure adequate blood pressure and oxygenation.
5. Provide adequate sedation and analgesia.
6. Avoid volume overload and hypovolemia.
7. Avoid hyperglycemia.

Data from Weinberg AD. Hypothermia. *Ann Emerg Med* 1993;22:370.

Outcome

The topic of outcome fits comfortably at the end of most clinical discussions. With submersion injury, however, outcome may have been more appropriately discussed first. As with any condition that includes hypoxic-ischemic brain injury as a primary part of its pathology, submersion injury has a tragically poor prognosis. It is within the context of this poor prognosis that decisions and management plans are made. A common question is, "How far should treatment go?" Much of the most recently published literature on submersion injury attempts to answer this difficult question.

Traditionally, all critically ill patients, including submersion victims, are approached with aggressive resuscitation and life support so that each potential survivor has the best chance of eventual recovery. This minimizes the risk of allowing a potential survivor to die because maximal support has been withdrawn. This approach, however, also ensures that many patients whose best possible outcome is persistent vegetative state will also survive. As early resuscitation is associated with improved outcomes, many studies have attempted to determine clinical, laboratory, or other variables to identify which patients would benefit from resuscitative efforts.[150,151] Although no individual characteristics have been found to predict survivability, the Orlowski score is an example of an attempt to identify the likelihood of neurologically intact survival.[149] In using the Orlowski score, one point is given for each item; scores of two or less are associated with a 90% likelihood of complete recovery, and submersion-injury patients with scores of three or more have only a 5% chance of survival. The items in the Orlowski score are as follows:

- Age 3 years or older
- Submersion time of more than 5 minutes
- No resuscitative efforts for more than 10 minutes after rescue
- Comatose on admission to the emergency department
- Arterial pH of less than 7.10

Habib and colleagues[152] predicted outcome in a retrospective case series. Patients arriving in the ED comatose and pulseless had a uniformly poor outcome, whereas those with a pulse and blood pressure in the ED completely recovered. In addition, patients who remained comatose longer than 200 minutes had poor outcomes, and those who were not comatose had normal recovery. A 48-hour period of observation in the pediatric ICU, in addition to the variables seen in the first hours after submersion, may improve our ability to predict outcome. Reliably predicting which patients will experience which outcome early in the clinical course would be helpful in counseling families regarding prognosis and in making decisions about initiating or withdrawing expensive or limited therapeutic resources.

The neuroprotective effects of cold-water drowning are poorly understood. We know that hypothermia profoundly decreases the cerebral metabolic rate. Neuroprotective effects seem to occur only if the hypothermia occurs at the time of submersion and only if rapid cooling occurs in water with a temperature of less than 5° C.[143,146,153] Intact survival of comatose patients after cold-water submersion injuries still is quite uncommon. Anecdotal reports of survival exist for children with moderate hypothermic submersion (core temperature less than 32° C), but most persons experiencing cold-water submersion do not develop hypothermia rapidly enough to decrease cerebral metabolism before severe, irreversible hypoxia and ischemia occur.[151]

PREVENTION

Prevention of unintentional injuries remains key to protecting children. Over time health care professionals have realized that expert trauma care alone cannot slow the injury epidemic that kills more children and young adults in the United States than any other cause. Motor vehicle accident injury and death have seen a decrease in incident however, prevention methods, such as car seats and seat belts, continue to be underutilized.[154] Submersion events and death from drowning are, in most cases, preventable. A majority of victims are young, previously healthy people. There have been no recent breakthroughs in medical technology or treatment modalities that have improved survival rates for submersion victims. As with all accidental injuries, prevention is the only effective means of reducing morbidity and mortality. This is especially true of submersion injury because outcomes are often poor regardless of therapy.[147] Health care professionals can play a major role in educating the public as a whole and individual patients and families. Efforts to prevent deaths from drowning are appropriately focused on improved supervision, proper fencing around pools, and CPR training. Children and adults should be instructed never to swim alone or unsupervised. A recent Cochrane Library review demonstrated that isolation fencing (self-closing latched gate around the pool) is superior to perimeter fencing (enclosing the house and yard together).[155] Pool alarms and covers have not been shown to prevent drowning. Lowering rates of alcohol use around bodies of water and educating parents on the importance of constant supervision of children in the bathtub are also important. Submersion injuries may even occur in toilets and water buckets.[123,125,126] Appropriate measures must be taken to ensure that children are never unsupervised in bathrooms, and water buckets must be emptied when not in use. Training families in CPR may decrease the duration of hypoxia experienced by a submersion victim. Infant swimming or water-adjustment programs do not prevent submersion injuries and are potentially hazardous, providing parents with a false sense of security if they believe their infant can swim.[126]

Children under the age of five tend to be injured within the home, whereas older children and young adults are injured outside the home. The four *Es* of injury prevention are often used as an organized structure for prevention strategies.

- *Education*
  Encourage safe behavior through information

- *Enactment/enforcement*
  Pass safety laws and encourage law officers to enforce them
- *Engineering*
  Designing safety into environment/products
- *Economic incentives*
  Make safety affordable and made risk expensive

Each strategy has evidence of effectiveness. Education is the strategy that health care providers can best support in their daily practice.[154] Providing education through face-to-face counseling, videos, and written materials on bicycle helmets, car seats, home safety, water safety, and poisoning prevention have shown to have positive outcomes leading to improved safety knowledge and behaviors.[152]

Safety and prevention require national, state, local, and individual support. Significant attention must be given to prevention to decrease the incidence of the leading cause of death in children. As stated by Cowden et al., in *Pediatric Emergency Medicine Practice,* the best-supported interventions are behavior change counseling and provision of safety devices with standardized education.[154]

CASE STUDY 1

J.K., a 16-year-old young woman, suffered severe blunt chest trauma when a horse from which she had fallen tripped and fell on her chest. She was intubated at the scene because of respiratory distress and was hand ventilated with 100% oxygen while transported.

On arrival her oxygen saturation was 83% on a ventilator (PIP 20 cm H_2O, PEEP 5 cm H_2O R12 and FIO_2 1.00). A chest radiograph demonstrated a large tension pneumothorax on the right side with bilateral pulmonary contusions. She had multiple rib fractures and fractures of T1 and T2 transverse processes. Bilateral chest tubes were placed immediately with improvement in saturations, but there was a continuous air leak from the right side.

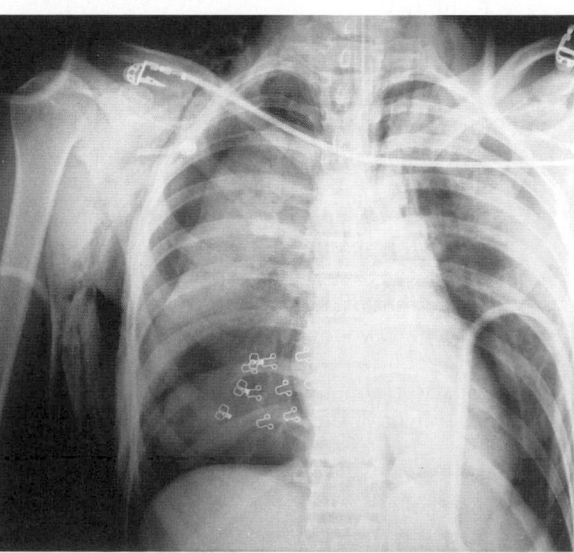

She was weaned to an FIO_2 of 0.23 in the next 12 hours. The patient underwent flexible bronchoscopy through the endotracheal tube, which demonstrated a laceration of the right bronchus intermedius. This was treated nonoperatively, but healed with a stricture, which subsequently required a sleeve resection.

1. Suspicion of a traumatic pneumothorax is best confirmed by which physical signs?
   A. Hyperexpansion of the ipsilateral chest
   B. Subcutaneous emphysema
   C. Diminished breath sounds on the ipsilateral chest
   D. Elevated jugular venous pressure
2. Treatment of an adolescent with a symptomatic tension pneumothorax secondary to blunt thoracic trauma is best accomplished immediately by:
   A. Insertion of a large-bore needle in the midclavicular line of the second to third intercostal space
   B. Insertion of a large-bore needle in the posterior axillary line of the second to third intercostal space
   C. Carefully monitored observation
   D. Insertion of a 12 Fr chest tube in the midclavicular line of the second to third intercostal space
   E. Insertion of a 12 Fr chest tube in the posterior axillary line of the second to third intercostal space

CASE STUDY 2

A 12-year-old boy is watching a golf match when a club slips out of a golfer's hand and strikes him on the left temporal region of his head. Answer the following questions about his injury and its treatment.

1. He falls to the ground unconscious and is not able to be aroused. He is breathing and nonresponsive to verbal stimuli (although he pulls away from pain). He exhibits tachycardia at 128; his pulse is full and bounding. His eyes are nonreactive and midline. There is no bleeding at the injury site. The patient's Glasgow Coma Scale score is:
   A. 10
   B. 15
   C. 6
   D. 8
2. Which of the following do you do next?
   A. Order stat head and spine CT scan and laboratory tests for electrolyte level; monitor pulse Oximetry; and order a spinal tap.
   B. Immobilize head and spine, cover with jackets, call EMS, and monitor vital signs.
   C. Move to the clubhouse on a golf cart, put ice on the impact point, and give aspirin for headache.
   D. Penalize the golfer two strokes for loss of club control and failing to call "fore."
   E. Start a large-bore IV line, insert airway, sit him up at a 45-degree angle, and monitor vital signs.
3. What is/are the most likely future actions with regard to the patient and his injury?
   A. Observe in the hospital for 24 to 48 hours.
   B. Vital signs and neurological checks Q1 × 4, Q2 × 2, Q4 × 4 until discharge.
   C. Order reduced activity level and observe at home for 2 days after discharge.
   D. All of the above are standard and appropriate actions.

KEY POINTS

- Three general causes of brain damage are trauma, genetic-developmental, and toxic-infective.
- The spectrum of thoracic injuries in pediatric patients includes birth trauma and blunt, penetrating, and iatrogenic thoracic trauma.
- Motor vehicle accidents, bicycle accidents, and falls are contributors to blunt thoracic injuries resulting in complications associated with pulmonary contusions and flail chest.
- Pneumothorax, hemothorax, airway injury, and vascular injury are included in the spectrum of penetrating thoracic injuries seen in children.
- The epidemiology of thermal injuries includes unintentional fire or burn-related events. In younger children scald injuries are common, whereas fireworks contribute to many of the thermal injuries in older children.
- Thermal injury management includes topical antimicrobial therapy, fluid resuscitation, nutritional support, airway support and management, grafting, and in some cases escharotomy.
- *Drowning* refers to all forms of submersion injury leading to respiratory impairment. *Immersion* describes the face and airway being covered by water or liquid, whereas *submersion* describes the entire body being under water.
- Respiratory management of drowning victims should begin before the victims is out of the water. Endotracheal intubation and positive-pressure ventilation with PEEP should be initiated upon arrival of emergency response personnel. Monitoring of oxygenation, ventilation, and severity of acidosis are vital. Treatment of hypothermia is also key. Using minimal tidal volumes and peak inspiratory pressure can reduce the risk of secondary lung injury. High-frequency oscillatory ventilation should be considered.
- Contributing factors to morbidity and mortality of drowning victims include witnessed or unwitnessed event, cold water, warm water, saltwater, or freshwater.
- Prevention strategies for unintentional injuries of children include education, enactment/enforcement, engineering, and economic incentives. Specific actions include the use of seat belts, car seats, proper fencing around pools, appropriate supervision, and CPR training.

ASSESSMENT QUESTIONS

1. What is the leading cause of death for children ages 1 to 19 years?
   A. Drowning
   B. Trauma
   C. Suffocation
   D. Burns
2. Which organ or organs could be injured in response to the Monro-Kellie doctrine?
   A. The brain
   B. The heart
   C. The lungs
   D. All of the above
3. The Glasgow Coma Scale (GCS) score includes the following variable(s):
   A. Eye opening, verbal response, motor response
   B. Temperature, pulse rate, SpO2, blood pressure
   C. Grip strength, Babinski response, eyes closed nose touch
   D. Children's soma scale score plus SpO2
4. Paralysis of the hemidiaphragm caused by birth trauma is secondary to:
   A. Distortion of the thoracic spine during delivery
   B. Distortion of the cervical spine during delivery
   C. Direct rupture of the diaphragm with increased intrathoracic pressure during delivery
   D. Damage from obstetrical forceps
5. What is the most appropriate treatment for congenital chylothorax?
   A. Institution of a high-fat diet
   B. Intubation and ventilation with a high MAP
   C. Intubation and ventilation with a high PEEP
   D. Place on nothing-by-mouth (NPO) status, with total parenteral nutrition
   E. Ligation of the thoracic duct at the base of the left neck
6. Children with penetrating thoracic trauma in the right anterior seventh intercostal space should have the following:
   A. Immediate thoracotomy and control of bleeding from the right lower lobe
   B. Chest CT scan
   C. Chest and abdominal CT scan
   D. Immediate bronchoscopy
   E. Immediate pericardiocentesis
7. What is the function of normal skin?
   I. Protect the body from infection and injury
   II. Prevent fluid loss
   III. Regulate hemodynamics
   IV. Provide mass and form
   V. Provide sensory input
       A. I, II, III
       B. II, III, IV
       C. III, IV
       D. I, II, V
       E. III, IV, V
8. How is *superficial partial-thickness burn* defined?
   A. The skin is red without blisters and very painful.
   B. It involves the epidermis and the entire dermis.
   C. It is also known as eschar.
   D. Dermal appendages, including hair follicles and sweat glands, are involved
   E. It involves the epidermis and part of the superficial part of the dermis.
9. What does the rule of nines estimate?
   A. The percent of body surface that is burned in infants and young children
   B. Fluid requirements for burn injury fluid resuscitation
   C. The weight of the patient for total body surface area
   D. Ideal body weight for ventilator management
   E. The PaO2 related to a specific oxygen saturation on the oxyhemoglobin dissociation curve

10. Carbon monoxide inhaled into the lungs and transferred to the bloodstream:
    A. Combines with hemoglobin and reduces the oxygen-carrying capacity
    B. Has a higher affinity for binding to hemoglobin than oxygen
    C. Shifts the oxyhemoglobin dissociation curve to the left and reduces the ability of hemoglobin to offload oxygen to the tissues
    D. Is responsible for the majority of immediate deaths occurring at the scene of building fires
    E. All of the above

11. The 2002 World Congress on Drowning consensus statement defines drowning as:
    A. Death from asphyxia caused by submersion in water
    B. Respiratory injury occurring when the whole body is underwater
    C. The process of experiencing respiratory impairment from submersion in a liquid medium
    D. A witnessed episode of submersion

12. Males are how many times more likely to die of unintentional drowning than females?
    A. No difference
    B. Two
    C. Four
    D. Ten

13. The primary determinant of neurological outcome after submersion injury is:
    A. Duration of hypoxia and cardiac arrest
    B. Duration of submersion in water
    C. Temperature of water in which victim was immersed/submerged
    D. Volume of water aspirated into the lungs

14. The major determinant of subsequent survival and long-term morbidity in drowning is:
    A. Initial body temperature
    B. Extent of central nervous system injury
    C. Severity of electrolyte abnormalities
    D. Presence of multiorgan system failure

15. Priorities in initial management of the drowning victim in the field include:
    A. Prompt initiation of airway management, rescue breathing, and CPR
    B. Stabilization of the cervical spine
    C. Administration of 100% oxygen when available
    D. Prevention of progressive hypothermia
    E. All of the above

16. Patients with hypothermia after submersion should be aggressively rewarmed to 37° C) as soon as possible.
    A. True
    B. False

17. Ventilator management for respiratory disease caused by submersion injury includes which of the following strategies?
    A. Aggressive hyperventilation
    B. Adequate use of PEEP
    C. Maintenance of FIO_2 above 50% to increase oxygen delivery to the brain
    D. Rapid reduction in PEEP when gas exchange improves

18. What is the organized structure for prevention strategies?
    A. Education and training
    B. Enforcement of current laws
    C. The four Es of injury prevention
    D. Improved parental supervision

References

1. Centers for Disease Control and Prevention, National Center for Injury Prevention and Control: *Vital signs.* Available at: http://www.cdc.gov/VitalSigns/pdf/2012-04-vitalsigns.pdf. Accessed February 23, 2013.
2. Centers for Disease Control and Prevention, National Center for Injury Prevention and Control, Office of Statistics and Programming. *Web-based Injury Statistics Query and Reporting System (WISQARS).* Available at: http://www.cdc.gov/injury/wisqars/. Accessed February 23, 2013.
3. Newsbytes. *Case Manager* 2001;12:6.
4. Faul M, Xu L, Wald MM, et al: *Traumatic brain injury in the United States: emergency department visits, hospitalizations and deaths, 2002–2006,* Atlanta, 2010, Centers for Disease Control and Prevention, National Center for Injury Prevention and Control.
5. Laskowski-Jones L, Salati DS: Responding to pediatric trauma, *Nursing* 31(9):37, 2001.
6. Norton PGW: Accidental falls don't often cause severe head injuries, *Pediatric News,* June 1, 2003. Available at: http://www.merckmedicus.com/pp/us/newsarticleprint.jsp?newsid=311832. Accessed January 26, 2006.
7. Rubin DM, Christian CW, Bilaniuk LT, et al: Occult head injury in high risk children, *Pediatrics* 111:1382, 2003.
8. Bergman DA, Baltz RD, et al: The management of minor closed head injury in children, *Pediatrics* 104:1407, 1999.
9. Greenes DS, Schutzman SA: Clinical indicators of intercranial injury in head-injured infants, *Pediatrics* 104:861, 1999.
10. Crocker JFS, Bagnell PC: Reye's syndrome: a clinical review, *CMA J* 124:375, 1981.
11. Morki B: The Monro-Kellie hypothesis: applications in CSF volume depletion, *Neurology* 56:1746, 2001.
12. Greitz D, Wirestam R, et al: Pulsatile brain movement and associated hydrodynamics studied by magnetic resonance phase imaging: the Monro-Kellie doctrine revisited, *Neuroradiology* 34:370, 1992.
13. Plum F, Posner JB: *The diagnosis of stupor and coma,* ed 3, Philadelphia, 1980, FA Davis.
14. Deshpande JK: *Anesthesia for neurosurgery in infants and children.* Available at: http://www.csaol.cn/img/2007asa/RCL_src/328_Deshpande.pdf. Accessed March 17, 2008.
15. Fenichel GM: *Clinical pediatric neurology,* ed 3, Philadelphia, 1977, Saunders, pp 93–95.
16. Finder JD, Yellon R, Charron M: Successful management of tracheotomized patients with chronic saliva aspiration by use of constant positive airway pressure, *Pediatrics* 107:1343, 2001.
17. Clifton GL, Miller ER, et al: Lack of effect of hypothermia after acute brain injury, *N Engl J Med* 22:556, 2001.
18. Narayan RK: Hypothermia for traumatic brain injury: a good idea proven ineffective, *N Engl J Med* 344:602, 2001, [editorial].
19. Hockenberry MJ, Wilson D: *Wong's nursing care of infants and children,* ed 9, St. Louis, 2010, Mosby Elsevier. Available at: Pageburst Online. Accessed April 13, 2013.

20. Ghajar J, Hariri RJ: Management of pediatric head injury, *Pediatr Clin North Am* 39:1093, 1992.

21. Plum F, Posner JB: *The diagnosis of stupor and coma*, ed 3, Philadelphia, 1980, FA Davis.

22. Deshpande JK: *Anesthesia for neurosurgery in infants and children.* Available at: http://www.csaol.cn/img/2007asa/RCL_src/328_Deshpande.pdf. Accessed March 17, 2008.

23. American Academy of Neurology: Position of the American Academy of Neurology on certain aspects of the care and management of the persistent vegetative state patient, *Neurology* 39:125, 1989.

24. Stafford PW, Harmon CM: Thoracic trauma in children, *Curr Opin Pediatr* 5:325, 1993.

25. Nakaqawa H, et al: Cervical emphysema secondary to pneumomediastinum as a complication of childbirth, *Ear Nose Throat J* 82:948, 2003.

26. Schullinger JN: Birth trauma, *Pediatr Clin N A* 40:1351, 1993.

27. Rodgers BM, Hawks P: Bilateral congenital eventration of the diaphragms: successful surgical management, *J Ped Surg* 21:858, 1986.

28. Johnstone DW, Ferns RH: Chylothorax, *Chest Surg Clin NA* 4:617, 1994.

29. Wolff AB, Silen ML, et al: Treatment of refractory chylothorax with externalized pleuroperitoneal shunts in children, *Annals Thor Surg* 68:1053, 1999.

30. Collins J: Chest wall trauma, *J Thorac Imag* 15:112, 2000.

31. Tsai FC, Chang Y, et al: Blunt trauma with flail chest and penetrating aorta injury, *Eur J Cardiothorac Surg* 16:374, 1999.

32. Bliss D, Silen M: Pediatric thoracic trauma, *Crit Care Med* 30:S409, 2002.

33. Bickell WH, et al: Immediate versus delayed fluid resuscitation for hypotensive patients with torso injuries, *N Engl J Med* 331:1105, 1994.

34. LeBlang SD, Dolich MO: Imaging of penetrating thoracic trauma, *J Thorac Imag* 15:128, 2000.

35. Mayberry JC: Imaging in thoracic trauma: the trauma surgeon's perspective, *J Thorac Imag* 15:76, 2000.

36. Barton ED: Tension pneumothorax, *Curr Opin Pulm Med* 5:269, 1999.

37. Self ML, Mangram A, et al: Nonoperative management of severe tracheobronchial injuries with positive end-expiratory pressure and low tidal volume ventilation, *J Trauma* 59:1072, 2005.

38. Kern JA, Tribble CG, et al: Thoracoscopy: a potential role in the subacute management of patients with thoraco-abdominal trauma, *Chest* 104:942, 1993.

39. Thakur A, Brickmiller T, et al: Bronchial perforation after closed-tube endotracheal suction, *J Pediatr Surg* 35:1353, 2000.

40. Sapin E, Gumpert L, et al: Iatrogenic pharyngo-esophageal perforation in premature infants, *Eur J Pediatr Surg* 10:83, 2000.

41. Bagwell CE, Salzberg AM, et al: Potentially lethal complications of central venous catheter placement, *J Pediatr Surg* 35:709, 2000.

42. Flores JC, Barja J, et al: Complications of central venous catheterization in critically ill children, *Pediatr Crit Care Med* 2:57, 2001.

43. Cordero AMG, Fernandes JC, et al: Possible risk factors associated with moderate or severe airway injuries in children who underwent endotracheal intubation, *Pediatr Crit Care Med* 5:364, 2004.

44. Redleaf MI, Fennessy JJ: Pneumomediastinum after rigid bronchoscopy, *Ann Otol Rhinol Laryngol* 104:955, 1994.

45. Ricard JD, et al: Ventilator-induced lung injury, *Curr Opin Crit Care* 8:12, 2000.

46. Safe Kids Worldwide (SKW): *Burn and scalds safety in the USA*, Washington, DC, 2011, SKW.

47. Toon MH, et al: Children with burn injuries-assessment of trauma, neglect, violence and abuse, *J Inj Violence Res* 3(2):98–110, 2011. doi: 10.5249/jivr.v3i2.91.

48. Joffe MD: Burns. In Fleisher GR, Ludwig S, editors: *Textbook of pediatric emergency medicine*, ed 4, Philadelphia, 2000, Lippincott Williams & Wilkins, pp 1427-1434.

49. Aub JC, Pittman H: The pulmonary complications: a clinical description, *Ann Surg* 117:834, 1943.

50. Barillo DJ, Brigham PA, et al: The fire-safe cigarette: a burn prevention tool, *J Burn Care Rehabil* 21:162, 2000.

51. Finkelstein JL, Schwartz SB, et al: Pediatric burns: an overview, *Pediatr Clin North Am* 39:1145, 1992.

52. O'Neill JA: Advances in the management of pediatric trauma, *Am J Surg* 180:365, 2000.

53. Granger JP: An evidence-based approach to pediatric burns, *Ped Emer Med Practice* 6(1), 2009.

54. Sole ML, Klein DG, et al: *Introduction to critical care nursing*, ed 6, St. Louis, 2013, Elsevier. Available at: http://pageburstls.elsevier.com/books/978-0-323-08848-0/id/B9780323088480000294_f0110. Accessed April 13, 2013.

55. Sheridan RL, Schnitzer JJ: Management of the high-risk pediatric burn patient, *J Pediatr Surg* 36:1308, 2001.

56. Ramzy PI, Barret JP, Herndon DN: Thermal injury, *Crit Care Clin* 15:333, 1999.

57. Henriques FC Jr: Studies of thermal injury: V. The predictability and significance of thermally induced rate process leading to irreversible epidermal injury, *Arch Pathol* 43:489, 1947.

58. Linares HA: A report of 115 consecutive autopsies in burned children: 1966–1980, *Burns* 8:270, 1982.

59. Brown JM: Respiratory complications in burned patients, *Physiotherapy* 63:151, 1977.

60. Clark WR Jr, Webb WR, et al: The pathophysiology of the acute smoke inhalation, *Surg Forum* 177, 1977.

61. Foley FD, Moncrief JA, Mason AD Jr: Pathology of the lung in fatally burned patients, *Ann Surg* 167:251, 1968.

62. Moylan JA: Inhalation injury: a primary determinant of survival, *J Burn Care Rehabil* 3:78, 1981.

63. Haponik EF, Summer WR: Respiratory complications in burned patients: Pathogenesis and spectrum of inhalation injury, *Crit Care* 2:49, 1987.

64. Pruitt BA Jr, DiVincenti FC, et al: The occurrence and significance of pneumonia and other pulmonary complications in burned patients, *J Trauma* 10:519, 1970.

65. Shirani KZ, BA Pruitt Jr, AD Mason Jr: The influence of inhalation injury and pneumonia on burned mortality, *Ann Surg* 205:82, 1987.

66. Thompson PB, Herndon DN, et al: Effects on mortality of inhalation injury, *J Trauma* 26:163, 1986.

67. Haponik EF, Lykens MG: Acute upper airway obstruction in burned patients, *Crit Care Rep* 2:28, 1990.

68. Waymack JP, Law E, et al: Acute upper airway obstruction in the post burn period, *Arch Surg* 120:1042, 1985.

69. Haponik EF, Munster AM, et al: Upper airway function in burn patients, *Am Rev Respir Dis* 129:251, 1984.

70. Haponik EF, Meyers DA, et al: Acute upper airway injury in burn patients; serial changes of flow volume curves and nasopharyngoscopy, *Am Rev Respir Dis* 135:360, 1987.

71. Wald PH, Balmes JR: Respiratory effects of short-term, high-intensity toxic inhalations: smoke, gases, and fumes, *J Intensive Care Med* 2:260, 1987.

72. Zirka BA, Budd DC, et al: What is clinical smoke poisoning? *Ann Surg* 181:151, 1975.

73. Moritiz AR, Henriques FC Jr, McLean R: The effects of inhaled heat on the air passages and lungs: an experimental investigation, *Am J Pathol* 21:311, 1945.

74. Head JM: Inhalation injury in burns, *Am J Surg* 139:508, 1980.

75. Walker HL, McLeoud CG, McManus WL: Experimental inhalation injury in the goat, *J Trauma* 21:962, 1981.

76. Demling RH: Initial effect of smoke inhalation injury on oxygen consumption (response to positive pressure ventilation), *Surgery* 115:563, 1994.

77. Z-Y Liu, Li N, et al: Pulmonary surfactant activity after severe steam inhalation in rabbits, *Burns* 12:330, 1986.

78. Rodkey F, O'Neal J, Collison H: Relative affinity of hemoglobin S and hemoglobin A for carbon monoxide and oxygen, *Clin Chem* 20:834, 1974.

79. Emmans HW: Fire and fire protection, *Sci Am* 231:21, 1974.

80. Zirka BA, Ferre JM, Floch HF: The chemical factors contributing to pulmonary damage, *Surgery* 71:704, 1972.

81. Parish RA: Smoke inhalation and carbon monoxide poisoning in children, *Pediatr Emerg Care* 2:36, 1985.

82. Barker SJ, Tremper KK, Hyatt J: The effect of carbon monoxide inhalation on pulse oximetry and transcutaneous Po_2, *Anesthesiology* 66:677, 1987.

83. Moylan JA, Chan CK: Inhalation injury an increasing problem, *Surgery* 188:34, 1978.

84. Stone HH, Martin JD Jr: Pulmonary injury associated with thermal injury, *Surg Gynecol Obstet* 129:1242, 1969.

85. Putman CE, Tummillo AM, et al: Radiological manifestations of acute smoke inhalation, *AJR Am J Roentgenol* 129:865, 1977.

86. Wanner A, Cutchauarece A: Early recognition of upper airway obstruction following smoke inhalation, *Am Rev Respir Dis* 108:1421, 1973.

87. Moylan JA, Adib K, et al: Fiberoptic bronchoscopy following thermal injury, *Surg Gynecol Obstet* 140:541, 1975.

88. Moylan JA, Wilmore DW, et al: Early diagnosis of inhalation injury using xenon scan, *Ann Surg* 176:477, 1972.

89. Whitener DR, Whitener LM, et al: Pulmonary function measurements in patients with thermal injury and smoke inhalation, *Am Rev Respir Dis* 122:731, 1980.

90. Petroff PA, Hander EW, et al: Pulmonary function studies after smoke inhalation, *Am J Surg* 132:346, 1976.

91. Garzon AA, Seltzer B, et al: Respiratory mechanics in patients with inhalation injury, *J Trauma* 10:5, 1970.

92. Mlcak RP, Desai MH, Nichols RJ: Respiratory care. In Herndon DA, editor: *Total burn care*, London, 1996, WB Saunders, pp 193–204.

93. Sirani KZ, Pruitt BA, Mason AD: The influence of inhalation injury and pneumonia on burn mortality, *Ann Surg* 205:82, 1986.

94. Pruitt BA Jr, Cioffi WG, et al: Evaluation and management of patients with inhalation injury, *J Trauma* 30:563, 1990.

95. Levine BA, Petroff PA, Slade CL: Prospective trials of dexamethasone and aerosolized gentamicin in the treatment of inhalation injury, *J Trauma* 18:118, 1978.

96. Nieman GF, Clark WR, Hakim T: Methylprednisolone does not protect the lung from inhalation injury, *Burns* 17:384, 1991.

97. Hirsh SR, Zastrow JE, Korg RC: Sputum liquification agents: a comprehensive in vitro study, *J Lab Clin Med* 74:346, 1969.

98. Brown M, Desai M, et al: Dimethylsulfoxide with heparin in the treatment of smoke inhalation injury, *J Burn Care Rehab* 9:22, 1988.

99. Desai MH, Brown M, et al: Reduction of smoke injury with dimethylsulfoxide and heparin treatments, *Surg Forum* 36:103, 1985.

100. Desai MH, Brown M, Mlcak RP: Nebulization treatments of inhalation injury in the sheep model with dimethylsulfoxide/heparin combinations and N-acetylcysteine, *Crit Care Med* 14:321, 1986.

101. Desai MH, et al: Reduction in mortality in pediatric patients with inhalation injury with aerosolized heparin/N-acetylcysteine therapy, *J Burn Care Rehabil* 19:210, 1998.

102. Reynolds EM, Ryan DP, Doody DP. Mortality and respiratory failure in a pediatric burn population. *J Pediatr Surg* 1993;28:1326.

103. Mammel MC, Boros SJ: Airway damage and mechanical ventilation: a review and commentary, *Pediatr Pulmonol* 3:443, 1987.

104. Ogura H, Cioffi WG, Okerberg C: *Effects of pressure-controlled, inverse-ratio ventilation on smoke inhalation injury in an animal model*, San Antonio, TX, 1991, US Army Institute of Surgical Research.

105. Sheridan RL, Kacmarek RM, et al: Permissive hypercapnia as a ventilatory strategy in burned children, *J Trauma* 39:854, 1995.

106. Arnold JH: High-frequency oscillatory ventilation: theory and practice in paediatric patients, *Paediatr Anaesth* 6:437, 1996.

107. Cioffi WG, Rue LW, et al: Prophylactic use of high-frequency ventilation in patients with inhalation injury, *Ann Surg* 213:575, 1991.

108. Rue LW, Cioffi WG, et al: Improved survival of burned patients with inhalation injury, *Arch Surg* 128:772, 1993.

109. Cioffi WG, Graves TA, et al: High-frequency percussive ventilation in patients with inhalation injury, *J Trauma* 29:350, 1989.

110. Cortiella J, Mlcak RP, Herndon D: High-frequency percussive ventilation in pediatric patients with inhalation injury, *J Burn Care Rehabil* 20:232, 1999.

111. Demarst GB, Hudson LD, Altman LC: Impaired alveolar macrophage chemotaxis in patients with acute smoke inhalation, *Am Rev Respir Dis* 119:279, 1979.

112. Gadek JE, Fells GA, et al: Antielastase of the human alveolar structures, *J Clin Invest* 68:889, 1981.

113. Mlcak RP, Desai MH, et al: Lung function following thermal injury in children: an 8-year follow-up, *Burns* 24:213, 1998.

114. Mlcak RP, Desai MH, et al: Increased physiological dead space: tidal volume ratio during exercise in burned children, *Burns* 21:337, 1995.

115. Smith G: *Global burden of drowning*. presented at the World Congress on Drowning, June 26-28, 2002, Amsterdam, the Netherlands.

116. In: Bierens JJLM, editor: *Handbook on drowning: prevention, rescue, treatment*, Amsterdam, 2005, Springer. Available at: http://www.drowning.nl. Retrieved October 2008.

117. Idris AH, Becker LB, et al: Recommended guidelines for uniform reporting of data from drowning: the "Utstein style." *Circulation* 108:2565, 2003.

118. Modell JH: Serum electrolyte changes in near-drowning victims, *JAMA* 253:253, 1985.

119. Harries MG: Drowning in man, *Crit Care Med* 9:407, 1981.

120. Modell JH: Drowning, *N Engl J Med* 328:253, 1993.

121. National Center for Injury Prevention and Control, Centers for Disease Control and Prevention. *Web-based Injury Statistics Query and Reporting System (WISQARS)* [online]. Available at: www.cdc.gov/ncipc/wisqars. Accessed October 2008.

122. Orlowski JP: Drowning, near-drowning and ice-water submersions, *Pediatr Clin North Am* 34:75, 1987.

123. Cohen RH, Matter KC, et al: Unintentional pediatric submersion-injury–related hospitalizations in the United States, *Inj Prev* 14:131, 2008.

124. Somers GR, Chiasson DA, et al: Pediatric drowning: a 20-year review of autopsied cases. I. Demographic features, *Am J Forensic Med* 26:316, 2005.

125. Lavelle JM, Shaw KN, et al: Ten-year review of pediatric bathtub near-drownings: evaluation for child abuse and neglect, *Ann Emerg Med* 25:344, 1995.

126. DeNicola LK, Falk JL, et al: Submersion injuries in children and adults, *Crit Care Clin* 13:477, 1997.

127. Quan L, Bennett E, et al: Ten-year study of pediatric drownings and near-drownings in King County, Washington, *Pediatrics* 83:1035, 1989.

128. Wintemute GJ: Childhood drowning and near-drowning in the United States, *Am J Dis Child* 144:663, 1990.

129. Brenner RA, Committee on Injury, Violence, and Poison Prevention: Prevention of drowning in infants, children, and adolescents, *Pediatrics* 112:440, 2003.

130. Bierens JJ, Knape JT, et al: Drowning, *Curr Opin Crit Care* 8:578, 2002.

131. Levin DL, Moriss FC, et al: Drowning and near-drowning, *Pediatr Clin North Am* 40:321, 1993.

132. Miyamoto O, Auer RN: Hypoxia, hyperoxia, ischemia, and brain necrosis, *Neurology* 54:362, 2000.

133. Causey AL, Tilelli JA, et al: Predicting discharge in uncomplicated near-drowning, *Am J Emerg Med* 18:9, 2000.

134. Leroy P, Smismans A, Seute T: Invasive pulmonary and central nervous system aspergillosis after near-drowning of a child: case report and review of the literature, *Pediatrics* 118:e509, 2006.

135. Giamona ST, Modell JH: Drowning by total immersion, effects on pulmonary surfactant of distilled water, isotonic saline and sea water, *Am J Dis Child* 114:612, 1967.

136. Orlowski JP, Szpilman D: Drowning: rescue, resuscitation, and reanimation, *Pediatr Clin North Am* 48:627, 2001.

137. Karch SB: Pathology of the lung in near drowning, *Am J Emerg Med* 4:4, 1980.

138. Ender PT, Dolan MJ: Pneumonia associated with near-drowning, *Clin Infect Dis* 25:896, 1997.

139. Donoghue AJ, Nadkarni V, et al: Out-of-hospital pediatric cardiac arrest: an epidemiologic review and assessment of current knowledge, *Ann Emerg Med* 46:512, 2005.

140. Modell JH, May F: Effects of volume aspirated fluid during chlorinated fresh water drowning, *Anesthesiology* 27:662, 1966.

141. Modell JH, Davis JH: Electrolyte changes in human drowning victims, *Anesthesiology* 30:414, 1969.

142. Rosen P, Stoto M, Harley J: The use of the Heimlich maneuver in near drowning: Institute of Medicine report, *J Emerg Med* 13:397, 1995.

143. Manolios N, Mackie I: Drowning and near-drowning on Australian beaches patrolled by life-savers: a 10-year study, *Med J Aust* 148:165, 1988.

144. Nolan P, Morley PT, et al: Therapeutic hypothermia after cardiac arrest: an advisory statement by the Advancement Life support Task Force of the International Liaison Committee on Resuscitation, *Resuscitation* 57:231, 2003.

145. Hickey RW, Kochanek PM, et al: Hypothermia and hyperthermia in children after resuscitation from cardiac arrest, *Pediatrics* 106:118, 2000.

146. International Liaison Committee on Resuscitation, American Heart Association: Guidelines for cardiopulmonary resuscitation and emergency cardiovascular care—an international consensus on science, *Resuscitation* 46(3), 2000.

147. Sarnaik AP, Preston G, et al: Intracranial pressure and cerebral perfusion pressure in near-drowning, *Crit Care Med* 13:224, 1985.

148. Bohn DJ, Biggar WD, et al: Influence of hypothermia, barbiturate therapy, and intracranial pressure monitoring on morbidity and mortality after near-drowning, *Crit Care Med* 14:529, 1986.

149. Spack L, Gedeit R, et al: Failure of aggressive therapy to alter outcome in pediatric near-drowning, *Pediatr Emerg Med* 13:98, 1997.

150. Graf WD, Cummings P, et al: Predicting outcome in pediatric submersion victims, *Ann Emerg Med* 26:312, 1995.

151. Orlowski JP: Prognostic factors in pediatric cases of drowning and near-drowning, *JACEP* 8:176, 1979.

152. Habib DM, Tecklenburg FW, et al: Near-drowning: morbidity and mortality, *Pediatr Emerg Med* 12:255, 1996.

153. Corneli HM: Hot topics in cold medicine: controversies in accidental hypothermia, *Clin Ped Emerg Med* 2:179, 2001.

154. Cowden JD, Dowd DM, et al: Preventing childhood injury: the role of the emergency physician, *Pediatr Emerg Med Prac* 4:10, 2007.

155. Thompson DC, Rivara FP: Pool fencing for preventing drowning in children, *Cochrane Database Syst Rev* 1: CD001047, 1998.

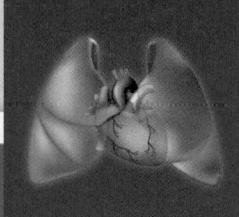

Chapter 32

Disorders of the Pleura

PAUL C. STILLWELL

LEARNING OBJECTIVES

After reading this chapter the reader will be able to:

1. Describe the normal function of the pleural space in healthy children
2. List the causes of pneumothorax in neonates and children
3. Recognize the causes of pleural effusions and empyema in children of all ages
4. Discuss the principles of managing abnormal air or fluid in the pleural space in children

KEY TERMS

Chest tube
Empyema
Pleural effusion

Pneumomediastinum
Pneumothorax
Thoracotomy

Video-assisted thoracoscopic surgery (VATS)

The pleura surround the outer surface of the lungs and the mediastinum as well as the inner surface of the chest wall and the diaphragm. This sliding surface provides minimal resistance between the lung and chest wall during respiratory movements. The pleural "space" is generally only a *potential* space with a normal fluid volume of 1 to 5 ml. The pleural membranes, however, are very thin and permeable to both liquid and gas; an estimated 5 to 10 L of fluid per day cross from the parietal pleura to the visceral pleura in a normal adult.[1-3]

The pleura lining the chest wall, mediastinum, and diaphragm is called the *parietal pleura*. Its blood supply is from the systemic circulation, and its venous drainage is through the azygos, hemiazygos, and internal mammary veins into the superior vena cava. The *visceral pleura* covers the surface of the lungs including the fissures, with its blood supply from bronchial arteries and its venous drainage through the pulmonary veins.[1] In the healthy subject a positive 9 cm H_2O of hydrostatic pressure drives fluid from the parietal pleura capillary bed into the pleural space, and a negative 10 cm H_2O of hydrostatic pressure favors absorption of fluid into the visceral pleura capillaries.[1-3]

Several factors determine the amount of fluid in the pleural space. The *intracapillary* hydrostatic pressures tend to drive fluid out of the capillaries, whereas the *pericapillary* hydrostatic pressures tend to counterbalance this force. The *plasma* colloid osmotic pressures exert a force to retain fluid within the capillaries, whereas the *pericapillary* colloid osmotic pressure tends to favor fluid movement out of the capillaries. Changes in the balance of these forces determine how much fluid is retained within the pleural space. Increased capillary permeability (e.g., acute respiratory distress syndrome), decreased intravascular colloid osmotic pressure (e.g., low serum albumin), and increased pulmonary venous pressure (e.g., heart failure) are common contributors to accumulation of fluid in the pleural space. Obstructed lymphatic drainage is another factor that favors accumulation of fluid in the pleural space.[1,2] *Chylothorax,* a collection of lymphatic fluid in the pleural space, is an uncommon cause of pleural effusion in children, except when they have undergone thoracic surgery with interruption of the thoracic duct.[1,2]

In healthy individuals the chest radiograph seldom demonstrates any pleural fluid.[3] An estimated 4% of normal

623

adults may have minor radiographic evidence of pleural fluid if the films are taken in the decubitus or Trendelenburg position. A pleural effusion has typical radiographic features (Figures 32-1 to 32-3). Ultrasound examination or computed tomography (CT) of the chest may be more sensitive in identifying small accumulations of pleural fluid.[2,4]

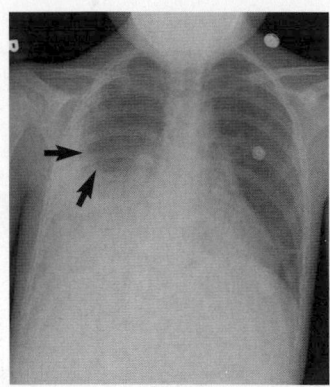

FIGURE 32-1 Upright chest radiograph of a 7-year-old child with a large pleural effusion on the right. The bottom third of the right hemithorax is white with a rounded superior margin (meniscus sign, *arrows*). The diaphragm is obscured, and there are air bronchograms in the right lower lung zone. This parapneumonic effusion was an empyema caused by *streptococcal* pneumonia.

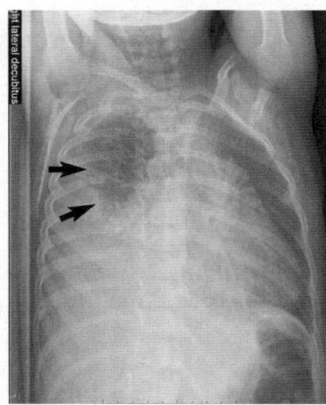

FIGURE 32-2 Right-side-down decubitus radiograph of the child in Figure 32-1. The fluid is more prominent on the lateral chest wall margin, indicating free movement of the fluid in the pleural space (*arrows*).

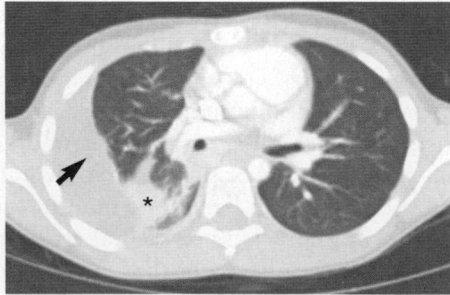

FIGURE 32-3 Chest CT scan showing a right-sided empyema along the right lateral wall (*black arrow*) and a right lower lobe infiltrate between the empyema and the spinous process (*asterisk*).

The CT scan may also provide more information about the underlying lung parenchyma than is available from the plain chest radiograph, especially when large amounts of fluid are present. However, ultrasound and CT usually are not required to identify a clinically significant effusion. Ultrasound may be used to facilitate finding the optimal location to perform a thoracentesis.[4]

PLEURAL EFFUSIONS

Pleural effusions may be suspected clinically when there is an area of decreased-intensity breath sounds on chest auscultation with an associated dullness to percussion over the corresponding area.[2,3] Comparison with the contralateral lung can help distinguish the normal boundaries of the thoracic cavity unless the effusion is bilateral. The patient may experience few symptoms from a small pleural effusion but usually has symptoms of respiratory distress with larger accumulations. Chest pain, chest wall tenderness, dyspnea, and pain with coughing or deep breathing are often associated with pleural effusions. In addition to decreased intensity of breath sounds with dullness to percussion, crackles may be appreciated immediately superior to the effusion, where the lung may be involved with underlying pneumonia, or the normal lung may be partially compressed by the effusion. The location of these abnormal examination findings may change when the position of the patient is changed if the fluid is flowing freely within the pleural space. The respiratory care practitioner may be the first to detect the findings of a pleural effusion during auscultation.[3]

When a suspected effusion is confirmed by a chest radiograph, the initial decision is whether it should be drained, either for diagnostic purposes or for therapeutic purposes, or both. In adult medicine and with older, cooperative children, a thoracentesis is often the initial approach to drainage.[3,5] This diagnostic procedure consists of placing a needle into the pleural space and withdrawing the pleural fluid. On occasion an underlying disease such as overt heart failure or nephrotic syndrome will leave little doubt as to the cause and nature of the pleural effusion, thereby decreasing the need for a diagnostic thoracentesis.[3,5] The pleural fluid is generally categorized as either a transudate or an exudate on the basis of specific criteria (Table 32-1 and Box 32-1). Disease processes associated with transudates and exudates in children are listed in Boxes 32-2 and 32-3.[2,3,5] In pediatric patients for whom prolonged drainage may be required, such as an empyema, a chest tube may be placed initially either by an interventional radiologist or by a surgeon, often after performing a video-assisted thoracoscopic surgery (VATS). If this is the case, thoracentesis is usually foregone and the fluid analysis is sent on a sample from the chest tube. In most children's hospitals the pleural drainage is increasingly done by an interventional radiologist with ultrasound guidance.[6]

Complications of thoracentesis include pneumothorax, hemorrhage, and infection. A *pneumothorax* may be created

TABLE 32-1

Distinguishing Transudate from Exudate

Measurement	Transudate	Exudate
Protein (g/dl)	<3	>3
Effusion/serum protein ratio	<0.5	>0.5
LDH (units/L)	<250	>250
Effusion/serum LDH ratio	<0.6	>0.6

LDH, Lactate dehydrogenase.

Box 32-1   Common Pleural Fluid Analyses

- Total protein
- Lactate dehydrogenase (LDH)
- Cell counts and differential cell count
- pH
- Cytology
- Studies for infection
- Gram stain, bacterial culture
- Acid-fast stain and culture
- Fungal stains and culture
- Glucose
- Amylase

Box 32-2   Causes of Transudative Pleural Effusions

- Congestive heart failure
- Nephrotic syndrome
- Cirrhosis or liver failure
- Acute glomerulonephritis
- Hypoproteinemia
- Myxedema
- Sarcoidosis
- Peritoneal dialysis

Box 32-3   Causes of Exudative Pleural Effusions

- Parapneumonic effusion or empyema
- Pulmonary embolism
- Neoplasm
- Collagen vascular disease
- Trauma
- Drug hypersensitivity
- Lung transplant rejection
- Chylothorax
- Gastrointestinal diseases
- Lymphatic disease
- Postcardiac surgery syndrome
- Acute chest syndrome (sickle cell disease)

---

by nicking the lung with the needle or by not maintaining a closed system and allowing air to enter the chest cavity from the atmosphere. *Hemorrhage* may result from nicking a vessel or the lung during needle insertion.[3] If sterile technique is not followed, *infection* can be introduced into the pleural space, or the sample sent for microbiology evaluation will be contaminated, or both. Other complications include an allergic reaction to the sedating medicines or hypoventilation resulting from oversedation. Because most pediatric patients receive sedation or anesthesia for chest tube placement and thoracentesis, a person skilled at providing and monitoring their sedation is usually in attendance. However, it is important for the respiratory care practitioner to be familiar with these complications because he or she may be monitoring the patient's cardiovascular and pulmonary status after completion of the procedure. Any deterioration in the patient's clinical status after the procedure immediately should be called to the attention of the appropriate care team for further assessment.

Several laboratory tests are performed on the pleural fluid to identify the cause of effusion.[2-5] The most common type of pleural effusion in pediatrics is a *parapneumonic effusion,*[2,4,6] which indicates that the pleural fluid is the result of an underlying pneumonia. Although typically a bacterial pneumonia, parapneumonic effusion can also result from a viral, fungal, or parasitic infection or from tuberculosis (Box 32-4).[6] If the

---

Box 32-4   Causative Organisms in Parapneumonic Pleural Effusions

AEROBIC BACTERIA
- *Streptococcus pneumoniae*
- *Staphylococcus aureus* (both methicillin sensitive and resistant)
- *Haemophilus influenzae*
- *Streptococcus pyogenes*
- Group A, β-hemolytic streptococci

ANAEROBIC BACTERIA
- *Bacteroides* species
- *Peptostreptococcus* species
- *Peptococcus* species
- *Fusobacterium* species

TUBERCULOSIS
- *Mycobacterium tuberculosis*

VIRUSES/MYCOPLASMA
- Adenoviruses
- Parainfluenza viruses
- *Mycoplasma pneumoniae*

FUNGI/FUNGAL ORGANISMS
- *Coccidioides immitis*
- *Actinomyces* species
- *Nocardia* species

PARASITES
- *Paragonimus* species
- *Cysticercus* species
- *Entamoeba histolytica*

pneumonia extends to infect the pleural space as well, the effusion is then termed an **empyema.**[4,6] The effusion is characterized as an empyema by the presence of frank pus in the pleural space, by a positive culture of the pleural fluid, by a positive Gram stain of the pleural fluid, or by a pleural fluid white blood cell count greater than 15,000/mm³. *Streptococcus pneumoniae* is the most common organism causing pneumonia and empyema in children.[2,4,6]

In adult patients the presence of an empyema suggests that a chest tube should be placed to prevent subsequent fibrous entrapment of the lung.[5] In children, lung entrapment seldom occurs after empyema. It is becoming less common for physicians to perform repeated thoracenteses or to wait for the antibiotic therapy alone (without chest tube drainage) to resolve both the pneumonia and the empyema (see Surgery in the Pleural Space later in this chapter).[6-8] In addition to chest tube drainage, prolonged antibiotic therapy is often administered (e.g., 4 to 6 weeks).[6-8] The availability of long-term indwelling intravenous catheters allows transition of intravenous therapy from hospital to home. The duration of combined intravenous and oral antibiotics necessary for successful resolution of an empyema is not well defined. Eventual healing of the pneumonia and pleural space with normal lung function and a normal chest radiograph is the usual outcome for children, although the chest radiograph may not return to normal for several months.[2,6-8] In addition to chest tube drainage alone, insertion of fibrinolytic agents (e.g., urokinase, tissue plasminogen activator, dornase alpha) into the pleural space to enhance drainage and perhaps hasten healing has been tried.[9,10] Studies in adults do not show a consistent benefit,[10] but there are no large controlled studies in children. In small series of pediatric patients for whom intrapleural fibrinolytic therapy has been tried, it has been achieved safely.[6,8,9] Because of the wide variation in success with different management strategies, the decision regarding whether to drain or not, what type of drainage, whether fibrinolytic therapy should be used, or whether surgery should be offered for the child with an empyema, management should be individualized.[6-9]

Although less common, other causes of pleural effusion besides infection should be considered; malignancy, acute chest syndrome from sickle cell disease, and postsurgical effusions can also create exudative effusions.[2,3]

Additional studies besides total protein and lactate dehydrogenase levels may help identify the cause of the effusion. Cell counts and special stains may be helpful. Malignant cells are found in 60% to 90% of effusions caused by malignancy.[2,3,5] The respiratory care practitioner may be asked to determine the pleural fluid pH, using a blood gas machine. The specimen must be collected anaerobically in a heparinized syringe and kept on ice until it is analyzed. A pH less than 7.0 or less than 0.15 pH unit below the arterial pH in a patient with parapneumonic effusion may indicate that the patient is at risk for prolonged effusion and subsequent lung entrapment. This has not been extensively studied in children.[2,3,5]

PNEUMOTHORAX

Air in the pleural space is called a **pneumothorax.**[2,11-14] It is termed a *tension pneumothorax* if the volume of intrapleural air increases with each breath, subsequently pushing the heart and mediastinal structures into the opposite hemithorax. This is generally a life-threatening situation unless the tension is relieved. The patient with a tension pneumothorax will subsequently go into shock from decreased venous return to the heart and from compromised cardiac output caused by the shift of the mediastinum.[2,12] Sometimes the pleural air is not under tension and causes only minimal or moderate respiratory distress. A small percentage of patients with a pneumothorax are asymptomatic or have only mild and vague symptoms; however, it is much more common for chest pain and shortness of breath to accompany the pneumothorax.[12] On examination, breath sounds will have decreased intensity on the affected side and the percussion note will be hyperresonant. With a mediastinal shift, the location of the heart's point of maximal impulse may change and the patient is usually cyanotic with severe respiratory distress. Air under the skin is called *subcutaneous emphysema,* which usually indicates a pneumothorax or pneumomediastinum.[2,11,12]

A pneumothorax has a characteristic radiographic appearance (Figures 32-4 and 32-5). Lung markings are lost toward the peripheral chest wall, with evidence of a collapse of the underlying lung. In diseases in which the lung is stiff from underlying disease, such as respiratory distress syndrome of the newborn or cystic fibrosis, the lung may stay partly expanded (see Figures 32-4 and 32-5). The pneumothorax is *spontaneous* if no trauma or procedural intervention preceded its occurrence. A *primary spontaneous* pneumothorax occurs in patients without known underlying lung disease, and a *secondary spontaneous* pneumothorax occurs in patients with known lung disease (such as cystic fibrosis).[11-14] The common causes of pneumothorax in neonates and children are listed in Boxes 32-5 and 32-6.

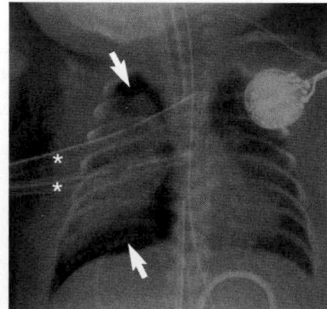

FIGURE 32-4 Chest radiograph from an extremely premature infant who has a right-sided pneumothorax (*arrows*) that persists despite two chest tubes (*asterisks*). The lung stays partially expanded because it has poor compliance (i.e., it is too stiff to collapse completely). The outline of the visceral pleura and lung is clearly seen due to air in the pleural space. An endotracheal tube and umbilical venous catheter are also present.

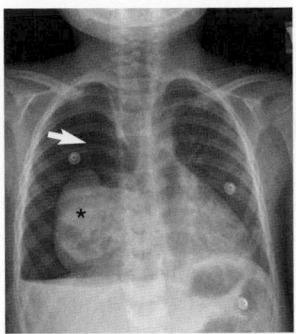

FIGURE 32-5 Chest radiograph of a 5-year-old boy with a right-sided pneumothorax caused by necrotizing pneumonia. There is a large volume of free air in the right pleural space (*arrow*) and the right lung is deflated and collapsed (*asterisk*). The right hemidiaphragm is flattened and the pneumothorax can be seen extending into the left chest. A chest tube has not yet been inserted.

Box 32-5	Causes of Pneumothorax in Neonates

- Respiratory distress syndrome (hyaline membrane disease)
- Meconium aspiration
- Barotrauma
- Spontaneous onset
- First breath
- Congenital anomaly (cystic pulmonary adenomatoid malformation)
- Congenital diaphragmatic hernia
- Pulmonary hypoplasia
- Congenital lobar overdistention or emphysema
- Iatrogenic

Box 32-6	Causes of Pneumothorax in Children

- Chronic obstructive lung disease
- Cystic fibrosis
- Bronchopulmonary dysplasia
- Asthma
- Trauma
- Surgery
- Foreign body with ball-valve effect
- Tumor
- Infection
- Pneumatocele
- Barotrauma
- Spontaneous onset
- Congenital anomaly
- Bronchogenic cyst
- Iatrogenic

Box 32-7	Conditions Associated with Air Leakage in Pneumothorax

- Interstitial emphysema
- Pneumomediastinum
- Pneumopericardium
- Pneumoperitoneum
- Subcutaneous emphysema

Other air leaks that may be associated with pneumothorax are listed in Box 32-7.

Treatment of the pneumothorax depends on whether it is under tension.[2,12-14] The tension pneumothorax is an emergency and should be relieved as soon as possible. The pleural space is drained by thoracentesis with a large-bore needle while awaiting more definitive therapy (see the next section). Some small pneumothoraces in patients with chronic lung disease (e.g., cystic fibrosis) might only be observed if there is no clinical deterioration. If the patient is stable, noninvasive therapy with 100% oxygen may be given a brief trial before a more definitive therapy is considered. In rare cases it may be appropriate to withdraw the air by thoracentesis, similar to removing pleural fluid but without resorting to thoracostomy tube drainage.[12-14]

THORACOSTOMY DRAINAGE

Tube thoracostomy drainage, or chest tube drainage, is the placement of a tube in the pleural space to drain air or fluid, or both, out of the pleural space. **Chest tubes** are routinely placed after many thoracic surgeries to ensure appropriate drainage of air, fluid, or blood.[15,16] A chest tube is usually placed to drain an empyema in adults, and they are often placed to drain empyemas in children as well.[6,8] The decision to place a chest tube for drainage of a pleural effusion is based on the patient's clinical status and whether the physician thinks that the respiratory system is compromised by the presence of the pleural fluid. Tension pneumothoraces almost always require chest tube drainage.

The insertion of a chest tube outside the operating room is generally done in an intensive care unit or in a specialized treatment area because of the seriousness of the underlying illness and the risk of complication. Sedation or anesthesia is usually needed, so a person skilled in providing these services (such as an anesthesiologist) is usually present during the procedure. The complications of chest tube insertion are similar to those of thoracentesis and may occur more commonly in small premature infants.[2] Some patients require more than one chest tube per side, especially if the pleural fluid is very viscous or loculated or if a pneumothorax persists.[17]

Once the chest tube is in the appropriate intrapleural location, the end is connected to commercially available devices that provide both a water seal and a collection chamber, the basic principles of which are demonstrated in Figure 32-6. There is a port for wall suction so that continuous negative pressure can be provided to the pleural space to help evacuate its contents. The level of water in the suction control chamber determines the amount of negative pressure applied to the pleural space. Bubbling in the water seal chamber indicates ongoing air leaks, which are usually from the pleural space.[15,16]

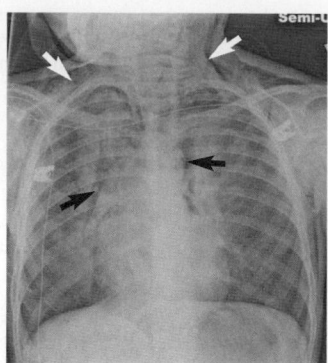

FIGURE 32-6 Chest radiograph of a 8-year-old asthmatic taken during an acute exacerbation. There is extensive mediastinal air evident around his heart and tracking upwards into his neck and supraclavicular soft tissues (arrows).

Modern pleural collection systems contain all three components in a single system that may not have liquid in the "suction control chamber" or in the "water seal chamber" (dry system). The interested student can learn more about chest tubes and pleural collection systems by watching the excellent animated video at the following site: www.youtube.com/watch?v=x_14I9ANZG8.

The respiratory care practitioner should be familiar with the features of the chest tube collection equipment commonly used in his or her institution to help monitor ongoing air leak and to ensure patient safety. While caring for the patient, the practitioner must not disrupt the chest tube and its attachments. A change in the patient's clinical status during evaluation by the respiratory care practitioner may indicate either a new problem with the lung or a malfunction of the chest tube system, which demands immediate evaluation. The practitioner should also anticipate patient discomfort at the site of the chest tube while manipulating the patient or surrounding equipment during chest physical therapy or ventilator tubing changes.[16]

The *bronchopleural fistula* presents a difficult management problem. When the integrity of the lung is not reestablished after an air leak or injury, a large portion of the volume of inspired gases may pass directly through the air leak, thus bypassing the gas-exchanging units of the lung. This can cause hypoventilation in the affected lung and a very large air leak through the chest tube. The bronchopleural fistula may be so severe that hypoventilation occurs despite increasing mechanical ventilatory support and the presence of several chest tubes.[17] Spontaneous healing of a bronchopleural fistula may take several days or even weeks. Surgical intervention may be required to oversew the air leak. In the interim, every attempt is made to reexpand the affected lung and minimize the interference with ventilation. In extreme cases, independent lung ventilation may be required or special valves inserted between the chest tube and wall suction to occlude the chest tube drainage intermittently during the inspiratory cycle

of the mechanical ventilator.[17] Special glues and patches have been used to seal the bronchopleural fistula.[17]

PNEUMOMEDIASTINUM

When air leaks into the mediastinum rather than the pleural space is it called a **pneumomediastinum**[12,18] (Figure 32-7). The patient usually experiences chest, back, or neck pain and, if the pneumomediastinum is large, shortness of breath. The most common finding on examination is subcutaneous emphysema (crepitus). Pneumomediastinum is caused by a high-pressure Valsalva maneuver such as occurs during violent coughing or lifting heavy objects. They occur most commonly in patients with underlying asthma. Other causes of air in the mediastinum include esophageal injury or infection in the mediastinum.[12,18,19] The chest radiograph (see Figure 32-7) demonstrates air in the mediastinum, which often tracks upward into the neck. Intervention is seldom needed but treatment of any underlying predisposing condition (such as asthma) should be offered.

SURGERY IN THE PLEURAL SPACE

The indications for surgery in the pleural space in pediatric patients with empyema are less well established than in adults.[19,20] Basic infectious disease tenets state that pus in a closed space should be drained. This is the basis for recommending closed-tube thoracostomy drainage for an empyema. The failure to drain the empyema adequately risks the development of a trapped lung, which subsequently may require pleural decortication.[19] In children treatment with appropriate antibiotic therapy usually avoids the need for subsequent decortication.[6,8,19] The child with an empyema who has had a slow clinical response to broad-spectrum intravenous antibiotics may benefit from a surgical procedure to evacuate the purulent material and consider a pleural decortication.[19] The use of fibrinolytics is an alternative option for children with slowly improving empyema despite chest tube drainage.[7,9]

No clear consensus exists on the most appropriate management of the difficult problem of surgery in the pleural space, so each patient should receive the benefit of an individualized multidisciplinary therapeutic plan with flexibility to change depending on therapeutic success or failure.[19,20]

If a chest tube placed to drain an empyema stops functioning, often the empyema fluid is loculated and the chest tube is in the wrong place. Repositioning the chest tube or adding another may allow better drainage. Injecting fibrinolytics (urokinase, dornase alpha, or tissue plasminogen activator) into the pleural cavity may facilitate drainage by liquefying the organizing empyema and dissolving the fibrin septations that are causing loculation of fluid.[6,7,9]

Thoracoscopy is the direct visualization of the pleural space through either rigid or flexible surgical equipment.[20] This technique has had increasing utilization for a variety of pediatric pulmonary problems since the initial use

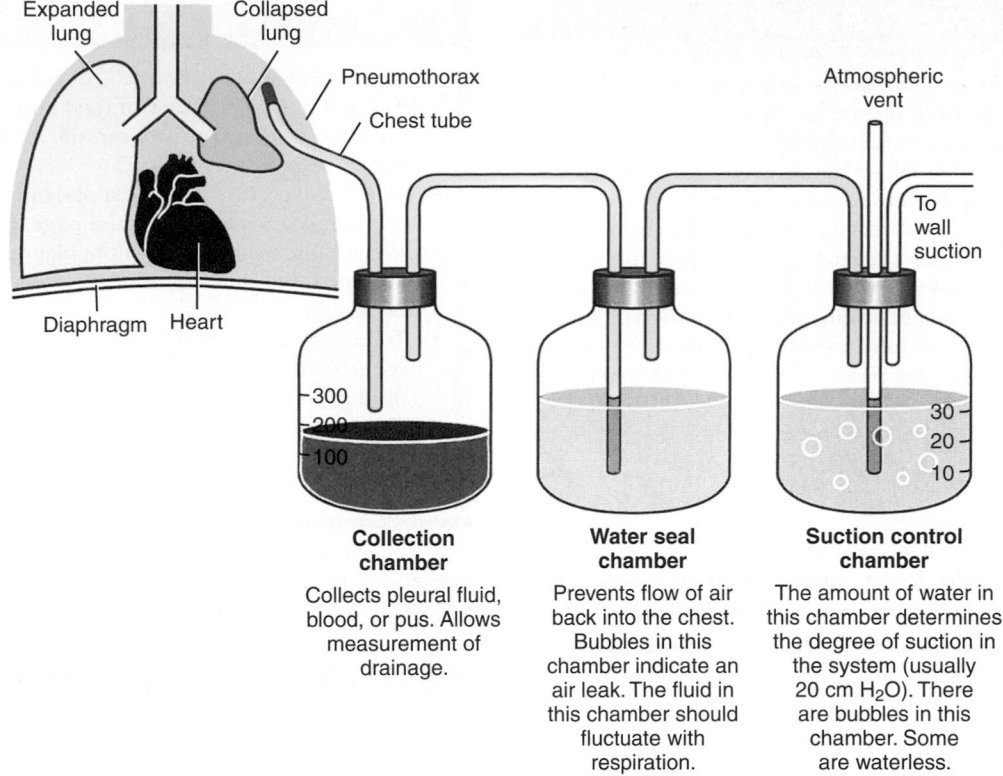

FIGURE 32-7 Example of the three-bottle system for thoracostomy drainage. Most current systems include all three components in a single plastic container rather than three separate bottles. Not all systems include the three components, and occasionally two components are combined (collection chamber and water seal chamber).

nearly 40 years ago.[20] Video-assisted thorascopic surgery technology is now commonly used for the following[20]:

· Biopsy in patients with diffuse lung disease
· Evaluation and biopsy of mediastinal masses
· Diagnosis and management of pleural disease
· Treatment of spontaneous pneumothorax
· Intrathoracic resections
· Evacuation of empyema fluid

In larger children, some surgical interventions are possible through the thoracoscope.[20] The major advantage of this approach is the avoidance of a **thoracotomy,** resulting in less postoperative pain and a shorter recovery period. Because the surgeon inserts a video camera into the pleural space to allow visualization of the surgical field, the procedure is called **video-assisted thoracoscopic surgery (VATS).**

The current size limitations of the equipment may limit the usefulness of thoracoscopy in premature infants and neonates, and some have recommended that it not be used in children less than 6 months of age or in those who weigh less than 8 kg.[20] General anesthesia is required, and unilateral lung ventilation must be used. This may be accomplished by using a double-lumen endotracheal tube in larger patients (adolescents) or by performing mainstem intubation or bronchial blocking with a balloon catheter in the smaller child.[20] However, some children younger than 4 years of age cannot tolerate unilateral ventilation and become hypoxic because of their relatively limited respiratory reserve. Pneumothorax, infection, and bleeding are the most often reported complications, although complications often depend on the patient's preoperative condition.[20]

Surgical intervention is seldom needed for persistent pneumothorax or bronchopleural fistula in children. Borrowing from the experience with malignant pleural effusions, *chemical pleurodesis* has been attempted in children who have persistent pneumothorax or recurrent pneumothorax due to cystic fibrosis.[21,22] This procedure uses agents such as tetracycline or talc to produce a pleural abrasion that results in the adhesion of pleural surfaces. There has been no clear consensus as to whether surgical intervention or chemical pleurodesis is the most appropriate approach to this problem, and both may be performed in some patients.[21,22] An individualized patient management plan should be offered, with flexibility to consider alternative options if the initial plan is unsuccessful. The use of chemical or surgical pleurodesis may complicate or prohibit consideration of subsequent lung transplantation.

The respiratory therapist should be aware of the variety of pleural space diseases that might compromise the patient's respiratory function. Familiarity with these diseases will help the practitioner understand the reason for the patient's deterioration or improvement and will contribute to the health care team's management of these problems.

CASE STUDY 1

A premature infant born at 24 weeks of gestation suffers immediate respiratory distress in the delivery room. She is intubated and given endotracheal surfactant replacement immediately. Despite the surfactant therapy and mechanical ventilation, she continues to have respiratory distress. Her chest radiograph demonstrates air in the right pleural space that persisted despite placement of two chest tubes (see Figure 32-4). The persisting air leak into the pleural space is likely from either tracheal trauma from intubation or pleural disruption from chest tube insertion in addition to hyaline membrane disease (respiratory distress syndrome) and mechanical ventilation.

Because her air leak has persisted despite chest tube placement, the next most appropriate intervention is:
- **A.** Chest CT scan
- **B.** Rigid bronchoscopy
- **C.** Alteplase instilled in the pleural space
- **D.** Pneumonectomy
- **E.** Chest tube replacement

See Evolve Resources for answers.

CASE STUDY 2

A 7-year-old girl complains of cough, right-sided chest pain, and fever. She has previously been well. Examination by her pediatrician reveals inspiratory crackles over the right lower lobe, so amoxicillin is prescribed for presumed bacterial pneumonia. Two days later her fever has persisted and she is increasingly short of breath. A chest radiograph (see Figure 32-1) demonstrates a right lower lobe infiltrate with right-sided pleural effusion. The right-side-down lateral decubitus radiograph (see Figure 32-2) confirms the effusion. Video-assisted thoracoscopic surgery (VATS) is performed to sample the pleural effusion and place a chest tube for drainage. Analysis of the pleural fluid reveals a white blood cell count of 22,000 per cubic mm with 96% segmented neutrophils. The total protein is 5.4 mg/dl and the lactate dehydrogenase (LDH) is 425 IU. Although the Gram stain and culture of the fluid is negative, a blood culture is positive for *Streptococcus pneumoniae*. In addition to chest tube drainage she is treated with intravenous amoxicillin. After 3 days the chest tube is removed and she completes a 10-day course of intravenous amoxicillin followed by 7 days of oral amoxicillin. She makes a full recovery and her chest radiograph returns to normal.

The most appropriate label for this patient's pleural fluid is:
- **A.** Empyema
- **B.** Chylothorax
- **C.** Hemithorax
- **D.** Transudative effusion

See Evolve Resources for answers.

KEY POINTS

- The pleural space is normally only a potential space that has a small amount of fluid and no air. The pleura facilitates movement between the lung and chest wall during respiration.
- When air accumulates in the pleural space (a pneumothorax), it usually requires drainage.
- When fluid accumulates in the pleural space (a pleural effusion), the cause of the fluid accumulation should be sought.
- Treatment of air or fluid in the pleural space often requires drainage by a chest tube, especially if the fluid is an empyema.
- If surgery is required in the pleural space, it is often achieved by video-assisted thoracoscopic surgery (VATS).

ASSESSMENT QUESTIONS

See Evolve Resources for answers.

1. Which of the following statements regarding the pleural space in a normal child is *true*?
   - **A.** There is usually no fluid in the pleural space.
   - **B.** There is normally a small amount of free air in the pleural space that can be seen only on a decubitus chest radiograph.
   - **C.** There is a small amount of fluid in the pleural space that represents a balance of the fluid flux between the parietal and visceral pleura.
   - **D.** The parietal pleura is thick and leathery to prevent penetration by sharp objects.
2. What is the most common cause of pneumothorax in the small premature infant with respiratory distress syndrome (hyaline membrane disease)?
   - **A.** Neonatal pneumonia
   - **B.** Barotrauma from mechanical ventilation and poorly compliant lungs
   - **C.** Complication from subclavian intravenous line placement
   - **D.** Meconium aspiration
3. The lung disease that is most commonly associated with spontaneous pneumothorax in adolescents is:
   - **A.** Langerhans cell histiocytosis (eosinophilic granuloma)
   - **B.** Pulmonary alveolar proteinosis
   - **C.** Congenital tracheoesophageal fistula
   - **D.** Cystic fibrosis
4. Which of the following pleural fluid measurements indicates the fluid is an exudate rather than a transudate?
   - **A.** Total protein = 5.0 g/dl
   - **B.** Lactate dehydrogenase (LDH) = 120 IU/L
   - **C.** White blood cell count (WBC) = 860 cells/mm^3
   - **D.** pH 7.30

5. When assessing the function of a chest tube draining air from the pleural space of a pediatric patient, which of the following suggests an ongoing intrapleural air leak?
   A. Bubbling in the water seal chamber
   B. Fluid in the collection chamber
   C. Fluctuating fluid in the chest tube
   D. Bubbling in the suction control chamber

6. Which of the following organisms most commonly causes empyema in toddlers and school age children?
   A. *Mycobacterium tuberculosis*
   B. Adenovirus
   C. *Streptococcus pneumoniae*
   D. *Aspergillus fumigatus*

7. Which of the following characteristics determines that the pleural fluid is an empyema?
   A. Appearance of thin, amber-colored fluid
   B. WBC count greater than 15,000 cells/mm^3
   C. pH equal to 7.32
   D. Lactic dehyrogenase of 150 U/dl

8. Which of the following statements about video-assisted thoracoscopic surgery (VATS) in the management of empyema is *true*?
   A. VATS often hastens the resolution of empyema compared with chest tube drainage alone.
   B. VATS requires the same skill level and equipment as standard chest tube insertion.
   C. VATS has been shown to be superior to the instillation of fibrinolytic agents (e.g., urokinase, streptokinase, or tissue plasminogen activator) in the management of pediatric empyema.
   D. VATS should be performed early in the evaluation and management of pleural effusion regardless of whether or not the fluid is a transudate, an exudate, or an empyema.

9. Which congenital anomaly is commonly associated with a pneumothorax in a neonate?
   A. Congenital diaphragmatic hernia
   B. Pulmonary sequestration
   C. Unilateral absence of the pulmonary artery
   D. Esophageal atresia

References

1. Pleura, lungs, trachea and bronchi. In Standring S, Borley NR, Collins P, et al, editors: *Gray's anatomy: the anatomical basis of clinical practice*, Spain, 2008, Churchill Livingstone Elsevier, pp 989–991.
2. Montgomery M: Air and liquid in the pleural space. In Wilmott RW, Chernick V, Boat TF, Deterding RR, Bush A, Ratjen F, editors: *Kendig and Chernick's disorders of the respiratory tract in children*, ed 8, Philadelphia, 2012, Elsevier, pp 976–994.
3. Sharma GD: Pleural effusion (nonbacterial). In Light ML, Blaisdell CJ, Homnick DN, Schechter MS, Wienberger MM, editors: *Pediatric pulmonology*, ed 1, Elk Grove Village, IL, 2011, American Academy of Pediatrics, pp 559–570.
4. Calder A, Owens CM: Imaging of parapneumonic pleural effusions and empyema in children, *Pediatr Radiol* 39:527, 2009.
5. Light RW: Pleural effusion, *N Engl J Med* 346:1971, 2002.
6. Walker W, Wheeler R, Legg J: Update on the causes, investigation and management of empyema in childhood, *Arch Dis Child* 96:482, 2011.
7. Carter E, Waldhausen J, Zhang W, Hoffman L, Redding G: Management of children with empyema: pleural drainage is not always necessary, *Pediatr Pulmonol* 45:475, 2010.
8. Walker W, Wheeler R, Legg J: Update on the causes, investigation and management of empyema in childhood, *Arch Dis Child* 96:482, 2011.
9. Krenke K, Peradzynska J, Lange J, Ruszczynski M, Kulus M, Szajewska H: Local treatment of emypema in children: a systematic review of randomized controlled trials, *Acta Paediatrica* 99:1449, 2010.
10. Sonnappa S, Cohen G, Owens CM, et al: Comparison of urokinase and video-assisted thoracoscopic surgery for treatment of childhood empyema, *Am J Respir Crit Care Med* 174:221, 2006.
11. Rahman NM, Maskell NA, West A, et al: Intrapleural use of tissue plasminogen activator and DNase in pleural infection, *N Engl J Med* 365:518, 2011.
12. Tauber D: Pneumothorax and pneumomediastinum. In Light ML, Blaisdell CJ, Homnick DN, Schechter MS, Wienberger MM, editors: *Pediatric pulmonology*, Elk Grove Village, IL, 2011, American Academy of Pediatrics, pp 571–581.
13. Johnson NN, Toledo A, Endom EE: Pneumothorax, pneumomediastinum, and pulmonary embolism, *Pediatr Clin N Am* 57:1357, 2010.
14. Sahn SA, Heffner JE: Spontaneous pneumothorax, *N Engl J Med* 342:868, 2000.
15. Robinson PD, Cooper P, Ranganathan SC: Evidence-based management of paediatric primary spontaneous pneumothorax, *Paediat Respir Rev* 10:110, 2009.
16. Miller KS, Sahn SA: Chest tubes: indications, technique, management, and complications, *Chest* 91:258, 1987.
17. Durai R, Hoque H, Davies TW: Managing a chest tube and drainage system, *AORN J* 91:275, 2010.
18. Baumann MH, Sahn SA: Medical management and therapy of bronchopulmonary fistulas in mechanically ventilated patients, *Chest* 97:721, 1990.
19. Caceres M, Ali SZ, Braud R, Weiman D, Garrett HE: Spontaneous pneumomediastinum: a comparative study and review of the literature, *Ann Thorac Surg* 86:962, 2008.
20. Kokoska ER, Chen MK, the New Technology Committee: Position paper on video-assisted thoracoscopic surgery as treatment of pediatric empyema, *J Pediatr Surg* 44:289, 2009.
21. Karpelowsky J: Paediatric thorascopic surgery, *Paediatr Respir Rev* 13:244, 2012.
22. Rolla M, D'Andrilli A, Rendina EA, Diso D, Venuta F: Cystic fibrosis and the thoracic surgeon, *Eur J Cardiothorac Surg* 39:716, 2011.

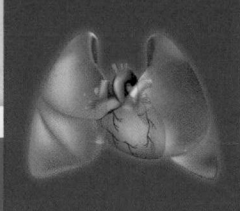

Chapter 33

Neurological and Neuromuscular Disorders

BRIAN K. WALSH

LEARNING OBJECTIVES

After reading this chapter the reader will be able to:

1. Discuss the components of the central and peripheral nervous systems that control normal respiration
2. Explain how the nervous system interacts with the muscles of respiration during normal and pathological breathing
3. Identify which muscle groups are enervated by the brainstem and how bulbar weakness interferes with protecting the airway and clearing secretions
4. Identify the most common central nervous system conditions that affect respiratory pattern and neuromuscular impairment
5. Identify the most common peripheral nervous system conditions that cause neuromuscular and respiratory impairment
6. Describe the important features of the respiratory physical examination for children with neuromuscular weakness
7. Describe the tests available to quantify respiratory compromise for children with neuromuscular weakness
8. Describe the respiratory aids available to support respiration for children with neuromuscular weakness
9. Explain the indications and proper use of respiratory aids for children with neuromuscular weakness
10. Identify the multisystem and nonrespiratory complications related to neuromuscular disease

KEY TERMS

Bulbar muscles
Disorders of the motor nerves
Disorders of the neuromuscular junction

Diurnal ventilation
Myopathy
Neuromuscular control of respiration
Neuromuscular disease

Poliomyelitis
Respiratory control system
Spinal muscular atrophy

Although there are many congenital and acquired neuromuscular conditions that present in childhood, the uniting feature of all these disorders is their effect on the respiratory system. The primary cause of morbidity and mortality for children with neuromuscular disease is respiratory compromise.[1] As such, health care providers should have a comprehensive understanding of the physiology of normal breathing, its derangements in neuromuscular disorders, the evaluation of patients with weakness, and specific aspects of their care.

NEUROMUSCULAR CONTROL OF RESPIRATION

Advances over the previous century provided detailed understanding of the control of respiration and the various components involved in breathing, but there remain significant gaps in our comprehension of the overall system.[2,3] The presence of a "neuromuscular respiratory system" was first recognized by the second-century anatomist and physician Galen.[4] Central and reflex control of breathing has been subsequently described by investigators, including Hering, Breuer, and Head, with significant contributions in the early twentieth century by Haldane and Priestley on the role of carbon dioxide in chemical respiratory control.[5] This chapter focuses on the present state of understanding of the **neuromuscular control of respiration**.

Central Nervous System

The respiratory system brings oxygen into the body to fuel energy production and removes carbon dioxide, a metabolic waste product. Central nervous system (CNS) control occurs in the cerebral cortex, which supports voluntary breathing actions, and incorporates input from the brainstem, which is involved with automatic breathing actions.[3,6] CNS signals are transmitted to the anterior horn cells of the spinal cord and then to the motor neurons that supply the respiratory muscles. Separate pathways in the spinal cord support both voluntary (corticospinal) and involuntary (reticulospinal) ventilation and transmit signals through descending pathways to motor neurons in the cervicothoracic portion of the spinal cord. These motor neurons transmit signals through peripheral nerves and across the neuromuscular junction to the muscles of respiration.[7] Dysfunction in any part of this control system, from brainstem to respiratory muscles, can result in respiratory failure.

Peripheral Nervous System

Each lower motor neuron arises from the cell body in the spinal cord (anterior horn cell) to supply the respiratory muscles. The efferent nerves extend to the diaphragm and intercostal muscles and to the accessory muscles of the neck. The diaphragm is supplied by the phrenic nerve, the intercostal muscles by the intercostal nerves, the accessory muscles of the neck from the cervical plexus, and the abdominal muscles from the lumbar nerve roots.[3,8]

The nerves divide into branches when reaching the muscle fiber and apply themselves to the muscle membrane at the motor endplates. At these junctions, the chemical transmitter acetylcholine is released to depolarize the muscle membrane and causes intracellular calcium release, which in turn serves to initiate contraction of the muscle fiber.[9]

Respiratory Muscles

The muscles of respiration are divided into three groups: inspiratory muscles, expiratory muscles, and accessory muscles. Although not formally classified as accessory muscles of respiration, the muscles of the upper airway are also important in maintaining airway patency and may lose function with certain neuromuscular disorders.

The main inspiratory muscle is the diaphragm, which contributes almost three quarters of the inspiratory capacity. Cervical nerves 3 to 5 contribute to form the phrenic nerve, which drives the diaphragm. Additional inspiratory force is provided by the external intercostal muscles, which contract to expand the rib cage during inspiration. The innervation of the intercostal muscles is via the intercostal nerves, which come off the thoracic spinal nerve roots.

The expiratory muscles include the internal intercostals, which help to reduce the thoracic volume, as well as the accessory abdominal muscles. These include the internal and external obliques and the transversus abdominus, which contract to displace the diaphragm into the thoracic cavity, and the rectus abdominus, which also contributes to increasing pleural pressure during exhalation.

The accessory muscles of respiration include the sternocleidomastoid, scalenes, trapezii, latissimus dorsi, and platysma and pectoralis groups. These groups are active predominantly with increased respiratory work, such as exercise, or loss of functional residual capacity, which occurs with infection or neuromuscular weakness. By contributing to rib cage expansion, these muscles support inspiration during active ventilation, although function during quiet breathing also exists.[3,6]

Respiratory Control System

Respiratory control is divided into both voluntary and metabolic control systems. Voluntary control originates in the cerebral cortex and is mediated by tracts in the dorsolateral spinal cord; voluntary control regulates ventilation affected by sleep, pain, or anxiety. Metabolic control, mediated by the ventrolateral pathways, incorporates inputs from central chemoreceptors within the medulla. Peripheral receptors in the carotid and aortic bodies respond to fluctuations in arterial oxygen pressure (PaO_2), arterial carbon dioxide pressure ($PaCO_2$), and pH. These various receptors operate via feedback loops that help to contribute to respiratory drive and regulate the ventilatory pattern in most normal physiological states.[3]

In addition, mechanical receptors in the lung and airways provide feedback to the respiratory centers as well as stimulate spinal reflexes that further regulate the breathing pattern. Examples of mechanical receptor control include the Hering-Breuer reflex, which prevents overinflation, coughing, bronchoconstriction, and the recruitment of accessory muscles during respiratory distress. Related mechanical receptors in the upper airway also induce coughing, glottic closure, vagal stimulation, and singultus (hiccups).

Bulbar Muscles

The **bulbar muscles** are not related to ventilation but are important in protecting the airway and secretion clearance. The bulbar muscles are enervated by the motor neurons emanating from the brainstem. This muscle group controls the epiglottis and other glottic structures, tongue, mouth, larynx, and throat. Bulbar muscle weakness impairs swallowing, coughing, speech, and other throat and pharyngeal activities. Bulbar muscle weakness also leads to severe fixed and variable extrathoracic upper airway obstruction on forced inspiratory and expiratory respiratory efforts. Examples of forced respiratory efforts include coughing, sneezing, respiratory distress, and pulmonary function testing.

NEUROMUSCULAR DISEASES THAT AFFECT THE RESPIRATORY SYSTEM

Neuromuscular disease is a broad term that encompasses many diseases that affect muscle function either directly, via muscle pathology, or indirectly, via nerve pathology. The diseases themselves are associated with a diverse range of muscle impairment from increased muscle tone with rigidity and spasticity to muscle weakness and flaccidity. This chapter covers primarily those affecting infants and children with muscle weakness or paralysis, because these conditions affect the respiratory system by impairing ventilation and airway clearance.

Central Nervous System

Conditions in the CNS that affect respiration include either those that affect the brainstem respiratory centers or the pathways connecting these centers to the motor neurons in the spinal cord.[3]

Disorders of the Brain

One of the best examples of a CNS disorder that affects breathing is congenital central hypoventilation syndrome (CCHS). Also known as "Ondine's curse," this represents a condition of hypoventilation associated with sleep. The name refers to the mythical character Ondine, who after professing his love "with every waking breath" was cursed by the water nymph he betrayed to stop breathing on falling asleep.[10] Although almost all cases of CCHS are congenital,

affecting approximately 1 in 200,000 live births, it can also be acquired through spinal cord or other central nervous system injury.[10] CCHS, manifested by nocturnal hypoventilation and respiratory arrest, is diagnosed by polysomnography and treated with lifetime nocturnal mechanical ventilation or phrenic nerve pacing.[10,11]

CASE STUDY 1

You are called to evaluate an otherwise healthy full-term neonate in the newborn nursery who appears to turn blue when sleeping. What steps would you take in evaluating this patient for a neuromuscular disease?

See Evolve Resources for answers.

Other cranial conditions affecting respiration in infants and children include congenital disorders such as hydrocephalus and anencephaly, along with genetic neurodegenerative disorders such as Tay-Sachs disease and Friedreich's ataxia.[3,12,13] Acquired CNS disorders include neoplasms, infarction, hemorrhage, and anoxic injury.[3] All these conditions are associated with multiple organ system symptomatology, resulting from diffuse neurological injury and loss of autonomic control. Respiratory symptoms of these conditions include changes in respiratory drive or pattern, respiratory and upper airway muscle weakness with loss of airway clearance ability, and chronic aspiration.

Disorders Affecting the Spinal Cord

Trauma. Almost 11,000 Americans sustain a spinal cord injury every year, costing an approximated 9.7 billion dollars in health care expenditure.[14] The spinal cord nerve roots that control diaphragm function exit the spine at the level of the cervical vertebrae.[8,15] Spinal cord injury above cervical vertebra 3 will require tracheostomy and mechanical ventilation or phrenic nerve pacing.[16] Spinal cord injuries between vertebrae 3 and 5 will have variable amounts of respiratory impairment, and those below the fifth vertebra almost always allow independent breathing.[3] However, the abdominal and intercostal rib muscles involved in cough function exit the spinal cord lower in the thoracic spine.[15] Therefore, lower spine injuries may permit spontaneous respiration but have significant impact on airway clearance mechanisms.[3]

Chiari Malformations. Chiari malformations are congenital malformations characterized by a small or misshapen skull, causing the cerebellum to protrude through the bottom of the skull into the spinal canal. Under these circumstances, the brainstem, spinal cord, cranial nerves, or the cerebellum may be stretched or compressed. In addition, the flow of cerebrospinal fluid around the brain and spinal cord can be obstructed, causing hydrocephalus or a cyst to form within the spinal cord, known as syringo-myelia.[17] Estimates indicate that between 0.5% and 1% of live births in the United States may be affected by a Chiari malformation.[17] Symptoms of Chiari malformations are variable and related to the affected areas. Many patients with Chiari malformations report no symptoms, but those who do complain of headaches, dizziness, vision changes, muscle weakness, or balance problems.[18] Younger children may present with difficulty swallowing, choking, irregular breathing patterns, or apnea.[17] Chiari malformations can be easily diagnosed by magnetic resonance imaging scan and are treated by surgical decompression.

Other Conditions. Less common causes of spinal cord impairment include spinal tumors, infections, and birth injury. Spinal tumors either originate locally in the CNS or are metastatic. Meningiomas are primary CNS tumors that develop from the meninges, the membrane that surrounds the brain and spinal cord. They are rare in children, with pediatric cases accounting for only 1.5% of all cases.[19] Metastatic spinal tumors are also rare in children but may be seen with invasive lymphomas and have been reported in other childhood cancers.[20] Central nervous system infections, such as epidural abscesses, can have both local inflammatory and mass effect on the spinal cord, causing neuromuscular symptoms to develop. Finally, spinal cord injury may be a rare complication of the birthing process. In this situation, traction applied to the infant's head while assisting delivery may result in nervous system trauma. These injuries include cervical spinal cord hematomas as well as direct nerve and nerve root stretch injury.

Peripheral Nervous System
Disorders of the Motor Nerves

Acute paralytic **poliomyelitis** was once the most common neuronopathy in the United States.[21] However, massive immunization campaigns have been effectively instituted and all but eliminated community-acquired poliovirus infections in the United States. As a result, the spinal muscular atrophies are now the most common cause of degenerative nerve cell disease in children.

Spinal Muscular Atrophy. The **spinal muscular atrophies** (SMAs) include a number of different disorders that clinically manifest as muscle weakness as a result of progressive destruction of the motor neurons of the spinal cord and brainstem.[22,23] The SMAs are hereditary disorders transmitted by autosomal recessive inheritance, with three recognized forms categorized by severity and age of onset.[22,23] All types are caused by defects at the same site on chromosome 5, and the overlap in clinical features is considerable.[24-26] SMA type I, also called Werdnig-Hoffmann disease, is the acute infantile form, which usually presents within the first 6 months of life.[27] In these children, limb weakness develops rapidly, whereas the facial muscles are slower to fail and the extraocular muscles are essentially spared. The result is a child who appears alert and

responsive but cannot move. The respiratory effects of SMA type I include weakness of the bulbar, abdominal, and intercostal muscles, which makes feeding difficult and leads to aspiration and a weak, ineffective cough. A weak cough results in recurrent pneumonias and poor airway clearance. Even relatively minor viral infections result in severe airway and ventilator compromise. Without intervention, most infants will die of respiratory insufficiency and infection before reaching 1 year of age.[26]

SMA type II, the chronic childhood form, has a later onset and often more insidious course.[27] Some affected children may be able to sit unsupported, but usually proximal muscle weakness prevents these children from standing or walking independently and leads to scoliosis; these children eventually become wheelchair dependent.[28] The course of SMA type II is unpredictable; long intervals without progression of weakness are expected and survival into adulthood is common.[29] SMA type III (Kugelberg-Welander disease) is the mildest form; affected patients are able to stand and walk independently and have much slower progression of muscle weakness compared with the other two forms.[27]

Poliomyelitis. Poliomyelitis is an infection caused by the polio virus and was one of the most dreaded childhood diseases of the twentieth century in the United States.[21] The vast majority of infected individuals are asymptomatic or experience only mild, nonspecific viral symptoms. However, in a small proportion of patients, the virus enters the central nervous system, where it infects and destroys motor neurons in the spinal cord, leading to muscle wasting and weakness.[30] Most commonly, this causes a self-limited case of nonparalytic viral meningitis, but in a small proportion of patients the infection causes permanent wasting and paralysis. Depending on the site of paralysis, paralytic polio is classified as spinal, affecting the nerves of the trunk and extremities; bulbar, affecting the nerves that control breathing, speaking, and swallowing; or bulbospinal, representing a combination of these two forms.[30] Bulbospinal polio is particularly problematic because it affects the nerves in the cervical spine region that control diaphragm function. Destruction of these nerves makes independent respiration, swallowing, and effective coughing impossible. Lifelong ventilator support and airway clearance is essential for the survival of these patients.[30]

Guillain-Barré Syndrome. Guillain-Barré syndrome (GBS), or acute inflammatory demyelinating polyradiculo-neuropathy, is an acute, autoimmune process that affects the peripheral nervous system. Guillain-Barré syndrome is not hereditary, affects persons of all ages, and has an approximate population incidence that ranges from 1 to 3 per 100,000 population.[31,32] Although its cause is not completely understood, GBS is probably triggered by an acute infectious process, which leads to antibody-mediated destruction of the myelin sheaths that coat peripheral nerves.[33] This demyelination leads to nerve conduction block, which causes weakness and often sensory and autonomic changes as well.[34] Guillain-Barré syndrome usually presents as an ascending weakness or paralysis that starts in the legs and spreads to the upper limbs and the face. The weakness is often preceded by sensory symptoms such as "pins and needles" and muscle tenderness, followed by a complete loss of deep tendon reflexes.[33] Patients often experience rapid progression of symptoms; more than three quarters of patients reach a nadir in strength within 3 weeks of symptom onset.[33] Autonomic dysfunction, characterized by arrhythmias, blood pressure lability, and gastrointestinal dysfunction, may also be present.[35] Respiratory paralysis occurs in roughly 14% to 18% of children with GBS, and approximately 20% of all patients with GBS require intensive care during the acute phase of illness.[32,33] Treatment is mainly supportive, although corticosteroids, plasmapheresis, and intravenous immunoglobulin have all been used with variable success.[32,36] Although plasmapheresis is considered the treatment of choice in adults, certain technical factors may limit its usefulness in children. Careful monitoring of patients' respiratory status, accompanied by intubation and mechanical ventilation when required, constitutes the mainstay of acute supportive care. If the child is well ventilated during the critical time of profound paralysis, complete recovery can be expected.[31] Most children fully recover within 6 months, and fewer than 10% have symptom recurrence.[31,34]

Disorders of the Neuromuscular Junction

Infantile Botulism. Human botulism results from eating food contaminated with the organism *Clostridium botulinum* or the toxin it produces.[37] The clinical spectrum of infantile botulism ranges from asymptomatic carrier states, mild hypotonia, and failure to thrive to severe with progressive, life-threatening paralysis or sudden death.[38] Most infants experience a prodromal syndrome of constipation and poor feeding, followed by progressive bulbar and skeletal muscle weakness and loss of tendon reflexes. Typical features on examination include diffuse hypotonia, ptosis, dysphagia, and a weak cry. Respiratory history and examination are often notable for respiratory insufficiency and apnea. Diagnosis is confirmed by the isolation of *C. botulinum* organisms from the stool. In general, botulism is a self-limited disease lasting 2 to 6 weeks, and even with the use of immunoglobulin therapy the infant requires meticulous supportive respiratory care. In severe cases, this support is lifesaving. Recovery is often complete, but relapse can occur in as many as 5% of affected infants.[39]

Myasthenia Gravis. Myasthenia gravis is an autoimmune disorder characterized by fluctuating muscle weakness and easy fatigability.[40] The pathophysiology of the disorder occurs at the neuromuscular junction, where circulating antibodies block synaptic receptors, inhibiting the effect of neurotransmitter chemicals, most notably acetylcholine; this prevents muscle contraction.[40] The current prevalence of myasthenia gravis in the United States is estimated to be about 20 per 100,000 population, although frequent misdiagnosis means that the true prevalence is likely higher.[41] Juvenile myasthenia describes the immune-mediated form of myasthenia gravis that occurs in late infancy through adult life.[42] Two forms are recognized[43]:

- *Ocular myasthenia*, in which the eye muscles are primarily or exclusively affected
- *Generalized myasthenia*, in which moderate to severe weakness occurs in bulbar, limb, trunk, and even respiratory muscles

The initial features of both the ocular and generalized forms are usually ptosis, diplopia, or both.[41] Prepubertal onset is associated with a slight male bias and ocular symptoms only, whereas postpubertal onset is associated with a strong female bias and generalized myasthenia.[44] Patients with myasthenia gravis often have little chronic respiratory compromise and are symptomatic only during periods of myasthenia crisis, when symptoms, particularly bulbar symptoms, suddenly escalate. During a crisis patients may have sudden paralysis of the respiratory muscles, temporarily requiring assisted ventilation. Treatment also includes using cholinesterase inhibitors to help transmission of acetylcholine and immune suppressants such as corticosteroids and cyclosporine. Exchange transfusions and intravenous immunoglobulin therapy rapidly restore function but are temporary measures.[41]

Congenital myasthenia and *familial infantile myasthenia* are terms used to describe clinical syndromes that are caused by several different genetic defects and are generally rare. Respiratory insufficiency and feeding difficulty may be present at birth or develop during infancy. Usually, ptosis and generalized weakness are present at birth. Many affected newborns require mechanical ventilation, but over a course of weeks most infants become stronger and no longer need ventilator support.[45]

A transitory myasthenic syndrome is observed in 10% to 15% of offspring of myasthenic mothers. The syndrome is believed to be caused by the transfer of antibody from the myasthenic mother to her normal fetus. Symptoms are generally observed within hours of birth. The severity of newborn symptoms correlates with the newborn's antibody concentration and not the severity of weakness in the mother, which is generally exacerbated during pregnancy.[46] Difficulty feeding and generalized hypotonia are the major clinical features; they are eager to feed, but suckling quickly causes fatigue. Respiratory insufficiency is uncommon, and weakness becomes progressively worse in the first few days of life and then improves. Recovery is complete, and transitory neonatal myasthenia does not develop into myasthenia later in life.

Other Conditions Affecting the Neuromuscular Junction. In the medical setting, there are a number of other causes of incomplete or failed transmission at the neuromuscular junction related to drug exposure. These medications include antibiotics, corticosteroids, antirheumatics, lidocaine, lithium, and anesthetic agents.[3]

Myopathies

Myopathies are diseases of the skeletal musculature causing muscle weakness and degeneration. Myopathies are caused by inherited genetic defects and by inflammatory, endocrinological, and metabolic disorders.

Duchenne and Becker Muscular Dystrophy

The muscular dystrophies are a group of genetic disorders with multisystem symptoms involving the cardiac, respiratory, gastrointestinal, endocrine, and nervous systems.[47] Although there are more than 100 diseases that have similarities to muscular dystrophy, the two most common muscular dystrophies that present in childhood are Duchenne and Becker muscular dystrophy.[47] Duchenne muscular dystrophy (DMD) is the most common childhood form of muscular dystrophy, occurring in roughly 1 in 3500 live male births.[47,48] The male preponderance is related to its inheritance pattern: DMD is an X-linked genetic disorder, resulting in female carriers and affected males. DMD presents in early childhood with proximal muscle weakness, which manifests as difficulty in running, climbing stairs, and standing.[47] The muscle weakness is progressive and eventually leads to profound skeletal and respiratory muscle weakness in all cases. By adolescence, all patients with DMD are wheelchair bound and require assistance with ventilation.[47] Becker muscular dystrophy is also an X-linked inherited muscular dystrophy, with a distribution of muscle wasting and weakness similar to that of DMD.[47] However, Becker muscular dystrophy typically has a milder course with symptom onset in the second decade or later.

There is no cure for any of the muscular dystrophies, and current therapy is supportive. Treatment goals are to maintain function, prevent contractures, and provide psychological support for the child and family. Traditional estimates suggest that up to 90% of patients with DMD die of respiratory failure before reaching 20 years of age.[49] Muscular dystrophy affects the heart as well, and the second leading cause of death in DMD is cardiomyopathy and cardiac failure, or arrhythmia.[48] However, aggressive intervention with noninvasive ventilation, airway clearance techniques, and surgical correction of spine deformation to improve lung volumes at the onset of respiratory symptoms has been demonstrated to significantly reduce morbidity and prolong life for patients with muscular dystrophy.[49]

Myotonic Dystrophies

Myotonic dystrophy is a highly variable inherited disease characterized by chronic, slowly progressive muscle wasting and weakness, cataracts, heart conduction defects, and endocrine disorders.[50] The muscles most commonly affected are the voluntary muscles in the face, neck, and lower arms and legs and, in more severe cases, the intercostal muscles and the diaphragm.[50] Myotonic dystrophy most commonly presents in adolescence or adulthood, but a severe congenital form exists and is associated with mental retardation, orthopedic problems, and other developmental delays.[50] Affected infants are extremely hypotonic and may have difficulty feeding. They often require ventilatory support, at least temporarily, because of muscle weakness and decreased central ventilatory drive.[50] Similar to the muscular dystrophies, the overwhelming majority of affected children die in infancy. However, supported ventilation, corrective surgery, and tube feeding have all extended the life span of patients and dramatically improved quality of life for these children and their families.[50] Refer to Chapter 12 for airway clearance techniques related to this patient population.

Glycogen Storage Diseases

The glycogen storage diseases are a family of 12 inherited errors of metabolism that result in enzyme defects in glycogen synthesis or breakdown. In general, clinical classifications can be made on the basis of whether affected organs include the liver only, or additionally the muscles, blood cells, connective tissue, heart, brain, and kidneys. In terms of respiratory involvement, glycogen storage disease type II (also called Pompe disease or acid maltase deficiency) has the most severe symptoms. Pompe disease is a rare, autosomal recessive disorder occurring in roughly 1 in 40,000 to 100,000 live births.[51,52] It is caused by a deficiency in the enzyme α-1,4-glucosidase, which causes glycogen accumulation in cellular lysosomes and leads to progressive weakness in all muscles.[52] Like all the congenital disorders, the severity of symptoms of Pompe disease are related to age at onset. Infantile onset is the most severe form and is characterized by the development of marked hypotonia, hepatomegaly, and severe cardiomegaly within several months of birth. Mental development is usually normal, although most children die of respiratory or cardiac complications before 2 years of age.[53] Late-onset Pompe disease occurs in patients with minimal—as opposed to absent—levels of the acid maltase enzyme.[51,52] Symptoms in these affected individuals present in adolescence or adulthood, tend to progress somewhat more slowly, and include primarily weakness of muscles in the trunk, lower limbs, and the diaphragm. A small number of adult patients live relatively normal lives without major limitations.[52]

Electrolyte Abnormalities

Less common causes of muscle weakness in the outpatient setting include electrolyte abnormalities—most commonly caused by insufficient dietary intake. Potassium is essential for many body functions, including muscle and nerve activity. Maintenance of the electrochemical gradient of potassium between the intracellular and extracellular space is essential for normal nerve function. Mild hypokalemia is often asymptomatic; however, moderate hypokalemia may cause diffuse muscular weakness, myalgias, and arrhythmias.[54] This is particularly important when attempting to liberate a patient from mechanical ventilation because the respiratory muscles could be in a weakened state (atrophy vs. fatigue) and electrolyte abnormalities will only add to this impairment. Severe hypokalemia has been associated with respiratory depression from severe impairment of skeletal muscle function.[55] Similarly, hypomagnesemia can cause weakness and muscle cramps and may contribute to impairments in respiratory muscle function.[54] Hypomagnesemia, which can be seen in the presence of hypokalemia, hypocalcemia, and hypophosphatemia, should prompt the evaluation of other electrolyte disturbances that can further exacerbate these clinical symptoms.[56]

RESPIRATORY EVALUATION OF CHILDREN WITH NEUROMUSCULAR DISEASE

Pulmonary Function Testing

Neuromuscular weakness affecting the respiratory system initially develops as impaired cough and airway clearance, with gradual progression to nocturnal and eventually daytime hypoventilation. Monitoring the respiratory status of a patient with neuromuscular weakness depends on the underlying disease, its rate of progression, and extent of involvement. Because most conditions involve weakness of the inspiratory and expiratory muscles, pulmonary function testing including muscle strength assessment is the main mode of testing, with polysomnography and noninvasive measures of hypoventilation as the disease progresses in severity.

The use of pulmonary function tests in diagnosing and monitoring the progression of the neuromuscular disease has been well established in adults, but pediatric testing remains a challenge. Although newer techniques in respiratory muscle strength testing are being introduced, the majority of school-age children and adolescents are best monitored by standard spirometry with maximal inspiratory and expiratory pressure monitoring (Figure 33-1).[57,58] Additional testing includes assessment of cough flows, because it is the main determinant of respiratory compromise. However, because peak cough flows have been well correlated with forced vital capacity (FVC) and forced expiratory volume at 1 second, these tests remain the mainstay of pulmonary function testing in this population.[8,59]

Standard spirometry is performed according to the standards of the American Thoracic Society (New York, NY). Measurements include FVC, forced expiratory volume at 1 second, and forced inspiratory volume displayed primarily as a flow–volume loop. Including forced inspiratory volume allows for separate evaluation of extrathoracic and upper airway obstruction in children with bulbar

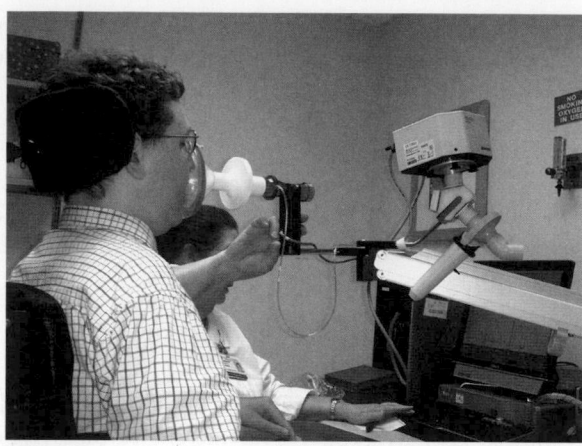

FIGURE 33-1   Spirometry. The majority of school-age children and adolescents are best monitored by standard spirometry with maximal inspiratory and expiratory pressure monitoring. In this image a mask has been substituted for a mouthpiece because of bulbar weakness and inability to use or create a seal around a standard mouthpiece.

weakness. Measuring maximal expiratory pressure and maximal inspiratory pressure and, in some instances, static mouth pressures allows monitoring of diaphragm and other cough-related strength.[60] For patients with Duchenne muscular dystrophy, a decline in FVC has been demonstrated to be a useful predictor of worsening respiratory muscle weakness and death, so that interventions such as pulmonary clinical monitoring, secretion clearance, and ventilatory assistance devices can be recommended to be initiated at specific rates of decline.[61] An FVC less than 20% of predicted, or 1 L, is associated with significant carbon dioxide retention and a limited survival rate past 3 years.[48] Last, static lung volume measurements in this population usually reveal restriction, which may be the result of multiple factors, including diminished chest wall compliance, reduced inspiratory muscle strength, and kyphoscoliosis if present.

Measuring carbon dioxide tension and oxygen analysis are useful adjuncts when determining whether an assisted ventilation device may be required. Noninvasive capnography and pulse oximetry are easily applied in the clinic, but arterial gas analysis should be performed if these are not available. In addition, noninvasive monitoring of cardiac output, using capnometry and a modified Fick equation, may be done to determine the cardiac function of patients with cardiac involvement but should not replace echocardiography for definitive analysis. Daytime monitoring should be performed every 3 months, or more frequently with diminished mucus mobilization, decline in lung function, and reduced peak cough flows.[48,62] With further progression of carbon dioxide retention and muscle weakness and advancing concerns regarding nighttime hypoventilation, home overnight oximetry or polysomnography may be useful in determining the early need for assisted respiratory support.

Measurement of cough effectiveness and lung volume, combined with monitoring for hypoventilation, may provide an assessment of trends that could facilitate the timeliness of initiating airway clearance and ventilatory support. With patient and caregiver education, these studies may help patients sustain more normal daily activities and direct the care needed to minimize the complications associated with respiratory muscle weakness.

CASE STUDY 2

You have just completed pulmonary function testing on a 5-year-old boy who has Duchenne muscular dystrophy and appears to be following to the usual disease course. Although he has difficulty running and climbing stairs, he has not progressed to need respiratory support at this time. Mom seeks your advice about when to have her son "trached" (a tracheostomy performed). What would you advise?

See Evolve Resources for answers.

Sleep Studies

Polysomnography must be performed and sleep-disordered breathing monitored in all patients with neuromuscular weakness. Nighttime sleep–disordered breathing often precedes diurnal respiratory failure in affected patients. Polysomnography is the most complete diagnostic test available to assess for the nature and severity of the sleep disturbance.[63] Sleep assessment allows for anticipatory evaluation and more timely recognition and management with assisted ventilation. Full polysomnography should include sleep stage recording, arousal documentation, and monitoring of oxygen saturation, hypoventilation, and hypercapnia.[64] Together, this testing allows for monitoring of sleep complaints and treatable conditions in an otherwise progressive disease process. See Chapter 25 for more details.

RESPIRATORY CARE OF CHILDREN WITH NEUROMUSCULAR DISEASE

General Considerations

The onset of pulmonary symptoms of children with neuromuscular disease largely depends on the underlying disease.[59] For example, a boy with Becker muscular dystrophy is likely to have few respiratory symptoms until late adolescence or adulthood, whereas an infant with SMA type I will almost certainly develop symptoms in the first few months of life. In either case, however, a predictable sequence of events will occur, leading each child to experience progressive respiratory insufficiency and eventually respiratory failure.[65] Initially, respiratory muscle weakness is manifested as

a weak cough and impaired airway clearance, which leads to recurrent atelectasis and chest infections.[59] As respiratory muscle weakness progresses, patients experience nocturnal hypoventilation and symptoms related to hypercapnia. These symptoms include nightmares, frequent wakening, early morning headaches, and daytime sleepiness.[47] At this point, most patients maintain relatively normal daytime respiration and are eucapnic while awake. However, further deterioration in respiratory muscle strength eventually leads to daytime respiratory insufficiency and daytime hypercapnia.[59] Complete respiratory failure follows shortly thereafter; the trajectory of this decline, however, is unique to each patient and disease and is usually hastened by serious illness or concomitant conditions such as scoliosis. With early and proactive institution of cough assist devices or mechanical ventilatory support, this trajectory may be effectively slowed.

Many of the interventions used to support airway clearance and ventilation in adults have also been used to assist children; however, limitations in size and the inability of young children to cooperate with or comprehend respiratory therapies can present unique challenges. Although respiratory insufficiency or some form of cardiopulmonary disease is the most common cause of death among children with almost any congenital or acquired neuromuscular disorders, innovations in pediatric ventilatory assistance have considerably extended survival and improved quality of life for affected children.[48,66] Although you may have to search hard for the appropriate-sized equipment and implementation, it does exist. The industry of pediatric assisted ventilation and airway clearance is growing year by year, so keep checking.

Airway Clearance Mechanisms

Airway clearance is achieved in a healthy individual via two mechanisms: mucociliary transport and cough clearance. The mucociliary escalator lining the bronchial tree moves a thin layer of mucus upward toward the proximal airway, where the mucus and entrapped particles are sensed and expelled via cough clearance. Normal coughing is a highly controlled reflex with defined phases. The initial phase is inspiration, when a maximal inspiration is performed in order to get air behind the mucus or debris that needs to be cleared. The next phase is the compressive phase, during which the glottis is closed and the abdominal muscles contract. This allows intrathoracic pressure to rise and narrows the central airways, making the velocity of the airflow higher. The last phase of coughing is expulsion, during which the glottis is opened and air is released at a high velocity, carrying with it collected mucus and debris.

Children with neuromuscular weakness may have trouble with each phase of coughing; inspiratory muscle weakness reduces vital capacity and maximal inhaled volume, bulbar muscle weakness can lead to impaired glottic closure, and expiratory muscle weakness reduces the maximal intrathoracic pressure and expulsive force.[59,67] The significance of this cannot be overstated: In patients with neuromuscular disease, most episodes of acute respiratory failure result from the inability to eliminate airway secretions and mucus during otherwise benign chest infections.[68] A peak cough flow less than 160 L/min is associated with impaired secretion clearance, but early intervention at 250 to 270 L/min is recommended for beginning cough assistance.[48]

Facilitating Clearance of Mucus

Mucus mobilization can be facilitated by good enteral hydration, use of humidity and medications that reduce mucus viscosity, and assisted maneuvers to clear secretions from the airways. These maneuvers include manual physiotherapy, mechanical or vibratory chest percussion, and postural drainage. The goal of these therapies is to transport secretions in the peripheral airways centrally to larger airways, where assisted coughing can more easily expel them from the respiratory tract. Commercially available mucolytics commonly used for this purpose include dornase alfa, bicarbonate (HCO_3^-), and N-acetylcysteine (NAC). Dornase alfa (Pulmozyme) is an aerosolized enzyme that hydrolyzes the extracellular DNA in infected or colonized sputum, reducing sputum viscoelasticity. If proper airway clearance is provided and pulmonary infections avoided, dornase alfa may not be helpful. Dornase alfa is only approved by the Food and Drug Administration (FDA) for cystic fibrosis. Similarly, NAC cleaves the disulfide bonds in mucoproteins, reducing their chain lengths and thinning lung mucus. All mucus has disulfide bonds. NAC has been known to cause bronchospasm, therefore limiting its success if pretreatment with a bronchodilator is not provided. The least used mucolytic is the oldest, and that is 2% to 4% bicarbonate. HCO_3^- has been instilled into the airway of intubated patients or aerosolize to reduce viscosity of mucus. The reduction in viscosity is created by the elevation in mucus pH. These medications can be used as daily maintenance therapy or on an as-needed basis during infections. If necessary, NAC can be used up to six times a day to facilitate mucus clearance.

Chest percussion is the manual clapping performed by a caregiver to the patient's thorax, alternating from the ventral, lateral, and dorsal aspects of the chest for periods usually lasting 10 to 20 minutes at a time.[68] Chest vibration is similar in application, but instead of manual clapping the thorax is vibrated via a handheld device or a circumferential chest vest. A third option is intrapulmonary percussive ventilation (IPV), in which high-frequency percussive ventilation is delivered through an IPV device used either alone or in conjunction with aerosol therapy.[69] Percussion and vibration maneuvers are often repeated several times every day, depending on the quantity of mucus, its viscosity, and its adhesiveness to the airway and the patient's health status.[68] In particular, more frequent use of percussion or vibration is an important component of therapy during respiratory tract

infections, when mucus production can often overwhelm a weak child's clearance mechanisms.[70] See Chapter 12 for more details on airway clearance or Chapter 20 for more details of inhaled medications.

Assisted Coughing

For effective coughing, sufficient strength is needed in bulbar, inspiratory, and expiratory muscles. For patients with generalized weakness, manually assisted coughing (MAC) can permit successful long-term use of noninvasive ventilatory support.[68] For effective MAC, the patient inspires maximally, augmented by either breath stacking or assisted insufflation, and an abdominal thrust or thoracic squeeze, timed to glottic opening, is applied by an assistant or caregiver.[68] For those using abdominal thrusts, a one-handed technique with counterpressure applied to the thorax with the other hand can further increase cough strength. If upper limb weakness is not involved, a patient can employ either maximal insufflation or abdominal thrust in isolation and augment cough peak flow.[67] There are some limitations to assisted cough, however; MAC requires a cooperative patient willing and able to provide adequate physical effort, and a committed caregiver, able to assist multiple times a day.[68]

Mechanical in-exsufflators are cough assist devices that attach to the patient via an oronasal interface. These work by helping to deliver deep insufflations until the lungs are fully expanded, followed by an immediate negative pressure exsufflation that helps to facilitate mucus mobilization (Figure 33-2).[68] When mechanical cough assist devices are used for secretion clearance, multiple cycles are given in one sitting, until no further secretions are induced.[68] Some patients with severe bulbar weakness may not tolerate mechanical assistance and require manual cough assistance.

Glossopharyngeal Breathing

Glossopharyngeal breathing (GPB), sometimes called "frog breathing," can be used to provide brief periods of normal alveolar ventilation for a patient with neuromuscular weakness who spends periods off a ventilator, or during times of unexpected ventilator failure.[68] The technique of GPB is to augment insufflation by "gulping" air in a series of breaths, closing the glottis between "gulps" to entrap air in the lungs.[68] Using this method, one glossopharyngeal "breath" often consists of six to nine gulps of air. Although severe bulbar muscle weakness can limit the effectiveness of GPB, previous reports of its use in patients with almost no independent breathing and no vital capacity have been published.[68] Bach[71] and Bach and Alba[72] reported that after a period of training to develop proficiency, even patients with ventilator dependence and no autonomous breathing capability have successfully used GPB to facilitate independent breathing for periods ranging from minutes to all day.

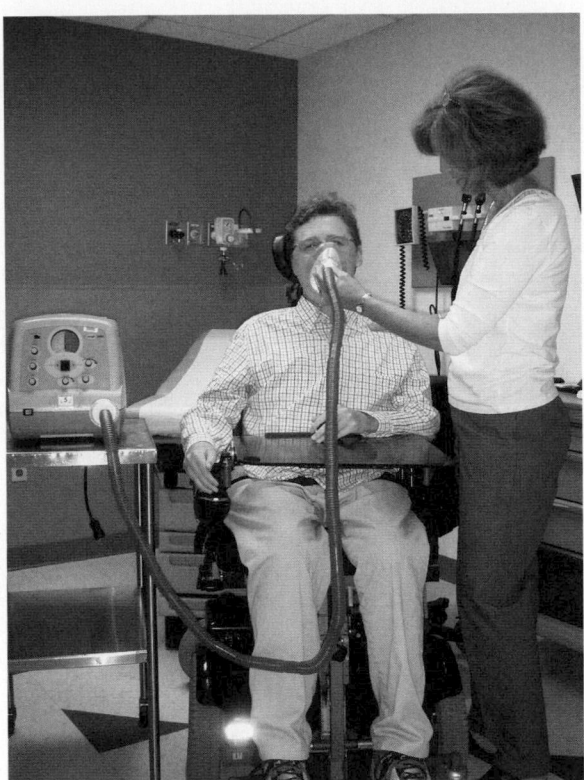

FIGURE 33-2 Mechanical cough assist. Mechanical cough assist devices attach to the patient via an oronasal interface and deliver deep insufflations until the lungs are fully expanded, followed by an immediate negative pressure exsufflation until the lungs are fully deflated.

Mechanical Ventilatory Support
Noninvasive Ventilation

In the early 1980s, noninvasive ventilation was pioneered first by Rideau and colleagues in France and subsequently by Bach and colleagues in the United States.[73] Since that time, several large studies have shown that noninvasive ventilation is not only effective and well tolerated but is a preferred method of respiratory support for patients with progressive neuromuscular disease.[68,73] Indeed, work has demonstrated that chronic noninvasive ventilation can extend the average life expectancy for patients with DMD by an average of 6 years and even restore normal life expectancy for older patients with static weakness, such as long-term polio survivors.[73] Noninvasive ventilation appears to succeed because it allows fatigued respiratory muscles to rest, improves pulmonary mechanics, and restores normal ventilatory sensitivity to carbon dioxide levels.[73]

The goals of assisted ventilation in children are to maintain pulmonary compliance and normal lung and thoracic growth and to maintain normal alveolar ventilation. (See Chapter 16 for more details on noninvasive ventilation.) Lung and thorax growth is particularly important when the onset of weakness is in infancy, as is the case with patients with SMA type I. In these cases

the lungs and chest wall do not grow normally because of the inability to take deep breaths. It is important for the caregivers of these children to move their thoracic cavity with large tidal volumes (mimic a sigh) several times a day to prevent abnormal growth and reduce atelectasis. Currently there are no ventilators on the market that offer a sigh, so this will need to be manually done. As children age and hypoventilation develops, assessment of pulmonary function determines when assisted ventilation support is indicated, usually with progression from nocturnal-only ventilation to around-the-clock assistance as muscle weakness progresses.

Nocturnal Ventilation

Generally accepted indications for initiating nocturnal ventilation include rapid progression of weakness, hypercapnia or end-tidal carbon dioxide levels exceeding 45 to 50 mm Hg during or at the end of sleep, arterial desaturation below 95% during sleep, and symptoms of respiratory insufficiency.[68,74] The level of nocturnal support is adjusted until there is satisfactory resolution of symptoms and saturations consistently remain greater than 95%.[75] Because of the thoracic deformities that are commonly present, tidal volume or pressure calculation may be inaccurate. In these cases auscultating the basilar lung regions provides a baseline for initial pressure or volume settings.

Initial means of respiratory support include a variety of noninvasive methods. In children, choice of assist device or ventilator mode and patient interface is likely to be dictated by patient age and size. Although the mouthpiece intermittent positive pressure ventilation (IPPV) with lip seal to minimize leak may be preferred in certain instances, these are available only in adolescent and adult sizes.[68] Therefore, nasal ventilation is the most practical means of noninvasive ventilatory support for small children. Younger children and infants can often be easily fitted with nasal interfaces such as adapted continuous positive airway pressure circuits or nasal pillows, nasal masks, or full face masks, although custom headgear might be necessary (Figure 33-3). With any of these designs, the clinician must ensure that a proper fit not only minimizes leaks but avoids pressure on the bridge of the nose and prevents future face deformity.[68] Nocturnal ventilation is often best instituted via IPPV with a portable volume ventilator.[68,75] Ventilator settings should be adjusted to mimic age- and weight-based norms for tidal volume and respiratory rate. In older children, bilevel respiratory assist devices may be used, but because pressure levels are set, they do not accommodate progressive changes in muscle weakness. However, new volume-targeted pressure devices offer a suitable, more compact alternative that can automatically accommodate increasing muscle weakness.

Often, nocturnal ventilatory assistance improves both nocturnal and **diurnal ventilation,** and the overnight rest allows the respiratory muscles to improve daytime stamina.[68] In fact, most patients use diurnal IPPV for the first time

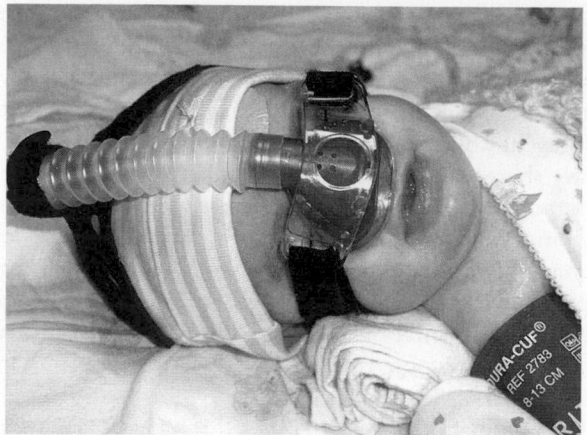

FIGURE 33-3 Infant nasal bilevel positive airway pressure. Nasal ventilation is the most practical means of noninvasive ventilatory support for small children. Although fittings for custom headgear may be necessary, younger children and infants can often be easily fitted with nasal interfaces such as adapted continuous positive airway pressure circuits or nasal pillows, nasal masks, or full face masks.

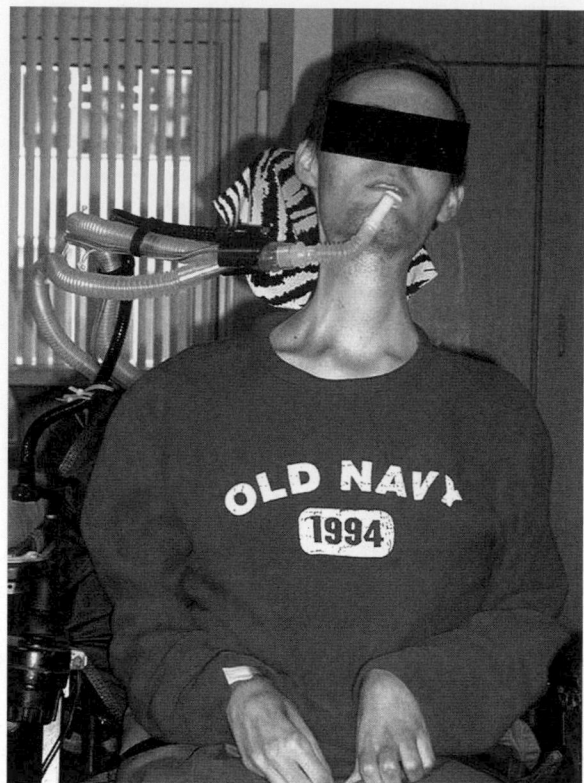

FIGURE 33-4 Mouthpiece ventilation. Mouthpiece intermittent positive pressure ventilation is a safe and effective means of chronic ventilation, even in patients with respiratory failure and no reserve. This mode of support is often preferred by adolescents and adults because it both provides adequate respiratory support and permits normal social interaction

during chest infections, weaning off and returning to isolated nocturnal use, for periods lasting up to several years.[75,76]

Diurnal Ventilation

Daytime use of ventilatory assistance becomes necessary when patients develop end-diurnal hypoventilation.[76] Again, the goal of ventilatory assistance is normalization of arterial blood gas and elimination of respiratory symptoms.[68,76] Ample evidence exists that children, adolescents, and adults who are able to cooperate overwhelmingly prefer noninvasive ventilation.[76,77]

Mouthpiece IPPV has now been studied in several cohorts of end-stage patients and has been demonstrated to be a safe and effective means of chronic ventilation, even in patients with respiratory failure and no reserve (Figure 33-4).[68,76] It is extremely well tolerated by patients, even in sleep,[68] is a user-friendly system during eating and social activities, and is also relatively inexpensive.[76]

Tracheostomy

Tracheostomy has long been a part of traditional management for patients with progressive neuromuscular weakness.[68,78] Often, tracheostomy tubes are placed during times of respiratory crisis, during or after bouts of respiratory failure triggered by chest infections.[79] Newer therapeutic approaches to patients with neuromuscular weakness discourage tracheostomy, not only because it is often unnecessary but also because noninvasive support is overwhelmingly preferred by patients. Tracheostomy tubes present numerous disadvantages by impeding normal swallowing and phonation and limiting social interactions; in addition, more advanced in-home health care assistance and intensive follow-up is required. Hygiene

issues are also a concern when considering a tracheostomy tube. Tube and stoma care can be uncomfortable, skin breakdown at the stoma site leads to cutaneous infections, and tracheostomy tubes risk sudden plugging with mucus, which can be life threatening.[68]

Although adolescents and adults prefer noninvasive ventilatory aids for all the reasons given previously, it is important to mention that tracheostomy has also been favorably viewed by many patients. For example, in a 2000 survey in which patients with DMD and amyotrophic lateral sclerosis were surveyed on their quality of life, more than two thirds were satisfied with their lives and 84% believed they had made the right choice.[80] In general, we recommend that as patients demonstrate a need for ventilatory assistance, noninvasive ventilation be pursued first. Tracheostomy is probably best reserved for those patients with severe bulbar weakness and chronic aspiration, if arterial blood gas tensions can no longer be controlled, if there are patient–interface difficulties, or if there is failure to thrive.[70] It is also important to remember that a subpopulation of patients—those with spinal cord injury and Guillain-Barré in particular—may benefit from temporary tracheostomies to facilitate hospital discharge and entry into a rehabilitation program. The long-term goal in these cases is to improve respiratory muscle strength, permitting successful decannulation.

Although more and more centers are developing expertise with chronic noninvasive ventilation, a survey of Jerry Lewis Muscular Dystrophy Association clinics from 1997 showed that few used any form of cough assist and only 20% used mouthpiece positive pressure ventilation.[81] The reasons for this are explained by a combination of family and practitioner unfamiliarity with noninvasive methods, and poor availability or uncertainty about how to use home cough assist devices. This underscores the importance of connecting patients and their families early in the course of the disease with an accredited center caring for a high volume of patients with neuromuscular disease.

Nonrespiratory Care

General medical concerns will cross all stages of growth and development for children with neuromuscular weakness, and attention must be paid to nutritional and cardiac status, extent of scoliosis and restrictive respiratory disease, the contribution of weakness to other organ system functioning, the need for communication assistance, and mental health care. Some of these concerns, such as cardiomyopathy and arrhythmias, relate to the multisystem effects of the neuromuscular conditions. Others, such as surgical correction of contractures and scoliosis, can be an important strategy in maintaining mobility and preserving lung function.[47]

End-of-life care issues are inevitable in the course of progressive neuromuscular disease. In the discussion of these events it is important to provide the facts and answer every question fully and in terms the parents or patient can understand, without frightening technical language. This communication is one of the most difficult tasks in providing care to these patients. It requires tact, skill, empathy, and complete support of any decisions made by the parents or patient. The three primary goals include deciding on end-stage pain and dyspnea control, providing spiritual and psychiatric support, and respecting choices concerning tests and treatments.[48]

TRANSITION TO ADULTHOOD

Improved technology and advances in respiratory care have significantly increased the life expectancy of children with neuromuscular weakness.[82] Transition to adulthood requires increasing reliance on ventilator assistance, nursing support, and assistive technologies to help achieve independent living.[59] Another issue that persists across all childhood chronic illnesses is the need for age-appropriate caregivers, so that older adolescents and adults can begin to receive care in an adult health care environment.[83]

Children with neuromuscular weakness require more life-sustaining equipment and assistance in achieving independence. More personal assistance, either from family or skilled nursing, is required in providing basic care needs.[68] Increased support has been associated not only with extended life expectancy but improved quality of life as well.[61,84] Unfortunately, the timing of instituting these assistive technologies and skilled nursing care remains dependent on the individual patient and clinical scenario.[64]

Successful transition requires attention to the challenges associated with providing ventilatory assistance to the young adult with neuromuscular weakness. Additional issues during the transition process include facilitating coordination of care among multiple subspecialists, establishing a cadre of skilled caregivers, and arranging support for maintaining activities of daily living. If successful, the transition is likely to result in continued maintenance of a high quality of life despite the physical limitations associated with the underlying condition.[84]

KEY POINTS

- Understanding neuromuscular control of respiration and airway clearance is important in avoiding associated complications and developing the best plan of therapy.
- Being proactive with assisted ventilation in a progressive neuromuscular disease can help avoid pulmonary infections and sequelae.
- Early monitoring of disease progression with pulmonary function testing can assist with proactive therapy before signs and symptoms of hypoventilation or ineffective airway clearance.
- Newer therapeutic approaches to patients with neuromuscular weakness discourage tracheostomy.
- Communication is one of the most difficult tasks in providing care to progressive neuromuscular disease patients. It requires tact, skill, empathy, and complete support of any decision made by the parents or patients.

ASSESSMENT QUESTIONS

See Evolve Resources for answers.

1. Which of the following are muscles of inspiration?
    I. Diaphragm
    II. Internal intercostals
    III. External intercostals
    IV. External oblique muscles
    V. Rectus abdominus
        A. I and II
        B. I and III
        C. I, III, and V
        D. II and IV
        E. I, IV, and V

2. Which condition(s) of the central nervous system affect(s) respiration?
   A. Tay-Sachs disease
   B. Congenital hydrocephalus
   C. Congenital central hypoventilation syndrome
   D. A, B, and C
   E. B and C
3. Which condition is the most common myopathy affecting respiratory muscle function in childhood?
   A. Spinal muscular atrophy
   B. Myasthenia gravis
   C. Muscular dystrophy
   D. Guillain-Barré
   E. Scoliosis
4. Guillain-Barré is an acute, autoimmune process that affects the peripheral nervous system and causes:
   A. Inevitable respiratory failure, tracheostomy, and mechanical ventilation
   B. Hereditary weakness that progresses from the legs to the arms
   C. Mild hydrocephalus and confusion along with chest wall weakness
   D. Demyelination of the peripheral nerve sheaths, leading to conduction abnormalities
   E. Pain, starting in the arms and chest and leading to arm and chest weakness
5. Which of the following is an autoimmune disorder of infancy and childhood, which occurs when antibodies block synaptic receptors at the neuromuscular junction?
   A. Myotonic dystrophy
   B. Pediatric botulism toxicity
   C. Infantile spinal muscular atrophy
   D. Juvenile myasthenia gravis
   E. Infantile transitional myasthenia gravis
6. A neuromuscular disease evaluation of the respiratory system of a child with neuromuscular weakness might include which of the following?
   I. Spirometry with a flow–volume loop
   II. Polysomnography
   III. Electroencephalogram
   IV. Mixed venous blood gases
   V. Maximal inspiratory and expiratory pressures
   A. I and V
   B. I, II, and V
   C. III and V
   D. II, III, and V
   E. II, III, and IV
7. There are several phases of a normal cough to create sufficient cough flow for effective pulmonary clearance. The patient with neuromuscular weakness:
   A. Is unable to produce peak cough flows
   B. May have difficulty with any of the phases of an effective cough
   C. Is able to produce high expiratory flows but does not generate enough volume for an effective cough
   D. Has impaired glottic closure and diaphragmatic force for an effective cough
   E. Does not have true impairment of cough flows, because it is relative to the reduced vital capacity

8. Glossopharyngeal breathing:
   A. Is known as "frog breathing," which inflates the lungs by gulping air
   B. Has limited effectiveness in patients with bulbar weakness
   C. May provide normal alveolar ventilation in the case of a malfunctioning mechanical ventilator
   D. A and B only
   E. All of the above
9. Select the two indications for initiating nocturnal ventilatory assistance for a pediatric patient with neuromuscular weakness:
   I. Supine negative inspiratory force of 60 to 90 cm H_2O
   II. Hypercapnia during sleep with end-tidal carbon dioxide levels in excess of 50 mm Hg
   III. Documented evidence of right-sided heart failure with peaked P waves on electrocardiogram (ECG)
   IV. Arterial oxygen tension less than 88 mm Hg during 20% of the sleep study
   V. Oxygen desaturation to less than 95% during sleep and symptoms of respiratory insufficiency
   A. I and III
   B. I and V
   C. II and IV
   D. II and V
   E. III and IV
10. Placing a tracheostomy tube to facilitate mechanical ventilation for progressive neuromuscular weakness:
   A. Is reserved only for patients with severe bulbar weakness, chronic aspiration, and inability to maintain acceptable blood gas values
   B. May be temporary in children with spinal cord injury or Guillain-Barré
   C. May be temporary to provide rest of the respiratory muscles and aggressive pulmonary hygiene
   D. A and B
   E. B and C

References

1. Shahrizaila N, Kinnear W, Wills A: Respiratory involvement in inherited primary muscle conditions, *J Neurol Neurosurg Psychiatry* 77:1108, 2006.
2. Widdicombe J: Reflexes from the lungs and airways: historical perspectives, *J Appl Physiol* 101:628, 2006.
3. Benditt JO: The neuromuscular respiratory system: physiology, pathophysiology, and a respiratory care approach to patients, *Respir Care* 51:829, discussion 837, 2006.
4. Derenne JP, et al: History of diaphragm physiology: the achievements of Galen, *Eur Respir J* 8:154, 1995.
5. Remmers JE: A century of control of breathing, *Am J Respir Crit Care Med* 172:6, 2005.
6. Phillipson E, Duffin J: *Hypoventilation and hyperventilation syndromes*, ed 4, Philadelphia, 2005, Elsevier Saunders.
7. Sivak ED, Shefner JM, Sexton J: Neuromuscular disease and hypoventilation, *Curr Opin Pulm Med* 5:355, 1999.
8. Robinson D, Esau S: Assessment of ventilatory function in patients with neuromuscular disease, *Clin Chest Med* 18:751, 1994.

9. Polkey MI, Moxham J: Clinical aspects of respiratory muscle dysfunction in the critically ill, *Chest* 119:926, 2001.

10. Gaultier C, et al: Genetics and early disturbances of breathing control, *Pediatr Res* 55:729, 2004.

11. Chen ML, et al: Diaphragm pacers as a treatment for congenital central hypoventilation syndrome, *Expert Rev Med Devices* 2:577, 2005.

12. Williams H: A unifying hypothesis for hydrocephalus, Chiari malformation, syringomyelia, anencephaly and spina bifida, *Cerebrospinal Fluid Res* 5:7, 2008.

13. Gravel RA, Triggs-Raine BL, Mahuran DJ: Biochemistry and genetics of Tay-Sachs disease, *Can J Neurol Sci* 18(3 suppl):419, 1991.

14. National Center for Injury Prevention and Control, Centers for Disease Control and Prevention: *Spinal cord injury (SCI): fact sheet*, Bethesda, MD, 2008, Centers for Disease Control and Prevention, Available at: www.cdc.gov/ncipc/factsheets/scifacts.htm. Retrieved October 2008.

15. Netter F: *Atlas of human anatomy*, ed 4, Philadelphia, 2006, WB Saunders.

16. Hirschfeld S, Exner G, Luukaala T, Baer GA: Mechanical ventilation or phrenic nerve stimulation for treatment of spinal cord injury–induced respiratory insufficiency, *Spinal Cord* 46:738, 2008.

17. Fenoy AJ, Menezes AH, Fenoy KA: Craniocervical junction fusions in patients with hindbrain herniation and syringohydromyelia, *J Neurosurg Spine* 9:1, 2008.

18. Halawa A, Krishnaswamy G: Tussive headache with weakness and atrophy of the right hand, *Rev Neurol Dis* 4:224, 2007.

19. Kumar V, Abbas AK, Fauto N: *Robbins and Cotran pathologic basis of disease*, ed 7, Philadelphia, 2004, WB Saunders.

20. Laningham FH, et al: Childhood central nervous system leukaemia: historical perspectives, current therapy, and acute neurological sequelae, *Neuroradiology* 49:873, 2007.

21. De Jesus NH: Epidemics to eradication: the modern history of poliomyelitis, *Virol J* 4:70, 2007.

22. Bach JR, et al: Spinal muscular atrophy type 1: management and outcomes, *Pediatr Pulmonol* 34:16, 2002.

23. Ioos C, et al: Respiratory capacity course in patients with infantile spinal muscular atrophy, *Chest* 126:831, 2004.

24. Munsat TL, et al: Phenotypic heterogeneity of spinal muscular atrophy mapping to chromosome 5q11.2-13.3 (SMA 5q), *Neurology* 40:1831, 1990.

25. Russman BS, et al: Spinal muscular atrophy: new thoughts on the pathogenesis and classification schema, *J Child Neurol* 7:347, 1992.

26. Kaindl AM, et al: Spinal muscular atrophy with respiratory distress type 1 (SMARD1), *J Child Neurol* 23:199, 2008.

27. Chng SY, et al: Pulmonary function and scoliosis in children with spinal muscular atrophy types II and III, *J Paediatr Child Health* 39:673, 2003.

28. Lunn MR, Wang CH: Spinal muscular atrophy, *Lancet* 371:2120, 2008.

29. Gozal D: Pulmonary manifestations of neuromuscular disease with special reference to Duchenne muscular dystrophy and spinal muscular atrophy, *Pediatr Pulmonol* 29:141, 2000.

30. Kasper DL, Braunwald E, Fauci AS: *Harrison's principles of internal medicine*, ed 16, New York, 2004, McGraw-Hill.

31. Hauck LJ, et al: Incidence of Guillain-Barré syndrome in Alberta, Canada: an administrative data study, *J Neurol Neurosurg Psychiatry* 79:318, 2008.

32. Ehroni E, et al: Guillain-Barré syndrome in Greece: seasonality and other clinico-epidemiological features, *Eur J Neurol* 11:383, 2004.

33. Kleyweg RP, et al: The natural history of the Guillain-Barré syndrome in 18 children and 50 adults, *J Neurol Neurosurg Psychiatry* 52:853, 1989.

34. Sarnat H: *Guillain-Barré syndrome*, Philadelphia, 2007, Elsevier Saunders.

35. Finkelstein JS, Melek BH: Guillain-Barré syndrome as a cause of reversible cardiomyopathy, *Tex Heart Inst J* 33:57, 2006.

36. Winer JB: Treatment of Guillain-Barré syndrome, *QJM* 95:717, 2002.

37. Tseng-Ong L, Mitchell WG: Infant botulism: 20 years' experience at a single institution, *J Child Neurol* 22:1333, 2007.

38. Sobel J: Botulism, *Clin Infect Dis* 41:1167, 2005.

39. Glauser TA, Maguire HC, Sladky JT: Relapse of infant botulism, *Ann Neurol* 28:187, 1990.

40. Conti-Fine BM, Milani M, Kaminski HJ: Myasthenia gravis: past, present, and future, *J Clin Invest* 116:2843, 2006.

41. Vern JC, Massey JM: Myasthenia gravis, *Orphanet J Rare Dis* 2:44, 2007.

42. Kothari MJ: Myasthenia gravis, *J Am Osteopath Assoc* 104:377, 2004.

43. Thanvi BR, Lo TC: Update on myasthenia gravis, *Postgrad Med J* 80:690, 2004.

44. Batocchi A, et al: Early-onset myasthenia gravis: clinical characteristics and response to therapy, *Eur J Pediatr* 150:66, 1990.

45. Misulis KE, Fenichel GM: Genetic forms of myasthenia gravis, *Pediatr Neurol* 5:205, 1989.

46. Djelmis J, et al: Myasthenia gravis in pregnancy: report on 69 cases, *Eur J Obstet Gynecol Reprod Biol* 104:21, 2002.

47. Emery AE: The muscular dystrophies, *Lancet* 359:687, 2002.

48. Birnkrant DJ, et al: American College of Chest Physicians consensus statement on the respiratory and related management of patients with Duchenne muscular dystrophy undergoing anesthesia or sedation, *Chest* 132:1977, 2007.

49. Bach JR, Ishikawa Y, Kim H: Prevention of pulmonary morbidity for patients with Duchenne muscular dystrophy, *Chest* 112:1024, 1997.

50. Cardamone M, Darras DT, Ryan MM: Inherited myopathies and muscular dystrophies, *Semin Neurol* 28:250, 2008.

51. Kishanni PS, Chen Y-T: *Glycogen storage diseases*, ed 15, Philadelphia, 1996, WB Saunders.

52. Katzin LW, Amato AA: Pompe disease: a review of the current diagnosis and treatment recommendations in the era of enzyme replacement therapy, *J Clin Neuromuscul Dis* 9:421, 2008.

53. Pellegrini N, et al: Respiratory insufficiency and limb muscle weakness in adults with Pompe's disease, *Eur Respir J* 26:1024, 2005.

54. Marino PL: *The ICU book*, ed 2, Philadelphia, 1998, Lippincott Williams & Wilkins.

55. McCarty M, Jagoda A, Fairweather P: Hyperkalemic ascending paralysis [report], *Ann Emerg Med* 32:104, 1998.

56. Pathare N, et al: Deficit in human muscle strength with cast immobilization: contribution of inorganic phosphate, *Eur J Appl Physiol* 98:71, 2006.

57. Nicot F, et al: Respiratory muscle testing: a valuable tool for children with neuromuscular disorders, *Am J Respir Crit Care Med* 174:67, 2006.

58. Koessler W, et al: Two years' experience with inspiratory muscle training in patients with neuromuscular disorders, *Chest* 120:765, 2001.

59. Panitch HB: Respiratory issues in the management of children with neuromuscular disease, *Respir Care* 51:885, discussion 894, 2006.

60. Steier J, et al: The values of multiple tests of respiratory muscle strength, *Thorax* 62:975, 2007.

61. Finder JD, et al: Respiratory care of the patient with Duchenne muscular dystrophy: ATS consensus statement, *Am J Respir Crit Care Med* 170:456, 2004.

62. Gauld LM, Boynton A: Relationship between peak cough flow and spirometry in Duchenne muscular dystrophy, *Pediatr Pulmonol* 39:457, 2005.

63. Dhand UK, Dhand R: Sleep disorders in neuromuscular diseases, *Curr Opin Pulm Med* 12:402, 2006.

64. Toussaint M, Chatwin M, Soudon P: Mechanical ventilation in Duchenne patients with chronic respiratory insufficiency: clinical implications of 20 years published experience, *Chron Respir Dis* 4:167, 2007.

65. Birnkrant DJ: The assessment and management of the respiratory complications of pediatric neuromuscular diseases, *Clin Pediatr* 41:301, 2002.

66. Simonds AK: Respiratory complications of the muscular dystrophies, *Semin Respir Crit Care Med* 23:231, 2002.

67. Panitch HB: Airway clearance in children with neuromuscular weakness, *Curr Opin Pediatr* 18:277, 2006.

68. Bach JR: *Management of patients with neuromuscular disease,* Philadelphia, 2004, Hanley & Belfus.

69. Toussaint M, et al: Effect of intrapulmonary percussive ventilation on mucus clearance in Duchenne muscular dystrophy patients: a preliminary report, *Respir Care* 48:940, 2003.

70. Simonds AK: Recent advances in respiratory care for neuromuscular disease, *Chest* 130:1879, 2006.

71. Bach JR: New approaches in the rehabilitation of the traumatic high level quadriplegic, *Am J Phys Med Rehabil* 70:13, 1991.

72. Bach JR, Alba AS: Noninvasive options for ventilatory support of the traumatic high level quadriplegic patient, *Chest* 98:613, 1990.

73. Rideau Y, et al: Prolongation of life in Duchenne's muscular dystrophy, *Acta Neurol* 5:118, 1983; and Bach JR, Alba AS, Saporito LR: Intermittent positive pressure ventilation via the mouth as an alternative to tracheostomy for 257 ventilator users, *Chest* 103:174, 1993. As cited in Simonds AK, et al: Impact of nasal ventilation on survival in hypercapnic Duchenne muscular dystrophy, *Thorax* 53:949, 1998.

74. Laub M, Berg S, Midgren B: Symptoms, clinical and physiological findings motivating home mechanical ventilation in patients with neuromuscular diseases, *J Rehabil Med* 38:250, 2006.

75. Tzeng AC, Bach JR: Prevention of pulmonary morbidity for patients with neuromuscular disease, *Chest* 118:1390, 2000.

76. Toussaint M, et al: Diurnal ventilation via mouthpiece: survival in end-stage Duchenne patients, *Eur Respir J* 28:549, 2006.

77. Bach JR, Alba AS, Saporito LR: Intermittent positive pressure ventilation via the mouth as an alternative to tracheostomy for 257 ventilator users, *Chest* 103:174, 1993.

78. Bach JR: Medical considerations of long-term survival of Werdnig-Hoffman disease, *Am J Phys Med Rehabil* 86:349, 2007.

79. Bach J, et al: Neuromuscular ventilatory insufficiency: effect of home mechanical ventilator use v. oxygen therapy on pneumonia and hospitalization rates, *Am J Phys Med Rehabil* 77:8, 1998.

80. Narayanaswami P, et al: Long-term tracheostomy ventilation in neuromuscular diseases: patient acceptance and quality of life, *Neurorehabil Neural Repair* 14:135, 2000.

81. Bach JR, Chaudhry SS: Muscular Dystrophy Association: standards of care in MDA clinics, *Am J Phys Med Rehabil* 79:193, 2000.

82. Scal P, et al: Trends in transition from pediatric to adult health care services for young adults with chronic conditions, *J Adolesc Health* 24:259, 1999.

83. Denboba D, et al: Achieving family and provider partnerships with children with special health care needs, *Pediatrics* 118:1607, 2006.

84. Kohler M, et al: Quality of life, physical disability, and respiratory impairment in Duchenne muscular dystrophy, *Am J Respir Crit Care Med* 172:1032, 2005.

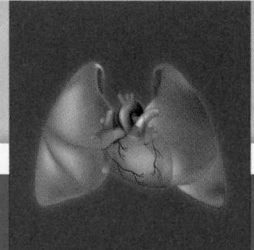

Chapter 34

Transport of Infants and Children

STEVEN E. SITTIG

LEARNING OBJECTIVES

After reading this chapter the reader will be able to:

1. Discuss and recognize the importance of team composition, roles, and education
2. Review and compare the caveats of each mode of transport
3. Explain the role of communication during a medical transport
4. List the specific equipment needed for pediatric transport
5. Demonstrate how to provide a patient assessment in a nontraditional environment
6. Review safety and accreditation requirements for pediatric transport agencies

KEY TERMS

Dedicated transport teams   UHF/AM transceiver   Unit-based transport teams

Since the late 1980s the care of the critically ill pediatric patient has seen rapid development in technology and improvement in patient outcomes. Today many infants and children who previously would have died are surviving. The cost of such care has necessitated regionalization of intensive care centers to larger tertiary care centers. This regionalization has led to the need for safe and effective patient transport systems. For neonatal transport, antenatal transport of the mother and high-risk fetus to a tertiary center is preferred unless contraindicated because of maternal complicating factors.[1,2] However, antenatal referral is not always possible and the critically ill neonate must often be transported after birth. In most states the operation of a neonatal/pediatric transport team will be based at neonatal/pediatric tertiary centers. Each state typically has its own specific rules and regulations for staffing, training, equipment, and safety. There are few things more challenging and yet rewarding to clinicians than transporting critically ill infants and children from a local hospital to a tertiary care medical center. Respiratory therapists must adjust their focus to monitoring the status of patients and performing procedures while operating in a dynamic environment, such as a moving ambulance or aircraft.

The ages, sizes, and diagnoses of transported neonatal and pediatric patients encompass virtually the entire scope of the critically ill population, from the 500-g infant to the 100-kg adolescent. The skilled, rapid transport of neonatal and pediatric patients suffering from serious illness or trauma to facilities specializing in the care of these patients has resulted in significantly improved outcomes.[3-6] The skilled transport of critically ill patients is an intervention of the highest value and an activity in which respiratory therapists should be proud, enthusiastic, and encouraged to participate.

TEAM COMPOSITION

Staffing

Critical care transport requires experienced personnel with advanced clinical skills, additional training, and education. If the team is to function autonomously, they must work together with others involved in the transport process. Personnel are the single most valuable assets of any transport system. Because the stabilization and critical care skills required for the critically ill pediatric patient are specialized, the composition of the team is important. Team composition varies among different health care institutions across the country. More important than the exact credentialing of the transport personnel is the training and skills of the team. A qualified transport team should consist of individuals who have typically 2 years pediatric/neonatal critical care experience and training in the special needs of children during transport and who have participated in the transport of these patients with the frequency to maintain their expertise.[7] Transport team members must often function with a high workload of critical tasks that are frequently evolving, and thus the team must adapt dynamically to achieve its goals.[8]

Most transport teams are composed of one or more of the following health care team members:

· A registered nurse
· A respiratory therapist
· An emergency medical technician
· A neonatal nurse practitioner
· A staff physician, resident, or fellow

Data show that most pediatric transport teams in the United States are led by a nurse and accompanied by a respiratory therapist. The use of a specialized pediatric transport team (registered nurse and respiratory therapist) has been shown to result in lower morbidity than the traditional emergency medical services (EMS) helicopter staffed with a flight/trauma nurse and a paramedic.[9-11] The bulk of the research on prehospital care has focused on the adult population. Consequently, little of the care provided by EMS to pediatric patients is based on evidence from prehospital care research.[12,13] A respiratory therapist is at an advantage because of the large number of transported pediatric patients who require respiratory support. The background and training of nurses and respiratory therapists are so different that such a team creates a broader scope of knowledge and experience when both are used. This combination works successfully in the majority of critical care and even routine transports.[14] A recent national survey showed that neonatal transport teams primarily are comprised of registered nurses and respiratory therapists.[15]

Although many nonneonatal pediatric teams may include a resident or attending physician, there is little published evidence that this team model offers improved outcomes compared with non–physician-based teams. All pediatric transport teams should have a mechanism to identify critical patient transports that may require the addition of a physician to the transport team. All team members should be cross-trained so that each member of the team can function at the other's skill level. The medical director of the pediatric transport program should be a critical care intensivist, anesthesiologist, or neonatologist with an interest in transport medicine.[16]

Though most exclusive neonatal/pediatric transport teams are affiliated with children's hospitals, the administrative home of the transport team varies with each institution. **Unit-based transport teams** are staffed and scheduled within the intensive care units (ICUs) or, in the case of respiratory therapists, within the respiratory care department. The transport staff are generally given a patient care assignment and then "pulled" from that assignment when a transport call is received. This patient assignment is then back filled by the department staff or an on-call person is used to fill the assignment until the transport is completed. From an administrative standpoint this is the most cost effective use of personnel resources.

Dedicated transport teams are scheduled and staffed separately from the ICU personnel. These staff members generally "float" throughout the hospital without a patient assignment when they are not on transport. They are there to assist other hospital personnel but can leave immediately when a transport call is received. A large volume of transports is necessary to justify a dedicated transport team. Most transport programs have found that once volumes exceed 1000 to 1200 transports per year, it is fiscally advantageous to allocate the resources for a dedicated transport team. Personnel accustomed to managing transport coordination are the best suited for accomplishing the relatively complex logistics of transporting critically ill patients.

The objective of adequate staffing is to ensure that each member of the transport team has the opportunity to participate in enough transports per month (15 to 20 per month) to maintain a high level of competency while at the same time making sure not to overwork the staff and create "burnout." Transport team professionals have unique responsibilities and are exposed to powerful demands. They cannot avoid incidents that pose personal threats to their own emotional well-being. Contact with dead or severely ill or injured children, for example, can be detrimental to the caregiver.[17]

Box 34-1   Minimal Requirements for Transport Team Members

TRANSPORT NURSE
- Licensed by the state
- Two years of experience as a registered nurse, including 12 months of neonatal intensive care unit/pediatric intensive care unit (NICU/PICU) experience
- Current basic cardiac life support (BCLS) certification
- Current neonatal resuscitation program (NRP) certification
- Current pediatric advanced life support (PALS) certification
- Current advanced cardiac life support (ACLS) certification
- Certificate of added qualification in neonatal pediatric transport (C-NPT)—National Certification Corporation (NCC)
- Has participated in a pediatric transport course and has demonstrated a working knowledge of transport equipment and transport supplies
- Has observed a program-specified number of transports and been checked off by preceptor and medical control physician before being released for transport duty

TRANSPORT RESPIRATORY THERAPIST
- Registered respiratory therapist (RRT) by the National Board for Respiratory Care (NBRC)
- Neonatal and pediatric specialty credentialed (RRT-NPS) by the National Board for Respiratory Care
- Licensed by the state
- Two years of NICU/PICU experience
- Current BCLS certification
- Current NRP certification
- Current PALS certification
- Current ACLS certification
- Certificate of Added Qualification in Neonatal Pediatric Transport (C-NPT)—National Certification Corporation (NCC)
- Has participated in a pediatric transport course and has demonstrated a working knowledge of transport equipment and transport supplies
- Has observed a program-specified number of transports and been checked off by preceptor and medical control physician before being released for transport duty

Training

The neonatal/pediatric transport team plays a vital role in the transport of critically ill children to tertiary pediatric facilities. Pediatric transport practitioners are experienced personnel requiring a wide range of high-level clinical competence dealing with many diseases affecting children. The team must be comfortable caring for critically ill patients, whether at a small referral hospitals or during the transport process itself by ground ambulance or air. The transport team is a vital component of successful patient care during transport to a tertiary care center. This highly specialized team brings the basic services of the neonatal intensive care unit (NICU) or pediatric intensive care unit (PICU) to the patient's bedside.

The qualities of the team members are as important as the team composition. The selection process should include interviews not only with the nursing and respiratory leadership but with the medical director of the transport team under whose license the person will operate. Ideal candidates should have exemplary clinical skills, leadership and decision-making abilities, flexibility, compassion, and assertiveness, all while working in a high-stress transport service.

See Box 34-1 for a list of minimal requirements for transport team members.

Inadequate training of pediatric caregivers has been correlated with increased morbidity.[8,9] Several different professional organizations have developed training/educational requirements for pediatric transport teams. The Air & Surface Transport Nurses Association (ASTNA, Greenwood Village, CO), American Association for Respiratory Care (AARC, Irving, TX), Commission on Accreditation of Medical Transport Systems (CAMTS, Anderson, SC), American Academy of Pediatrics (AAP, Elk Grove Village, IL), and National Certification Corporation (NCC, Chicago, IL) are commonly recognized. In general, they recommend that transport nurses and respiratory therapists have at least 2 years of pediatric critical care experience. Annual recurrent training should include didactic material and hands-on training in procedures that are used during transport (Box 34-2). The use of high-fidelity patient simulation has also grown in acceptance of neonatal and pediatric transport team members.

Additional courses such as Pediatric Fundamental Critical Care offered by the Society of Critical Care Medicine and the neonatal-focused S.T.A.B.L.E. program also offer didactic training options.

Simulation-Based Medical Education

Simulation-based medical education (SBME) is believed to be superior to the traditional style of medical education

Box 34-2   Annual Recurrent Training Topics*

- Advanced airway management
- Central line/umbilical artery line insertion
- Peripheral intravenous catheters/interosseous placement (IO)
- Thermoregulation
- Identification and treatment of pneumothorax
- Stabilization of critically ill pediatric patients
- Acid-base balance
- High-altitude physiology (for air transport)
- Stress factors in transport (e.g., noise, vibration)
- Transport equipment operation
- Transport-based simulation scenarios
- Aircraft/ambulance safety procedures
- Aircraft evacuation drills
- Community relations

*Not exclusive.

from the viewpoint of the active and adult learning theories. SBME can provide a learning cycle of debriefing and feedback for learners as well as evaluation of procedures and competency. SBME offers both learners and patients a safe environment for practice and error. Effective team performance in complex environments requires that team members hold a shared understanding of the task, their equipment, and their teammates. Therefore many of the simulation-based training (SBT) systems and programs have been designed (partly) to enhance shared/team cognition.[18-20]

MODES OF TRANSPORTATION

The single largest expense of a transport program is in the operation and maintenance of its transport vehicles. The selection of specific vehicles is an important decision that must include many different factors. The vehicles must be safe and have the operational characteristics appropriate for the program requirements. All vehicles used to transport patients must comply with local, state, and federal guidelines for both air and ground ambulances. The vehicles must have 110-volt AC electrical power available for the medical equipment used during transport. There should be sufficient medical gas (medical air and oxygen) capacity for all transport operations plus reserve capacity for use in the event of mechanical breakdown. The vehicles must also have provisions for suction equipment. The medical equipment used in transport, as well as the stretcher/incubator, must be safely secured within the vehicle during transport. The vehicle must have interior room that will allow the transport team to treat and assess the patient and, on occasion, perform procedures safely during transport.[21] All transport vehicles must have two-way communication capability, using radios or cellular phones. Each mode of transport—ground, rotor wing (helicopter), and fixed wing (airplane)—has advantages and disadvantages. The vehicle chosen should be appropriate for the patient population and geographical area served.

Ground Transport

Ground transport should be considered when distances are 30 miles or less one way for critical patients and less than 80 miles one way for stable patients. The ground transport vehicle should be an ambulance equipped with the special equipment needed for intensive care transport. The ambulance should have a hydraulic or electrical lift for loading the heavy transport incubators used in neonatal transport (Figure 34-1). The incubator should be secured by a designed floor-securing system or at minimum with four-point restraint straps.[22] The ambulance interior should be large enough to secure two transport incubators for transport of twins and room to seat the transport team members required for the care of two patients.

Advantages and disadvantages of ground transportation are listed in Box 34-3.

Air Transport
Rotor Wing

Helicopters are effective for rapid transport of critical patients within a 30- to 150-mile radius.[23] The size of the helicopter and the corresponding size of the cabin within the helicopter must be adequate to handle the equipment and transport team members. The transport team must be able to access and treat the patient during flight should an emergency arise. A neonatal transport

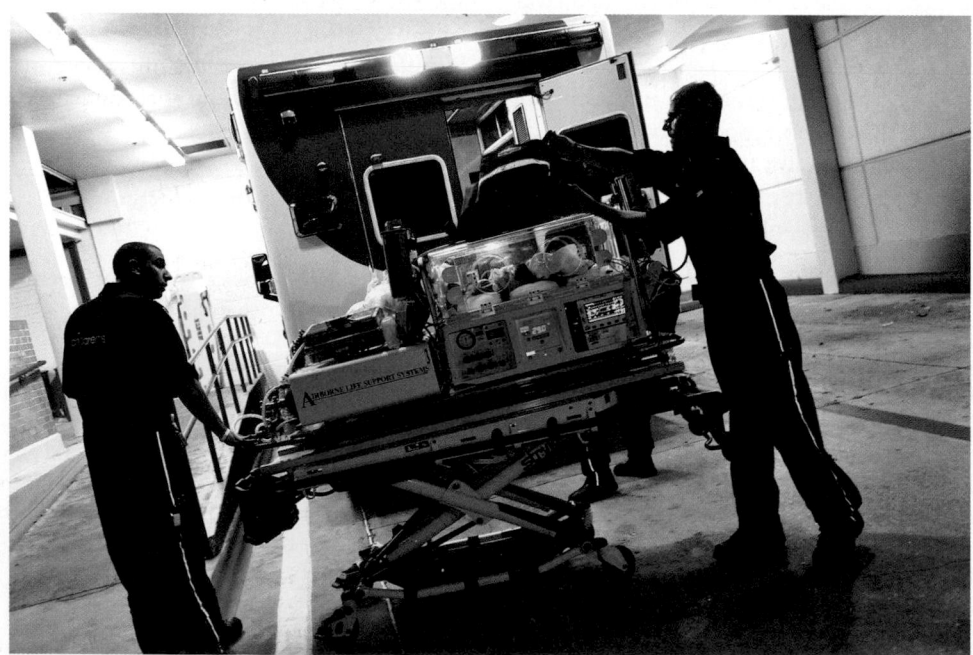

FIGURE 34-1   Ambulance with stretcher mounted neonatal transport incubator.

Box 34-3 | **Advantages and Disadvantages of Ground Transportation**

ADVANTAGES
- Lowest operating cost
- Ability to go directly from hospital to hospital
- Ability to carry a large number of staff and equipment
- Ability to transport in poor weather

DISADVANTAGES
- Slower response time over greater distances
- Can be slowed or stopped by traffic congestion
- Road noise and vibration

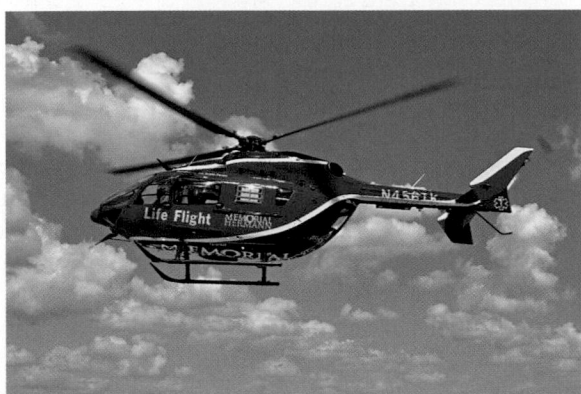

FIGURE 34-2 Memorial Hermann Life Flight® operates a mid-sized twin-engine helicopter that has the capacity to transport a neonatal transport team with a transport incubator.

Box 34-4 | **Advantages and Disadvantages of Rotor Wing Transportation**

ADVANTAGES
- Rapid response time within a 30- to 150-mile radius
- Ability to fly directly from hospital to hospital

DISADVANTAGES
- High operating and capital expenses
- Small operating radius without refueling
- Small cabin area allows limited medical procedures (no cabin pressurization)
- Limited payload for personnel and equipment
- Inability to fly in inclement weather

---

team with a transport incubator will typically require a midsized twin-engine aircraft in order to have enough room for proper patient care (Figure 34-2).

Advantages and disadvantages of helicopters are listed in Box 34-4.

Fixed-Wing Aircraft

Airplanes are effective for long-distance patient transport. Because airplanes fly from airport to airport, the increased coordination of ground ambulances for two airports, the time required to load and unload at both airports, and the additional ground transport time must be balanced against the time required to drive from hospital to hospital. Under normal circumstances the time needed to drive 120 miles is greater than the fixed-wing aircraft transport time for the same distance. All airplanes used for critical patient transport should have the ability to control the cabin altitude (pressurization), which makes the transport of critically ill patients with marginal arterial oxygenation possible (Figure 34-3).

Advantages and disadvantages of airplanes are listed in Box 34-5.

EQUIPMENT

The equipment, both communication and medical, carried on board an ambulance, helicopter, or airplane will need to meet various standards. In general, the equipment should be as lightweight as possible, both electrical and battery operated, and should not interfere electromagnetically with aircraft navigation or communication equipment.[24] It should be as ruggedly constructed as possible. All equipment should be well secured for the duration of transport.[22]

Communications

The transport team should always have the ability to communicate with the online medical control physician who is supervising the transport. This communication has traditionally been accomplished via radio for both ground and air transport. However, the use of cellular phones in ground ambulances has steadily increased, especially with more cellular companies offering a "walkie-talkie"–type option. Both helicopters and airplanes are equipped with VHF radios for communicating with air traffic control. EMS helicopters are generally equipped with another type of radio, called a **UHF/AM transceiver.** This additional radio allows communication with ground support agencies (fire, police, etc.) and their dispatch centers. The transport teams on the helicopter can contact their online medical control via this UHF radio. Because of the short-range limitations of UHF radios, fixed-wing air ambulances should be equipped with a satellite-type cell phone for air-to-hospital communication. This will allow communication from just about any location around the world.

Medical
Monitoring Equipment

Electrocardiogram monitoring, pulse oximetry monitoring (SaO_2), and blood pressure monitoring are standard practice during the transport of critically ill patients. Most modern transport monitors incorporate the following:
- Electrocardiograph (ECG)
- SaO_2 (pulse oximeter)
- Noninvasive blood pressure monitoring (blood pressure cuff)

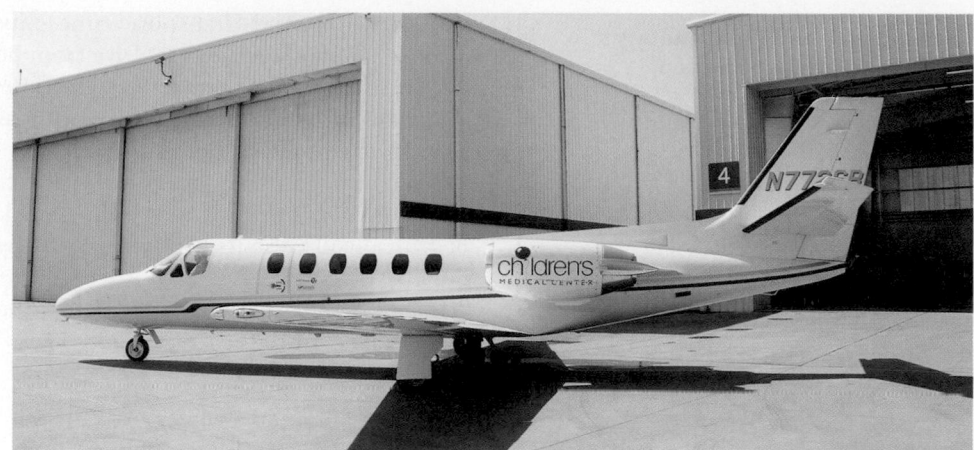

FIGURE 34-3   A jet-engine aircraft that has the ability to transport two patients and five medical crew members within a pressurized cabin.

Box 34-5	Advantages and Disadvantages of Airplanes

ADVANTAGES
- Rapid response time for distances greater than 120 miles
- Ability to fly long distances
- Larger cabin area to allow for more medical procedures
- Ability to control cabin altitude (pressurization)
- Larger payload for equipment and personnel including family members
- Ability to fly in inclement weather

DISADVANTAGES
- Moderate operating and capital expenses
- Requires an airport to land, and thus an ambulance transfer at both ends of the flight

- Invasive blood pressure monitoring (pressure transducers)
- Patient temperature monitoring (skin probes)

End-tidal carbon dioxide ($ETCO_2$) monitoring is a valuable option on most transport monitors; monitoring $ETCO_2$ provides the transport team with a visual method to ensure effective ventilation in the intubated patient during transport. Alarm limits should be set for each transport. Because of the high noise levels found in the transport environment, visual alarm indicators are usually more helpful than audible alarms.[25-27] Monitors with interchangeable battery packs allow for quicker turnaround times as an alternative to waiting for batteries to recharge.

Ventilator

Use of a transport ventilator will allow the transport team to provide the same level of care given or already established in an ICU. Transport ventilators are now available with most of the intensive care parameters (i.e., positive end-expiratory pressure, synchronized intermittent mandatory ventilation, noninvasive ventilation,

adjustable fraction of inspired oxygen, and pressure support) in small, portable, lightweight cases. Ventilators with external battery packs allow for quicker turnaround times compared with waiting for an internal battery to recharge. Many newer models now have "hot swappable" batteries that allow the operator to change out batteries while the ventilator continues to function. The decision to use a volume-limited or a pressure-limited ventilator should be based on the patient's size and ventilatory requirements. A manual resuscitation bag should always be carried on transport in the event of ventilator malfunction. Transport team members should be reminded that studies have shown there are tendencies to hyperventilate the patient while using a manual resuscitator.[28,29]

Transport Incubator

The ability to transport an infant with a body weight of 5 kg or less in a neutral thermal environment requires the use of a transport incubator. There are several commercially available transport incubators at present. They are modular units that allow customers to select among different models of heart monitors, ventilators, infusion pumps, and oxygen/air sources. When considering the purchase of a transport incubator, the first concern should be the type of vehicle in which the incubator will be transported. For example, the primary factor if planning to use the incubator in an aircraft (especially a helicopter) would be the weight and size of the incubator. Other factors to consider include battery power, which should be able to power the incubator for 2 to 3 hours; easy access to the infant without excessive heat loss; ability to visually monitor the infant at all times; and adequate lighting of the patient in dark areas.

Infusion Pumps

The syringe pump–type infusion pump is popular with transport teams because it requires no special tubing or cassette. A standard syringe (anywhere between 1 and 60 ml) is loaded onto the pump. The pump applies constant pressure to the plunger of the syringe and can be programmed for infusion rates from 0.1 to 999 ml/hr. These pumps are lightweight and battery powered, capable of running for 3 to 4 hours between charges. There are now also small portable infusion pumps that can use premixed bags of medication or fluid for larger volume infusions. These infusion pumps may even have built-in drug libraries in them.

Point-of-Care Testing

Pediatric transport teams are gradually moving to the use of a commercially available portable blood gas analyzer. Studies have shown that point-of-care testing reduces stabilization times and can have the potential to improve the quality of care during transport.[30-32] Most analyzers have a small, battery-powered, handheld unit and a variable set of testing cartridges. Transport teams are able to do blood analysis either during transport or at small outlying hospitals, which do not have the ability to analyze small blood samples. The following parameters can be determined with three or four drops of blood: pH, carbon dioxide pressure (PCO_2), oxygen pressure (PO_2), sodium (Na), potassium (K), ionized calcium (iCa), glucose (Glu), hematocrit (Hct), and hemoglobin (Hb).

Medications

The type and quantity of medications carried by the transport team should meet the requirements for care of the various patients transported. If the team operates under medical protocols, each medication carried should have its own protocol for use. Proper attention should be given to the storage of medication as well as a system to check for expiration of stored medications. Medications should be stored to prevent exposure of extreme temperatures of heat or cold. A process must also be developed to handle drugs requiring refrigeration, such as surfactant.

Medical Gas Supply

Pediatric transport teams who transport low birth weight infants will need to have both medical oxygen and medical air available while on transport. This will allow for the use of a blender to titrate the inspired oxygen of low-birth-weight infants. It is critical that the amounts of gas needed be calculated on the basis of projected use. The amount of gas taken should be approximately double that required. This allows for emergency usage in the event of mechanical breakdown of a vehicle. In ground ambulances, where weight is less of a consideration, additional medical gas supplies are usually provided by size H cylinders. This additional gas source allows the team to conserve the gas supply found on the incubator. In aircraft, where weight is a significant consideration, the use of aluminum and Kevlar cylinders has become the standard because of their low weight. Most fixed-wing aircraft have electrical air

compressors to provide medical air and liquid oxygen systems for medical oxygen, thus providing gases over a long duration. A small portable oxygen supply such as a D-sized cylinder should also be available for emergency use or equipment failure.

Supplies

The type and quantity of disposable supplies carried by the transport team should be sufficient for the proper care of the various patients transported. Weight and portability of the system to carry the needed supplies should be assessed.

PATIENT ASSESSMENT AND STABILIZATION

Assessment of the patient begins with the first phone call from the referring hospital. The basic information required to initiate a transport should include the following[33]:

- Name
- Weight
- General description of the patient's condition
- Any relevant medical history
- Current vital signs, including oxygen saturation, heart rate, respiratory rate, and blood pressure
- Any current major clinical problems
- Status of current lines, fluids, medications, treatments, etc.

The referring hospital should be given any recommendations for changes in medical management and the estimated time of arrival of the transport team. The referring hospital should also be given phone numbers and instructions to call back with any questions or significant changes in the patient condition before the transport team's arrival.

On arrival, assessment of the patient by the transport team should be thorough yet rapid. Stabilization at the referring hospital has become a much-discussed topic. The question of "stay and play" or "scoop and run" is debated in transport conferences across the country. The goal of the transport team should be to transport the patient in the most stable condition possible. Proper stabilization should be designed to minimize the number of adverse incidents (e.g., hypoxic or hypotensive events) that may occur during the transport. At the same time, the team should avoid the temptation to perform time-consuming therapeutic testing procedures while on transport. Before departure it is very helpful to briefly discuss with the family what has been done to stabilize their child and where the child will be admitted once the transport is completed. Directions and contact information for the receiving facility is also helpful for the family of the patient.

ADVANCED TRANSPORT

High-Altitude Physiology

A complete understanding of flight physiology is essential in order to provide optimal patient care in the air–medical environment.[34,35] Normal physiological responses to changing altitude are further complicated when transporting an already compromised patient.

Boyle's law states that at constant temperature, volume is inversely proportional to pressure. As the aircraft and patient rise in altitude, the volume of contained gases expands. This expansion has the following clinical implications for patient care:

- Increased respiratory rate and depth
- Changes in intravenous flow rates
- Nausea and vomiting
- Increased need to urinate
- Increased pain
- Endotracheal tube cuff expansion (prevented by filling the cuff with normal saline)
- Increased sinus pressure in the case of those with head colds or blocked sinuses

Dalton's law of partial pressure states that the pressure of a gas mixture equals the sum of the partial pressures of gases making up the mixture. As the aircraft climbs to altitude, the barometric pressure within the aircraft drops; the fraction of inspired oxygen remains the same (21%), but the delivery of oxygen to the patient is reduced because of decreased partial pressure.

Cabin pressurization allows the transport team to compensate for the decreased barometric pressure at flight altitude. Each aircraft manufacturer designs a maximal pressurization limit for their aircraft. This limit is based on the maximal pressure differential between cabin pressure and actual barometric pressure at flight altitude, which is expressed as a ratio of flight altitude to cabin pressure, each expressed as pounds per square inch (psi). Cabin pressurization creates an artificial atmospheric pressure inside the aircraft, known as *cabin altitude*. The cabin altitude can be adjusted from sea level to a maximal differential (usually 5000 to 6000 ft) depending on patient requirements and aircraft operations. An aircraft flown with a sea-level cabin altitude will not experience any of the effects of high altitude, but this could have a negative effect on the operation of the aircraft. Because of the pressure differential, the aircraft might need to be flown at a lower flight altitude to allow for the sea-level cabin pressurization. This lower flight altitude might increase the fuel burn (possibly requiring a fuel stop), slow the aircraft and thus increase transport time, and expose the aircraft to more severe weather concerns. Documentation of the cabin altitude during the patient transport should be included in the patient transport record. If for any reason flight cabin altitude may compromise the patient's condition, medical control should be contacted.

Most large twin-engine airplanes have pressurization systems. There are no helicopters with pressurization systems. It is imperative that the transport team be aware of an aircraft's abilities and limitations before employing the vehicle in patient care.

Nitric Oxide

The use of nitric oxide for the treatment of some congenital cardiac diseases and pulmonary hypertension in the neonatal and pediatric population is well established in the literature.[36] At many community hospitals, nitric oxide may also be administered to some very low birth weight premature infants to potentially lower the risk of lung and brain damage. Therefore it is likely that the number of requests to transport a patient already receiving nitric oxide will continue to increase. Furthermore, the beneficial effects of nitric oxide in the stabilization and transport of critically ill neonatal and pediatric patients may require transport teams to initiate the use of nitric oxide before transport.[37] The transport respiratory therapist must be able to integrate the nitric oxide delivery device with the patient's ventilator and monitor the various gas levels. As with all transport equipment, the nitric oxide delivery device should be as lightweight as possible, should be both electrically and battery operated, should not interfere electromagnetically with aircraft navigation or communication equipment, and should be ruggedly constructed.[34] The nitric oxide delivery device and the cylinder should be well secured for the duration of transport. A considerable amount of study has been focused on the exposure of the transport team to exhaled nitric oxide and on the scenario of a catastrophic release of gas from a nitric oxide cylinder within the small working area of an ambulance or aircraft. The results have shown that the high air exchange rates within ambulances and aircraft and the low doses of nitric oxide used make environmental nitric oxide toxicity unlikely.[38]

SAFETY OF TRANSPORT

Every transport program (air or ground) must provide a safe work environment. There should be a structured safety program in place to protect both the patient and the transport team members.[16] This program should include the following:

- A safety officer
- An incident reporting process
- Strict safety policies that are enforced
- Annual safety training
- Regularly scheduled transport safety committee meetings
- Regular safety assessments

Recommendations and actions from the transport safety committee must be linked to the transport program's performance improvement program. Safe performance in the transport environment starts with properly trained and educated personnel.[39] Didactic education should include the following:

- Disease physiology and how it relates to transport
- Safety
- Communications
- Stress management
- Survival training
- Legal aspects of transport

Whenever possible, opportunities to practice classroom instruction in the back of an aircraft/ambulance during actual operations are invaluable. Many programs now have mockups of vehicles in which to practice patient care in a transport environment.

The use of red lights and sirens (RLS) should be monitored and addressed because overuse has been shown to increase risk to the patient, public, and caregivers.[40-42] Every transport program should have a post–accident/incident action plan (PAIP).[16] The plan should include the process for notification of the following in the event of an accident involving the transport team:

· Transport team management
· Hospital administration
· Physicians
· Risk management
· Transport team members
· Transport team families
· Public affairs
· Media

ACCREDITATION

The transport program must be in compliance with local, state, and federal regulations related to the transport of neonatal and pediatric patients. Regulations that involve the following all have an effect on the transport of patients, documentation requirements, team composition, equipment and supplies, and transfer/transport consent forms.

· Certificates of need
· City/county/state/federal licensure
· Emergency medical services state health departments
· Consolidated Omnibus Budget Reconciliation Act (COBRA)
· Emergency Medical Treatment and Active Labor Act (EMTALA)
· Centers for Medicare and Medicaid Services (CMS)
· Federal aviation regulations (FARs)
· Federal Aviation Administration (FAA)

The program director must be knowledgeable about all these regulations and requirements. The transport staff must also be aware of and understand the regulations that influence the day-to-day operations of the program.

The Commission on Accreditation of Medical Transport Systems (CAMTS) is a peer-review organization comprised of 21 transport-related organizations that offers a program of voluntary evaluation of compliance with a set of accreditation standards. The core elements of the standards include aircraft/ambulance configuration, communications, legal requirements, maintenance, management, pilots and drivers, medical direction, scope of care, safety program, scheduling, and training and education of personnel. By participating in the voluntary accreditation process, transport teams can verify their adherence to quality standards to themselves, their peers, medical professionals, insurance companies, and the general public. At present several different states and counties require the CAMTS standards as the minimal standards required of transport teams for state and county licensing.

KEY POINTS

- The transport of critically ill neonates and pediatric patients is a very specialized level of care requiring extensive training as well as clinical experience of the staff. Team composition may vary but typically these teams are staffed by specially trained registered nurses and respiratory therapists. Each team member brings a needed level of critical care found in neonatal and pediatric intensive care units to the patient. Discuss and recognize the importance of team composition, roles, and education.

- The transport of critically ill neonates and pediatrics patients can occur via ground or air depending on the distance needed to be traveled. Ground ambulances are common transport vehicles as they are the least expensive to operate versus any aircraft. They offer the advantage of direct hospital-to-hospital transfer and large space for transport staff as well as equipment. Disadvantages included road noise/vibration, potential slow response due to road conditions including traffic and weather. Rotor wing aircraft offer fast transport in distances less than 150 miles and often can provide hospital-to-hospital transfer. Disadvantages of rotor wing aircraft include high cost of operation and limited cabin space for medical team and patient. Fixed wing aircraft are typically less expensive to operate than rotor wing aircraft. Fixed wing aircraft are typically utilized for distances over 120 miles and can fly long distances. Disadvantages of fixed wing aircraft include the need for an airport to land, and thus an ambulance transfer at both ends of the flight. Review and compare the caveats of each mode of transport.

- Communication is extremely important during medical transport. As technology has improved the ability to contact medical control in any mode of transport had become easier. The use of cell phones, radios, and even Internet-capable tablet device offer multiple advantages Explain the role of communication during a medical transport.

- The equipment needed for transport of critically ill neonates and pediatric patients needs to provide critical care found in intensive care units but must be portable and lightweight. Equipment should have a long battery life or have the capability to interchange batteries while the equipment is in operation, List the specific equipment needed for pediatric transport.

- Patient assessment in the transport environment can be a challenge versus hospital-based care assessments. Utilization of monitors, alarm conditions, and visual assessment of the patient is very important. Demonstrate how to provide a patient assessment in a nontraditional environment.

- Safety during medical transport of neonate and pediatric patients is imperative not only for the patient but also for the medical crew. Utilization of red lights and siren during ground ambulance transport needs to be evaluated as this can significantly increase the danger to the public as well as patient and medical crew. Safe operations also must be conducted around aircraft.
- Accreditation of transport program services is primarily provided by the Commission on Accreditation of Medical Transport Services (CAMTS). This organization offers peer-reviewed standards vetted by multiple specialists involved in medical transport. Review safety and accreditation requirements for pediatric transport agencies.

ASSESSMENT QUESTIONS

See Evolve Resources for answers.

1. Rapid transport of a neonate or a pediatric patient with a serious illness or trauma to a specialty facility can result in which of the following?
   A. Improved outcomes
   B. No difference
   C. Worse outcomes
   D. Unknown
2. Which of the following is the single most important asset in transport?
   A. Aircraft
   B. Lifesaving equipment
   C. Ambulance
   D. Personnel
3. How many transports are typically required to justify a dedicated team?
   A. 300 to 500
   B. 500 to 700
   C. 700 to 900
   D. 1000 to 1200
4. What is the single largest expense of a transport team?
   A. Personnel
   B. Transport vehicles
   C. Transport ventilators
   D. Cardiopulmonary monitors
5. What types of alarms are preferred in transport?
   A. Audible
   B. Visual
   C. Both audible and visual
   D. None
6. Why should mechanical ventilators be used during transport?
   A. Many of them offer the same level of support as ICU ventilation.
   B. They help prevent hyperventilation associated with manual ventilation.
   C. Monitoring of pressure, tidal volume, and minute ventilation can be achieved with appropriate alarm functions.
   D. All of the above

7. Many transport teams are offering point-of-care testing with a portable blood gas analyzer for what reasons?
   A. It reduces stabilization times and improves quality of care.
   B. Many blood gas analyzers are small and battery powered.
   C. It compensates for clinical assessment skills.
   D. A and B
8. The simple goal of the transport team is to:
   A. Transfer the patient in the most stable condition possible
   B. Transfer the patient within the "golden hour"
   C. Scoop and run
   D. None of the above
9. According to Boyle's law, what will the endotracheal tube cuff pressure do when the aircraft climbs in altitude?
   A. Remain the same
   B. Increase in pressure
   C. Decrease in pressure
   D. The pilot balloon pressure will increase, but the ETT cuff pressure will remain constant
10. Every transport program should have a:
    A. Rescue plan
    B. Backup plan
    C. Post–accident/incident action plan
    D. Media coverage plan

References

1. Queenan JT, Hobbins JC, Spong CY, editors: *Protocols for high-risk pregnancies,* ed 5, Hoboken, NJ, 2010, Wiley Blackwell, pp 491–499.
2. Hohlagschwandtner M, Husslein P, Klebermass K, Weninger M, Nardi A, Langer M: Perinatal mortality and morbidity. Comparison between maternal transport, neonatal transport and inpatient antenatal treatment, *Arch Gynecol Obstetr* 265(3):113, 2001.
3. Reynolds M, Thomsen C, Black L, et al: The nuts and bolts of organizing and initiating a pediatric transport team, *Crit Care Clin* 8:465, 1992.
4. Pon S, Notterman DAI, et al: The organization of a pediatric critical care transport program, *Pediatr Clin North Am* 40:241, 1993.
5. Johnson CM, Gonyea MT: Transport of the critically ill child, *Mayo Clin Proc* 68:982, 1993.
6. Loehr AB, Messmer PR: The case for specialized transport teams, *AJN Am J Nursing* 111:11, 2011.
7. Kronick JB, Frewen TC, Kissoon N, et al: Pediatric and neonatal critical care transport: a comparison of therapeutic interventions, *Pediatr Emerg Care* 12:23, 1996.
8. Eppich WJ, Brannen M, Hunt EA: Team training: implications for emergency and critical care pediatrics, *Curr Opin Pediatr* 20:255, 2008.
9. Orr R, Wenkatarama S, Seidberg N, et al: Pediatric specialty care teams are associated with reduced morbidity during pediatric interfacility transport, *Crit Care Med* 27;30A, 1999.
10. Orr RA, Felmet KA, Han Y, et al: Pediatric specialized transport teams are associated with improved outcomes, *Pediatrics* 124:40, 2009.
11. Stroud MH, Prodhan P, Moss MM, Anand KJ: Redefining the golden hour in pediatric transport, *Pediatr Crit Care Med* 9:435, 2008.

12. National Research Council: *Emergency medical services: at the cross-roads*, Washington, DC, 2007, The National Academies Press.

13. Sayre MR, et al: The National EMS Research strategic plan, *Prehosp Emerg Care* 9:255, 2005.

14. Warren J, Fromm RE Jr, Orr RA, Rotello LC, Horst HM: Guidelines for the inter- and intrahospital transport of critically ill patients, *Crit Care Med* 32(1):256, 2004.

15. Karlsen KA, Trautman M, Price-Douglas W, Smith S: National survey of neonatal transport teams in the United States, *Pediatrics* 128:685, 2011.

16. Commission on Accreditation of Medical Transport Systems: *Accreditation standards of the Commission on Accreditation of Medical Transport System*, ed 9, Anderson, SC, 2012, CAMTS, pp 20.

17. Freehill KM: Critical incident stress debriefing in health care, *Crit Care Clin* 8:491, 1992.

18. Deering S, Johnston LC, Colacchio K: Multidisciplinary teamwork and communication training, *Semin Perinatol* 35:89, 2011.

19. Akaike M, Fukutomi M, Nagamune M, et al: Simulation-based medical education in clinical skills laboratory, *J Med Invest* 59:28, 2012.

20. Salas E, Rosen MA, Burke CS, et al: Markers for enhancing team cognition in complex environments: the power of team performance diagnosis, *Aviat Space Environ Med* 78:B77, 2007.

21. Scott S, Smith C, O'Connor T, et al: A multidisciplinary approach to neonatal ambulance design, *Neonatal Netw* 13:13, 1994.

22. Kempley ST, Ratnavel N, Fellows T: Vehicles and equipment for land-based neonatal transport, *Early Human Develop* 85:491, 2009.

23. Brink LW, Neuman B, Wynn J, et al: Air transport, *Pediatr Clin North Am* 40:439, 1993.

24. Nish WA, Walsh WF, Land P, et al: Effect of electromagnetic interference by neonatal transport equipment on aircraft operation, *Aviat Space Environ Med* 60:599, 1989.

25. Kinsella JP, Griebel J, Schmidt JM, Abman SH: Use of inhaled nitric oxide during interhospital transport of newborns with hypoxemic respiratory failure, *Pediatrics* 109:158, 2002.

25a. Macnab AJ, Chen Y, Gagnon F, et al: Vibration and noise in pediatric emergency transport vehicles: a potential cause of morbidity? *Aviat Space Environ Med* 66:212, 1995.

26. Sittig SE, Nesbitt JC, Krageschmidt DA, et al: Noise levels in a neonatal transport incubator in medically configured aircraft, *Int J Pediatr Otorhinolaryngol* 75:74, 2011.

27. Korniewicz DM, Clark T, David Y, et al: A national online survey on the effectiveness of clinical alarms, *Am J Crit Care* 17:36, 2008.

28. Niebauer JM, White ML, Zinkan JL, et al: Hyperventilation in pediatric resuscitation: performance in simulated pediatric medical emergencies, *Pediatrics* 128:e1195, 2011.

29. O'Neill JF, Deakin CD, et al: Do we hyperventilate cardiac arrest patients? *Resuscitation* 73:82, 2007.

30. Di Serio F, Petronelli MA, Sammartino E: Laboratory testing during critical care transport: point-of-care testing in air ambulances, *Clin Chem Lab Med* 48:955, 2010.

31. Macnab AJ, Grant G, Stevens K, et al: Cost benefit of point of care blood gas analysis vs. laboratory measurement during stabilization prior to transport, *Prehosp Disaster Med* 18:24–8, 2003.

32. Kost GJ, Sakaguchi A, Curtis C, et al: Enhancing crisis standards of care using innovative point-of-care testing, *Am J Disaster Med* 6:351, 2011.

33. Reimer-Brady J: Legal issues related to stabilization and transport of the critically ill neonate, *J Perinat Neonatal Nurs* 10:59, 1996.

34. Raszynski A: Aviation physiology and international transport of infants and children, *Int Pediatr* 14:99, 1999.

35. McAdams RM, Dotzler SA, Pole GL, Kerecman JD: Long-distance air medical transport of extremely low birth weight infants with pneumoperitoneum, *J Perinatol* 28:330, 2008.

36. Hill KD, Lim DS, Everett Ad, et al: Assessment of pulmonary hypertension in the pediatric catheterization laboratory: current insights from the Magic registry, *Cathet Cardiovasc Interv* 76:865, 2010.

37. Lowe CG, Trautwein JG, et al: Inhaled nitric oxide therapy during the transport of neonates with persistent pulmonary hypertension or severe hypoxic respiratory failure, *Eur J Pediatr* 166:1025, 2007.

38. Kinsella JP, Griebel J, Schmidt JM, Abman SH: Use of inhaled nitric oxide during interhospital transport of newborns with hypoxemic respiratory failure, *Pediatrics* 109;158, 2002.

39. Ratnavel N: Safety and governance issues for neonatal transport services, *Early Hum Dev* 85:483, 2009.

40. O'Brien DJ, Price TG, Adams PI, et al: The effectiveness of lights and siren use during ambulance transport by paramedics, *Prehosp Emerg Care* 3:127, 1999.

41. Bigham BL, Buick JE, Brooks SC, et al. Patient safety in emergency medical services: a systematic review of the literature. *Prehosp Emerg Care* 2012 (16):20-35.

42. King BR, Woodward GA, et al: Pediatric critical care transport—the safety of the journey: a five-year review of vehicular collisions involving pediatric and neonatal transport teams, *Prehosp Emerg Care* 6:449, 2002.

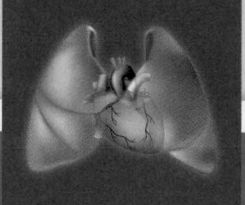

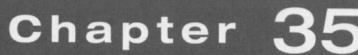
Chapter 35

Home Care

ANN-JANETTE GRIFFIN

OUTLINE

LEARNING OBJECTIVES

After reading this chapter the reader will be able to:

1. Discuss the critical components of a discharge plan for the child who is respiratory technology dependent
2. Recognize barriers that may delay the hospital discharge of a child who is respiratory technology dependent
3. Compare the three types of oxygen systems available for use in the home
4. Describe the procedure used to attach the apnea–bradycardia monitor and the scenarios in which a monitor is indicated

5. List the essential components of a trach-to-go bag
6. Recognize the need for decannulation and changing the tracheostomy tube
7. Discuss how caregivers are best prepared in caring for a ventilator-dependent child at home
8. Discuss the considerations needed in selecting the home ventilator and the home medical equipment provider

KEY TERMS

Decannulation
Discharge planner

Durable medical equipment (DME)
Home assessment

Medicaid
Plan of care

Advances in pharmaceuticals and medical devices have now made it possible for parents and health care professionals to care for infant and pediatric patients who are technology dependent. Today an unprecedented amount of that medical care is being provided in the child's home. The reasons are many for this shift toward care at home.

Medical equipment is now more portable and better able to accommodate home care needs. There is also the ever-increasing pressure to reduce health care costs and shorten hospital stays by expediting the transition from hospital to home. Perhaps most important is the growing belief that prolonged hospitalizations have a negative impact on the development of infants and children and therefore the home is the optimal setting for the medically stable, technology-dependent patient.[1]

In 1981 the move toward caring for technology-dependent children at home caught national attention when, during a press conference, President Ronald Reagan cited the case of 3-year-old Katie Beckett. Katie had been hospitalized since she was admitted at 3 months old with viral encephalitis. Regulations at that time mandated that she remain in the hospital in order for Medicaid to cover her medical bills. Two days after that press conference, the Secretary of Health and Human Services waived the rules that were preventing Katie from being discharged to her home, where she could be treated far less expensively. Only a few months after that, a waiver program was established that enables a child living at home to receive Medicaid-funded long-term care services. That program remains in place today and is often referred to as the *Katie Beckett waiver*.[2]

DISCHARGE PLANNING: THE DECISION TO GO HOME

Discharge planning is defined as a plan for a patient's continuum of care during transition to home or other facility. Upon arrival, neonatal and pediatric intensive care facilities are moving toward planning for discharge to an alternative site of care.

Alternative sites may include the child's home, foster care, long-term care facilities, and hospice care. The intent for discharge planning is to reduce the hospital stay, which minimizes medical costs and risk of additional infection. These infections could include ventilator-associated pneumonia (VAP), methicillin-resistant *Staphylococcus aureus* (MRSA), and vancomycin-resistant enterococci (VRE).

Central to the discharge planning process is a multidisciplinary team of health care professionals who work together to establish an appropriate discharge plan (Box 35-1). Extensive collaboration between the team and the parents is necessary to ensure that discharge planning is achieved

---

Box 35-1	Multi-disciplinary Health Care Professional Team Members Involved in a Discharge

1. Discharge planner
2. Social worker
3. Physician (On-service in unit)
4. Postdischarge physician
5. DME provider
6. PDN services
7. Insurance case management
8. Occupational therapist
9. Physical therapist
10. Respiratory therapist
11. Speech therapist

DME, Durable medical equipment; *PDN*, private duty nursing.

---

properly.[3] This team of health care professionals may include a discharge planner—a medical staff member designated to assist in the discharge planning, social worker, and physician on-service in unit and postdischarge physician, as well as private duty nursing (PDN) services and, if applicable, insurance case management. Another important role is provided by the **durable medical equipment (DME)** provider. Durable medical equipment is the medical equipment used by patients in the home or in a facility to aid in providing a better quality of living. Additional team members may also include the occupational therapist, physical therapist, respiratory therapist, and speech therapist. All these members are integral parts of the team and are helpful in establishing the home plan of care.

Before making the decision to provide home care for a child dependent on technology, a discharge plan is developed.[4] This plan is often referred to as a plan of care, which is defined as a written and detailed plan implemented to meet the medical needs of the patient. Critical components of this plan of care include the following:

· Social: Assessment of patient and family needs as well as identification and education of in-home caregivers.
· Financial responsibility: Assessment of available financial resources, such as private insurance versus state Medicaid programs. A Medicaid program is a health insurance plan provided by the state and federal government for qualifying low-income individuals and families.
· **Home assessment:** An evaluation of the home environment in which a ventilator-dependent child is to reside.
· Providers in home: Identification and availability of medical equipment and health care resources.
· Communication: Open communication between the parent/caregivers and the discharge planning team.
· Barriers: Recognition of barriers that may delay the discharge home.

Patient and Family Assessment

The entire discharge planning team should meet and assess the needs of both the child and family. Before the discharge home, the child must be medically stable and receiving optimal ventilatory, nutritional, and developmental support.[5] Assessment includes evaluation of the family's ability, availability, and commitment to care for their child as well as a psychosocial assessment for parenting risk factors that could potentially result in adverse outcomes.[6] Limitations, including language, physical, and cognitive, may delay discharge until appropriate support can be provided to family to help overcome these barriers.

The family's involvement is critical to the health and well-being of the child.[7] Involvement of bedside care is critical for the parent or caregiver so that a "norm" can be established. Involvement may include tracheostomy changes, following established feeding regimens, and evaluation of alarms that may occur. Additional time is required for the DME provider to conduct caregiver training regarding equipment and supplies needed in the home.

After training is complete, the parent or caregiver should be able to return demonstration of the equipment by explaining usage and cleaning procedures. All progress on training must be reported back to the discharge planning team. The private duty nursing agency must also meet with the family to familiarize themselves with the caregiver, patient, and plan of care.

Checklists have been found to be a useful tool so that all discharge planning team members may see the status of the parent or caregiver skill base. Some facilities use contracts with caregivers to outline expectations in the home.

Identification and Education of In-Home Caregivers

In most situations at least two people, usually the parents, are identified as the primary caregivers. These caregivers must have the ability and commitment to learn and actively participate in the child's care at home. The educational component of the discharge plan includes training not only the primary caregivers but also any other individuals who identify themselves as a support person for the child (i.e., grandparents, extended family, and close friends) and even the child to the greatest extent possible. Because there are many aspects to consider as part of the discharge planning process, the DME provider begins the training of home care equipment and supply at the time the referral is made. This is done to ensure that all necessary paperwork, insurance verifications, and home assessments are completed. Also, a planned emergency escape route from the home will need to be discussed with the caregiver.

All education, whether knowledge or skill based, must be consistent and at the level of understanding of each participant.[9] Keep in mind that the level of care that parents of technology-dependent children are expected to provide is far beyond that normally expected of parents. Mastery of the skills requires both material knowledge and practical experience. Training should be provided by an experienced professional who can also recognize unvoiced needs of the primary caregivers. A training manual that includes a detailed checklist is a useful tool to organize the required skills and help avoid missing any essential steps. It also assists in providing consistent education while serving as a resource for the caregivers (Box 35-2). Because most individuals obtain more information by actually performing procedures, it is imperative that the caregivers be given the opportunity to perform hands-on care with the child in a controlled hospital environment. With the hospital staff assuming a supportive role, the caregivers should provide as much hands-on care of the child as possible. Participating in mock scenarios also provides opportunities to problem solve and practice skills and emergency techniques.[10]

Caregivers, especially those with children who require a tracheostomy or ventilator, are required to participate in an in-hospital trial or rooming-in period in which they are responsible for the total care of their child. The goal of this period is to build confidence in their ability to care for their child while also offering an opportunity for backup assistance and coaching. While rooming-in, the caregivers are responsible for all routine care (i.e., feeding, bathing, dressing), respiratory care (i.e., treatments, ventilator checks, suctioning), medication delivery, equipment cleaning and troubleshooting, and arranging for relief periods with co-caregivers. Before discharge, they must have demonstrated knowledge and competency as well as be independent in successfully handling all aspects of their child's care.[11-13]

Financial Resources

In today's managed care arena, high cost and inadequate funding of care are usually the major obstacles to providing quality care at home. Funding necessary to provide long-term care to the technology-dependent child varies, depending on the complexity of care required, the level of parental capability, and responsibilities the parents may have (e.g., other children, work outside the home). Although home care costs are usually less than the cost for care in the hospital, parents often find that their insurance does not cover 100% of the cost at home as it did in the hospital. These nonreimbursable costs may be for home equipment and supplies, transportation to and from the hospital and clinics, and even changes made to the home in order to accommodate the child and equipment. Inadequate reimbursement creates a financial hardship for families and may be cause for DME providers and nursing agencies to refrain from providing services to the child. Limited payment for home care equipment and personnel has in many cases limited the scope and practice of mechanical ventilation in the home and delayed discharge for months. This has led professional societies to work together to create expert guidelines for mechanical ventilation outside the intensive care unit.[14]

Because professional care can be costly, it is essential to establish a solid financial plan to fund this care long before discharge. It should be determined early whether the insurance policy has a limit on medical equipment, supplies, and home care resources. The funding source must cover the cost of equipment, supplies, and professional services, such as skilled nursing and physical, occupational, and speech therapies. In most cases, insurance

---

Box 35-2	**Essentials of a Home Care Training Manual**

- Basics of anatomy and physiology
- Orientation checklist
- Supply list of equipment and supplies
- Special care procedures (tracheostomy care cleaning, emergency procedures)
- Equipment manuals

will fund these needs as long as the patient meets the criteria of medical stability, and the physician certifies a plan of care and completes a certificate of medical necessity. There should be continued communication with the child's insurers. A case manager is usually assigned by the payer to monitor care and ensure it is cost effective. Notifying the case manager early in the discharge process is essential in order to maximize the available dollars. In many cases, the home medical equipment provider is the expert on reimbursement for home medical supplies.[15,16]

Home Assessment

Depending on the home equipment needed, an on-site evaluation of the patient's home may be required before discharge to address any concerns or problems in the home environment. The evaluation includes assessment of the physical space, electrical capabilities, heating/cooling system, in-house water supply, availability of 24-hour telephone access, and geographic location of the home (Box 35-3). With many modern families only having cellular phones and financial limitations restricting some families' access to landlines, the DME and PDN companies meet many limitations regarding communication with caregivers. It is best to address these issues early in the discharge planning process so that adequate time is available to make any necessary changes.

It is essential that the house be fully accessible for the child and the home care staff. There must be enough room for the child and equipment to be easily moved in and out of the home. Children who are ventilator dependent ideally need a bedroom of their own so that family members are not disturbed by the care needed during sleep or the nursing staff. The bedroom must be large enough to accommodate the medical equipment as well as a comfortable chair for the nurse to use. An area for supplies and equipment storage should be designated and counter space made available for cleaning small equipment and reusable items. The room must be climate controlled, with proper ventilation, and free of drafts. The amount of medical equipment in the room can cause a small room to heat up quickly, and some mechanical ventilators will shut down if the temperature exceeds a certain level.

The electrical circuitry of the home must be evaluated to determine whether there are a sufficient number of grounded electrical outlets to provide safe operation of the equipment. Because multiple pieces of equipment may be running simultaneously, the household circuitry must support the total amperage of the equipment to be supplied. If not, another circuit breaker must be installed.

Durable Medical Equipment and Supply

Durable medical equipment includes any product or device (Box 35-4) that is used by patients in the home or in a facility to aid in providing a better quality of living. The equipment required depends on the child's medical condition. The company that supplies this equipment is referred to as the DME provider. Additional equipment may be needed at each site that the child attends (i.e., daycare, school). Equipment that will be used at home should be used in the hospital first so that caregivers can become familiar and proficient with its use. Any differences in its use at home should be addressed before discharge.[8]

When selecting a DME provider, the following must be considered:

1. *Does the provider supply all the equipment needed?* Many providers are no longer supplying apnea monitors. It may also prove difficult to find one that provides tracheostomy and ventilator supplies.
2. *Does the provider have a contract with the child's health care insurer, or is it considered out-of-network?* Caregivers are required to pay much less for the equipment and supplies when an in-network provider is selected.
3. *Does it employ respiratory therapists who are trained to provide the patient/caregiver with education, psychosocial support, and physical assessment needed for children who require specialized respiratory equipment and supplies?*
4. *Does it provide service to the area in which the child lives?* It is essential that the selected DME provider have a pediatric staff that is available for consultation and emergency coverage 24 hours a day, 7 days a week.

Box 35-3	Checklist for Home Assessment

- Adequate electrical power and wiring
- Appropriate heating/cooling system
- Working smoke detectors
- Satisfactory lighting
- Sufficient space in bedroom for equipment
- Counter space to clean equipment
- Storage space for equipment
- Ample physical space for nurse/caregiver to work
- Door sizes to accommodate child and equipment entry
- Steps or wheelchair ramps to access home
- Telephone service to initiate 9-1-1 service
- Emergency escape route planned
- Fuse/breaker box labeled

Box 35-4	Examples of Durable Medical Equipment

1. Air compressor
2. Oxygen concentrator
3. Mechanical ventilator
4. Continuous positive airway pressure (CPAP) systems
5. Bilevel positive airway pressure (BiPAP) systems
6. Wheelchairs
7. Infusion pumps
8. Suction machines
9. Pulse oximeter
10. Apnea bradycardia monitor

HOME CARE PERSONNEL AND COMMUNITY RESOURCES

Home care involves cooperation and collaboration between the hospital and the home nursing and community services. The visiting nurse or home care agency that will be supporting the child at home is contacted before discharge and given therapy and medication regimens, a follow-up appointment schedule, and instructions on general care of the child. These instructions include recognizing signs that would indicate the child is becoming ill and how to seek medical help. Acknowledgment of the parents as experts in the care of the child is an essential point during the education of the nursing and DME providers. Some caregivers may even choose to assist in teaching the home care staff about the needs of their child. Home care nurses must be educated on use of the medical equipment that will be in the home. This training is most often made available by the DME provider. If the child is of school age, the teachers and school nurse also need to understand any special needs and limitations the child may have. Respite services and emergency staffing in case the caregiver is ill should also be included in the discharge plan.[8]

Before discharge, a primary care provider is identified and an initial appointment scheduled. It is imperative that the designated primary care provider be one who is agreeable to caring for a technology-dependent child. Not every physician is willing to assume responsibility for a medically fragile child who is moving into the home environment. Unfortunately, failure to obtain a primary care provider can delay discharge home. Appointments for follow-up care with each physician specialist (e.g., surgery, pulmonary, otolaryngology) should also be arranged before discharge, with every effort made to schedule the appointments together on the same day. This not only decreases the burden on the family but has also proven to improve compliance. Each family is given a telephone list that includes the office and emergency phone numbers of the child's physicians and community resources (Box 35-5).

Box 35-5 **Health Care and Community Resources Telephone List**

The resource telephone list should include phone numbers for the following:
- Listing of physicians involved in care, including specialties
- Hospital to which patient would be transported to in case of emergency
- Pharmacy
- Durable medical equipment provider
- Private duty nursing agency
- Therapies: occupational, physical, speech
- School and daycare
- Insurance contact
- Utility companies

Public awareness is a vital part of the technology-dependent child's acceptance back into the community. The local utility company must be informed that for medical reasons the child is dependent on electricity. This information is provided through a letter signed by the physician. Having the letter on file allows the company to make it a high priority to restore electricity to the home in the event of a power outage and may even qualify the family for a discounted rate. A similar letter stating that the child needs a functioning communication system is sent to the telephone company. The water and sewage company as well as the local emergency medical service providers are also contacted and provided with information concerning the child's medical condition. Some emergency medical service or volunteer departments have little or no experience in caring for a child with a tracheostomy or who is ventilator dependent. In that case special training should be arranged and a plan developed for the child's needs before discharge. Such community awareness allows for a smooth transition from the hospital to the home and to the school environment.

Communication with the Discharge Planning Team

When parents are overwhelmed by the uncertainty of their child's condition and future, they often develop unrealistic expectations of outcomes, time frames, and discharge dates. Open communication with the discharge planning team is key to providing a successful discharge home and preventing readmission to the hospital. The purpose of the initial meeting is often simply to determine whether or not home care is suitable and manageable for the child. Patient care conferences in which the family and the discharge planning team candidly discuss the needs of the child and what they will face at home should continue at strategic points during the discharge process. These conferences provide an opportunity for the family to meet the home health providers, including nurses and respiratory therapists, and to voice any questions or concerns they may have. The meetings should focus on establishing the needs of the family and the child as well as providing a detailed plan for discharge and discussing any problems that may affect its success. It is during these meetings that the home care therapist clarifies the time frame in which training and equipment setup must be completed. Because the child and family's needs often change over time, this also provides an opportunity to review the family's needs, how they are managing, and progress toward the home care goals.[8]

Barriers That Delay Discharge

Many technology-dependent children remain hospitalized for extended periods even though they are considered medically stable. Unfortunately, it is often a nonmedical reason that delays the discharge. These barriers may include the inability to obtain a safe home environment or alternative care site, lack of financial resources, or uncooperativeness within the family. Diverse sociocultural backgrounds, including problems stemming from language, can impact communication and the learning needs of the caregivers. Delays in obtaining medical equipment or a provider for the equipment will in turn delay beginning the education for the caregivers. Other barriers to discharge include the inability to provide home nursing or community resources as well as failing to identify all pertinent problems or needs.[4,17-19]

OXYGEN THERAPY AT HOME

Unlike adults, in whom measurement of the arterial partial pressure of oxygen is considered critical, the need for home oxygen therapy for infants and children is established on the basis of oxygen saturation as measured by pulse oximetry.[1,20] Although some children will require oxygen for many years, the majority who are discharged home with oxygen need it for a limited period. Eventually they will require it only at night, and then wean off completely.

The three types of oxygen systems available for the home environment are liquid oxygen, oxygen concentrators, and compressed oxygen cylinders. Selection of the system is commonly the responsibility of the DME provider. Regardless of the type of oxygen system provided, it is essential that the DME provider be advised of the specific flow rate the child requires. This will determine which flow meter to use with the system. Although there are flow meters available that provide "microflows" with readings as low as 0.025 L/min, some clinicians do not advocate using them. When weaning from oxygen begins, the majority of infants are often decreased to 0.1 L/min and do not require lower flows before going to room air. There is also some concern that a caregiver could become confused by the decimal points and inadvertently administer the incorrect flow.[20]

Before discharge home, the child's caregivers must receive the oxygen equipment and successfully complete training in its use. If the child attends daycare or school, then arrangements should also be made to instruct responsible staff and teachers in use of the equipment.

Liquid Oxygen System

The liquid oxygen system consists of a base unit reservoir and a small, portable canister used for patient transport (Figure 35-1). The canister weighs 8 to 10 lb and is carried with a shoulder strap or rolling cart. When the canister becomes empty it is refilled from the base unit. The base unit has a flow meter that can deliver oxygen at low to high flow rates. Most systems have interchangeable flow meters that range from 0.08 to 15 L/min.

Advantages to this system are that no electricity is required and little noise is produced. Also, some caregivers prefer to use the canister for transport rather than an oxygen

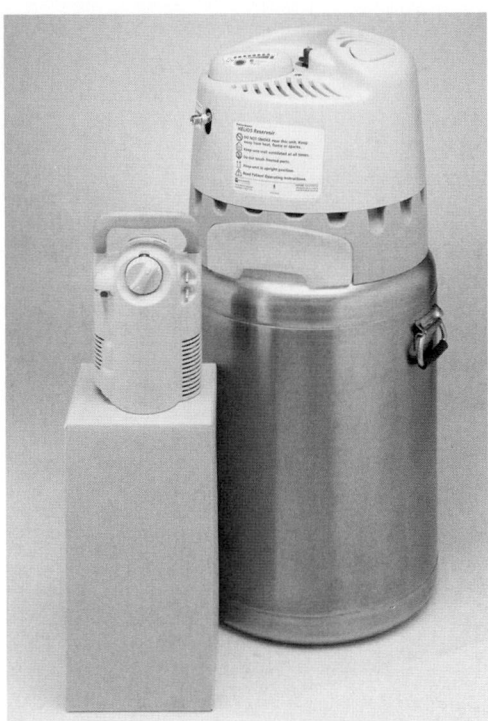

FIGURE 35-1 Stationary liquid oxygen (LOX) system with a portable system capable of being refilled by the patient or family.

cylinder. A disadvantage to using this system is that the base unit requires regular refilling by the DME provider. Frequency depends on both the oxygen flow rate and the size of the reservoir and can be as often as once a week to every other month. Another disadvantage to the liquid oxygen system is that it vents continually to prevent pressure from building within the reservoir, resulting in a loss of oxygen regardless of whether the flow is on or off. Caregivers must therefore be reminded that liquid oxygen will evaporate and portable units should be checked for contents and filled just before use.

Oxygen Concentrators

First produced in the 1960s, the oxygen concentrator is an electric device capable of separating oxygen from nitrogen in room air, collecting the oxygen, and then dispensing it through a flow meter (Figure 35-2).[22] Most concentrators provide greater than 90% oxygen. On some concentrators the flow meters can be changed to provide low flow rates (Figure 35-3), whereas others have dual flow meters to accommodate the varied needs of the patient (Figure 35-4). The DME provider needs to evaluate each concentrator's specifications before use with pediatric patients to ensure it can be used with low flows. When using concentrators, oxygen cylinders are provided for the patient to use for transport and for backup in the case of an electrical power outage.

As long as there is an electrical source, an oxygen concentrator provides an unlimited supply of oxygen and does not need to be refilled. It can be easily moved from room to

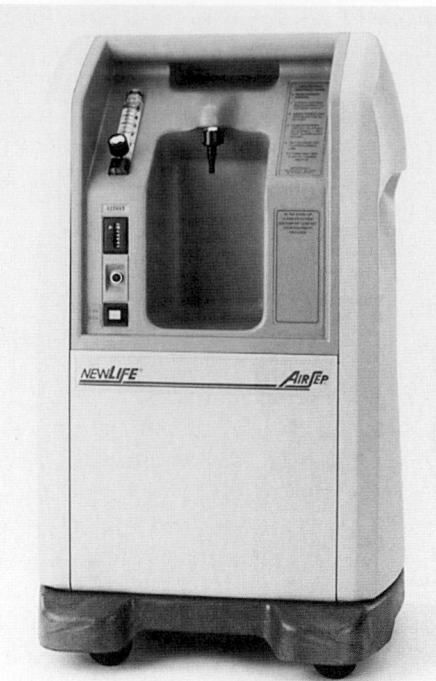

FIGURE 35-2   Oxygen concentrator.

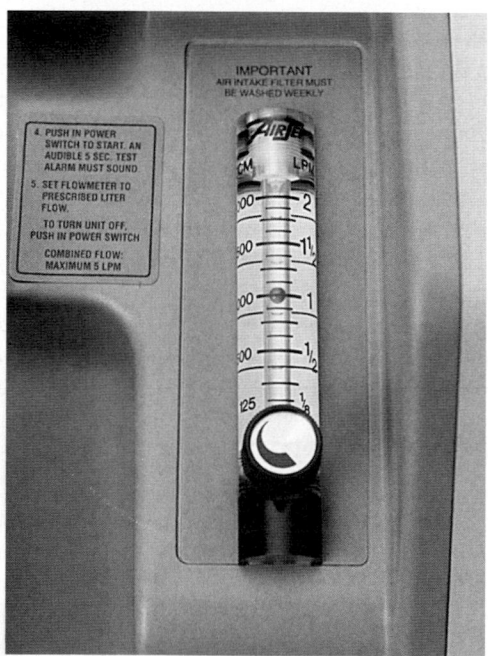

FIGURE 35-3   Close-up view of the low-range flow meter on an oxygen concentrator.

room and requires minimal maintenance. However, the concentrator's motor may produce additional heat and noise. Caregivers may notice that use has resulted in an increase in their monthly electrical bill.

Oxygen Cylinders

A compressed gas cylinder is usually made of seamless aluminum or fiberglass so that it can be as lightweight as

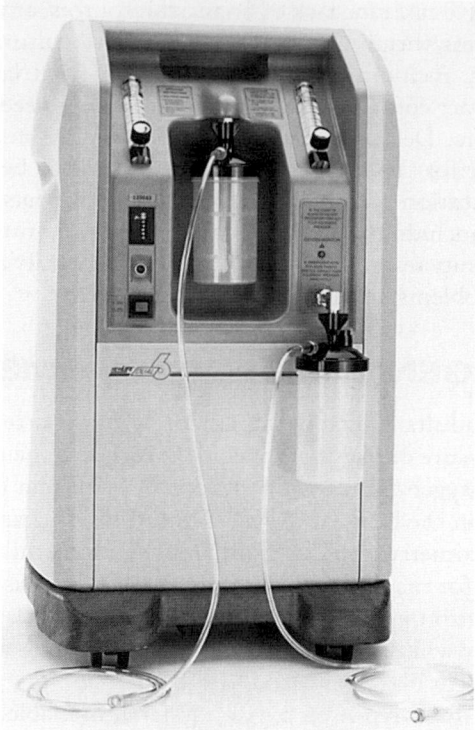

FIGURE 35-4   Oxygen concentrator with dual flow meters set at different flow rates.

possible. Oxygen cylinders are considered a cost-effective method of providing oxygen because they do not require electricity and can be stored for a long period without leakage. The major disadvantages of cylinders are the storage space required and the potential safety hazards as a result of the gas being contained under high pressure. Although the cylinders are smaller, they may still seem a bit more bulky than the liquid oxygen canister.

Portable cylinders are available in a variety of sizes and are identified by letter designations. At one time the E cylinder was the smallest available in portable cylinders, making liquid oxygen the number one choice for pediatric patients. Today, however, compressed gas cylinders are gaining in popularity thanks to the availability of smaller cylinders with custom carrying cases and regulators that allow flows as low at 1/32 lpm. This is ideal for patients who are graduates of the NICU and needing the smallest amount of flow.

APNEA–BRADYCARDIA MONITORS

An apnea–bradycardia monitor, more commonly referred to as an *apnea monitor,* is a portable machine that noninvasively monitors an infant's respiratory rate and heart rate. When there is apnea beyond a preset time limit, or when the infant's heart rate falls below or exceeds preset limits, an alarm will sound to notify the caregivers. Rather than being purchased by the caregiver, an apnea monitor is usually rented from a DME provider, because they are usually only needed for a short time. There are various apnea–bradycardia monitors that also incorporate a pulse oximeter.

For effective monitoring, monitors should be equipped with an event recorder that is able to capture and store cardiopulmonary events. The events are provided in a printout, commonly known as a download. Downloading is the process by which the information stored in the monitor is retrieved. At one time, the DME provider could perform a download for the information over the phone. This would require a hard-wired phone line or landline to download the appropriate software via a modem from the DME provider. With the majority of people using cellular phones and no longer having a hard-wired phone, the option of downloading via modem is obsolete. This requires the DME provider to go to the patient's home or physician's office and complete the download with a direct connection. A laptop is used to store the information, which is then sent on to the physician. The download contains a printout of waveforms; a log of the events, including the frequency of alarms and how low the heart rate dropped; and the frequency of monitor use. The information obtained can be used to distinguish the type of apnea, decide the type of medical treatment needed, and determine compliance and when to discontinue the monitor. If a child lives a long distance from the DME provider, a second monitor may be placed in the home for convenience of the DME provider and is not usually covered by the insurance. To have consistent, consecutive data when downloading the memory, it is recommended that only one monitor be used and the other kept solely for backup in case of monitor malfunction.

Monitor Placement

An apnea monitor may be considered medically necessary for infants who meet the following conditions:

- Have apnea of prematurity, which is defined as documented episodes of periodic breathing that result in prolonged apnea (20 seconds or greater) or bradycardia (heart rate less than 80 beats/min). Because the neurological breathing control mechanisms may not have matured by the time a newborn is ready for discharge home, an apnea monitor may be required to monitor the infant when a caregiver is not in constant attendance. It is up to the physician to decide when the monitor is no longer needed.
- After receiving theophylline for treatment of apnea or bradycardia. The monitor is considered medically necessary until the infant is event free for 2 weeks after the medication is discontinued.
- Have experienced an apparent life-threatening event (ALTE), which is defined as an episode characterized by a combination of apnea, color change, choking, gagging, or muscle tone change that required mouth-to-mouth resuscitation or vigorous stimulation. The

monitor is used until the infant is event free for 2 to 3 months.
- Have pertussis with positive cultures. The monitor is used for 1 month after the diagnosis.
- Are diagnosed with gastroesophageal reflux disease accompanied by apnea, bradycardia, or oxygen desaturation. The monitor is indicated until the infant is event free for 6 weeks.
- Have neurological or metabolic disorders affecting respiratory control.
- Have chronic lung disease and are requiring noninvasive or invasive ventilatory support.
- Have two siblings who died of sudden infant death syndrome (SIDS). These infants may be monitored until they have remained event free and are 1 month older than the age at which their siblings died. Because there is no proof that apneic episodes are related to SIDS, the American Academy of Pediatrics (Elk Grove Village, IL) released a policy statement in 2003 that does not recommend apnea monitoring in infants with only one SIDS sibling.[23] However, this diagnosis is not usually covered by insurance.

Although an apnea–bradycardia monitor may be a helpful adjunct to monitoring the infant requiring mechanical ventilation, use of this monitor is redundant and caution should be advised when interpreting alarm conditions. The reverse is also true: As long as heart rate is maintained and minimal chest excursion occurs, the alarm on the monitor will not be activated. However, this does not necessarily indicate that the ventilator is functioning properly. An infant with a tracheostomy is often prone to mucous plugging or decannulation. During these potentially life-threatening events, the apnea alarm will not be activated as long as the infant can struggle against an occlusion in the tracheostomy tube or breathe through an open stoma after accidental decannulation. Likewise, the bradycardia alarm usually becomes activated late during this type of event. When monitoring an infant with a tracheostomy, the clinician and parents must be aware of the potential hazards and the limitations of the monitor.

Caregiver Education

The DME provider usually trains the parents in the use and care of the monitor. Parents are instructed to use the monitor whenever the infant is sleeping (naps and at night), riding in the car, and anytime the infant is not being held or closely watched. To monitor the infant, electrodes are either stuck on the infant's chest or held in place with a soft belt and the heart rate and respiratory pattern are measured by means of a method known as impedance pneumography (Box 35-6). The monitor should be placed on a table near the infant, not on the floor, and at least 1 ft away from electrical devices such as televisions, air conditioners, telephones, electric water bed heaters, nursery monitor intercoms, oscillating fans, and humidifiers. Interference from these devices, although uncommon, may

Box 35-6	Lead Placement for Apnea Monitors

1. Wash and dry infant's chest. Do *not* use lotions, oil, or powders.
2. Connect electrodes to lead wires, making sure metal tips of lead wires are pushed all the way in.
3. Place foam belt on a flat surface, then place infant's back on the belt. Line the belt up with infant's nipples.
4. Position electrodes on belt (smooth side up) with each electrode under an armpit lined up with infant's nipples. White lead is on infant's right side, *not* the caregiver's right (hint: "White is Right") and black is on the infant's left side, *not* the caregiver's left.
5. Wrap belt around infant's chest and fasten with Velcro tab. Check belt to make sure it is tight, so caregiver can fit only one finger between belt and infant's chest wall. Belt may be shortened by cutting it.
6. Connect lead wires to patient cable. White lead goes to cable for right arm (marked *RA*). Black lead goes to cable for left arm (marked *LA*).
7. Turn monitor to "ON."

affect the monitor's performance. If items (e.g., diapers, toys) are near the monitor, they should be placed so that they do not block the displays or muffle the alarms. Caregivers should be advised not to allow the infant to sleep with adults, children, or pets at any time as well as while being monitored because their movement may prevent the monitor from working properly. Parents should check daily that the monitor's alarms sound by disconnecting the leads from the infant. They should also perform a daily inspection of the electrodes, lead wires, and power cords as well as a cleaning procedure. A logbook should be provided for parents to record the date and time of all events, unique observations about the monitor, and any intervention required (i.e., stimulation, resuscitation). The Velcro belt can be washed by hand in soapy water, rinsed well, and hung to air dry. Moving the patches just slightly can help minimize skin irritation. The belt should be tight enough to fit only one finger between the belt and the infant's chest. If the belt is too loose, signals for breathing and heart rate will not be picked up and may result in frequent loose lead or false alarms. If the belt is too tight, it may interfere with the infant's breathing. Powder, oil, and lotion can disrupt the monitor's conduction and result in false alarms. If skin irritation should become an issue, the parent should contact the referring physician for directive. Unless traveling outside the home, the apnea monitor should be plugged into an electrical outlet so that the batteries can remain fully charged.

Education for parents also includes infant cardiopulmonary resuscitation (CPR) and recognizing the signs of apnea. Parents should be instructed to respond to alarms by turning on the light if the room is dark and immediately checking the infant for signs of breathing. If the infant is breathing and skin color is good, parents should check the electrode placement, lead wires, and cable. If the infant is pale, cyanotic, or not breathing, stimulation is immediately required. It is essential that parents be taught not to shake their infant as a form of stimulation because vigorous shaking may result in severe head and neck injury and even death. If the infant does not respond, then CPR is indicated immediately. Any time CPR is performed, the infant should be seen immediately by a physician.

Most monitors have built-in algorithms that differentiate precordial movement from chest wall movement, but false alarm conditions are frequent. The most common reason for a false alarm is shallow breathing. An infant may be having abdominal breathing and the chest wall is not moving enough to be recognized as a breath. Lead wires that connect the electrodes to the monitor can become loose during vigorous infant activity, often resulting in false alarms. There is an increased chance of obtaining false alarms when the infant is playing, burping, being fed, and moving. Other causes of false alarms are crying, the Valsalva maneuver, incorrect lead or belt placement, poor skin contact, broken lead wires, and a low battery. Although there is no way for a parent to distinguish between a real and a false alarm when it initially sounds, especially if the infant is breathing by the time the parent arrives, information obtained from a download will include the amount of time the infant did not breathe and what the heart rate was at that time. The download can allow for differentiation between real apneas and loose lead wires, because there is an abrupt drop in the heart rate with a loose lead wire instead of the gradual drop that occurs with a true apneic event.

Changes in heart rate may be the source of annoying intermittent alarms for which a cause is difficult to find. Usually this is from an apneic episode that may not be long enough to alert the parents of apnea but that causes the heart rate to decelerate and briefly activate the bradycardia alarm. A rare cardiac arrhythmia may also cause a similar situation. Proper settings to minimize false alarms are important because parents become conditioned to most alarms being false. They must be constantly reminded of this phenomenon and encouraged not to delay in responding to the monitor when it alerts them.

PULSE OXIMETERS

The pulse oximeter is used for continuous monitoring as well as "spot checks." Its use in the home is indicated for infants and children who require continuous oxygen therapy and whose oxygen need varies from day to day or with activities, including feeding, sleeping, and playing. By monitoring the oxygen saturation, the caregiver has the ability to increase or decrease the oxygen flow rate to maintain a specific oxygen saturation range.[1] Use of a pulse oximeter may also be indicated during the process of weaning from oxygen therapy and to monitor infants and children who have a tracheostomy and/or are using mechanical ventilation at home. Potential inaccuracies associated with oximeter readings may result from poor perfusion and excessive movement of the child.[24]

For infants with hypoplastic left heart syndrome, daily pulse oximetry spot checks along with daily weighing is often part of the home surveillance program after stage 1 of the Norwood procedure. On discharge from the hospital, parents are given a notebook to record their infant's daily weights and oxygen saturations. They are also provided with guidelines about when to notify the health care provider with concerns, including contacting their physician if the oxygen saturation is less than 70%, if the infant's weight drops more than 30 g in 24 hours, or if the infant fails to gain at least 20 g during a 3-day period. The daily home surveillance of both oxygen saturation and weight in infants who are at increased risk of death before they return for stage 2 of the Norwood procedure has resulted in improved interstage survival.[25]

THE CHILD WITH A TRACHEOSTOMY

Although children receive a tracheostomy for a variety of medical conditions, there are three primary indications for placement: to provide a stable airway for children with upper airway obstruction, to provide an interface for long-term invasive mechanical ventilation, and to allow for more effective pulmonary toilet in children with excessive secretions or aspiration. Placement of a tracheostomy in a child may be a life-saving maneuver, but it has a significant impact on the family as well as on socialization and health of the child. Parents are concerned that they will never hear their baby cry or their child speak. Because of the small diameter of the infant and pediatric tracheostomy tube, there remains the potential hazard of airway obstruction and the child requires constant observation. To minimize this risk, adequate humidification, effective suctioning, CPR, tracheostomy care with regular tube changes, and decannulation are essential components of home care management. Because there is little research to guide the care of a child at home with a tracheostomy, in the absence of scientific data many recommendations are based on consensus, the care performed in the hospital, and local clinical practice. Unfortunately, many times procedures are determined by insurance coverage policies when payment limits the type and amount of supplies that will be reimbursed.[26]

At least two family members—usually the parents—must be identified as primary caregivers and education should begin as early as possible. Caregivers must understand basic airway anatomy, recognize the signs of respiratory distress, and demonstrate how to respond to an emergency. They must also be able to demonstrate proper use of the home medical equipment (Box 35-7), suctioning technique, how to

clean and change out the tracheostomy tube, and proper placement and care of the speaking valve. The DME provider will educate the caregivers on the respiratory and tracheostomy equipment. The hospital staff will provide the remaining education. Caregivers are encouraged to frequently visit the hospital and to participate in as much of their child's bedside care as possible. The child with a tracheostomy must have emergency supplies readily available at all times. An emergency bag, or trach-to-go bag, should accompany the child at all times (Box 35-8). The contents of this bag should

---

Box 35-7 — **Home Medical Equipment and Supplies Needed for a Child with a Tracheostomy**

- Self-inflating manual resuscitation bag
- Oxygen supplies
  - Stationary and portable oxygen supply systems
  - Oxygen tubing and bleed-in adapters
- Heated humidifier with a tracheostomy collar (to use at night)
- Air compressor or high-pressure concentrator to power humidifier
- Heat and moisture exchangers (to use during day)
- Suction supplies
  - Portable and stationary suction machines
  - Suction collection canister and connecting tubing
  - Suction catheter kits
  - Single-dose normal saline units
  - Sterile water
  - Gloves
- Tracheostomy supplies
  - Tracheostomy tubes: current size
  - Tracheostomy tubes: next smaller size
  - Tracheostomy ties: Velcro or twill tape
  - Cotton-tipped applicators or gauze
  - Tracheostomy cleaning kits
  - Water-soluble lubricant
- Disinfectant solution
- Monitoring systems
  - Pulse oximeter (optional)
  - Apnea monitor (optional)

Box 35-8 — **Contents of a "Trach-to-Go" Bag**

- DeLee suction trap to use if suction machine fails
- Suction catheters and gloves
- Small bottle of sterile water for cleaning suction catheter
- Single-dose normal saline units for irrigation
- Lubricant for tracheostomy tube insertion
- Two tracheostomy tubes (current size, one size smaller)
- Extra obturator
- Tracheostomy ties (Velcro or twill tape)
- Blunt-nosed scissors for cutting tracheostomy ties
- Self-inflating resuscitation bag with mask
- Heat and moisture exchangers
- Stethoscope

not be used at the bedside but instead used only when the child is away from the home. Caregivers must attend a CPR class that includes training with an emphasis on emergency management of the airway and tracheostomy tube. They must be able to recognize respiratory distress, such as accidental decannulation and a plugged tube, and respond to emergency situations quickly, including changing the tube.[27]

Airway Suctioning

Simplicity is an essential component of successful home medical management, especially with suctioning. Home suctioning differs from the aseptic, sterile technique used in the hospital, where a sterile glove and a sterile catheter are used for each suctioning procedure. Two methods are used at home: one is referred to as the modified clean technique, defined as using a sterile catheter with clean, nonsterile, disposable gloves. The other is the clean technique and is defined as the use of a clean but nonsterile catheter with clean, nonsterile gloves or freshly washed, clean hands.[28] When performing suctioning by the clean technique, the hands are washed thoroughly before beginning the procedure. The suction catheter begins as a sterile catheter but instead of being discarded, it is washed, disinfected, and reused (Box 35-9). There is some variation among caregivers regarding how long a catheter is used before it is cleaned. Some clean the catheter after every suctioning procedure, whereas others change the catheter ever 8 to 24 hours. Should the catheter be contaminated (i.e., dropped on the floor), it should be cleaned at that point.[28] If other individuals in the home are ill, the modified clean technique, using a sterile catheter and clean glove, should be used temporarily. Some professional clinicians may choose to use sterile technique in the home while the child is ill.

In addition to learning the suctioning techniques, caregivers must be able to recognize the need for suctioning. Suctioning is based on clinical assessment and should be performed on an as-needed basis rather than scheduled. Typically caregivers are taught to suction when the child wakes up in the morning or after a nap because secretions accumulate in the airway during sleep. They should suction after chest physiotherapy and respiratory treatments when indicated and when secretions can be heard in the tube. Suctioning should be performed if the child seems restless or uncomfortable or exhibits signs and symptoms of respiratory distress. If the child has an effective cough, suctioning is performed infrequently. If the child exhibits copious amounts of secretions or is ill, more frequent suctioning may be required, as often as every 2 to 4 hours.

Caregivers should be taught to note the amount, color, and consistency of the secretions and to report significant changes to their physician. To prevent injury to the tracheal mucosa, the suction catheter is inserted in the tracheostomy to only ¼ to ½ inch beyond the tip of the tube.[29] A suction catheter should be premeasured and marked and then set aside for caregivers to use as a measuring guide. Routine use of normal saline for lavage is not recommended.[28] Caregivers must demonstrate proficiency at suctioning when the child is in the hospital, before the rooming-in period.

All children with a tracheostomy should have a stationary and portable suction machine (Figure 35-5). In addition to an internal battery that can be charged from AC power, the portable suction unit must have a cigarette lighter adapter to charge off of the car battery. The caregiver is advised to take the trach-to-go bag with the patient whenever leaving the house. A DeLee suction trap should be kept in the bag for use in case the suction unit fails. Suction catheters, oral suction tubes, and suction canisters are supplied by the DME provider. A manual self-inflating resuscitation bag with external PEEP valve, appropriate-size mask, oxygen, and extra suction canisters should be kept in the home and readily available in case of an emergency (Box 35-10).

Box 35-9	Cleaning Suction Catheters in the Home

1. Using a 20-ml syringe, flush the catheter clean with either sterile/boiled water or 3% hydrogen peroxide.
2. Soak in one (not all) of the following to disinfect:
   A. 1:50 dilution of bleach for 3 minutes (1 teaspoon of bleach to 1 cup of water)
   B. 70% isopropyl alcohol for 5 minutes
   C. 3% hydrogen peroxide for 30 minutes
   D. Commercial disinfectant, such as Control III, for 15 to 20 minutes
3. Rinse the inside and outside of catheter with sterile/boiled water.
4. Place on a clean paper towel to air dry and then store in a clean, sealed plastic bag.

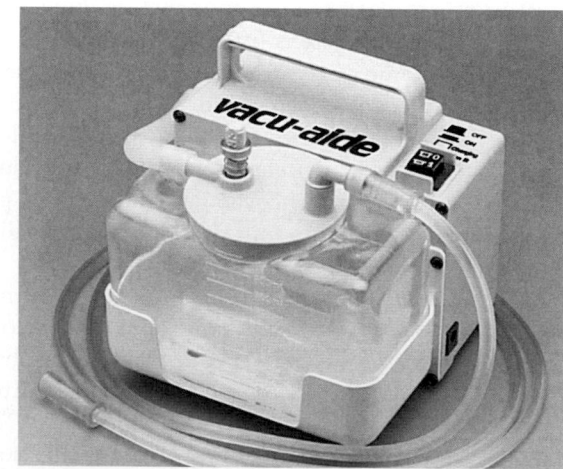

FIGURE 35-5 Battery-powered portable suction machine.

Box 35-10	Emergency Tracheostomy Supplies Kept at the Bedside

- Extra tube, same size currently using
- Extra tube, one size smaller
- Obturator
- Tracheostomy tube ties
- Scissors
- Manual resuscitator bag, external PEEP valve, and appropriate-size mask
- Standby oxygen, if ordered

PEEP, Peak end-expiratory pressure.

Box 35-12	Steps in Performing Tracheostomy Change

1. Wash hands.
2. Gather equipment.
3. Suction patient, then wash hands again.
4. Arrange workspace with adequate lighting.
5. Place obturator in the extra identical tracheostomy tube; thread ties or collar through one side of tube.
6. Lightly coat tip of tube with water-soluble lubricant.
7. Place child on back with a rolled towel under the shoulders.
8. Cut and remove old ties and pull tube out with a curved, downward motion.
9. Gently insert tube into the stoma, using a downward and forward motion that follows the curve of the tube.
10. Remove the obturator immediately after inserting the tube.
11. Using a syringe with sterile water, inflate the pilot balloon to the prescribed amount.
12. Secure the ties.
13. Suction as needed.
14. Assess the child's respiratory status.

Decannulation and Tube Changes

The purpose of changing the tracheostomy tube in the home is to minimize infection and the formation of granulation tissue.[30] As a general rule for children, the tube is changed once a week or as needed should it become obstructed. All caregivers must be taught to change the tube routinely and during an emergency if the child suddenly experiences signs and symptoms of respiratory distress (Box 35-11).[31] Before the rooming-in period and before a child can be discharged home, both primary caregivers are required to demonstrate that they can correctly and independently change the tracheostomy tube. Caregivers are strongly encouraged to be available to change the tracheostomy tube as often as possible while the child is in the hospital.

If at all possible, tube changes should be performed in the early morning before the child eats (Box 35-12). It is best for two caregivers to be present when changing the tracheostomy tube: one to remove the tube and the other to insert the clean one. All equipment, including the emergency supplies, should be gathered and readily available at the bedside. To change the tube, a blanket or towel roll is placed under the child's shoulders to extend the neck. While one caregiver holds the tube in place, loosens the ties, and then removes the tube, the other caregiver inserts the clean tube. The clean tracheostomy ties are attached, the child's work of breathing is assessed, and assurance is made that the airway is intact.

Two tracheostomy tubes should always be available at the bedside and in the trach-to-go bag. One tube should be

the size the child is currently using and the other tube should be one size smaller. The smaller tube is available in case a situation exists in which the current size cannot be reinserted. If resistance is met when attempting to replace the current tube, then the smaller tube is placed until further medical assistance can be obtained. A child's stoma can close quickly, so placement of a smaller tube will preserve the opening. Cuffless tubes are preferred in children; however, a cuffed tube may be required if the child is being mechanically ventilated.

Humidification Systems

Several types of humidification systems can be used in the home care environment. Humidification during mechanical ventilation is necessary to prevent destruction of airway epithelium, hypothermia, atelectasis, and thickening of secretions. The humidification system chosen should provide a minimum of 30 mg of H_2O/L of delivered gas at 30° C /86° F and meet specifications of the American National Standards Institute (Washington, DC). These are especially important in the pediatric population requiring continuous mechanical ventilatory support that uses high peak inspiratory flow rates.[32]

A portable, 50-psig air compressor or a 20-psig high-flow/high-pressure oxygen concentrator with a heated humidifier and tracheostomy collar is an excellent humidification system. The humidifier should be stabilized near the child's bed, either attached to the bed or to a table located nearby. They will also instruct the parents in preparing sterile water and normal saline at home (Box 35-13). The tracheostomy collar is often bulky and limits the child's mobility. Therefore it is suggested that

Box 35-11	Indications for Changing a Tracheostomy Tube

- Scheduled change is due
- Suction catheter does not pass freely (plugging)
- Respiratory distress is unresolved by suctioning or other interventions
- Oxygen desaturation is unresolved by suctioning or other interventions
- Accidental decannulation

Box 35-13	Preparing Sterile Distilled Water and Normal Saline at Home

1. Buy distilled water from a local store.
2. Obtain clean glass jars with lids. Baby food jars work well for saline.
3. Boil the distilled water for 15 minutes.
4. For normal saline, add 1 tablespoon of noniodized salt to 1 quart of distilled water (or ¼ teaspoon of salt to 1 cup of distilled water) and boil for 15 minutes.
5. Sterilize the jars by completely immersing them in water and boiling for 15 minutes.
6. Sterilization must be done on a stove. Do not use a dishwasher or a microwave.
7. Pour the water out of the pan and allow the jars and lids to cool in the pan.
8. Remove the jars and lids from the pan without touching the inside of the jars or lids.
9. Place the jars and lids upright on a clean towel.
10. Pour the boiled distilled water into the jars and place the lids on tightly.
11. Do not pour any used solution back into the jar.
12. After 3 days, discard any leftover solution and resterilize the jar and lid.

unless the child is being mechanically ventilated, the collar and heated humidity should be used during sleep at night and that a heat and moisture exchanger (HME) be used during transport and daytime hours. The first attempt at using the heat and moisture exchanger should take place in a controlled setting several days before the child is discharged home. The caregivers should be taught to observe for signs and symptoms of respiratory distress associated with the lack of humidification. The heat and moisture exchanger should never be used with another humidification system. The added moisture will wet the exchanger and increase the child's work of breathing through the exchanger. The caregiver should understand that airway obstruction may occur if secretions are trapped in the heat and moisture exchanger. If the child requires oxygen, the addition of a T-ring adapter, side ring adapter, or HME with O_2 port placed around the tracheostomy tube can reduce the amount of oxygen flow necessary to maintain the child's oxygen saturation levels. These adapters can be used with the heat and moisture exchanger and with the tracheostomy collar.

Communication and Speaking Valves

Children begin to communicate from the moment they are born. Communication is an innate component of every human who interacts with the environment and is part of the bonding process for parents and caregivers. Research also shows that speech and language development is interdependent on and interactive with motor and cognitive development. The child with a tracheostomy is limited in

his or her ability to vocalize, and speech therapy becomes an essential part of the home care plan. The goal of speech therapy is to improve deficits in speech and language development. Therapy assists in developing oral motor skills, maximizing language, and encouraging nonvocal behavior. Many forms of communication are used with the pediatric tracheostomy patient, including computers, sign language, and speaking valves. The benefits of combining all forms of effective communication are critical to the child's development.

A tracheostomy tube not only causes the child's vocal cords to remain in the open position, resulting in a diminished ability to vocalize and cough, but it also impacts a child's swallowing function. These factors can lead to a higher susceptibility to aspiration, subsequent pneumonia, and atelectasis, which can in turn result in longer placement of the tracheostomy tube and need for mechanical ventilation.[33] Use of a speaking valve provides a form of communication, enhances the ability to cough effectively, and also filters and protects the airway from particles.[34] The effective cough reduces the need for suctioning and the potential for infection and airway trauma.[31] Restoration of airflow through the upper airway also restores sensation to the oropharynx as well as the sense of smell and taste. In turn this improves appetite, overall nutritional intake, and swallowing efficiency.[35]

The Passy-Muir tracheostomy swallowing and speaking valve (PMV) allows a child to speak without occluding the tracheostomy stoma. The valve was developed in the 1980s by David Muir, a patient with muscular dystrophy who had a tracheostomy. Opening only during inspiration, the PMV allows air to enter the airway. On expiration the valve closes, which results in air being forced out of the airway through the vocal cords, nose, and mouth (Figure 35-6). The patient can resume speaking, which enhances social interaction and decreases frustration by making it easier to vocalize spontaneously. Ideally the speaking valve should be placed within a few days of receiving the tracheostomy so that the child will consider it part of the tracheostomy tube. Successful transitioning techniques used when placing the valve include play therapy and distractions such as coloring books, whistles, and toys. Techniques for training children to exhale through the valve include blowing whistles, bubbles, and feathers. If the tracheostomy tube does not allow the child to exhale through the valve, then the tube should be downsized. A speaking valve is contraindicated in patients who have severe tracheal stenosis or excessive secretions, require continuously inflated cuffed tubes, or are unconscious or heavily sedated.

Activities of Daily Living

Pediatric patients with a tracheostomy should be treated as normal children.[36] A child with a tracheostomy can take part in most play activities suitable for that age. With an infant or small child, all small toy parts or objects should be removed from the play area because the child might put

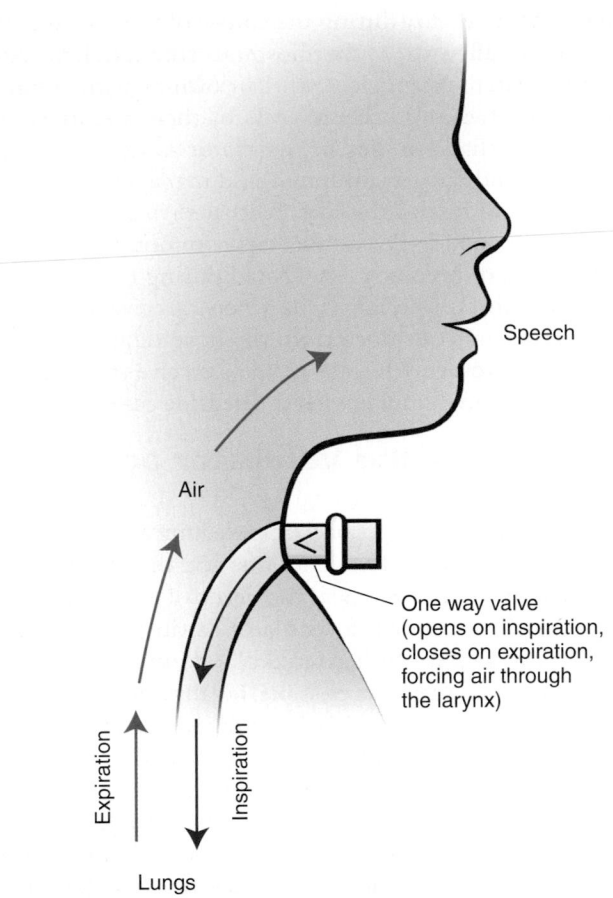

Speech

Air

Expiration   Inspiration

Lungs

One way valve
(opens on inspiration,
closes on expiration,
forcing air through
the larynx)

FIGURE 35-6 Tracheostomy speaking valve enables speech by redirecting exhaled air around the tracheostomy tube and through the larynx and upper airway.

these into the tube. During outdoor play the caregivers must protect the child's tracheostomy from extreme temperatures and dirt in the air. Extremely cold or hot air may be irritating to the child's lungs. Heat and moisture exchangers are used to protect the airway from such irritants.

When bathing a child with a tracheostomy, the child may be placed in a tub but care must be taken not to allow water into the tube. To wash a child's hair, hold the child on his or her back over a sink or tub. Wash and rinse the hair with a cup of water and washcloth, or spray the hair carefully. The child can play in the water, but never submerge the child in the water or leave the child alone in the tub. An older child can take a shower as long as the tracheostomy is protected.

There is no need to buy special clothing for the child with a tracheostomy. However, parents are instructed to buy clothes that do not cover the tracheostomy. Items to avoid include turtlenecks, necklaces, scarves, or any type of material with fibers that could be released into the tracheostomy opening. The home environment should be kept as free of lint, dust, and animal hair as possible. It is imperative that no one smokes, uses powders, or sprays aerosols

around or on the child. Particles and fumes can enter the lungs through the tube and cause breathing problems.

The primary caregiver may become ill and be unable to care for the child for an extended time. This is a major reason why more than one caregiver should be trained to care for the child. Qualified providers, or respite care, should be available to care for the child in the absence of the primary caregiver.

Transporting the child may require extra precautions and planning (Box 35-14). It is recommended that another individual besides the driver be in the vehicle with the child. Standard car seat restraints may not work for the child with a tracheostomy. A survey on the methods of transporting technology-dependent children found that the children were restrained appropriately; however, in 66% of the cases the heavy medical equipment was not secured.[37]

MECHANICAL VENTILATION IN THE HOME

As neonatal and pediatric respiratory care continues to evolve, we have seen an increase in the number of children with chronic respiratory failure who are medically stable. Many of these children require some level of ventilatory assistance, ranging from noninvasive nighttime ventilation to 24-hour ventilatory support. The clinical conditions resulting in respiratory failure and chronic ventilatory support are varied and include chronic lung disease, acquired or congenital neuromuscular impairment, airway abnormalities, and ventilatory control disorders. And even though the number of ventilator-assisted children is relatively small compared with other groups, the cost of care is substantial when specialized equipment and education are required and especially when hospital stays are prolonged. There is no argument that the hospital is an unsuitable environment for the ventilator-assisted child who is medically stable. The benefits of having the child at home are many, including an enhanced quality of life. Yet the discharge process for a ventilator-assisted child can be long and complicated. In few other situations does it require a more coordinated multidisciplinary team approach.

Family Preparation

The decision to provide care at home must be family centered, not staff generated. Successful home management of the ventilator-assisted child depends largely on the parents' willingness and capacity to meet the needs of their child.[32] Care at home is time consuming, labor intensive, and expensive. Parents should be told that care at home will require more than normal parenting skills. It will impact every aspect of each family member's lifestyle and quality of life. Siblings often feel neglected, and marriages are challenged. An even heavier burden is imposed on single-parent families. But time and again families agree that overcoming the challenges and finally arriving home is justified and worthwhile.

Before the discharge process begins for a ventilator-assisted child, the following criteria must be met:

· At least two adult caregivers must be willing to commit to participate in the necessary training and the child's ongoing care.
· Parents must be in agreement on taking the child home.
· Caregivers must be physically and mentally capable of providing home care for the child.

Once a family makes the decision to commit to caring for their ventilator-assisted child at home, a formal discharge process begins. One of the first steps to be done is to meet with all of the members of the discharge planning team. Parents should be informed that the discharge process may take several weeks or even months, depending on the individual child's needs. Identification of the two primary caregivers is essential at this point. Because transition to home for a ventilator-assisted child involves such an extensive commitment from the caregivers, they may be asked to sign contracts agreeing to the education/training, hospital rooming-in period, and the steps involved in discharge home. The caregivers should be given an overview of the discharge process with projected dates and time lines for certain steps in the process.

Moving the child from the intensive care unit to an area where the caregivers can be more involved in their child's care is an enormous step in beginning the discharge process. Even though formal teaching by the DME provider may not have begun, the caregivers can learn a great deal about the care of their child from the respiratory therapists, nurses, physical therapists, speech therapists, and occupational therapists who care daily for the child. Once teaching begins, the caregivers have more time to begin practicing their skills in their child's room. Quite often the most successful transitions home are with those families who have spent the most time at their child's bedside, taking an active part in the daily care.

Parents with ventilator-assisted children have commented on how they initially feel shocked and crushed by the uncertainty of their child's illness and their family's future. It may be helpful for the caregivers to be in contact with other parents who have a similar experience. The parents' ability and commitment to be involved in their child's care may vary during the course of the hospitalization, especially when the hospital stay extends into months. Parents struggle with their own adjustment and coping abilities and other aspects of their life. Research has shown that families of ventilator-assisted children face profound burdens in household management, social relations, and financial issues.[38] Because many caregivers must work outside the home, it is common for employment issues to become complicated during the discharge process. This is especially true when caregivers live and work quite some distance from the hospital, yet they are being asked to be with their child to receive training and to become more familiar with the bedside care.

Selection of the Ventilator and DME Provider

There is no standard approach for selecting a ventilator for the pediatric patient. The ventilator and the settings chosen must be tailored to meet the needs of each child. The overall goal is to choose a ventilator capable of maintaining clinical stability with arterial blood gas levels as close to physiological values as possible. Ideally, ventilators chosen for home care should be user friendly, compact, and portable and operate on a variety of power sources.[4,39] The device should incorporate a reliable alarm system and should be trouble free for extended periods. Home care ventilators should have hidden controls or a locked panel to prevent pediatric patients or siblings from inadvertently altering the settings.

Always consider the child's needs when selecting a suitable ventilator. Factors to be considered include, but are not limited to, home versus public school, distance to the health care provider, and how well it will meet the growing needs of the child. If the ventilator selected for home mechanical ventilation is not available in the hospital, the DME provider may be asked to supply the appropriate machine for a trial period before discharge.

Another factor to be considered when selecting a home ventilator concerns the compatibility of the circuit and the positive end-expiratory pressure (PEEP) valve. PEEP is often accomplished by using an external PEEP valve, which can be heavy and may also have exhalation ports that can be easily blocked. The combination of the PEEP valve and circuit must have minimal exhaled resistance. The PEEP valve must also be able to function at any angle; this precludes gravity and water columns for home use.

A major advantage of a portable ventilator is the ability to use a variety of power sources, including house current, an internal battery for short periods, and an external battery for extended periods. Some portable ventilators can operate from a car battery by connecting to the cigarette lighter. A 12-V battery should be available for use during trips away from home and as an extended backup during an electric power failure. A 12-V 74-A/hour, deep-cycle battery can power a ventilator for about 20 hours without recharging. A 12-V 34-A/hour, gel-cell battery can power a ventilator for about 10 hours before recharging is required. It is important to note how heavy the battery is and whether the combined weight of the battery and ventilator still allows portability. In rural areas where power outages frequently occur, or where it may take extensive time for electricity to be restored, it is often advisable to purchase a backup electricity generator. Another alternative is to have portable backup batteries or power packs.

The DME provider should be selected as soon as it is determined that the child will go home. Caregivers should be given the option of selecting the provider; however, there may be few choices, because many may not provide ventilators for children. To obtain one that is an in-network provider with the child's insurance carrier or one that will accept Medicaid reimbursement may narrow the field even more. It is essential, though, that the chosen DME provider have home care personnel who are familiar with the care of infants and children with tracheostomies and who are also familiar with pediatric mechanical ventilation. If the provider agrees to accept the patient, then the home assessment can be scheduled and a list of needed supplies provided. The supply list should be given to the provider as soon as possible so that equipment can be ordered (Box 35-15).

A second ventilator, or backup ventilator, should be provided in the home for the child who meets the following conditions[40]:

· Cannot maintain spontaneous ventilation for 4 or more consecutive hours
· Lives in an area where a replacement ventilator cannot be provided within 2 hours
· Requires mechanical ventilation during mobility

Box 35-15 | **Home Medical Equipment and Supplies for Ventilator-Assisted Children**

- Mechanical ventilator
  - Primary ventilator
  - Backup ventilator
  - 12-volt battery and connecting cable
  - Ventilator circuits
- Humidification supplies
  - Humidifier and heater
  - Heat and moisture exchangers
- Tracheostomy supplies
- Suctioning supplies
- Self-inflating manual resuscitation bag
- Oxygen
  - Oxygen concentrator
  - Stationary oxygen system with regulator able to support resuscitation (½-15 lpm regulator)
  - Portable oxygen system with regulator able to support resuscitation (½-15 lpm regulator)
- Monitoring systems
  - Pulse oximeter (optional)
  - Apnea monitor (optional)

An emergency backup/transport ventilator must be available in the event of a ventilator malfunction. Without a backup/transport ventilator in the home, the home care company must assume the responsibility for providing immediate service. It is also best to have extra ventilator circuits and a spare temperature probe in the home. Although it is not practical to duplicate all equipment, it may be reasonable to have a second suction machine and oxygen source to use at the school or at daycare.

User and clinician manuals should be available from the manufacturer, along with training materials. The user information manual should be left in the home for parents to use as a reference. All educational materials should be well organized and easy to understand. Various factors must be considered to achieve the goals of pediatric ventilatory support in the home environment (Box 35-16).

Common Delays to Discharge Home

In spite of the most valorous attempts at organization, communication, and planning within the discharge process, obstacles to discharge will still occur. The major barriers for chronically ventilated children include failure to obtain qualified nursing staff, delays in approval for home care funding, an unsuitable home environment, complex family issues, and arrangements for out-of-home placement.[41,42]

Recruitment of qualified nursing is a problem no matter where the child's home may be. Some areas are better staffed than others, but there always tends to be a shortage of nurses who can care for the ventilator-assisted child. In some cases, the discharge date is set, the caregivers have completed all training and assessments, and the parents have roomed-in; and then, for various reasons, nursing staff is no longer available and the child cannot go home. When nursing shortage is an issue, some families have resorted to advertising for their nurses. Although it is not an option for most families, some have just opted to go home without nursing care.

Funding delays are often the greatest hurdle to getting the child home. Without reimbursement, home equipment cannot be obtained. The greatest difficulty arises when there is little or no reimbursement for the ventilator. Community resources, such as nursing, speech therapy,

---

Box 35-16 | **Goals of Pediatric Home Mechanical Ventilation**

- Enhance quality of life
- Extend life
- Provide an environment that promotes individual growth
- Improve psychological function
- Improve physical function
- Reduce morbidity
- Be cost beneficial

physical therapy, and occupational therapy, are also unattainable without funding. Without reimbursement, discharge is delayed indefinitely.

The sooner it is known that housing is unsuitable, the more likely solutions can be made. That is why it is so important that the DME provider obtain the home assessment as soon as it is determined that the child intends to be sent home. Many times the problems are simply that electrical outlets are not in compliance, or a ramp needs to be built to accommodate the wheelchair/adaptive stroller. There are situations in which the home is in an area that the nurses or DME provider refuses to travel to, because it is too far away or it is unsafe. Other situations include not having electricity or air conditioning, not enough space for the child's equipment, or even extreme situations in which the caregivers have been evicted. The social worker is an invaluable member of the discharge planning team when these issues arise.

Family issues are all too often the most difficult barriers to overcome. The longer the hospital stay, the more likely that family dynamics will change. Strained finances, guilt, fatigue, worry, and emotional distress are all issues faced by most families of ventilator-assisted children. However, issues such as divorce, which often results in loss of one of the primary caregivers, and drug abuse and mental illness are the types of issues that tend to result in the longest delays.

Although it is not a commonly faced obstacle, making arrangements to discharge the ventilator-assisted child to an alternative site often leads to extensive delays. It may take weeks if not months to find a medical foster home for the child, which in turn requires home assessment and education of the foster parents. Locating an institution that accepts ventilator-assisted children may be difficult if the child resides in a state that does not have such a facility. It is often difficult for parents to agree to send their child to a facility that is hours away, much less in another state. It may be even more difficult to find a facility that has an opening available for the child.

Home at Last

Before a ventilator-dependent child can be discharged home, the following criteria must be met. Ventilator settings must be stable for at least 1 week. The oxygen concentration must be less than 40%, and blood gas analysis must be stable and within normal limits.[32] The home environment must be acceptable and the home equipment available either at the hospital or at the child's home. It is also essential that there be adequate home care available. This includes two primary caregivers who have successfully completed all of the training and the rooming-in period, as well as adequate home nursing staff. On the day of discharge, transportation home or to the alternative site of care may be provided by the caregivers vehicle or by an ambulance. It is recommended that the respiratory therapist from the DME provider either follow the child home

Box 35-17	Problems Associated with Home Mechanical Ventilation

- Disconnected ventilator circuit
- Leaks in ventilator circuit
- Obstructions in ventilator circuit
- Water in ventilator circuit
- Water in exhalation valve
- Water in external PEEP valve
- Dirty filter
- Leak around tracheostomy tube
- Ventilator autocycling
- Power surge
- Increased suctioning requirement
- Increased oxygen requirement
- Change in child's pulmonary status
- Change in child's nutritional status
- Change in child's activity level
- Development of infection
- Extensive time required to adjustment to home/ environment

PEEP, Positive end-expiratory pressure.

in a separate vehicle or meet the child when he or she arrives home and assist the family with "settling in" at home.

Children requiring mechanical ventilation have not only complex medical problems but home medical equipment that requires frequent evaluation (Box 35-17). Although equipment malfunction may be minimal, there can be no delay in troubleshooting when problems arise. For this reason it is imperative that these children be provided with appropriate medical expertise. This includes 24-hour availability of the DME provider's staff as well as nurses and respiratory therapists from a physician group managing the ventilator at home.

Ventilator-assisted children should be evaluated by a pulmonologist every 3 to 6 months. During the visits, the child's ventilatory status and oxygenation requirements are evaluated to determine optimal ventilator settings and the potential for weaning. Because children often have large leaks associated with uncuffed tubes, the child's tracheostomy is assessed for correct size and placement. In fact, studies have shown that 9 of 11 children with uncuffed tubes are inadequately ventilated, resulting in chronic hypercapnia and fatigue.[43-48] Problems with equipment are addressed, and continuing education of the caregivers is provided if necessary.

A SUCCESSFUL TRANSITION HOME

Caring for technology-dependent children in the home often presents challenges for their families, their community, and the health care system. Every caregiver of a technology-dependent child is at risk of physical burnout, financial and emotional stress, depression, and social isolation, especially when support and resources are insufficient or inaccessible.[49,50] Many of these challenges can be resolved by interdisciplinary discharge planning, the use of discharge protocols, case management approaches, respite care, psychological counseling, and adequate financial provisions for sustaining home care.[51] A successful transition home often depends on when the discharge process begins. Waiting until the last minute often ends in failure. The advances in care and equipment that make a child's survival possible in the first place are many times the greatest challenges in the transition home. The family's central role in the discharge planning process must be recognized and supported because in the end, successful transitions may have less to do with the child's medical condition than with the family's commitment to the child and their ability to adapt, work as a team, and persevere.

CLINICAL HIGHLIGHT

Home Care Ventilator for Premature Patient with Chronic Lung Disease

MEDICAL HISTORY

Your patient is a baby boy born at 23 weeks of gestation with chronic lung disease (CLD) complicated by supraglottic airway obstruction. History summary includes tracheostomy placement with ventilator dependency on control mode ventilation (CMV) and converted to high-frequency oscillatory ventilation (HFOV) because of worsening ventilation and oxygenation. Patient was able to be weaned to CMV and then weaned further to synchronized intermittent mandatory ventilation (SIMV). After 3 months of endotracheal intubation, the tracheostomy was placed. Patient was stabilized on ventilator settings for 4 weeks.

DISCHARGE PLANNING

The discharge planning referral to a durable medical equipment (DME) company and private duty nursing (PDN) was initiated to begin planning for home. The DME provided home ventilator for patient to be placed on and be evaluated for tolerance of changeover while patient remained in the neonatal intensive care unit (NICU). Tracheostomy cardiopulmonary resuscitation (CPR) training was completed by parents and additional caregivers who will be in the home (grandparents). The primary bedside nurse continues working with the caregivers for trach changes, suctioning, and bagging metered-dose inhaler (MDI) treatments to trach. A social worker is involved to assist with the financial resources because the family has limited access to funds. Commercial insurance is not available at either parent's work; therefore the patient will be eligible for state Medicaid program.

Nutritional support is stable because patient is able to take all feedings orally. No gastrostomy tube has been placed at this time. The home therapy referral was made and will be established once discharge is complete with patient stable at home. A discharge planning meeting is scheduled with ventilator discharging team. This was initiated to bring all parties together and discuss plan of care and discharge.

HOME ASSESSMENT

The DME provider performed the home assessment at the current address and found electrical limitations in the bedroom where the patient will reside. Minimum width of doorways found to be in an acceptable range, and accessibility to bath, kitchen, and laundry were all acceptable. Telephone service is not available in the home, but caregivers do have cellular phones available. An emergency escape route is planned with an alternate route established. Parents are asked to inform all possible caregivers about the escape route to ensure the plan is understood and enforced if necessary. The fuse box is labeled for ease in accessing in an emergency. The number of individuals in the home beside the patient includes the mother of baby, father of baby, two sisters, and one brother. General cleanliness and condition of the home met needed criteria. The family recently moved into the home and is still unpacking. The home is kept clean but organization of personal effects is needed. This should be completed before the medical equipment or supply is brought into the home. Once this is complete, it will reduce possibility of misplacing medical supplies. The DME provider has the following recommendations for the family before patient discharge:

- Two power strips to be used only for medical equipment
- Two flashlights for emergency lighting and charging of backup/transport ventilator with additional batteries in a room other than where patient resides

The DME provider reported back to ventilator the discharge team that assessment passed with some minor limitations.

DURABLE MEDICAL EQUIPMENT TRAINING

A meeting is set with parents for training on medical equipment. Caregivers, including both parents, are present for orientation. Training material presented to caregivers include training manuals, cleaning instructions, and necessary reference sheets. Basic anatomy and physiology are discussed in relation to the patient's current medical condition. Monthly supplies were provided; caregivers were educated on the use of each item and were given an explanation of the quantity of supply to expect per month as dictated by covered benefits from the insurance provider. When education is completed a competency-training summary is documented, signed, and dated by the respiratory therapist and caregivers. An update of progress is reported back to the ventilator discharge team. They are informed that orientation has been completed.

PARENT CARE UNIT

The parents check in and attended parent care unit (PCU) for 48 hours. This task was able to be successfully completed and all care is delivered to the patient by the parents without the assistance of nursing staff. The DME provider was contacted by parents during PCU with questions regarding the suction machine. Troubleshooting was done over the phone with the parents and the issue was able to be resolved; it was discovered that the charger was not completely engaged with the unit to provide a charge. Parents were able to complete PCU without incident. Information regarding the fact that the parents successfully completed PCU is sent to all providers involved and a plan is set to discharge the following morning.

DAY OF DISCHARGE

Time of discharge is set for 11:00 AM. A full assessment of the patient is completed by the rounding physician team, discharging ventilator team, and pulmonary team. The PDN and respiratory therapist from the DME provider were present for the discharge. The parents worked with the respiratory therapist to get all equipment on the adaptive stroller, including placing the patient on the transport ventilator and placing a heat and moisture exchanger (HME) inline to the ventilator circuit; other supplies for the bedside were loaded for travel home. Discharge orders were signed by the discharging physician and instructions provided to caregivers. Parents loaded the patient into the car, and the DME provider followed caregivers to their home. Upon arrival to home, parents and the DME provider carried the patient in while the patient remained on the ventilator circuit. Upon arrival to the patient's room, the patient was placed on the home ventilator. The PDN completed an assessment of the patient while the DME provider completed the transfer to home. This included plugging in all equipment, assessing saturations, verifying ventilator settings, and confirming the comfort level of parents and other caregivers. Reinforcement of on-call phone numbers to the caregivers was done. A follow-up call is placed to parents once the patient is home for a few hours.

FOLLOW-UP

The DME provider did an in-home follow-up daily for the remainder of the week. At the end of the week, parents were reinstructed on how to reach the DME provider on call as well as the home ventilator team physicians. When the DME provider returned to work the following week, an additional trip to the home was completed to ensure that the parents were comfortable and confident in the use of the equipment and supplies and to discuss with the parents any questions that may have arisen since the last time the DME provider had been in the home. A complete ventilator check is documented, ensuring that orders correlate with the present settings. The DME provider continues to communicate with the family throughout the first month to verify the parents have what is needed to care for their child as well as answer all questions. Per the policy of the DME provider, the therapist evaluated the need to continue returning to the home on a daily basis. The parents were doing well, and DME provider opted to make a weekly call to the parents. Upon completion of the first month at home, the DME provider assisted parents with ordering of the first month's supplies. This entailed a full inventory done with one of the parents. Reinstruction of monthly supply quantities was discussed, and a date and time were set with parents for delivery of the monthly order. The DME provider continued to do ventilator checks per policy and assisted parents with questions and concerns that arose. The patient remained on continuous ventilation for approximately 7 months. The weaning process then began, allowing the patient to come off the ventilator for 5 to 10 minutes at a time, as tolerated. This time increased until the patient was off the ventilator all waking hours and then on to being off the ventilator at all times. After 21 months of being at home with a ventilator, the patient was able to be decannulated with minimal medical needs from the DME provider.

KEY POINTS

- Critical components of discharging a child to home with technology dependency are excellent communication by all parties involved, timely planning to have all necessary roles and expectations established, overcoming possible barriers that may cause delay in discharge, and awareness to the needs of not only the child but the parents/caregivers as well.
- Recognizing, understanding, and addressing the possible barriers that may be present, either in the home, with the parents/caregivers or issues related to finances will assist the entire team insure a successful discharge.
- With multiple oxygen systems available on the market, finding the best suited for the child's needs is extremely important. Liquid oxygen, oxygen concentrators, and compressed gas sources are most commonly used in a home environment. The patient's oxygen liter flow should be the determining factor for selecting a modality source.
- To ensure the child has all the key components needed when traveling outside the home, a list is generated for a designated trach-to-go bag. This is an essential part of caring for a child with technology needs.
- Understanding when a child needs his or her trach tube changed is key for caring for a child with a trach. Child will have clinical signs to be aware when the need is present for a trach change.
- Preparing a parent/caregiver for attending to a child with a ventilator takes a great deal of time, understanding and patience, as well as preparation. Parents/caregivers training never ceases, it is done daily from the time the child is still inpatient and continues even after they have discharged home.
- Things to consider when selecting a home ventilator include the portability of the unit, weight and battery capabilities of the unit, and how the unit will be used for the child. Determining which DME provider is best suited for child is always important as well. In considering providers, the family should consider what insurance companies are in network with provider, the distance of the provider to where the child will reside, and ensure the provider is capable of managing the pediatric population.

ASSESSMENT QUESTIONS

See Evolve Resources for answers.

1. After a home assessment, what is the most common barrier that may delay a patient's discharge?
   A. Electrical issues
   B. Not owning a home
   C. Need for flashlights
   D. Width of the doorway too large

2. "A medical staff member designated to transition a patient from hospital facility to home or other level of care" is the definition for which of the following?
   A. Social worker
   B. Discharge planner
   C. Speech pathologist
   D. DME provider

3. What is an indication for changing a tracheostomy tube?
   A. Respiratory distress
   B. Weekly tracheostomy change
   C. Suction catheter does not pass freely
   D. All of the above

4. In a home care setting, how often should a routine tracheostomy change be performed?
   A. Monthly
   B. Daily
   C. Weekly
   D. Bi-weekly

5. In the home, what equipment is needed for a ventilator-dependent child?
   A. Heater/humidifier unit
   B. Wall flow meter
   C. Sterile gloves
   D. Microwave

6. The goal of having caregivers stay for an in-hospital trial is to:
   A. Give an opportunity for backup assistance from hospital staff
   B. Give caregivers a chance to relax
   C. Allow caregivers to assist with finances
   D. Take patients away from bedside nurse so they can admit new patients

7. Prolonged hospital stays can cause emotional stress on families. Which would not be a stressor for a family with a premature child that has required a prolonged stay?
   A. Strained finances
   B. Feeling of guilt
   C. Exhaustion
   D. All of the above

8. A 12-year-old male with Duchenne muscular dystrophy is admitted to the hospital for a planned tracheotomy and preparation for home mechanical ventilation. Discharge planning should begin for this child and his family:
   A. Immediately after placement of the tracheostomy tube
   B. On admission to the hospital
   C. After transition to the home mechanical ventilator
   D. Once the child is medically stable

9. The parents of an infant who is ventilator dependent have missed several educational sessions that are required before discharge home. They have also been sporadic in visiting their child and practicing bedside skills. What action should the discharge planning team take next?
   A. Submit a report to the local child neglect hotline.
   B. Ask the infant's physician to counsel with the parents.
   C. Provide the parents with a discharge contract/agreement.
   D. Suggest that the parents attend a parenting class together.

10. Which of the following is usually the major obstacle to providing quality care in the home of a technology-dependent child?
    A. High cost and inadequate funding of home care services
    B. DME providers that do not employ respiratory therapists
    C. Inability to provide home nursing
    D. Lack of two committed in-home caregivers

11. The need for home oxygen therapy for infants is most often established by:
    A. Arterial blood gas analysis
    B. Oxygen saturation measured by pulse oximetry
    C. Sleep scoring from polysomnography studies
    D. Capillary blood gas analysis

12. An infant requires oxygen with a nasal cannula at 0.5 L/min. The mother states that because of financial difficulties they have moved to a one-bedroom house. Which of the following oxygen systems would be most appropriate to provide in this home?
    A. Liquid oxygen with a base unit reservoir
    B. An oxygen concentrator
    C. A compressed gas H cylinder of oxygen
    D. Multiple compressed gas E cylinders of oxygen

13. An infant will be discharged home with an apnea–bradycardia monitor. Which of the following instructions should the parents be given?
    A. "Your baby only needs the monitor during naps and when sleeping at night."
    B. "The belt is tight enough if you can fit two fingers between it and your baby's chest."
    C. "When the monitor alarms, immediately check for correct electrode placement."
    D. "Do not place lotion on your baby's chest."

14. During use of a home apnea–bradycardia monitor, which of the following is the most common cause of a false alarm?
    A. The baby is crying.
    B. The lead wires are loose.
    C. The baby is breathing shallowly.
    D. The baby is burping.

15. How often should a cuffless tracheostomy tube in a child be changed when at home?
    A. Once a day
    B. Once a week
    C. Once each month
    D. Only when it becomes obstructed

16. After placing a speaking valve on a child with a 4.5 cuffless pediatric tracheostomy tube, the child exhibits signs of difficulty in exhaling. Which of the following changes should be made?
    A. Change to a 4.5 cuffed tracheostomy tube.
    B. Replace the tracheostomy tube with a fenestrated tube.
    C. Change to a 4.0 cuffed tracheostomy tube.
    D. Downsize to a 4.0 cuffless tracheostomy tube.

17. In which of the following situations should a second (backup/transport) ventilator be placed in a child's home?

   A. The child requires the ventilator only at night while sleeping.

   B. The child's home is within a 1-hour drive of the DME provider.

   C. The child is sprinting from the ventilator for 2 hours twice each day.

   D. The home nursing agency can provide nurses only at night.

References

1. American Thoracic Society: Statement on the care of the child with chronic lung disease of infancy and childhood, *Am J Respir Crit Care Med* 168:356, 2003.

2. Social Security Administration: Supplemental security income for the aged, blind, and disabled; deeming of income and resources [20 CFR Part 416], *Fed Regist* 47:24274, 1982.

3. Gracey K, et al: The changing face of bronchopulmonary dysplasia. 2. Discharging an infant home on oxygen, *Adv Neonatal Care* 3:88, 2003.

4. American Association for Respiratory Care: Clinical practice guidelines: discharge planning for the respiratory care patient, *Respir Care* 40, 1995.

5. DeWitt PK, et al: Obstacles to discharge of ventilator-assisted children from the hospital to home, *Chest* 103:1560, 1993.

6. American Academy of Pediatrics: Statement on hospital discharge of the high-risk neonate—proposed guidelines, *Pediatrics* 102:411, 1998.

7. Gilmartin MR: Transition from the intensive care unit to home: patient selection and discharge planning, *Respir Care* 39:456, 1994.

8. American Academy of Pediatrics Committee on Children with Disabilities: Guidelines for home care of infants, children, and adolescents with chronic disease, *Pediatrics* 96:161, 1995.

9. Czervinske MP: Ensuring quality care for infant tracheostomy patients: part 1, *AARC Times* 2331, 1999.

10. Fiske E: Effective strategies to prepare infants and families for home tracheostomy care, *Adv Neonatal Care* 4:42, 2004.

11. American Association for Respiratory Care: Clinical practice guidelines: providing patient and caregiver training, *Respir Care* 41, 1996.

12. Glenn KA, Make BJ: *Learning objective for positive pressure ventilation in the home,* Denver, 1993, National Center for Home Mechanical Ventilation and National Jewish Center for Immunology and Respiratory Medicine.

13. American Medical Association Home Care Advisory Panel: *Physicians and home care: guidelines for the medical management of the home care patient,* Chicago, 1992, American Medical Association.

14. American Academy of Pediatrics, Committee on Children with Disabilities: Managed care and children with special health care needs: a subject review, *Pediatrics* 102:657, 1998.

15. Hill L, Thompson M: Case management of technology-dependent children: a family-centered approach, *J Home Care Pract* 6:37, 1994.

16. McCarthy M: A home discharge program for ventilator-assisted children, *Pediatr Nurs* 12:331, 1986.

17. American Academy of Pediatrics, Medical Home Initiatives for Children with Special Needs Project Advisory Committee: The medical home, *Pediatrics* 110:184, 2002.

18. American Academy of Pediatrics, Committee on Child Health Financing: Guiding principles for managed care arrangements for the health care of newborns, infants, children, adolescents, and young adults, *Pediatrics* 105:132, 2000.

19. American Academy of Pediatrics, Committee on Children with Disabilities: Managed care and children with special health care needs: a subject review, *Pediatrics* 102:657, 1998.

20. Balfour-Lynn IM, Primhak RA, Shaw BNJ: Home oxygen for children: who, how, and when? *Thorax* 60:76, 2005.

21. Harris ND, Stamp JM: Current developments in oxygen concentrator technology, *J Med Eng Technol* 11:103, 1987.

22. American Academy of Pediatrics, Committee on Fetus and Newborn: Policy statement 2003: apnea, sudden infant death syndrome, and home monitoring, *Pediatrics* 111:914, 2003.

23. American Association for Respiratory Care: Clinical practice guidelines: pulse oximetry, *Respir Care* 36:1406, 1991.

24. Ghanayem NS, et al: Home surveillance program prevents interstage mortality after the Norwood procedure, *J Thorac Cardiovasc Surg* 126:1367, 2003.

25. Lewarski J: Long-term care of the patient with a tracheostomy, *Respir Care* 50:534, 2005.

26. Fiske E: Effective strategies to prepare infants and families for home tracheostomy care, *Adv Neonatal Care* 4:42, 2004.

27. American Thoracic Society: Care of the child with a chronic tracheostomy, *Am J Respir Crit Care Med* 161:297, 2001.

28. Hodge D: Endotracheal suctioning and the infant: a nursing care protocol to decrease complications, *Neonatal Netw* 97, 1991.

29. Fitton CM: Nursing management of the child with a tracheotomy, *Pediatr Clin North Am* 41:513, 1994.

30. Miyasaka K, et al: Interactive communication in high-technology home care: video phones for pediatric ventilatory care, *Pediatrics* 99:1, 1997.

31. American Association for Respiratory Care, Mechanical Ventilation Guidelines Committee: Clinical practice guidelines: humidification during mechanical ventilation, *Respir Care* 37:887, 1992.

32. Torres LY, Sirbegovic DJ: Problems caused by tracheostomy tube placement, *Neonatal Intensive Care* 1652, 2004.

33. Miyasaka K, et al: Interactive communication in high-technology home care: video phones for pediatric ventilatory care, *Pediatrics* 99:1, 1997.

34. Dettelbach MA, et al: Effect of the Passy-Muir valve on aspiration in patients with tracheostomy, *Head Neck* 17:297, 1995.

35. Keen SE, et al: Effect of in-home nursing care on distress and coping resources in caregivers of ventilator-assisted children at home, *Am Rev Respir Dis* 143A:257, 1991.

36. Jansen MT, et al: Caregiver's safety restraint practices for technology-dependent children during motor vehicle transportation, *Am Rev Respir Dis* 147A:410, 1993.

37. Tsara V, et al: Burden and coping strategies in families of patients under noninvasive home mechanical ventilation, *Respiration* 73:61, 2006.

38. University of Illinois: *Conference proceedings: strategies for success in home for medically fragile children,* Springfield, IL, 1989, University of Illinois, Division of Services for Crippled Children.

39. American Association for Respiratory Care: Clinical practice guidelines: long-term invasive mechanical ventilation in the home, *Respir Care* 52:1056, 2007.

40. DeWitt PK, et al: Obstacles to discharge of ventilator-assisted children from hospital to home, *Chest* 103:1560, 1993.

41. Edwards EA, O'Toole M, Wallis C: Sending children home on tracheostomy dependent ventilation: pitfalls and outcomes, *Arch Dis Child* 89:251, 2004.

42. Kacmarek RM, et al: Imposed work of breathing during synchronized intermittent mandatory ventilation (SIMV) provided by five home care ventilators, *Respir Care* 35:405, 1990.

43. Robert P, et al: Work of breathing imposed during spontaneous breathing in the SIMV mode of home care ventilators [abstract], *Respir Care* 37:1358, 1992.

44. Gilgoff IS, Peng RC, Keens TG: Hypoventilation and apnea in children during mechanically assisted ventilation, *Chest* 101:1500, 1992.

45. Chatburn RL, Volsko TA, El-Khatib M: The effect of airway leak on tidal volume during pressure- or flow-controlled ventilation of the neonate: a model study, *Respir Care* 41:728, 1996.

46. Bach JR, Alba AS: Tracheostomy ventilation: a study of efficacy with deflated cuffs and cuffless tubes, *Chest* 97(8):679, 1998.

47. Keens TG, et al: Frequency, causes, and outcomes of home ventilatory failure, *Am Rev Respir Dis* 147A:408, 1993.

48. Leonard BJ, Brust JD, Nelson RP: Parental distress: caring for medically fragile children at home, *J Pediatr Nurs* 8:22, 1993.

49. Thyen U, Kuhlthau K, Perrin JM: Employment, child care, and mental health of mothers caring for children assisted by technology, *Pediatrics* 103:1235, 1999.

50. Capen CL, Dedlow ER: Discharging ventilator-dependent children: a continuing challenge, *J Pediatr Nurs* 13:175, 1998.

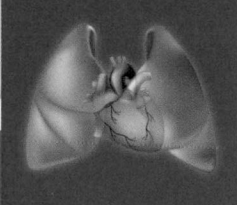

Chapter 36

Quality and Safety

LISA TYLER, LINDA NAPOLI

OUTLINE

LEARNING OBJECTIVES

After reading this chapter, the reader will be able to:

1. Define *quality* and *patient safety*
2. Describe the evolution of the quality movement and its importance to health care
3. Discuss the elements of teamwork and the effects on quality outcomes
4. Explain the impact of leadership support on quality and the use of a just culture to facilitate accountability
5. Describe how quality outcomes are measured and compared both internally and externally
6. Discuss the aspects of high reliability organizations as related to key concepts, evidenced-based practice, patient safety indicators, and the Agency for Health Care Research and Quality (AHRQ)
7. Explain how information technology can have both positive and negative impacts on health care organizations and quality outcomes
8. Identify the various processes used to build safety practices and tools used to define problems
9. Discuss James Reason's culture of safety theory and how it relates to errors
10. Recognize different methods used to support safety behaviors to prevent errors

KEY TERMS

Agency for Health care Research and Quality (AHRQ)
Benchmarking
Crew resource management (CRM)
Error
Evidence-based practice
Failure Modes and Effects Analysis (FMEA)
Health Failure Modes and Effects Analysis (HFMEA)

High reliability organizations (HRO)
Institute of Medicine (IOM)
Just culture
Kaizen
Lean methodology
Near miss
Negligence
Plan-Do-Study-Act (PDSA)
Precursor
Quality

Quality indicator
Root cause analysis (RCA)
SBAR
Sentinel event
Serious safety event
Six Sigma
Ventilator-associated pneumonia (VAP)

Quality and safety in health care are two key factors facing health care providers today. Internally there is a focus on improving quality and safety, which starts at the CEO and board level and continues throughout the organization. Externally there is emphasis on how measures of quality and safety are reported and shared across health care systems. Children differ in many ways compared with adults in regard to health care delivery and the relationship to medical errors and harm. Primary contributing factors include children's characteristics and development stages, demographics, dependency on parents and other caregivers concerning care and legal status, and varying epidemiology of medical conditions.[1] In addition, many devices and drugs are used "off-label," which means they have not been tested or approved for use in pediatrics. This can create a burden for health care providers to render services and deliver medications as discrepancies arise between what the patient needs and what is approved to be used. For this reason, patient-safety problems and solutions for children are multifaceted with unique attributes. Therefore understanding the main safety strategies in the pediatric population is vital. They are (1) epidemiology of errors and identification of the source of the issue; (2) understanding the science and safety aspects behind the culture; and (3) having a core source of safety solutions that are incorporated into risk assessment and solutions for each unique characteristic.[2]

Pediatric errors in the inpatient setting have been researched and described in a variety of studies. It has been reported that approximately 13 adverse events per 1000 hospital discharges occur in patients newborn through 15 years old.[3] **Negligence** (described as a lack of skills and/or failure to follow or deviation from standard practices and procedures) was determined to be the cause in 27.6% of events. Adverse drug events were identified in 2.3% of hospitalizations, and 19% were deemed preventable. Serious errors occurred more often in the critical care setting, and adverse drug events occurred three times more often among pediatric patients than among adults. Neonatal intensive care unit (NICU) data revealed 47% of errors were medication related, 11% patient misidentification, 7% delay or errors in diagnosis, and 14% involved errors in the administration or methods of using a treatment.[4]

WHAT IS QUALITY IN HEALTH CARE?

A variety of theories of quality care have been discussed with continued development across different health care platforms. The **Institute of Medicine (IOM),** a nonprofit organization whose purpose is to provide advice on issues related to science, medicine, and health, defines health care **quality** as the "degree to which health services for individuals and populations increase the likelihood of desired health outcomes (quality principles) and are consistent with current professional knowledge (professional practitioner skill), and meet the expectations of the market place."[5] Patient safety is defined by the IOM as "the prevention of harm to patients." Emphasis is placed on a system of care delivery that prevents errors; learns from the errors that do occur; and is built on a culture of safety involving health care professionals, organizations, and patients.[6] For that reason, safety is the foundation upon which all other aspects of quality care are built.

Quality practices and processes must be embedded in the foundation of health care institutions for both patient care and financial well-being. The public's increasing awareness of quality care through the reporting of high-profile reports on safety failures has had a significant impact on the focus of quality outcomes. A commitment to total quality is a necessary part of an organization's journey toward improvement. The philosophy of total quality consists of an attitude that is infused into the entire organization, both internally and externally. Those who work in organizations dedicated to the concept of total quality constantly strive for excellence and continuous improvement in everything they do.

HEALTH CARE QUALITY EVOLUTION

The awareness and subsequent scrutiny of quality care evolved through massive reporting processes and evaluation of landmark events. Released in 2000, the United States Institute of Medicine issued *To Err Is Human: Building a Safer Health System.* This report estimated up to a million patients experienced some type of preventable error, with 44,000 (120 patients per day) to 98,000 (268 patients per day) Americans dying as a result of preventable medical errors.[7] To put this into perspective, it is equivalent to one Boeing 737 or 747 crashing and killing everyone on board every day.[8] The typical consumers would never tolerate such odds. It further reported that adverse events occur in 2.9% to 3.7% of hospitalizations, with 7000 deaths per year from medication errors alone.[7]

Error is an act producing a preventable adverse outcome compared with the natural progression of disease leading to injury or death. More people die in a given year as a result of medical errors than from motor vehicle accidents (43,458), breast cancer (42,297), and AIDS (16,516).

The report made several suggestions to improve patient safety:

· Improve leadership and knowledge
· Identify and learn from errors
· Set performance standards and expectations for safety
· Implement safety systems in health care organizations[7]

The second major report from the IOM committee, *Crossing the Quality Chasm: A New Health System for the 21st Century* (2003), expanded the work outlined in *To Err Is Human* to an industry-wide process redesign, targeting a culture of improving the quality of care. The report focused on the quality of care currently present in the U.S. health care system. *Crossing the Quality Chasm* included a call for action to improve the American health care delivery system as a whole, in all its quality dimensions, and found too often health care failed to deliver its potential benefits. Other problem areas include gaps or chasms (wide differences) in patient care, performance variability, and the inability to use resources effectively (fragmented delivery systems/waste and overuse of services) because of system structures.

The committee defined six concrete components of high quality care:

· Safe—The patient is not harmed or injured by any care or procedure.
· Effective—The patient receives the desired or expected result from the care or procedure administered.
· Patient-centered—Care is provided to a patient with respect and awareness of his or her preferences, needs, and values, with the patient involved in clinical decisions.
· Timely—Care is provided at the right time, avoiding harmful delays.
· Efficient—Care is performed in an organized and capable way, achieving desired results, with minimal waste in time, effort, or supplies.
· Equitable—Patient receives care characterized by justice and fairness with impartiality toward all.[6]

Even with hospitals focusing on quality and attempting to integrate these guidelines into care, 3 years later an estimated 380,000 to 450,000 preventable adverse drug events occurred in hospitals each year.[9] In a more recent report, the Centers for Disease Control and Prevention noted that another 100,000 deaths could be attributed to infections. Newer studies from Health Affairs in April 2011 suggest the rate of preventable harm may be up to 10 times higher than the IOM estimates.[10] If this estimate is correct, preventable deaths may also be greater than the IOM estimates.

In 2008, medical errors cost the United States $19.5 billion with $17 billion directly associated with additional medical cost. This cost is attributable to increased hospital cost (length of stay), malpractice, and lost income for households. [11]

Errors are also costly by creating a loss of trust in the medical system. In October 2011, Health Grades reported that patients being treated in a 5-star rated hospital, as compared with a 1-star rated hospital, had a 73% lower mortality rate and 54% lower risk of dying. Distinction among type of hospital, patient, or procedure is not always available for further analysis.

TEAMWORK

Developing teams of caregivers for multidisciplinary communication was described early on by IOM as a necessary component of change that needed to occur to improve patient safety. The traditional health care model is hierarchical, with physicians giving orders and others doing what they say. The airline industry had this same problem; pilots were given the ultimate authority. When the airline industry embarked on a campaign to improve safety, they promoted a concept known as **crew resource management (CRM).** It is reminiscent of a "stop the line" philosophy employed in many factory operations to decrease defects in manufacturing. With CRM, crews were taught to function as a team, with each member having equally important roles and responsibilities regarding safety.[12] The expectation is for every member to appropriately assert concerns for safety. The culture of health care organizations must shift to emulate the importance of teamwork. This can be especially difficult because many units, departments, or locations of a given organization may have very different cultures. Every member of the team has to be valued and be able to contribute. This will result in better coordination of care, early recognition of errors, and more rapid interventions.[12] Additionally, there will be an improvement in employee satisfaction with a decrease in turnover, increasing the number of skilled providers performing care.

LEADERSHIP

Willingness to admit everyday errors is important in designing the work environment to be able to permit errors so as to improve on processes. Before the IOM report *To Err Is Human,* individual personal blame had been attributed to errors. This made people unwilling to come forward and admit errors because disciplinary action would be applied. In an attempt to counteract this concern, there was a move toward a "blame-free" environment. The reality is no one can offer a blame-free system in which any conduct can be reported without acceptance of responsibility at some level. There is a balance between the need to learn from our mistakes and the need for accountability.

Just Culture

The concept of a just culture in lieu of no blame has been introduced to address the concept of accountability and unsafe behavior. A **just culture** focuses on identifying and addressing systems issues leading individuals to engage in unsafe behaviors while maintaining individual accountability by establishing a zero tolerance for reckless behavior. It distinguishes between human error, at-risk behavior, and reckless behavior (ignoring a safety step). As stated by the AHRQ, "in a just culture, the response to an error or near miss is predicated on the type of behavior associated with the error, not the severity of the event."[13]

Let's take as an example the process of confirming patient identification before performing procedures. The therapist neglects to do this and performs the treatment on the wrong patient. If the organizational system allows for inconsistency of providing identification bands for patients, it needs to be addressed as a system issue. Focus would be placed on the improvements in the system and not the individual. If on the other hand the therapist neglected to perform patient identification when the system sufficiently supports the placement of identification bands, and gave a treatment to the wrong patient, then the therapist has been reckless and has to be held accountable for the error.

MEASURING QUALITY IMPROVEMENT

Various systems for classifying errors are used today. According to Health Performance Improvement (HPI),[14] safety events can be classified in three ways: near misses, precursor events, and serious safety events.

Near misses are those errors that do not reach the patient because they are detected before they do. An example would be morphine being ordered at a higher dose than should be given; the pharmacist checks the order before preparing the drug, recognizes it is outside normal dosing guidelines, and informs the physician.

The second classification is a **precursor** safety event, an event that reaches the patient but results in minimal to no detectable harm. If that same morphine dose error is not detected by the pharmacist or nurse and gets delivered to the patient but the patient does not have any adverse response, then it is a precursor safety event.

A **serious safety event** is an event that reaches the patient and results in moderate to severe harm or death. If the overdose of morphine is given and the patient experiences a depression in respiratory effort resulting in apnea or death, this becomes a serious safety event. Serious safety events must be reviewed through a root cause analysis (RCA) to determine if a gap in care or a deviation from normally accepted practice has occurred. This is an important determination because harm can even occur when normally accepted practices have been followed. Such events would not be classified as serious safety events.

It has been suggested that for every one serious safety event, there are hundreds of precursor safety events and thousands of near misses. It is important for health care organizations to not only analyze serious safety events but also review and report near misses and precursor events. Thorough reporting and analysis of near misses, precursor safety events, and serious safety events will identify systems needing improvement.

The Joint Commission on the Accreditation of Healthcare Organizations (JCAHO) also reviews errors that are classified as **sentinel events.** The Joint Commission defines a sentinel event as "an unexpected occurrence involving death or serious physical or psychological injury, or the risk thereof."[15] Organizations voluntarily report events after having completed an RCA. They then track categories for what has been submitted and reviewed. This allows us to see trends in patient safety. They also will report sentinel events on their website and encourage organizations

to apply learning techniques to prevent similar events from occurring. As an example, in their Sentinel Alert 38, tubing misconnections were highlighted.[16] Tubing misconnections are a potentially common area of concern for respiratory therapists. There have been reports of feeding tubes being connected to cuff pilot balloons of artificial airways and suction ports on inline suction catheters. After this report, organizations should have internally identified all possible tubing misconnections that could occur and implemented processes to eliminate the potential for this error.

Through reviewing sentinel events, The Joint Commission sets national safety patient goals annually with the purpose of improving patient safety. The 2013 goals are listed in Table 36-1.

Demonstrating improvements in quality outcomes encompasses measuring whether efforts made lead to change toward the primary goal or at least moving in the desired direction. Further analysis must define whether efforts could contribute to unintended results in different parts of the system and require additional resources to bring a process back into acceptable range.[17] Quality measure reporting should reflect quality practices, encourage better performance, and identify areas of improvements compared with other similar organizations. Reporting of quality measures may be mandatory or voluntarily reported. State-to-state mandated reporting varies. In addition, other regulatory organizations may direct certain reporting obligations. Voluntary reporting is used to help the consumer search for high-quality health care. *U.S. News and World Report* magazine uses voluntary reporting to identify its best hospitals.

Benchmarking—Internal/External

Measures of quality and safety can track progress of improvement initiatives using reporting benchmarks. **Benchmarking** in health care is defined as the continual and collaborative discipline of measuring and comparing the results of key work processes with those who have what are considered best practices.[18] This process enables organizations to continuously measure services, practices, costs, and products using best practices to improve care. There are two types of comparative benchmark models, internal and external.

Internal benchmarks are used to identify best practices within the organization over time. It is important to understand that what is considered best practice within the organization over time may not be reflected in other institutions.[7] To be effective at internal benchmarking, implementing a process designed to promote idea sharing is required. Steps for the process include the following:

1. Identify processes to benchmark.
2. Organize efforts by conducting audits of current processes, determining what tools are most appropriate for the analyzing processes.
3. Identify a similar internal process for comparison.

TABLE 36-1

Joint Commission 2013 National Patient Safety Goals

Goal	Specifics
Identify patients correctly	Use at least two ways to identify patients.
	Make sure the correct patient gets the correct blood.
Improve staff communication	Get important test results to the right staff on time.
Use medications safely	Label medications before a procedure.
	Take extra care with patients who take medicines to thin blood.
	Record and pass along correct information about a patient's medicines.
Prevent infections	Use hand cleaning guidelines from the CDC.
	Use proven guidelines to prevent infections that are difficult to treat.
	Use guidelines to prevent infection of the blood from central lines.
	Use proven guidelines to prevent infection after surgery.
	Use proven guidelines to prevent infections of the urinary tract caused by catheters. Use hand cleaning guidelines from the CDC.
	Use proven guidelines to prevent infections that are difficult to treat.
	Use guidelines to prevent infection of the blood from central lines.
	Use proven guidelines to prevent infection after surgery.
	Use proven guidelines to prevent infections of the urinary tract caused by catheters.
Identify patients at risk	Identify patients at risk for suicide.
Prevent mistakes in surgery	Make sure the correct surgery is done on the correct patient and at the correct place on the patient's body.
	Pause before surgery to make sure that a mistake is not being made.

CDC, Centers for Disease Control and Prevention.

4. Prioritize ideas from the team and turn them into projects with time lines for adopting best practices.
5. Evaluate outcomes of the two processes to determine what causes the significant differences between them.
6. Evaluate transferability of those aspects leading to improved performance.
7. Transfer the aspects and monitor results.[19]

External benchmarking requires a comparison of work with other organizations with the intent to find new ideas, methods, products, or services. The objective is to continuously improve one's own performance by measuring how it performs by comparing it with others.[20] External benchmarking involves using comparative data between organizations to scale performance and to identify processes that have been proven successful in other organizations. External benchmarking is usually performed through some type of intermediary, such as National Association of Children's Hospitals and Related Institutions (NACHRI) or Children's Hospital Association (CHA). Organizations must be able to define who to benchmark against. Most reporting is general and does not account for differences across the health care continuum. For example, evaluating results for community hospitals and tertiary care facilities may not provide a reasonable comparison.

Some experts believe internal benchmarking is the most important type of comparison. Internal benchmarking may provide several advantages over its external counterpart because access to information is more readily available. One drawback of external benchmarking is that target companies may be reluctant to share information for fear of losing competitive distinctions.[20]

This is typically not the case with internal functions. Another advantage is the transferability of practices. Although there may be geographical and process differences within an organization, a cohesive infrastructure provides a common basis for benchmarking standards. External benchmarking can be difficult with cultural diversity of organizations, practices that may work for one but not another because of varying organizational operations. Finally, internal benchmarking can provide a seemingly safe training environment in which skills and processes can be developed. This process prepares organizations for external benchmarking processes.[20] A disadvantage of internal benchmarking is that set targets may fall short of actual best practice in the industry.

There are known discrepancies in the way in which organizations confirm the existence of **ventilator-associated pneumonia (VAP),** a subtype of hospital-acquired pneumonia that can occur when a person is receiving mechanical ventilation via an artificial airway. This makes is it difficult to use external benchmarking data in setting goals for rate reduction. Most organizations are currently using internal VAP rate to set goals for improvement.

RELIABILITY

High Reliability Organizations

High reliability organizations (HRO) consistently minimize adverse events despite complex and hazardous work by maintaining a commitment to safety at all levels, from the frontline clinician to upper executives. To improve the ability to provide the highest quality care, health

TABLE 36-2

High Reliability Organization Attributes

Sensitivity to operations	There has to be constant awareness of the state of the systems and processes that affect patient care. If errors occur, quickly identify and fix them. People should be familiar with operations beyond their own job. People communicate clearly so there is a clear picture of any given situation. Implementing patient care rounds and safety huddles is a strategy for accomplishing this.
Preoccupation with failure	Systematically study potential problems instead of only reacting to actual problems. Analyze near misses and precursor safety events as failures that reveal potential danger rather than as evidence of success and ability to avoid danger.
Reluctance to simplify	Accept that the work is complex and don't expect simplistic solutions to work. Take nothing for granted. Listen to different points of view. Develop clinical guidelines, protocols, and rapid response teams.
Deference to expertise	In order to provide quality health service to increase the likelihood of desired health care outcomes, recognize available knowledge and defer to most relevant expertise. Listen to all team members physicians, nurses, respiratory therapists, parents, patients, etc.
Commitment to resilience	Cultivate the ability to detect, contain, and respond to system failures.

care must apply these concepts, which are described in Table 36-2.

Because many of these concepts are very different than the way we have practiced in the past, we have to conceptualize ways to apply them. If tasks are too complex, it becomes impossible to distinguish doing the work right from doing it wrong. If there are no opportunities to talk about issues with other staff, there is little chance people will be exposed to other views or information and little opportunity to discuss near misses. If leaders aren't routinely observing and talking with staff providing direct patient care, they will not understand the operations for which they are responsible. Some approaches that have been tried successfully include the following:

Simplifying work processes. To be successful in making your system more reliable, reduce what staff are expected to do into a limited set of clearly defined behaviors. Encourage staff to incorporate error prevention techniques into their work.

Daily check-ins. These are short and focused meetings between the unit leadership and staff. This supports the importance of any effort that leadership is involved in and allows for staff to raise questions.

Executive rounds. Leadership within an organization is the driving force behind the culture that exists within it. In order for quality and safety to be a priority, the message must come from the CEO and board. Having executives around in the clinical environment will create an opportunity for leaders to model the behavior that they want staff to perform. During rounding, hospital leaders are able to retain an awareness of operations that will assist them in good decision making. Rounds allow staff to raise issues with leaders and it solidifies the importance of quality and safety behaviors. Leaders must follow up on any issues that are raised so continual feedback can occur.

Safety huddles. Safety huddles are used as a way to gather the clinical team together throughout the day. An example is to have huddles on units every 12 hours in order to raise safety issues with the entire team. The huddles are usually very short but allow anyone to raise concerns about safety.

Performance management. This is extremely important to reward staff for desired behavior and identify and resolve any unwanted behaviors.[21]

Implementation of these concepts will result in patient safety being an intrinsic part of how organizations operate all the time. This is proven based on results from other industries similar to health care, in that they are complex, high-risk systems that have accomplished great safety improvements by doing so. They have driven themselves to become HROs. As a definition, "reliability depends on the lack of unwanted, unanticipated and unexplainable variance in performance."[22] What can we learn from other similar industries? In the United States in 1980 there were 7.3 unplanned nuclear reactor shutdowns per 7000 hours. In 2000 there was none (Figure 36-1).

The nuclear power industry worked hard on safety culture and error prevention and was able to achieve this dramatic improvement in safety statistics. The airline industry was able to reduce their accident rate over 30 years from about 25 accidents per year to near zero. This was accomplished using the same principles applied to nuclear power. Despite being complex and high-risk industries, they have successfully developed processes to remain safe.

Evidence-Based Practice

Health care organizations consist of diverse levels of experience pertaining to clinical process innovations, and staff tolerance for change involving incorporation of evidence into practice differs. **Evidence-based practice (EBP)** can facilitate quality improvement efforts as on ongoing process. Primarily EBP is the multidisciplinary approach to decision making in which the practitioner systematically finds, appraises, and uses the most current and valid research findings as the basis for clinical decisions. These theories can be applied to the health care organizational structure and processes. A generalized

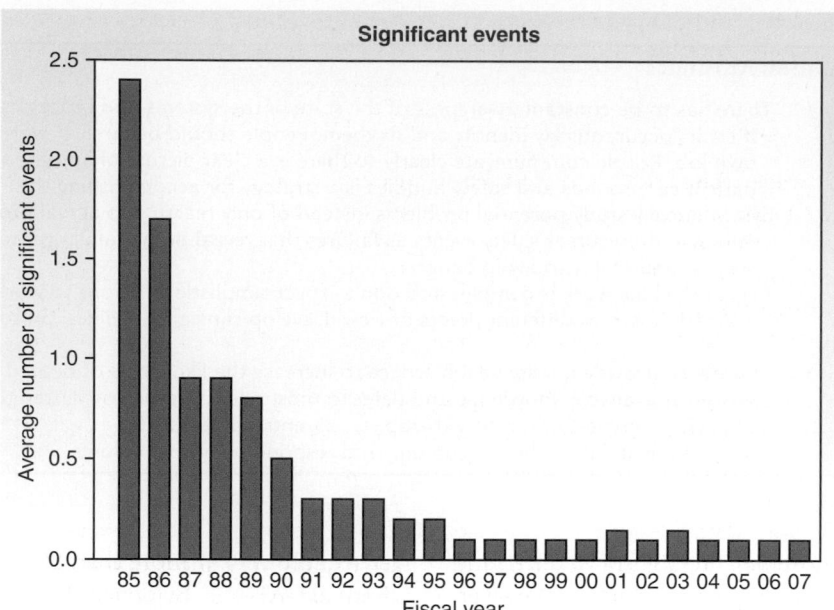

FIGURE 36-1 Nuclear reactor significant events (1985-2007). (Source: U.S. Nuclear Regulatory Commission New Release No. 09-033, February 2009.)

approach for constructing quality improvement processes should include the following:

· Identification of a problem and executive visibility
· Designation of clinical champion and team
· Process flow chart prepared before and after implementation of the intervention or change, to identify responsibility and ensure resource needs are transparent
· Mapping out of necessary tools to support changes that are developed and used to track outcomes built into decision support and information systems and education training materials
· Monitoring with feedback if provided to involved staff on a regular basis
· Continual detailing of the intervention, which is reviewed for ongoing improvement and maintenance
Figure 36-2 conceptualizes what is required when incorporating evidence into practice.

Clinical care guidelines should be established using evidence to improve clinical outcomes. Challenges in pediatric evidence-based practice are present because of limited accessibility and readiness of applicable data.

Practitioner Skills

Achieving high-quality care on a consistent basis in a reliable way requires all health care team providers to make right decisions about the appropriateness of services as well as the skills, judgment, expertise, and timely execution of care provided.[5] The decision-making process should include focus on utilization of resources, quantity and necessity of treatment and test ordered, and appropriateness of therapy with a thorough evaluation of risk–benefit analysis. Once the treatment plan is in place, duty falls on the performance or skill—that is, how well actions were carried out—of the individual to provide care in

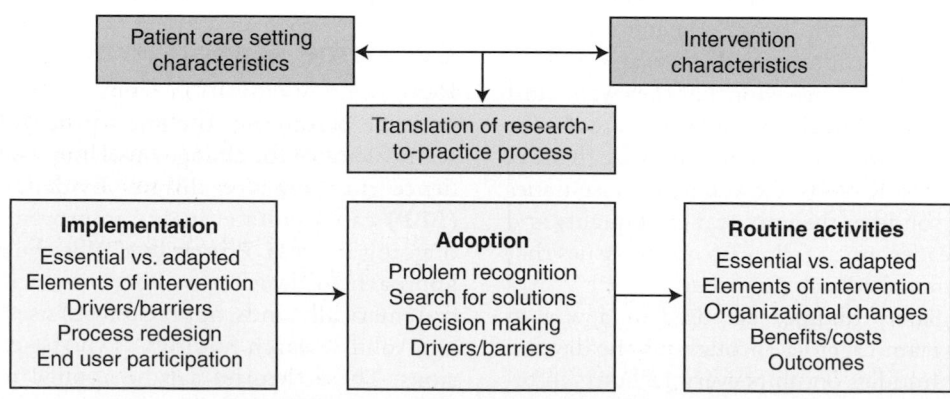

FIGURE 36-2 Transferring evidence into practice.

the manner that fits the policies and standards in place to reduce errors and optimize patient safety.

Agency for Healthcare Research and Quality

The **Agency for Healthcare Research and Quality (AHRQ)** is a federal authority for patient safety and quality care. The AHRQ is a leader, particularly in pediatrics, funding safety and quality improvement efforts, formulating information, and distributing those findings to health care practitioners and the public to optimize awareness.[23] The reports and assessments provide organizations with comprehensive, evidence-based information on typical medical conditions and new health care technology. More recent reviews of potential pediatric safety issues reveal that the hospitalized child who experiences a safety event, as compared with those who do not, have a length of stay 2 to 6 times longer, hospital mortality 2 to 18 times greater, and hospital charges 2 to 20 times higher. In addition, the severity of illness and type of hospital, outside of birth trauma, are directly associated with patient safety incidents. After extensive review, 18 **quality indicators** for both provider level and diagnostic area were recommended as measurable components. Because these indicators have the most potential to cause an adverse event in hospitalized children, safety systems targeting these areas should reduce length of stay and any additional events in this patient population[23] (Box 36-1).

As part of AHRQ's safety mission and initiatives, this federal agency actively provides information, tools, and grants to improve the statistics for health care–associated infections (HAIs). Action alerts are posted monthly, keeping the health care community up to date with the latest research. The goal is to identify and prevent infections at the point of care.

Health care–associated infections are infections patients acquire while receiving treatment for another condition in some type of health care facility. Millions of infections and thousands of deaths occur annually, making HAIs the most common complication of hospital care. Financially, HAIs add $28 to $33 billion to health care costs. AHRQ researches barriers and challenges in preventing the most common and therefore most costly HAIs. These infections cause extended hospital stays and increased cost and risk of mortality. Types of infections include bloodstream infections (BSIs), catheter-associated urinary tract infections (CATIs), surgical site infections (SSIs), and ventilator-associated pneumonia, which together account for more than 80% of all HAIs.[24]

In an AHRQ Evidence Report/Technology Assessment, *Prevention of Healthcare Associated Infections,* researchers identified proper hand-washing hygiene as a major intervention for all HAIs. The report suggests printed or electronic reminders and staff education as successful methods for improving patient outcomes.[24]

According to the U.S. Department of Health and Human Services (HHS), AHRQ is a leader in collaborating and aligning its efforts with cross agencies in developing comprehensive short- and long-term goals to reduce and eliminate HAIs nationwide. The Partnership for Patients is one of those agencies. Their shared goal is to "improve the quality, safety, and affordability of health care for all Americans."[24] This will result in more than 1.8 million fewer injuries with more than 60,000 lives saved over a 3-year period. Working with Partnership for Patients, the AHRQ prioritized safety measures include the following:

Reduction of Health Care–Associated Infections

Appropriate timing of antibiotics for surgical patients will help reduce wound infections after surgery, a common occurrence. If successful, postoperative sepsis, a severe bloodstream infection occurring after surgery, will decrease. Receiving the right antibiotic at the right time on the day of surgery is most effective in preventing HAIs postoperatively. Additionally, "ensuring good glycemic control, using appropriate hair removal methods, continuing beta blocker therapy when appropriate, and administering appropriate thromboembolism prophylaxis can reduce morbidity and mortality."[24]

Central Line–Associated Bloodstream Infections

Because children who require central lines are often already in critical condition because of their medical condition, which can include trauma or premature birth, any new infections can negatively affect their chances of recovery.

Box 36-1	Pediatric Quality Indicator Set

Provider Level Indicators	**Area Level Indications**
Accidental Puncture or	Asthma Admission Rate
Laceration	Diabetes Short-Term
Decubitus Ulcer	Complication Rate
Foreign Body Left During	Gastroenteritis
Procedure	Admission Rate
Iatrogenic Pneumothorax	Perforated Appendix
in Neonates at Risk	Admission Rate
Iatrogenic Pneumothorax	Urinary Tract Infection
in Non-neonates	Admission Rate
Pediatric Heart Surgery Mortality	
Pediatric Heart Surgery Volume	
Postoperative Hemorrhage	
or Hematoma	
Postoperative Respiratory Failure	
Postoperative Sepsis	
Postoperative Wound Dehiscence	
Selected Infections Due to	
Medical Care	
Transfusion Reaction	

From Pediatric Quality Indicators: Software Documentation, Version 3.2 SAS. Table 1. Pediatric Quality Indicator (PDI) Variables. Department of Health and Human Services Agency for Healthcare Research and Quality, www.qualityindicators.ahrq.gov, Accessed September 23, 2013.

Great emphasis needs to be placed on the proper insertion and management of central lines, which will result in a significant lowering of infection rates.[24]

Reduction of Severe Adverse Events

Serious adverse events (SAEs) are situations arising from medical and surgical procedures or adverse drug reactions, which are commonly treated in outpatient settings—physician offices, hospital outpatient departments, and hospital emergency departments. If successfully prevented, ambulatory care visits as a result of adverse effects of medical care will diminish.

Mechanical adverse events are SAEs for the homebound patient caused by the placement or use of catheters. Bleeding, hematomas, or knotting of the catheter are examples of these events. Patients often visit an ambulatory care center for assistance.

Respiratory Failure

Respiratory issues are not uncommon after surgery. Reintubation or prolonged mechanical ventilation may be necessary. "Causes include: over-sedation, exacerbation of underlying cardiovascular or respiratory conditions, and ventilator-associated pneumonia."[24] Close attention should be paid to these risk factors.

Preventable and Premature Mortality Rates

Rapid identification and aggressive treatment of complications may prevent deaths after hospital care. Death may occur from "pneumonia, thromboembolic events, sepsis, acute renal failure, gastrointestinal bleeding or acute ulcer, shock, or cardiac arrest."[24]

30-Day Mortality Rates

Reducing deaths within 30 days of admission, especially from pneumonia and acute myocardial infarction, is another safety initiative.

INFORMATION TECHNOLOGY

The role of information technology is crucial to the quality and patient safety movement. Pediatric-specific technology is evolving but is challenged because of the fact that most computerized systems are designed for adults. Limited effectiveness in preventing medication errors without significant additional improvement processes make for specific localized institutional needs. Health information technology systems enable more reliable, effective communication within and across health care settings. Accessibility to patient information at the point of care assists clinicians with decisions and can reduce error potential.[25] A variety of IT health systems are currently available that perform checks in real time, assisting with calculations and alerting providers of potential adverse events. Additional system benefits may include recommended treatment decisions based on evidence-based medicine, prescription systems where orders are checked for accuracy, and patient records that can be accessible to both health care practitioner and patients.

Technology can be an efficient solution for facilitating prescription orders, where the paper-based process often leads to errors resulting from illegible handwriting, incorrect dosing, or missed drug-drug interactions and allergy alerts. As meaningful use stages are defined and increased focus is placed on the ability to exchange health information across health care settings, improved coordination of care is enabled. Health IT systems are tools that have been recognized to prevent medication errors and provide solutions to communication and accountability gaps. IT solutions provide the ability to assist clinical decision making. Although effective IT systems within a health care setting are important in realizing better quality of care, expanding these practices beyond the primary and acute care setting increases the opportunity to detect potential adverse events through access to current, accurate, and complete patient health information.

There are potential drawbacks to IT implementation. If it is not optimally integrated into the workflow of the organization, it can generate extra work for the clinical team. Another barrier to the adoption of IT is the extreme cost of implementation and maintenance of the system. In addition, the cultural adjustment associated with the adoption of a new system such as electronic health records can be challenging if people resist practice change.

DESIGNING SAFE PROCESS

Six Sigma

Six Sigma was developed by Motorola as a quality improvement (QI) strategy. The term itself is derived for the Greek letter *sigma,* which statisticians use to measure standard deviations or known variance and the degree to which almost perfect production can occur.[26] Six Sigma is based on scientific method and involves improving, designing, and monitoring processes to minimize or eliminate waste while optimizing satisfaction and increasing financial stability. There are two main methods Six Sigma uses to measure processes. One inspects process outcomes by counting defects and uses a statistical conversion rate. The second method predicts process performance by estimating process variation.[27]

Six Sigma employs a five-step strategic process: define, measure, analyze, improve, and control approach.[28] Goals, stakeholders, and process owners of an improvement activity are identified in the define stage of the Six Sigma strategic process. A task is identified, historical data are reviewed, and a scope of expectations is defined. Various tools such as focus groups, mapping, and cause–effect diagrams are employed to define improvement process.[29] Next, standards are selected and performance objectives and sources of variability are defined. During the measure step, quantitative measurements of current practices are compiled. Collected data are analyzed and validated to determine the capability of the new process. In addition, objective data are used to identify ways to eliminate gaps between the current state and the desired state and statistical tools are used to guide improvement plans. In the improve stage, planned changes are implemented and evaluated. Quantitative data are collected again and used to evaluate the outcome of the implemented change. The final step of the process is the control step. This step is considered the most important in the process— requirement identification and construction of formal plans and processes for maintaining control of the new system.[26]

Although created for the manufacturing industry, Six Sigma is successfully used to decrease defects and variations, decrease operating costs, and improve outcomes in a variety of health care settings and processes.[27] Standardizing processes to improve efficiency and outcomes should be a focus of patient safety efforts in health care organizations.

Lean production

The **Lean methodology**, derived for the Toyota production system, targets customer needs and aims to improve processes by removing activities that are considered no-value-added. The basic principles of Lean are to minimize waste in all aspects of production. The critical components of Lean include identifying exactly what defines "value" to the customer and then creating a value map, similar to a process map but with the addition of a value-added or no-value-added step from the customer's perspective.

Successful application of the Lean methodology in the health care system includes eliminating unnecessary activities associated with overcomplicated processes and work-arounds with frontline staff.[27] The goal of the methodology is to maximize value added, activated in the best possible sequence, to enable continuous operations. In essence this will improve quality and prevent errors.[27] In addition, Lean methodology can be used to develop applications for evidence-based practice processes and needs.[26]

Root Cause Analysis (RCA)

Another extensively used technique to identify and understand the underlying causes of an event as well as potential associated events is called a **root cause analysis (RCA)**. The RCA technique is a retrospective, systematic process using information from an unplanned event to identify and understand the underlying causes of the event.[26] It is used to identify trends and assess risk when human error is suspected, with the understanding that the system issues, not individual factors, are likely the root cause of most problems.[6] It is important to understand in health care that a problem often has more than one cause and that errors as a result of those causes can be interrelated.

A multidisciplinary team completely examines the event, aims to uncover underlying causes, and identifies causal, situational, enabling, and contributing factors, both active and latent, of the incident. The final step of the RCA is developing recommendations for system and process improvement based on the findings of the investigation.[27] RCA has been shown to be a useful technique to report errors and differentiate between active and latent errors, identifying the need for change to policies and procedures and serving as a basis to suggest system changes, including improving the communication of risks.[27]

The Joint Commission now requires an RCA be performed in response to all sentinel events (significant harm to a patient) and expects the organization to develop an action plan aimed at reducing future risks based on the findings, as well as to monitor the effectiveness of the action plan.[26]

Failure Modes and Effects Analysis

Failure Modes and Effects Analysis (FMEA) is a prospective risks assessment tool used to identify and eliminate known and potential failures, problems, and errors for a system, design, process, or service before they actually occur. This technique was developed by the U.S. military and is used by the National Aeronautics and Space Administration (NASA) to predict and evaluate potential failures and unrecognized hazards and to proactively identify steps in a process to reduce or eliminate future failures. It was adapted for health care by the Department of Veteran Affairs and the National Center for Patient Safety.[26]

In health care the goal is to use a multidisciplinary team to evaluate a process from the quality improvement perspective.[27] The estimated effect of each process failure is determined by how likely it is to occur, how visible the failure is, and how catastrophic the failure would be if it happened. Information learned from the FMEA process can be used to provide data for prioritizing improvement strategies, serve as a benchmark for improvement efforts, educate and provide a rationale for practice change, and increase the ability of the team to facilitate change across all services and departments within a hospital.[27] This tool is most effective when new processes are being designed.[26]

Health Failure Modes and Effects Analysis (HFMEA) is used to provide detailed hazard analysis of smaller processes and develop specific recommendations. It is important to list all possible and potential failure modes of each process and determine if they warrant further action.[27]

How are these quality improvement strategies similar? Can they work together in synergy or should they be done in isolation? Although these QI systems were developed from outside the medical field, they have successfully been adapted to health care processes. The terms of Lean and Six Sigma are often used together; though different in approach, their complementary processes can be used simultaneously. Six Sigma can be used to identify variation of practice, then measure the scope of the problem. Lean can identify the voice of the customer and the defined value to formulate the clinical question to ask. A part of Lean is **Kaizen,** which means continuous quality improvement, emphasizing the philosophy that poor quality arises from bad systems rather than bad people, which is part of the Lean principles.[30]

Plan-Do-Study-Act

The **Plan-Do-Study-Act** (PDSA; Figure 36-3) method is aggressively used to make constructive changes in the health care industry as a rapid-cycle improvement process.[31] It is one of the most commonly used methodologies in health care. Introduced by Shewart and Deming as a continuous quality improvement business practice, PDSA moved into health care when the Institute for Healthcare Improvement (IHI) recommended it for implementing a process for quick change.[26] This method uniquely implements small and frequent changes that are analyzed for effectiveness before they are implemented on a large-scale basis.[31] The PDSA quality improvement efforts aim to establish a functional relationship between changes in behavior and capability and outcomes. To establish targeted constructive changes, three questions are posed before implementing a PSDA cycle:

1. What is the goal of the project?
2. How will one know whether the goal was reached?
3. What will be done to reach the goal?

The PDSA method aims to determine the nature and scope of the problem, the necessary changes, a plan to implement those changes, who should be involved, and what should be measured to determine the impact of the change. Once data and information are collected, key measures are reviewed to indicate the success or failure of the implementation.[27] In the **P**lanning phase, current situations and root causes are evaluated. The hypothesis is developed about what will occur with the change. The **D**o phase includes small-scale testing or pilots being carried out. The **S**tudy or check phase examines the results. It is in this phase where the assessment of the change is based on quantitative or qualitative data. In the **A**ct phase, the decision to enact or abandon the planned change is made from the analysis of data in the previous stage. This includes whether the change will be moved to larger scale implementation. Ideally multiple PDSA cycles are used in succession, starting with the easiest and then moving to more difficult.[26] The majority of PDSA quality improvement efforts find greater success using a series of small and rapid cycles to achieve the goals of intervention.[27]

TOOLS FOR PROCESS EVALUATION

A variety of tools ranging from basic to complex are used to define and analyze distinct processes that typically produce quantitative data. This section provides a few examples of quality tools used by organizations to facilitate improvement processes.

Flowcharts are used to map each step of a process showing logical sequencing for completion of an operation. A flowchart is a good starting point for a team seeking to improve an existing process or planning a new process or system. Check sheets are simple tools to measure the frequency of events or defects over a time interval. This process is used for information gathering and can be used easily while providing immediate data to help understand processes.

In cause-and-effect diagrams, commonly known as fish-bone diagrams, the problem (effect) is stated in a box and the likely causes (bones) are listed around the heading that leads to the effect. This is often used to identify contributing factors of a complex problem. The spaghetti diagram is a visual way to depict the material or information flow through a process in a diagrammatic form (Figure 36-4). The spaghetti diagram helps identify waste that is often not even recognized as such—for example, walking to and from a medication dispensing machine that is located too far away for staff using it. This diagram helps determine the physical flow and distance that information and people travel to process work (see Figure 36-4).

Tree diagrams help to identify the tasks and methods needed to solve a problem and reach a goal. These diagrams entail creating a detailed list of tasks that need to be accomplished to achieve a goal. One example of a tree diagram is a driver diagram. Figure 36-5 is an example of the driver diagram process used to outline reducing HAI through the reduction of VAP.

Quality tools are different than the improvement process. Multiple tools might need to be used for any given process improvement project.

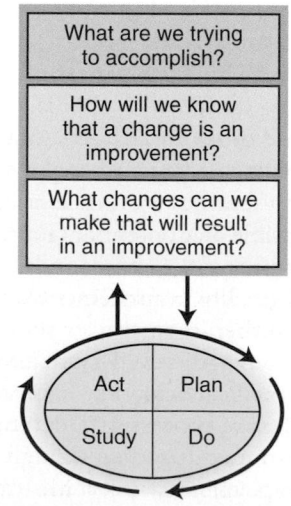

FIGURE 36-3   Plan-Do-Study-Act cycle.

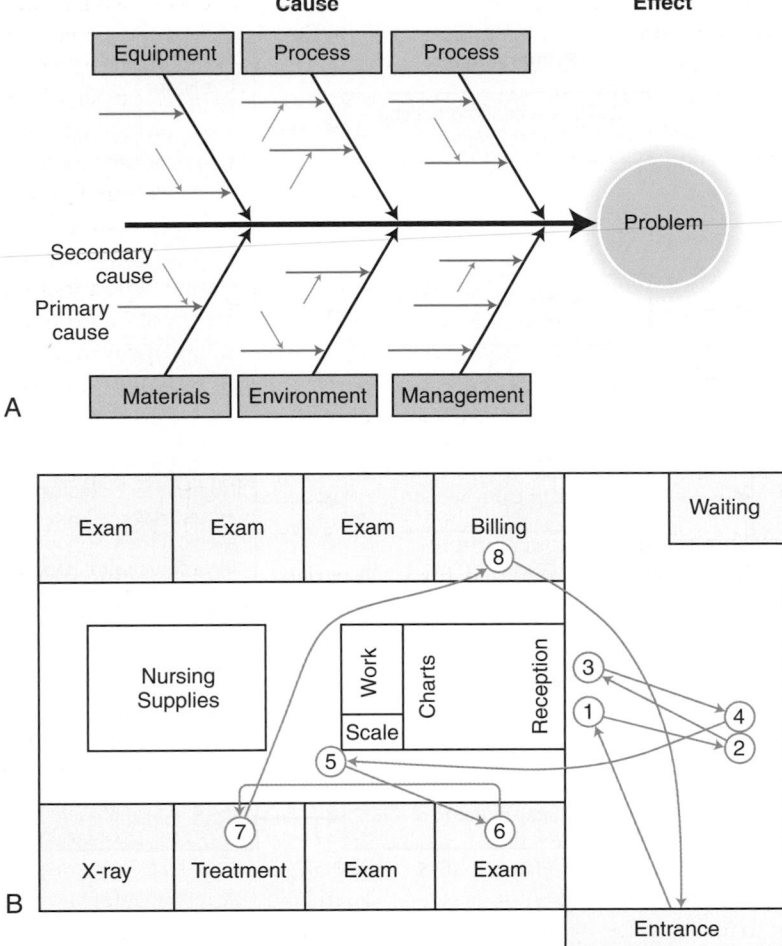

FIGURE 36-4   A, Fishbone diagram. **B,** Spaghetti diagram.

HANDOFF COMMUNICATION

Handoff communication is a high-risk process causing errors that lead to ineffective care and patient safety breaches. It is estimated that 80% of serious medical errors involve miscommunication among caregivers when a patient is transferred or handed off to another area. Improving the accuracy, completeness, and accessibility of patient information can reduce ineffective handoff communication. In 2006 the Joint Commission added a handoff-related goal to its expanding set of national patient safety goals and made specific expectations that health care organizations implement a standardized approach to handoff communication. One way to improve communication processes is the use of a standardized method of handoff.

CULTURE OF SAFETY

A study by Taylor et al. showed the incident report system used in children's hospitals does not always support quality care. Their study showed that incidents of actual harm to the child were reported but not "near misses." Quality improvement comes from the "near misses" as well as the

harmful events. Improving education of staff concerning what should be reported and how to report an incident is a priority. They summarized that a reporting system should be "easily accessible, require a small amount of time and be in electronic format, where possible."[32] As Taylor's team states, ultimately, reporting medical errors should be seen not as a punitive exercise but as an essential ingredient in providing optimal patient care.[32]

James Reason, a well-known professor and expert on the practice and theory of safety, describes safety cultures as shared values and beliefs that interact with an organization's structures and control system to produce behavioral norms. An ideal safety culture is the necessary driver in sustaining efforts to reduce operational hazards. Two kinds of fallibility are present: individual and systems. Individual accidents are ones in which specific persons or groups are both the agent and the victim.[33]

There are many layers of defense, barriers, and safeguards that are a part of a systems approach to prevent errors. They include alarms, physical barriers, and alerts, as well as procedural and administrative controls. Their function is to protect patients from hazards or harm. Most often they work effectively, but many systems have weaknesses or gaps.

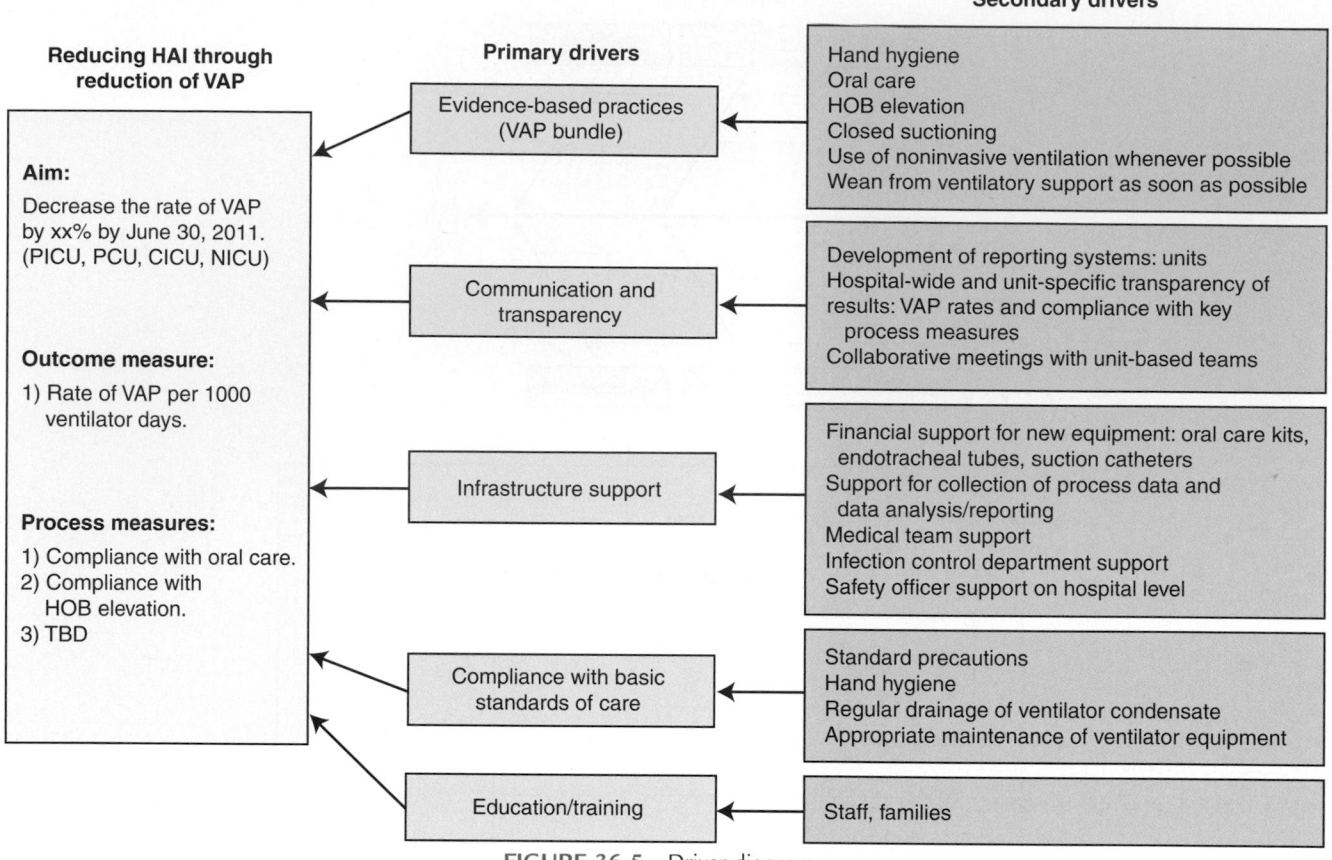

FIGURE 36-5 Driver diagram.

These gaps are created by active failures and latent conditions. Nearly all adverse events involve a combination of these two factors. Active failures are unsafe acts committed by those people who are in direct contact with the patient or system. Latent conditions are the inevitable flaws within the system caused by failures in design and or process and management's inability to anticipate all possible scenarios. The Swiss cheese models shown in Figure 36-6 illustrate both how layers work to prevent errors from reaching patients and how at times the holes line up in sequence to allow harm to patients and produce what can be a serious adverse event.[34]

SAFETY BEHAVIORS FOR ERROR PREVENTION

A key area for improving safety is to promote behaviors that prevent errors. Most organizations have implemented methods to do this based on an analysis of their own needs and what will work best within their internal culture to obtain the best improvement results. Techniques for preventing errors may include coaching and cross-checking, speaking up for safety by incorporating an organizational phrase that should make everyone stop and listen, critical thinking development, effective communication techniques, and paying attention to details. Everyone must incorporate coaching and cross-checking into the way an organization functions. It must be viewed as a positive intervention. It is important to look out for one another to catch possible mistakes and build a greater sense of accountability of the team. This helps everyone perform at their best and promotes team performance. Encouraging safe and productive behaviors and discouraging those behaviors that are not a part of the peer coaching process. Often a 5:1 positive feedback ratio is used to reinforce good habits and eliminate bad ones.

Speaking up for safety normally encompasses using smart words to guide practices and avoid resistance; verbiage typically includes phrases like "I have a concern," "I need clarification," and "Help me to understand." It will also provide a means for going up the chain of command if necessary.

Thinking critically about observations made during the course of the workday, asking questions, and listening to your "gut" enable practitioners to practice with a questioning attitude. It is important to reflect on practices and processes that one may have issues with and resolve any questions that one may have with source verification, content expert substantiation, and other confirmation processes.

Paying attention to detail can be very effective in avoiding slips during patient care. Self-checking by making yourself stop and think before acting can reduce the probability

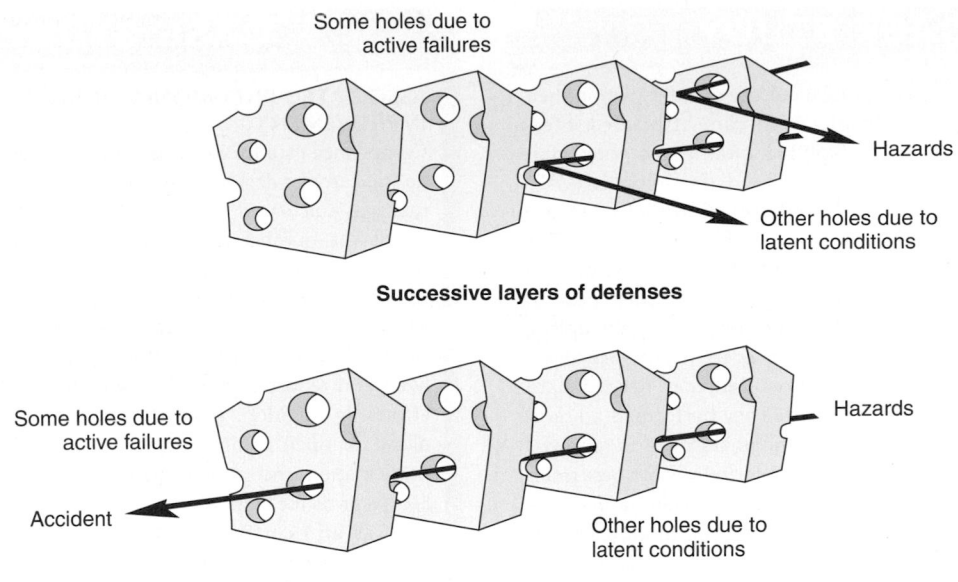

FIGURE 36-6 Swiss cheese models.

of making an error. This process should only take a few seconds and is especially critical when you are asked to perform a task that you have not done in a while.

Communicating effectively entails a variety of safety practices to ensure accurate communication and understanding. Phonetic clarification is a tool to ensure that correct information is being transmitted. When communication involves a letter, the letter is followed by a word that begins with the letter—for example, "C Charlie, A Alpha, T Tango." In addition, numerical clarification is used to ensure that accurate numbers are being communicated. For 50, one would say, "50, that's five-zero." Implementation of leading zero placement and following zero elimination when using decimals is another effort in place to improve communication.

Handoff communication using **SBAR** (Situation/ Background/Assessment/Recommendation) has become a widely accepted sign-out strategy because of the support of the Joint Commission and the IHI. It uses a structured method for all communication practices between providers.[24]

Situation: Who or what you are calling about and the immediate problem

Background: A brief description of the relevant history related to the condition

Assessment: Your view of the situation and your perception of the urgency of action

Recommendation: Your suggestion about the action that should be taken or your request for guidance on what action to take

SBAR originated at Kaiser Healthcare but can also be credited to the nuclear U.S. Navy. The Joint Commission then expanded the strategy to include interactive communication that allowed for questions between givers and receivers of information, a process for verification of the information exchanged, and an opportunity to review historical data and finally a process that limited interruptions.[35]

A three-way repeat back is another method to ensure that important information is transferred in a clear, complete, and accurate manner. This involves the sender providing an order, request, or information in a clear and concise format; the receiver acknowledges by repeating back the order, request, or information, and then the sender acknowledges the accuracy of the repeat back. If the information is incorrect, the process is repeated.

Patient safety has to become second nature and an intrinsic part of how we practice as respiratory therapists. As part of the multidisciplinary team we have a responsibility to perform the techniques mentioned in this chapter to reduce errors and improve practice. As public awareness has increased and continues to do so, all health care organizations will need to be able to provide evidence of improvements in safety. In order to accomplish this, there will be many exciting changes in the future. Respiratory therapists need to be involved in and lead such changes in areas related to our practice. In 1859 Florence Nightingale said, "It may seem a strange principle to enunciate as the very first requirement in a Hospital that it should do the sick no harm."[36] Although this concept was never fully understood at the time, the time is now to do so. We have a long way to go, but by embracing proven quality and safety techniques, health care can be as safe as other high-risk, complex industries.

CASE STUDY

As hospitals engage in creating a culture of safety within their organizations, elimination of health care–associated infections has been a focus. In Tyoli Hospital it was noted that there had been 5 ventilator-associated pneumonias (VAP) per 1000 ventilator days confirmed using Centers for Disease Control and Prevention criteria over the past month. The hospital realized an improvement effort must be initiated. A multidisciplinary team was assembled to consider how to move forward. The team consisted of respiratory therapists, nurses, physicians, and infection prevention specialists. When the team convened, they realized they needed data and information to move forward. They performed a literature review of VAP, did external benchmarking, and reviewed practices across all intensive care units to look for best practices. Specific care elements for patients on ventilators were clustered into a bundle. A bundle is a group of independent steps that when implemented collectively and reliably result in significantly better patient outcomes than when individually applied. An example of a bundle to reduce VAP is provided in the following list:

- Elevation of head of bed
- Daily assessment of readiness to extubate
- Comprehensive oral care
- Daily assessment of readiness to wean/extubate
- Keep ventilator circuit free from condensate
- Inline suction catheters
- Peptic ulcer disease prophylaxis
- Deep venous thrombosis prophylaxis

When all these things were completed, the team developed a driver diagram (see Figure 37-5). The diagram identified factors that would affect accomplishing the goal of reducing VAP, along with the specific reduction goal and the process measures used to monitor compliance with implemented changes.

The next phase was educating all staff involved in care of patients on ventilators, with the expectation everyone would follow the same care bundle, and included all disciplines. Clinical champions were identified for each area and discipline to lead the process change. The implementation process can be launched successfully if the health care system is effectively designed, with champions from administration, leadership, and frontline staff maintaining the initiative's momentum. Before implementing the standardized care delivery process, staff members were introduced to evidence-based information about VAP. They also were oriented to the ventilator bundle and daily goal sheets at staff meetings and in-services, through poster presentations and one-to-one individual sessions. Ongoing education, reeducation, and reinforcement provided ample opportunity for staff to voice concerns, ask questions, and offer feedback about the initiative.

CASE STUDY

ASSOCIATED PNEUMONIA MOVEMENT TOWARD IMPROVEMENT

Compliance rate for identified process measures were used as an indicator of degree of bundle implementation. Compliance rate was calculated as the number of interventions delivered versus the number of possible interventions. Weekly audits were conducted to collect data and track compliance with the use of the daily goal sheet and the bundle interventions, reeducating and reinforcing, as necessary, to address any noncompliance issues. Once data were available, findings were analyzed and reported graphically to visually reinforce the staff's efforts. In addition, a weekly schedule for team meetings to allow for open communication occurred, which encouraged participation and gained buy-in from the frontline clinicians. Storyboards for emphasis of implementation and current VAP rate (as an example, "Days VAP free") were useful tools in making these changes to standard operating procedure.

The following figure displays the process measure compliance over the next year.

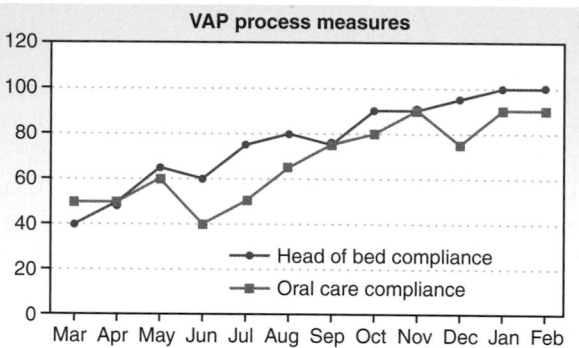

Tyoli hospital continued its focus on VAP prevention and monitored VAP rates per 1000 ventilator days monthly. Their VAP rates are depicted in the following figure.

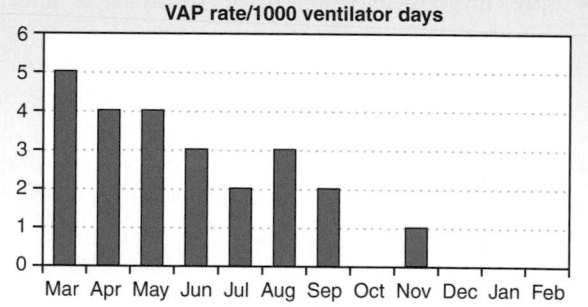

After review of these data, Tyoli hospital's efforts at VAP reduction would be best affected by implementing which of the following?
1. Reeducation of staff on head of bed to influence VAP rates.
2. Implementation of oral care kits to improve compliance.
3. Continuation of current activities while monitoring compliance.
4. Selection of other process measures to improve VAP rates.

See Evolve Resources for answers.

KEY POINTS

- Health care quality is defined as the degree to which health services for individuals and populations increase the likelihood of desired health outcomes (quality principles), are consistent with current professional knowledge (professional practitioner skill), and meet the expectations of the marketplace. Patient safety is the foundation upon which all aspects of quality care are built.

- The awareness and subsequent scrutiny of quality care evolved through massive reporting processes and evaluation of landmark events. In 2000 the U.S. Institute of Medicine issued *To Err Is Human: Building a Safer Health System*. The second major report from the IOM committee, *Crossing the Quality Chasm: A New Health System for the 21st Century* (2003), expanded the work, calling for action to improve the American health care delivery system as a whole.

- The culture of health care organizations must shift to emulate the importance of teamwork.

- The concept of a just culture in lieu of no blame has been introduced to address the concept of accountability and unsafe behavior. A just culture focuses on identifying and addressing systems issues leading individuals to engage in unsafe behaviors while maintaining individual accountability by establishing a zero tolerance for recklessness.

- Demonstrating improvements in quality outcomes encompasses measuring whether efforts made lead to change toward the primary goal or at least moving in the desired direction. Internal and external benchmarking are two methods used to calculate outcomes.

- High reliability organizations (HRO) consistently minimize adverse events despite complex and hazardous work by maintaining a commitment to safety at all levels, from the frontline clinicians to upper executives. This is accomplished by sensitivity to operations, preoccupation with failure, reluctance to simplify, deference to expertise, and commitment to resilience.

- Information technology provides accessibility to patient information at the point of care, assists clinicians with decisions, and can reduce error potential. Drawbacks include the generation of extra work for the clinical care providers, the extreme cost of implementation, and a cultural adjustment associated with the adoption of a new system.

- Safety processes include Six Sigma, Lean methodology, root cause analysis, Failure Modes and Effects Analysis, and Plan-Do-Study-Act process. Tools include fishbone diagrams, spaghetti diagrams, and flowcharts.

- James Reason describes the many layers of defense, barriers, and safeguards that are part of a systems approach to prevent errors, but gaps or holes are present that may lead to patient harm. Nearly all adverse events involve a combination of these two factors. Active failures are unsafe acts committed by those people who are in direct contact with the patient or system. Latent conditions are the inevitable flaws within the system caused by failures in design or process and management's inability to anticipate all possible scenarios.

- Methods health care practitioners can use to prevent errors include the following:
  Coaching and cross-checking
  Speaking up for safety
  Thinking critically about observations
  Paying attention to detail
  Communicating

ASSESSMENT QUESTIONS

See Evolve Resources for answers.

1. The IOM defines what as the foundation upon which quality care is built?
   a. Safety
   b. Situational awareness
   c. Errors
   d. Research

2. *To Err is Human* said approximately how many patients were injured per year as a result of medical errors in the United States?
   a. 25,000
   b. 150,000
   c. 77,000
   d. 100,000

3. When using a crew resource management philosophy in health care, who would be considered able to ask questions to anyone on the team?
   a. Physician
   b. Nurse
   c. Respiratory therapist
   d. Anyone

4. Using the concept of a just culture, if a respiratory therapist fails to follow proper procedure when the system supports such procedures, the therapist would be dealt with in what way?
   a. System improvement
   b. Employee accountability and discipline
   c. Employee termination
   d. System interruption and reengineering

5. Benchmarking is a common practice in comparing results (quality) both internally and externally. Which of the following statements is true about benchmarking?
   a. External benchmarking is an easy way to compare organizations.
   b. Internal benchmarking provides more access to information.
   c. External benchmarking always specifies differences between types of hospitals.
   d. Internal benchmarking makes it difficult to affect change.

6. What types of work can evidence-based practice help support?
   a. Care protocols/guidelines
   b. Safety error resolution
   c. Staff callout procedures
   d. Management education

7. The use of electronic medical records can improve patient care by providing which of the following?
   a. Workflow between different areas of the hospital
   b. Making it less expensive to provide care
   c. Enhancing accuracy of prescriptions
   d. Giving the clinician less patient information

8. What attribute do Six Sigma and Lean methodology have in common?
   a. Process and efficiency improvement
   b. Fishbone diagram implementation
   c. Clinical outcome variation
   d. Employee and management development

9. The Swiss cheese model by James Reason is used to describe which of the following concepts?
   a. There are no defenses to prevent errors.
   b. Quality improvement can only be based on serious safety events.
   c. Employees to not fear punitive responses to errors.
   d. There are defenses against errors but errors still occur.

10. Which of the following is the most important thing we can improve to enhance patient safety?
    a. Communication
    b. Detail orientation
    c. Staffing levels
    d. Orientation

References

1. Steering Committee on Quality Improvement and Management and Committee on Hospital Care: Principles of pediatric patient safety: reducing harm due to medical care, *Pediatrics* 127(6)1199-1212, 2011.
2. Woods DH: Child-specific risk factors and patient safety, *J Patient Safety* 1(1):17–22, 2005.
3. Leape LL, Brennan, TA: The nature of adverse events in hospitalized patients: results of the Harvard Medical Practice Study II, *N Engl J Med* 324(6):377–384, 1991.
4. Suresh GHJ: Voluntary anaymous reporting of medical errors for neonatal intensive care, *Pediatrics* 133(6):1609–1618, 2004.
5. Buttell P, Hendler R, Daley J: Quality in healthcare concepts in practice. In Cohn KH, editor: *The business of healthcare*, vol. 1, Westport, CT, 2007, Preager, pp 61–95.
6. America CO: *Crossing the quality chasm: a new health system for the 21st century*, Washington DC, 2001, National Academy Press.
7. Kohn L, Corrigan J, editors: *To err is human: Building a safer health system*, Institue of Medicine, Committee on Quality of Health Care in America, Washington DC, 2000, National Academy Press.
8. Nance JJ: *Why hospitals should fly*, Bozeman, MT, 2008, Second River Healthcare Press.
9. Institute of Medicine: *Preventing medication errors*. Available at: http://www.iom.edu. Accessed: September 2012.
10. Andel CD: The economics of health care quality and medical errors, *J Health Care Finance* 39(1):39–50, 2012.
11. Shreve J, ven Dan J: *The economic measurement of medical errors*, Schaumberg, IL, 2010, Society of Actuaries/Milliman.
12. Ransom ER, Joshi MS, Nash DB, Ransom SB: *The healthcare quality book*, ed 2. Chicago, 2008, Health Administration Press.
13. Marx D: *Patient safety and the "just culture": A primer for health care executives*, National Heart, Lung, and Blood Institute; National Institutes of Health, 2001, AHRQ, pp 1–28.
14. Healthcare Performance Improvement. www.HPIresults.com: Available at: http://www.hpi.com. Accessed: September 2012.
15. The Joint Commission: *Sentinel Event*. The Joint Commission. [Online] 2013. http://www.jointcommission.org/sentinel_event.aspx. Accessed October 2012.
16. The Joint Commission: Tubing misconnections—a persistent and potentially deadly occurrence, *Sentinel Event Alert*, The Joint Commission (36): April, 2006.
17. Varkey P, Reller MK: Basics of quality improvement in health care, *Mayo Clin Proc* 82:735–739, 2007.
18. Gift RG: *Benchmarking in health care*, ed 5, Chicago, 1994, American Hosptial Publishing.
19. Southard PB, Parente DH: A model for internal benchmarking: when and how? *Benchmarking Int J* 14(2):161–171, 2007.
20. Kay JF: Health care benchmarking, *H K Med Diary* 12(2), 2007.
21. Hines S, Luna, K, Lofthus J, et al: *Becoming a high reliability organization: operational advice for hospital leaders*. Contract No. 290-04-0011. The Lewin Group, 2008, Agency for Healthcare Research and Quality. http://www.ahrq.gov/professionals/quality-patient-safety/quality-resources/tools/hroadvice/hroadvice.pdf.
22. Hollnagel E: Simplification of complexity: the use of simulation to analyze the reliability of cognition. In Aldemir S, MA, Cacciabue PA, editors: *Reliability and safety assessment of dynamic process systems*, Berlin, 1993, Springer Verlag.
23. Lacey S, Smith JB, Cox K: Pediatric safety and quality. In Hughes R, editor: *Patient safety and quality: an evidence based handbook for nurses*, Rockville, MD, 2008, Agency for Healthcare Research and Quality, pp 1–30.
24. Agency for Healthcare Research and Quality: *Patient Safety Primers. Safety Culture*. U.S. Department of Health and Human Services. [Online] September 2012. http://psnet.ahrq.gov/primer.aspx?primerID55. Accessed January 2013.
25. Cortelyou-Ward K, Swain A, Yeung T: Mitigating error vulnerability at the transition of care through the use of health IT applications, *J Med Syst* 36:3826, 2012.
26. Seidi KL: The intersection of evidence-based practice with 5 quality improvement methodologies, *JONA* 42(6):301, 2012.
27. Hughes RG: Tools and strategies for quality improvement and patient safety. In Hughes RG, editor: *Patient safety and quality: an evidence based handbook for nurses*, Rockville, MD, 2008, Agency for Healthcare Research and Quality, pp 1–20.
28. Barry R, Murcko A: *The Six Sigma book for healthcare: improving outcomes by reducing errors*, ed 1, Chicago, IL, 2003, Health Administration Press.
29. Lanham B, Maxson-Copper P: Is Six Sigma the answer for nursing to reduce medical errors and enhance patient safety? *Nurs Econ* 21(1):39–41, 2003.
30. Graban M, Swartz JE: Change for health. *Management Services*, 56(2):35–39, 2012.
31. Berwick, D: Developing and testing changes in delivery of care, *Ann Intern Med* 128(8): 651–656, 1998.
32. Taylor JA, Brownstein D: Use of incident reports by physicians and nurses to document medical errors in pediatric patients, *Pediatrics* 114:729–735, 2004.
33. Reason J: Achieving a safe culture: theory and practice. In *Work & stress*, vol. 3, Taylor & Francis Ltd, 1998, Abingdon, Oxford, UK, pp 293–306.
34. Reason J: Human error: models and management, *BJM* 320:768–770, 2000.
35. Freitag M, Carroll VS: Handoff communication: using failure modes and effects analysis to improve the transition in care process, *Qual Manag Health Care* 20(2):103–109, 2011.
36. Nightingale F: *Notes on hospitals*, London, 1863, Longman, Green, Longman, Roberts, and Green.

Glossary

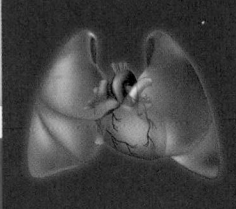

A

Acrocyanosis Blue hands and feet with decreased perfusion.

Acute respiratory distress syndrome A severe form of acute lung injury characterized by pulmonary edema and alveolar collapse secondary to the disruption of the alveolar-capillary membrane and surfactant dysfunction. Subsequently, hypoxemia and widespread infiltrates on chest radiographs can occur after a variety of predisposing pulmonary and nonpulmonary insults.

Adaptive control ventilation Uses a pressure setting as the main determinate of lung inflation; however, it adjusts the pressure to maintain a desired tidal volume based on a preset algorithm.

Adaptive pressure ventilation A mode of ventilation that can provide either support or control modes of ventilation and adjust to lung physiology based on measured parameters determined by a preset closed-loop algorithm.

Aerosol A suspension of solid or liquid particles suspended in a gas.

Aerosol output The rate at which the volume or mass of drug formulation is emitted by the aerosol generator.

Aerosol therapy Delivery of medical or bland aerosols generated by an aerosol device such as the nebulizer, the pressurized metered-dose inhaler or the dry-powder inhaler for the treatment of patients with pulmonary or systemic diseases.

Agency for Health Care Research and Quality (AHRQ) A federal authority for patient safety and quality care.

Aging Refers to changes in aerosol particles that occur after they are generated.

Agonist A chemical substance capable of activating a receptor to induce a pharmacological response.

Air bronchogram The radiographic appearance of the air-filled bronchus against surrounding opacified alveoli.

Airway clearance technique (ACT) Sometimes called *airway clearance therapy*. A therapy or technique designed to improve secretion or mucus management.

Airway resistance The pressure difference per unit flow as gas flows into or out of the lungs (flow/pressure).

Allele One member of a pair of genes that controls the same trait.

Allograft rejection The rejection of tissue transplanted between two genetically different individuals of the same species.

Alveolar volume The tidal volume that interacts with the alveolar-capillary membrane and is involved in gas exchange.

Amnioinfusion Injection of normal saline into the amniotic sac.

Anaphylaxis Systemic immunoglobulin E–mediated hypersensitivity response resulting from exposure to foreign antigen.

Anencephaly Congenital absence of the cranial vault, with the cerebral hemispheres completely missing or reduced to small masses.

Anesthetic gas mixtures Volatile gases designed to provide inhalational anesthesia. Anesthetics such as isoflurane, halothane, desflurance, enflurance, and sevoflurane.

Angiogenic clusters Small cellular pools that supply nutrition to the growing embryo. Also called *blood islands*.

Aorticopulmonary septum Formed by ridges between the bulbus cordis and truncus ultimately developing into separate aortic and pulmonary arteries.

Apgar Score Evaluation of newborns based on five factors heart rate, respiratory effort, muscle tone, reflex irritability, and skin color.

Apnea Pathological condition in which breathing ceases for longer than 20 seconds.

Apnea of infancy (AOI) Generally refers to infants with a gestational age of 37 weeks or more at the onset of apnea.

Apnea of prematurity (AOP) Sudden cessation of breathing that lasts for at least 20 seconds or is accompanied by bradycardia or oxygen desaturation (cyanosis) in an infant younger than 37 weeks of gestation.

Apparent life-threatening event (ALTE) An episode that is frightening to the observer and is characterized by some combination of apnea (central or occasionally obstructive), color change (usually cyanotic or pallid but occasionally erythematous or plethoric), marked change in muscle tone (usually marked limpness), choking, or gagging.

Arachidonic acid A polyunsaturated fatty acid present in cell membranes of brain, muscles, and liver.

Arterial blood gas Blood gas analysis of an arterial sample obtained via arterial puncture or directly from an arterial catheter.

Assist control ventilation Similar to control; however, it attempts to support patient efforts with fully control breaths. Frequency is then driven by the patient's effort.

Asthma Asthma is a reversible obstructive lung disease created by chronic inflammation of the airways. These inflamed airways often hyper-react (bronchospasm) to various triggers.

Asthma action plan A written management plan with information that a patient or family can refer should the patient become symptomatic.

Asthma education Disease-specific education designed to improve self-management.

Asthma triggers Exposure to allergen or aggravating agents that worsen asthma symptoms.

Atelectasis An absence of air in the lung parenchyma.

Atelectrauma Ventilator-associated lung injury that is also associated with the opening and closing of alveoli.

Atomizer A simple aerosol pneumatic aerosol generator without baffle.

Atrial bulge One of three identifiable structures in the primitive heart.

Atrioventricular septal defect Also known as *AV canal* or *endocardial cushion defect*, refers to an anomaly in which there is absence of the septa between the atria and ventricles.

Atypical or new bronchopulmonary dysplasia Often develops in preterm newborns who may have required minimal or even no ventilator support and relatively low inspired oxygen concentrations during the early postnatal days.

Azoospermia A condition in which a male does not have a detectable number of sperm in his semen.

B

B₂ agonist Otherwise known as *bronchodilators* or *airway smooth muscle relaxants*.

Baffle Any surface on which gas containing aerosol impacts with larger particles depositing on the surface while smaller particles remain suspended.

Ballard Score Postnatal examination score for determining gestational age based on external physical findings.

Barium swallow A fluoroscopic evaluation of the esophagus using a barium sulfate contrast agent; same as esophogram

Barotrauma Ventilator-associated lung injury that is associated with inappropriate use of pressure that does not recruit or improve ventilation or oxygenation.

Benchmarking Continual and collaborative discipline of measuring and comparing the results of key work processes with those who have what are considered best practices.

Betamimetic Stimulating, mimicking, or referring to β-adrenergic receptors of the sympathetic nervous systems.

Bilateral choanal atresia Incomplete opening into the nasopharynx caused by membranous or bony structures

Biophysical profile (BPP) Technique for evaluating fetal status using fetal heart rate monitoring and ultrasound assessment of amniotic fluid volume, fetal muscle tone, gross fetal movement, and fetal breathing motion.

Blastocyst The ball of cells that results from repeated cellular shortly after fertilization.

Breath-actuated nebulizer (BAN) Aerosol generator that produces aerosol from liquid formulation only during inhalation.

Breath-enhanced nebulizers Jet nebulizers that use one-way valves to control ambient gas entering the nebulizer and on the mouthpiece or mask to direct exhaled gas.

Bronchial fremitus Vibrations of the chest resulting from movement of air through airways partially obstructed by mucus.

Bronchiectasis A chronic condition resulting in the abnormal dilation of the bronchial airways.

Bronchiolitis Swelling and inflammation of the bronchioles, which are the smallest airways in the lung.

Bronchiolitis obliterans An inflammatory lung disease of the small airways, or bronchioles.

Bronchomalacia Increased flaccidity of the brochial cartilage that leads to airway narrowing and collapse during respiration.

Bronchopulmonary dysplasia (BPD) A form of chronic lung disease that develops in preterm neonates treated with oxygen and positive-pressure ventilation (PPV).

Bulbar muscles A muscle group that controls the epiglottis and other glottis structures, tongue, mouth, larynx, and throat and is important for airway protection and secretion clearance.

Bulboventricular loop Formed during early fetal development when the bulbus cordis and ventricular bulge merge, it is a one-ventricular structure that is the precursor of the ventricles.

Bulbus cordis One of three identifiable structures in the primitive heart eventually merges with the ventricular bulge to form the bulboventricular loop.

C

Calorimetry Clinically, the quantification of energy expenditure of a patient.

Capillary blood gas Blood gas analysis obtained via capillary puncture.

Capnography Refers to the measurement and display of carbon dioxide values during the respiratory cycle over time.

Carbon dioxide production The sum volume of carbon dioxide produced by cells in the body as a result of metabolism per unit of time.

Carboxyhemoglobin Hemoglobin that has carbon monoxide instead of the normal oxygen bound to it.

Cardiac output The amount of blood ejected from the heart over the course of 1 minute.

Cardiac index The ratio of the cardiac output to the body surface area.

Cardiomyopathy A chronic disease of the heart muscle (myocardium) in which the muscle is abnormally enlarged, thickened, and/or stiffened.

Cation Any positively charged atom or drug molecule.

CCAM Congenital cystic adenomatoid malformation.

Central venous catheter A catheter inserted in the central venous system.

Central venous oxygen saturation The percentage of oxygenated hemoglobin in central venous blood. This can be measured via blood sample or by fiberoptic catheters in vivo.

Central venous pressure The blood pressure of the central venous system, typically measured in the superior vena cava.

Centrifugal pump A type of pump used in ECMO—blood is propelled forward by a constrained vortex.

Cervical cerclage A procedure to suture close a cervix that has painlessly dilated in the second trimester of pregnancy. The most common method is a pursestring suture placed transvaginally at the level of the internal cervical os.

Cervical dilation Opening of the cervix as a result of painful uterine contractions in labor. It is assessed by vaginal examination and expressed in centimeters or finger breadths; one finger breadth is approximately 2 cm. At full dilation the diameter of the cervical opening is 10 cm.

Cervical effacement Thinning of the cervix associated with dilation of the cervix in labor.

Cervical insufficiency Painless dilation of the cervix early in the pregnancy. Depending on what point in pregnancy this occurs, cervical insufficiency can lead to miscarriage, stillbirth, or preterm delivery. Cervical insufficiency tends to be a recurring problem.

CHARGE A syndrome of defects including *c*olobomas, congenital *h*eart defects, choanal *a*tresia, *r*etarded development, *g*enital hyperplasia, and *e*ar anomalies.

Chest physical therapy Sometime called chest physiotherapy. In general a group of therapies that focus on chest wall compression, percussion, or vibration in order to clear secretions.

Chief complaint Reason the child is presenting for treatment.

Cholelithiasis Stones in the gallbladder that can be of different compositions depending on disease process.

Chorion Structural part of the placenta facing the fetus serving as the vascular connection to the fetus through the umbilical cord.

Chorionic membrane Sac-like structure that surrounds the growing fetus.

Chorionic villi Capillary network within the chorion that allows gas and nutrient exchange between the mom and the fetus.

Chronic lung disease The initial diagnostic criteria mandated continuing oxygen dependency during the first 28 days of life with compatible clinical and radiographic findings to label an infant as having BPD. Later, it was proposed to use the need for supplemental oxygen at 36 weeks postmenstrual age (PMA) as the diagnostic criterion especially in preterm very low birth weight (VLBW) infants.

Chronic pulmonary insufficiency of prematurity Is diagnosed in very immature babies who have made at least a partial recovery from RDS but then go on to develop apnea and increasing oxygen requirements. They have low lung volumes and respond well to CPAP.

Churg-Strauss syndrome A syndrome described as a blood vessel autoimmune vasculitis that can lead to necrosis.

Chylothorax Abnormal collection of lymph in the pleural space.

Classic bronchopulmonary dysplasia Was first described by Northway as a severe chronic lung injury in premature infants who survived hyaline membrane disease after treatment with mechanical ventilation and oxygen.

Clubbing Pathological changes in the nail beds of the fingers and toes, typically a manifestation of chronic diseases (e.g. cardiopulmonary, gastrointestinal, inflammatory).

CO_2 elimination The sum volume of exhaled carbon dioxide.

Coarctation of the aorta Severe narrowing of the thoracic aorta in the proximity of the ductus arteriosus.

Compliance Ability of lungs and thorax to expand; expressed as the volume change per unit of pressure change.

Computed tomography A medical imaging procedure that creates sectional images that can be viewed in multiple imaging planes.

Congenital heart disease A malformation of the heart, aorta, or other large blood vessels that is the most common form of major birth defect in newborns.

Continuous positive airway pressure (CPAP) Refers to application of continuous pressure during both inspiration and expiration in a spontaneously breathing neonate.

Contraction stress test (CST) Assessment of changes in the fetal heart rate (FHR) Especially decelerations in the face of uterine contractions induced by administration of intravenous dilute oxytocin solution. Repetitive decelerations in the FHR are called a *positive CST* and suggest that the fetus will not experience repetitive hypoxemic stress during labor.

Control ventilation Likely the oldest mode of ventilation designed to control ventilation with either pressure or volume targeting; however, does not determine patient interaction.

Cor pulmonale Right-sided heart failure as a result of chronically elevated pulmonary artery pressures.

Corticosteroids An anti-inflammatory agent that is used to block late phase reaction to allergens, reduce airway hyperreactivity, and inhibit anti-inflammatory cell migration and activation.

Cough The process of expelling air forcefully in an effort to clear the airway.

Cough assistance An ACT designed to support a weak cough by increase expiratory flow rates.

Crew resource management (CRM) CRM was first developed in the airline industry to improve safety. CRM training encompasses a wide range of knowledge, skills, and attitudes including communications, situational awareness, problem solving, decision making, and teamwork.

Croup A common cause of upper airway obstruction resulting from inflammation of the larynx, trachea, and bronchi.

Cutdown method Placement of a catheter via surgical stoma that allows direct visualization and cannulation of the target vessel.

Cystic fibrosis A hereditary chronic disease of the exocrine glands, characterized by the production of viscid mucus that obstructs the pancreatic ducts and bronchi, leading to infection and fibrosis.

D

Deadspace volume The portion of tidal volume that is not involved in gas exchange.

Decannulation Permanent removal of a trach tube.

Dedicated transport teams A transport team whose primary responsibility is to the transport of patients. These are usually higher volume transport programs, but these staff may assist in the intensive care units when normal transport duties are completed.

Deoxyhemoglobin Hemoglobin that does not have oxygen bound to its structure.

Deposition Aerosol particles leaving suspension with delivery to surfaces of the device, airway, or lung.

Dextral looping A process that occurs between days 23 and 28 of gestation whereby the ventricular bulge balloons into a C-shaped loop that pushes the atrial bulge in a superior direction.

Difficult pediatric airway management Proper use of resources and tools to properly obtain and maintain a pediatric airway with its unique aspects.

Difficult pediatric airway recognition Proper and early recognition of a difficult airway by using history and anatomy scoring systems.

Diffusing capacity A test performed to determine the overall ability of the lung to transport gas into and out of the blood.

Diplopia Double vision caused by a defective function of the extraocular muscles or a disorder of the nerves that innervate (stimulate) the muscles.

Direct calorimeter Refers the measurement of heat produced by a subject, usually to calculate energy expenditure.

Discharge planner Medical staff member designated to transition a patient from hospital facility to home or other level of care.

Disorders of the motor nerves Disorders that affect the motor neurons of the spinal cord and brainstem.

Disorders of the neuromuscular junction A disorder that occurs at the neuromuscular junction affecting neurotransmitting capabilities.

Diurnal ventilation Daytime use of ventilator assistance.

Doppler effect In medicine this phenomenon is used most often to measure flow of blood within blood vessels.

Doppler ultrasonography The detection of moving objects, such as intravascular blood exploiting shifts in frequency between emitted ultrasonic waves and their echoes.

Drowning All forms of submersion injury leading to respiratory impairment, including nonfatal injury resulting from filling of the lungs with water or other substance.

Dry powder inhaler (DPI) An aerosol device designed to deliver drug in a powder form.

Durable medical equipment (DME) Medical equipment used in the home to aid in a better quality of living.

Dysphasia Any impairment in the ability to speak.

E

ECMO Extracorporeal membrane oxygenation.

Ectoderm One of the three germ layers. Responsible for the development of the central and peripheral nervous systems, sensory epithelia, skin and special components of the skin, and teeth.

Electrocardiography The measurement and interpretation of the electrical activity of the heart over time.

Embryonic disk Structure making up the three germ layers the ectoderm, the endoderm, and the mesoderm.

Emitted dose The volume or mass of aerosol leaving the aerosol device.

Empyema (pleural) Pleural effusion that has evidence of bacterial infection by evidence of pus, high white blood cell count (e.g., > 15,000 per mm³), or a positive Gram's stain.

Encephaloceles Defect resulting from failure of the embryonic neural tube to form correctly around the brain.

Encephalopathy A condition characterized by altered brain function and structure.

End tidal CO₂ The partial pressure of carbon dioxide at end exhalation.

Endocardial cushions The structure that separates the atria from the ventricles in the developing heart.

Endoderm One of the three germ layers. Responsible for the development of the digestive system, respiratory system, urinary system, liver, pancreas, tonsils, thymus, thyroid, parathyroid, and epithelial lining of the auditory tube and tympanic cavity.

Endomyometritis Bacterial infection of the lining of the uterus and the underlying muscle after delivery of the newborn and placenta. Before the advent of affective antibiotics, a common cause of maternal morbidity and mortality.

Energy expenditure The quantity of energy, typically measured in kilocalories per day (kcal/day) resulting from metabolic processes.

Epiglottitis A life-threatening condition in which the epiglottis is inflamed.

Error An act of producing a preventable adverse outcome compared with the natural progression of disease leading to injury or death.

Escharotomy Surgical incision of the eschar and superficial fascia of the chest or a circumferentially burned limb in order to permit the cut edges to separate and restore blood flow to unburned tissue.

Esophageal atresia A serious birth defect in which the esophagus, which connects the mouth to the stomach, is segmented and closed off at any point. This condition usually occurs with tracheoesophageal fistula, in which the esophagus is connected to the trachea. Esophageal atresia occurs in approximately 1 in 4000 live births.

Esophogram A fluoroscopic evaluation of the esophagus using a barium sulfate contrast agent; same as barium swallow.

Evidence-based practice The multidisciplinary approach to health care in which the practitioner systematically finds, appraises, and uses the most current and valid research findings as the basis for clinical decisions.

Exhaled nitric oxide A biomarker of airway inflammation.

Expiratory positive airway pressure (EPAP) Expiratory positive airway pressure setting raises end-expiratory lung volume and impedes upper airway collapse.

Extracorporeal membrane oxygenation (EMCO) A medical-surgical technique in which blood is drained from the body—extracorporeal—and mechanically pumped through an artificial lung—membrane oxygenator.

Extremely low birth weight (ELBW) infant Infant born with birth weight less than 1000 g.

Exudative effusion A pleural effusion that has high protein or a high lactate dehydrogenase (LDH); often associated with infection in children.

F

Failure Modes and Effects Analysis (FMEA) A prospective risks assessment tool used to identify and eliminate known and/or potential failures, problems, and errors for a system, design, process, and/or service before they actually occur.

Fetal alcohol syndrome (FAS) The sum total of the damage done to the child before birth as a result of the mother drinking alcohol during pregnancy. FAS always involves brain damage, impaired growth, and head and face abnormalities.

Fetal fibronectin (fFN) A protein produced by fetal cells and a type of fibronectin. fFN is found at the interface of the chorion and the decidua (between the fetal sac and the uterine lining). It can be thought of as an adhesive or "biological glue" that binds the fetal sac to the uterine lining.

Fetal lung fluid An intraluminal lung fluid important for the proper growth and development of the fetal lung.

Fine-particle fraction (FPF) The proportion of aerosol particles between 1 to 5 microns (or 0 to 3.5 microns), with high likelihood of depositing in the lung.

Flexible fiberoptic bronchoscopy Bronchoscopy allows examination of the lower airways by a trained bronchoscopist. The flexible fiberoptic bronchoscope contains fiberoptic light bundles that places a light source at the tip of the instrument and allows examination of the lower airways. The flexible fiberoptic bronchoscope comes in a variety of sizes that are appropriate to the pediatric airway.

Flow–volume loop A graph of the flow rate as a function of lung volume during a complete respiratory cycle consisting of a forced inspiration followed by a forced expiration.

Focal biliary cirrhosis A medical condition characterized by areas of localized fibrosis in the biliary ducts as a result of obstruction.

Fontanel A "soft spot" of the skull. The cartilage has not yet hardened into bone between the skull bones.

Fontan procedure The third and final stage of surgical palliation for single-ventricle cardiac lesions. It involves connecting the superior vena cava and the inferior vena cava directly to the pulmonary artery.

Foramen ovale One of the fetal shunts allowing blood to flow from the right atrium to the left atrium without traversing the pulmonary circulation in the fetus.

Functional residual capacity The volume of air remaining in the lungs at the end of passive expiration.

Funnel chest Deformity in pectus excavatum of the cartilaginous ends of the rib that causes an inward curve of the sternum.

G

Gastroschisis Defect in the abdominal wall lateral to the midline with protrusion of the intestines.

Gentle ventilation A descriptive term for respiratory support for preterm infants using a low-tidal-volume strategy to decrease lung injury, with the acceptance of higher values for $PaCO_2$.

Geometric standard deviation (GSD) An expression of the range of particle diameters in an aerosol of a specific MMAD.

Germinal matrix The highly cellular and highly vascularized region in the brain from which cells migrate out during brain development. The germinal matrix is the source of both neurons and glial cells and is most active between 8 and 28 weeks of gestation.

Glasgow Coma Scale score An assessment tool used to communicate the severity and depth of coma in a patient who has suffered traumatic brain injury.

Glenn procedure Second stage of surgical palliation for single ventricle cardiac lesions. It involves connection of the superior vena cava directly to the pulmonary artery. Pulmonary blood flow is supplied by venous return from the upper body, while blood from the lower body returns to the single ventricle.

Global Lung Initiative European Respiratory Society task force charged with strengthening the science and statistical methodology of all pulmonary function reference values.

Group B *Streptococcus* (GBS) A common bacterium that often colonizes the intestines and secondarily the lower genital tract. GBS is usually harmless in adults. In newborns, however, it can cause a serious illness known as group B streptococcal disease.

Grunting Audible expiratory noise caused by closure of the glottis during expiration.

H

Head bobbing Occurs when the sternocleidomastoids contract during inspiration, pulling the head down and the clavicles and rib cage up.

Health Failure Modes and Effects Analysis (HFMEA) A tool used to provide detailed hazard analysis of smaller processes and develop specific recommendations.

Heart-lung transplantation Surgical procedure carried out to replace both heart and lungs in a single operation.

Heart transplantation Surgical procedure involving the replacement of a patient's diseased or injured heart with a healthy donor heart.

Helium dilution test A method of measuring the functional residual capacity of the lungs using a closed-circuit system in which a spirometer is filled with a mixture of helium and oxygen.

Helium-oxygen gas mixture Otherwise known as *heliox*. Heliox is a mixture of helium and oxygen offered in two tank concentrations, 80%/20%, = and 70%/30%. Heliox blenders approved by the Food and Drug Administration can be used to mix various concentrations.

Hemofiltration An adjunct device used to regulate fluid management during ECMO. Similar to a dialysis-type filter, a hemofilter can be used to remove large volumes of fluid to increase the volume of red blood cells—hemoconcentration—or small amounts of fluid to augment urine output.

Hepatitis B virus (HBV) One of many viruses that infect the liver (hepatitis). HBV is endemic in parts of the world and results from "sharing" body fluids. In North America and Europe it is associated with unprotected intercourse and needle sharing. HBV is an acute disease in most cases, with as much as a 5% mortality; it can infrequently progress to a chronic disease. The chronic form of HBV results in continuous shedding of the virus and high risk of cirrhosis and cancer. HBV can be contracted by the newborn of the individual shedding the HBV.

Herpes simplex virus (HSV) A very common sexually transmitted infection; type 2 HSV causes genital herpes and type 1 HSV usually causes cold sores but also can cause genital herpes; congenital HSV can be transmitted to the fetus during birth if the mother has an active infection.

Heterozygote Containing two different alleles of a gene.

HFOV High-frequency oscillatory ventilation.

High-flow nasal cannula (HFNC) A means of respiratory assistance that uses a soft nasal cannula interface and high humidified flow source to raise the intraluminal pharyngeal pressure.

High-flow nasal cannulae There is no single universally accepted definition. A reasonable definition would be a flow rate between 2 and 8 L/min.

High-flow oxygen therapy Oxygen delivery strategy that uses a delivery device that provides flows that exceed the patient's inspiratory flow requirements. The excessive flows allow the device to provide a fixed amount of fraction of delivered oxygen.

High-frequency jet ventilation A mode of ventilation that combined with a low frequency ventilator provided short pulsed jets using an endotracheal tube (ETT) adapter, peak end-expiratory pressure (PEEP), and sigh breaths.

High-frequency oscillatory ventilation A mode of ventilation that provides small tidal volumes at very fast rates of 5 to 15 Hz with a piston and provides continuous distending pressure. To maintain such high rates, expiratory gas flow is enhanced by an active exhalation phase.

High-frequency percussive ventilation Delivers short bursts of gas to a sliding Venturi valve. The burst may entrain air to deliver high-frequency distending pressure at peak inspiratory pressure (PIP) and peak end-expiratory pressure (PEEP). High-frequency breaths are active at both levels of pressure.

High-frequency ventilation Pressure mode of ventilation at a frequency of 150 breaths per minute or higher.

High position A placement position for an umbilical artery catheter. This position overlies the sixth through eighth thoracic vertebrae.

High-reliability organization (HRO) An organization that has succeeded in avoiding catastrophes in an environment where normal accidents can be expected because of risk factors and complexity.

Hila The area adjacent to the heart where the pulmonary bronchi, arteries, and veins enter and exit the right and left lungs.

Hirsutism Excessive or abnormal hair growth involving the face and body.

Home assessment An evaluation of the home environment in which a ventilator-dependent child is to reside, meeting electrical criteria and accessible for adaptive strollers.

Horizontal fissure A fissure separating the middle lobe from the right upper lobe of the lung; same as *minor fissure*.

Human immunodeficiency virus (HIV) A lentivirus (a member of the retrovirus family) that causes acquired immunodeficiency syndrome (AIDS), a condition in humans in which progressive failure of the immune system allows life-threatening opportunistic infections and cancers to thrive.

Humidified high-flow nasal oxygen Medical gas conditioned at or near body temperature, saturated with water vapor, and delivered at flows higher than traditionally acceptable flow rates via a nasal cannula interface. More specifically, flows should be adequate to provide for high fractions of oxygen and ventilatory support as per the mechanism of deadspace washout and exceeding the inspiratory flow requirements of the patient.

Hydrofluoroalkane (HFA) Propellants used in modern pressurized metered-dose inhalers (pMDIs).

Hydrops fetalis Massive edema in the fetus or newborn, usually in association with severe erythroblastosis fetalis. Severe anemia and effusions of the pericardial, pleural, and peritoneal spaces also occur. The condition often leads to death, even with immediate exchange transfusions after delivery. Also called *fetal hydrops*.

Hygromas Sacs of fluid resulting from a blockage in the lymphatic system.

Hyperinflation therapy In general a group of supportive therapies that increases functional residual capacity (FRC) by encouraging the patient to take deep breaths or by assisting with positive pressure.

Hypertonic A solution that has a higher osmotic pressure than a physiological concentration.

Hypochloremic metabolic alkalosis An acid-base disorder characterized by alkalosis related to increased serum bicarbonate levels with compensatory low chloride levels.

Hypoplastic left heart syndrome A spectrum of lesions involving abnormal development of left-sided cardiac structures including the mitral valve, left ventricle, aortic valve, and aortic arch.

Hypothalamic-pituitary-adrenal axis Part of the neuroendocrine system that controls the immune system. This axis is a direct influence and feedback interaction between the hypothalamus, pituitary gland, and the adrenal gland.

Hypothermia Occurs when body temperature falls below 95 °F (35 °C).

Hypoxemia Medical condition that is characterized by a reduced level of oxygen determined by arterial blood gas.

Hypoxia The reduction of oxygen supply to the body or region of the body. The deprivation of adequate oxygen.

I

Ileus A disruption of the typical motility of the gastrointestinal tract.

Impulse oscillometry Measurement of resistance and reactance using a loudspeaker to produce pulsations within the airway during normal quiet breathing.

Indirect calorimeter Refers to the approximation of heat resulting from metabolism through the measurement of oxygen consumption and carbon dioxide production, with the clinical goal of determining a patients energy expenditure.

Inhaled mass The mass of drug that enters the airway, typically into the upper airways.

Inhaled nitric oxide Nitric oxide delivered in parts per million mixed with nitrogen and added to a breathing circuit mixed with oxygen.

Inspiratory positive airway pressure (IPAP) Inspiratory positive airway pressure setting determines the tidal volume.

Institute of Medicine (IOM) American nononprofit, nongovernmental organization founded in 1970, under the congressional charter of the National Academy of Sciences. Its purpose is to provide national advice on issues relating to biomedical science, medicine, and health, and its mission to serve as adviser to the nation to improve health.

Intimal mounds Endothelial tissue within the lumen of the ductus arteriosus that assist in postgestational closure of the ductus.

Intracranial pressure The pressure of cerebrospinal fluid (CSF) within the cranium.

Intrauterine growth retardation (IUGR) Occurs when the estimated weight of the fetus is at or below the tenth weight percentile for his or her age (in weeks).

Intraventricular hemorrhage (IVH) Bleeding into the fluid-filled areas (ventricles) inside the brain. The condition is most often seen in premature babies.

J

Just culture Identifies and addresses system issues leading individuals to engage in unsafe behaviors while maintaining individual accountability by establishing a zero tolerance for reckless behavior.

K

Kaizen Continuous quality improvement, emphasizing the philosophy that poor quality arises from bad systems rather than bad people.

Kyphosis Abnormal lateral curvature of the spine; also called *hunchback*.

L

Lamellar bodies A storage apparatus for surfactant consisting of concentric layers of lipid and protein and contained within the cytoplasm of alveolar type II cells.

Laminaria tent Used to expand the cervix in pregnant women to "ripen" (expand) the cervix to make labor and delivery easier and also to cause abortions during the first half of pregnancy.

Lanugo Fine hair that covers premature infants mostly over the shoulders, back, forehead, and cheeks.

Laryngeal web A common laryngeal malformation that consists of accessory tissue between the vocal cords at the anterior commissure.

Laryngomalacia The inward collapse of the soft cartilage of the upper airway during inspiration.

Lean method The concept of streamlining processes and eliminating waste to keep costs low while maintaining high-quality products or services.

Left-to-right shunt Type of shunt n which oxygenated blood mixes with deoxygenated blood.

Leukocytosis White blood cell (WBC) greater than $25,000/mm^3$.

Leukopenia White blood cell count (WBC) less than $3500/mm^3$.

Listeria monocyogenes A group of bacteria capable of causing illness, including potentially fatal infections in the elderly, newborns, pregnant women, and persons with a weakened immune system. *Listeria monocytogenes* is the form of *Listeria* most commonly responsible for infections.

Low-birth-weight (LBW) infant Infant born weighing less than 2500 g.

Lower airway The trachea and distal structures. The trachea divides into the mainstem bronchi, which divide into smaller divisions called subsegmental bronchi.

Lower inflection point The point on the pressure–volume loop where the shape changes from concave to exponential. This point represents the start of alveolar expansion during inspiration.

Low-flow oxygen therapy An oxygen delivery strategy that uses a delivery device that provides flows that are less than the patient's inspiratory flow requirements. This mixing of room air gases dilutes the high concentration of low-flow oxygen and provides a variable faction of delivered oxygen.

Low-frequency ventilation Generic term for modes of ventilation that provide breath rates of less than 150.

Low position A placement position for an umbilical artery catheter. This position overlies the third to fourth lumbar space.

Low tidal volume ventilation A strategy of mechanical ventilation in which tidal volumes are limited (often targeted to 6 ml/kg based on the available adult acute lung injury data) while also limiting the plateau pressure.

Lung compliance A measure of the ease of expansion of the lungs and thorax, determined by pulmonary volume and elasticity.

Lung transplantation A surgical procedure involving the removal of one or both diseased lungs from a patient and the replacement of the lungs with healthy organs from a donor.

M

Macrosomia Abnormally large size of the body.

Mainstream capnography A method of measuring carbon dioxide during the breathing cycle that uses a sensor placed directly in the breathing circuit to analyze carbon dioxide.

Major fissures A fissure separating the upper and lower lobes of the lungs; same as *oblique fissures*.

Malpractice Illegal, unethical, negligent, or immoral behavior by somebody in a professional or official position, resulting in a failure to fulfill the duties or responsibilities associated with that position.

Mass effect A displacement of normal anatomy because of a pathological abnormality.

Mass median aerodynamic diameter (MMAD) A measurement of particle size based on the distribution of mass of drug that deposits on various stages of an impactor.

Maximal respiratory pressures Measures the amount of pressure your inspiratory and expiratory muscles can exert. It is helpful in evaluating possible respiratory muscle weakness.

Mean arterial pressure An indicator of left ventricular afterload. Estimated using the equation.

Mechanical ventilation A technique through which gas is moved toward and from the lungs through an exogenous device connected directly to the patient.

Mechanism of injury (MOI) The method in which the injury occurred. This includes the object causing the injury and/or the reason for the injury, the amount of force applied, and the vector or direction of that force.

Meconium The green-tinged bowel content of an infant, which is usually passed within 48 hours after delivery.

Meconium aspiration The inhalation of meconium by a fetus or newborn. It can block the air passages and cause failure of the lungs to expand or other pulmonary dysfunction, such as pneumonia or emphysema.

Mediastinum The area in the midline chest cavity that is composed of the heart, aorta, main pulmonary artery and proximal branches, origins of the great vessels from the aorta, the superior vena cava, and thymus.

Medicaid U.S. health care plan for qualifying patients with low incomes and resources.

Meningitis Inflammation of the overlying membranes of the brain and spinal cord, known as the meninges.

Mesoderm One of the three germ layers. Responsible for the development of the cardiovascular system, lymphatic system, connective tissues, muscle tissue, skins, kidneys, and reproductive tissues, among other areas.

Micrognathia Small lower jaw.

Microstomia Small mouth.

Minimum inhibitory concentration The lowest antimicrobial concentration that will inhibit visible growth of a microorganism

Minor fissure A fissure separating the middle lobe from the right upper lobe of the lung; same as *horizontal fissure*.

Modified Allen's test A test used to verify the presence of collateral circulation to the hand and/or foot via selective manual occlusion of the arteries feeding the extremity.

Mottling Irregular areas of dusky skin alternating with areas of pale skin.

Mucolytic Pharmacological agent capable of dissolving, digesting, or liquefying mucus.

Myelomeningoceles Defect resulting from failure of the embryonic neural tube to form correctly around the spine.

Myopathy A disease of the skeletal musculature causing muscle weakness.

N

Nasal cannula A variable performance medical gas delivery interface that is designed with one or two prongs that inject gas into one or both nares.

Nasal flaring Contraction of muscles in the nasal passages during inspiration causes a widening of the nostrils.

Near miss An unplanned event or events that had potential to cause injury, illness, or harm but did not because it was detected before reaching the patient.

Nebulizer An aerosol device producing aerosolized suspension of liquid drug particles used for aerosol therapy.

NEC Necrotizing enterocolitis

Necrotizing enterocolitis (NEC) A serious bacterial infection in the intestine, primarily of sick or premature newborn infants. It can cause the death (necrosis) of intestinal tissue and progress to blood poisoning (septicemia).

Negative pressure assisted ventilation (NPAV) A method of respiratory assistance based on intermittent application of subatmospheric pressure external to the chest wall through a tank or mold.

Negligence Lack of skills, failure, or deviation from standard practices/procedures.

Neuromuscular control of respiration The central and reflex neurological control system of breathing driven largely by chemical respiratory control (*neuro*) that interacts with the muscles of respiration (*muscular*).

Neuromuscular disease Broad term used to describe a diseases that directly or indirectly affect the muscle function via nerve pathology.

New or atypical bronchopulmonary dysplasia Often develops in preterm newborns who may have required minimal or even no ventilator support and relatively low inspired oxygen concentrations during the early postnatal days.

Nitrogen washout test A method of measuring the functional residual capacity of the lungs using the open circuit system in which the subject breaths 100% oxygen.

Nonaccidental trauma A euphemism for child abuse; the injury or maltreatment of a child.

Noninvasive positive-pressure ventilation (NPPV) A method of respiratory assistance that involves an external interface and cyclical positive pressure device.

Nonstress test (NST) A screening test for fetal well-being used in the second half of pregnancy. The mother depresses an event marker when fetal movement is perceived. Acceleration of fetal heart rate with movement is a "reactive" test and is considered reassuring.

Norwood procedure The first stage of surgical palliation for single ventricle cardiac lesions. It consists of consists of reconstructing the aorta and adding a shunt to provide pulmonary blood flow.

O

Oblique fissure A fissure separating the upper and lower lobes of the lungs; same as *major fissures*.

Oligohydramnios A reduced quantity of amniotic fluid for an extended period; associated with lung hypoplasia.

Omphalocele Protrusion of the membranous sac that encloses abdominal contents through an opening in the abdominal wall into the umbilical cord.

Open lung strategy The clinical application of recruitment maneuvers followed by maintenance with appropriate level of positive end-expiratory pressure (PEEP) to prevent alveolar collapse.

Oxygen consumption The sum volume of oxygen that is consumed by the body as a result of metabolism, per unit of time.

Oxygen delivery Delivery of oxygen to body tissues as a function of oxygen content and cardiac output.

Oxygen hood A fixed-performance oxygen delivery device designed to surround the entire head of a neonate or infant.

Oxygen therapy The therapeutic administration of oxygen.

Oxygenation index A calculation used in critical care medicine to aid in determining the severity of illness and probable mortality associated with severe respiratory failure. The equation is:

$$OI = (F_{IO_2})(mPaw)/Pa_{O_2} \times 100.$$

Oxyhemoglobin The structure that is formed when oxygen is bound to hemoglobin in red blood cells.

Oxytocin A hypothalamic hormone stored in the posterior pituitary that has uterine-contracting and milk-releasing actions; it may also be prepared synthetically or obtained from the posterior pituitary of domestic animals. Used to induce active labor, increase the force of contractions in labor, contract uterine muscle after delivery of the placenta, control postpartum hemorrhage, and stimulate milk ejection.

P

Papilledema A swelling of the optic nerve, at the point where this nerve joins the eye, that is caused by an increase in fluid pressure within the skull (intracranial pressure).

Parenteral A route of administration in a manner other than through a digestive canal; that is, intravenous, intramuscular, or subcutaneous.

Parietal pleura The pleura that cover the surface of the chest wall and mediastinum.

Partial pressure of carbon dioxide in arterial blood Pa_{CO_2} is a measurement of carbon dioxide in arterial blood.

Partial pressure of oxygen in arterial blood *Partial pressure* is a way of describing how much of a gas is present and refers to the pressure exerted by a specific gas in a mixture of other gases. Pa_{O_2} is a measurement of oxygen in arterial blood.

Patent ductus arteriosus The failure of the connection between the aorta and the pulmonary artery (ductus arteriosis) to close at birth.

Pectus carinatum Protruding xiphisternum or xiphoid process; also called *pigeon chest*.

Pectus excavatum Sunken or funnel chest.

Pediatric airway anatomy The anatomy (normal and abnormal) of the pediatric airway at different stages of growth.

Pediatric intubation techniques The standardized and acceptable insertion of an endotracheal tube within the trachea.

Percutaneous method Insertion of a catheter through the skin to a target vessel.

Periodic breathing Irregular pattern of intermittent respiratory pauses longer than 5 seconds.

Peripheral artery catheter An indwelling catheter placed in a peripherally located artery.

Permissive hypercapnia Ventilation that allows Pa_{CO_2} to rise slowly over time as the pH becomes normalized. The goal is to reduce tidal volume and rate while preventing volutrauma during mechanical ventilation.

Persistent vegetative state Condition of profound nonresponsiveness in the wakeful state caused by brain damage.

Pharmacokinetic The way a drug is absorbed, distributed, metabolized, and eliminated from the body.

Picture archiving and communication system (PACS) A digital image management network system consisting of acquisition systems, display workstations, and storage devices.

Piezo A form of ceramic that vibrates in response to electric input.

Placenta Vascular interface between the mom and the fetus allowing gas and nutrient exchange through the chorionic villi and the umbilical cord.

Placenta previa The location of the placenta so that it covers the cervical os (complete previa) or is located adjacent to or partially covers the os (partial previa). One of the most common causes of life-threatening hemorrhage in pregnancy.

Placental abruption Separation of the placenta from the wall of the uterus before the birth of the baby. This can result in severe, uncontrollable bleeding (hemorrhage).

Plan-Do-Study-Act (PDSA) Method to determine nature and scope of a problem.

Plan of care A detailed plan implemented for the medical needs of an individual.

Plasticity Describes how experiences and injury reorganize neural pathways in the brain.

Plethsymography A device (body box) that measures the volume of gas in the lungs, including that which is trapped in poorly communicating air spaces.

Pleural effusion Abnormal collection of fluid in the pleural space.

Pleural space A potential space between the lung, mediastinum, and chest wall.

Pneumatocele A thin-walled, air-filled cavity within the lungs.

Pneumomediastinum Abnormal air in the tissue of the mediastinum, often tracking up into the neck.

Pneumonia A lung infection that primarily affects the alveoli and distal airways.

Pneumopericardium The presence of air in the pericardial cavity.

Pneumoretroperitoneum and pneumoperitoneum Air tracks downward to the extraperitoneal fascial planes of the abdominal wall, mesentery, and retroperitoneum and eventually ruptures into the peritoneal cavity.

Pneumothorax An accumulation of free air within the pleural space that compresses the lungs.

Poliomyelitis Infection caused by the polio virus.

Polyhydramnios The presence of excess fluid in the amniotic sac. By definition, polyhydramnios is diagnosed if the deepest vertical pool is more than 8 cm or amniotic fluid index (AFI) is more than ninety-fifth percentile for the corresponding gestational age. With a deep pocket of 8 cm as criteria of polyhydramnios, the incidence is 1% to 3% of all pregnancies. About 20% are associated with fetal anomalies.

Portal hypertension A medical condition characterized by abnormally high blood pressures in the portal vein system, typically associated with chronic liver disease.

Position The arrangement of the patient's body when obtaining a radiographic image.

Positive expiratory pressure (PEP) therapy designed to restrict expiratory flow and thereby creating backpressure designed to increase functional residual capacity and dilate secretion-filled airways.

Postductal Relating to that part of the aorta distal to the aortic opening of the ductus arteriosus.

Postductal oxygen saturation Measurement of oxygen saturation (of an infant's blood) occurring before the ductus arterious.

Potter's syndrome/sequence Potter syndrome/sequence and Potter phenotype refer to a group of findings associated with a lack of amniotic fluid and kidney failure in a fetus or infant.

Precipitous delivery Delivery of infant anywhere unintended or without a provider.

Precursor Somebody or something that comes before, and is often considered lead to the development of, another person or thing.

Preductal Right radial artery.

Preductal oxygen saturation Measurement of oxygen saturation of the blood taken after the ductus arteriosis.

Preeclampsia Multiorgan dysfunction of late pregnancy, most often diagnosed by hypertension, proteinuria, and edema. The disorder is of uncertain origin but is most commonly associated with first pregnancies, multifetal pregnancies, and underlying vascular and rheumatological conditions.

Premature delivery The birth of an infant after the period of viability but before 37 completed weeks of gestation.

Premature rupture of membranes (PROM) Premature rupture of membranes (PROM) is an event that occurs during pregnancy when the sac containing the developing baby (fetus) and the amniotic fluid bursts or develops a hole before the start of labor.

Pressure ventilation Uses a pressure setting as the main determinate of lung inflation.

Pressurized metered-dose inhaler An aerosol device with pressurized cartridge and valves that emits precise dosages of drugs (between 10 and 100 μg) in suspension or solution.

Primary germ layers The endoderm, mesoderm, and ectoderm. Individual layers of specialized embryonic cells responsible for production of all tissues within the developing fetus.

Projection The path of the X-ray beam describing the body surfaces the beam enters and exits.

Provocation test A procedure to elicit a hyperreactive airway response to either direct or indirect stimulation.

Prune belly syndrome Congenital lack of abdominal musculature.

Pseudoglandular Refers to a stage of fetal lung development identified by the appearance of multiple round structures resembling glands.

$P_{TC}CO_2$ Partial pressure of carbon dioxide as measured using a transcutaneous monitor.

$P_{TC}O_2$ Partial pressure of oxygen as measured using a transcutaneous monitor.

Pulmonary acinar units Formed during the canalicular period, each unit consists of a respiratory bronchiole, alveolar ducts, and alveolar sacs.

Pulmonary artery catheter A catheter inserted into the pulmonary artery via the central venous system and right side of the heart. This catheter can provide direct intracardiac and pulmonary pressure monitoring along with cardiac output measurement.

Pulmonary artery pressure The blood pressure measured in the pulmonary arteries. Normally 15 to 30 mm Hg systolic and 5 to 15 mm Hg diastolic, with a mean pressure of 10 to 20 mm Hg.

Pulmonary capillary wedge pressure The pressure measured in a pulmonary capillary after wedge occlusion via balloon catheter. Normally 5 to 15 mm Hg.

Pulmonary hypertension A rare lung disorder characterized by increased pressure in the pulmonary artery.

Pulmonary hypertrophic osteoarthropathy A medical condition characterized by digital clubbing and inflammation of the outer surface (periostium) of the long bones in the upper and lower extremities; associated with cystic fibrosis and other chronic lung conditions.

Pulmonary hypoplasia An incomplete development of the lungs characterized by an abnormally low number and/or size of bronchopulmonary segments and/or alveoli.

Pulmonary interstitial emphysema A lung anomaly characterized by an increase in the air spaces distal to the terminal bronchioles with destruction of the alveolar walls.

Pulmonary mechanics Study or measurement physiological parameters (e.g. resistance, compliance, etc.) that affect a subject's work of breathing.

Pulmonary surfactant Complex mixture of phospholipids and proteins produced by type II pneumatocytes whose function is to lower surface tension proportionally to alveolar size.

Pulmonary vasodilation Vasodilation of the pulmonary vasculature by smooth muscle relation.

Pulse oximetry Noninvasive measurement of the saturation of hemoglobin, usually referring to the proportion of hemoglobin bound with oxygen.

Pulse pressure The difference between systolic and diastolic blood pressure.

Q

Quality The extent to which health services provided to individuals and patient populations improve desired health outcomes.

Quality indicator Measurement that provide a quantitative basis for clinicians, organizations, and planners aiming to achieve improvement in care and the processes by which patient care is provided.

R

Racemic A chemical compound or mixture that possesses an equal amount of enantiomers.

Reactance Represents the "out of phase imaginary part" of impedance and encompasses both the elastance and inertia, which along with resistance define the mechanical characteristics of the equation of motion model.

Recurrent aspiration syndrome Aspiration of gastrointestinal tract caused by lack of control of airway protective mechanisms or abnormal anatomy.

Reduced alveolar recruitment Known as *atelectasis*.

Residual drug volume (or mass) The volume (or mass) of drug solution remaining in a nebulizer at the end of nebulization.

Respirable mass The mass of drug that can (or does) reach the lung.

Respiratory control system Control of the respiration divided into both voluntary and metabolic (involuntary) control systems.

Respiratory distress syndrome (RDS) A syndrome in premature infants caused by developmental insufficiency of surfactant production and structural immaturity in the lungs.

Resting energy expenditure The amount of energy required by the body during resting conditions (usually expressed in kilocalories per day, kcal/day).

Retinopathy of prematurity (ROP) A condition in which premature babies experience disorganized blood vessel growth in their eyes. Although milder cases of ROP may spontaneously correct themselves, in the worst cases, ocular scarring caused by retinopathy of prematurity can result in blindness.

Retropharyngeal cellulitis Inflammation of the tissues behind the pharynx.

Rh isoimmunization One of the causes of hemolytic disease of the newborn (also known as HDN). The disease ranges from mild to severe. When the disease is mild, the fetus may have mild anemia with reticulocytosis. When the disease is moderate or severe, the fetus can have a more marked anemia and erythroblastosis (erythroblastosis fetalis). When the disease is very severe it can cause morbus haemolyticus neonatorum, hydrops fetalis, or stillbirth.

Right atrial pressure The blood pressure in the right atrium of the heart. This pressure indicates the filling pressure of the right atrium; normally 2 to 7 mm Hg.

Right-to-left shunt Type of shunt in which desaturated systemic venous blood bypasses the lungs and enters the systemic circulation.

Roller pump A type of mechanical pump used in extracorporeal membrane oxygenation (ECMO). Blood is compressed and displaced by a roller heads through durable tubing.

Root cause analysis (RCA) A retrospective systematic process using information for an unplanned event to identify and understand the underlying causes or the event.

Rule of nines A method of estimating the extent of body surface that has been burned in an adult, dividing the body into sections of 9% or multiples of 9%.

S

Saccules An anatomical description of the lung parenchyma at about 26 weeks of gestation; the terminal structures of the lung at this stage of development are relatively smooth-walled, cylindrical structures.

Scoliosis Abnormal "sideways" curvature of the spine.

Secondary crests Anatomical description of the ridges that subdivide saccules during the embryological development of the lung.

Sentinel event Another name for serious safety event.

Sepsis Systemic evidence of infection characterized by temperature change, increased heart rate, increased respiratory rate, and leukocytosis or leukopenia.

Septum primum The structure that divides the primitive atria into left and right chambers.

Septum secundum A structure between the atria in the developing heart, which together with a flap from the septum primum for the foramen ovale.

Serious safety event An event that reaches the patient and results in moderate to severe harm or death.

Serum lactate Measurement of lactate in a blood sample. This value is indicative of anaerobic metabolism. Normally 0.7 to 1.3 mmol/L.

Shock Inadequate tissue oxygen delivery.

Sickle cell A disease of an autosomal recessively inherited disorder of the hemoglobin structure.

Sidestream capnography A method of measuring carbon dioxide during the breathing cycle that uses a small sample line that aspirates a sample of gas from a T-piece placed at the breathing tube to the main unit where the gas is analyzed.

Silhouette sign The radiographic appearance two normal structures lose their distinct edges and blend imperceptibly into one structure.

Simple oxygen mask A variable-performance, low-flow oxygen delivery device designed to surround the nose and mouth.

Six Sigma A process improvement set of tools and strategies developed by Motorola.

Spacer A valveless device used to collect emitted aerosol, typically from a pressurized metered-dose inhaler (pMDI), placed in a circuit between the aerosol generator and the patient airway.

Specific airway conductance The reciprocal of airway resistance; 1/Raw measured at a specific lung volume.

Spinal muscular atrophy Include a number of different disorders that clinically manifest as muscle weakness as a result of progressive destruction of the motor neurons.

Spine sign An increased density of the lower thoracic vertebral bodies on a lateral chest radiograph caused by increased tissue density from an adjacent collapsed lower lobe.

Spirometry Measurement of breath air.

Status epilepticus A seizure that lasts more than 30 minutes, constituting a neurological emergency.

Steatorrhea Loose, greasy stools.

Sternocleidomastoids Neck muscles that serve to flex and rotate the head.

Strabismus A disorder in which the two eyes do not line up in the same direction and therefore do not look at the same object at the same time; also known as "crossed eyes."

Stretor A low-pitched, wet sound similar to snoring.

Stridor A high-pitched, monophonic, audible noise that may occur during inspiration or expiration or may be biphasic.

Subcutaneous emphysema Air in the fascial planes of the neck and skin.

Subgaleal hemorrhage Tearing of the emissary veins where edema from blood loss can extend from the eyes to the nape of the neck.

Suctioning The process of cleaning the airway with a negative pressure device that removes liquids and solids.

Sudden infant death syndrome (SIDS) SIDS is the sudden death of an infant under 1 year of age that remains unexplained after a thorough case investigation, including performance of a complete autopsy, examination of the death scene, and review of the clinical history.

Support ventilation A mode of ventilation designed to support a patient respiratory effort; however, it cannot fully support or control ventilation.

Surface tension Forces created by the attraction of water molecules at the alveolar air–fluid interface that tend to collapse the alveolus.

Surfactant A surface-active phospholipoprotein formed by alveolar type II cells important in reducing alveolar surface tension and ultimately the work of breathing in the newborn; critical to the extrauterine survival of the immature fetus.

Surfactant proteins Pulmonary surfactant-associated proteins produced by type II pneumatocytes.

Surfactant replacement therapy Intratracheal administration of exogenous (natural or synthetic) surfactant for the treatment of various respiratory conditions associated with surfactant deficiency and/or inactivation.

Sweep gas The fresh gas supplied to a membrane oxygenator, usually composed of a combination of oxygen and carbon dioxide, and titrated to achieve clinically acceptable blood gases.

Sympathomimetic An agent that mimics the physiological effect when the sympathetic nervous system is stimulated.

Syphilis A chronic infectious disease caused by a spirochete (*Treponema pallidum*), either transmitted by direct contact, usually in sexual intercourse, or passed from mother to child in utero, and progressing through three stages characterized respectively by local formation of chancres, ulcerous skin eruptions, and systemic infection leading to general paresis.

T

Tactile fremitus Vibrations of the chest produced by the spoken voice.

Tension pneumothorax Abnormal collection of air in the pleural space with increasing pressure causing significant shift of the mediastinal structures.

Tension time index The product of the inspiratory time-to-cycle time ratio and the integrated area under the pressure curve throughout the respiratory cycle.

Teratogen Any agent or factor that induces or increases the incidence of abnormal prenatal development.

Tetralogy of Fallot Congenital heart defect that includes four components (1) pulmonary artery stenosis, (2) ventricular septal defect, (3) overriding aorta to the right, and (4) right ventricular hypertrophy.

Therapeutic gas mixtures Gas delivered by inhalation for a specific purpose such as pulmonary vasodilation, bronchodilation, drug delivery, or to reduce work of breathing.

Tocolytic Of or being an agent that arrests uterine contractions in labor.

Tolerance The lack or low level of response to a pharmacological agent.

Toxoplasmosis An infection caused by a single-celled parasite named *Toxoplasma gondii* that may invade tissues and damage the brain, especially of the fetus and newborn.

Tracheoesophageal fistula An abnormal opening between the trachea and the esophagus.

Tracheomalacia A condition in which the thoracic trachea abnormally collapses during expiration, leading to an expiratory wheeze.

Tracheostomy The hole created by the tracheotomy procedure.

Tracheotomy The surgical procedure that consist of process of opening the trachea from the anterior aspect of the neck and inserting a tubes used to assist with breathing, secretion removal, or airway patency.

Trach tube Short for tracheostomy tube.

Transcutaneous monitor A device or method that measures carbon dioxide or oxygen in the tissues just beneath the skin.

Transillumination Placing a high-energy or fiberoptic device on an infant's chest wall in a darkened room.

Transposition of the great arteries One of the most common congenital heart defects. The positions of the aorta and the pulmonary artery are reversed, with the aorta arising from the right ventricle and the pulmonary artery arising from the left ventricle.

Transpulmonary pressure The difference between the alveolar pressure and the intrapleural pressure in the lungs.

Transudative effusion A pleural effusion that has low protein or low lactate dehydrogenase; often associated with low cardiac output or renal dysfunction in children.

Trigger The link between the patient's respiratory effort and the ventilator. There are three types of triggers to ventilator support flow, pressure, and electrical activity of the diaphragm.

Trophoblast The outer layer of the blastocyst, which combines with the endometrium to for the chorionic membrane.

Truncus arteriosus Rare defect in which a single great artery arises from the ventricles of the heart, supplying the systemic, pulmonary, and coronary arteries.

Tuberculosis A chronic bacterial disease caused by infection with *Mycobaterium tuberculosis*.

U

UHF/AM transceiver An ultra high frequency/amplitude modulation (UHF/AM) transceiver is a device comprising both a transmitter and a receiver that are combined and share common circuitry or a single housing. This communication device is capable of communicating over two different frequency ranges.

Ultrasonic nebulizer (USN) Electronic nebulizer using piezo crystal to make standing waves in the medication to generate aerosol particles.

Umbilical artery catheter An indwelling catheter placed in one of the two arteries in an infant umbilicus.

Unit-based transport teams A transport team assigned to an intensive care unit that responds to transport requests when they are received.

Upper airway Consists of all the structures connecting the mouth and nose with the glottis.

V

VACTERL A syndrome of defects including *v*ertebral, *a*nal, *c*ardiac, *t*racheal, *e*sophageal, *r*enal, and *l*imb anomalies.

Valved-holding chamber A spacer with a system of one-way valves used to reduce oropharyngeal deposition and reduce the need for hand–breath coordination, most commonly used with pressurized metered-dose inhalers (pMDIs).

Vaporizer Because most anesthetics are a liquid at room temperature, a vaporizer designed for each chemical makeup must be used to carefully deliver a percent gas mixture accurately.

Vascular ring An encircling of the trachea and esophagus by connected segments of the aortic arch and its branches.

Velamentous cord insertion An abnormal condition during pregnancy. Normally the umbilical cord inserts into the middle of the placenta as it develops. In velamentous cord insertion, the umbilical cord inserts into the fetal membranes (choriamniotic membranes), then travels within the membranes to the placenta (between the amnion and the chorion).

Venoarterial A method of extracorporeal membrane oxygenation (ECMO) support in which blood is drained from the venous system and returned to the arterial system; both heart and lung function are supported.

Venous blood gas Blood gas analysis obtained from a venipuncture or directly from a venous catheter.

Venovenous A method of extracorporeal membrane oxygenation (ECMO) support in which blood is drained and returned form and to the venous system; only lung function is supported.

Ventilator-associated pneumonia (VAP) A sub-type of hospital-acquired pneumonia (HAP) that occurs in people who are receiving mechanical ventilation via an artificial airway.

Ventricular bulge One of three identifiable structures in the primitive heart eventually merges with the bulbus cordis to form the bulboventricular loop.

Venturi mask A fixed-performance, high-flow oxygen delivery device design to provide a specific amount of oxygen via a Venturi entrainment device.

Vernix caseosa Gray-white cheeselike substance present in the skin folds of a term infant and more abundant in a preterm infant.

Very low birth weight (VLBW) infant Infant born weighing less than 1500 g.

Vibrating mesh nebulizer (VMN) An electronic device using an aperture plate or mesh to pump medications through aperture to generate aerosol particles.

Video-assisted thoracoscopic surgery (VATS) Minimally invasive surgery in the thorax with a video camera inserted in one aspect of the chest wall and operating instrument(s) inserted though other aspects of the chest wall. The surgeon views the operative field on a monitor.

Visceral pleura The pleura that covers the surface of the lungs.

Vocal cord dysfunction A condition characterized by full or partial vocal fold closure that usually occurs during inhalation.

Volume median diameter (VMD) Measurement of aerosol particle size as measured with a laser diffraction device.

Volume ventilation Uses a preset tidal volume as the main determinate of lung inflation.

Volumetric capnography A method by which exhaled gas flow and carbon dioxide measurements are made in order to calculate and display relevant parameters and waveforms such as airway dead space volume, alveolar volume, and carbon dioxide elimination.

Volutrauma Ventilator-associated lung injury that is associated with large tidal volumes.

W

Wharton's jelly A gelatinous substance contained within the umbilical cord that serves to protect umbilical vasculature and prevent the cord from becoming kinked.

Wilson-Mikity syndrome Preterm infants with respiratory distress in the first days of life, which appears to resolve. Then 1 to 5 weeks later, the tachypnea and cyanosis return. Radiologically, there are diffuse pulmonary infiltrates that in some infants change to a cystic emphysematous pattern.

Work of breathing The effort required to inspire air into the lungs.

Z

Zygote Fertilized egg.

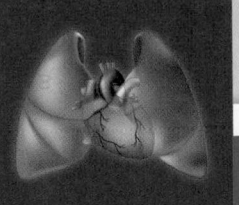

Credits List

Chapter 1

Figure 1-1 From Moore KL, Persaud TVN: *The developing human,* ed 5. Philadelphia, 1993, WB Saunders.

Figure 1-2 Langston C, Kida K, Reed M, et al. Human lung growth in late gestation and in the neonate. *Am Rev Respir Dis* 1984 Apr; 129(4):607-13.

Figure 1-3 Langston C, Kida K, Reed M, et al. Human lung growth in late gestation and in the neonate. *Am Rev Respir Dis* 1984 Apr; 129(4):607-13.

Figure 1-4 Langston C, Kida K, Reed M, et al. Human lung growth in late gestation and in the neonate. *Am Rev Respir Dis* 1984 Apr; 129(4):607-13.

Figure 1-5 Langston C, Kida K, Reed M, et al. Human lung growth in late gestation and in the neonate. *Am Rev Respir Dis* 1984 Apr; 129(4):607-13.

Chapter 2

Figure 2-1 From Blechschmidt E, editor: *The stages of human development before birth.* Philadelphia, 1961, WB Saunders.

Figure 2-2 From Moore KL, editor: *The developing human: clinically oriented embryology,* ed 3. Philadelphia, 1982, WB Saunders.

Figure 2-3 Modified from Moore KL, editor: *The developing human: clinically oriented embryology,* ed 3. Philadelphia, 1982, WB Saunders.

Figure 2-4 Modified from Moore KL, editor: *The developing human: clinically oriented embryology,* ed 3. Philadelphia, 1982, WB Saunders.

Figure 2-5 From Moore KL, Persaud TVN: *The developing human: clinically oriented embryology,* ed 8. Philadelphia, 2008, WB Saunders.

Figure 2-6 Modified from Moore KL, editor: *The developing human: clinically oriented embryology,* ed 3. Philadelphia, 1982, WB Saunders.

Chapter 3

Figure 3-3 From McKinney E, James S, Murray S, Nelson K, Ashwill J. *Maternal-child nursing,* ed 4, WB Saunders: Philadelphia, 2012.

Figure 3-4 Courtesy Frank Fox, RDMS.

Chapter 4

Figure 4-1 From Price D, Gwin J. *Pediatric nursing: an introductory text,* ed 11. Philadelphia: Saunders, 2012.

Figure 4-3 From Ballard JL: New Ballard score, expanded to include extremely premature infants. *J Pediatr* 1991; 119:417-423.

Figure 4-4 Adapted from Lubchenco L.: *The high risk infant.* Philadelphia, 1976, WB Saunders.

Figure 4-5 From Hockenberry M, Wilson D. *Wong's essentials of pediatric nursing,* ed 8. St. Louis: Mosby, 2013.

Figure 4-6 From Price D, Gwin J. *Pediatric nursing: an introductory text,* ed 11. Philadelphia: Saunders, 2012.

Figure 4-7 From Wilkins RL, Stoller JK, Kacmarek RM: Egan's fundamentals of respiratory care, ed 9, 2009, Mosby. Modified from Silverman WA, Anderson DH: A controlled clinical trial of effects of water mist on obstructive respiratory signs, death rate and necropsy findings among premature infants. *Pediatrics* 17:1-6, 1956.

Figure 4-8 From Price D, Gwin J. *Pediatric nursing: an introductory text,* ed 11, Philadelphia: Saunders, 2012.

Figure 4-10 From Hockenberry M, Wilson D. *Wong's essentials of pediatric nursing,* ed 8. St. Louis: Mosby, 2013.

Figure 4-11 From Price D, Gwin J. *Pediatric nursing: an introductory text,* ed 11, Philadelphia: Saunders, 2012.

Chapter 5

Figure 5-1 CareFusion.

Figure 5-4 Courtesy Katrina Hynes.

Figure 5-8 From Mottram C. *Ruppel's Manual of Pulmonary Function Testing,* ed 10, St. Louis: Mosby, 2012.

Figure 5-12 Courtesy Katrina Hynes.

Figure 5-13 From Mottram C. *Ruppel's Manual of Pulmonary Function Testing,* ed 10, St. Louis: Mosby, 2012.

Figure 5-15 Courtesy Katrina Hynes.

Figure 5-16 Courtesy Katrina Hynes.

Chapter 8

Figure 8-8 From Understanding hemodynamic measurements made with the Swan-Ganz catheter. Irvine, Calif, Baxter Edwards Laboratories, 1989.

Figure 8-9 From Oski FA: Fetal hemoglobin, the neonatal red cell, and 2,3-diphosphoglycerate. Pediatr Clin North Am 1972; 19:907-917.

Chapter 9

Figure 9-1 From *Pulse oximetry,* note 7. Image used by permission from Nellcor Puritan Bennett, LCC, Boulder, CO, part of Covidien.

Figure 9-2 From *Clinical reference card,* no 1. Hayward, Calif, Nellcor, 1988.

Figure 9-6 From *Advanced concepts in capnography.* Image used by permission from Nellcor Puritan Bennett, LCC, Boulder, CO, part of Covidien.

Figure 9-7 From Stock MC: Non-invasive carbon dioxide monitoring. *Crit Care Clin* 1988; 4:511.

Figure 9-8 From Stock MC: Non-invasive carbon dioxide monitoring. *Crit Care Clin* 1988; 4:511.

Figure 9-9 From Stock MC: Non-invasive carbon dioxide monitoring. *Crit Care Clin* 1988; 4:511.

Figure 9-10 From Curley MA, Thompson JE: End tidal CO2 monitoring in critically ill infants and children. *Pediatr Nurs* 1990; 16:397.

Figure 19-4 Redrawn from Short BL: Physiology of extracorporeal membrane oxygenation. In Polin RA, Fox WW, editors: *Fetal and neonatal physiology*. Philadelphia. WB Saunders, 1992.

Figure 19-5 Redrawn from Meyer A, Struber M, Fischer S. Advances in extracorporeal ventilation. *Anesthesiol Clin* 2008; 26:381.

Chapter 21

Figure 21-7 From Moodie DS, Stillwell PC: Thoracic organ transplantation in children: the state of heart, heart-lung, and lung transplantation. *Clin Pediatr* 1993; 32:322-328.

Chapter 22

Figure 22-1 From Paetzel M. Respiratory distress syndrome (grade 1-4) of the premature and newborn. Available at: http://www. radiologyteacher.com/index.cgi?&nav5view&DatID5127. Accessed January 1, 2013.

Figure 22-2 From Bancalari E: Bronchopulmonary dysplasia and neonatal chronic lung disease. In: Fanaroff AA, Martin RJ, editors. Neonatal-perinatal medicine diseases of the fetus and infant, ed 9. St Louis: Mosby-Elsevier, 2011.

Figure 22-3 From Viscardi RM: Prenatal and postnatal microbial colonization and respiratory outcome in preterm infants. In: Bancalari E, editor. The newborn lung: neonatology questions and controversies, ed 2. Philadelphia: Saunders, 2012.

Figure 22-4 From Arthur R. The neonatal chest x-ray. Paediatr Respir Rev 2001;2:311.

Figure 22-5 From Arthur R. The neonatal chest x-ray. Paediatr Respir Rev 2001;2:311.

Figure 22-6 From Harris TR, Herrick BR. Pneumothorax in the newborn. Biomedical Communications, Tucson: Arizona Health Sciences Center, 1978.

Figure 22-7 Redrawn from Wiswell TE, Bent RC: Meconium staining and the meconium aspiration syndrome. Pediatr Clin North Am 1993; 40:957; modified from Bacsik RD: Meconium aspiration system. *Pediatr Clin North Am* 1977; 24:467.

Figure 22-8 From Arthur R. The neonatal chest x-ray. Paediatr Respir Rev 2001;2:311.

Figure 22-9 From Steinhorn RH, Abman SH. Persistent pulmonary hypertension. In: Gleason CA, Devaskar SU, editors. Avery's disease of the newborn, ed 9. Philadelphia: Saunders, 2012.

Figure 22-10 From Arthur R. The neonatal chest x-ray. Paediatr Respir Rev 2001;2:311.

Figure 22-11 From Arthur R. The neonatal chest x-ray. Paediatr Respir Rev 2001;2:311.

Figure 22-12 From Arthur R. The neonatal chest x-ray. Paediatr Respir Rev 2001;2:311.

Figure 22-13 From Arthur R. The neonatal chest x-ray. Paediatr Respir Rev 2001;2:311.

Figure 22-14 From Bancalari E: Bronchopulmonary dysplasia and neonatal chronic lung disease. In: Fanaroff AA, Martin RJ, editors. Neonatal-perinatal medicine diseases of the fetus and infant, ed 9. St Louis: Mosby- Elsevier, 2011.

Figure 22-15 From Narasimhan R, Papworth S.: Pulmonary hemorrhage in the neonate., Paediatr Child Health 2009;19:171, 2009.

Chapter 23

Figure 28-10 From Kumar V, Abbas A, Nelson F. Robbins and Cotran: *Pathologic basis if disease*, ed 7, Saunders, 2005, Philadelphia.

Chapter 24

Figure 24-1 From Mullin CE, Mayer DC: *Congenital heart disease: a diagrammatic atlas*. New York. This material used by permission of Wiley-Liss, Inc., a subsidiary of John Wiley & Sons, Inc. 1988.

Figure 24-2 From *Congenital heart abnormalities*. Clinical Education Aid No. 7. Columbus, Ohio. Ross Products Division, Abbott Laboratories, 1970.

Figure 24-3 From Mullin CE, Mayer DC: *Congenital heart disease: a diagrammatic atlas*. New York. This material used by permission of Wiley-Liss, Inc., a subsidiary of John Wiley & Sons, Inc 1988.

Figure 24-4 From *Congenital heart abnormalities*. Clinical Education Aid No. 7. Columbus, Ohio. Ross Products Division, Abbott Laboratories, 1970.

Figure 24-5 From Mullin CE, Mayer DC: *Congenital heart disease: a diagrammatic atlas*. New York. This material used by permission of Wiley-Liss, Inc., a subsidiary of John Wiley & Sons, Inc.1988.

Figure 24-6 From *Congenital heart abnormalities*. Clinical Education Aid No. 7. Columbus, Ohio. Ross Products Division, Abbott Laboratories, 1970.

Figure 24-7 Modified from Mullin CE, Mayer DC: *Congenital heart disease: a diagrammatic atlas*. New York. This material used by permission of Wiley-Liss, Inc., a subsidiary of John Wiley & Sons, Inc.1988.

Figure 24-8 From Mullin CE, Mayer DC: *Congenital heart disease: a diagrammatic atlas*. New York. This material used by permission of Wiley-Liss, Inc., a subsidiary of John Wiley & Sons, Inc 1988.

Figure 24-10 From: Park MK, Troxler RG. *Pediatric cardiology for practitioners*. Mosby. St. Louis. 2002:386.

Figure 24-11 Redrawn from Sano S, Ishino K, Kawada M, et al. Right ventricle-pulmonary artery shunt in first-stage palliation of hypoplastic left heart syndrome. *J Thorac Cardiovasc Surg*. 2003 Aug;126(2):504-9.

Figure 24-12 Redrawn from Castaneda AR, Jonas RA, Mayer JE, Hanley FL. *Cardiac surgery of the neonate and infant*. W.B. Saunders. New York 1994:377.

Figure 24-14 From Mullin CE, Mayer DC: *Congenital heart disease: a diagrammatic atlas*. New York. This material used by permission of Wiley-Liss, Inc., a subsidiary of John Wiley & Sons, Inc 1988.

Figure 24-15 From Mullin CE, Mayer DC: *Congenital heart disease: a diagrammatic atlas*. New York. This material used by permission of Wiley-Liss, Inc., a subsidiary of John Wiley & Sons, Inc. 1988.

Figure 24-16 From Mullin CE, Mayer DC: *Congenital heart disease: a diagrammatic atlas*. New York. This material used by permission of Wiley-Liss, Inc., a subsidiary of John Wiley & Sons, Inc.1988.

Figure 24-17 From Mullin CE, Mayer DC: *Congenital heart disease: a diagrammatic atlas*. New York. This material used by permission of Wiley-Liss, Inc., a subsidiary of John Wiley & Sons, Inc. 1988.

Figure 24-18 From Mullin CE, Mayer DC: *Congenital heart disease: a diagrammatic atlas*. New York. This material used by permission of Wiley-Liss, Inc., a subsidiary of John Wiley & Sons, Inc.1988.

Figure 24-19 From Mullin CE, Mayer DC: *Congenital heart disease: a diagrammatic atlas*. New York. This material used by permission of Wiley-Liss, Inc., a subsidiary of John Wiley & Sons, Inc.1988.

Figure 24-20 From Mullin CE, Mayer DC: *Congenital heart disease: a diagrammatic atlas.* New York. This material used by permission of Wiley-Liss, Inc., a subsidiary of John Wiley & Sons, Inc. 1988.

Chapter 26

Figure 26-11 Modified from Denny FW, Clyde WA: Acute lower respiratory tract infections in nonhospitalized children. *J Pediatr* 1986; 108:635.

Chapter 31

Figure 31-2 From Nolte J: *The human brain: an introduction to its functional anatomy.* St Louis, Mosby, 2002; modified from von Economo C: *The cytoarchitectonics of the human cerebral cortex.* Oxford. Oxford University Press, 1929.

Figure 31-3 From MacGregor J: *Introduction to the anatomy and physiology of children,* London. Routledge, 2000.

Figure 31-4 From Hockenberry M, Wilson D: Nursing care infants and children, ed 9. St. Louis: Mosby, 2011.

Figure 31-5 From Heuer A. Wilkins' clinical assessment in respiratory care, ed 7. St. Louis: Mosby, 2014.

Figure 31-6 From Hess DR, MacIntyre NR, Mishoe SC, et al: *Respiratory care: principles and practice.* Philadelphia. WB Saunders, 2002.

Figure 31-7 Courtesy University of Michigan Trauma Burn Center, Ann Arbor, MI. From Sole et al. Introduction to critical care nursing, ed 6. Philadelphia: Saunders, 2013.

Figure 31-8 Data from Weinberg AD. Hypothermia. Ann Emerg Med 1993;22 (Pt 2):370-377.

Chapter 33

Figure 33-3 Reprint permission from Dr. Howard Panitch, Children's Hospital of Philadelphia.

Chapter 34

Figure 34-1 Courtesy Texas Children's Medical Center.

Figure 34-2 Courtesy Memorial Hermann Hospital, Houston, Texas.

Figure 34-3 Courtesy Texas Children's Medical Center.

Chapter 35

Figure 35-1 Image used by permission from Nellcor Puritan Bennett, LCC, Boulder, CO, part of Covidien. With permission Paul Bowen Photography.

Figure 35-2 Courtesy AirSep, Buffalo, NY.

Figure 35-3 Courtesy AirSep, Buffalo, NY.

Figure 35-4 Courtesy AirSep, Buffalo, NY.

Figure 35-5 Courtesy Sunrise Medical, Longmont, Colo.

Chapter 36

Figure 36-1 Data from U.S. Nuclear Regulatory Commission New Release No. 09-033, February 2009.

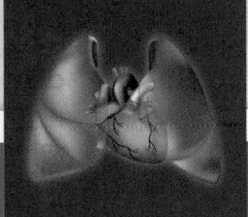

Index